D1609013

FISH
MEDICINE

FISH MEDICINE

MICHAEL K. STOSKOPF, D.V.M., Ph.D.

Professor and Head
Department of Companion Animal and Special Species Medicine
College of Veterinary Medicine
North Carolina State University
Raleigh, North Carolina

Original Illustrations
by

Timothy H. Phelps, M.S., F.A.M.I.

and

Brent A. Bauer, M.F.A., F.A.M.I.
Department of Arts as Applied to Medicine
The Johns Hopkins University School of Medicine
Baltimore, Maryland

W.B. SAUNDERS COMPANY
Harcourt Brace Jovanovich, Inc.
Philadelphia   London   Toronto   Montreal   Sydney   Tokyo

W. B. SAUNDERS COMPANY
Harcourt Brace Jovanovich, Inc.

The Curtis Center
Independence Square West
Philadelphia, Pennsylvania 19106

Library of Congress Cataloging-in-Publication Data

Stoskopf, Michael K.
Fish medicine / Michael K. Stoskopf.

   p. cm.

Includes index.

ISBN 0–7216–2629–7

1. Fish—Diseases.   I. Title.

SH171.S78 1992

639.3—dc20   91-41386

FISH MEDICINE   ISBN 0–7216–2629–7

Printed in Mexico.

Last digit is the print number: 9   8   7   6   5   4   3   2   1

*This book is dedicated to the clinicians and scientists
who will build on it to improve our understanding of fish medicine;
to my grandfather,
a devoted fisherman who would have found it interesting;
and particularly to my wife, Suzanne,
who has cheerfully and graciously endured the tribulations
of having a preoccupied and remiss husband these past few years.*

CONTRIBUTORS

DOUGLAS P. ANDERSON, Ph.D.
Immunologist (Fisheries), U.S. Fish and Wildlife Service, Department of the Interior, National Fish Health Research Laboratory, Kearneysville, West Virginia

MARSHALL H. BELEAU, D.V.M., M.S.
Abbott Laboratories, North Chicago, Illinois

BRAD N. BOLON, D.V.M., M.S.
Chemical Industry Institute of Toxicology, Research Triangle Park, North Carolina

PAUL R. BOWSER, Ph.D.
Associate Professor, Department of Avian and Aquatic Animal Medicine, College of Veterinary Medicine, Cornell University, Ithaca, New York

LYDIA A. BROWN, Ph.D., B.V.Sc., F.R.C.V.S.
European Technical Manager, Aquaculture and Animal Health, Abbott Laboratories, West Gomeldon, Salisbury, United Kingdom

ROBERT A. BULLIS, D.V.M., M.S.
Research Associate in Microbiology, Department of Pathobiology, School of Veterinary Medicine, University of Pennsylvania, Laboratory for Marine Animal Health, Marine Biological Laboratory, Woods Hole, Massachusetts

A. JIM CHACKO, Ph.D.
Professor of Aquaculture, Division of Environmental Sciences Programs, Unity College, Unity, Maine

PAUL CHEUNG, Ph.D.
Osborn Laboratories of Marine Sciences, New York Aquarium, New York Zoological Society, Brooklyn, New York

RUTH FRANCIS-FLOYD, D.V.M., M.S.
Department of Large Animal Clinical Sciences and Department of Fisheries and Aquaculture, University of Florida, Gainesville, Florida

MARGIE LEE GALLAGHER, Ph.D.
Professor/Senior Scientist, East Carolina University, Institute for Coastal and Marine Resources, Greenville, North Carolina

BEVERLY A. GOVEN-DIXON, Ph.D.
Associate Professor, Department of Biological Sciences, California State University, Hayward, California

JOHN B. GRATZEK, D.V.M., Ph.D.
Professor and Head, Department of Medical Microbiology, College of Veterinary Medicine, University of Georgia, Athens, Georgia

SAMUEL H. GRUBER, Ph.D.
Professor, Rosenstiel School of Marine and Atmospheric Sciences, Division of Marine Biology and Fisheries, University of Miami, Miami, Florida

BRUCE G. HECKER, B.A.
Curator of Fishes, National Aquarium in Baltimore, Baltimore, Maryland

RICHARD A. HECKMANN, Ph.D.
Professor of Zoology, Ezra Taft Benson Agriculture and Food Institute, Zoology Department, Brigham Young University, Provo, Utah

GLENN L. HOFFMAN, Ph.D.
Parasitologist, U.S. Fish and Wildlife Service, Department of the Interior (retired); Fish Parasitology Consultant, Kearneysville, West Virginia

BARBARA HORNEY, D.V.M., PH.D., DIPL. A.C.V.P.
: Adjunct Faculty, Atlantic Veterinary College, Department of Pathology and Microbiology, University of Prince Edward Island, Charlottetown, Prince Edward Island, Canada

GERALD JOHNSON, D.V.M.
: Associate Professor, Department of Pathology and Microbiology, Atlantic Veterinary College, University of Prince Edward Island; Fish Health Coordinator, Charlottetown, Prince Edward Island, Canada

SUZANNE KENNEDY-STOSKOPF, D.V.M., PH.D., DIPL. A.C.Z.M.
: Department of Microbiology, Pathology, and Parasitology, College of Veterinary Medicine, North Carolina State University, Raleigh, North Carolina

J. HOWARD KERBY, PH.D.
: Fish Culture and Ecology Laboratory, National Fisheries Research Center, U.S. Fish and Wildlife Service, Department of the Interior, Kearneysville, West Virginia

JOSEPH V. KITZMAN, D.V.M., PH.D.
: Associate Professor of Pharmacology, College of Veterinary Medicine, Mississippi State University, Mississippi State, Mississippi

GEORGE W. KLONTZ, M.S., D.V.M.
: Professor of Aquaculture, Department of Fish and Wildlife Resources, University of Idaho, Moscow, Idaho

SANTOSH P. LALL, PH.D.
: Department of Fisheries and Oceans, Biological Sciences Branch, Halifax, Nova Scotia, Canada

CHARLES A. MANIRE, D.V.M.
: Rosenstiel School of Marine and Atmospheric Science, Division of Marine Biology and Fisheries, Miami, Florida

ERIC B. MAY, PH.D.
: Assistant Professor, College of Veterinary Medicine; Adjunct Assistant Professor, School of Medicine, University of Maryland; Pathologist, National Aquarium in Baltimore, Baltimore, Maryland; Coordinator of Fish Health/Disease Programs, Maryland Department of Natural Resources, Cooperative Oxford Biological Laboratory, Oxford, Maryland

FOSTER L. MAYER, PH.D.
: U.S. Environmental Protection Agency, Environmental Research Laboratory, Gulf Breeze, Florida

PHILIP E. McALLISTER, PH.D.
: U.S. Fish and Wildlife Service, Department of the Interior, National Fish Health Research Laboratory, Kearneysville, West Virginia

CAROL M. MORRISON, PH.D.
: Research Scientist, Biological Sciences Branch, Department of Fisheries and Oceans, Halifax Fisheries Research Laboratory, Halifax, Nova Scotia, Canada

THOMAS G. NEMETZ, D.V.M., PH.D.
: Post-doctoral Associate, Department of Genetics, University of Georgia, Athens, Georgia

EDWARD J. NOGA, M.S., D.V.M.
: Associate Professor of Aquatic Medicine, College of Veterinary Medicine, North Carolina State University; Aquatic Animal Veterinarian, North Carolina State University Veterinary Teaching Hospital, Raleigh, North Carolina

CHARLES S. PIKE, III, M.S.
: Rosenstiel School of Marine and Atmospheric Sciences, Division of Marine Biology and Fisheries, University of Miami, Miami, Florida

JOHN A. PLUMB, PH.D.
: Professor, Department of Fisheries and Allied Aquacultures, International Center for Aquaculture, College of Agriculture, Auburn University, Auburn, Alabama

GEORGE W. POST, PH.D.
: Professor of Fishery and Wildlife Biology and Professor of Microbiology (ret.), Rio Rico, Arizona

SARAH L. POYNTON, PH.D.
: Lecturer, Division of Comparative Medicine, The Johns Hopkins University School of Medicine, Baltimore, Maryland

RENATE REIMSCHUESSEL, V.M.D., PH.D.
: Assistant Professor, Department of Pathology, University of Maryland School of Medicine, Baltimore, Maryland

JEROME V. SHIREMAN, PH.D.
: Professor, Department of Fisheries and Aquaculture, University of Florida, Gainesville, Florida

EMMETT B. SHOTTS, JR., PH.D.
Professor of Medical Microbiology, College of Veterinary Medicine, University of Georgia, Athens, Georgia

CHARLIE E. SMITH, B.A.
U.S. Fish and Wildlife Service, Fish Technology Center, Bozeman, Montana

LYNWOOD S. SMITH, PH.D.
Professor, School of Fisheries, University of Washington, Seattle, Washington

STEPHEN A. SMITH, M.S., D.V.M., PH.D.
Former: Department of Companion Animal and Special Species Medicine, College of Veterinary Medicine, North Carolina State University, Raleigh, North Carolina
Current: Assistant Professor, Department of Pathobiology, Virginia-Maryland Regional College of Veterinary Medicine, Virginia Polytechnic Institute and State University, Blacksburg, Virginia

LAURA JANE STEWART, M.S.
Nutritionist, San Antonio Zoological Gardens and Aquarium, San Antonio, Texas

MICHAEL K. STOSKOPF, D.V.M., PH.D., DIPL. A.C.Z.M.
Professor and Head, Department of Companion Animal and Special Species Medicine, College of Veterinary Medi-cine, North Carolina State University, Raleigh, North Carolina

RONALD L. THUNE, PH.D.
Professor, Department of Veterinary Microbiology and Parasitology, Louisiana State University School of Veterinary Medicine, and Department of Veterinary Science, Louisiana Agricultural Experiment Station, Louisiana State University Agricultural Center; Director, Louisiana Aquatic Animal Disease Laboratory, Baton Rouge, Louisiana

JOSEPH R. TOMASSO, JR., PH.D.
Professor, Department of Aquaculture, Fisheries, and Wildlife, Clemson University, Clemson, South Carolina

OLE J. TORRISSEN, PH.D.
Ministry of Fisheries, Institute of Marine Research, Matre Aquaculture Research Station, Matredal, Norway

CRAIG S. TUCKER, PH.D.
Professor, Mississippi State University, Mississippi State, Mississippi. Fishery Biologist, Mississippi Agriculture and Forestry Experiment Station, Stoneville, Mississippi

RICHARD E. ZURBRIGG, D.V.M., M.SC.
Research Associate, Royal Ontario Museum, Department of Zoology, University of Guelph; Supervisor, Diagnostic Serology, Health of Animals Laboratory, Guelph, Ontario, Canada

PREFACE

I present to you, the reader, what my section editors, authors, artists, and I hope will be a valuable tool in the development of clinical fish medicine. It is a timely offering. The production of food fishes continues to gain ever greater acceptance worldwide as an effective and valuable means of providing high-quality protein to mankind. Increased efficiency of commercial fishing has brought the stocks of many wild fisheries to critical points where their management, including medical management, will determine whether they can be sustained. The demand for recreational fisheries continues to increase, requiring the production and stocking of millions of fish each year in the United States alone. Meanwhile, home hobbyists are becoming more sophisticated in their understanding of the roles that diseases play in their hobby and industry. The value of veterinary care for hobby fishes is rapidly gaining acceptance. The popularity of large display aquaria has never been greater, as the general public recognizes the aesthetic beauty of the aquatic world and seeks the opportunity to explore it. The importance of medical management of these collections is also being recognized.

Fish Medicine comes to you as clinical fish medicine is emerging as a discipline in its own right, distinct from fish pathology, fisheries biology, and fisheries management. The book is intended to provide a foundation for the further development of that young discipline, which incorporates aspects of each of the others into the traditions of clinical veterinary medicine. This is not a fish pathology text. It does not dwell exclusively on the postmortem appearance of disease, although good clinicians need to understand that aspect of illness. In recent years, several excellent texts have been produced that provide a pathologist's view of fish disease. This book, on the other hand, is designed to focus on clinical approaches to living fishes, both as individuals and as populations.

The first section of *Fish Medicine* is a book in itself. Its 17 chapters cover basic clinical knowledge applicable to fishes in general. It is intended to serve as an introduction to fish medicine and to be used as a text for courses in fish medicine taught in veterinary schools and colleges. You may find that this section includes chapters you would not expect in a clinical text. The first two chapters, for example, are designed to bridge the gap between a reader's in-depth knowledge of terrestrial animal anatomy and histology and the morphology of fishes. As the clinical management of fishes becomes more accepted and integrated into the mainstream of veterinary medical education, hopefully the appearance of these chapters in a clinical text will become as unnecessary as a chapter on dog anatomy in a book on canine medicine. For now, however, the diversity of fish morphology as it applies to clinical practice is treated by addressing themes and working generalizations, supplemented with detailed illustrations drawn from careful dissections of many previously unstudied but clinically important fish species. Other chapters in the general medicine section focus on techniques and methodology that can be applied to a wide variety of fish species. The didactic emphasis is on guiding the clinically trained individual in understanding the approaches needed to treat aquatic patients.

The remainder of the book, the special medicine section, is intended as a reference source and takes the reader several steps further into the intricacies of clinical fish medicine related to specific groups of fishes. The eight sections and 85 chapters in this part of the book are designed with the clinician, rather than the fish taxonomist, in mind. Fishes are grouped into sections by the factors that relate most directly to their clinical management.

The goal was to split out the groups of fishes to the extent that the clinical knowledge base allowed. This has created some rather broad groupings on a taxonomic basis. As our medical knowledge of these fishes expands, it may become more appropriate to separate them further, but for now, grouping the less studied fishes by environmental requirements allows the medically oriented reader to find them by simply knowing their preferred habitat. Once the appropriate section is found, the clinician has access to a rather concise review of the vast array of information that is widely scattered in the periodic literature pertaining to that group of fishes.

Throughout the book, the text is designed to be familiar to the clinician. Technical medical terminology is applied freely without apology, whereas taxonomic names of fishes are relegated to appendices, and standardized common names are used throughout the book. Tables and artificial keys are used extensively to speed the retrieval of clinically important information. The concise style, and even the selection of the typeface, are intended to make reading for specific facts stimulating and effective. Appendices provide thorough conversion tables and summarize drug dose information in tables to facilitate the rapid retrieval required in acute clinical cases.

So here it is—a systematic and comprehensive review of the state of a clinical art. Use it wisely and it will help you answer important questions, discover new knowledge, and, most important of all, ask new questions.

MICHAEL K. STOSKOPF, D.V.M., PH.D., DIPL. A.C.Z.M.
April 1992

ACKNOWLEDGMENTS

The creation of a work of this magnitude would not be possible without the help of many generous and hard-working souls. Most certainly, many more have contributed than are named here, and their talents are no less appreciated. Certainly, first and foremost, my gratitude must be expressed to my authors, section editors, and particularly my artists, Tim Phelps and Brent Bauer. They have tolerated my editorial idiosyncrasies and produced great results. Linda Mills, of W.B. Saunders Company, has valiantly championed the book, shepherding it through the publishing process. Darlene Pedersen, Linda's predecessor, got it past several early hurdles. Gina Scala and Kathleen McCullough have managed to copy-edit out most of the syntactical quirks and have taught me considerable in the process. Designer Paul Fry created an elegant look for the book, and Joe Dieter was always willing to lend me his talents in design and composition.

A number of people have helped with the typing and preparation of the manuscript. Particular thanks are due to Margaret Hemingway, Debra Collins, and Sharon Eldridge, who have prepared and re-prepared the final manuscript of the entire book. Tammy Crafton, Sharon Dappie, Pamela Lomas, Kim Evans, Polly Moniz, Lora McKenzie, Joyce Man, and Violet Catrow also deserve thanks for working on the manuscript for individual chapters. Equally important, many colleagues have contributed their time and expertise by reading and reviewing the manuscript for various chapters. I want to thank D. Scarratt, Anne Moore, John Seamer, John Harsbarger, E.L. Bousfield, Eugene M. Burreson, Jacqueline Madill, Hugh W. Ferguson, R.A. Khan, Gary McClelland, F. Rafi, Phil Sannes, Stewart C. Schell, W.B. Scott, Rosalie A. Schnick, and Ed Smallwood for valuable review efforts. The index, a daunting task, was ably provided by Nancy Matthews.

Technical assistance to produce some of the original data presented in this book has been provided by Bernie Dappie, Vivian Marryatt, Jocelyn Carter, Stephen Smith, Tom Arrow, Tim Phelps, Jill Arnold, Susan Nevy, Erika Faulk, Larry Peiper, Marshall Judges, Juan Sabalones, and Bruce Hecker, among others. E.J. Crossman and F.W.H. Beamish also contributed facilities and equipment.

A number of institutions provided support for authors and editors working on this book, and deserve special thanks. These include Johns Hopkins University, the National Aquarium in Baltimore, the Osborne Laboratory of the New York Zoological Society, the Maryland Department of Natural Resources, the University of Florida, the Department of Zoology of the University of Guelph, the Royal Ontario Museum, Huntsman Marine Laboratory, the University of Georgia, Auburn University, the U.S. Fish and Wildlife Service, Louisiana State University, and, particularly, the College of Veterinary Medicine, North Carolina State University.

CONTENTS

PART I

GENERAL MEDICINE

Chapter 1

ANATOMY

MICHAEL K. STOSKOPF

In fish medicine, as in any other clinical specialty, a basic knowledge of anatomy is important. Unfortunately, the structural diversity of fishes and the lack of basic anatomic information on even relatively common fish species make obtaining this knowledge difficult. This chapter focuses on clinically important aspects of fish anatomy and is intended to serve as a reference for the clinician on specific organs in a variety of fishes. Some clinically important aspects of vascular anatomy and organology are also presented. There is no question that one picture is worth at least a thousand words, so the topographic anatomy of fish species with divergent body forms is illustrated (Fig. 1–1). The information presented in this chapter by no means represents the limits of diversity found in fishes, but within the confines of a single chapter it should go a long way toward preparing the clinician for the surprises in store.

Nearly everyone's concept of a typical fish is what is known as a fusiform fish. These fishes include most of the sportfishes and commercially important species, such as trout, salmon, and bass. The reason to cover this type of fish in some detail is that the majority of fishes seen in clinical practice fall into this category. It is also the type of fish we know the most about. In particular, the rainbow trout is perhaps the most extensively studied species of fish. Of course, there actually is no single, "typical" fusiform fish, and each species has certain adaptations that allow it to succeed in its particular environmental niche. While exploring the anatomy of the trout, some common variations in other fusiform fishes will be noted. Important specializations of other fusiform fishes will also be covered in more detail in the appropriate sections of the special medicine part (Part II) of this book.

THE RAINBOW TROUT, A FUSIFORM TELEOST

External Anatomy

In describing the gross anatomy of a fish, most anatomists divide it into three body regions, the head, the trunk, and the tail (Fig. 1–2). The head extends to the caudal margin of the gill covering or operculum. The trunk continues from the head to the most caudal point of the peritoneal cavity, which

in many fusiform fishes is indicated externally by the urogenital and anal openings. The muscular tail begins at this point and extends caudally. The term *fusiform* refers to the overall shape where the head is smaller than the trunk, with a taper from the mouth to a point behind the pelvic fins that is usually the deepest (dorsal to ventral) point of the fish (see Fig. 1–1). From this point, the body tapers again to the end of the caudal peduncle.

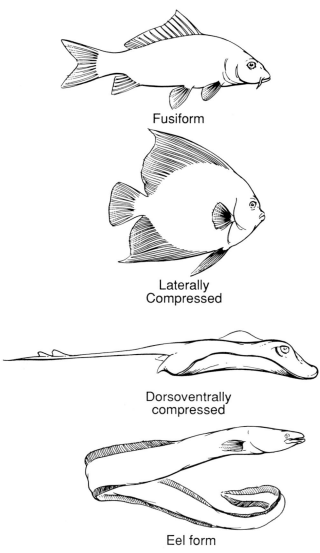

Fusiform

Laterally
Compressed

Dorsoventrally
compressed

Eel form

FIGURE 1–1. Morphological types of fishes.

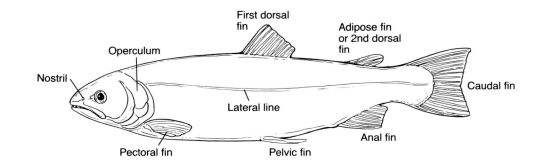

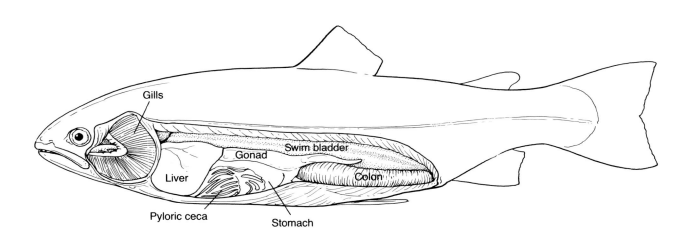

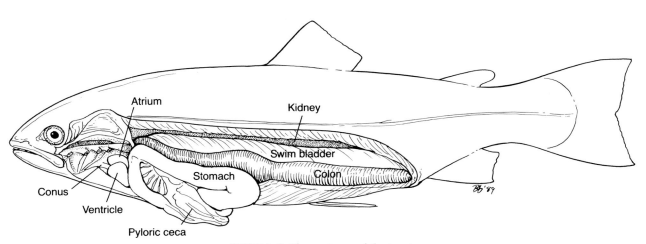

FIGURE 1–2. The anatomy of the trout.

Scales

A major difference between the rainbow trout and the majority of other fusiform fishes is the relatively light scale pattern of the trout. Scales are translucent plates of dermal origin that project into the epidermis, forming a protective environmental barrier for the fish. Trout have oval-shaped cycloid scales with smooth borders (Fig. 1–3) that are considered more primitive than the ridged ctenoid scales found on many fusiform fishes.

Scale types have some clinical significance, dictating handling and treatment procedures. Lightly scaled fishes like trout, particularly scaleless fishes such as catfishes, can be much more sensitive to drugs and toxins in the water. This affects some treatment protocols. Very finely scaled fishes like herrings, jack, and tunas are easily damaged, even in simple procedures, such as capture and transfer. These fishes often require anesthesia for examinations and simple procedures, including injections. At the other extreme, large-scaled fishes such as sturgeons, bonefish, and tarpons can be very difficult to inject with remote injection devices like pole syringes, and large scales may complicate surgical efforts.

Fins

The fins of fishes are often used as clinical landmarks or to locate lesions so that they can be monitored over time. A basic knowledge of fin nomenclature and how it varies on different types of fishes is useful. The trout has a fairly complete complement of fins. The paired pectoral fins originate high on the sides of the trunk just behind the gill openings. The musculoskeletal girdle for these fins is attached to the skull. The other paired set of fins on the trout are the pelvic fins, which are set close together on the ventral surface, cranial to the urogenital and anal openings. The trout also has the four unpaired fins found in most fusiform teleosts. The cranial or first dorsal fin begins further caudally on the dorsal surface of the trout than in other fusiform fishes like perches, basses, swordtails, and guppies. The caudal or second dorsal fin of the trout is located behind the first dorsal fin and is sometimes known as the "adipose" fin. The anal fin is found just caudal to the genital and anal openings of the fish on the ventral surface. The caudal fin is the terminal fin and is commonly referred to as the "tail."

Internal Anatomy

Musculoskeletal System

For a clinician, the musculoskeletal anatomy of a fish is perhaps most easily accessible through radiography. Teleost fishes have axial and appendicular skeletons of true bone with the same basic components of mammalian skeletons. Although skeletal patterns vary considerably, the clinician evaluating a case can usually rely on the conservation of symmetry and functional design. For additional insight into the structure of the fish skeleton, study the radiographic plates in Chapter 5.

One of the most clinically important aspects of the muscular system is demonstrated in the trout, but is more consequential in many marine pelagic fishes. This is the difference between dark and light muscle. The dark, or red, muscle in the trout and most other fusiform fishes is located just beneath the skin. In the trout this is a middle band of muscle, but in tunas and other fishes it can be much more extensive. The dark muscle of fish is thought to be involved in sustained swimming activity. It has a higher lipid content and is histologically distinct from the white muscle. The clinical importance of the location of dark muscle on a fish is that there are distinct differences in drug kinetics when injections are made into dark muscle. Anesthetics, for example, tend to distribute much differently when injections are made into the dark muscle compared with injections into the white muscle. This aspect of anatomy and pharmacology warrants considerable study with other drugs, but it should be kept in mind when a clinician is selecting injection sites and angles in larger fish.

Cardiovascular System

The circulatory system of fishes is relatively simple (Fig. 1–4). Poorly oxygenated blood circulates from the cranially placed heart to the gills, where it is oxygenated by a countercurrent system in the gill lamellae. It then continues through the dorsal aorta to the arteries supplying the various organs and tissues and then returns to the heart via the venous system. The heart of any teleost, including trout, is considered a two-chambered heart, although four

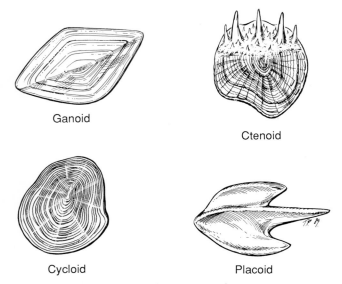

Ganoid

Ctenoid

Cycloid

Placoid

FIGURE 1–3. The four major scale types.

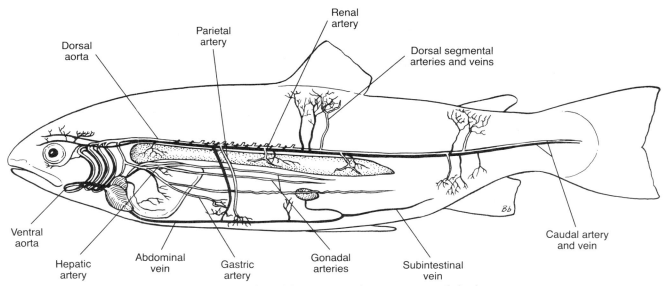

FIGURE 1–4. The relationship of the trout vasculature system to skeletal structures.

distinct regions are readily distinguishable. The thin-walled sinus venosus receives venous blood from hepatic veins and the common cardinal veins and empties into the somewhat thicker atrium through paired sinoatrial valves. The atrium, usually considered the first chamber of the fish heart, transfers blood to the muscular ventricle through the nonmuscular atrioventricular valve. The fourth component of the trout heart is the bulbus arteriosus, which contains no cardiac muscle but consists entirely of elastic connective tissue and smooth muscle. The bulbus arteriosus receives blood from the ventricle through semilunar ventriculobulbar valves and, via its elastic recoil, pushes the blood through the ventral aorta to the gills. In the lungfishes and coelacanth, the atrium and ventricle are partially divided into two symmetric chambers and are much like amphibian hearts.

The physiology resulting from the vascular patterns in the tail and flank regions of fishes is clinically important (Fig. 1–5). A renal portal system can have major effects on the pharmacokinetics of drugs ad-

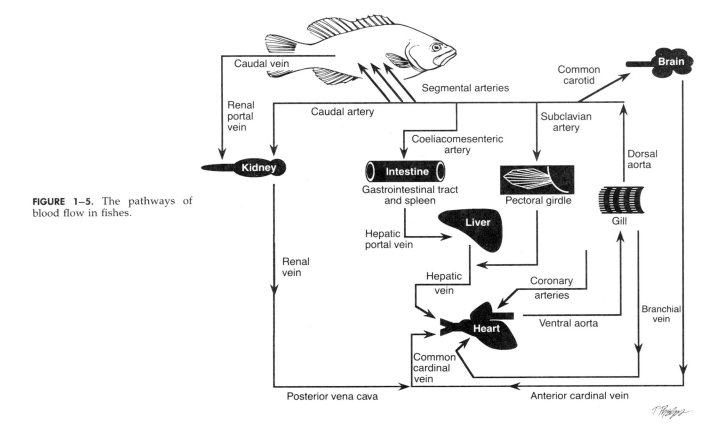

FIGURE 1–5. The pathways of blood flow in fishes.

ministered intramuscularly or at various intravenous sites. Anatomists have identified eight anatomical patterns of blood flow in the caudal region of various fishes. These can be categorized into four clinically significant physiological groups (Fig. 1–6).

Most fishes have a venous return system in which the majority of the blood returning from the tail and sides of the body passes through the kidney before going to the heart. The caudal vein divides into right and left renal portal veins that pass along the dorsal surface of each respective kidney, sending

branches into the renal parenchyma. Segmental veins from the flank also empty into the renal portal veins and subsequently into the kidney. Blood is carried away from the kidney by the caudal cardinal veins. This complete renal portal system occurs in pike, all of the sharks, skates, and rays, the lungfishes, ciscos, whitefish, burbot, tiger barb, sculpins, porcupinefishes, balloonfish, mullets, sea robins, cusk-eels, rockfishes, ocean perch, redfish, cowcod, chilipepper, goatfishes, mackerels, polypterids, and soles.

Other fishes, particularly the cyprinids and an-

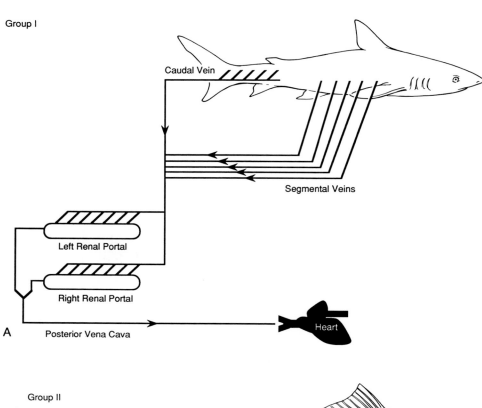

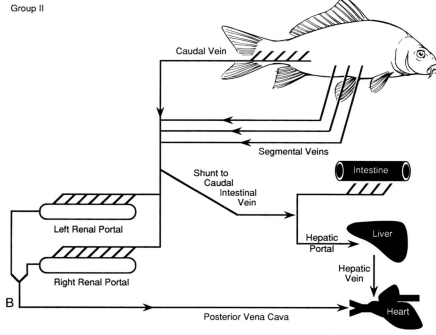

FIGURE 1–6. Portal systems in fish. *A.* Group I (sharks, lungfish, flatfish, sea robins, etc.). *B.* Group II (cyprinids and anguillaform eels).

guilliform eels, have systems in which only some blood passes through the renal portal system, and a portion passes directly to the hepatic portal system. In cyprinids, this occurs through a communication between the caudal vein and the caudal intestinal vein. In eels, special venous arcades occur between the renal portal veins and the intestinal vasculature. With this system, some blood from the tail goes to the renal portal system, and some goes to the hepatic portal system.

The second most common caudal venous pattern in fishes is found in tench, cod, grenadiers, eelpouts, ide, daces, rudd, and some members of the cyprinid family. In this system, some blood from the caudal vein is taken directly to the heart, completely bypassing all portal systems. In the tench, only blood

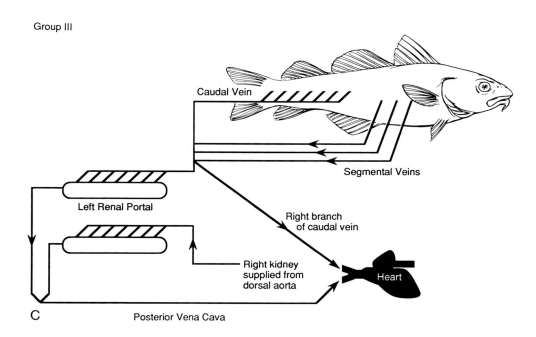

Group III

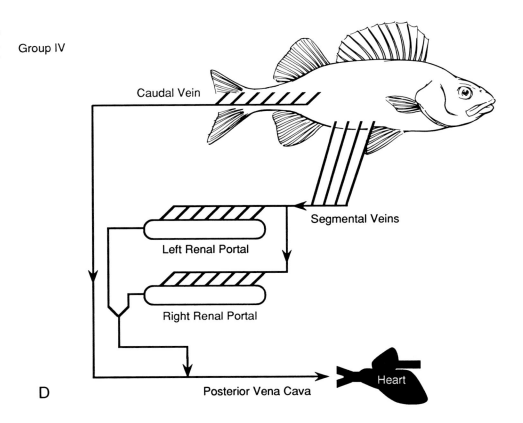

FIGURE 1–6 *Continued C.* Group III (cod, grenadiers, eelpouts, etc.). *D.* Group IV (perch, salmonids, tunas, lumpfish, etc.).

Group IV

from the ventral portion of the tail goes to the kidneys. In the other fishes, the caudal vein branches into a left renal portal vein that goes to the left kidney and a right branch that goes directly to the heart.

In the fourth pattern of caudal venous return, all blood from the caudal vein is taken directly to the heart, and the kidneys are supplied only from segmental veins from the flank musculature. This pattern is found in the salmonids, perches, including yellow perch, tunas, lumpfish, and lumpsucker. In these fishes, no blood from the tail is filtered through a portal system before being recirculated by the heart.

Fish have a well-developed lymphatic system (Harder, 1975) consisting of lymph vessels that start as blind ducts near the submucosa of the gastrointestinal tract, the spleen, liver, and other parenchymal organs. These vessels join to form larger ducts that parallel the venous system and eventually empty into it. Fish do not have lymph nodes; however, lymphoid tissue is found in several places. It is probably best termed lymphomyeloid tissue, since it is multipotential. In lampreys and sharks, as well as in many other fishes, this tissue is found in the cranial kidney. In bony fishes, it can be located in the mesentery.

The Respiratory System

The pharynx of trout and most teleosts can be divided into three cavities, the buccal cavity and two opercular cavities. The entrances of the opercular cavities from the buccal cavity are guarded by mandibular and maxillary valves. This differs from the sharks (elasmobranchs), which have a single orobranchial cavity and five or more parabranchial cavities on each side of the fish. The presence or absence of the mandibular and maxillary valves is important clinically when it is desirable to ventilate a fish artificially. Many teleost fishes must have their mouth moved in order to open the valves and allow water to ram over the gills.

Trout have four gill arches with holobranchs and one with a hemibranch, called the pseudobranch. These arches are supported by cartilaginous rods extending from the floor to the roof of the opercular cavities of the pharynx. The cranial aspects of the gill arches are modified into gill rakers, which help prevent food and debris from reaching the respiratory components of the gills. The structure of the gill rakers is different enough among species to have been employed as a taxonomic tool. Gill raker structure seems to parallel the feeding habits of the species (Hughes, 1984).

The arrangement and form of the actual gills on the posterior aspects of the gill arches have also been used as taxonomic features even to the level of differentiating individual species of trout. Each gill arch has two rows of gill filaments. Each row is called a hemibranch, and two hemibranches form a holobranch. Each hemibranch consists of a row of gill filaments that stand up like teeth on a comb. Abduc-

tor and adductor muscles allow the fish to spread and collect hemibranchs on an individual gill arch.

Gill filaments, often referred to as primary lamellae, or just lamellae in the older literature, are formed on the caudal edges of the gill arches. Each gill filament has secondary lamellae (respiratory platelets) that run perpendicular to the axis of the primary lamella. In some fishes, there is only one row of secondary lamellae on each side of the filament, whereas in others there are two rows on each side. New secondary lamellae are formed at the tip of the gill filaments in bony fishes, and the oldest secondary lamellae are, therefore, located at the base of the gill filament. In sharks, new secondary lamellae are developed in a growth zone at the base of the gill filament, and the secondary lamellae at the tip of the gill filament are the oldest. The gills are supplied by a dual arterial system, with one artery providing for oxygenation of blood by the gill, and the other supplying the arch and lamellae (Laurent and Dunel, 1978; Laurent, 1984) (Fig. 1–7).

Most teleost fishes, including the trout, have a pseudobranch. The pseudobranch arises embryologically from the caudal hemibranch of the mandibular gill arch, is supplied with oxygenated blood, and, therefore, has no respiratory function (Harder, 1975); thus, the name *pseudobranch*. As early as 1839, two morphological types of pseudobranchs were recognized, those with distinguishable lamellae in contact with the water and those that were covered and had no close water contact (Muller, 1839). Free pseudobranchs are essentially identical to normal gills. They are true hemibranchs that may be shorter than a normal gill hemibranch. This kind is found in blennies, herrings, and flounders. Covered pseudobranchs have some connective tissue overlying them. This kind of pseudobranch is found in individual species from a number of orders of fishes. Embedded pseudobranchs are covered by the mucous membrane of the opercular cavity and are separated from the opercular cavity by folds of tissue. These may be located in the tissues at the base of the skull rather than on the operculum. Covered pseudobranchs have been graduated into four types based on their degree of isolation from water, but the clinical usefulness of this classification is not clear (Leiner, 1938; Bertin, 1958).

The pseudobranch is distinct from the carotid labyrinth of some air-breathing fish. In the trout, the pseudobranch is located on the underside of each operculum. In a striped bass, on the other hand, it is attached to the hyoid arch and resembles a gill. The pseudobranch lies deep in the roof of the opercular cavity in carps.

The function of the pseudobranch is unknown. Efferent blood from the organ passes to the brain and the eyes, and a direct vascular connection exists to the choroid of the eye in salmonids (Yatsutake and Wales, 1983). A variety of functions have been proposed based upon the histological structure of the organ, including a primary osmoregulatory function. Connections to the vascular rete of the swim

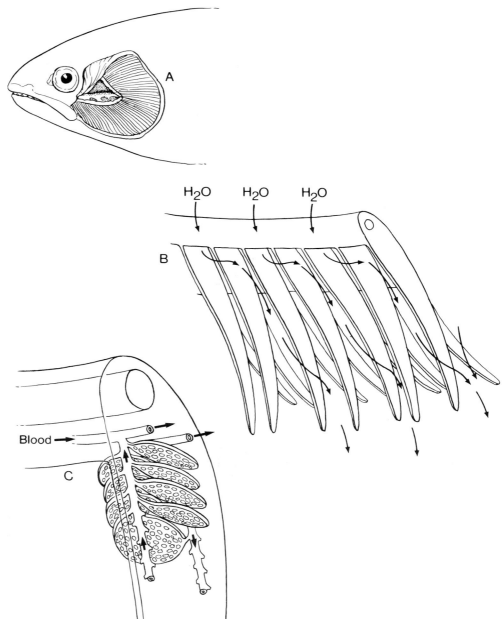

FIGURE 1–7. The hemodynamics and hydrodynamics of the gills of a salmonid fish. *A.* The gills lie flat in the opercular chamber with the leading edge of the branchial arch facing craniad. *B.* Water rushes over the leading edge of the branchial arch and through the primary lamellae on its way out of the opercular cavity. *C.* The water floods secondary lamellae that are supplied by a recurrent blood supply.

bladder in some species have also led to the postulation that it may be involved in filling the swim bladder (Lagler et al., 1977).

Digestive System (Fig. 1–8)

The rainbow trout is a carnivorous fish and, therefore, has a relatively short and simple digestive tract. Teeth are present but are not particularly prominent. As in most fishes, the mouth is devoid of distinct consolidated salivary glands (Anderson and Mitchum, 1974), although considerable mucus is produced by the buccal glands. The short esophagus enters a J-shaped stomach that has both cardiac and

pyloric regions, which can be distinguished on the mucosal surface but not on the serosal surface. The intestines have been assigned a variety of names by various investigators, but we shall adopt the terms small intestine and large intestine. Alternative terms that may be encountered in the literature include intestine and rectum (Burnstock, 1959; Bullock, 1963), ascending and descending intestines (Weinreb and Bilstad, 1955), and anterior and posterior intestines.

There is no real problem in identifying the structures as bowel, but some fishes, such as the goldfish and carp, do not have a defined stomach. This occurs in species from a number of orders. If fish do have a stomach, it is either straight, as is found in pikes,

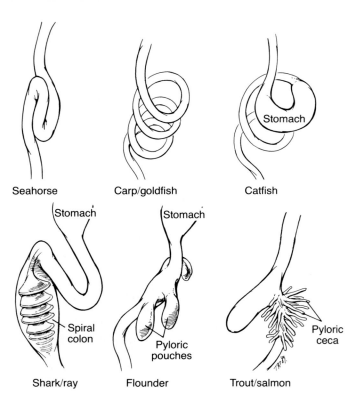

Seahorse   Carp/goldfish   Catfish

Shark/ray   Flounder   Trout/salmon

FIGURE 1–8. Comparative gastrointestinal morphology.

or U- or J-shaped, as in the sharks and most fishes with stomachs, or it has a gastric diverticulum that pouches off the U-shaped stomach, as in the freshwater angelfish. The demarcation between the stomach and small intestine may be completely lacking, or the pylorus may be dramatically marked by numerous pyloric diverticula. There may or may not be a demarcation between the small bowel and the large intestine. The entire bowel can be no more complicated than a straight tube, or it can be looped in various numbers of coils. The variations are many, but they all end at the anus.

In the trout, as the small intestine originates from the pylorus, pyloric diverticula arise. These blind sacs are encased in adipose tissue that encompasses the diffuse pancreas of the trout, which can be identified histologically. No discrete pancreas will be found on gross examination, and the multiple small ducts from the pancreatic tissue emptying into the small intestine are difficult, if not impossible, to appreciate grossly. In other fishes, the pancreas is also diffusely distributed, usually along the portal veins as they emerge from the intestinal serosa. The exocrine tissue is more diffusely distributed than the endocrine tissues, which are usually located near the liver or embedded within hepatic tissue. Islets are not numerous. The pancreas is present as a discrete organ only in the sharks, lungfishes, and some catfishes.

The exocrine ducts of the pancreas in fishes develop from three anlagen, with usually only one persisting late in development. However, all three can be found in many salmonids. In the majority of fish species, the single persistent duct develops from the right ventral anlage and is designated in some literature as Wirsung's duct. In skates, the persistent duct develops from the dorsal anlage and is called Santorini's duct.

The liver of the trout is not distinctly divided into lobes. It is located in the cranial coelomic cavity originating just caudal to the transverse septum that separates the peritoneal and pericardial cavities. It is located predominantly on the left side of the abdomen and is supplied by a hepatic portal system. The liver is connected to a prominent gallbladder via a hepatic duct. The gallbladder in turn empties into the pyloric end of the stomach through a bile duct.

The livers of various fishes can be quite pigmented. This is due to the presence of so-called melanomacrophage centers, which are sometimes considered indicative of inflammatory response. The opposite extreme is a light, almost white appearance of the liver, particularly in captive-reared animals fed prepared diets. This condition can be seen occasionally in wild fish, but it is prevalent in captive-reared fish.

The swim bladder (gas bladder, air bladder, pneumatic tract) is actually derived from the digestive system. In some fishes (physostomes), including trout, the swim bladder maintains an active communication with the esophagus through the pneumatic duct. In late embryonic and early postembryonic development, the swim bladder forms as a diverticulum of the esophagus. Young trout can gulp air from the surface to fill this pouch. Food can accidentally enter the swim bladder in very young trout, where it will not be digested, but will instead cause future swim bladder infections (Ross et al., 1975).

The swim bladder is a retroperitoneal organ. Its course of development varies in different fish species, resulting in a variety of final adult forms (Fig. 1–9). The simplest form of the swim bladder itself is found in the sturgeons and salmonids, including trout. In these fishes, the swim bladder is a wide, short duct with only one chamber. In the carp group, the swim bladder is divided into cranial and caudal compartments with a connecting isthmus. In the codfishes, the swim bladder is divided into three chambers (Mclean and Nilsson, 1981).

In trout, the opening to the esophagus is eventually closed by a sphincter muscle that controls the pneumatic duct, allowing rapid gas uptake or dispersal. The pneumatic duct in salmonids and catfishes arises from the right side of the esophagus. In carp, the duct develops from the left side of the esophagus. In contrast, the "lungs" of lungfishes and polypteruses originate from the ventral side of the foregut.

Other fishes that do not maintain a connection between the digestive system and the swim bladder (pysoclistous fishes) develop one or more prominent retia mirabilia associated with the bladder. These complex counter-current capillary systems are often found in the cranial wall of the bladder and may be found in the cranial wall of each chamber in multichambered species (Grizzle and Rogers, 1976). The retia are thought to enhance the availability of oxygen and, to a lesser extent, other gases to the epithelium of the swim bladder for concentration in the bladder itself. The rete mirabile of the swim bladder may be associated with the structurally similar choroid body of the eye, which is present in some, but not all, fishes (Lagler et al., 1977). In addition to the rete mirabile, many, but not all, fishes with prominent cranial capillary retia also have an anterodorsal capillary network called the oval. The oval is derived from the prevesicle of the embryonic pneumatic duct and is thought to function in the removal of gases from the swim bladder. Some fishes, including the carps, catfishes, and many eels, have both a pneumatic duct and a rete mirabile associated with their swim bladders.

In some fishes, such as in the freshwater butterflyfish, the swim bladder is highly complicated and penetrates into the centra and both transverse processes of many vertebrae, creating pneumaticized vertebrae (Schwartz, 1969). The freshwater butterflyfish floats on the surface and gulps air frequently, and its swim bladder may participate in respiration.

The swim bladder is missing entirely in many pelagic and deep sea fishes. The organ can be located in embryos of mackerels, tunas, and flounders, but flounders lose their swim bladders when they begin to live on the bottom, and adult mackerels and tunas do not have a swim bladder. On the other hand, over half of the benthic fishes have very large swim bladders. Some of these deep sea species have their swim bladders filled with lipids rather than gas.

The actual function of the swim bladder remains somewhat speculative. It is certainly involved in the maintenance of hydrostatic equilibrium. In some fishes, it may be involved in respiration, sound production, and possibly perception of pressure fluctuations, including sound waves (Reyer, 1977; Ross, 1979).

Hematopoietic Organs

Fish do not have bone marrow to serve as a hematopoietic organ. Their erythrocyte production is accomplished by the same tissues that produce their lymphoid response, lymphomyeloid tissue, located diffusely in the mesentery. The primary site of hematopoiesis in the trout is the cranial kidney (Yatsutake and Wales, 1983). The gross anatomy of the kidney is discussed later under the urogenital system. The trout spleen is an accessory hematopoietic organ.

Much of the lymphomyeloid tissue of the fish is found in the spleen. The trout spleen is adjacent to the greater curvature of the stomach. In other fishes, it is often found near the lesser curvature of the stomach or, in stomachless fishes, near that part of the intestine that passes where the stomach would be. The position of the spleen is similar to what would be expected in mammalian anatomy, with some exceptions. The lampreys do not have a spleen but instead have a fat-body or sheath. In the lungfishes, the spleen and pancreas are together but are well delineated. In other teleosts, the capsule of the spleen often contains considerable pancreatic tissue. Fish spleens can be pigmented. Pigment nodules result in a spotted appearance of the spleen in some fishes.

The trouts, like most fishes, have a distinct thymus that is a highly vascular, paired, bilateral organ found under the dorsal edge of the operculum just dorsal to the gill arches. In contrast with the mammal thymus, the fish thymus is difficult to locate

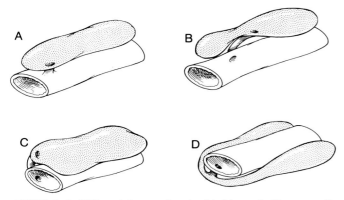

FIGURE 1–9. Different types of swim bladders. *A.* Sturgeon. *B.* Charachin. *C.* Australian lungfish. *D.* Pike.

in young fish, but it can be seen grossly in fish older than 5 months (Yatsutake and Wales, 1983). In some fishes, the thymus is found within the cranial kidney. In air-breathing catfishes, the thymus is caudal to the accessory respiratory organ, much more caudal than in most fishes. In the sharks, the thymus is fairly distinct and is located on the dorsal inner edges of the gill slits.

The Endocrine System (Fig. 1–10)

The pituitary of the trout is located ventral to the diencephalon, similar to that in a mammal. Compared with that in other fishes, the pituitary in the trout is foreshortened craniocaudally and deep dorsoventrally. Otherwise, it is unremarkable.

The thyroid gland of the trout is diffuse, a common situation in many species of fishes. It cannot be identified as a discrete organ. Follicles are found throughout the course of the ventral aorta and the branchial arteries. Follicles can even be found in the retro-orbital tissues.

Fish do not have discrete adrenal organs. The two types of adrenal tissue are distributed in the kidneys and along larger blood vessels. The component found in the kidney is sometimes called the "interrenal organ." In trout, this organ is located in the lymphoid portion of the cranial kidney. In most fishes, it is found in a layer around the posterior cardinal vein and its tributaries.

The second component of fish adrenal tissue, the suprarenal organ, is homologous to the adrenal medulla. It develops from the nerve tissue of the sympathetic ganglia and remains in close contact with them. These are sometimes called the paraganglia. Suprarenal tissue may contain a large number of neurons along with chromaffin cells. In sharks and rays, the suprarenal organs are found along the aorta and form larger complexes referred to as corpora axillaria. This is the origin of the term *suprarenal organ,* since in sharks the corpora axillaria is found on the dorsal side of the caudal kidney. In bony fishes, the suprarenal organ is almost always located in the region of the cranial kidney.

The kidney also contains the corpuscles of Stannius. These are found only in bony fishes, not in the sharks. These corpuscles are piles of cells arranged in alveoli, usually located dorsally and in the midline of the caudal kidney, where the left and right kidneys come together. Sometimes they are located on the ventral side of the kidney. Most fishes have two corpuscles of Stannius. Some catfishes have three to seven such corpuscles scattered along the ventral surface of the caudal third of the kidney. Trout and other salmonids have 4 to 14 of these structures. Removal of these organs affects electrolyte balance. The corpuscles become very active when fish have external damage that breaches the epithelial osmotic barrier. The corpuscles are considered endocrine organs, since they do not have ducts.

The ultimobranchial bodies are also called the postbranchial or suprapericardial bodies. They are located near the gill slits. In mammals, the ultimobranchial bodies are fused into the thyroid. In fish, they produce calcitonin. They are *not* anlagen of parathyroid glands. Fish do not have discrete parathyroid organs.

In trout and salmons, the ultimobranchial bodies are bilateral, located ventral to the esophagus, near the sinus venosus. In the rays, the ultimobranchial bodies are also paired, but they are found in the caudal wall of the pericardial cavity. In sharks, they are found only on the left side of the body on the dorsal wall of the pericardial cavity between the elements of the last gill arch.

Urogenital Organs

Kidneys in fishes vary considerably. Classically, they are described as they occur in trout species, as a fused, single, long, thin organ lying retroperitoneally just ventral to the spinal column, occupying the dorsal wall of the coelomic cavity along its entire length. This is an oversimplification. The pronephros and the cranial portion of the mesonephros, often designated as the cranial, anterior, or head kidney, can be topologically distinct from the caudal portion

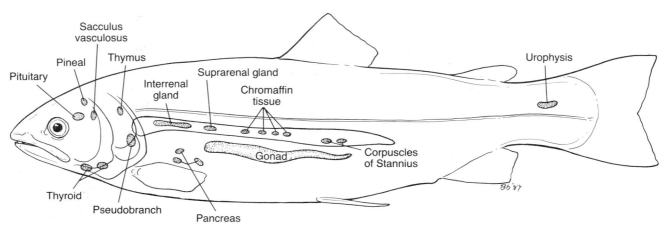

FIGURE 1–10. The location of endocrine organs in the trout.

of the mesonephros, designated as the caudal, posterior, or tail kidney. Even when the organs are continuous, the cranial portions of the kidneys usually remain separate, but the caudal portions are most often fused to some degree. Numerous authors have classified fish kidneys into various groups and subgroups, none of which are particularly relevant in diagnostic efforts. What is important is to be sure to sample both the cranial and the caudal kidney when performing a postmortem examination. Not only is the gross morphology quite variable, but the histology can be startling, particularly in species that have completely aglomerular kidneys.

The genital organs of the male trout have been well studied (Robertson, 1958; Henderson, 1962). The elongate testis bound in a thick white capsule of connective tissue is supported by a distinct mesorchium arising from the swim bladder peritoneum. The testis consists of elongate, blind, branching seminiferous tubules that produce spermatozoa that are discharged into a short deferent duct at the posterior pole, which carries the sperm to the genital pore. The reproductive and urinary systems are completely separate in both male and female trout (Henderson, 1962).

The ovaries of the trout are not as well studied as the male gonads but are very similar to those in other fish species (Yamamoto et al., 1965). Trout ovaries are long, paired organs that develop a beaded texture and enlarge significantly as oocytes mature during spawning season (Fig. 1–11). They are supported by a mesovarium, and their vascular supply enters along the dorsomedial aspect of the gonad. The tunic of the ovary is very thin and transparent compared with the tunic of the testis. After ovulation, a number of oocytes remain behind and are eventually resorbed. These have been called transitory corpora lutea and corpora atretica, but all evidence suggests that these are merely unovulated oocytes (Dodd, 1960).

The trout develops oviducts from a modified müllerian duct during embryonic development, but these nearly disappear in the adult. Ova are shed into the coelomic cavity before being passed through the remaining caudal portions of the oviducts at the genital pore.

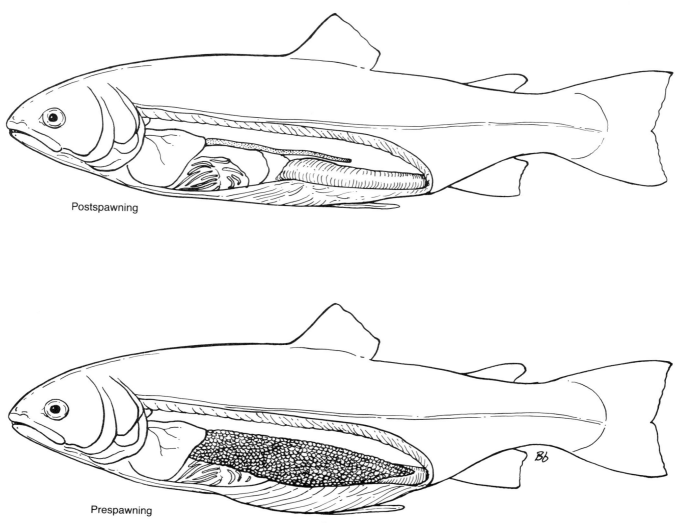

Postspawning

Prespawning

FIGURE 1–11. Seasonal gonadal variations in the trout.

Sensory Organs

The eyes of the trout are somewhat similar to those of other fishes. They are bilaterally placed in bony sockets of the skull, where they are independently moveable by three paired extrinsic oculomotor muscles. Although most fish are described as having no eyelids, trout have a single fatty membrane around the eye. The presence of a modified eyelid is common in fishes. The sclera of the cranially com-

pressed globe of the trout eye is supported by an annular ring of cartilage continuous with the nasal and temporal plates of true bone (Fig. 1–12). The trout cornea is elliptical and considerably thinner at the nasally located center, a common finding in rapidly swimming fish (Prince, 1956). An annular ligament connects the cornea to the outer rim of the iris (Prince, 1956). This ligament, along with the protrusion of the spherical lens through the pupil, appears to severely limit iris movement (Ali, 1959).

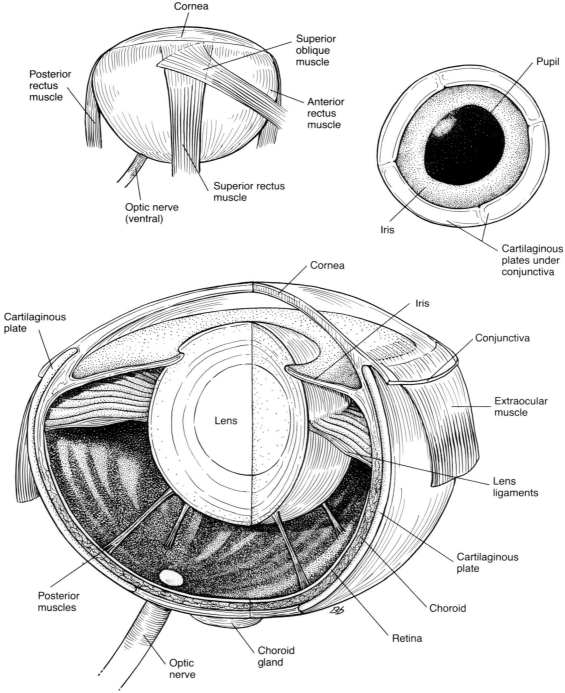

FIGURE 1–12. Diagrams of the globe and retrobulbar structures of the trout eye.

The pupil in most bony fishes is circular with some elongation in the direction required for acquiring food. In the trout the pupil elongation is ventromedial (Anderson and Mitchum, 1974). Some fishes that inhabit deep water where light levels are extremely low technically have no pupil, since their entire iris is missing (Harder, 1975).

To accommodate, the inelastic lens of the trout must be moved toward the retina by a special retractor lentis muscle (Pumphrey, 1961). This is the common mode of accommodation in fish eyes (Walls, 1942). Funduscopic examination of the trout reveals a lack of a fovea for binocular vision. This would be expected, considering the lateral placement of the eyes on the head of trout.

Olfaction in the trout is centered in the nasal passages, where water is circulated between the pairs of nasal openings as the fish swims (Watling and Hillemann, 1964). Likewise, taste organs in trout are centered in the buccal cavity and esophagus. Some similar sensory organs are found on the surface of the head, but not to the extent found in species like the catfish.

The lateral line system of trout consists of bilateral supraorbital, suborbital, mandibular, and temporal canals on the head (Fig. 1–13). These are continuous with the lateral line that runs the length of the body at about halfway between the dorsal and ventral limits of the trunk (Weber and Schiewe, 1976).

The pineal organ lies between the midbrain and dorsal forebrain in most fish species including the trout. It is often considered a sensory organ. In young fish it is visible through the cartilage of the cranium. The pineal is thought to be sensitive to light and may have an important secretory function for trout. A complete understanding of the function of this tubular organ that is connected to the third ventricle remains elusive (Dodt, 1963; Falcon and Meissi, 1981).

Contrary to popular belief, fish do have ears (Fig. 1–14). The ear of the trout consists of semicircular canals and three endolymph-filled ampullae—the utriculus, the sacculus, and the lagena. Each of these ampullae contains a calcareous otolith. The bilateral endolymph-filled labyrinths of fish are encased in the bone and cartilage of the posterior part of the cranium. They are thought to maintain muscle tone, balance, and perception of gravity as well as to serve in the reception of sound (Lowenstein, 1971).

CHANNEL CATFISH

The external appearance of the channel catfish varies depending on the age, sex, and geographical location of the fish (Fig. 1–15). Generally, a channel catfish is slender with a slightly depressed head that is approximately one-fifth its total length. The skin is devoid of scales. Eight barbels are present around the subterminal mouth, four dorsal and four ventral. The maxillary barbels located on the upper lip are the largest. Much smaller nasal barbels are found on

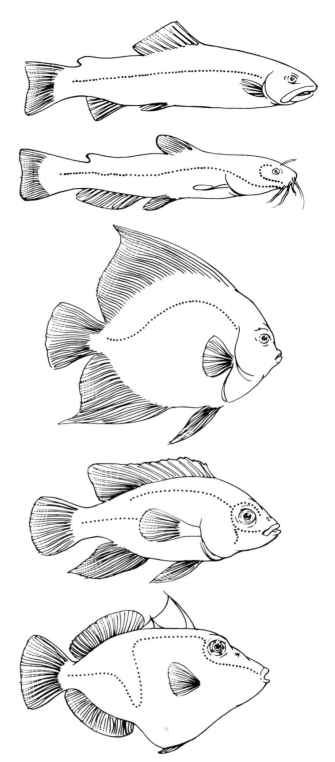

FIGURE 1–13. Comparative lateral line locations.

the cranial margins of the caudal nares. The two pairs of barbels on the lower lip are the larger outer mandibular barbels and the smaller central mental barbels.

Experienced practitioners can usually determine the gender of a mature channel catfish on the basis

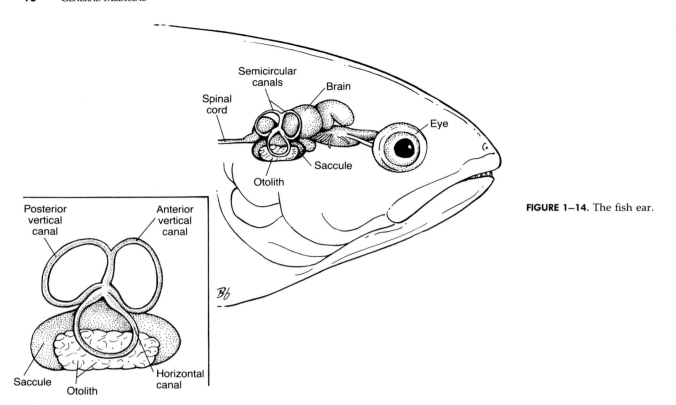

FIGURE 1–14. The fish ear.

of the wider flat head and pigmented underbody and jaw of the males. Females have a fuller body and lighter color during spawning. Mature males also have a distinct urogenital papilla. The female genital opening is separate from the urinary opening and has small flaps over it.

The fins of the channel catfish are relatively unremarkable. It has paired pectoral fins, which each have one hard ray with a serrated posterior edge and nine soft rays. The dorsal fin begins about one-third of the body length from the rostrum and has one serrated spine and six soft rays. The second dorsal fin is an adipose fin with no rays, being supported only by fibrous connective tissue. The paired pelvic fins each have eight soft rays and are found immediately cranial to the anal and urogenital openings near the halfway point of the body. The anal fin is caudal to the anus and is a taxonomic feature in the catfishes, with each species having different numbers of rays. The caudal fin of the channel catfish is deeply forked.

The lateral line apparatus of the channel catfish is readily visualized. On the body, it runs from the base of the caudal fin to the head along the midbody. Near the head it arches dorsad. Branches extend from the main lateral line to the adipose fin. On the head, branches form the supraorbital canal cranial and medial to the cranial nares, proceeding caudad above the eye. An infraorbital canal is present caudal and lateral to the cranial nares running below the eye. Just caudal to the eye, the infraorbital canal turns dorsad and joins the supraorbital canal to form the postocular commissure, which proceeds caudally. A preoperculomandibular canal starts on the lower jaw and runs caudally from just cranial and lateral to the mandibular barbel. This canal joins the postocular commissure and helps form the cephalic lateralis, which connects with the lateral line of the body just behind the posttemporal bone. Small pit organs (ampullary organs) are also abundant on the head and less so on the body. They form a depression or pit in the dermis that is readily visible to the naked eye. The function of these pit organs is not known, although there is some thought that they might be electroreceptors.

Internal Topology

The most remarkable aspect of the catfish skeleton is the absence of several bones in the skull, but this is of more taxonomic interest than clinical interest. Channel catfish have four pairs of gill arches, which are covered by opercula. Gill filaments are present on each arch along with two rows of gill rakers. Catfish have an oral valve consisting of flaps of skin that jut caudally into the mouth from the upper and lower jaws to prevent respired water from exiting through the mouth.

The channel catfish is omnivorous (Jearld, 1970; Cross, 1967). It has an alimentary canal that is from one to three times the length of its body (Gammon, 1970) and a U-shaped stomach with discernible fundic and pyloric regions. There are no pyloric ceca (Gammon, 1970). An intestinal sphincter, visible only on opening the gut, separates the large and small intestines.

The liver of the channel catfish is relatively small.

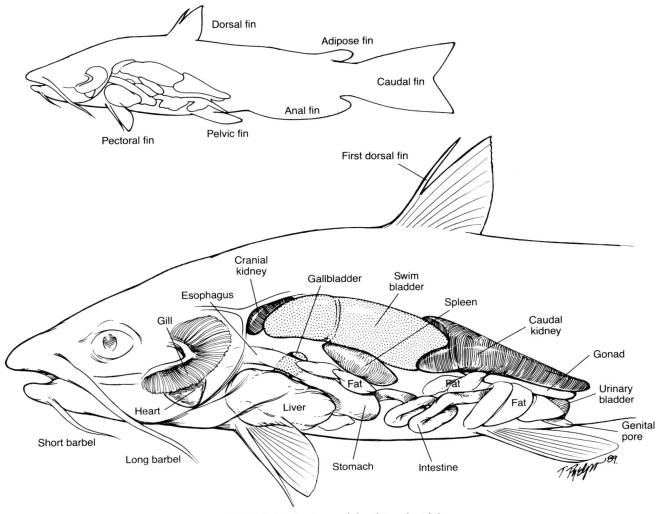

FIGURE 1–15. Anatomy of the channel catfish.

It can be yellowish brown to dark red and is not divided into distinct lobes. The liver extends only a few millimeters caudal to the ventral pectoral girdle. The caudal edge ends at the level of the caudal edge of the base of the pectoral fin on the right side. It extends a few millimeters further caudally on the left. The gallbladder is on the right caudal aspect of the liver, and a common bile duct enters the cranial small intestine just caudal to the liver.

The pancreas of the channel catfish is scattered as white nodules, sometimes referred to as Brockman bodies, in the mesentery around the bile duct and the hepatic portal vein, and between the spleen and liver. There are multiple pancreatic ducts that run parallel to the common bile duct, but they dump separately into the small intestine. The spleen is located on the left side of the catfish, above the stomach. It is usually translucent and sits just cranial to the gonads.

The swim bladder of the channel catfish is located retroperitoneally, sitting between the completely divided cranial and caudal kidneys. It is semirigid and opaque white and has three chambers, one cranial and two caudal. The transverse septum, which divides the cranial chamber from the caudal pair, is incomplete. Both longitudinally separated caudal chambers communicate freely with the cranial chamber. The channel catfish is physostomous, with a pneumatic duct between the midventral aspect of the cranial swim bladder chamber and the dorsolateral right side of the esophagus very close to the stomach. The cranial chamber also comes in direct contact with the skin, forming lateral cutaneous areas.

Although the kidneys are fused laterally, the cranial and caudal kidneys of the channel catfish are completely separated by the interposing swim bladder. The cranial kidney is composed of endocrine and hemopoietic tissue and is substantial. It generally extends caudad to just behind the gills. The caudal kidney has lateral margins, which can wrap around the posterior swim bladder chambers. The caudal kidney extends cranially to the middle of the dorsal fin and has two corpuscles of Stannius located laterally. Two ureters (opisthonephric, or wolffian, ducts) go through the length of the caudal kidney and open at the urogenital pore into the urinary bladder. The urinary bladder is in the caudal body cavity just ventral to the caudal kidney.

The gonads of the channel catfish are immediately ventral to and attached by mesenteries arising from the peritoneum covering the caudal kidney and swim bladder. Short ducts extend from the caudal ends of the gonads to the genital pore. The testes are lobate with numerous fingerlike projections. There are distinct differences in the gross appearance of the cranial and caudal regions of the testes. The cranial portion is composed of the seminiferous tubules. The paired ovaries are tubular and enclosed in a tunica albuginea.

GOLDFISH

The external appearance of goldfish is extremely varied (Fig. 1–16). Like the various breeds of dogs, goldfish have been bred into a myriad of forms and shapes at the whim of goldfish "fanciers." Some of these forms are discussed in Chapter 42. The more extreme forms have their own particular problems based upon the deformations of their anatomy. For example, breeds of goldfish with protruding eyes are prone to ocular trauma and infections. Rotund breeds like lion heads and orandas are difficult to evaluate for ascites or abdominal distention, an important sign of viral and bacterial diseases affecting goldfish. Similarly, breeds with peculiar scale formations, such as the pearl-scale breeds, can be falsely diagnosed as

suffering from external parasitism or pathological abdominal distention.

Goldfish, like other cyprinids, have no teeth in their jaws. They do generally have three rows of pharyngeal teeth on the lower pharyngeal bones. These pharyngeal teeth are true teeth and are used to crush food against a masticating or carp stone on the basioccipital bone. This carp stone is also called the pharyngeal process. It surrounds several major vessels to the head and is covered with a horny epithelium.

Goldfish have the classic four gill arches. The greatest number of gill filaments is on the first gill arch, as is typical of most fishes. The pseudobranch of the goldfish lies deep in the roof of the opercular cavity. The heart of the goldfish lies under and just caudal to the gills. A distinct transverse septum separates the pericardial cavity from the abdominal cavity.

The abdominal cavity of goldfish is dominated by a long complex gastrointestinal system compatible with their primarily herbivorous gustatory preference. The esophagus appears to enter the coiling intestines directly. There is no distinct stomach or even a dilatation of the gastrointestinal system, nor are there any pyloric ceca. Usually three coils of intestine nestle a prominent spleen in the center of the intestinal coil.

The swim bladder of goldfish is two-chambered with an isthmus and distinct cranial and caudal compartments. The two chambers cannot be closed off from each other unless the isthmus is damaged; however, each chamber has its own rete in its cranial wall. The size of the chambers can be nearly equal

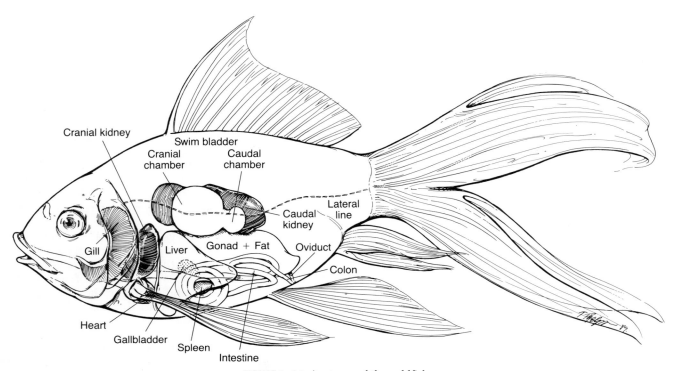

FIGURE 1–16. Anatomy of the goldfish.

or quite disparate in the heavy-bodied breeds of goldfish. These fish are prone to swim bladder disorders, which affect their ability to maintain proper equilibrium in the water. The two chambers of the swim bladder are nearly equal in volume in koi and traditional forms of goldfish.

The cranial and caudal kidneys of the goldfish are distinctly separated. The cranial kidney is located retroperitoneally, just in front of the cranial chamber of the swim bladder. The caudal kidney lies between the cranial and caudal swim bladder chambers. The gonads of the goldfish lie just ventral to the swim bladder. They change size dramatically with the reproductive cycle. The testes fuse posteriorly to form a Y-shaped organ.

The goldfish liver has two main lobes that unite cranially, dorsal to the esophagus. A deep indentation in the cranial dorsal surfaces of the liver accommodates the cranial swim bladder chamber. The gallbladder is surrounded by the right liver lobe. The left lobe of the goldfish liver is occasionally referred to as the splenic lobe, since it protects the spleen in a caudal ventral impression. There are usually two additional small accessory liver lobes in goldfish, one just caudal to each of the two main lobes. The left accessory caudal lobe of the liver can be rudimentary (Weber, 1827). Similar liver structure is found in the koi, ide, and pomfret.

The dorsal mesentery of the goldfish forms a sagittal septum that separates the two main liver lobes and contains the hepatic vasculature. Occasionally the liver will be completely divided by this septum, forming two distinct livers that are never joined cranially during embryonic development. The hepatic septum contains three hepatic veins, one arising from the left liver lobe and two from the right liver lobe, which carry blood from the liver to the heart.

STURGEONS (Figs. 1–17 and 1–18)

The sturgeon's individual, large, shieldlike scales give it a primitive, armored appearance. The heterocercal tail fin, where the backbone runs along the dorsal edge of the caudal fin, gives the tail a shape reminiscent of the sharks. The sturgeons are obviously designed for bottom feeding, with the prominent ventral mouth and barbels common in other bottom dwellers. Sturgeon can grow to immense size and are extremely important economically for their production of caviar. The species found in the United States are relatively uncommon and are the focus of considerable effort to restock them.

The operculum of the sturgeon does not completely cover the gills. Four gill arches have two hemibranchs each. The heart is located in a heavily protected pericardial cavity that is separated from the abdomen by a thick connective tissue septum.

Young sturgeons have teeth, but adults are toothless. Their digestive tract is relatively short. The strong muscular esophagus is lined with longitudinal folds and delivers food to a U-shaped stomach. The opening of the pneumatic duct into the stomach is prominent. The pyloric region is a distinctive structure. It consists of a complex network of pyloric ceca that open into each other, forming a spongelike structure that obscures much of the stomach from view. The small intestine is very short and almost a saccule that runs cranially from the pylorus to the intestinal valve, demarcating the beginning of the spiral intestine. The spiral intestine is similar to the spiral valve found in sharks and rays. It begins at the most cranial reach of the gastrointestinal tract and runs caudally to the anus.

The right lobe of the liver of the sturgeons is much more extensive than the left lobe, extending caudally to approximately the level of the caudal tip

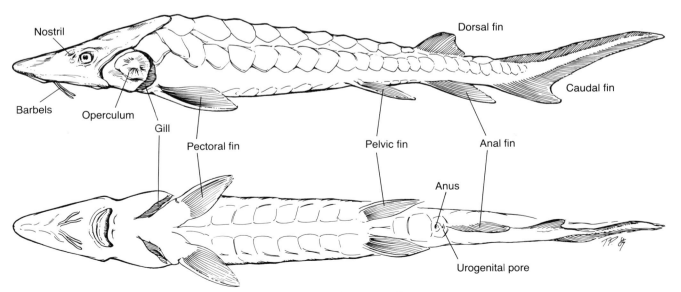

FIGURE 1–17. External anatomy of the sturgeon.

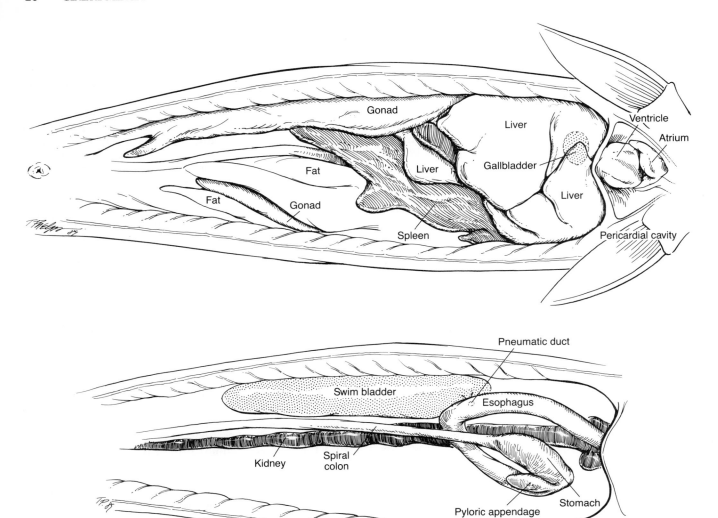

FIGURE 1–18. Internal anatomy of the sturgeon. Note the asymmetrical location of the swim bladder.

of the pectoral fin. The left lobe of the liver is much smaller than the right lobe and extends only to the level of the caudal margin of the origin of the pectoral fin. The gallbladder is visible in the cranial ventral portion of the right hepatic lobe. The spleen is long and has multiple lobes. It lies on the left side of the abdomen next to the stomach and is rather large compared with the spleen of other fishes. The pancreas of the sturgeon is found as dispersed bits of tissue throughout the abdomen.

The swim bladder of the sturgeon is a simple single ellipsoid chamber with a prominent pneumatic duct that opens into the stomach. The swim bladder is displaced to the right side of the abdomen and is not located along the midline as would be expected. The wall of the swim bladder is opaque and relatively thick.

The gonads and kidneys of the sturgeons are in intimate contact. The testes run from the pericardial region to a point near the anus. Cranially, they are attached directly to the peritoneum, and caudally they are suspended by a mesorchium. Sperm pass through the kidneys to reach the primary urinary ducts. Male sturgeon also have a patent oviduct, which appears structurally identical to that seen in females. The function of this duct in males is not known. The ovaries are also connected to the kidneys, but the connection is reduced and apparently nonfunctional. Ova are released into the body cavity and taken up by the oviducts (müllerian ducts), which carry them to the urogenital opening that is just caudal to the anal opening.

The eyes of the sturgeon have two crescent-shaped bony lamellae, one ventral and one dorsal, which are located between the sclera and the cornea to lend support to each globe. These lamellae are distinct from the subconjunctival ossicles that are also present.

FRESHWATER ANGELFISH

The freshwater angelfish are very popular aquarium fish. These cichlids have a very striking appearance, being laterally flattened and presenting a large lateral body surface. Their anatomy is not well studied (Fig. 1–19). Externally, their most striking features are their modified body form and fins.

The operculum and gills of the freshwater angelfish are similar to those of other cichlids. The heart of the freshwater angelfish is hidden under the cranial ventral tip of the liver. It lies in a triangular pericardial cavity, which is bounded cranially by the bony limit of the gill chamber.

The abdomen of most freshwater angelfish is filled with considerable fat. The liver is the most prominent organ in the abdomen. There are two major lobes, one on each side of the abdomen, which join cranially. The cranial ventral portion of the liver lies over the cardiac atrium. The stomach is moderately indistinct and usually hidden under the liver. It is U-shaped, often with a gastric cecum. The intestines are relatively long, arranged in coils in the lower abdomen. The spleen lies at the ventral caudal tip of the liver in the midabdomen. It is usually round or bean-shaped.

The swim bladder of the freshwater angelfish is thin-walled and transparent. It is a single chamber cranially, which is split into two fingers caudally, lying deep in the tail musculature. The two fingers of the caudal swim bladder are separated by three to four ventral vertebral processes. The kidneys of the freshwater angelfish are located retroperitoneally and are not separated into distinct cranial and caudal organs; however, the cranial kidney fills the space between the cranial aspect of the swim bladder and the skull and is a prominent organ. The kidneys run the entire length of the abdomen and are fused, lying just below the spinal column.

LEFT-EYED FLOUNDERS

The external anatomy of an adult flounder is a dramatic departure from the anatomy of other fishes (Fig. 1–20). The flounder lives its life on its side. During early development, the right eye migrates completely to the left side of the flounder's head, and the animal assumes a position with its right side down and left side up. The pectoral fins remain on each side of the animal, positioned high at the level of the middle of the operculum. The flounders have strong teeth in both jaws and a distinct fleshy tongue that is continuous with the gill isthmus and has a spadelike distal tip. There are four pairs of gill arches covered completely by the operculum. The cloaca opens on the ventral (right) side of the fish under the anal fin.

As might be expected, the abdominal contents of the flounder are asymmetrical. The liver is essentially a single lobe that occupies most of the left, or upper, side of the fish. On the right side, or down side, of the fish, only two small portions of the liver are visible, protruding around the gallbladder. A short, thick-walled esophagus empties directly into the stomach, which is approximately twice the length of the esophagus. The stomach has a small pyloric pouch. Three large, thick pyloric ceca, about half as long as the stomach, branch off the small intestine. Two branch off on opposite sides of the small intestine, about 1.5 cm after the pylorus. The third cecum branches off the intestine another 1.5 cm after the first two ceca. The intestinal tract is short, approximately the same total length as the stomach, with the rectum emptying into the cranial aspect of the cloaca.

The bean-shaped spleen of the flounder is found in the lesser curvature of the stomach. It is generally half the size of the pyloric ceca. Paired gonads are nestled into a pocket in the tail musculature. The oviducts are prominent and end in an opening in the caudal aspect of the cloaca. The cranial and caudal kidneys are continuous, located retroperitoneally under the vertebral bodies. There is no swim bladder, as might be expected in a bottom-dwelling species.

The heart is located approximately one-third of the body width dorsal to the base of the anal fin. It is most superficial on the upper, or left, side of the flounder. There is a well-developed bulbus arteriosus, which receives the blood from the ventricle and sends it to the gills.

Locating the brain of a flounder can be a challenge. The eyes are used as landmarks. In the flounder, the brain is located approximately 1.5 eye diameters caudal to the right, or upper, eye. It is interesting that the optic nerves of the flounder do not appear to cross.

MARINE ANGELFISHES

The tropical marine angelfishes are another group of laterally compressed fishes with a distinct body form (Fig. 1–21). They are quite colorful and have a modified fin structure with a single dorsal fin running along the majority of the dorsal surface and a single ventral fin rather than separate pelvic and anal fins. Externally, the lateral line is prominent. In the blue angelfish, the lateral line begins just behind the dorsal commissure of the opercular arches. From there it follows the line of the back, running about one-fifth of the total body depth below the dorsal limit of the body, to the base of the caudal peduncle. The lateral line of the gray angelfish begins about 1 cm above the dorsal commissure of the operculum and parallels the dorsal ridge of the body about one-quarter of the body width down. The lateral line continues to the caudal peduncle, where it runs in a straight line, slightly above horizontal midline, to the beginning of the caudal fin. There are six sensory pits around the eye and the top of the mouth in the gray angelfish. The pupil of the gray angel fish is

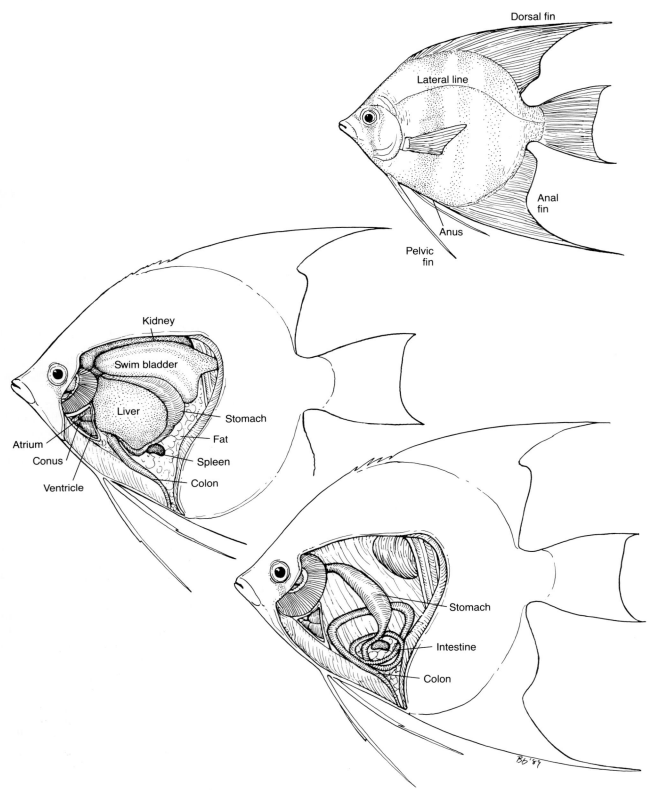

FIGURE 1–19. Anatomy of the freshwater angelfish.

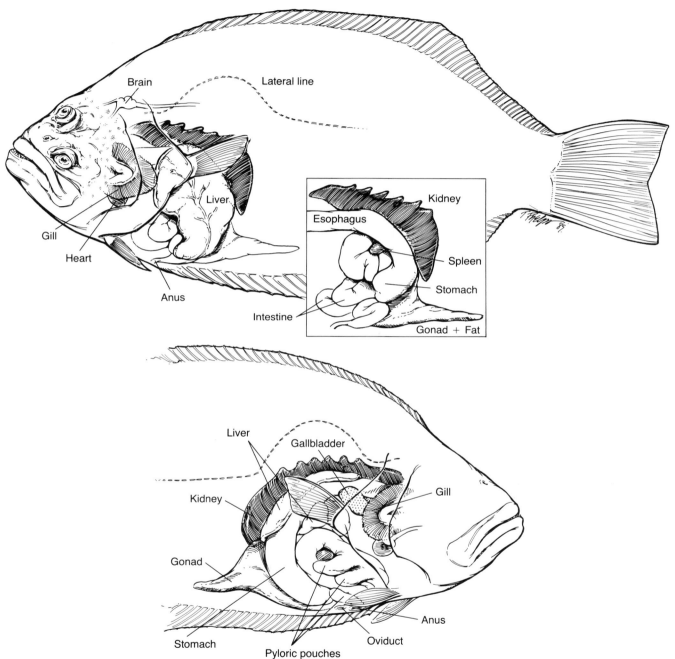

FIGURE 1–20. Anatomy of the flounder.

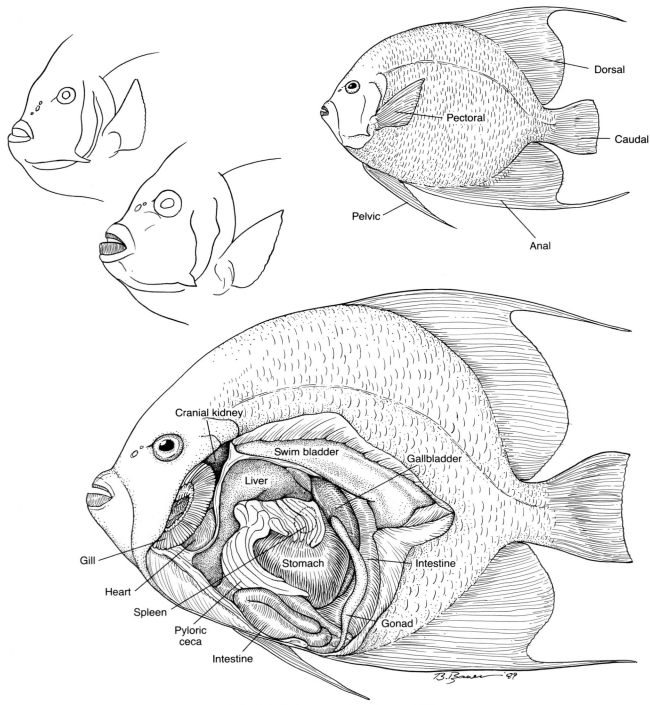

FIGURE 1–21. Anatomy of marine angelfish.

asymmetric, and elliptical, with the narrow radius of the ellipse toward the nasal canthus.

The operculum of marine angelfishes can have prominent spines, usually on the ventral caudal aspect. Some marine angelfishes will also have bony spines on their chin. Additional defensive spines occur on the ventral body, caudal to the anus at the start of the ventral fin.

Under the operculum there are four pairs of complete gill arches with two hemibranchs each. The heart of the marine angelfishes lies in a well-defined pericardial cavity nearly obscured by the gills above the bony ventral notch formed by the cleithrum and coracoid bones. In a full-grown specimen, the heart is a full 4 cm deep from the ventral surface of the fish. The heart is a typical fish heart with a very large and prominent thin-walled atrium.

In the abdomen of the marine angelfishes, the liver is usually nearly symmetrical but extends slightly further caudally on the left side. There is a single ventral lobe, which cradles the stomach and joins the rest of the liver with a broad isthmus. The gallbladder is prominent and lies dorsal to the stomach, often extending caudally to lie between the origins of the gonads.

The esophagus is extremely large, approaching 3 cm in diameter in larger specimens, with distinct corrugations in the serosal surface. The esophagus empties into a large distinct C-shaped stomach, which occupies much of the abdominal cavity. The pylorus of the stomach lies adjacent to the cardia. A distinct cardiac and fundic region of the stomach can be identified grossly. In the French and gray angelfishes there are 18 small thin pyloric ceca radiating from the beginning of the small intestine. The blue angelfish has between 20 and 24 pyloric ceca. The small intestine is long, up to 75 cm, and is over five times as long as the colon into which it empties.

The pancreas is diffuse and not identifiable as a discrete organ. The very flat spleen of the marine angelfishes is technically on the right side of the fish, but it lies nestled in the fold where the esophagus enters the stomach, nearly on midline. Its location is similar to the location of the spleen in the lesser curvature of the stomach in mammals. The spleen is usually darkly pigmented by melanocytes in its capsule. It is well protected by the stomach and bowel from accidental damage from intraperitoneal injection.

The swim bladder of the marine tropical angelfishes is thick and fibrous with a thin endothelial lining. It is a single chamber cranially, which is split into two fingers caudally, lying deep in the tail musculature. The two fingers of the caudal swim bladder are separated by six prominent ventral vertebral spines in the French and gray angelfishes and by three enlarged ventral processes in the blue angelfish.

The cranial kidney of marine angelfishes is very prominent and well separated from the caudal kidney. The large cranial kidney lies dorsal to and directly behind the gill chamber as a single mass. It extends caudally the width of one or two vertebrae and is nearly spherical. The caudal kidney, on the other hand, is extremely thin and very minor, appearing simply as blotches in the ventral view of the vertebrae. Ureters from the caudal kidney enter a very thinly walled urinary bladder, which lies in the caudal ventral quadrant of the abdomen behind the bowel. The urethra is extremely short, running from the ventral aspect of the urinary bladder to open into the cloaca, just caudal to the rectal opening. The gonads run ventrad from the origin of the gallbladder to the level of the cloaca, forming a Y-shaped organ. The sexual ducts empty into the cloaca.

The brain of marine angelfishes can be difficult to locate because of the disc-like shape of the head and body. The best method for locating the brain is to use the eye as a landmark. The brain lies on midline, just at the dorsal limit of the globe or the orbit if the eye has been removed. The optic nerve runs nearly directly medially, to cross just under the cranial portion of the brain.

SEA HORSES (Fig. 1–22)

The sea horses are often mistaken for invertebrates, probably because of their hard platelike exteriors. Sea horses are bony or teleost fishes, however, and possess backbones. The hard outer skin of sea horses complicates clinical procedures and simple injections. The sea horse swims in a vertical head-up position using its pectoral fins to stabilize itself. These fins are located high on its body, essentially on the head, where one might expect to find ears. The sea horse propels itself through the water with the help of a single dorsal fin. There is a small pelvic fin, which is of no value in locomotion.

Sea horses are sexually dimorphic, and their gender can easily be determined by examining their genital openings near the pelvic fin. Females have a small inverted crescent-shaped anus just cranial to a very small punctate reproductive opening. Both openings are located cranial to the pelvic fin. The male sea horse has a similar crescent-shaped anus above the pelvic fin but has an elongated genital opening below the pelvic fin rather than above it. This is the opening to the pouch.

The gills of the sea horse are relatively inaccessible because the operculum has a nearly complete membranous attachment to the body. The modified tail is suitable for grasping and holding to anchor the seahorse in position.

The internal anatomy of the sea horses is nearly as unusual as the external anatomy. An esophagus leads to a stomach, which is merely a dorsal pouch, at the crook of the neck. The pylorus is inapparent or missing, making it very difficult to appreciate the stomach. The intestines of the male sea horse are nearly 50% longer than those of the female. There is a gallbladder, a discrete organ at the most cranial portion of the liver, just below the crook of the neck. The liver is most evident on the right side of the

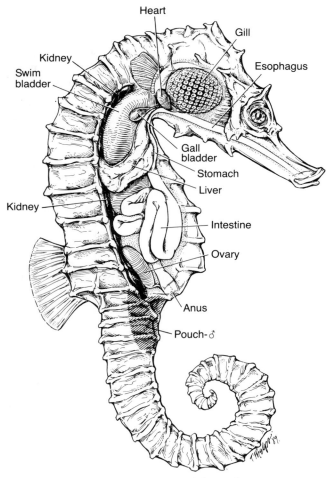

FIGURE 1–22. Anatomy of the sea horse.

animal, where it takes a bend caudally about halfway down the abdomen.

The sea horse kidneys are paired and located retroperitoneally, with no separation between the cranial and caudal portions. The gonads can be quite variable. The testes often appear as thin white lines running on the ventral surface of the kidneys. The ovaries are low, paired orange structures.

The heart of the sea horse is a dark triangular organ in the apex of the neck, just behind the gills. It surrounds the esophagus with three major vessels on each side, one coursing cranially to the gills and two running caudally, bringing return blood from the liver and kidneys. The gills of the sea horse are quite striking structures, quite distinct from those of other fishes. Sea horse gills are hemispherical organs with many individual gill projections, giving the organ the appearance of a small chrysanthemum. They lie in a closed gill chamber, making gill biopsy impractical.

SHARKS (Fig. 1–23)

The sharks are elasmobranchs, members of the class Chondroichthys. Their entire skeleton consists of cartilage rather than bone, although the jaws are heavily mineralized. Externally, they are covered by small placoid scales that give the skin a rough sandpaper texture. The placoid scale is derived from the same embryonic progenitor as the teeth of sharks. These scales, which are histologically identical to the shark's teeth, are also found in the mouth and throat, extending down the pharynx to the level of the caudal gill chamber. The teeth of sharks are replaced in sets as they are used and broken or lost.

The fins of sharks are distinctive, being considerably more substantial than the transparent membranes supported by thin rays and spines found in most bony fishes. Nevertheless, the same fin nomenclature is applied. The majority of shark species have very streamlined fusiform body conformations. They may or may not have a complete complement of fins. The variation seen most frequently is the absence of a dorsal fin. The tough fibroelastic properties of shark skin allow it to hold sutures very well but, at the same time, rapidly dull surgical needles. The lateral line of most sharks is quite prominent.

Most sharks have five pairs of individual gill slits. The gills are located within the gill slits, which can be closed off by highly developed gill septa. The thymus is fairly distinct, located in the upper inner edges of the gill slits. The ultimobranchial bodies are found only on the left side of the body, on the dorsal wall of the pericardium between the elements of the last gill arch rather than on both sides (Harder, 1975).

Internally, the clinically significant comparative anatomy points for a shark are its large liver, the presence of a spiral valve, the absence of a swim bladder, and the presence of a rectal gland. The liver of the shark is extremely large and may make up nearly 25% of the animal's body weight. It has two nearly equally sized lobes that run nearly the entire length of the abdomen. The gallbladder is in the cranial part of the left liver lobe. Not all sharks have gallbladders.

The esophagus of the brown shark empties through a well-developed esophagogastric sphincter into a J-shaped stomach that has a distinct pylorus. Many sharks do not have the esophagogastric sphincter of the brown shark, which probably inhibits regurgitation. The small intestine of the brown shark is relatively short, emptying through an intestinal valve into the spiral colon, sometimes called the spiral valve. The spiral colon provides a greatly increased surface area for nutrient absorption in the otherwise short digestive tract of the shark.

The rectal gland is found dorsal to the colon, opening into that part of the intestine just before the cloaca. The gland is suspended by a mesentery of the colon. It has also been called the cecal gland, anal gland, supra-anal gland, or digitiform appendix. It is a thick-walled tube with a narrow central lumen. The glandular tissue of the tube gives rise to many tubules that are arranged running radially to the lumen (Harder, 1975). Blood from the rectal gland is fed into the hepatic portal system. It is thought that this gland has a major role in sodium chloride excretion and sodium balance.

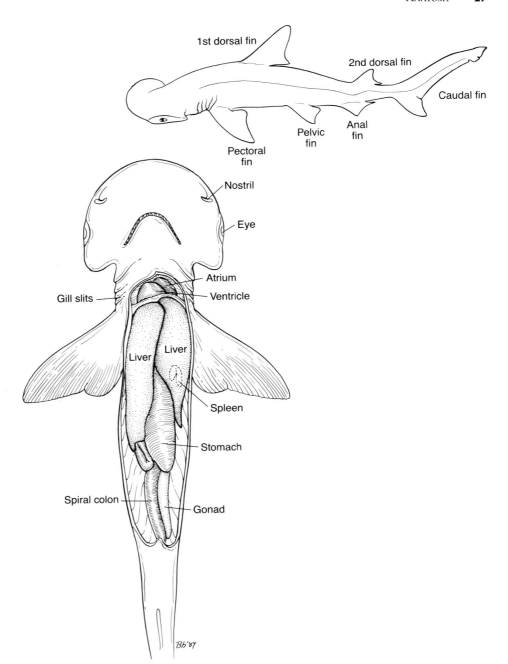

1st dorsal fin

2nd dorsal fin

Caudal fin

Anal
fin

Pelvic
fin

Pectoral
fin

Nostril

Eye

Atrium

Ventricle

Gill slits

Liver Liver

Spleen

Stomach

Spiral colon

Gonad

FIGURE 1–23. Anatomy of the bonnethead shark.

The pancreas is a discrete organ in sharks. It wraps around the small intestine near the pylorus. The spleen is usually elongated and essentially bilobed. Sharks frequently have accessory spleens, which are not the result of any traumatic event. The kidneys of the shark are located retroperitoneally, and the left and right kidneys are completely separate. The cranial edge of the kidney is usually just below the base of the front edge of the first dorsal fin. Directly underneath the kidney are the gonads. In the male shark, the cranial portion of the kidney serves as an epididymis. Just caudal to this portion of the kidney is a region that produces liquid to accompany the sperm as it runs caudally through the seminiferous tubules and the sperm duct. This is sometimes called the Leydig gland.

Two masses of lymphomyeloid tissue, the epigonal organs, run along the dorsal abdomen, nearly obscuring the kidneys and testis in the male and the kidneys, uterus, oviduct, and ovary in the female shark.

In sharks and rays, the suprarenal organs are found along the aorta, forming large complexes referred to as corpora axillaria. This is the source of the term *suprarenal organ*. In sharks, the corpora axillaria are found on the dorsal side of the caudal kidney.

The brown shark has eyelids and a nictitans. The wall of the eye is strengthened by a cartilage layer, which is thick at the posterior part of the globe and thins as it nears the limbus of the cornea. There is a tapetum lucidum.

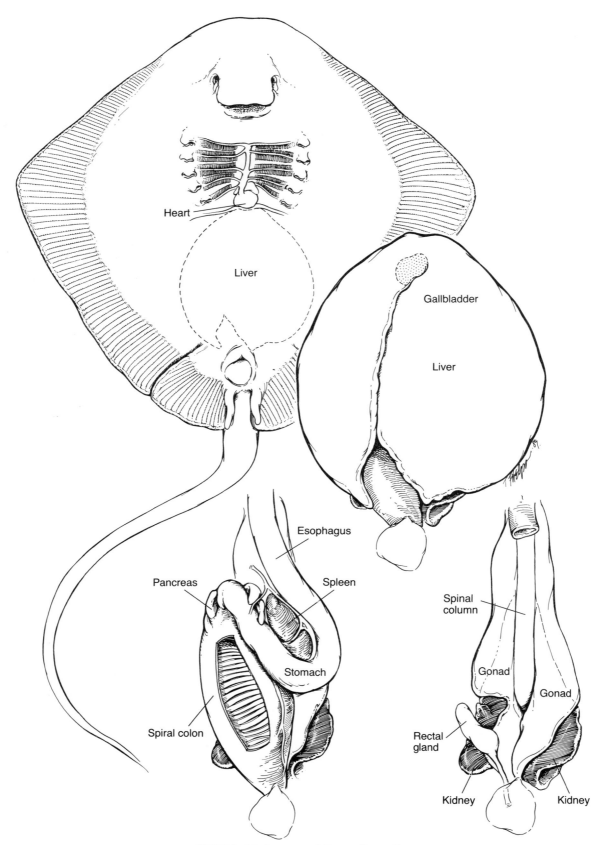

FIGURE 1–24. Anatomy of the southern stingray.

SKATES AND RAYS

The rays are also elasmobranchs, or cartilaginous fishes, but they have a very distinct body form, quite different from that of the sharks (Fig. 1–24). Rays and skates are flattened dorsoventrally, maintaining normal dorsal ventral orientation in their environment, as opposed to the laterally flattened flounders, which lie on their sides. The rays are covered by placoid scales much like those found covering the sharks. The mouth of a ray is oriented downward to facilitate bottom feeding. The mouth is a crushing type, with broad crushing plates suitable for diets based primarily upon mollusks and crustaceans.

An important adaptation in the skates and rays to bottom feeding is the spiracle system, which allows water for respiration to be taken in on the dorsal side of the fish, moved past the parabranchial gill cavities, and expelled underneath through the five pairs of ventral gill slits. This minimizes the intake of silt and bottom debris but also complicates gill biopsy. The spiracle is a remnant of the gill slit between the first and second gill arches. The true spiracle has a short hemibranch that is the same as the pseudobranch in bony fishes (Harder, 1975).

The thyroid gland of the skates and rays is a disc-shaped compact organ located in the ventral throat region similar to that found in sharks. It is not diffusely distributed like those in the bony fishes. The ultimobranchial bodies are paired and found caudal to the pericardium.

The internal organs of the rays are similar to those of the sharks. When the abdomen is opened, essentially all abdominal organs are obscured by the massive liver. Only the caudal aspect of the stomach and the spiral colon peek out from under the large liver. The digestive system consists of a short esophagus with an esophageal valve just above a series of transverse rugae in the cranial stomach. There is a transition zone, and then the rest of the true stomach is lined with deep longitudinal rugae. The stomach ends at a pylorus that dumps into a very short, sacculelike intestine that leads to the spiral valve. The spiral valve empties into the short rectum, which in turn empties into the cloaca. The ray has a true cloaca.

The spleen of the rays is on the left side of the abdomen, well covered by the large liver. The pancreatic duct develops from the dorsal anlage, just as it does in sharks and skates (Harder, 1975). This duct is commonly called the Santorini duct. The kidneys run retroperitoneally along the spine as in other fishes. In the rays, as in the sharks, the suprarenal organs are found along the aorta and form larger complexes referred to as corpora axillaria. The interrenal glands are paired and enclosed in a connective tissue capsule between the caudal ends of the kidneys. There is no swim bladder. The gonads are located ventral to the kidneys.

Male rays have copulatory organs that are modifications of the medial edges of the pelvic fins, called claspers. They have a dorsal longitudinal groove. During copulation the distal end of the clasper is inserted into the oviducts, opening the female's cloaca. Rays also have a clasper gland beneath the ventral skin of the claspers that produces a white viscous secretion that coagulates in water and may serve to seal off the clasper groove and help in semen transport (La Marca, 1963).

Rays and skates have a rectal gland similar to that in sharks. The gland is a thick-walled tube with a central lumen. The glandular tissue is divided into lobes, and the ducts run parallel to the length of the organ rather than radially as they do in the sharks. The gland receives blood from a branch of the caudal mesenteric artery, which divides to form a vascular network. There is apparently no countercurrent principle involved in the relationship of the ducts and the vascular supply (Harder, 1975). Blood from the rectal gland goes into the hepatic portal system. In some of the rays, the rectal gland has an S shape rather than the usual finger shape.

Skates have a paired bilateral organ of unknown function. It is found lateral to the vas deferens of the testicle and opens near the genital opening into the cloaca. It can be quite large and consists of many folds of epithelium. It secretes a clear liquid that is essentially free of protein and complex polysaccharide with a pH of 9.2 and a carbon dioxide content of 210 mmol/L (Harder, 1975). This gland is called the alkaline gland, or sometimes Marshall's gland.

Rays have no eyelids but instead are able to pull their eyes back into their head for protection. There is a choroidal tapetum lucidum between the lamina vasculosa and the lamina choriocapillaris, which is different from the usual teleost eye (Harder, 1975).

LITERATURE CITED

Ali, M.A. (1959) The ocular structure, retinomotor and behavioral responses of juvenile Pacific salmon. Can. J. Zool. 37:965–996.
Anderson, B.G., and Mitchum, D.L. (1974) Atlas of Trout Histology. Wy. Game Fish Dept. Bull. 13:1–110.
Bertin, L. (1958) Organes de la respiration aquatique. In: Traité de zoologie. Vol. 13 (Grassé, P.P., ed.). Masson, Paris, pp. 1303–1341.
Bullock, W.L. (1963) Intestinal histology of some salmonid fishes with particular reference to the histopathology of acanthocephalan infections. J. Morphol. 112:23–44.
Burnstock, G. (1959) The morphology of the gut of the brown trout, *Salmo trutta*. Q.J. Microsci. Sci. 100:199–220.
Cross, F.B. (1967) Handbook of Fishes of Kansas. University of Kansas Museum of Natural History, Lawrence, Misc. Publ. 21.
Dodd, J.M. (1960) Gonadal and gonadotrophic hormones in lower vertebrates. In: Marshall's Physiology of Reproduction 3rd ed. Vol. I (Parkes, A.S., ed.). Longmans, Green, New York, pp. 417–582.
Dodt, E. (1963) Photosensitivity of the pineal organ in the teleost, *Salmo irideus* (Gibbons). Experientia 19:642–643.
Falcon, J., and Meissi, H. (1981) The photosensory function of the pineal organ of the pike (*Esox lucius* L.). Correlation between structure and function. J. Comp. Physiol. 144A:127–138.
Gammon, R.L. (1970) The Gross and Microanatomy of the Digestive Tract and Pancreas of the Channel Catfish, *Ictalurus punctatus*. M.S. Thesis, Kansas State University, Manhattan, Kansas.
Grizzle, J.M., and Rogers, W.A. (1976) Anatomy and Histology of the Channel Catfish. Auburn University Agricultural Experiment Station, Auburn, Alabama.
Groman, D.B. (1982) Histology of the Striped Bass. American Fisheries Society Monograph No. 3. Bethesda, Maryland.
Harder, W. (1975) Anatomy of Fishes. Schweizerbart'sch Verlagsbuchhandlung, Stuttgart, Germany.

Henderson, N.E. (1962) The annual cycle in the testes of the eastern brook trout, *Salvelinus fontinalis* (Mitchill). Can. J. Zool. 40:631–641.

Hughes, G.M. (1984) General Anatomy of the Gills in Fish Physiology. Vol. XA (Hoar, W.S., and Randall, D.J., eds.). Academic Press, New York, pp. 1–72.

Jearld, A., Jr. (1970) Fecundity, Food Habits, Age and Growth, Length-weight Relationships and Condition of Channel Catfish, *Ictalurus punctatus* (Rafinesque), in a 3300 Acre Turbid Oklahoma Reservoir. M.S. Thesis, Oklahoma State University, Stillwater, Oklahoma.

Lagler, K.F., Bardach, J.E., Miller, R.R., and Passino, D.R.M. (1977) Ichthyology. 2nd ed. John Wiley & Sons, New York.

La Marca, M.J. (1963) The functional anatomy of the clasper and clasper gland of the yellow sting ray, *Urolophus jamaicensis* (Cuvier). J. Morphol. 114:303–323.

Laurent, P. (1984) Gill Internal Morphology in Fish Physiology. Vol. XA (Hoar, W.S., and Randall, D.J., eds.). Academic Press, New York, pp. 73–184.

Laurent, P., and Dunel, S. (1978) Relations anatomiques des ionocytes (cellules à chlorure) avec le compartiment veineux branchial: définition de deux types d'épithélium de la branchie des Poissons. C.R. Acad. Sci. [D] (Paris) 286:1447–1450.

Leiner, M. (1938) Die Physiologie der Fischatmung. Akad. Verlagsges, Leipzig.

Lowenstein, O. (1971) The labyrinth. In: Fish Physiology. Vol. 5 (Hoar, W.S., and Randall, D.J., eds.) Academic Press, New York, pp. 207–240.

McLean, J.R., and Nilsson, S. (1981) A histochemical study of the gas gland innervation in the Atlantic cod, *Gadus morhua*. Acta Zool. 62:187–194.

Muller, J. (1839) Vergleichende Anatomie der Myxinoiden. III. Uber das Gefassystem. Abh. Akad. Wiss., Berlin, pp. 175–303.

Prince, J.H. (1956) Comparative Anatomy of the Eye. Charles C Thomas, Springfield, Illinois, p. 355.

Pumphrey, R.J. (1961) Concerning Vision in The Cell and the Organism (Ramsay, J.A., and Wigglesworth, V.V., eds.). Cambridge University Press, New York, pp. 193–208.

Reyer, H.U. (1977) The role of the swim-bladder in vertical movement of fishes (*Carassius auratus, Salmo gairdneri*, and *Tilabia mariae*). Biol. Behav. 2:109–128.

Robertson, O.H. (1958) Accelerated development of testis after unilateral gonadectomy with observations on normal testis of rainbow trout. U.S. Fish Wild. Serv. Fish. Bull. 58:9–30.

Ross, A., Yatsutake, J.W.T., and Leak S. (1975) *Phoma herbarum*, a fungal plant saprophyte as a fish pathogen. J. Fish. Res. Board Can. 32:1648–1652.

Ross, L.G. (1979) The haemodynamics of gas resorption from the physoclist swimbladder: The structure and morphometrics of the oval in *Pollachius virens*. J. Fish Biol. 14:261–266.

Schwartz, E. (1969) Luftatmung bei Pantodon buchholzi und ihre Beziehung zur Kiemenatmung. Z. Vergl. Physiol. 65:324–339.

Walls, G.L. (1942) The Vertebrate Eye and Its Adaptive Radiation. Hafner, New York, pp. 563–591. (Reprinted 1963.)

Watling, H., and Hillemann H.H. (1964) The development of the olfactory apparatus of the grayling *Thymallus arcticus*. J. Fish. Res. Board Can. 21:373–396.

Weber, D.D., and Schiewe, M.H. (1976) Morphology and function of the lateral line of juvenile steelhead trout in relation to gas-bubble disease. J. Fish Biol. 9:217–233.

Weber, E.H. (1827) Uber die Leber von Cyprinus carpio, die zugleich die Stelle des Pancreas zu vertreten scheint. Arch. Anat. Physiol. 2:294–299.

Weinreb, E.L. and Bilstad, N.M. (1955) Histology of the digestive tract and adjacent structures of the rainbow trout, *Salmo gairdneri irideus*. Copeia 1955:194–204.

Yamamoto, K., Oota, I., Takano, K., and Ishikawa T. (1965) Studies on the maturing process of the rainbow trout, *Salmo gairdnerii* irideus—I. Maturation of the ovary of a one-year old fish. Bull. Jpn. Soc. Sci. Fish. 31:123–132.

Yatsutake, W.T., and Wales, J.H. (1983) Microscopic Anatomy of Salmonids: An Atlas. U.S.D.A. Fish and Wildlife Service, Resource Publication 150, Washington, D.C.

Chapter 2

FISH HISTOLOGY

MICHAEL K. STOSKOPF

A chapter on histology is an uncommon inclusion in a clinical text; however, like anatomy, the information is important to clinicians, yet relatively unavailable. Although the processing and reading of biopsy and necropsy materials is generally the domain of pathologists and technicians, the final responsibility for interpreting the results rests with the clinician. A good clinician must separate normal individual variation and age-related or seasonal changes from clinically important pathology. This requires a strong grounding in normal tissue and cell morphology. Fortunately, much of the histology of fishes is very similar to that in terrestrial mammals, providing a very good framework for comparative assessment. Since a complete treatment of the histologic details of fishes is beyond the scope of this chapter, particular care will be taken to emphasize differences from terrestrial mammalian tissues of similar function and tissues with no obvious mammalian analogue.

SKIN

The skin of fish is analogous to that of terrestrial mammals. It usually is composed of an epidermis and dermis supported by a hypodermis or subcutaneous layer. The thickness of the skin and of each of its layers varies between and even within species, depending upon age, season of year, and location on the body. Fish skin and the mucous layer it produces provide the first defense against invasion by infectious agents, osmotic pressures, and mechanical injury. Knowledge of the skin histology of fishes is particularly important to clinicians because cytologic examination of skin scrapings is a common diagnostic procedure.

Epidermis

The epidermis of fish is usually composed of stratified squamous epithelium arranged in the three layers familiar to terrestrial histologists. The stratum basale or germinativum is a single layer of columnar epithelium situated on a basement membrane. The basement membrane is not usually visible by light microscopy without special staining. The basal cells contain ovoid nuclei that are large and have more diffuse chromatin than nuclei in cells in other skin layers.

On top of the stratum basale lies a stratum of variable numbers of layers of fusiform cells with rigid walls, tonofibrils, and irregularly shaped dense nuclei (Anderson and Mitchum, 1974; Burton, 1978; Leonard and Summers, 1976). The cells in these layers vary from cuboidal to squamous as they approach the outer cuticular layer of the epithelium.

The outer cuticular layer of fish epidermis is generally defined to include the most stratified layers of epithelium and the outermost mucous coating. The outer epidermal cells of fish are usually living and do not have keratinized skeletons, although in some fish there are keratinized surface cells (Mittal and Whitear, 1979). The keratinized cells are usually found only on breeding tubercles. For this reason, some authors consider the cuticle to consist of the mucus alone unless there are keratinized cells. This is less common usage. In either case, the cuticle is often removed during routine processing for histological sections and is best examined through direct smears.

In addition to typical epithelial cells, a wide variety of unique cell types have been described in fish epidermis from different species of fishes. Although these cell types are not yet commonly used in clinical diagnosis, their presence can be confusing to observers unaware of their nature. Examples include the filament, or malpighian, cells that remain unkeratinized but contain 7.5-nm filaments in aggregates (Bullock and Roberts, 1975; Henrikson and Matoltsy, 1968a; Downing and Novales, 1971a, b), club cells (Henrikson and Matoltsy, 1968c), chemosensory cells (Whitear, 1971), granule cells (Roberts et al., 1971; Blackstock and Pickering, 1980), chloride cells (Henrikson and Matoltsy, 1968c; Lasker and Threadgold, 1978), mucous or goblet cells (Henrikson and Matoltsy, 1968b; Harris et al., 1973; Pickering, 1974; Pickering and Macey, 1977), and a wide variety of other glandular cells.

The layer of mucus covering the squamous epithelium of teleosts is secreted from mucous cells throughout the epidermis. These mucous cells differentiate in the stratum germinativum and migrate to the surface of the skin, where they discharge their secretions (Hawkes, 1983). Some histologists feel that at the skin surface, the mucous cell pushes between the spindle-shaped epithelial cells, discharges its entire contents, and dies (Van Oosten, 1957; Brown and Wellings, 1970). Mucous cells have basal, compact nuclei and are filled with membrane-enclosed packets of glycoproteins that are positive for sialomucins and sulfomucins when stained by alcian blue-PAS. The sulfomucins possibly protect fish from bacterial and fungal infections (Gona, 1979).

In addition to mucous cells, a few families of fishes, including the armored catfishes, trout, sharks, and a number of genera of the order Perciformes, have glandular cells called serous cells. Although these cells are lumped into a single group, they are not well studied and have a variety of different shapes and products. In the sharks, skates, and rays, they are sometimes called albuminoid or acidophilic gland cells (Harder, 1975).

Other cells found in fish epidermis are the inappropriately named club cells. These are not club-shaped in all or even most species of fishes and are not related to the mucous cells of the lamprey that are called club cells. They are sometimes called giant cells (Mittal and Munshi, 1970) since they are multinucleate in some fishes. They are also called alarm substance cells (Fig. 2–1). In the carp, the alarm substance cells produce pterin, which initiates alarm reactions when perceived by the olfactory organs of other fish in the school (von Frisch, 1941; Pfeiffer, 1970; Pfeiffer et al., 1971). These cells do not open to the surface of the epithelium and are found in the middle of the epidermis. They are completely distinct from the mucous cells and are not associated with them. In different fish species, alarm substance cells vary considerably in size and number of nuclei.

Scales

Scales also provide protection to the outer surface of the epithelium in many fish. Histologically, scales are acellular dermal bone composed of mineralized matrix around collagen. Scales are anchored in dermal pockets between layers of collagen in the stratum spongiosum of the dermis and the epidermal basement membrane, with parts of the upper and lower scale surface covered by epidermis. The entire scale is covered by a thin cellular layer distinct from other epidermal tissues. On the underside of the scale, or the surface close to the body, are two or three layers of hyposquamal cells. These are connected to a layer or layers of episquamal cells on the external side of the scale by radius cells that penetrate through the scale matrix. These connecting cells get their name from the scale radii that they form.

Dermis

Underneath the epidermis, the dermis of fish can vary from a narrow stratum compactum of dense white connective tissue to a more extensive dermis consisting of an outer stratum compactum and an inner stratum spongiosum of loose connective tissue. The inner portion carries blood vessels and lymphatic ducts that nourish the skin (Harder, 1975). In clear fishes, such as the glass catfish and glass eel, the arrangement of the collagen fibers in the dermis is extremely regular, much in the fashion of the collagen in the cornea, allowing light to pass through the dermis unreflected (Harder, 1975). In these fish, the peritoneum is often pigmented to protect abdominal organs from light. In most fish, the dermis contains pigment cells that can occur in layers at different levels.

The coloration of fish is a complex subject, but of clinical interest because of the many color changes associated with different disease conditions. Pigment cells in fish skin can contain a wide variety of pigments or substances other than melanin. These include the carotenoids, pterin, guanine crystals, which impart silvery color and many others (Junqueira et al., 1978; Harder, 1975). As a result, a variety of terms for specialized cells have arisen. Melanophores containing melanin absorb the entire visible range of light. Xanthophores contain rodopterin and carotenoid granules and appear yellow to orange. Cells that contain platelets of guanine or hypoxanthine are called iridophores. These cells reflect light, rather than absorb it, giving fish their shiny appearance (Bagnara and Hadley, 1973).

Iridophores are clustered in groups, often associated with melanophores, with the cell body of the pigmented cell deep to the iridophores. Dendritic processes of the melanophores project up and enclose the iridophores. In normally shiny fish, pigment in the melanophores is collected in the melanophore cell bodies, and light is reflected after striking the guanine or hypoxanthine platelets of the iridophores. When the skin of a fish becomes dark, melanin is being dispersed into the dendritic processes of the melanophores, where the melanin absorbs light before it can strike the iridophores. Xanthophores, like melanophores, are often found at

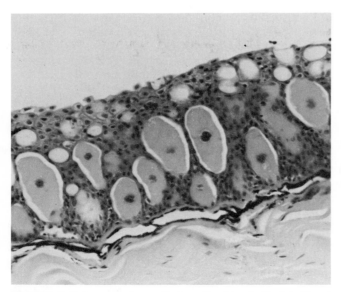

FIGURE 2–1. Cutaneous alarm cells from the skin of a black bullhead catfish. In some cells the double nuclei can be discerned (H&E, 200×).

several levels in the dermis but are not necessarily associated with clusters of iridophores.

Hypodermis

The hypodermis lies between the stratum spongiosum of the dermis and skeletal or muscular elements beneath the skin. It consists primarily of areolar connective tissue and is usually most prominent along the flanks. In some areas, for example the head region, the hypodermis is indistinguishable from the stratum spongiosum.

Fins

In many fish, fins can be considered as large folds of skin with special support. Fins are usually covered by stratified squamous epithelium continuous with the epidermis of the body. This squamous epithelial covering is usually specialized. The underlying dermis has a reduced stratum compactum and increased hypodermis compared with skin covering the body. All fins are linked to the musculoskeletal system through their special support, which can consist of soft segmented rays, hard unsegmented rays commonly referred to as spines, or combinations of both. Soft segmented rays in teleosts contain paired lepidotrichia composed of dermal bone that develops from the same primordia as the scales.

Hard spines are singular mineralized structures (Harder, 1975; Grizzle and Rogers, 1976).

MUSCULOSKELETAL TISSUES

Muscle

Like terrestrial vertebrates, fish have three major histologic classifications of muscle tissues. Involuntary smooth muscle in fish is composed of unbranched, long-tapering, mononucleate cells devoid of striations, similar to the tissue in more familiar land vertebrates. Fish also have the two striated forms of muscle common to terrestrial vertebrates, cardiac and skeletal muscle. These cells contain myofilaments organized in myofibrils visible by light microscopy. Cardiac muscle in fish is similar to cardiac muscle in terrestrial species. It consists of striated, branched, multinucleate cells with nuclei near the center of the cell. Occasionally, inexperienced histologists will confuse the nuclei of endothelial cells lining the heart with peripheral nuclei in fish cardiac muscle. Striated skeletal muscle in fish is unbranched, multinucleate, with nuclei just under the sarcolemma, or cell membrane, just as in other vertebrates.

The skeletal muscles of fish can be divided into two types, dark or red muscles and light or white muscles, on the basis of morphology and physiology (Fig. 2–2). Light muscles are the most plentiful mus-

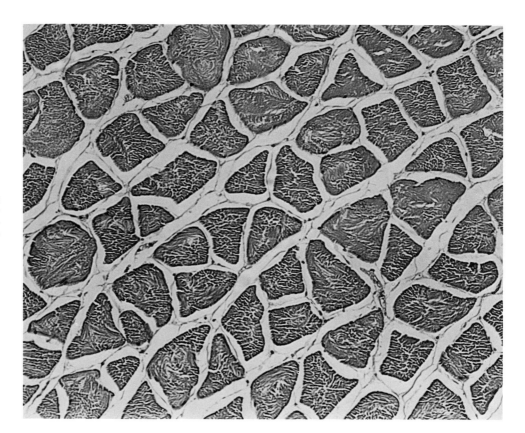

FIGURE 2–2. Skeletal muscle from a killifish. It is striated and non-branching and has peripheral nuclei similar to mammalian skeletal muscle (H&E, 100×).

cles in most fishes, making up the deep skeletal muscles in the epaxial and hypaxial myomeres. These light muscles are relatively poorly perfused but are considered useful in short, strong bursts of swimming, during which they rapidly become anaerobic (Nag and Nursall, 1972).

The term *myomere* is commonly used in fish anatomy and refers to a separate muscle bundle, with parallel fibers running along the long axis of the body of the fish, connected by myosepta to a vertebra. There is an epaxial and a hypaxial myomere for each vertebra in most fishes.

Dark or red muscle is generally found superficial to the epaxial and hypaxial white skeletal muscles of fish. This muscle tissue has a higher lipid content than do white muscle cells and more mitochondria per cell. These narrower muscle cells are also supported by a better vascular supply than that of white muscle (Grizzle and Rogers, 1976). Dark or red muscle is usually most prominent in the areas underlying the fins of major propulsion. In salmonids, this is under the lateral line in a configuration to move the tail. In perch and other species that utilize their pectoral fins for locomotion, dark muscle is abundant in the areas under these fins. In sea horses that use their dorsal fin for continuous propulsion, dark muscle is more prominent under the dorsal fin. Dark muscle is thought to be utilized for continuous slower swimming.

Cartilage

Cartilage plays an important structural role in fish. Cartilaginous skeletons are expected in the sharks and rays, but the skeleton of many young teleost fish also consist primarily of hyaline cartilage similar to that found in mammals. In addition, fish have a variety of specialized cartilages that are somewhat different from those found in terrestrial species. One example is the cartilage commonly found supporting the gill filament. This cartilage has an acidophilic matrix and less matrix per cell than is found in most cartilage. The chondrocytes in gill filament cartilage are basophilic. Some fish also have a chondroid covering of the opercular bone, consisting of closely spaced, round cells in a matrix with scattered fibers. This is considered a very primitive form of cartilage. Another primitive form of cartilage can be found in the barbels of some fish, including catfishes.

The notochord within the vertebral column of fish contains another special form of cartilage that is composed of noncalcareous tissue intermediate between cartilage and cellular connective tissue. It contains very tumescent chondrocytes with fluid-filled vacuoles that displace other elements, including the nucleus, to their periphery. These cells are reminiscent of fat cells in the way they accumulate intracytoplasmic fluid and in the presence of the large, single vacuole occupying most of the cell. Some histologists classify this cartilage as a distinct tissue because it contains intracellular matrix unlike carti-

lage or bone (Grizzle and Rogers, 1976). The notochord is surrounded by an elastic, connective tissue sheath.

Bone

Fish bones are generally formed by one of two processes similar to those known in mammals, direct ossification of dermal bone or perichondrial ossification of hyaline cartilage. Similarly, fish bones tend to be one of two types, cellular or acellular. However, teleost and elasmobranch fishes have a variety of tissues intermediate between cartilage and bone, based on the definitions used in other vertebrates, and these can confuse the issue (Harder, 1975). Acellular bones are devoid of osteocytes (Roberts, 1978) and can be formed either by dermal ossification or by a perichondrial ossification, which does not leave cavities for osteoblasts during bone formation. Perch and higher orders of fish tend to have acellular bones. These bones are surrounded by a fibrous connective tissue periosteum and an osteogenic layer of osteoblasts. These osteoblasts are irregularly shaped and acidophilic and contain large, round nuclei with diffuse chromatin. They are widely spaced in newly formed ground substance and become flattened and degenerate distal to the supporting periosteum.

Cellular fish bone contains osteocytes in lacunae within the ossified matrix of the bone (Fig. 2–3). This type of bone is generally found in the older orders of fish, such as the salmonids, in which it is found in the gill arches. In these bones, osteoblasts and osteoclasts generally appear similar to those in mammals (Lopez, 1970).

A type of bone in fishes termed mixed bone is a result of both dermal and chondral bone formation. It may have hyaline cartilage associated with it but is commonly acellular bone in areolar or dense white connective tissue. A subtype of mixed bone is the spongy bone, which forms the jaw bones, gill arches, and some other head bones in many fishes. Spongy

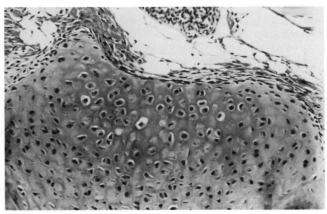

FIGURE 2–3. Cellular bone from the vertebral body of a silver salmon (200×).

bone is laminated with spaces that give it a sponge-like appearance.

CARDIOVASCULAR TISSUES

The arteries and veins of fishes are similar to those in other animals. Elastic arteries can be found near the heart, and muscular arteries more peripherally. Semilunar valves are found in fish veins and also in the segmental arteries of many fishes. It is thought these endothelial valves are used to allow muscle contractions to aid in blood circulation in fishes. Specialized vascular structures are found in fishes. In the spleen, for example, capillaries have a very large bore and are essentially endothelium-lined sinusoids.

Lymphatic vessels in fish are smaller than their corresponding blood vessels and may consist exclusively of an endothelial lining. Larger lymphatics have a layer of connective tissue with scattered smooth muscle cells, rather than the three sharply defined layers found in blood vessels. Lymphatics also have numerous valves to prevent backflow. Lymph hearts, similar to those found in amphibia, are often found in the fork of the caudal vein. Lymph hearts occur in some eels, tench, pike, and trout. The lymph heart of fish is two-chambered, with a distinct atrium and ventricle. The lateral system of lymph vessels opens into the anterior atrium of the lymph heart in those fish that have one.

The hearts of fishes consist of the three layers of tissue familiar to students of terrestrial histology, the epicardium, myocardium, and endocardium. The external epicardium consists of a layer of epithelium on a thin connective tissue layer that merges with the pericardial cavity lining. The myocardium varies in thickness in different parts of the heart. It is thin in the sinus venosus, but it is contractile and is thought to be responsible for the small electrocardiographic wave sometimes designated as the v wave (Satchell, 1971). The muscular layer is somewhat thicker in the cardiac atrium, where pectinate muscles radiate from the roof of the atrium forming a star-burst muscular net. The bulbus arteriosus also contains cardiac muscle that has an independent contraction rhythm. The bulbus of the fish heart is not homologous to either the conus arteriosus or the bulbus aortae found in mammals (Harder, 1975). It often contains longitudinal rows of valves, which are closed by contractions of the circumferentially arranged cardiac muscle. The ventricle, as expected, has the thickest layer of cardiac muscle. The endocardium in fishes consists of an endothelial layer supported on a thin layer of connective tissue and is similar to that found in mammals.

RESPIRATORY TISSUES

A good basic knowledge of normal histology of the gill is important to the clinician, since changes in

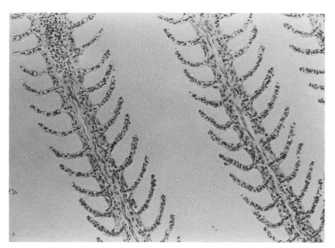

FIGURE 2–4. Gill lamellae from a guppy (H&E, 100×).

the gill epithelium are a very good early warning of environmental and infectious disease processes. The epithelium covering the gill arches is continuous with the epithelium of the pharynx and buccal cavity. It often contains taste buds and mucous cells. Abductor bundles of striated muscle can often be found along the lateral sides of the gill arch and between the hemibranchs. The supporting gill arch bone or cartilage changes with the age of the fish and with the species. Adult fish have less cartilage and more bone.

Gill filaments or primary lamellae are supported by a central core of cartilage, contain both supply and exchange blood vessels, and are covered by epithelium that is continuous with that of the secondary lamellae (Fig. 2–4).

The secondary lamellae of the gill are covered with a squamous epithelium, usually at least two layers thick. This epithelium is thickest in air-breathing fishes. The layers of the epithelium are occasionally separated by intercellular spaces that contain macrophages. Rather than normal variation, as described in various histology texts, this is possibly an indication of inflammation. Chloride cells are intensely acidophilic and are found in the epithelium at the base of the secondary gill lamellae of marine fishes. They are very rare in freshwater species. Mucous cells also occur on some parts of the secondary gill lamella, particularly near the base.

Pseudobranchs have quite variable structure in different fish species. In some fishes, the pseudobranch has a glandular appearance, owing to consolidation of the filaments of the primordial gill (Fig. 2–5). There are usually many capillaries, numerous large acidophilic cells with abundant mitochondria, and nuclei that have indistinct boundaries and very little chromatin.

DIGESTIVE TISSUES

The digestive system of fishes consists of structures similar to those found in terrestrial vertebrates.

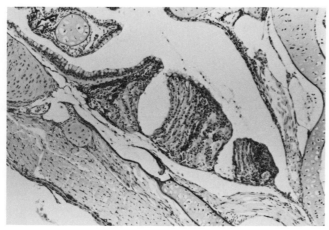

FIGURE 2–5. The pseudobranch of a young brook trout showing the nearly glandular appearance of the modified gill (H&E, 100×).

The histologic patterns are also similar, and the same nomenclature can be applied in most cases. The tunica mucosa usually consists of an epithelial mucosa overlying a layer of loose connective tissue or the lamina propria. The lamina propria may have a stratum compactum of dense connective tissue, such as is found in the stomach of salmonids, or a stratum granulosum consisting of granular eosinophilic cells found in the intestines of many fish. Underneath the lamina propria is usually a muscularis mucosae. The three layers of the tunica mucosa are supported on a connective tissue tunica submucosa, which is in turn surrounded by the tunica muscularis. The tunica muscularis usually has both a circular and a longitudinal layer of muscles, although the relationship between these layers can be quite variable. When considering a viscus, the final layer is a cuboidal epithelial serosa, overlying a bit of loose connective tissue and many blood vessels and nerves.

Teeth

The mouth of fishes is often highly adapted to their feeding behavior and diet. Most fishes have teeth. In most cases, they are true teeth, joined by connective tissue to bones. On section, the pulp of the fish tooth is primarily connective tissue with odontoblasts arranged on the outer perimeter to secrete dentin. Fish dentin is mostly collagen with calcium salts, similar to bone. Projections from the odontoblasts enter the dentin proper through dentin tubules. The surface of the dentin is covered with enamel secreted, while the tooth is still in the germ phase, by an enamel organ consisting of two layers of epithelial cells.

Tongue

In most fishes, the tongue is poorly developed. Often it is little more than connective tissue covered

with epithelium that contains many unicellular glands. For example, the elephantnose fish has a groove-shaped tongue, which is entirely connective tissue with no muscle at all (Mikuriya, 1972). There are exceptions. The polypterus has a well-developed tongue with considerable smooth muscle on its edges, radiating to the center of the tongue (Marcus, 1934). The archerfish also has a muscular tongue, but it is not attached to floor of the mouth. Instead, it lies in the middle of the roof of the mouth and can be furrowed to make a tube for shooting streams of water.

Pharynx

In most fishes the pharynx is lined with stratified epithelium, containing mucous cells in crypts. There is usually a lamina propria, but no muscularis mucosae. The tunica muscularis is composed of a thick, outer circular layer and an inner longitudinal layer of striated muscle. Some fishes have distinct pharyngeal pads, which are muscular bulges in the roof of the mouth. Histologically, pharyngeal pads consist of stratified, mucous membrane epithelium containing many goblet cells and numerous taste buds covering a thick layer of connective tissue. The pharyngeal pad epithelium has no basal membrane in most cases, but elastic fibers in the connective tissue seem to serve the same function. Beneath the connective tissue layer is a thick layer of striated muscles and nerves. It is postulated that the pharyngeal pad assists swallowing by pressing food against the gill rakers to squeeze out excess water. Alternatively, the pharyngeal pad might substitute as a special salivary gland (Harder, 1975).

Esophagus

In most fishes the esophagus is lined by stratified squamous epithelium (Fig. 2–6). Perch and some sharks have esophagi lined with ciliated columnar or cuboidal epithelium. At the entrance to the esophagus, the mucosa contains many mucous cells and, frequently, numerous taste buds. There is no basal layer at this point, and the mucosa lies directly on the lamina propria, a thick layer of loose connective tissue not subdivided into separate layers. In bony fish, there are usually no lymph vessels in this layer. The esophagus usually lacks a muscularis mucosae. The tunica submucosa may or may not have a stratum compactum and granulosum. The tunica muscularis of the esophagus consists of an inner longitudinal layer and an outer circular layer of striated muscle, with a few oblique fibers that form a woven basket pattern with the other muscle layers. This is distinctive from the rest of the digestive tract, which has a tunica muscularis consisting of smooth muscle. As the esophagus continues caudad, the striated muscle is gradually replaced with smooth muscle, beginning with the outer layers, progressing inward.

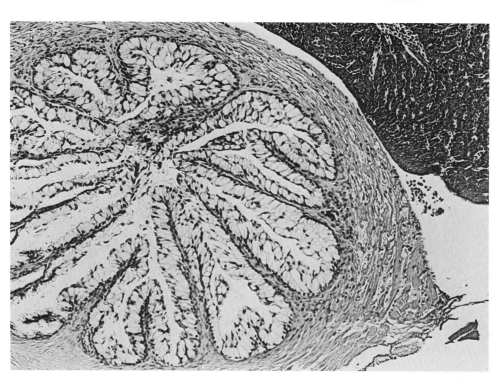

FIGURE 2–6. The esophagus of a female red swordtail (H&E, 100×).

Also, the orientation of the layers of muscle in the tunica muscularis begins to reverse. The inner longitudinal layer becomes thin and disappears as a new longitudinal layer of smooth muscle is laid down externally. Where the esophagus enters the coelom, it is covered with a two-cell thick tunica serosa.

Swim Bladder

The histology of the swim bladder is extremely variable between species but, nevertheless, very important clinically. In some fishes, the swim bladder has essentially the same histology as its origin, the digestive tract. In other fishes, the anatomy of the swim bladder is greatly reduced. There may be no more than an inner mucous membrane layer with a thin outer connective tissue covering.

In sturgeon, pepsin-secreting and mucus-secreting glands are still found in the swim bladder, which has all of the components of a digestive viscus. Most species have swim bladders covered with a simple squamous epithelium over a layer of dense fibrous connective tissue with longitudinal, circular, and oblique fibers arranged in layers. Guanine crystals, shaped like thin platelets embedded in this connective tissue, give the swim bladder of some species a distinctive silver color. The outer layers of connective tissue are joined to the inner layers of the structure by a loose, elastic, connective tissue layer. The inner epithelium of the swim bladder is commonly cuboidal and may be ciliated, partially ciliated, or completely devoid of cilia. The epithelial layer can include pigment cells. It is supported by a muscularis of smooth muscle in most fishes.

Rainbow trout have a thin muscularis of smooth muscle with many elastic fibers arranged with the outer layer of fibers running longitudinally and inner fibers circumferentially (Eissele, 1922). Perch have a thin-walled swim bladder covered with a peritoneum containing numerous melanocytes. Underneath is a fibrous tunic that covers an inner layer of circular connective tissue fibers. The only evidence of a muscularis is in the region of the oval or gas gland. Some groups of the catfish and loach families have their swim bladder protected within a bony capsule derived from the vertebrae.

The gas gland (oval, red gland, red body) varies widely in shape and form. It is often oval or round but can be a torus or stellate or dendriform. It can occupy a small or large percentage of the swim bladder wall. The gas gland is a highly vascular organ that usually consists of parallel venous and arterial rete mirabile arranged in a counter-current fashion. There are many versions of these glands in different species. In the codfish and the stickleback, only a single pair of retia is formed between the venules and arterioles of the gland. As many as three sets of retia can occur in other species, with retia forming at the capillary, venule/arteriole, and vein/artery levels.

Stomach

Three distinct regions of the stomach can be identified in those fish that have stomachs: the cardia, fundus, and pyloric regions. Not all of these regions can be identified in every fish species. The cardia is the region immediately around the entrance of the esophagus (Fig. 2–7). It is usually lined with cuboidal epithelium, which becomes taller and more columnar as the mucosa approaches the fundic region. The fundic and pyloric regions are lined with tall columnar epithelium. Also, the shallow folds in the gastric mucosa of the cardia usually deepen and become more extensive towards the pyloric region (Harder, 1975; Hybia, 1982). Characteristically, the cardia has numerous acid-secreting cells in its complex mucosa, but few or no gastric glands. There are no specialized cardiac glands reported in fish. The muscularis mucosae of the cardia is thin or nonexistent, and the stratum compactum and stratum granulosum are often not present. The outer tunica muscularis varies in different species.

The fundic region of the stomach is often a blind sac, lined with tall columnar epithelium pouching off from the main tube of the stomach. The fundus is characterized by numerous gastric glands, which empty into the troughs of the gastric folds. The gastric glands are found deep in the propria mucosae as single or forked tubes of cuboidal epithelium. The epithelial cells have central nuclei and many acidophilic granules (Krause, 1923). They are not differentiated into chief or parietal cells as in mammalian stomachs. The glands produce a secretion that does not contain mucus and is considered more analogous to, but not identical to, the secretions of mammalian chief cells. The tunica propria of the fundus contains connective tissue fibers that form a net around the gastric glands, numerous nerve plexuses, blood vessels, and lymph vessels. Large numbers of mast cells between the bundles of connective tissue are considered normal by many histologists. The muscularis mucosae of the fundus is usually thick, and the stratum compactum and stratum granulosum are often prominent. When the muscularis mucosae is very prominent, the stomach is sometimes inaccurately called a gizzard. The gizzard analogy is strengthened by a thick keratin-like mucopolysaccharide layer deposited over the mucosa of the stomach in some fish species.

The pyloric region of the fish stomach may be devoid of gastric glands or may contain specialized glands. Glands in the pyloric region of trout, pike, eels, and perch produce only a mucous substance similar to neck cells in mammalian gastric glands (Harder, 1975). Considerable work remains to be done on the description of gastric gland distributions in the stomachs of various fishes.

The actual pyloric valve of the fish stomach can vary from a circular muscular sphincter to a simple mucous membrane fold that acts more like a valve. In several species, the pyloric valve is either extremely poorly developed or missing altogether.

The small intestine in fish is usually identified by the landmark of the pylorus, if one is present. It is difficult to distinguish even histologically where a small intestine would become a large intestine in most fish. It is impossible to reliably distinguish duodenum, jejunum, and ileum. Arbitrary designations have been published, but these do not agree and are of little or no value.

The small intestine is lined with a single layer of columnar epithelium characterized by central nuclei and scattered goblet cells. With the notable exception of the pike, the muscularis mucosae is usually missing. Most fishes have no special mucous glands that go deep into the submucosa. Codfishes are an exception, with deep glands found at the base of surface folds that resemble crypts of Lieberkühn. These are found along the entire length of the bowel. The

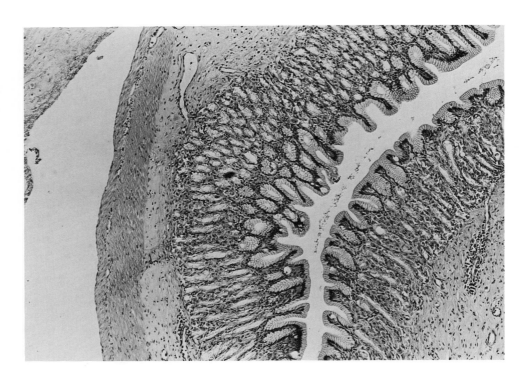

FIGURE 2–7. Cardiac portion of the stomach of a dusky squirrel fish (H&E, 100×).

epithelium in these crypts is tall cuboidal with basal nuclei. Brunner's glands have not been reported in fish.

The stratum compactum of the anterior bowel varies in thickness in different species of fish but is usually slightly elastic. The musculature throughout the intestines is usually smooth muscle, but it is almost entirely striated fibers in the tench (Baumgarten, 1965). Movement of the tunica muscularis is controlled by a nerve plexus in the submucosa, which does not contain any nerve cell bodies, and Auerbach's plexuses located between the longitudinal and circular layers of muscle. The plexus submucosus of fish is not identical to Meissner's plexus in mammals, since there are no nerve cell bodies in the fish plexus. The serosa of the anterior intestine consists of a thin layer of connective tissue, covered with a simple epithelium continuous with the mesentery. Pyloric ceca, when they occur, have histologic structures similar to those of the small intestine. There are no special glandular cells or tubules or any sphincters in these structures.

The large intestine of fishes is difficult to discern. Sometimes, the mucosal relief is a bit simpler than that in the small intestine. In the goldfish, the mucosal folds are deeper in the small intestine. In the rainbow trout, the opposite is the case, so extrapolation between species is difficult. True ceca at the junction of the small intestine with the large intestine or colon are rare. They have been described in three species of flatfish but are very small and apparently occur in only some individuals of the species.

Usually, the large intestine of fishes is not differentiated into colon and rectum. Occasionally, as the large intestine nears the anus, a mucosal valve is present that some histologists feel demarcates the rectum. This valve, Bacuhin's valve or the ileorectal valve, consists of a circular fold of mucous membrane that appears to prevent backflow of feces. In addition, when the valve is present, the tunica muscularis is notably thicker distal to the valve (Bishop and Odense, 1966).

Most fishes have a separate anus rather than a true cloaca. The anus of fishes is equipped with a muscular sphincter. Its epithelium undergoes a transition from columnar to stratified squamous. A true cloaca is found in only coelocanths, lungfish, sharks, and the embryos of some species such as the sturgeons and salmonids. The embryonic cloaca rarely persists.

Liver

The liver of fishes is similar histologically to other vertebrate livers. It is a reticulotubular gland covered with a serous membrane. Some species have a considerable amount of connective tissue forming a capsule for the liver. The lobular architecture of the fish liver is similar to that in other vertebrates. Fish hepatocytes are polygonal cells with spherical nuclei and usually a single nucleolus (Fig. 2–8). Fish hepa-

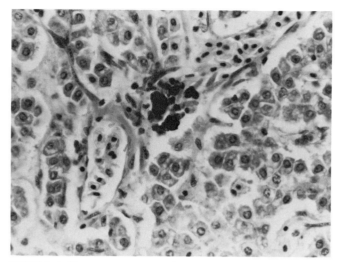

FIGURE 2–8. Hepatocytes surrounding a melanomacrophage center located near small hepatic blood vessels in the liver of an American eel (H&E, 400×).

tocytes often contain considerable lipid and glycogen, without showing the nuclear degeneration seen in fatty degeneration of the liver in terrestrial species. Considerable hypertrophy of hepatocytes occurs during vitellogenesis. The African lungfish (*Protopterus*) is reported to have hepatocytes with two separate nuclei (Szarski and Cybulska, 1967). In carp and some other fishes, pancreatic tissue is found within the liver along the portal vein (Fig. 2–9). Many fishes have a gallbladder made up of an inner layer of simple columnar epithelium over a layer of connective tissue and smooth muscle, covered by an outer serosal layer.

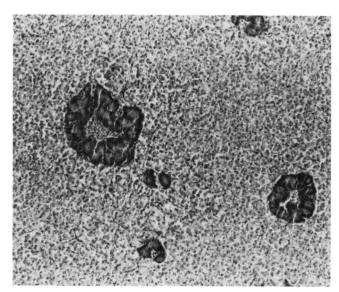

FIGURE 2–9. Darkly staining pancreatic tissue following vessels coursing through the normal liver parenchyma of a channel catfish (H&E, 100×).

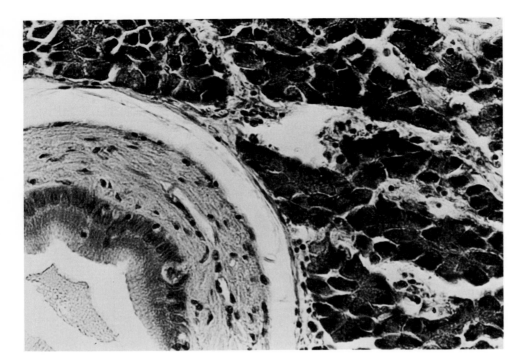

FIGURE 2–10. Pancreatic tissue surrounding the anterior intestine of a northern pike (H&E, 400×).

Pancreas

The exocrine pancreas of fishes consists of numerous tubuloalveolar glands that empty into main excretory ducts lined by secretory cells (Fig. 2–10). Thin intercalated ducts or isthmuses open into the excretory ducts. The intercalated ducts are lined by simple cuboidal epithelium with many goblet cells. The secretory cells of the exocrine pancreas have basal nuclei and many zymogen granules in their luminal cytoplasm. Islets of Langerhans with typical appearance are scattered among the exocrine glands, along with numerous nerves and blood vessels. Usually, the endocrine pancreas is not as diffusely distributed as the exocrine pancreas.

RENAL TISSUES

Histologically, the fish kidney is extremely variable. If present, fish glomeruli are structurally similar to mammalian glomeruli (Fig. 2–11). They are composed of a complete renal corpuscle with a Bowman's capsule and juxtaglomerular cells in the afferent arterioles. The juxtaglomerular cells are thought to secrete renin. The size of a glomerulus is highly variable between species. Freshwater fishes have larger and more numerous glomeruli than marine fishes. Several marine species, including the sea horses, pipefishes, and frogfishes, have completely aglomerular kidneys.

The renal tubule begins with a short neck portion characterized by low cuboidal epithelium with long cilia. The neck brings urine to the proximal convoluted tubule, which has been divided into segments I and II. In some fish species, these segments are easily differentiated on the basis of the height of the epithelial cells. Segment I has an eosinophilic cuboidal to columnar epithelium with a distinct brush border in the tubular lumen. The large, round nuclei of these epithelial cells are central or basal, and the apical cytoplasm has an extensive tubular system and many lysosomes and vesicles. Epithelial cells of segment II are columnar and taller than those of segment I. They have a centrally located oval nucleus, are intensely acidophilic, have a prominent brush border, but lack the extensive tubular system seen in epithelium from segment I. The intermediate segment is a specialized part of segment II seen in some fishes. It is absent in many species but is well-developed in carp and their allies. In the intermediate segment, the epithelium becomes lower and more cuboidal, and the brush border becomes intermittent and ciliated.

Fishes do not have a loop of Henle. Also, the distal convoluted tubule occurs only in kidneys of freshwater fishes. The distal convoluted tubule differs from the proximal tubule by having epithelial cells, which are less eosinophilic and have no brush border.

Urine continues to the collecting duct and ureter. The ureter is lined with a columnar epithelial layer. The lamina propria consists of connective tissue and circular, smooth muscle fibers. The outer layer of the ureter consists of dense connective tissue and is called the tunica adventitia. In some fishes, an enlarged portion of the distal ureter looks like and is called a urinary bladder. This structure is not homologous to urinary bladders of mammals that derive from the embryonic anlage of the rectum. The urinary bladder of fishes is a thin-walled sac with the same three distinct histologic layers seen in the ureter. The

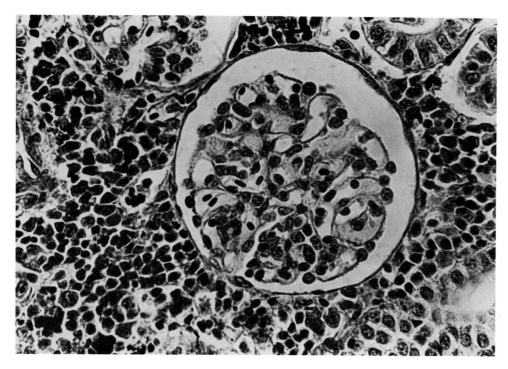

FIGURE 2–11. The renal glomeruli of brown trout resemble those of terrestrial vertebrates. The size of renal glomeruli varies considerably in different species of fish. Some fishes have completely aglomerular kidneys (H&E, 400×).

inner layer consists of one or two layers of cuboidal to columnar epithelium lining tunica media and tunica adventitia essentially identical to those found in the ureter.

The urinary function of the fish kidney is primarily in the caudal kidney. The cranial kidney contains a variety of tissues that have no function in the urinary system. Lymphoid tissue is quite prominent in this portion of the fish kidney, as is hematopoietic blast cells. The mitotic index of this tissue is normally high. The cranial kidney is highly vascular and contains considerable mature blood in its capillaries. In carp and goldfish, thyroid follicles are also commonly located in the interstitial tissues of the cranial kidney.

GENITAL TISSUES

The Ovary (Fig. 2–12)

Most fishes are cystovarian, but trout and salmon have a pocket structure that opens into the abdominal cavity (semicystovarian). Eggs move through a supporting groove that leads to the genital pore. The eel ovary is even more simple. It is a gymnovarian ovary where the ovarian tissue hangs down like a curtain and releases mature eggs directly into the body cavity.

Ova maturity has been studied and classified in many different ways, each emphasizing different histologic points. A commonly used system divides ovum maturation into seven stages (Srivastava and Rathi, 1970). The initial stage is called the *chromatin-nucleolar stage.* It is characterized by small oocytes with a central nucleus, several deep-staining nucleoli, and a thin layer of cytoplasm. This initial stage is followed by the *perinucleolar stage*, in which the nu-

cleus enlarges and the nucleoli move to the periphery of the nucleus. The cytoplasm becomes less basophilic, and a dark circular body, the yolk body, appears in the cytoplasm near the nucleus. In this stage, the oocyte is also surrounded by a thin layer of flat follicular cells.

In the subsequent *yolk vesicle stage*, vesicles begin to form in a thin layer beneath the oocyte membrane, and the oocyte elongates. Then the nucleoli lose their peripheral arrangement in the nucleus, and some are

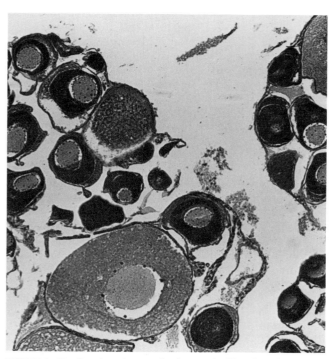

FIGURE 2–12. Ovarian tissue of a brown bullhead catfish (H&E, 400×).

lost. The follicular layer becomes more distinct, and this is defined as the fourth stage of maturation, the *transition stage*. In the *yolk granule stage* of development, the oocyte is full of yolk granules. At this point, the nucleus is large and central with a few nucleoli visible, and the follicular layer is thick and somewhat polar. When the nuclear membrane disappears and the nucleoli cannot be located, the ovum has entered the *maturation stage*. At this stage, the micropyle becomes visible, and the first polar body is extruded. At the end of this stage, the ovum itself is extruded to lay in the lumen of the ovary where it will become a *ripe egg* characterized by a translucent, PAS-positive cell membrane, and distinct animal pole with the nucleus at the micropyle.

Just after spawning, many postovulatory follicles, immature oocytes, and mature eggs are left in the ovary. Follicular cells hypertrophy and phagocytose debris formed from unspawned eggs becoming atretic.

It is important to remember that while some fishes reproduce in total synchrony with only a single spawn, as salmon do, most fishes have multiple spawns. Many fishes, like herrings, exhibit group synchrony with two groups of oocytes in the ovary near spawning season: one large and maturing, and the other small and immature, preparing for next season. Other fishes show complete asynchrony, with eggs in all stages of development at any time. These fishes, such as the sardines, mackerel, and goldfish, have long spawning seasons or several spawnings per season.

Testes

Fish testes have been divided into two large morphologic groups by histologists (Hybia, 1982). Some fishes have testes that do not have readily identifiable seminiferous tubules, which would have central lumens connected to the sperm duct. These gonads have a very short sperm duct and appear to be lobular structures with distinct connective tissue trabeculae. It is thought that maturing sperm are pushed into contact with the duct and somehow enter it. Other fishes have distinct seminiferous tubules in their testes, although these tubules differ somewhat from mammalian seminiferous tubules because they do not have a permanent germinal epithelium. Germinal cells move into the walls of the seminiferous tubules from the blind ends of the tubules only during the reproductive season. Fishes with testes with distinct seminiferous tubules have a longer sperm duct that leads from the seminiferous tubules to the seminal duct, which empties through the urogenital pore. Several species of fish have a seminal vesicle. Leydig cells exist in the connective tissue interstitium of fish testes and secrete sex steroids (Hybia, 1982). Other interstitial testicular cells in fish include Sertoli's cells and sustentacular interstitial cells.

Spermatogonia undergo a maturation process similar to the maturation process of ova. Male reproductive gametes undergo proliferation, maturation, and reduction division without the growth stage prior to maturation seen in ova development. After reduction division, the haploid spermatids undergo a stage of transformation during which they take on the typical sperm appearance. In different fishes, these stages of development can be long and gradual or very short.

Hermaphroditism

It is important to mention that various fish species demonstrate every type of sexuality known in zoology. Many species exhibit normal individual sexual development of a single gonad type or gonochorism. However, other species exhibit hermaphroditism. It is not unusual to see true hermaphroditism where both testicular and ovarian tissue are present simultaneously. Some fish are protandrous hermaphrodites, with testicular development preceding development of ovarian tissues, or the converse, protogynous hermaphrodites, in which female organs develop first, followed by testicular development.

ENDOCRINE TISSUES

Pituitary

The pituitary is similar in all vertebrates in its development from two distinct origins. Fishes are no exception. They have both an adenohypophysis and a neurohypophysis. These two components are developed to different degrees and forms in different fish species, and nomenclature based on relative locations of the tissues can be confusing. Histologically, however, the tissues are readily identifiable by criteria established for terrestrial vertebrates.

The adenohypophysis is made up of three histologically distinct parts: the proadenohypophysis (analogous to the rostral pars distalis), the mesoadenohypophysis (proximal pars distalis), and the meta-adenohypophysis (pars intermedia). The proadenohypophysis contains prolactin cells, corticotropic cells, and thyrotropic cells. Prolactin cells are found in a follicular arrangement in eels and salmonids, but not in carp and many other fish groups. Prolactin cells are very acidophilic, with many secretory granules in their cytoplasm, and do not stain with PAS or aldehyde fuchsin stains.

The corticotropic cells produce adrenocorticotropic hormone (ACTH). They are found in the dorsal region of the adenohypophysis in two or three layers. Corticotropic cells have many secretory granules, do not stain with PAS, but do stain with aldehyde fuchsin.

Thyrotropic cells produce substances similar to thyroid-stimulating hormone (TSH). They can be found among follicles of prolactin cells or sometimes (in eels) formed into cords. They are more often found as single cells or in clusters within the mesoadenohypophysis. Thyrotropic cells are basophilic with many secretory granules in the cytoplasm. They stain with both PAS and aldehyde fuchsin stains.

The mesoadenohypophysis has two distinct cell types. The somatotropic cells, sometimes called growth hormone cells, comprise the majority of the cells in the mesoadenohypophysis. These cells are acidophilic but will not stain with PAS or aldehyde fuchsin stains. The second type of cell in the mesoadenohypophysis is the basophilic gonadotropic cell, which produces gonadotropic hormone. These cells increase in number with maturity and sometimes invade the proadenohypophysis. They stain positive with both PAS and aldehyde fuchsin stains.

The meta-adenohypophysis contains a PAS-negative cell type of unknown function and a PAS-positive cell that seems to release melanophore-stimulating hormone. This portion of the adenohypophysis of the fishes has been less studied than the rest of the pituitary.

The neurohypophysis contains a variety of different neuron types and neuroglia. One distinct nerve fiber type is from the neurosecretory cells of the preoptic nucleus of the hypothalamus. These axons contain secretory granules, sometimes called herring bodies, which stain with aldehyde fuchsin stain. The ends of these fibers are usually in contact with capillary walls in the neurohypophysis or with cells in the meta-adenohypophysis. Another neuron type contains secretory granules that are acidophilic but do not stain with aldehyde fuchsin. These appear to originate in the median eminence. Other neurons identified in fish neurohypophyses include axons of the nucleus lateralis tuberis and axons of other hypothalamic secretory neurons.

Another structure related to the pituitary in fishes is the saccus vasculosus. The function of the saccus vasculosus is unknown, but it may serve as a depth indicator or in spinal fluid production. It is located just posterior to the pituitary and consists of a thin-walled sac formed by an evagination of the wall of the infundibulum. The lumen of the saccus vasculosus connects with the third ventricle of the brain and is covered by meninges on its outer surface.

A cell called the coronet cell extends through the entire thickness of the wall of the saccus vasculosus, much in the manner of ependyma cells in mammals. Coronet cells are narrow and attach to the basal lamina of the saccus and bulge out on their meningeal side. Coronet cells have papillary protrusions with modified cilia, containing typical outer doublets of microtubuli but no central pair. About 20 of these cilia form a crown on the surface of the cell. Nonmyelinated nerve fibers at the bases of coronet cells do not appear to form synapses. A more slender cell type, similar to the coronet cell, has been named the pseudocoronet cell.

Epiphysis

The epiphysis, or the pineal, is well developed in many fishes. The organ consists of a broadened base that corresponds to the pineal of primates. This continues in the fish as a tube with a distal thickening. The location of the distal end of the stalk varies among species. Several fishes, including trout, carp, tuna, and mackerel, have what amounts to a pineal window in the skull, directly over the distal end of the stalk. The entire epiphysis is contained within a connective tissue sheath. The hollow tube of the stalk is lined with ependymal cells and communicates with the third ventricle. The distal protuberance contains several cell types, including sensory cells reminiscent of photoreceptor rods found in the retina (Hybia, 1982) and a variety of glial cells. These include glycogen-storing cells and cytosome-rich cells. Also present are neurons with nonmyelinated axons.

Urophysis

Most species of fish have a ventral thickening of the spinal cord at the beginning of the last caudal vertebra called the urophysis. The ventral portion of the organ is highly vascular, supporting projections of neurosecretory cells. The organ is not grossly visible in eels but can be found in trout and is easy to locate in carp. Tuna have several separate bodies, rather than one discrete organ, and in the goosefish, the urophysis is completely separate from the spinal cord. In sharks, neurosecretory cells are distributed in the region, but their axons are short, and no urophysis is formed.

Three cell types are usually identified in the urophysis. A few small cells lie close to the central canal of the spinal cord. Elongated binuclear cells run parallel to the ventral surface of the urophysis. The actual neurosecretory cells are spindle-shaped or polyhedral with eccentric nuclei. Neurosecretory giant cells, two to three times as large as normal neurosecretory cells, are found in some larger species of fish. These cells have very pleomorphic nuclei. The structure of the urophysis is very reminiscent of the hypothalamic neurosecretory system in other vertebrates.

Thyroid Tissue

In most fishes, thyroid tissue is found as accumulations of vesicles or follicles on the floor of the gill chamber. Thyroid follicles can also be found in many other areas, including behind the eye and in the cranial kidneys. In the carp, thyroid tissue can be found in the spleen, along numerous blood vessels, and even in the heart. Compact thyroid glands, rather than disseminated islands of tissue, can be found in sharks, parrotfish, and tuna. As in mammals, the follicle is the functional and histologic unit of the fish thyroid. Each follicle consists of a lumen filled with acidophilic colloid and lined with simple cuboidal epithelium.

Ultimobranchial Bodies

The histology of the ultimobranchial bodies appears to vary considerably between species. The tissue is derived from the branchial pouches and is probably analogous to tissues incorporated into the mammalian thyroid gland as parafollicular cells (Hybia, 1982). In carp, the gland is a singular mass composed of many small follicles of glandular epithelium. No central cavity is present in the gland. The epithelial cells making up the follicles have round nuclei and no cytoplasmic secretory granules visible at the light microscopic level. In eels and trout, there are paired glands that are not made up of follicles but instead have a single, central cavity lined with pseudostratified columnar epithelium and occasional goblet cells.

Thymus

The thymus in fishes usually has a defined cortex and medullary regions. It is a highly vascular organ. Large stellate epithelial cells embedded in a wide-meshed lattice make up the cortex along with smaller reticular cells. The mesh of the lattice in the thymic medulla is tighter and made up of faintly striated reticular cells, sometimes called myoid cells. Deep-staining lymphocytes and mucous cells are present in the medulla. The intercellular vesicular spaces in the thymus increase in number and size with age, which may be an indication of degeneration of the organ.

Adrenal Tissues

Fish do not have adrenal glands but instead have interrenal organs and suprarenal organs. The interrenal organs develop from the mesothelium, which forms the peritoneum. The interrenal cells stain deeply eosinophilic. They have a well-developed endoplasmic reticulum and numerous tubulovesicular mitochondria. Their nucleus is round with a distinct nucleolus. Lipid inclusions are common in some species and stain well with Sudan black. These cells hypertrophy dramatically in some species when the fish are sexually active and synthesize steroids.

The suprarenal organs develop from nerve tissue of sympathetic ganglia and are sometimes referred to as paraganglia. They consist of chromaffin cells that stain strongly with chromic acid but otherwise stain poorly by routine methods. These cells have an oval or irregular nucleus with an indistinct nucleolus. Lipid inclusions are rare in these cells that secrete epinephrine and norepinephrine.

Corpuscles of Stannius

These endocrine organs consist of an envelope of connective tissue that encloses a parenchyma divided into lobules. Each lobule contains many large glandular epithelial cells with many coarse eosinophilic secretory granules in the basal portion of the cells (Fig. 2–13). There are no excretory ducts, but each lobule has a central cavity or pseudolumen. A reninlike substance can be obtained from these cells that also lowers serum calcium levels (Hybia, 1982).

NERVOUS TISSUES

Because of extensive efforts in comparative neurology, the nervous tissues of the fishes are perhaps the best studied. They are often used as model systems in studies of brain and nerve physiology. The brain of fishes is most commonly divided into five regions: telencephalon, diencephalon, mesencephalon, metencephalon, and myelencephalon. The structure of the fish brain is very similar to that of other vertebrates. Differences include the lack of lateral ventricles, and the presence of two large cells in the medulla referred to as Mauthner cells. The Mauthner cells may be part of the reticular formation concerned with rapid movements of the tail or perhaps information coming from the lateral line system.

The spinal cord of fishes consists of gray matter in the center that appears as an inverted Y in cross section. In the center of the gray matter is a central canal lined with ependymal cells and filled with spinal fluid. The gray matter can be divided into two regions. The trunk musculature is controlled primarily by cells in the dorsal gray matter. Fins and other structures are controlled by gray matter in the ventral

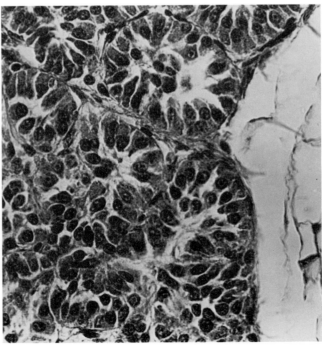

FIGURE 2–13. Corpus stannius tissue from a brown trout. Lobules of glandular epithelial cells contain many coarse eosinophilic secretory granules (H&E, 400×).

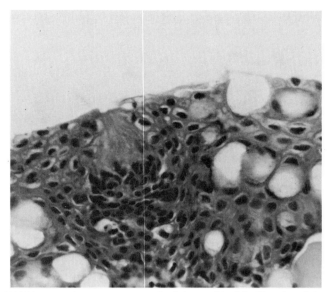

FIGURE 2–14. A cutaneous taste bud from a black bullhead catfish, which is nearly identical in structure to a mammalian taste bud (H&E, 400×).

layers found in most vertebrate eyes (Fig. 2–15). It varies in thickness from less than 100 to more than 500 μm in various fish species, primarily on the basis of the thickness of the photoreceptor cell layer and the outer layer of pigmented epithelial cells (Harder, 1975). There are a few unique features of the fish retina, but their clinical significance is unknown. For example, in addition to routine rods and cones, many fishes have twin cones. It is controversial whether any fishes have a fovea. If a fish species has a pseudobranch (see Chapter 1), a special rete mirabile can be found behind the retina. There is also often a unique glandular structure between the retina and the sclera, designated the choroid gland or choroid body. It is present in fish that have a pseudobranch. The choroid gland is often U-shaped and partially surrounds the optic nerve. It contains many tightly packed capillaries that appear to form a rete similar to that used for gas striping in the swim bladder. The function of this tissue is unknown, as is its potential role in exophthalmic conditions related to retrobulbar and subchoroid gas accumulations.

portion of the spinal cord. The gray matter is surrounded by white matter, and the entire spinal cord is protected in a meninx similar to that of other vertebrates.

SENSORY TISSUES

Taste Buds

The taste buds of fishes are similar to those of mammals and other vertebrates (Fig. 2–14). They consist of sensory cells, basal cells, sustentacular cells, marginal epithelium, and a nerve plexus that form a bulb-shaped structure. The sensory cells are barrel-shaped with short microvilli covering their apex, which extends into the sensory pit formed by the sustentacular cells. Sensory cells have basal nuclei and granular cytoplasm. The sustentacular cells are large fusiform cells with pale oval nuclei. The histology of the taste buds of fishes is essentially identical to the descriptions provided in mammalian histology texts.

Eyes

The histology of the fish eye is remarkably similar to mammalian histology. The cornea is organized in the same manner as mammalian corneas. The lens of fishes is usually spherical and consists mostly of carefully arranged lens fibers underneath a layer of lens epithelium. The lens is supported by ligaments and a retractor lentis muscle that functions to move the lens in the eye to allow accommodation.

The fish retina has the typical organization of

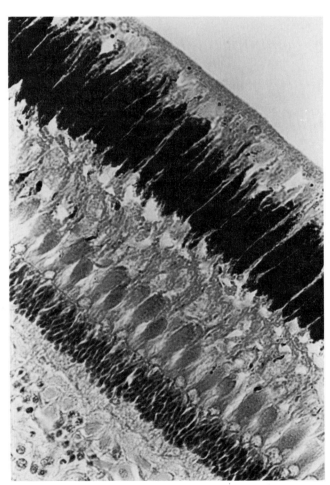

FIGURE 2–15. The basal layers of the retina of a largemouth bass showing the pigmented epithelium and basilary layers, and indistinct outer limiting membrane, rods and cones, the outer nuclear layer, the outer plexiform layer, and some of the inner nuclear layer (H&E, 400×).

Auditory Apparatus

Classification of the lateral line system as a component of the auditory sensory apparatus is controversial. I place it here because of the proposed function of reception of low-frequency wave forms in the environment. The lateral line apparatus consists of numerous tactile sensors referred to as neuromasts. Most fishes have neuromasts that are individually distributed on the skin surface, in addition to the neuromasts enclosed in the channels of the lateral line system. The channels of the lateral line system are usually lined with simple squamous epithelium, except in areas around the sensory neuromasts where it becomes cuboidal. Goblet cells, lymphocytes, and occasional eosinophils may be present in the canal.

Neuromasts consist of a sensory hillock with pear-shaped sensory hair cells supported by columnar sustentacular cells. Sensory hair cells have a tapered apex and can have both kinocilia and stereocilia, which act as sensory hairs of the receptor. These cells are in the center of the hillock. Their nucleus is round to ovoid and in the apical half of the cell. The basal surface of the sensory hair cells synapses with nerve axons. The sensory hairs of the lateral line receptor are embedded in a gelatinous substance that forms the cupula. Many feel the cupula is secreted by the sustentacular cells to separate the individual sensory hair cells. The sustentacular cells are elongated columnar cells with basal ovoid nuclei that are often indented. They surround and separate the receptor cells. The interdigitation of sustentacular cells between sensory receptor cells is the main histologic distinction between a lateral line neuromast and a taste bud. Some histologists have observed two additional supportive cell types in the neuromast hillock: basal cells, which line the basal portion of the neuromast, and mantle cells, which separate the neuromast from the epithelium lining the lateral line canal.

The ear apparatus of fishes is commonly referred to as the statoacoustic organ. These inner ears are similar in most fishes, although modifications do occur (Fig. 2–16). Each ear has three semicircular canals, analogous to those in mammals, and three otolith chambers that interconnect and contain endolymph. Each semicircular canal is lined with simple squamous epithelium and has an ampulla, which contains a structure similar to the neuromasts of the lateral line system. These otolith chambers are lined with simple sensory hair cells supported by sustentacular epithelium. A membrane lies over the sensory epithelium and supports the otoliths, forming an organ of Corti (Hybia, 1982).

Electric Receptors

Electric receptors are found in the "electric" fishes, including electric eels, electric catfish, and electric rays. They are also found in some fishes that do not have electric organs. For example, the electric receptors of sharks, commonly called ampullae of Lorenzini or ampullary canals, are not confined to electric rays and torpedoes. These organs are usually visible with the naked eye and are structurally similar in various fishes. They are not particularly important clinically. However, descriptions are rare, and electric receptors may be mistaken for other other tissue, so a brief description is warranted.

In the sharks, electric receptors are essentially tubes sunk into the body through the epidermis and dermis. At the bottom of each tube, ampullae lie in nests, surrounded by connective tissue that contains nerve axons. Sometimes the tubes are long, or they may branch in a stellar fashion with an ampulla at the end of each branch. There are six to eight chambers in each ampulla, lined with special epithelium. Each ampulla is innervated by 4 to 15 nerve fibers, which effectively form a nerve plexus around the structure (Harder, 1975).

In electric rays, the electric receptors are called vesicles of Savi. They consist of round vesicles, two or three mm in diameter, attached in groups of three to tendinous bands. Hundreds are present near the nostrils and between the electric organs of the fish. The vesicles are lined with a single layer of epithelium, which thickens at the base (Harder, 1975).

In catfish, the electric receptor organs are very similar to the lateral line organs, consisting of innervated sensory hillocks distributed around the body (Sato, 1956). These are sometimes referred to as pit organs. The size and arrangement of pit organs vary, depending on the species of fish. Sometimes, small ones are embedded in the epidermis, but larger ones are usually found in a depression with a raised rim of epithelium. The mormyrids or elephantnose fish have a number of different types of electric receptors that have been well described and reviewed (Harder, 1975). They are for the most part buried in the epidermis. Some have ducts, and others do not. They vary in the number of sensory cells and the

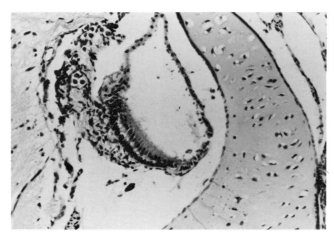

FIGURE 2–16. The inner ear of a young brook trout showing the crista ampullaris. The supporting cell and sensory cell layers can be discerned (H&E, 100×).

exact structure, but all are surrounded by a distinct capillary loop and nerve plexus.

Olfactory Organ

The olfactory apparatus is usually located in the nostrils of the fish. The olfactory tissue of fishes consists of ciliated supporting cells and slender sensory cells, which may be scattered along the nasal epithelium or may be grouped in olfactory buds. The primary sensory cell is bipolar with a central and a peripheral process. The peripheral process terminates in the surface of the olfactory epithelium as an olfactory hair. This is thought to be the actual sensory part of the cell. The central process is similar to an axon and often bends 90 degrees to track to the olfactory bulb where it synapses.

LITERATURE CITED

Anderson, B.G., and Mitchum, D.L. (1974) Atlas of Trout Histology. Wyoming Game and Fish Commission Bulletin 13.

Bagnara, J.T., and Hadley, M.E. (1973) Chromatophores and Color Change. Prentice-Hall, Englewood Cliffs.

Baumgarten, H.G. (1965) Uber die Muskulatur und die Nerven in der Darmwand der Schleie (Tinca vulgaris Cuv.). Z. Zellforxch. 68:116–137.

Bishop, C., and Odense, P.H. (1966) Morphology of the digestive tract of the cod, Gadus morhua. J. Fish. Res. Bd. Can. 23:1607–1625.

Blackstock, N., and Pickering, A.D. (1980) Acidophilic granular cells in the epidermis of the brown trout, Salmo trutta L. Cell Tissue Res. 210:359–369.

Brown, G.A., and Wellings, S.R. (1970) Electron microscopy of the skin of the teleost Hippoglossoides ellassodon L. Z. Zellforsch. Mikrosk. Anat. 103:149–169.

Bullock, A.M., and Roberts, R.J. (1975) The dermatology of marine teleost fish I. The normal integument. Oceanogr. Mar. Biol. Annu. Rev. 13:383–411.

Burton, D. (1978) Melanophore distribution within the integumentary tissues of two teleost species, Pseudopleuronectes americanus and Gasterosteus aculeatus form leiurus. Can. J. Zool. 56:526–535.

Downing, S.W., and Novales, R.R. (1971a) The fine structure of lamprey epidermis. I. Introduction and mucous cells. J. Ultrastruct. Res. 35:282–294.

Downing, S.W., and Novales, R.R. (1971b) The fine structure of lamprey epidermis. II. Club cells. J. Ultrastruct. Res. 35:295–303.

Downing, S.W., and Novales, R.R. (1971c) The fine structure of lamprey epidermis. III. Granular cells. J. Ultrastruct. Res. 35:304–313.

Eissele, L. (1922) Histologische Studien an der Schwimmblase einiger Knochenfische. Biol. Zbl. 42:125–138.

Gona, O. (1979) Mucous glycoproteins of teleostean fish: a comparative histochemical study. Histochemistry 11:709–718.

Grizzle, J.M., and Rogers, W.A. (1976) Anatomy and Histology of the Channel Catfish. Auburn University Agricultural Experiment Station, Auburn, Alabama.

Harder, W. (1975) Anatomy of fishes. E. Schweizerbart'sche Verlagsbuchhandlung (Nagele v. Obermiller), Stuttgart, Germany.

Harris, J.E., and Hunt, S. (1973) The fine structure of iridophores in the skin of the Atlantic salmon (Salmo salar L). Tissue Cell 5:479–488.

Harris, J.E., Watson, A., and Hunt, S. (1973) Histochemical analysis of mucous cells in the epidermis of brown trout (Salmo trutta L.). J. Fish. Biol. 5:345–351.

Hawkes, J.W. (1983) Skin and Scales in Microscopic Anatomy of Salmonids: An Atlas (Yasutake, W., and Wales, J., eds.) U.S. Dept. of Interior, Fish and Wildlife Service, Washington, D.C. pp. 14–17.

Henrikson, R.C., and Matoltsy, A.G. (1968a) The fine structure of teleost epidermis. I. Introduction and filament-containing cells. J. Ultrastruct. Res. 21:194–212.

Henrikson, R.C., and Matoltsy, A.G. (1968b) The fine structure of teleost epidermis. II. Mucous cells. J. Ultrastruct. Res. 21:213–221.

Henrikson, R.C., and Matoltsy, A.G. (1968c) The fine structure of teleost epidermis. III. Club cells and other cell types. J. Ultrastruct. Res. 21:222–232.

Hybia, T. (1982) An Atlas of Fish Histology, Normal and Pathological Features. Kodansha Ltd., Tokyo.

Junqueira, L., Alves Lima, M.H., and Farias, E.C. (1978) Carotenoid and pterin pigment localization in fish chromatophores. Stain Technol. 53:51–94.

Krause, R. (1923) Mikroskopishe Anatomie der Wirbeltiere in Einzeldarstellungen. IV. Fische. De Gruyter, Berlin, Leipzig.

Lasker, R., and Threadgold, L.T. (1978) Chloride cells in the skin of the larval sardine. Exp. Cell Res. 52:582–590.

Leonard, J.B., and Summers, R.G. (1976) The ultrastructure of the integument of the American eel, Anguilla rostrata. Cell Tissue Res. 171:1–30.

Lopez, E. (1970) Los Cellulaire dun Poisson Teleosteen Anguilla anguilla L. II. Action de Lablation des Corpuscules de Stannius. Z. Zellforsch 109:566–572.

Marcus, H. (1934) zur Stammesgeschichte der Zunge. II. Uber die Muskulatur der Polypteruszunge. Anat. Anz. 77:357–362.

Mikuriya, B.A. (1972) The gross anatomy and microscopic anatomy of the tongue and lower jaw of Gnathonemus petersii (Gthr. 1862) (Mormyridae, Teleostei). Z. Morph. Tiere 73:195–208.

Mittal, A.K., and Munshi, J.S.D. (1970) Structure of the integument of a fresh-water teleost, Bagarius bagarius (Ham.) (Sisoridae, Pisces). J. Morph. (Philad.) 130:229–235.

Mittal, A.K., and Whitear, M. (1979) Keratinization of fish skin with special reference to the catfish Bagarius bagarius. Cell Tissue Res. 202:213–230.

Morrison, C.M. (1987) Histology of the Atlantic Cod, Gadus morhua: An Atlas, Part One. Digestive Tract and Associated Organs. Department of Fishereies and Oceans, Ottawa, Canada.

Nag, A.C., and Nursall, J.R. (1972) Histogenesis of white and red muscle fibres of trunk muscles of a fish, Salmo gairdneri. Cytobios 6:227–246.

Pfeiffer, W. (1970) Uber die Schreckstoffzellen der Siluriformes (Ostariophysi, Pisces). Anat. Anz. 126:113–119.

Pfeiffer, W., Sasse, D., and Arnold, M. (1971) Die Schreckstoffzellen von Phoxinus phoxinus und Morulius chrysophekadion (Cyprinidae, Ostariophysi, Pisces). Z. Zellforsch. 118:203–213.

Pickering, A.D. (1974) The distribution of mucous cells in the epidermis of the brown trout, Salmo trutta L., and the char, Salvelinus alpinus L. J. Fish Biol. 6:111–118.

Pickering, A.D., and Macey, D.J. (1977) Structure, histochemistry and the effect of handling on the mucous cells of the epidermis of the char Salvelinus alpinus (L.). J. Fish Biol. 10:505–512.

Roberts, R.J. (1978) Fish Pathology. Bailliere Tindall, London.

Roberts, R.J., Young, H., and Milne, J.A. (1971) Studies on the skin of plaice Pleuronectes platessa L. I. The structure and ultrastructure of normal skin. J. Fish Biol. 3:87–98.

Satchell, G.H. (1971) Circulation in fishes. Cambridge Monogr. In Exp. Biol., Cambridge Univ. Press. 18:10–131.

Sato, M. (1956) Studies on the pit-organs of fishes. IV. The distribution, histological structure and development of the small pit organs. Annot. Zoo. Jpn. 29:207–212.

Srivastava, P.N., and Rathi, S.K. (1970) Effect of radiation on the reproductive system of the Indian catfish, Heteropneustes fossilis Bloch. I. Annual cycle in the development of ovarian eggs. Acta Anat. (Basel) 75:114–125.

Szarski, H., and Cybulska, R. (1967) Liver size in Protopterus dolloi Blngr. (Dipnoi). Bull. Acad. Pol. Sci. Biol. 15:217–220.

Van Oosten, J. (1957) The skin and scales. In: The Physiology of Fishes, Vol. 1 (Brown, M.E., ed.). Academic Press, New York, pp. 207–244.

von Frisch, K. (1941) Uber einen Schreckstoff der Fischhaut und seine biologische Bedeutung. Z. Vergl. Physiol. 29:46–145.

Whitear, M. (1971) Cell specialization and sensory function in fish epidermis. J. Zool. (Lond.) 163:237–264.

Yasutake, W.T., and Wales, J.H. (1983) Microscopic Anatomy of Salmonids: An Atlas. United States Department of the Interior Resource Publication 150, Washington, D.C.

Chapter 3

CLINICAL PHYSIOLOGY

MICHAEL K. STOSKOPF

It is somewhat ambitious to attempt a single chapter on fish physiology, considering the incredible diversity among species and the amount of information accumulated by basic researchers over the years. Whole series of volumes have been written about fish physiology that do not approach complete coverage of the subject (Hoar and Randall, 1969–1990). This chapter will focus on a few select areas of fish physiology that are particularly important to the clinical management of diseases in fish. It cannot be comprehensive but hopefully will provide the background needed in the more common clinical problems. For more in-depth coverage, readers should refer to dedicated fish physiology texts (Smith, 1982; Pickering, 1981; Atema et al., 1988).

BODY COMPARTMENTS

Many clinical activities involve some knowledge of effective body compartment sizes. This causes some difficulties for clinicians expanding their clinical involvement with different types of animals. For example, a common question is how much blood loss an animal can tolerate. The usual answer of 10% of the blood volume is applicable to most vertebrates. The problem comes with the next question. What is the blood volume of a fish? Again, the extreme variability among fishes makes this difficult, but luckily some generalizations are possible.

The fish has body compartments that are, on the whole, similar in relative size to those of other vertebrates. A generalized range for a variety of clinically useful compartments is listed in Table 3–1. The fluid compartments and blood volume are somewhat similar to what would be expected from mammalian physiology. Low blood volumes are generally seen in sedentary fish and larger blood volumes in active fish. Much more study of these parameters is required, but Table 3–1 can provide a starting place for the fish clinician.

OSMOTIC HOMEOSTASIS AND ELECTROLYTE BALANCE

Perhaps one of the more confusing areas in veterinary physiology is the study of electrolyte homeostasis mechanisms and the consequences of failure to maintain homeostasis. Unfortunately, the problem becomes even more complex in fish and is equally critical to understanding and developing critical care for fish patients. Therefore, it deserves some attention here.

The homeostatic organs in electrolyte balance in fishes are the gills, kidneys, urinary bladder, and gut, and in the sharks and rays, the rectal gland. These organs work in concert in very different ways to maintain electrolyte stability in marine versus freshwater fishes. In addition, the sharks and rays have developed a distinctive mechanism for dealing with osmotic pressures from the environment.

Marine Fishes

In marine fishes, the major factor working against electrolyte homeostasis is the osmotic loss of water (Fig. 3–1). The general tendency is for a marine fish to dehydrate, losing water to the external environment, in a manner analogous to, but not identical to, water loss in terrestrial mammals. In addition, the marine fish faces the diffusional entry of salts from the environment, further complicating the problem of balanced hydration.

Marine fishes apparently drink salt water. Although they cannot absorb water directly from ingested seawater because the osmotic gradient is in the wrong direction, marine fishes can reduce the water absorption gradient in the stomach and intestine by allowing sodium and chloride to diffuse into

TABLE 3–1. Relative Body Compartment Dimensions of Fishes

Biochemical Compartments	
Component	% of Total Body Weight
Lipid	3–20
Protein	12–15
Carbohydrate	2.5–4.0
Minerals	2.5–4.0
Water	67–80

Fluid Compartment Volumes	
Compartment	% of Total Body Volume
Extracellular fluid	27–33
Tissue fluid	20–27
(Extracellular—plasma)	
Cellular fluid	67–80
Blood	2.5–6.0
Erythrocytes	1.0–2.5
Plasma	2–4

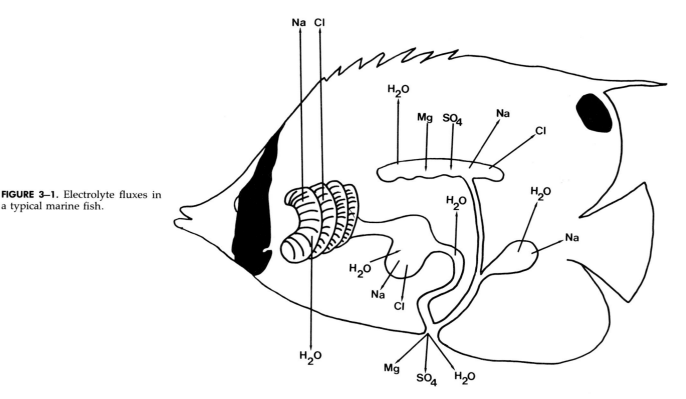

FIGURE 3–1. Electrolyte fluxes in a typical marine fish.

the body across the esophageal and gastric epithelial linings. Naturally, this results in a salt-linked water uptake from the ingested seawater. This causes a tremendously high sodium and chloride loading of the fish.

Considerable energy is expended to reduce this excessive salt load. Students of mammalian physiology might be surprised to learn that the kidneys are not the primary site of this electrolyte management. Excess sodium and chloride are excreted by mitochondria-rich cells in the gills called chloride cells. These cells in marine fishes have sodium-potassium adenosine triphosphatase (ATPase) activities 4 to 10 times greater than gill epithelial cells from freshwater fishes (De Renzis and Bornancin, 1984). This is felt to be the major route of sodium efflux in marine fish. The enzymatic drive of sodium excretion may also supply the energy for chloride efflux in marine teleosts. The sodium-potassium ATPase pump is activated by cortisol and is blocked by ouabain. Potassium concentrations in the water help to drive the sodium efflux through both a diffusional component and an impact on the active transport mechanism. Magnesium ions contribute to the potential across the gill epithelium and may contribute to sodium efflux by effects on the diffusional gradient. The alkaline nature of seawater does not provide many hydrogen ions to generate diffusion potentials, so hydrogen ion effects on sodium uptake and the rate of sodium loss at the gill are thought to be minimal in marine fishes.

Bicarbonate ions in the water stimulate chloride efflux (Potts, 1984). This effect is not due to effects on pH, since the impact of alkalinization on chloride

flux is to decrease transport (Zadunaisky, 1984). Chloride effluxes from the gills are also stimulated by β-adrenergic activators like isoproterenol and inhibited by epinephrine and α-adrenergic activators. Furosemide specifically inhibits chloride transport in the kidney of marine fishes and may have a similar effect on gill chloride efflux. Ouabain blocks the chloride efflux from the gills, as it does the sodium efflux. Acetylcholine and other cholinergic agonists cause a dose-dependent decrease in chloride efflux from the gill. Muscarinic agonists, such as carbachol, methacholine, and muscarine, also cause dose-dependent decreases in chloride efflux. Nicotine does not affect the chloride efflux. The hormone prolactin has been used to adapt teleosts to fresh water. Its short-term effect reduces active transport of chloride from the gills. Long-term effects of prolactin therapy include the dedifferentiation of the chloride cells (Zadunaisky, 1984).

Obviously, the impact of electrolyte movement across the gills is clinically tied to situations characterized by water retention, edema, and ascites. The skin of marine teleosts is relatively impermeable to water. The majority of water efflux is across gill membranes (Rankin and Bolis, 1984). Cortisol and adrenocorticotropic hormone (ACTH) increase water efflux from marine fishes, as does furosemide therapy.

The kidneys of marine fishes do play a role in electrolyte excretion; however, their function is more important in the balance of magnesium and sulfate levels and not, as might be assumed, in sodium and chloride elimination. Chapter 2 discusses the fact that glomeruli of marine fishes are smaller and less numerous than those in the kidneys of freshwater fishes (Nash, 1931). This reduction in filtration reaches its maximum in several species of marine fishes such as the anglerfishes, sea horses, and goosefish, which have completely aglomerular kidneys. It is perhaps easier to examine the electrolyte fluxes of marine fishes in those kidneys that prepare urine entirely by tubular secretion.

The renal electrolyte mechanisms in the marine fishes with aglomerular kidneys contrast dramatically with the classic filtration, reabsorption, and secretion model, which describes the function of most vertebrate nephrons. Without glomeruli, no filtration process is involved, and secretion is followed by reabsorption rather than vice versa. In marine fish kidneys, iso-osmotic sodium and chloride secretion into the forming urine does occur initially. However, passive water transport from the renal tubular cells to the urine to maintain urine flow is proportional not to urine sodium or chloride levels but rather to the urine concentrations of divalent cations, particularly magnesium. Magnesium and other divalent cations and anions are actively secreted in a process linked to the reabsorption of sodium and chloride from the urine. Magnesium levels in the urine of marine fishes are proportional to the serum concentrations of magnesium, and water is drawn by osmosis into the tubular lumen in response to the gradients established by magnesium ions. In the marine fish kidney, the secretion of ions and fluids is of major importance in urine formation; however, the hormonal control of these mechanisms is not understood.

The same process occurs in marine fishes with glomeruli in their kidneys (Beyenbach, 1982). These fishes do have a filtration process that provides the initial urine, which is effectively iso-osmotic with the serum. Sodium and chloride are secreted, to be resorbed during the active transport of magnesium ions into the urine. Water loss in the urine is related to the magnesium loading of the fish, and urine water content is maintained proportional to magnesium concentrations.

The clinical implication of marine fish electrolyte and water homeostasis mechanisms is that any breech of the barriers to the external environment or failures of the homeostatic mechanisms tend to result in dehydration of the patient. Marine fish with large epithelial wounds or major gill damage rapidly lose water, and clinical management should involve fluid replacement.

Sharks, Skates, and Rays

The sharks, skates, and rays have a unique method of dealing with hyperosmotic environments. In addition to their epithelial barriers to environmental water loss, these animals maintain plasma that is slightly hyperosmotic to the environment. This permits them to benefit from a slight passive water influx to balance metabolic water losses. The plasma osmolality of sharks and their allies is maintained by high extracellular concentrations of urea and trimethylamine oxides. These compounds are produced in the liver and are managed with some very unique adaptations to the metabolism of nitrogenous wastes.

In addition to the kidney, sharks, skates, and rays have a gland called the rectal gland (Fig. 3–2) that assists in the elimination of excess body sodium. It is located near and empties into the rectum of the shark. It is a tubular gland that functions much like the salt glands of seabirds.

The kidneys of sharks, skates, and rays are also important in electrolyte balance. While ammonia and ammonium are excreted mainly across the gills and not by the kidneys (Goldstein, 1982), this process is associated with monovalent ion uptake and has severe implications in acid-base balance (Evans, 1982).

The kidneys of sharks are relatively typical of marine species, consisting of a few long nephrons. Small volumes of urine that are nearly iso-osmotic with plasma, but contain very low concentrations of urea, are excreted. The urea is conserved to maintain the high plasma urea levels for osmotic maintenance of the plasma. This is thought to be accomplished by an active tubular reabsorption process linked to sodium transport (Schmidt-Nielsen et al., 1972); however, it is possible that the process is not active but passive, requiring little or no energy expenditure (Boylan 1972). In either case, it is felt that sharks adjust their urine more by alterations in tubular permeability than by adjustments in glomerular filtration rate. Large gradients are maintained for phosphate, sulfate, calcium, and magnesium (Henderson et al., 1987). The hormonal control of these mechanisms in sharks is not well understood.

Freshwater Fishes

In freshwater fishes, the major problem is to eliminate excess water that tends to accumulate by osmotic diffusion through exposed epithelial surfaces. Freshwater teleosts do not have the chloride cells that figure so prominently in ion fluxes of marine teleosts. Marine and estuary fish adapted to fresh water lose their chloride cells. In most freshwater fishes, sodium and chloride move across the gill membrane as an influx, rather than the efflux seen in marine fishes.

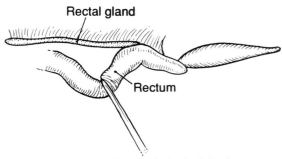

FIGURE 3–2. The rectal gland of sharks.

Sodium is taken up in exchange for hydrogen ions in a process many researchers feel is active transport and many others feel is passive. Chloride ions are exchanged for bicarbonate ions, generated metabolically from carbon dioxide in an active transport process. These two transport processes are not linked, and sodium and chloride flow can be in opposite directions for prolonged periods of time.

If the diffusional nature of hydrogen ion exchange for sodium is correct, and hydrogen ions act as counter ions to sodium uptake, it is reasonable that sodium uptake is inhibited in low pH water. The diffusional path for efflux of metabolically generated hydrogen ions does not exist in water with high hydrogen ion content (low pH), but it can have a high potential in alkaline water. Even though the concentration of hydrogen ions is very low in most natural fresh water, the hydrogen ion is much more permeable than sodium and, therefore, has a major impact on diffusion potentials. This is particularly true at acid pH.

This factor can become clinically important in species of freshwater teleosts that are normally adapted to high hydrogen ion content water (Fig. 3-3). When these fish are placed in neutral or alkaline water for any period of time, they develop ascites and tissue edema, which can be ameliorated with furosemide therapy. The mechanism for this water accumulation could be simply an accumulation of sodium through a greatly increased influx, in exchange for protons that have a very high diffusional gradient. The condition is routinely seen in electric eels that have been held in alkaline waters for periods of 6 to 12 weeks. The condition is completely reversible, if the pH of the water is adjusted to 6.0 to 6.5. Changing the pH of water two logs (i.e., from pH 8 to 6) doubles the rate of overall sodium loss (Potts, 1984) and corrects the condition.

Of course, fresh water is a broad category. Fresh water varies dramatically in sodium, chloride, hydrogen, and calcium ion content, and each of these has effects on the direction of diffusional ion movement. High water calcium content reduces membrane permeability to sodium and hydrogen ions, which reduces any sodium flux. Magnesium ions exert effects similar to but less dramatic than those of calcium. Sulfate ions can have an impact on chloride flux.

In freshwater fishes, urine generated by the kidneys is primarily water, and the urine flow rate varies with the osmotic gradient established across the gill epithelium and the glomerular filtration rate. Any changes in glomerular filtration rate are balanced by changes in the reabsorption rate across the tubular epithelium, which keeps the ratio of these two processes relatively constant (Rankin et al., 1980); however, the tubular resorption rate in freshwater fishes is always very low, favoring large volumes of urine. Therefore, in freshwater fishes, control of blood pressure and flow are major determinants of urine flow, and circulating catecholamines play a major role in osmotic homeostasis (Wahlqvist and Nilsson,

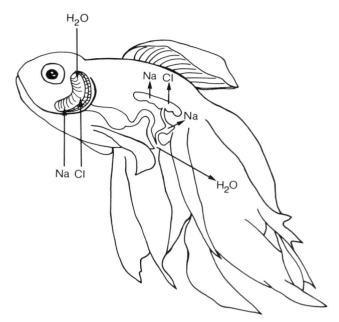

FIGURE 3–3. Electrolyte fluxes in a typical freshwater fish.

1977). In addition, the neurohypophyseal hormones have a complex role in urine production in freshwater fishes. Experimental evidence indicates that low doses of neurohypophyseal hormones exert an antidiuretic effect and high doses are diuretic (Henderson and Wales, 1974; Babiker and Rankin, 1978). Clinically, the end result is that any damage to the environmental barriers of a freshwater fish, or to its homeostatic mechanisms, tends to result in water accumulations, which cause tissue edema and swelling. Freshwater fishes should be managed entirely differently from marine fishes with regard to fluid and electrolyte therapy.

Lungfishes

Lungfishes are a special case among the freshwater fishes (Sawyer et al., 1982). They estivate for long periods in mud cocoons during dry seasons. These fish may spend years in a state of suspension. During these estivations, urine production ceases completely (Delaney et al., 1977) and water loss is limited to the gradual loss by evaporation from the lungs. During these times, urea is accumulated through catabolism of proteins, and the plasma osmolality rises significantly. When lungfish are reimmersed in water, they rapidly absorb water and swell. Glomerular filtration increases dramatically and a diuresis occurs. This appears to be controlled largely by a balance between dorsal aortic blood pressure and the tone of the renal vasculature. The hormonal basis is probably neurohypophyseal and not due to antidiuretic hormone mechanisms.

In the Australian lungfish, arginine vasotocin increases the dorsal aortic pressure and the glomerular filtration rate synchronously. In the African lungfish, the reimmersion diuresis considerably outlasts the pressor response, but this is thought to be possibly due to a slow return of the glomerular arterioles and renal vessels to resting states.

GAS EXCHANGE

Fish consume oxygen faster than most other aquatic organisms, but their maximum oxygen uptake is only between 1 and 10% of that of birds and mammals of the same size. Fish can sprint, using energy at 100 times their basal rate, for about 20 seconds (Holeton, 1979), at which time they are using an aerobic capacity comparable to a similar-sized mammal. Internal respiration mechanisms in fish are generally similar to those of mammals. Most, but not all, fish utilize an iron-based, oxygen-binding porphyrin or hemoglobin. Most fish have this porphyrin contained in erythrocytes. There are a wide variety of fish hemoglobins and some are fairly specialized.

Just as in mammals, the purpose of respiration in fishes is to get oxygen from the environment to the various cells in the body that need it for metabolic reactions. A major factor in accomplishing this is the thickness of the gill epithelium that usually serves as the environmental barrier, where the vascular system most closely approaches the external environment. Oxygen must traverse the gill epithelium and bind to hemoglobin contained in erythrocytes, which are then circulated to the rest of the fish's body where oxygen is delivered to tissues.

Some fishes have developed very specialized respiratory adaptations. For example, bettas, or Siamese fighting fish, are air breathers with a highly modified first epibranchial (labyrinth organ) and suprabranchial chamber (Peters, 1978). The labyrinth organ is a cavity in the roof of the mouth that has many epithelium-covered bony plates arranged in a complex pattern. The organ has an excellent blood supply, and it serves in oxygen absorption from air.

The labyrinth fishes (bettas, gouramis, climbing perch) rely predominantly on a diphasic respiratory pattern, but can utilize a monophasic pattern (Hughes and Singh, 1970). In the diphasic pattern, air is emptied from suprabranchial chamber as the fish rises. When the mouth leaves the water, the air is expelled. The fish then fills its buccal cavity with air and sinks, compressing the air into the suprabranchial chamber. In this pattern, exhalation precedes inhalation. There is total evacuation of the suprabranchial chamber and that air is expelled while the mouth is in the air.

In monophasic respiration, the fish surfaces and takes air into the buccopharyngeal cavity before sinking. As the fish sinks, the newly taken air is compressed and forced into the suprabranchial chamber while the old air is forced out of the chamber into the water. In this pattern, inhalation precedes exhalation, and the suprabranchial chamber never changes size throughout the respiration. Air is expelled out of the operculum rather than the mouth.

Mangrove mudskippers are gobies that use modified pectoral fins to climb about tide pools. These fish have highly vascularized depressions in the mouth and gill cavity that are always kept filled with water for oxygen exchange. Climbing perch move up to 250 m across land in a few minutes, using a labyrinth organ kept moist with water held in the mouth.

Lungfishes have two mechanisms of survival during drought. The Australian lungfish never leaves the water. It has a single lung that opens into the pharyngeal region. This fish remains in its puddle, breathing air. If the pool dries up, the fish dies. African and South American lungfishes have a pair of complex lungs that can be used to survive in mucous cocoons in mud burrows during times of drought. They respire air through a small aperture near their mouth and, in a state of estivation, can survive up to 4 years in this way.

HEPATIC FUNCTION

The role of the liver in fish is much like that in any terrestrial animal. It has a major role in the metabolism of lactate to pyruvate, a biochemical pathway that also occurs in the muscles and gills of fish. The liver of fish can store up to one-eighth the total glycogen stores in a fish. These stores are relatively unaffected during exercise but are depleted during starvation.

The biliary metabolism of fishes varies to some extent. Much as in mammals, most bile salts in fish are resorbed from the intestine and recycled. In general, cholesterol is converted to bile salts. In sharks, lungfishes, and the coelacanth, the bile also contains bile alcohol sulfate esters as sodium salts. In carp, the principal bile salt is in the form of alcohol sulfates (Haslewood, 1968). In most bony fishes, taurine conjugates of bile acids are also present.

DIGESTIVE PHYSIOLOGY

In fishes, environmental temperature affects gastrointestinal transit time significantly. As the temperature increases, transit time decreases in a relationship that is not quite log normal (Table 3–2). Near the upper physiological limit of temperature, this trend reverses itself and further increases in temperature increase the transit time. There is also a relationship to the size of the meal taken; larger meals take longer to digest (Jobling et al., 1977).

PANCREAS

The fish pancreas has been the subject of considerable study (Epple, 1969; Brinn, 1973). It has been used as a model to study the basic mechanisms of pancreatic function. Fish show a hypoglycemic response to insulin injections (Epple, 1969). The re-

TABLE 3–2. Total Gastrointestinal Emptying Times for Fishes at Various Temperatures

Fishes	Temperature (°C)	Transit Time (hours)	Reference
Sardine	18	12	Lasker (1970)
Rainbow trout	11	46	Grove et al. (1978)
	18	30.5	
Northern pike	12	72	Lane and Jackson (1969)
Goldfish	12	36–48	Lane and Jackson (1969)
	20	60–72	
Carp	12	60	Lane and Jackson (1969)
	23	48	
Channel catfish	12	24–36	Lane and Jackson (1969)
Yellow perch	12	30–60	Lane and Jackson (1969)
Tilapia	25	7–15	Moriarty (1973)
Sculpin	10	100	Western (1971)
Pumpkinseed	12	84	Lane and Jackson (1969)
Bluegill	22	36	Lane and Jackson (1969)
	17	48	Lane and Jackson (1969)

sponse is prolonged at low temperatures and short at higher temperatures (Murat and Serfaty, 1975). In a given fish species, the magnitude and duration of the hypoglycemic response to insulin also depend on the type of insulin injected, the dose, route of injection, season, nutritional state of the fish, and its previous nutritional history.

The primary controlling stimuli for insulin release into the plasma of fishes appear to be the dietary protein level, nutritional state, and season. Interestingly, circulating amino acids provide more stimulus than does glucose. Somatostatin strongly inhibits the release of insulin (Ince, 1980). Catecholamines both inhibit and stimulate the release of insulin. α-Adrenergic stimulation suppresses insulin release, and β-adrenergic stimulation increases insulin release (Plisetskaya et al., 1976).

Insulin is essentially an anabolic hormone in fish. In addition to a role in oxidative clearance of glucose, insulin in fish is involved in the regulation of protein metabolism. Insulin decreases the plasma amino nitrogen content and regulates individual amino acid and protein turnover in fishes. Generally, it functions to increase the incorporation of amino acids into muscle and liver by enhancing proteogenesis. At the same time, fish insulin suppresses gluconeogenesis from amino acids.

Insulin enhances the activity of the lipogenic pathways in fish, resulting in reduced plasma fatty acids and cholesterol (Lewander et al., 1976) as a result of a preferential effect on lipogenesis from glucose in muscle. Fish insulins are generally much more efficacious than mammalian insulins in this regard (Ince and Thorpe, 1974).

Insulin levels are higher in recently fed fish than in fasted fish, and they correlate more with plasma amino nitrogen than glucose levels. In fasting fish, blood glucose levels are maintained through gluconeogenesis (Cowey and Sargent, 1979). Seasonal changes are observed. Nonmigratory fishes, such as the scorpionfish, experience lower plasma insulin levels in the winter that are not entirely due to fasting. In this species, feeding continues just before and during spawning, and insulin levels are elevated.

Spawning is initiated with water temperature changes, and when this occurs, pancreatic islets hypertrophy and hyperinsulinemia is seen, along with improved glucose and amino acid tolerance. This is in contrast to many migratory species that fast during spawning.

NERVOUS SYSTEM

By and large, the nervous system physiology of fishes is typically vertebrate. The knowledge gained about mammalian nervous systems serves well in assessing, evaluating, and treating the nervous systems of fishes.

The iris aperture, blood pressure, gill blood flow, heart performance, gastric motility, swim bladder control, and color change all are under autonomic control in fishes. In bony fishes, the adrenergic system is predominantly mediated by epinephrine (Nilsson et al., 1983). The adrenergic neurons of sharks and rays are responsive to norepinephrine (von Euler and Fange, 1961).

Both teleost and cartilaginous fishes have α-adrenoceptors that function in the constriction of smooth muscle. These are also involved in melanocyte pigment aggregation (Holmgren and Nilsson, 1982), coeliac artery control, swim bladder sphincter control, and pupillary control (Nilsson et al., 1983). β-Adrenoceptors in fish mediate smooth muscle relaxation and increased heart activity, although in salmon the receptors are β₂ type, in contrast to mammalian systems where β₁-receptors predominate (Ask et al., 1980).

Acetylcholine is the mediator in the autonomic ganglia of fish between preganglionic terminals and postganglionic neurons. The postganglionic neuron receptors are of the nicotinic type, at least in codfishes. They can be blocked with hexamethonium or mecamylamine. Muscarinic receptors are found in effector organs in all fishes studied, with the exception of the lampreys, which have nicotinic receptors in their effector organs (Lukomskaya and Michaelson, 1972).

VISION

The color of water is related to its optical properties. Deep-blue water has little phytoplankton to contribute green chlorophyll and few yellow products of organic decay (Lythgoe, 1988). The major factor limiting underwater visibility in shallow water is scattering, rather than absorption (Lythgoe, 1988). In deeper water, absorption plays a much greater role.

There appears to be a relationship between the depth a freshwater species inhabits and the pigments in its retinal cones (Levine and MacNichol, 1979). Freshwater fishes that live in deep water or are active at twilight have cones matched to 550 and 620 Å or longer wavelengths. These fishes lack blue-sensitive cones. Fishes that live in shallower water have cones that are sensitive to a broader spectral band than deep-water fishes. For example, the roach and dace can see both shorter and longer wavelengths of light than man. Diurnal fish that live close to the surface may lack long-wave sensitivity.

Some shallow-water fishes use mechanical adaptations to their advantage as well. Yellow filters in the cornea and lens of shallow-water diurnal fishes effectively counter camouflage coloration of animals swimming above them and reduce the amount of short-wave light that is scattered in the eye and perceived as noise. The cost of such a mechanism is a reduction of sensitivity in low light levels. This effect is minimized by the ability of corneal chromatophores to become virtually transparent at night to avoid loss of sensitivity.

Visual Pigments

The visual pigments of fish are chromoproteins, a protein molecule (opsin) embedded in a chromophoric group. This light-sensitive group can be retinal (vitamin A_1 aldehyde) or dehydroretinal (vitamin A_2 aldehyde). Pigments containing retinal are rhodopsins, and those containing dehydroretinal are porphyropsins. The active state of the visual pigments of fish is the 11-*cis* isomer. When a photon is absorbed, the retinal pigment straightens to a trans-configuration. This shape change may result in calcium and cyclic nucleotide mobilization, which would change the plasma membrane permeability to sodium. This in turn would change the polarity of the photoreceptor and generate a nerve pulse (Lythgoe, 1988).

The porphyropsins have longer maximum wavelength absorption than the rhodopsins, and cones with higher porphyropsin content are sensitive to longer wavelengths. Porphyropsins are found primarily in freshwater fishes and occur only rarely in marine species. Porphyropsins are not found in mammals or birds.

In fishes with both types of pigment, the proportion of two pigments varies with the season and the developmental stage of the animal. Migration from fresh water to marine water is accompanied by a change in the rhodopsin-to-porphyropsin ratio, but this change occurs before the fish enters the new environment. The change is visually significant to the fish, but it is not triggered directly by water chemistry or the spectral quality of the water. It is possible that these changes are related to circulating thyroxin levels.

Optical Properties and Accommodation

For most fishes, the focal length and aperture diameter of the eye are related to the lens diameter, since the iris does not cover any part of the lens. This means retinal illuminance is directly proportional to the intensity of the light source and inversely proportional to the square of Matthiessen's ratio for the species. Matthiessen's ratio equals the focal length divided by the lens radius and is a constant (Fernald, 1988). Therefore, retinal illuminance is independent of eye size, and larger fish do not see brighter images even though their eyes continue to grow through life.

However, resolution does increase with eye size on the basis of an increased focal length if the receptor spacing stays the same. If the receptor spacing changes in proportion to the increase in eye size, the resolving power of the eye remains constant.

Under water, fish do not have the benefit of an air-cornea interface, and the refractive power of the cornea is neutralized. This interface provides about 43 diopters (D) of refractive power in humans. Fish must depend entirely on the refractive power of the spherical lens. A spherical lens provides the maximum refractive power available but eliminates the use of lens distortion to accommodate. Fish adjust the distance of the lens from the retina to accommodate. The distance of travel is very small. A retractor lentis muscle moves the lens nearer the retina and slightly ventrally to allow for distance vision. The flattened shape of most fish eyes and the normal protrusion of the lens in front of the iris apparently contribute to a wide-angle effect in fish vision.

Managing Different Light Intensities

The fish iris contracts or expands in direct response to light intensity shifts in a manner similar to that seen in mammals. The process is just much slower. Contraction resulting in miosis is typically faster (2 to 15 minutes) than relaxation, resulting in pupil dilation (30 or more minutes). Unfortunately, the length of time required to observe these reflexes reduces their clinical usefulness, but they are present.

In addition to iris responses, cone cells in the fish retina will contract when exposed to bright light. Conversely, rod cells contract during dark adaptation, and pigment migrates distally in the rod. This uncovers an occluded reflective tapetum in some fishes. In other fishes, the tapetum is always visible, and some fishes do not have a reflective tapetum.

Retinal Growth

Fish eyes continue to grow throughout the life of the fish. Eye growth can be very significant in fishes. African cichlids may triple the radius of their eye in 2 months (Fernald, 1985). This results in fundamental differences in the biology of fish retinas compared to mammalian retinas. In most vertebrates, postnatal eye growth is accommodated by stretching existing neural tissue. Some birds and a few mammals add some retinal cells immediately after birth, and many amphibians add retinal neurons after metamorphosis, but these additions are limited. In fish, retinal area enlargement occurs through both cell addition and neuronal stretching. The proportions of each mechanism used vary with the species of fish, but in all fishes cells are apparently added to the retina from a germinal zone around the outer margin of the retina (Muller, 1952). New cones are added throughout life, and the cone density per degree of visual angle increases slightly with eye size, resulting in increased visual acuity.

OLFACTION

Fish olfaction receptors are essentially the same as those found in mammals. The only real difference is that there is a thicker layer of water over the surface of the fish receptor. Also, though olfaction receptors in fish are usually located in the rostrum and nostrils, there is usually no connection between the nostrils and the mouth. Fish are capable of following very minute concentrations of chemicals in the water. The homing process of salmons is thought to be a result of the ability of these fishes to detect homing substances from their hatch place. In addition to homing to olfactory cues, fish use smell to signal retreat. L-Serine, for example, causes rapid avoidance in salmonids, whereas other amino acids have no such effect. The sense of smell in fish is acute, and their receptors function in much the same manner as those in mammals.

TASTE

The receptors of taste in fish are histologically similar to mammalian taste receptors. As discussed in Chapter 1, most of the taste receptors of fish are not located on the tongue. Fish taste receptors can be found on any part of the fish. Each species has a distinct pattern of receptor distribution.

Fish taste receptors have a response to stimuli that is slightly different from those of mammals. The response to glucose or sucrose is usually faint. Most fish have strong responses to bitter (quinine) and sour (acetic acid) stimuli. Catfishes have a strong

response to cysteine but no response to cystine or homocysteine. Adaptation of the taste receptors usually occurs within 10 to 20 seconds of initial exposure to the stimulus. Various ions in low to moderate concentrations can affect the taste response in fish. Iron, calcium, and magnesium ions depress taste responses in catfishes, but polyvalent anions usually enhance their taste responses to monovalent salts. At higher concentrations, these ions do not appear to cause enhancement of taste reception. Heavy metals will reduce taste receptor responses in fish. Exposure to mercury or lead will block taste reception for extended periods. Interestingly, fish exposed to mercury can have their taste reception restored by rinsing in a dilute solution of copper sulfate. Apparently a metal ion exchange mechanism is involved.

LATERAL LINE SYSTEM

The sensors of the lateral line system of fish are mechanoreceptors that operate on the same principle as the semicircular canals of mammals. In sharks and rays and some teleosts, the neuromasts of the lateral line system project from the body surface. In most fishes, the organs are partly enclosed in a groove or a tube with openings to the surface of the fish.

The neuromast organs of the lateral line system produce a constant spontaneous electrical potential output when no stimulus is present. External stimulation moves the kinocilium and cupula in an oscillating motion that results in nerve discharge rates that are proportional to the bending of the kinocilium. These discharges alter the output potential of the nerve cell, resulting in oscillations in the number of nerve pulses per unit time sent to the brain. The mechanism is probably similar to what occurs with hair cells in the mammalian inner ear. The result is a frequency-modulated signal, the same mechanism used in an FM radio transmission. The unique aspect of the lateral line system is that while most receptors respond only to an increasing stimulus, the neuromast of the lateral line responds to decreasing stimulus as well. Fish lateral line neuromasts respond to a range of frequency in the range of 1 to 100 or 200 Hz. The upper limit of detection varies from species to species (Smith, 1982).

HEARING

Fish lack a cochlea and have therefore been considered functionally deaf to sound by many workers. This is not the case. Fish detect waveform stimuli at frequencies well above those detected by their lateral line systems. The range of frequencies they detect varies with the species. Herrings hear sounds between 30 and 2000 Hz. The lower limits of fish hearing usually range between 25 and 100 Hz. The upper limits vary between 400 and 4000 Hz.

Swim bladders serve as mechanical amplifiers for fish hearing. Herrings and anchovies have tubular extensions of their swim bladders that extend close to their labyrinth and presumably serve as amplification conductors. Air-breathing eels use another system of amplification. They hold air bubbles in the roof of their mouth to enhance hearing as well as to serve in respiration. Carps have a special series of bones known as the weberian apparatus that connect the anterior swim bladder to the cranium and serve to mechanically transmit vibrations detected in the swim bladder.

ELECTRIC ORGANS AND ELECTRORECEPTION

Six families of fishes, including skates, the electric catfish, and the electric eel, are able to produce electricity at potentials far above those generated in normal muscular contraction. They accomplish this with an electroplax organ that has apparently evolved through parallel evolution in the variety of species. These organs occur only in fish. The electrical conductivity of water may have been a requirement for the evolution of electrical signals as purposeful communication.

The electroplax is a modified muscle cell. When it is stimulated, no contraction occurs; instead, the polarity of one face of the cell reverses momentarily, allowing current to flow. Each cell contains a large amount of ATPase, and considerable energy is expended in the generation of large electric potentials. A single electroplax cell can generate 70 to 100 mV. With many of the flat cells stacked upon each other, voltages up to 600 V can be generated by electric eels. The electric catfish generates up to 300 V, electric rays around 60 V, and the elephant-nosed fish only a maximum of about 25 V.

Fishes that produce these electric potentials also have specialized electroreception organs. These are located in canals or pits filled with a mucoid substance and are relatively well isolated from the external environment. Their structure is similar to that of a modified neuromast organ. These electroreceptors can respond to very low level electric fields, such as those produced by ordinary muscle contractions. Their sensitivity varies with the species of fish and with the conductivity of the fish's environment. For example, the elephant-nosed fishes detect fields as low as $0.25 \mu V$ in 2000-Ohm water. They have nearly twice the threshold in 10,000-Ohm water. Electric eels are capable of detecting a threshold of from 2 to 30 mV and can discriminate changes of 1.5 to 5.0 mV in currents above their threshold. Some fishes that do not produce high electric fields can sense them. The Atlantic salmon and many eels detect electricity in the microvolt range in ocean environments. Sharks are renowned for their ability to detect very small electric fields.

STRESS RESPONSE

Whole books have been written on the stress responses of fish (Pickering, 1981). The stress re-sponse in fish is very similar to that in man. A primary stress response is a spike in circulating cortisol levels with many of the same consequences seen in man. The stress response most studied in fish is that due to transport. For example, when large-mouth bass are transported from one location to another in tank trucks, there is a cortisol peak during the transport, accompanied by increases in serum glucose and serum osmolality. This is followed by decreased serum osmolality and low chloride levels (Carmichael et al., 1984). The decreases in serum osmolality are also seen in many fish diseases (Robertson et al., 1987).

The syndrome of delayed capture mortality has been extensively investigated in the skipjack tuna. It is characterized by myopathy, weakness, poor vision, and incoordination (Bourke et al., 1987). Behavioral signs seen include increased swimming speed with no "coast then glide" pattern. The affected fish swims in figure-of-eight patterns, often scraping the sides of its tank. Hematological changes include a decreased hematocrit that returns to normal in about 9 hours after capture. Cholesterol, glucose, triglycerides, total protein, calcium, and iron decrease in moribund fish. Uric acid and chloride levels increase. The serum alkaline phosphatase, bilirubin, and urea nitrogen do not change. Fish with the syndrome lose up to 10% of their body weight in 9 to 49 hours after capture. The cause of mortality has been attributed to disseminated intravascular coagulopathy (Smith, 1980), loss of osmotic homeostasis (Sleet and Weber, 1982), myopathy and renal tubular damage (Roberts et al., 1973), secondary bacterial or viral infections (Mazeaud et al., 1977), and lactic acid build-up (Wood et al., 1983). All that is certain is that the mechanism for the syndrome is not simple trauma or a reaction to hypoxia.

LITERATURE CITED

Ask, J.A., Stene-Larsen, G., and Helle, K.B. (1980) Atrial beta-adrenoceptors in the trout. J. Comp. Physiol. 139B:109–116.

Atema, J., Fay, R.R., Poper, A.N., and Tavolga, W.N. (eds.) (1988) Sensory Biology of Aquatic Animals. Springer-Verlag, New York.

Babiker, M.M., and Rankin, J.C. (1978) Neurohypophysial hormonal control of kidney function in the European eel (Anguilla anguilla L.) adapted to sea-water or fresh water. J. Endocrinol. 76:347–358.

Beyenbach, K.W. (1982) Direct demonstration of fluid secretion by glomerular renal tubules in a marine teleost. Nature 299:54–56.

Bourke, R.E., Brock, J., and Nakamura, R.M. (1987) A study of delayed capture mortality syndrome in skipjack tuna, Katsuwonus pelamis (L.). J. Fish Dis. 10:275–287.

Boylan, J.W. (1972) Model for passive urea reabsorption in the elasmobranch kidney. Comp. Biochem. Physiol. 42A:27–30.

Brett, J.R. (1972) The metabolic demand for oxygen in fish, particularly salmonids and a comparison with other vertebrates. Respir. Physiol. 14:151–170.

Brinn, J.E., Jr. (1973) The pancreatic islets of bony fishes. Am. Zoologist 13:653–665.

Carmichael, G.J., Tomasso, J.R., Simco, B.A., and Davis, K.B. (1984) Characterization and alleviation of stress associated with hauling largemouth bass. Trans. Am. Fish. Soc. 113:778–785.

Cowey, C.B., and Sargent, J.R. (1979) Nutrition. In: Fish Physiology. Vol. VIII (Hoar, W.S., Randall, D.J., and Brett, J.R., eds.). Academic Press, New York, pp. 1–69.

Delaney, R.C., Lahiri, S., Hamilton, R., and Fishman, A.P. (1977) Acid-base balance and plasma composition in the estivating lungfish (Protopterus). Am. J. Physiol. 232:R10–R17.

De Renzis, G., and Bornancin, M. (1984) Ion transport and gill ATPases. In: Fish Physiology. Vol. X. Gills Part B, Ion and Water Transfer. (Hoar,

W.S., and Randall, D.J., eds.). Academic Press, New York, pp. 65–104.

Epple, A. (1969) The endocrine pancreas. In: Fish Physiology. Vol. 2 (Hoar, W.S., and Randall, D.J., eds.). Academic Press, New York, pp. 275–310.

Evans, D.H. (1982) Salt and water exchange across vertebrate gills. In: Gills (Houlihan, D.F., Rankin, J.C., and Shuttleworth, T.J., eds.). Cambridge University Press, Cambridge, Massachusetts, pp. 149–171.

Fange, R., and Grove, D. (1979) Digestion. In: Fish Physiology. Vol. 8 (Hoar, W.S., Randall, D.J., and Brett, J.R., eds.). Academic Press, New York, pp. 161–260.

Fernald, R.D. (1985) Growth of the teleost eye: Novel solutions to complex constraints. Environ. Biol. Fishes 13:113–123.

Fernald, R.D. (1988) Aquatic adaptations in fish eyes. In: Sensory Biology of Aquatic Animals (Altema, J., Fay, R.R., Popper, A.N., and Tavologa, W.N., eds.). Springer-Verlag, New York, pp. 435–466.

Goldstein, L. (1982) Gill nitrogen excretion. In: Gills (Houlihan, D.F., Rankin, J.C., and Shuttleworth, T.J., eds.). Cambridge University Press, Cambridge, Massachusetts, pp. 193–206.

Grove, D.J., Lozoides, L., and Nott, J. (1978) Satiation amount, frequency of feeding and gastric emptying rate in Salmo gairdneri. J. Fish Biol. 12:507–516.

Haslewood, G.A.D. (1968) Evolution and bile salts. In: Handbook of Physiology (Code, C.F., ed.). Sect. 6, Vol. 5. American Physiological Society, Washington, D.C., pp. 2375–2390.

Henderson, I.W., and Wales, N.A.M. (1974) Renal diuresis and antidiuresis after injections of arginine vasotocin in the freshwater eel (Anguilla anguilla L.). J. Endocrinol. 61:487–500.

Henderson, I.W., Brown, J.A., Oliver, J.A., and Hayward, G.P. (1987) Hormones and single nephron function in fishes. In: Comparative Endocrinology (Gaillard, P.J., and Boer, H.H., eds.). Elsevier/North Holland, Amsterdam, pp. 217–222.

Hoar, W.S., and Randall, D.J. (eds.) (1969–1990) Fish Physiology. Vols. I–XII. Academic Press, New York.

Holeton, G.F. (1979) Oxygen as an environmental factor of fishes. In: Environmental Physiology of Fishes (Ali, M.A., ed.). Plenum Press, New York, pp. 7–32.

Holmgren, S., and Nilsson, S. (1982) Minireview. Neuropharmacology of adrenergic neurons in Teleost fish. Comp. Biochem. Physiol. 71C:141–153.

Hughes, G.M., and Singh, B.N. (1970) Respiration in an air-breathing fish, the climbing perch Anabas testudineus Bloch. I. Oxygen uptake and carbon dioxide release into air and water. J. Exp. Biol. 53:265–280.

Ince, B.W. (1980) Amino acid stimulation of insulin secretion from the perfused eel pancreas: Modification by somatostatin, adrenalin and theophylline. Gen. Comp. Endocrinol. 40:275–282.

Ince, B.W. (1983) Pancreatic control of metabolism. In: Control Processes in Fish Physiology (Rankin, J.C., Pitcher, T.J., and Duggan, R., eds.). Wiley Interscience, New York, pp. 89–102.

Ince, B.W., and Thorpe, A. (1974) Effects of insulin and metabolite loading on blood metabolites in the European silver eel (Anguilla anguilla L.). Gen. Comp. Endocrinol. 23:460–471.

Jobling, M., Gwyther, D., and Grove, D.J. (1977) Some effects of temperature, meal size and body weight on gastric evacuation time in the dab, Limanda limanda (L.) J. Fish Biol. 10:291–298.

Lane, T.H., and Jackson, H.M. (1969) Voidance time for 23 species of fish. Invest. Fish Control No. 33, cited in Fange and Grove (1979), Vol. 8 of Hoar and Randall.

Lasker, R. (1970) Utilization of zooplankton energy by a Pacific sardine population in the Californian current. In: Marine Food Chains (Steele, J.H., ed.). Oliver and Boyd, Edinburgh, pp. 265–284.

Levine, J.S., and MacNichol, E.F., Jr. (1979) Visual pigments in teleost fishes: Effects of habitat, microhabitat and behavior on visual system evolution. Sensory Processes 3:95–130.

Lewander, K., Dave, G., Johansson-Sjobeck, M.L., Larsson, A., and Lidman, U. (1976) Metabolic effects of insulin in the European eel (Anguilla anguilla). Gen. Comp. Endocrinol. 29:455–467.

Lukomskaya, N.J., and Michaelson, M.J. (1972) Pharmacology of the isolated heart of the lamprey, Lampetra fluviatilis. Comp. Gen. Pharm. 3:213–225.

Lythgoe, J.N. (1988) Light and vision in the aquatic environment. In: Sensory Biology of Aquatic Animals (Altema, J., Fay, R.R., Popper, A.N., and Tavologa, W.N., eds.). Springer-Verlag, New York, pp. 57–83.

Mazeaud, M.M., Maseaud, F., and Donaldson, E.M. (1977) Primary and secondary effects of stress in fish: Some new data with a general review. Trans. Am. Fish. Soc. 106:201–212.

Moriarty, D.J.W. (1973) The physiology of digestion of blue-green algae in the cichlid fish Tilapia nilotica. J. Zool. 171:15–23.

Muller, H. (1952) Bau un Wachstum der Netzhaut des Guppy (Lebistes reticulatus). Zool. Jb. Allgemein Zool. Physiol. Tier. 63:275–324.

Murat, J.C., and Serfaty, A. (1975) Effect of temperature on carbohydrate metabolism responses to epinephrine, glucagon, and insulin in the carp. C.R. Soc. Biol. (Paris) 169:228–232.

Nash, J. (1931) The number and size of glomeruli in the kidneys of fishes with observations on the morphology of the renal tubules of fishes. Am. J. Anat. 47:425–445.

Nilsson, S., Holmgren, S., and Fange, R. (1983) Autonomic nerve functions in fish. In: Control Processes in Fish Physiology (Rankin, J.C., Pitcher, T.J., and Duggan, R., eds.). Wiley Interscience, New York, pp. 1–22.

Peters, H.M. (1978) On the mechanism of air ventilation in anabantoids (Pices: Teleostei). Zoomorphology 89:93–124.

Pickering, A.D. (ed.) (1981) Stress and Fish. Academic Press, New York.

Pickering, A.D. (1984) Cortisol-induced lymphocytopenia in brown trout, Salmo trutta L. Gen. Comp. Endocrinol. 53:252–259.

Pickering, A.D., and Duston, J. (1983) Administration of cortisol to brown trout, Salmo trutta L. and its effects on the susceptibility to Saprolegnia infection and furunculosis. J. Fish Biol. 23:163–175.

Pickford, G.E., Srivastava, A.K., Slicher, A.M., and Pang, P.K.T. (1971) The stress response in the abundance of circulating leucocytes in the killifish, Fundulus heteroclitus. J. Exp. Zool. 177:109–118.

Plisetskaya, E.M. (1968) Brain and heart glycogen content in some vertebrates, and effect of insulin. Endocrinol. Exp. 2:251–262.

Plisetskaya, E.M., Leibush, B.N., and Bondareva, V. (1976) The secretion of insulin and its role in cyclostomes and fishes. In: The Evolution of Pancreatic Islets (Grillo, T.A.I., Leibson, L., and Epple, A., eds.). Pergamon Press, Oxford, England, pp. 251–269.

Potts, W.T.W. (1984) Transepithelial potentials in fish gills. In: Fish Physiology. Vol. X. Gills Part B, Ion and Water Transfer (Hoar, W.S., and Randall, D.J., eds.). Academic Press, New York, pp. 105–128.

Rankin, J.C., and Bolis, L. (1984) Hormonal control of water movement across the gills. In: Fish Physiology. Vol. X. Gills Part B, Ion and Water Transfer (Hoar, W.S., and Randall, D.J., eds.). Academic Press, New York, pp. 177–201.

Rankin, J.C., Logan, A.G., and Moriarty, R.J. (1980) Changes in kidney function in the river lamprey, Lapetra fluviatilis L., in response to changes in external salinity. In: Epithelial Transport in the Lower Vertebrates (Lahlou, B., ed.). Cambridge University Press, Cambridge, Massachusetts, pp. 171–184.

Rankin, J.C., Henderson, I.W., and Brown, J.A. (1983) Osmoregulation and the control of kidney function. In: Control Processes in Fish Physiology (Rankin, J.C., Pitcher, T.J., and Duggan, R., eds.). Wiley Interscience, New York, pp. 66–88.

Roberts, R.J., McQueen, A., Shearer, W.M., and Young, H. (1973) The histopathology of salmon tagging. II: Chronic lesion in returning adult fish. J. Fish Biol. 5:615–621.

Robertson, O.H., Hane, S., Wexler, B.C., and Rinfret, A.P. (1963) The effect of hydrocortisone on immature rainbow trout (Salmo gairdneri). Gen. Comp. Endocrinol. 3:422–436.

Robertson, L., Thomas, P., Arnold, C.R., and Trant, J.M. (1987) Plasma cortisol and secondary stress responses of red drum to handling transport, rearing density, and a disease outbreak. Progressive Fish Culturist 49:1–12.

Sawyer, W.H., Uchiyama, M., and Pang, P.K.T. (1982) Control of renal function in lungfishes. Fed. Proceed. 41:2361–2364.

Schmidt-Nielsen, B., Truniger, B., and Rabinowitz, L. (1972) Sodium-linked urea transport by renal tubules of spiny dogfish, Squalus acanthias. Comp. Biochem. Physiol. 42A:13–25.

Sleet, R.B., and Weber, L.J. (1982) The rate and manner of seawater ingestion by a marine teleost and corresponding water modification by the gut. Comp. Biochem. Physiol. 72A:469–475.

Smith, A.C. (1980) Formation of lethal blood clots in fishes. J. Fish Biol. 16:1–4.

Smith, C.J., and Grau, E.G. (1986) Ultrastructural changes in the parrotfish thyroid after in vitro stimulation with bovine thyrotropin. Fish Physiol. Biochem. 1:153–162.

Smith, L.S. (1982) Introduction to Fish Physiology. T.F.H. Publications, Neptune, New Jersey.

von Euler, U.S., and Fange, R. (1961) Catecholamines in nerves and organs of Myxine glutinosa, Squalus acanthias and Gadus callarias. Gen. Comp. Endocrinol. 1:191–194.

Wahlqvist, I., and Nilsson, S. (1977) The role of sympathetic fibres and circulating catecholamines in controlling the blood pressure and heart rate in cod, Gadus morhua. Comp. Biochem. Physiol. 56C:65–67.

Western, J.R.H. (1971) Feeding and digestion in two cottid fishes, the freshwater Cottus gobio and the marine Enophrys bubalis. J. Fish Biol. 3:225–246.

Wood, C.M., Turner, J.D., and Graham, M.S. (1983) Why do fish die after severe exercise? J. Fish Biol. 22:189–201.

Zadunaisky, J.A. (1984) The chloride cell. In: Fish Physiology. Vol. X. Gills Part B, Ion and Water Transfer. (Hoar, W.S., and Randall, D.J., eds.). Academic Press, New York, pp. 129–176.

Chapter 4

CLINICAL GENETICS

MICHAEL K. STOSKOPF

The clinical implications of genetics in fish medicine are not well studied. However, as genetic manipulation of fish stocks becomes more common and clinicians become involved with a wider variety of fish species, basic knowledge of fish genetics becomes valuable. Certainly, it is probable that chromosomal anomalies play an important role in fish reproductive failure, and the use of genetics and karyology will become more commonplace in breeding program evaluations.

Several problems complicate the study of fish genetics. Techniques commonly used in other animal groups are frequently not very successful in fish. In terrestrial species, chromosomes for study are usually collected from blood leukocytes to avoid tedious methods required to separate individual cells from other tissues. These leukocytes are then stimulated with mitogens to induce cell mitosis. Unfortunately, leukocytes of fish do not respond to many commonly used mitogens. In addition, the many forms of reproduction in fish make fish gene studies exciting but confusing.

REPRODUCTION

Different fish species use a variety of reproductive strategies. These include simple bisexuality, unisexuality, hermaphroditic unisexuality, and bisexual gonochorism where functional reproductive tissues of both genders coexist in a single individual.

The majority of fish reproduce bisexually and have separate sexes of approximately equal numbers. This pattern suggests the presence of sex chromosomes or heterosomes. Unfortunately, some of the generalizations made about heterosomy in mammals or birds cannot be made for fishes.

The sex chromosomes of most fishes have remained relatively undifferentiated. For example, the green swordtail, several other Caribbean poecilids, and some anabantids show no evidence of sex chromosome heterogamety (Kosswig, 1964). This of course suggests that sex determination in fish may be polyfactorial with epistatic sex genes playing a large role.

The mammalian pattern of male heterogamety, with female XX and male XY chromosome patterns, has been confirmed in 25 species of fish. These include four species of smelt, the black spotted stickleback, the California killifish, and the banded kil-

lifish. There are several other fish species that show no heterogamety but exhibit genetic evidence for this sort of reproductive pattern. These include two species of guppy, several species of swordtail, Siamese fighting fish, goldfish, and medaka.

A very extreme form of heterogamety is found in several fishes where males have only one X chromosome, and females maintain two X chromosomes. There is no Y chromosome. Fishes with this reproductive genome pattern include the hatchetfish, two species of lanternfishes, and the blackcheek tonguefish.

The female heterogamety pattern seen in birds (WZ:ZZ) is also found in fish. European eels, mosquitofish, rudd, and four-spined sticklebacks all have confirmed female heterogamety (Chiarelli et al., 1969). This pattern is suggested by genetic evidence in Mozambique tilapia (Hickling, 1960), sphenops molly, and the majority of the hermaphrodites in the order Perciformes (Atz, 1964; Yamamoto, 1969). Genetic evidence exists for female heterosomy in the southern platyfish, which can also be male heterogametic. This fish has three different heterosomes that can lead to both male and female heterogamety.

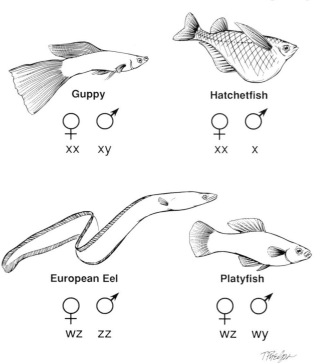

FIGURE 4–1. Strategies of genetic gender determination.

Hermaphroditism

Hermaphroditic Unisexuality

Hermaphroditic unisexuality, or a reproductive pattern where female individuals produce exclusively female offspring, occurs in some fishes (Fig. 4–2). One process by which this occurs is termed hybridogenesis (Schultz, 1969). Sperm of closely related sympatric species are used to stimulate egg division, with the male pronucleus degenerating and making no genetic contribution to the offspring. Normally, proper ploidy is maintained by either apomixis where meiosis is abortive, or automixis where meiosis is normal. However, before or after meiosis, a division occurs to reduce the chromosome complement. In either case, a male from a bisexual species is required to provide the sperm needed to initiate the process.

The first completely female species of fish discovered was appropriately named the Amazon molly (Hubbs and Hubbs, 1932). These fish breed with several different closely related species, but produce only female progeny. No paternal characteristics are transmitted; only maternal genes are inherited. The offspring are identical to their mothers and sisters (Kallman, 1970) with a diploid complement of 46 chromosomes. A triploid population has been identified in laboratory stocks of these fish, which resemble the shortfin molly, and probably arose from the incorporation of a haploid complement of the shortfin molly with the diploid Amazon molly (Balsano et al., 1972). The method of ploidy maintenance used by the Amazon molly is not known.

Other all female fish populations are documented. Some populations of silver crucian carp and Japanese goldfish are unisexually hermaphroditic. One gynogenetic population of goldfish is triploid (Cherfas, 1966, 1972), as a result of an aborted reductional division following an equatorial division prior to ovulation.

Synchronous Hermaphroditism

Synchronous hermaphroditism, where both sexual tissues are present in the same individual and are functional at the same time, occurs in several species of fish (Yamamoto, 1969) (see Fig. 4–2). Some of these are capable of self-fertilization, including belted sandfish (Clark, 1959, 1965), rivulus (Harrington, 1961), members of the sea bass family, and an Alaskan population of three-spined stickleback (Atz, 1964).

Asynchronous Hermaphroditism

Asynchronous hermaphroditism, where an individual fish transforms from one sex to another with changes in age, is also seen in fishes. In these fishes, juveniles possess both testicular and ovarian tissues. Sexual reversals in heterogametic fish are well documented, and suggest that polyfactorial sex deter-

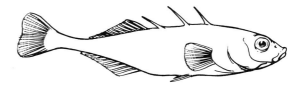

Synchronous
Three spined stickleback

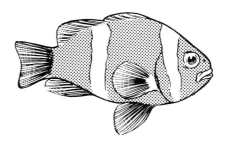

Protandrous
Clownfish

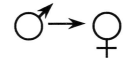

Protogynous
Haplochromis Cichlid

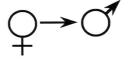

FIGURE 4–2. Types of hermaphroditism in fishes.

mination may occur through the influence of epistatic sex genes on the sex chromosomes. Protandrous hermaphrodites are first males, transforming, later into females. This form of hermaphroditism occurs in sea breams and porgies. Protogynous hermaphrodites are initially females and become males later in their lives. This pattern of hermaphroditism occurs in other members of the porgie family, some members of the sea bass family, and swamp eels (Liem, 1963; Chan, 1970).

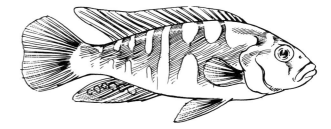

KARYOTYPIC DIVERSITY

Karyotypic diversity in fishes is not as extreme as might be expected. Many orders are relatively uniform with 24 acrocentric chromosome pairs. This chromosome number occurs in about 35 to 40% of the fish species that have been examined, including the relatively ancient hagfish and the recently evolved perches. Three-quarters of the fish species examined have between 22 and 24 chromosome pairs. In the cyprinid fishes, the median number of chromosome pairs is 25. Salmonid fishes have a median chromosome number of 36 pairs.

Although most fish have similar chromosome numbers, the range of chromosome numbers is very broad (Fig. 4–3). The lowest number, eight pairs, is found in the fire killifish. Several fishes have high numbers of chromosomes. Some salmonids, cyprinids, and catostomids have 40 to 52 pairs of chromosomes. Several species of lamprey have the highest recorded number of chromosomes for a fish with 84 pairs.

Some scientists suspect that the high chromosome number in lampreys is the result of ancestral polyploidy. Polyploidy is common in higher plants, but rare in bisexual vertebrates. In fish, triploid female unisexual populations have been reported, as well as male and female triploid and tetraploid goldfish populations in Japan. Triploid rainbow trout and triploid western roaches occur rarely, but are expected to be sterile. Triploid eastern brook trout also have been reported (Davisson et al., 1972). Interestingly, not everything that appears to be polyploidy is. The clown loach with 49 pairs of chromosomes and the related Khulli loach with 25 pairs of chromosomes have about the same amount of deoxyribonucleic acid (DNA) (1 pg per haploid nucleus). This tends to support the hypothesis that the disparity in chromosome number between these two closely related species is not due to polyploidy.

Fish chromosomes are smaller than those of most other vertebrates. They are routinely 2 to 5 μ long and often are less than 2 μ long. Lungfishes are exceptions, having large chromosomes on the order of 15 to 35 μ long. Trout and most salmonids have very symmetrical karyotypes, with chromosomes that are all about the same size and shape and have medially located centromeres. In contrast, the karyotypes of minnows and other cyprinids are often highly asymmetric, with considerable difference in chromosome size and placement of the centromere (Stebbins, 1971).

ESTABLISHING INBRED LINES

A variety of special techniques are being used to establish inbred lines of fish for specific uses. One approach has been to take advantage of the fish ova's susceptibility to artificial parthenogenesis (Purdom and Lincoln, 1973). In these techniques, eggs are activated with sperm and then subjected to temperature shocks that interfere with either the first or second meiotic division of the egg, or the first mitotic division of the embryo. Temperature shocking eggs fertilized with normal sperm has been used successfully to produce polyploidy lines of tilapia, plaice, plaice/flounder crosses, and sticklebacks. The common result is a triploid line of fish with increased growth rate (Purdom, 1973) that is expected to be sterile. These fish are useful in stocking programs where it is important to preserve the genetic integrity of wild populations.

Similar treatment of eggs that have been fertilized with sperm inactivated with radiation produces a high frequency of diploid gynogenomes. If the temperature shock interferes with the first meiosis, a line with 50% inbreeding is obtained. If the failure of first mitosis is accomplished, inbreeding is effective 100% in these diploid lines. This technique has been used in carp, loaches, sturgeon, and plaice, although the survival of embryos is very low.

LITERATURE CITED

Atz, J.W. (1964) Intersexuality in fishes. In: Intersexuality in Vertebrates Including Man (Armstrong, C.N., and Marshall, A.J., eds.). Academic Press, New York, pp. 145–232.

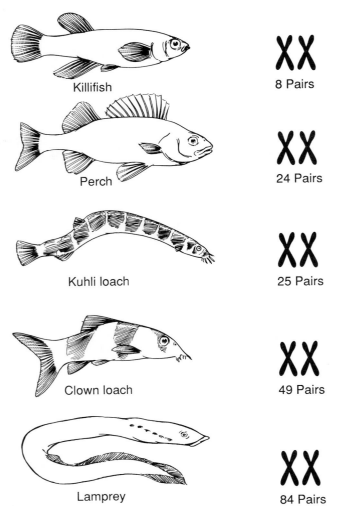

Killifish — 8 Pairs

Perch — 24 Pairs

Kuhli loach — 25 Pairs

Clown loach — 49 Pairs

Lamprey — 84 Pairs

FIGURE 4–3. Variations in chromosomal numbers between fishes.

Balsano, J.S., Darnell, R.M., and Abramoff, P. (1972) Electrophoretic evidence of triploidy associated with populations of gynogenetic teleost Poecilia formosa. Copeia 2:292–297.

Chan, S.T.H. (1970) Natural sex reversal in vertebrates. Philos. Trans. R. Soc. Lond. (Biol.) 259:59–71.

Cherfas, N.B. (1966) Natural triploidy in females of the unisexual forms of the goldfish (Carassius auratus gibelio Bolch). Sov. Genet. 2(5): 9–13.

Chiarelli, A.B., Ferrantelli, O., and Cucchi, C. (1969) The karyotype of some Teleostea fish obtained by tissue culture in vitro. Experientia 25:426–427.

Clark, E. (1959) Functional hermaphroditism in a serranid fish. Science 129:215–216.

Clark, E. (1965) Mating of groupers. Nat. Hist. 74:22–25.

Davisson, M.T., Wright, J.E., and Atherton, L.M. (1972) Centric fusion and trisomy for the LDH-B locus in brook trout, Salvelinus fontinalis. Science 178:992–994.

Gold, J.R. (1979) Cytogenetics. In: Fish Physiology. Vol. 8 (Hoar, W.S., Randall, D.J., and Brett, J.R., eds.). Academic Press, New York, pp. 353–406. 1979.

Harrington, R.W., Jr. (1961) Oviparous hermaphroditic fish with internal self-fertilization. Science 134:1749–1750.

Hickling, C.F. (1960) The Malacca tilapia hybrids. J. Genet. 57:1–10.

Hubbs, C.L., and Hubbs, L.C. (1932) Apparent parthenogenesis in nature in a form of fish of hybrid origin. Science 76:628–630.

Kallman, K.D. (1970) Genetics of tissue transplantation in Teleostei. Transplant. Proc. 2:263–271.

Kosswig, C. (1964) Polygenic sex determination. Experientia 20:190–199.

Liem, K.F. (1963) Sex reversal as a natural process in the synbranchiform fish Monopterus albus. Copeia 2:303–312.

Purdom, C.E. (1973) Induced polyploidy in plaice (Pleuronectes platessa) and its hybrid with the flounder (Platichthys flesus) Heredity 29:11–24.

Purdom, C.E., and Lincoln, R.F. (1973) Chromosome manipulation in fish. In: Genetics and Mutagenesis of Fish (Schroder, J.H., ed.). Springer-Verlag, Berlin, pp. 83–89.

Schultz, R.J. (1969) Hybridization, unisexuality, and polyploidy in the teleost Poeciliopsis (Poeciliidae) and other vertebrates. Am. Nat. 103:605–619.

Stebbins, G.L. (1971) Chromosomal Evolution in Higher Plants. Addison-Wesley, Reading, Massachusetts.

Yamamoto, T. (1969) Sex differentiation. In: Fish Physiology. Vol. 3 (Hoar, W.S., and Randall, D.J., eds.). Academic Press, New York, pp. 117–175.

Yamamoto, T, and Kajishima, T. (1969) Sex-hormonic induction of reversal of sex differentiation in the goldfish and evidence for its male heterogamety. J. Exp. Zool. 168:215–222.

Chapter 5

CLINICAL EXAMINATION AND PROCEDURES

MICHAEL K. STOSKOPF

TAKING THE HISTORY

The history remains the most important aspect of a clinical examination in fish medicine. Despite the advent of new, sophisticated diagnostic methods, no tool is more effective in narrowing the search for the underlying cause of a problem. The technique and objectives of taking a history in fish practice are identical with those in other types of veterinary practice, and the experienced practitioner will have a significant advantage in using this tool. While the skill of taking a history develops with practice and experience, a few basic skills can dramatically expedite that development.

At the risk of stating the obvious, it is usually easier to learn something by listening than by talking. Certainly, the history-taking time can be used to establish your credentials and inspire your client with confidence, but keep in mind that the client should be doing the majority of the talking. You should be asking clear, succinct questions that will cause your client to talk, and then you should be listening critically to the information being provided. Your questions should not be directive, steering the client to a particular conclusion, nor should they be small sermons. The time for education is after you have some idea of the problem at hand, not during the history. Keeping your questions open and short is more difficult than it seems.

For example, a common error is to ask a question with an attached answer, such as "Have you noticed any differences in feeding behavior lately? Are they slower to rise to the feed?" Although it might seem that you are only lending the client additional explanation or assistance to help them communicate relevant observations, this type of question runs the risk of providing false data. The hazard is greatest when questioning issues the client may not have considered previously. It is human nature to be agreeable. This is not necessarily obvious with some clients, but usually, if presented with a question in this form, a client who has not considered the answer to the question will provide you with the answer you are telegraphing you expect. After all, you are the expert they have hired to examine their problem, and if you expect a certain reply, there must be a reason. Of course, this defeats any collection of real information.

Avoid the temptation to take off on a minilecture after each response to one of your questions. Unless a client asks a direct question that can be answered in a sentence or two, a client's reply should be followed with another question from you. It is important to keep the history taking on track and to complete it in a reasonable amount of time. Within the limits of social graces, keep the history-taking session moving by asking your questions one after the other in a sequence that helps you consider the analysis of the problem.

Usually, the private fish owner is more comfortable if questions about the fish are asked first. Occasionally, such clients become anxious if the history jumps directly to issues of water quality or husbandry. So, it is a good idea to begin by asking what fish are affected, and what signs they are showing. This information may be volunteered before any questions can be asked. Follow up on the answers to these questions to determine the time course of the signs and the time course of the spread through individuals in the system or between systems. Once you have established the relative acuteness or chronicity of the situation, whether the problem is affecting particular species or age classes, the typical pattern of signs, and the timing of any new additions of fish to the system, you can move to an assessment of husbandry practices.

The first issue in husbandry is generally water quality, and I start my next round of questioning there. I want to know the source of the water and how it is being changed and/or filtered. I am particularly interested in any water changes or modifications of the system that have occurred in the time frame of the observed signs of the problem. Ask specific questions about the husbandry operations. For example, a private pet fish owner should be asked, "How do you make your water changes?" If the client fails to volunteer the source of the water for the change, that question should be asked after they have gone through the procedure.

The question "How is your water quality?" is too open-ended. Most clients say that they do not know, or that it is good. I have been trapped more than once by allowing clients to tell me that their water quality is good or that it is "rock steady." It may be "rock steady" but very poor for the species being kept. It is better practice to ask specifically about each water-quality parameter you are concerned about. Private fish owners in particular, but even some production fish managers, become confused about the nitrogenous waste assays. Often, they are not measuring a complete panel of ammonia, nitrite, and nitrate levels. If they are measuring anything, they most commonly are measuring nitrate levels. They will frequently confuse or not realize the difference in the words nitrite and nitrate until you have asked both questions. They may even respond that they just answered that question when you ask about the two parameters sequentially. It is important to determine what they are measuring and how they are doing it.

Other husbandry issues that must be explored in the history include nutrition and feeding practices, use of any additives for any purpose, occurrence of equipment sharing between facilities, day/night cycling, changes in caretakers of the system, and any events occurring in the atmosphere over the system or near the intake of any air pumps. The collection of the history may continue throughout the remote examination, if the practitioner is experienced enough to keep the history collection from interfering with the direct observation. It is usually better to complete the history, as much as possible, before beginning the remote examination. Any time savings accrued through combining the two will be lost if important data from either procedure is lost in the process of trying to do two complex things at once.

REMOTE EXAMINATION

In many situations, it will be possible to perform a remote examination of your patient before the hands-on examination. When this is possible, it can guide the hands-on examination and may even determine a physical examination is not appropriate. The best situation, of course, is to be able to see the patient in its normal habitat. This will be possible in certain types of practice; for example, when caring for fish kept in display aquaria or properly designed research aquaria facilities. Veterinarians providing care for these types of operations generally work on site, and the large viewing areas allow examination of the patient in a relatively undisturbed state. Similar advantages can be found in ambulatory visits to clients with home aquaria.

When the fish can be viewed in its routine habitat, it is important to examine the entire picture before you. Do not fail to examine the system and the environment of the system at the same time you observe your patient. Pay attention to the entire community interaction within the tank and do not focus only on the patient or patients you are being asked to examine. It is important to note the attitude of the fish in the water and the interaction of each fish with other fish in the tank. Where are the fish in the water column? Are the fish calm, active, or depressed? Wounds and trauma are usually easily

identified at the remote examination, even in relatively tiny fish. The remote examination is also the time to study respiration rates and fin positioning.

In addition to observing the fish, the remote examination should look at the system and the system environment. What is the air quality around the tank? Is the air musty? Can you detect solvent odors? Air quality can be an important factor in fish health.

What does the floor around the system look like? Is it dirty? Is there evidence that the floors are flooded frequently or constantly wet? If nothing else, this will give you a good idea of the owner's or operator's attitude toward cleanliness and maintenance.

Listen to the environment around the system as well. Fish are affected by sound. Loud continuous noise, or repetitive noise that disturbs you, is more than likely affecting the fish. High-pitched whines from failing pump bearings are uncomfortable for you, but low rumbles affect fish feeding and may be a major stressor. In addition, sudden, loud, intermittent noise can be a negative factor in fish health, through repetitive activation of startle responses. More work needs to be done in this area, but a good rule of thumb is that noise levels or patterns that make it uncomfortable for you to be near the system are equally disturbing to the fish that are being maintained in the system.

CLINICAL EXAMINATION AND PROCEDURES

A remote examination in an aquaculture facility rarely provides the opportunity to see the fish themselves. Nevertheless, the remote examination can be valuable. Observe the ground and levy conditions in pond facilities. Look at pond levels. Are they lower than usual? What plants are growing near the pond site? What is the predominant wind direction? What, if anything, is located upwind? What evidence is there of other animals (birds, reptiles, etc.) in the vicinity of the ponds? Is all mechanical equipment functional? How does the water smell? In net pen operations, observe the docks, pen floats, and surrounding water condition. When examining floating pens, many of the same observations are required. In addition, try to observe tidal conditions and examine the shores nearby for any indications of die-offs in wild species.

HANDS-ON PHYSICAL EXAMINATION

A close examination of any fish patient generally requires anesthesia. Any of a variety of anesthetic techniques discussed in Chapter 6 are suitable. Experienced fish practitioners and handlers may be able to perform a variety of examinations on unanesthetized fish, but this requires practice and skill to accomplish without injuring the fish.

Fish are commonly handled with bare hands, although this can be quite precarious (Fig. 5–1). The

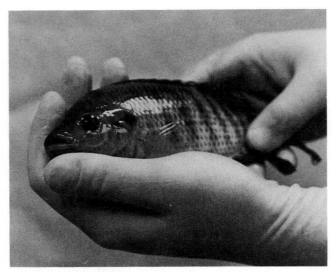

FIGURE 5–1. Handling a small unanesthetized fish for a "hands-on" physical examination. Note the latex gloves, which help restrain the fish without damaging it.

mucus produced by the fish can make it very difficult to maintain a safe hold on the patient. Over time, it is possible for the practitioner to develop allergies to the mucus. Latex surgical gloves are very useful for holding fish without damaging their skin. Techniques using cotton gloves or paper towels are thought to damage the skin of the fish and may be entirely unsuitable for delicate species.

Traditionally, the hands-on examination has been performed out of the water, and for many determinations this remains necessary. It is beneficial, however, to do much of the exam directly over the water, holding the fish so that your hand and the down side of the fish remain submerged. This allows the fish to respire on one side and prolongs the time available for the examination. It is also convenient to resubmerge the fish periodically for a few breaths. A common question is, "How long can you hold a fish out of water?" This varies a great deal with species, individual fish, and the condition of the fish. It is always safe to assume the shorter the time the fish is out of the water the better. I often try holding my breath during the examination, returning the fish to the water when I find it necessary to breathe. This limits my ability to talk to students during the procedure, but seems to provide a good practical guide. As I get older, I get a bit more humane in this regard. It may be that my examination skills have improved, making me much faster, but it is more likely that I just cannot hold my breath as long. Generally, I try to have the examination completed in 2 to 3 minutes, breaking at 45- to 60-second intervals to let the fish respire. There is no question that most fish can tolerate much greater times out of water than this, but rarely do I find it necessary, nor do I find it appropriate to do so.

The hands-on examination allows the clinician to manipulate the fish. Usually, if the remote examination has given any indications for cultures, these should be taken first, before the fish has been manipulated extensively. Likewise, mucus smears should be taken immediately upon removing the fish from the water. Then take the opportunity to lift the operculum and examine the gills. The gills should be red, with a completely symmetrical outer, or caudal, edge. A ragged caudal limit, excessive mucus, or paleness are indications for a gill biopsy. The fins should be spread and examined carefully. Any redness should be studied and attributed to either vascular congestion or hemorrhages, by determining whether discrete blood vessels are distinguishable. Any white or cloudy areas on the skin or fins should be examined to determine if they are raised. The eyes should be examined for any signs of corneal or lens opacity. In larger fish, the oral cavity should be examined for parasites or lesions. Usually, both sides of the fish can be examined in less than a minute. The fish can then be resubmerged. Biopsies should be taken at this time by lifting the fish again after it has taken a few breaths. Finally, any medications indicated by the remote examination should be applied, and the fish recovered from its anesthetized state. The complete hands-on examination should be quick, efficient, and comprehensive.

BLOOD AND BODY FLUIDS COLLECTION

Examination of blood and body fluids from fish patients is a valuable diagnostic tool. Blood adequate for a complete blood count can be collected safely from clinical patients weighing 100 g or more. With experience, samples can be taken from smaller fish without compromising their survival.

When taking blood samples from a fish, plastic syringes are routinely recommended. This avoids the rapid clotting that can occur with the use of glass syringes (Smith et al., 1952). I prefer to use a heparinized syringe coated with a light film of ammonium or lithium heparin solution, to further decrease the chance for interfering microcoagulation in the sample. This is controversial because of the possibility of dilution effects on small samples and purported morphology changes induced by the heparin, but in practice, these have not been major problems. Usually, the needle need not be heparinized.

The site preferred by many veterinarians for blood sampling from clinical patients is the tail. The veins running beneath the vertebrae of the fish can be sampled, using a lateral or a ventral approach (Fig. 5–2). In the more popular lateral approach, the needle is inserted under the scales, usually just below the lateral line on the middle portion of the tail (Fig. 5–3). The needle is directed cranially, parallel with the lateral line, and inserted to the level of the vertebral bodies near midline. The needle is usually held at about a 45-degree angle from the surface of the tail.

The ventral approach to the caudal vessels in-

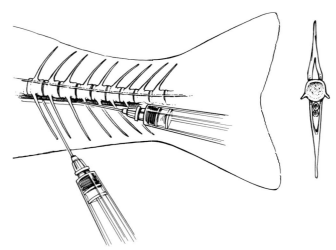

FIGURE 5–2. Ventral and lateral approaches to blood sampling from the vessels just ventral to the vertebral column.

volves inserting the needle at the ventral midline of the fish in the middle portion of the tail, and directing the needle slightly craniad and dorsad until it encounters the vertebral bodies. The needle can be backed off a tiny fraction of a millimeter and blood drawn. With practice, either of these approaches can be used to obtain reasonable clinical blood samples. The ventral approach is very successful for sampling sharks that have large caudal vessels encased in cartilage.

For research projects that require frequent blood sampling, it is more reliable in many fish species to install a cannula into the dorsal aorta through the buccal cavity rather than to try to sample the caudal vein. The technique for implanting these catheters is illustrated in Chapter 7.

Cardiac puncture is used by some researchers and, occasionally, by clinicians to obtain blood samples from fish. Cardiac puncture is usually approached from the ventral aspect of the fish. A needle is inserted just caudal to the bony notch formed by the bones creating the posterior margin of the oper-

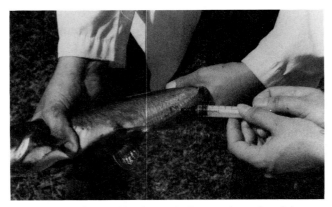

FIGURE 5–3. Taking a blood sample from a channel catfish using the lateral approach. (Courtesy of P.R. Bowser.)

cular cavity. The needle is moved directly dorsally until the heart is punctured and blood flows into the syringe. The cardiac puncture is most commonly accomplished in the ventricle or the bulbus arteriosus. This approach is usually successful in fusiform fishes but is not often successful in laterally compressed species. In these species, it is often advantageous to approach the cardiac puncture through the operculum. A needle is inserted into the caudal margin of the operculum, medial to the edge of the opercular bony structure, about one-third of the distance from the floor of the operculum to the roof. The needle is directed caudally and slightly toward midline until the bulbus arteriosus is encountered and blood flows into the syringe.

In some situations, it is appropriate to sacrifice a fish for pathologic and hematologic examinations, in which case additional blood collection methods are available. A common method is to cut off the tail of the anesthetized fish and allow the blood to drain from the caudal vessels into a collection tube. This technique has the advantage of being quick and maximizing sample size but suffers the disadvantages of contamination of the sample with tissue proteins and fluids and requiring the sacrifice of the fish.

There are additional blood sampling sites available on certain larger fish species. The sharks have a very useful vein that can be found on the dorsal midline, cranial and caudal to the cranial dorsal fin. It is a very superficial vessel but can be useful for fluid administration and blood sampling in larger animals.

Another very useful diagnostic fluid available to the clinician is ascitic fluid. Abdominocentesis in cases suspected of peritoneal effusions is very rewarding. A hypodermic needle is inserted into the abdominal cavity and directed into the ventral lateral abdomen. The fish is rotated to place the point of the needle in the dependent position, and ascitic fluid is easily withdrawn into a sterile syringe. Bacterial cultures of this fluid are often diagnostically useful and cytologic examination rewarding.

Urine collection from fish is difficult. In research situations, fish can be catheterized and urine collected continuously from the swimming fish. Certainly, clinical catheterization would be possible, and significant urine volume could be obtained from a fish that has a functional urinary bladder, but the technique is not often applied. An alternate method of urine collection has been used, where a small plastic reservoir is glued with methacrylate glue to the vent of the fish. What seems like a clever idea is actually a bit difficult in practice. For one thing, the glue used can cause severe skin irritation in some fish species. Second, getting the collection bag off of the fish without damage is tedious at times. Better methods need to be devised for routine clinical collection of urine if urinalysis is going to be used in diagnostic efforts. I have not found urinalysis particularly useful, but this may be only because I find it so difficult to collect.

Lymph can be collected from many species of fish from a dorsal lymph duct that runs above the spinal cord (Wardle, 1971). An appropriate-sized needle can be inserted along the dorsal midline and directed ventrally to the spinal column. In some fish, this can be accomplished in the tail region. In others, the sampling must be done cranial to the position of the cranial dorsal fin. The clinical usefulness of these samples is not well established, but lymph is abundant in most species, and its diagnostic potential should be further explored.

BIOPSY TECHNIQUES

Mucus Smear

A mucus smear is perhaps the most common biopsy technique used in fish medicine. A clean microscope slide can be pressed on an area of interest, or the edge of the slide can be moved from cranial to caudal to collect mucus from the surface of the skin (Fig. 5–4). Only gentle pressure is necessary. This is not analogous to performing a skin scraping for *Demodex* mites on a dog. Even very light motions will remove epidermis and even dermis in small fish. Too vigorous an approach can severely damage a fish.

Smears or impressions should be done whenever an ectoparasitic disease is suspected. If frank wounds are visible, the most fruitful examination will be of smears from smaller developing wounds as opposed to larger, older wounds, which may be overgrown with a variety of secondary invaders. If bacterial cultures are desired, they are usually performed prior to the mucus biopsy to avoid contamination of the wound.

Mucus biopsies, whether smears or impressions, should be examined immediately. Usually, a drop of tank water is added to the smear and a coverslip applied. The biopsy can be stored in a humidified transport container for short periods. A simple transport container can be made from a sealable plastic food container and moist paper towels or gauze. Vaseline in a syringe can also be used to preserve a smear for the time it takes to get it back to a lab. A bead of Vaseline can be applied around the sample and the coverslip seated on the bead of Vaseline.

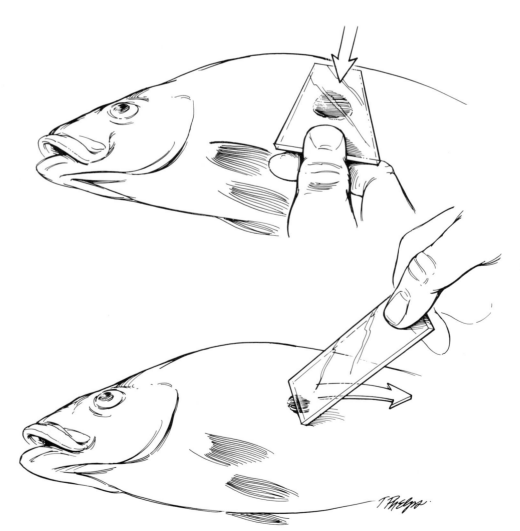

FIGURE 5–4. Making a skin impression smear.

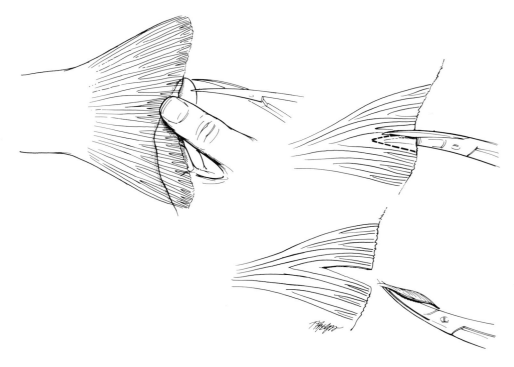

FIGURE 5–5. Taking a fin biopsy. First a pair of curved iris scissors is used to cut parallel to a fin ray. Then the scissors are reversed, and the second cut is made to remove a triangle of fin tissue. No fin rays are cut. The tissue is supported on the blades of the scissors and transferred to a clean slide.

Fin Biopsy

A fin biopsy is an extremely simple procedure (Fig. 5–5). The fin is spread, usually by the fingers or over the surface of a finger tip in the case of small tropical species. A fine-tipped iris scissors is used to cut a triangular wedge of fin tissue from between the fin rays. It is not necessary to cut the fin rays or spines. The cut fin rays will only complicate examination of the biopsy by making it difficult to seat the coverslip. The small clean wound made by the biopsy will heal readily. The small wedge of tissue should be placed on a slide with a drop of water of appropriate salinity, coverslipped, and examined immediately for the presence of protozoal parasites, heavy bacterial colonization, or abnormalities of the epithelial tissues.

Gill Biopsy

A gill biopsy is easily obtained by inserting the tip of a pair of iris scissors into the operculum (Fig. 5–6). In larger fish, the thumb can be inserted into the opercular opening and moved to the ventral aspect of the opening, to lever the operculum open for visualization. In smaller species, the tips of the scissors themselves can be used to open the operculum and observe the gills. The blades of the scissors are then inserted with the blades open to allow a few tips of primary lamellae to lap into the jaws of the scissors. Only a few tips of the primary lamellae need be taken. Bleeding should be minimal. It is not necessary to cut deep into the base of the lamellae.

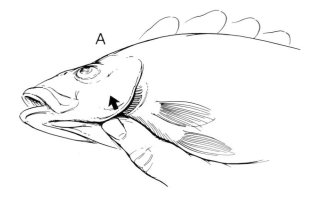

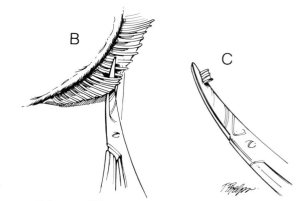

FIGURE 5–6. Taking a gill biopsy. *A.* The operculum is gently lifted with the thumbnail. *B.* Curved iris scissors are inserted into the operculum. *C.* The distal tips of three to six gill filaments are cut and supported on the scissors.

The cut lamellar tips are balanced on the tip of the scissor as it is withdrawn from the operculum. With practice, this procedure can be accomplished in a few seconds, always obtaining a good sample.

Kidney Biopsy

A number of diagnostic techniques for infectious and noninfectious diseases center on examination or culture of kidney tissue. It is possible to biopsy the cranial kidney of trout, and perhaps other species without sacrificing the patient. The most common sampling is a simple aspiration, using a plastic syringe and standard needle (Noga et al., 1986). Biopsy needles can also be used. A kidney biopsy is performed by lifting the operculum and inserting the needle, directing it first dorsally, then dorsocaudad to a level just ventral to the vertebrae and caudal to the last branchial arch. In this position, a syringe can be used to aspirate the cranial kidney for culture, or the biopsy needle can be closed for histological specimens. Cultures taken with this technique correlate well with cultures taken at necropsy, and the procedure is relatively safe (Noga et al., 1986). The major hazard with the procedure is the potential for damaging spinal nerve roots. This is a rare occurrence in the hands of experienced practitioners, but when it happens the fish generally dies within the first 24 hours of the biopsy, showing skin darkening.

Thyroid Biopsy

A wide variety of captive marine species develop thyroid disease. It is usually manifested as a hypertrophy and can be quite extensive. Marine reef fishes can develop large masses that may protrude from the operculum. Captive sharks frequently develop large goitrous swellings under the chin owing to thyroid hyperplasia. Biopsy of the thyroid is relatively simple in a fish with a large mass protruding into the opercular cavity. The mass can be readily visualized and a small piece of tissue collected with scissors or a biopsy punch. Electrocautery is often useful to stop bleeding. Coagulation powders and silver nitrate can be used if care is taken to avoid spilling any on the gills.

Thyroid biopsy in the shark is a bit more difficult (Fig. 5–7). It is best done under ultrasound guidance to avoid large blood vessels in the area of the thyroid. A standard biopsy needle is used to obtain the tissue specimen. The anesthetized shark is placed in dorsal recumbency and the ventral chin lifted out of the water. Routinely, the biopsy site is prepared with a povidone-iodine solution, and a small nick is made in the skin at the posterior edge of the thyroid on midline with a number 15 Bard-Parker blade. The biopsy needle is inserted through the skin and directed cranially at a shallow angle through the main mass of the thyroid gland. The small wound usually does not require a suture, although a single polyglycolic acid suture or closure with methacrylate is sometimes used.

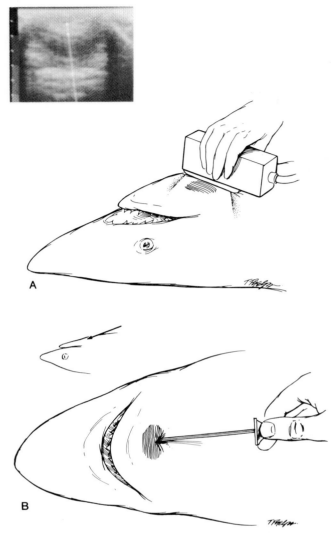

FIGURE 5–7. Thyroid biopsy of the shark. *A.* The thyroid is located by real-time ultrasonography. *B.* A biopsy needle is inserted at a shallow angle through a small skin incision.

IMAGING TECHNIQUES

Radiographs

Routine plain film radiographs of fish are easily obtained. High-detail techniques similar to those developed for avian patients are most valuable. Abdominal detail is best observed in those species that have appreciable intra-abdominal fat. A fish is less stressed when the radiograph can be taken without removing it from the water. This can be accomplished with a variety of restraint devices (Fig. 5–8). A simple box with adjustable panels used to confine the fish in a smaller space is quite useful. In this method, the depth of the water in the box, rather than

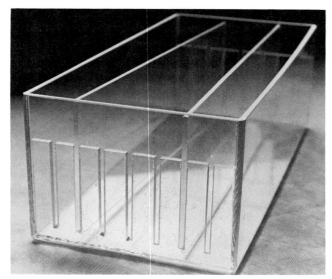

FIGURE 5–8. A restraint device for radiographing a fish that remains in water.

measurement of the patient, determines the radiographic technique required. There is some loss of detail when radiographs are shot through water, and considerably more x-ray energy is required than when fish are radiographed out of the water (Fig. 5–9). For this reason, many clinicians prefer to prepare their radiographic equipment carefully before bringing an anesthetized fish out of the water to sit on the radiographic plate (Fig. 5–10). If done quickly, this technique is not unduly stressful to a fish that is not critically compromised with disease.

Ultrasound (Figs. 5–11 to 5–13)

Ultrasound is an imaging modality that is particularly useful in fish medicine. Both real-time and static images are extremely valuable in a variety of applications. Ultrasound diagnostic equipment works by computing images from echoes received from high-frequency sounds sent into the body. The sound waves reflect and refract at interfaces between tissues of different acoustic density, in a fashion very similar to that of light passing through a variety of media of different refractive indices. The technique has the advantages of high biologic safety and the opportunity for observation of anatomic detail rendered in real time. Real-time ultrasound imaging uses rapid computer updating of the viewing screen to present new images in a cinematic fashion. This allows visualization of organ movements, including the observation of the beating heart. It is particularly useful in situations where exact anatomic knowledge is not available and in evaluation of dynamic organs such as the heart.

Other major advantages of ultrasound imaging are its sensitivity to differences in soft tissues and its relative portability. Units suitable for imaging fish

can be easily carried to fish-holding facilities. Limitations of ultrasound imaging include somewhat less resolution capability compared to conventional radiography and difficulties posed by air and bone imaging. The acoustic properties of air are so dramatically different from most tissues that the refraction and reflections of sound that occur at an air-tissue interface distort and disrupt the imaging process beyond interpretable limits. Similar problems can occur with very dense tissues or objects such as bone or mineralized lesions. Also, the depth of tissues that can be imaged is somewhat limited, with resolution becoming poorer as lower-frequency transducers are used to achieve greater imaging depth. This factor limits the use of ultrasound in very large animals to the examination of superficial structures.

The size limitations related to examining fish with ultrasound are usually due to the other extreme in patient size. Specific lesion or organ imaging in small fish is impractical because of the rather coarse resolution limits of ultrasound equipment. Even beating hearts smaller than 4 mm in diameter are difficult to detect reliably, and static organs or lesions 4 mm or smaller are essentially impossible to discern with currently available equipment. On the positive side, however, the problem of acoustic coupling to avoid interference from gases and air is essentially eliminated in the examination of aquatic patients. The water of the patient's environment can serve to couple the transducer to the fish's body, eliminating the need to use special ultrasound gels. Medical ultrasound transducers are not designed for operation underwater, but they are reasonably well protected for cleaning with damp wipes. They can be submerged if the transducer is placed in a watertight container, often a plastic bag, which can be tightly sealed around the transducer cable. Water-soluble coupling gels can be used within the bag to couple the transducer to the bag itself, and exclusion of most of the air in the bag also facilitates working underwater with a real-time or static imaging transducer. The submerged bag is then coupled to the patient with the water of the environment.

Selection of a transducer frequency is dependent upon the size of the patient and the degree of detail desired. Although 1- and 2-MHz transducers can be useful for examining structures deeper than 20 cm in large patients, a 5.0-MHz transducer is generally more functional in fish imaging. A real-time 5.0-MHz transducer allows reasonably good imaging to a depth of at least 13 cm. This, of course, varies with the design of the transducer, and equipment from different manufacturers will have slightly different capabilities even when utilizing the same ultrasound frequency range. Special transducers working at 7.0-MHz and 10.0-MHz are available. These are designed for ophthalmic work, but they can be extremely valuable for the examination of fish. They provide more resolution and are able to achieve depths of imaging suitable for examination of fish up to 0.5 or 1 kg body weight.

Sharks are perhaps the ideal subject for ultra-

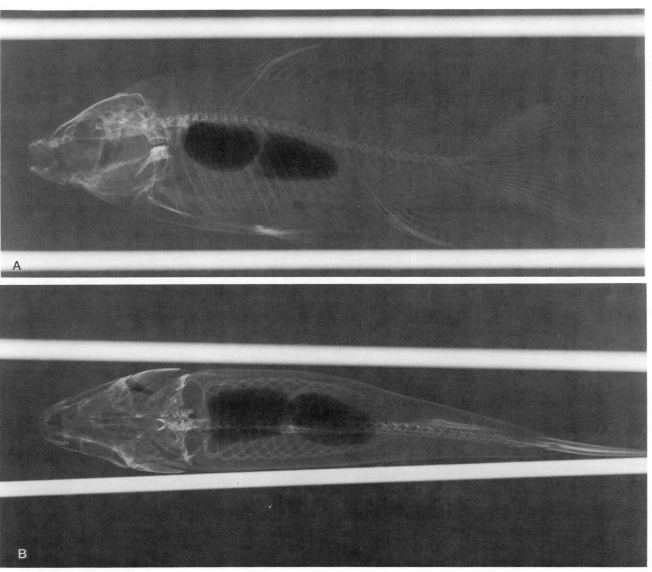

FIGURE 5–9. Radiographs of a koi taken using the device illustrated in Figure 5–8. Notice the lack of contrast due to the x-ray blocking capacity of the water. *A.* Lateral. *B.* Dorsoventral. (Courtesy of S. Smith.)

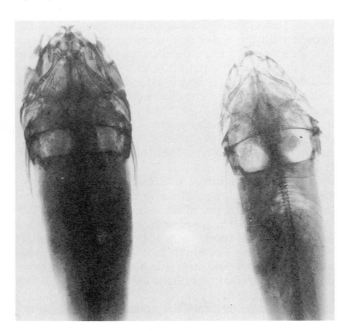

FIGURE 5–10. Radiographs of an Asian catfish taken with the fish out of water. *A.* Normal. *B.* Ascorbic acid deficient. (From Roberts, R.J. [1989] Fish Pathology, 2nd ed. Baillière Tindall, London.)

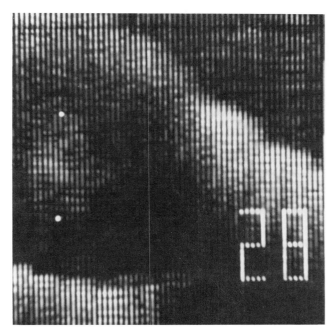

FIGURE 5–11. Ultrasonograph of a red-bellied piranha with a sonodense abdominal mass and severe ascites. (5-MHz linear array realtime, Polaroid.)

sonographic examination. They have essentially no mineralized bone and no gas-filled swim bladder to interfere with examination. Ultrasound can be used to examine skeletal problems, including trauma, in these animals. The entire shark is acoustically trans-

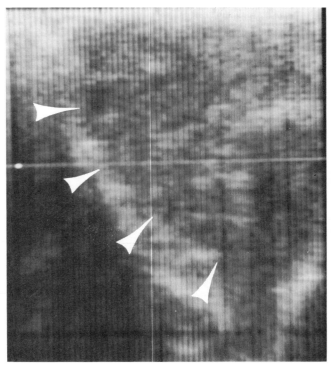

FIGURE 5–12. Anterior midline sagittal ultrasonograph of a hepatocellular tumor in a koi. (5-MHz linear array real time, Polaroid.)

parent to examination, and the large liver provides excellent acoustic windows to the bowel (Fig. 5–14).

Bottom fishes that do not have swim bladders are also excellent candidates for ultrasonographic examination. Luckily, with knowledge of the location of the swim bladder in other fishes, it is very easy to examine the abdominal organs, heart, or muscles for parasitic cysts by directing the ultrasound transducer away from the swim bladder. Unfortunately, the kidney remains difficult, if not impossible, to examine in this way. The bones of many smaller fishes are so thin and small that the ribs and vertebral processes do not interfere significantly with the imaging process. The axial skeleton, on the other hand, is a major obstruction to ultrasound imaging.

Xeroradiography

Xeroradiography is a technique that provides much better contrast and detail in fish radiography than plain film radiographs (Fig. 5–15). Unfortunately, the process is not commonly available to practitioners. Radiographs are taken using standard radiographic equipment and a special cassette. The cassette is processed in a developer that produces a paper hard-copy image that can represent bones as either light or dark. Although the process is inexpensive, the processing equipment is a major investment, and most fish practitioners will not have the advantage of xeroradiography.

Computed Tomography Scan

Computed tomography (CT) of fish is not as unlikely as it might seem. The economic basis for such extensive imaging work-ups exists with the high-priced ornamental koi and certain marine tropical species. Routine techniques can be used on fish anesthetized in water-filled restraining containers. It is important to provide water exchange and oxygenation to the fish while it is being held in the smaller restraining chambers. Oxygen depletion of small volumes of water can be very dramatic. Flow of water from an external water source does not cause a problem in the CT imaging.

The major advantage of CT technology is that deep objects are imaged without interference from images of overlying structures, as occurs in radiography. CT also provides better contrast resolution because the detector system rejects scatter and is more efficient at distinguishing soft tissues from one another. Better geometric accuracy, free of distortion, is also possible. The collection of data as CT numbers or values relative to the radiodensity of each voxel, or unit of digitized data, allows tissue characterization based on electron density (Hendee, 1988). If images are taken at two different x-ray tube potentials, it is possible to perform bone densitometry by calculating total bone mineral content from the CT numbers (Moss et al., 1983; Greenberg, 1983).

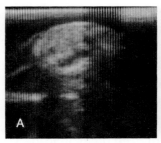 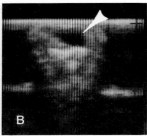 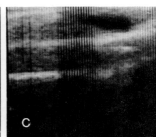

FIGURE 5–13. Ultrasonographs of an African Lungfish. (5 MHz linear array realtime, Polaroid.) *A.* Cross-section of the head at the level of the eyes. *B.* Cross-section 2 cm caudal to the opercular opening, showing modified swim bladder (lung) (arrow). *C.* Transverse longitudinal midline of same region.

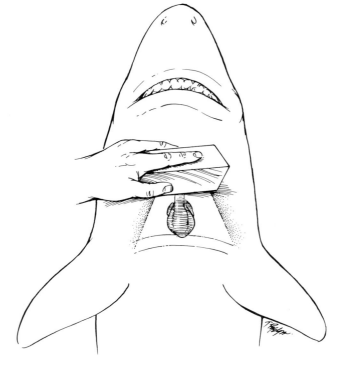

FIGURE 5–14. Positioning a real-time ultrasound array for monitoring the heart rate of a shark.

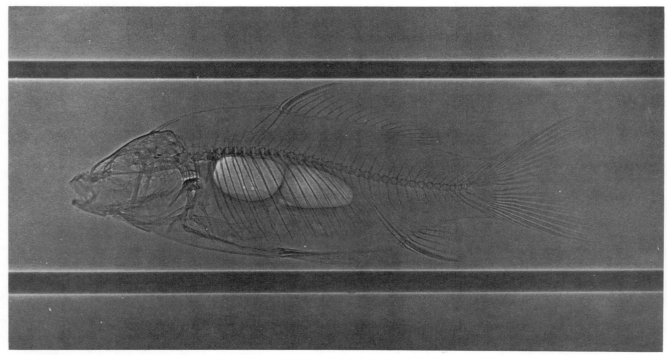

FIGURE 5–15. Xeroradiograph of the same koi as that in Figure 5–9. Note the improved visualization of cephalic bone structures.

The major disadvantages of CT technology center on the limitations of imaging only a narrow slice of the body. It is possible to miss pathology if slices are taken too far apart, or if data windows are too broad or narrow in the computer reconstruction, resulting in poor contrast. Even when slices are taken close together, the divergence of the x-ray beams may result in a disc-shaped region in the core of the patient being overlooked (Wagner et al., 1986). In addition, the computer reconstruction method can create artifacts. For example, when tissues of widely disparate radiopacity occur within the same voxel, their differing opacities are averaged, giving a CT number for that voxel that does not reflect the actual tissue radiopacity. At bone–soft tissue interfaces, this effect causes bones to appear thicker and makes soft tissues difficult or impossible to visualize. In imaging fish, this makes the skeletal elements easier to visualize but decreases the contrast of the already low contrast abdominal organs.

Magnetic Resonance Imaging (MRI)

The rapid development of nuclear magnetic resonance (NMR) imaging has created an important tool for examining clinical fish cases (Blackband and Stoskopf, 1990). The combination of magnetic resonance imaging (MRI) and NMR spectroscopy techniques, both localized and unlocalized, provides in vivo biochemical information that is otherwise unobtainable with current technology (Figs. 5–16 to 5–18). The special abilities of MRI to demonstrate cartilaginous structures and differentiate between tissues of similar radiographic density make MRI exceptionally suited to morphologic studies of teleosts, elasmobranchs, and invertebrates. Both conventional two-dimensional Fourier transform spin echo and inversion recovery imaging pulse sequences are effective. Localized spectra can be obtained using the STEAM technique (Frahm et al., 1987).

In MRI, particularly when using volume rf coils, the amount of water surrounding the animal must be minimized to reduce the loading of and the required diameter of the rf coil and obtain optimal sensitivity. In surface coil studies, the volume of water surrounding the fish continues to be limiting because of the fixed-bore diameter of the magnets. A flowing, multicompartment water system, similar to those used for CT scanning, avoids the need for large volumes of water around the specimen, preserving an adequate effective volume of water. These support systems can be constructed as open systems, allowing ready access to the specimen for manipulation. The total volume of water needed depends heavily on the mass of the animal involved and the time required to generate the image. A 10-L system with minimal water processing other than aeration operating at 22°C will maintain small (300–450 g) sharks for 6 hours without signs of compromising the animal. Larger reservoirs prolong the time the system can be utilized without water changes, and smaller animals can be safely maintained in systems longer than larger animals.

The advantages of a multicompartment system are purchased at the expense of flow. Although continuous flow over the breathing apparatus is preferable for maintaining the fish, even very slow

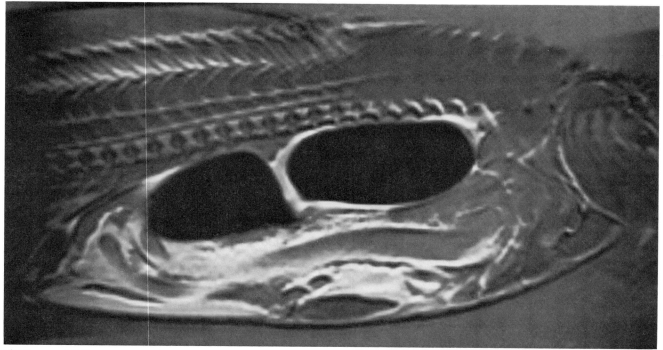

FIGURE 5–16. Midline sagittal magnetic resonance image of a koi (1.5 tesla, G.E. knee coil). Spinal column, gill arches, cranial and caudal swim bladders, cranial kidney, caudal kidney, ureters, liver, gonad, bulbus arteriosus, ventricle.

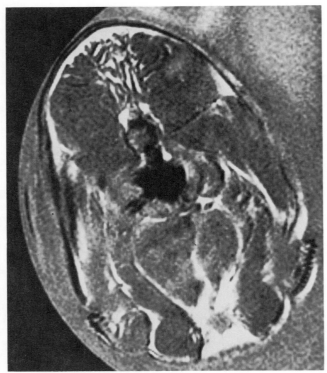

FIGURE 5–17. Cross-sectional magnetic resonance image of a koi at the level of caudal margin of the opercular opening (1.5 tesla, G.E. knee coil). Medulla, esophagus, liver, caudal tip of ventricle.

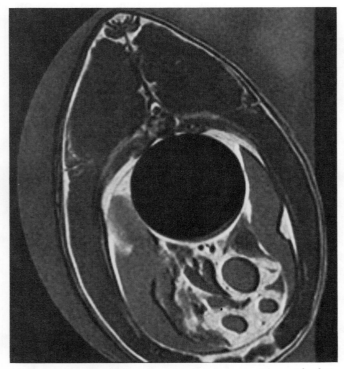

FIGURE 5–18. Cross-sectional magnetic resonance image of a koi 36 mm caudal to Figure 5–17 (1.5 tesla, G.E. knee coil). Spinal canal, vertebral body, aorta, cranial swim bladder, liver, gonad, intestines, caudal kidney.

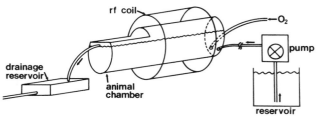

FIGURE 5–19. Life support system for use in magnetic resonance imaging of fish (see also Table 5–1).

flow in a life-support system during MRI causes distortions in the images (Fig. 5–19; see also Table 5–1). Consequently, protocols are used that image with the flow in the system turned off during image acquisition and interrupt data collection at short intervals to allow reoxygenation of the water.

The sensitivity of the MRI techniques is dependent upon the salinity of the water. Natural sea water is a conductive solution that contains paramagnetic ions. It makes a very noisy sample, reducing the efficiency of the radio frequency coil. The signal-to-noise differentiation available for animals held in salt water is consequently much less than that for animals maintained in freshwater. This, of course, translates into reduced resolution and/or increased imaging times for marine specimens. Removal of paramagnetic ions from salt water or reduction of salinity is not a practical approach to improving resolution in marine specimens.

An important issue in imaging fishes in vivo is the requirement to position them without movement for the time the data are being collected. Although the use of multicompartmentalized life-support systems tends to minimize the area available for the fishes to move in, it does not preclude and may even exacerbate movement of positional adjustment or acoustic startle reactions as the scan is initiated. General anesthesia is, therefore, necessary in most situations.

TABLE 5–1. Practical Considerations and Methods

A primary requisite in any in vivo study is the provision of suitable life support to maintain a physiologically stable subject. Life support requirements are similar for terrestrial and aquatic species, although aquatic species require the additional provision of adequate water volume of appropriate salinity and composition. We developed both closed and open life support systems to use in MR imaging studies addressing the following practical considerations:

a. Water Volume: Maintained over the gills with a flowing system.

b. Flow Artifacts: Eliminated by turning off the flow during acquisition. Data acquisition paused at intervals to allow reoxygenation.

c. Salinity: Causes heavy coil loading. Reducing salt content to the physiologically tolerable limit has no effect. Must therefore minimize water volume.

d. Anesthesia: Tricaine, 0.001 mg/L in water. Large safety margin if oxygenation maintained.

e. Pressurization: Provided by pump and tank system. A closed animal chamber then used. Pressure used simulates a depth of 0.1 mile.

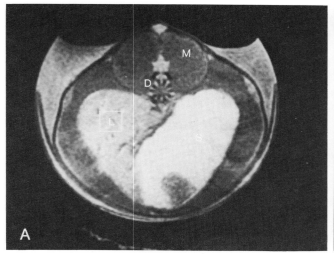
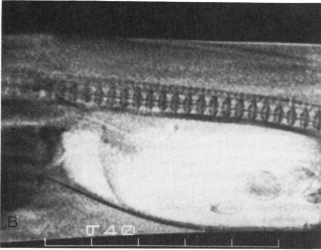

FIGURE 5–20. *A.* Cross-sectional magnetic resonance image of a spotted bamboo shark showing the liver (L), stomach (S), vertebral disk (D), and lumbar musculature (M) (1.5 tesla, G.E. knee coil, axial spin echo TR = 1500 msec, imaging time 6.4 min). *B.* Image along the length of the same shark. The spine is clearly evident. (Courtesy of S. Blackband.)

ELECTROCARDIOGRAM COLLECTION AND INTERPRETATION

Routine electrocardiogram (ECG) collection in clinical fish patients remains a thing of the future; however, the procedure is relatively simple (Fig. 5–21). A differential preamplifier fitted with high- and low-frequency noise filters can be used to filter out respiratory and swimming movements. Waveforms can be taken with direct or indirect leads. Miniature ultrasonic (frequency-modulated) radio transmitters have also been developed to deliver the complete waveform of the ECG. These transmitters can be attached to the dorsal surface of a fish or placed in the stomach. More commonly, direct leads are attached to the fish to obtain a clinical ECG.

Direct leads are implanted subcutaneously at the pectoral bases and near the anus with the ground to the water. Alternately, all three leads are placed in the heart region. Usually, short (1 mm), narrow electrodes are used (Oets, 1950; Labat, 1966). These are insulated from the water with silicone, polyester urethane, epoxy resin, or shrink-fit tubing. A high-gain, AC coupled, differential input preamplifier with ground to the water is used to boost the signal. Most of the ECG signal power is below 30 Hz. Noise can be reduced by using shielding or a Faraday cage, but a band pass filter between 20 and 40 Hz gives a reasonably clean and informative signal (Gehrke and Fielder, 1988). Problems with 60-cycle interference can be eliminated with the use of a narrow band 60 Hz notch filter.

The heart rate of unanesthetized fishes is generally in the wide range of 1 to 4 beats per second. There is normally a sinus arrhythmia. The heart rate varies with temperature, being slower at lower water temperatures (Gehrke and Fielder, 1988). The QRS component of the ECG is generally in the 1 millivolt range of amplitude. Anesthetized fish usually have a tachycardia during induction, followed by a pro-gressive bradycardia with increasing depth of anesthesia. Hypoxic conditions are characterized by irregular rhythm and increased T wave amplitude, as well as a bradycardia with shortening of the T-P interval and the P-T interval (Gehrke and Fielder, 1988).

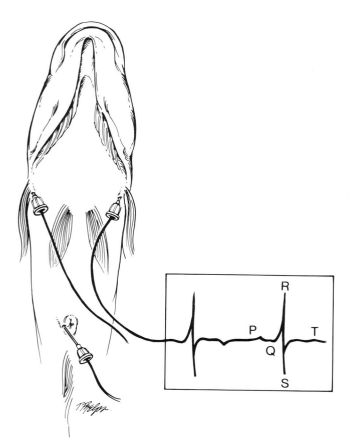

FIGURE 5–21. Electrocardiography of fish. Small needle electrodes are placed under the skin at the base of the pectoral fins and near the anus. P, QRS, and T waves can be discerned.

Interpretation of electrocardiograms in clinically ill fish is still in its early infancy. The wave form of the ECG in fish is similar to that in mammals. Conduction velocities of excitation are a bit slower. There is a P wave, a QRS complex, and a T wave. Another wave, the V wave has been recorded in some fish preceding the P wave. It is thought to be associated with the contraction of the sinus venosus.

BACTERIAL AND FUNGAL CULTURE SAMPLING

Most bacterial and fungal culture work from fish has been done on necropsy specimens. Other texts and manuals describe in detail methods for obtaining cultures from internal organs for population diagnostic studies (De Guzman and Shotts, 1988). Ideally, cultures for these purposes should be taken from recently euthanatized fish. If fish are being submitted to a laboratory for bacterial or fungal sampling, they should be shipped alive whenever possible. Once the fish is euthanatized, kidney cultures are routinely taken. The dorsal fin is clipped off, and the dorsum of the fish seared with a heated spatula. A cut is made into the middle of the seared area with sterile scissors until the spinal column is severed. The wound is opened by bringing the tail and head of the fish together, tearing tissues, and exposing the dark kidney.

An alternate method sterilizes the fish by dipping it in alcohol and opening the abdominal cavity with sterile technique. Samples are taken from specific organs with a sterile loop. This method has the advantage of allowing access to multiple abdominal organs. It is slower than sampling through the back and has a greater chance of contamination of samples.

Unfortunately, little or no work has been done to establish standardized methods for bacterial culturing from patients that must survive the diagnostic procedure. What little is written about clinical bacterial culturing of individual fish is steeped in dogma that may not be particularly accurate.

One such belief is that the results obtained from sampling the surface of a fish will not be significantly different from sampling the water the fish lives in. Studies cited to support this tenet deal with healthy fish and the quantitative bacterial populations recorded from their skin and surrounding water (Horsley, 1973; Gillespie and Macrae, 1975). Proponents of this position claim it is less stressful to the fish and, therefore, better to take samples from the filter bed or the water in a tank rather than from the fish itself.

On the other hand, studies using scanning electron microscopy have failed to provide evidence of significant bacterial colonization on the surface of healthy fish (Austin and Austin, 1987). This implies that studies on healthy fish fail to discriminate between colonizing bacteria and transient residents or bacteria merely in the layer of water immediately adjacent to the fish. In unpublished clinical trials

with captive display marine tropical fish, an examination of this approach led to surprisingly clear results. In 57 cases, including a wide variety of fish species, where superficial bacterial infections were suspected, bacterial cultures were taken with sterile swabs from both skin lesions and from the water. All cultures were handled identically and plated on the same media. In none of the cases were the bacterial isolates cultured from the water good representations of the bacterial isolates obtained from the lesions on the diseased fish. In most cases, the bacteria considered clinically most significant in the case were not isolated from the water sample. In all cases, the distribution and quantitative assessment of the bacterial water cultures were distinctly different from bacterial skin cultures. The variety of organisms cultured from the water often obscured the importance of the organisms felt to be actively involved in the pathology occurring in the fish. Further work needs to be done in this area before any definitive information will be available, but the clinician dealing with valuable fish should not discard the superficial wound bacterial culture as useless. It can be quite valuable in guiding antimicrobial therapy and assessing therapeutic efficacy.

To take a superficial bacterial culture, the fish can be captured and a sterile swab rubbed in the area of a skin wound without the use of any anesthetic. A clean and disinfected net or capture container should be used if possible. Care should be taken to a avoid handling the lesion site before the culture is taken. In many fish, the use of an anesthetic will improve the procedure. Little or no work has been done on the impact of immersion in common fish anesthetics on bacterial populations of the skin and wounds. Without this knowledge, any interpretation of results from an anesthetized fish should take into account the possibility that bacterial recoveries may not be complete, and important information may be lost. However, if anesthesia is required to safely accomplish the procedure in a fish, it should be used.

Gills can be cultured for bacteria by rubbing a small sterile swab gently against the gills through the open operculum (Fig. 5–22). Rolling the swab helps it pick up some of the mucus from the gills. The gill chamber and mucus on the gills harbor a relatively high bacterial population (Trust, 1975). Unfortunately, it is difficult to interpret the importance of these high bacterial loads. Insufficient work has been published in this area to give a good guide to the clinician. In general, evaluation techniques, similar to those used to evaluate gastrointestinal cultures in terrestrial mammals, may be useful in interpretation of gill cultures. Pure cultures of a single organism may be more indicative of a pathologic condition than a broad, mixed culture.

Bacterial and fungal cultures can be taken from several other sites. Clinically useful information can be obtained from culturing ascitic fluid obtained from abdominocentesis or abdominal gavage. Fecal bacterial cultures can be taken by inserting a small micro-

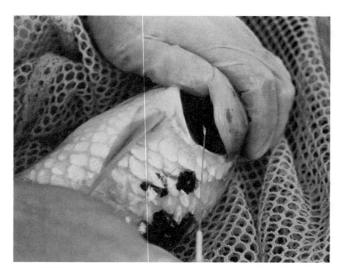

FIGURE 5–22. Taking a bacterial culture from the gill.

swab into the anal opening. Retrobulbar bacterial cultures are difficult to obtain reliably. These have been done by needle aspiration. Blood cultures are only feasible on relatively large fish. It is difficult to get an uncontaminated blood culture because of the difficulty of disinfecting the skin site where the needle is inserted and the difficulty in getting an adequate-sized blood sample. It is easier in sharks, where the caudal vein can be used to good advantage.

A variety of transport media have been used successfully for bacterial and fungal cultures taken from fish. Commercial swabs, which come with their own transport media, can be used for specimens that will reach the lab within 24 hours and have the opportunity to remain refrigerated. Samples should not be allowed to freeze. If longer transport times will be required, it may be beneficial to inoculate trypticase–soy agar broth with the swab before transport. If the sample is from a marine fish, it is beneficial to supplement the broth with artificial sea salts prior to sterilization.

The initial plating of bacterial cultures from fish is a controversial subject. Nearly as many opinions exist on how this should be done as there are fish microbiologists. The American Fisheries Society Blue Book recommends initial plating on trypticase soy agar and on *Cytophaga* agar and incubation at 20 to 25°C. Samples from marine fishes can be plated on salt-supplemented media. Ordinary blood agar serves remarkably well in the absence of specialized media.

VIRAL CULTURE SAMPLING

If a lesion is of suspected viral origin, and it is desirable to attempt to culture the virus for identification purposes or other reasons, a sterile biopsy is the preferred method. The biopsy sample should include the edge of the lesion and some of the apparently healthy tissue around the limits of the obviously affected tissue. Excessively large biopsies are not particularly beneficial to the culture efforts. Samples should be no more than 4 mm in diameter for explants. Adequate preparation will reduce problems with bacterial or fungal overgrowth of the tissue explants from the biopsy. Alternate application of 70% alcohol and povidone-iodine solution in the immediate area for biopsy is beneficial. Care should be taken to avoid prepping a wide area, as fish skin can be severely damaged by too severe an approach to disinfection. Some clinicians prefer to avoid extensive biopsy site disinfection, and rely on antibiotics and antifungal drugs in the collection and transport media.

A suitable transport medium consists of Hanks' balanced salt solution without calcium and magnesium, which has been fortified with penicillin (100 U/ml), streptomycin (100 μgml), and amphotericin B (2.5 μg/ml). It is preferable to keep the sample cold on ice (4°C). Samples in this media remain viable for 12 to 24 hours.

OPHTHALMIC EXAMINATION

Fish develop a large number of ocular problems, particularly in captivity. Considerable information can be obtained to support diagnosis and prognostication of these problems with a thorough ophthalmic examination. This examination need not take a great deal of time or special equipment. Much can be learned about a fish's eye with a thorough examination with a simple penlight. Initially observe the eye in the good illumination provided by the penlight. Pupillary reflexes are difficult to assess because they are quite slow in most fish, but they can be seen in many species. Examine both eyes and observe any variation in size or symmetry. Exophthalmos from a variety of causes is a common problem in fish, and early detection requires close assessment of normal fish of the same species. If the cornea is cloudy, it is important to determine whether the epithelium is intact. Illuminating the eye from an acute angle to the side will often reveal the depth of ulcers or penetrating wounds. Fluorescein dye and cobalt blue penlights can be used in fish, just as in terrestrial mammals.

If the cornea is transparent, the iris and lens can be evaluated in the identical manner that you would use for a terrestrial patient. Proper positioning of the penlight will allow detection of severely detached retinas, which appear as a white backing to the lens.

Even though a penlight examination can reveal considerable diagnostic information, examination with an ophthalmoscope and/or a slit lamp can provide a more refined assessment of the condition of the eye (Fig. 5–23). These examinations require anesthesia, and the unusual characteristics of the cornea and lens of various species of fish can require considerable adjustment on the part of the clinician.

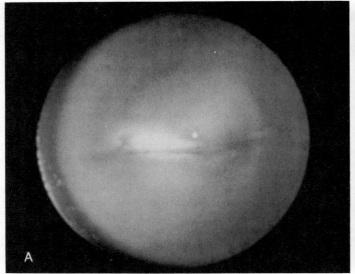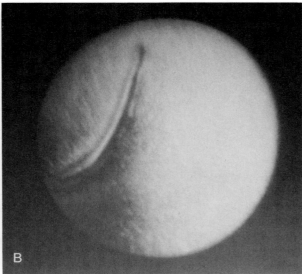

FIGURE 5–23. Fundus photographs of *(A) Tilapia,* and *(B)* Atlantic menhaden. A prominent falciform process is seen in each fundus. Fish fundus photographs may be taken by direct ophthalmoscopy using an optical interface provided by either immersing the eye in water or covering the cornea with a contact lens. Using an indirect method, the fish is suspended in air, and the inverted image produced by illuminating the fundus through a 28-D indirect ophthalmoscopy lens and photographing from a distance of 12 to 18 inches. For both methods the Kowa RC 2 hand-held fundus camera is convenient. (Courtesy of M. Nasisse.)

Ophthalmoscopic examination using a traditional terrestrial ophthalmoscope is sometimes aided by examining the fish with the eye under water. Other clinicians find this unnecessary and even a hindrance to the examination. This preference may be related to the species of fish being examined.

LITERATURE CITED

Austin, B., and Austin, D.A. (1987) Bacterial Fish Pathogens. Ellis Horwood, New York.

Blackband, S. J., and Stoskopf, M. K. (1990) In vivo nuclear magnetic resonance imaging and spectroscopy of aquatic organisms. Magn. Reson. Imaging 8:191–198.

De Guzman, E., and Shotts, E.B. (1988) Bacterial Culture and Evaluation of Diseases of Fish. In: Tropical Fish Medicine (Stoskopf, M.K., ed.). Vet. Clinics North Am., Small Anim. Pract. 18(2):365–374.

Frahm, J., Merboldt, K. D., and Hanicke, W. (1987) Localized proton spectroscopy using stimulated echos. J. Magn. Reson. 72:502–508.

Gehrke, P.C., and Fielder, D.R. (1988) Effects of temperature and dissolved oxygen on heart rate, ventilation rate and oxygen consumption of spangled perch, Leioptherapon unicolor (Gunther, 1859) (Percoidei, Teraponidae). J. Comp. Physiol. B 157:771–782.

Gillespie, N.C., and Macrae, I.C. (1975) The bacterial flora of some Queensland fish and its ability to cause spoilage. J. Appl. Bacteriol. 39:91–100.

Greenberg, M. (ed.) (1983) Essentials of Body Computed Tomography. W.B. Saunders, Philadelphia.

Hendee, W.R. (1988) Fundamentals of Diagnostic Imaging. In: Textbook of Diagnostic Imaging (Putman, C.E., and Ravin, C.E., ed.). W.B. Saunders, Philadelphia, pp. 1–70.

Horsley, R.W. (1973) The bacterial flora of the Atlantic salmon (Salmo salar L.) in relation to its environment. J. Appl. Bacteriol. 36:377–386.

Labat, R. (1966) Electrocardiologie chez les poissons Teleosteens: Influence de quelques facteurs ecologiques. Ann. Limnol. 2:1–175.

Moss, A.A., Gamsu, G., and Genant, H.K. (Eds). (1983) Computed Tomography of the Body. W.B. Saunders, Philadelphia.

Noga, E.J., Levine, J.F., Townsend, K., Bullis, R.A., Carlson, C.P., and Corbett, W.T. (1986) Kidney biopsy for the diagnosis of enteric redmouth disease. Proceedings, 17th Annual IAAAM Conference and Workshop, pp. 14a–14b.

Oets, J. (1950) Electrocardiograms of fishes. Physiol. Comp. Oecol. 2:181–186.

Smith, L.S., and Bell, G.R. (1964) A technique for prolonged blood sampling in free swimming salmon. J. Fish. Res. Bd. Can. 21:711–717.

Smith, G.C., Lewis, W.M., and Kaplan, H.M. (1952) A comparative morphologic and physiologic study of fish blood. Progressive Fish Culturist 14:169–172.

Trust, T.J. (1975) Bacteria associated with the gills of salmonid fishes in freshwater. J. Appl. Bacteriol. 38:225–233.

Wagner, H.N., Buchanan, J.W., and Espinonla-Vassallo, D. (1986) Diagnostic Nuclear Medicine: Patient Studies. Year Book, Chicago.

Wardle, C.S. (1971) New observations on the lymphatic system of the plaice and other teleosts. J. Mar. Biol. Assoc. U.K. 51:977–990.

Chapter 6

ANESTHESIA AND RESTRAINT

LYDIA A. BROWN

This chapter outlines the principles of anesthesia and restraint in fish. The question of whether or not fish feel pain does not yet have a clearly defined physiological answer. However, even without definitive proof that fish feel pain, anesthesia should be offered to fish for any painful or extremely stressful procedure. Anesthesia is a necessary tool in fish medicine.

Anesthesia is required for procedures in fish that do not require it in other domestic animals. A fish's reaction to adverse stimuli is as a series of reflex responses (Pickering, 1981) that can interfere with clinical diagnosis. Therefore, a clinician who wishes to examine a fish patient in detail must be prepared to tranquilize or anesthetize it. Immobilization, prolonged transport, and minor surgery for topical lesions all require some degree of tranquilization. General anesthesia is required for more complex surgery, laparotomies, and in some situations injections.

MANUAL RESTRAINT

It is possible to manually restrain fish, although it takes patience and skill. Restraint may be necessary to quickly move a fish from one facility to another. It may also be preferred in some instances, for example, minor examinations, when the time taken to administer anesthesia is longer and more stressful than competent manual restraint of the fish. When Koi broodfish need to be moved from one pond to another, fish handlers are frequently able to hold them immobile while they are being transferred. The fish is held under the pectoral fins in the palm of the hand, with the other hand holding the tail (Fig. 6–1). This type of restraint is less stressful than it appears and is appropriate for short-distance transfers between ponds.

When fish are manually restrained, they must be held firmly, yet gently. Larger fish may be held by the head and tail. Smaller fish may be gently compressed between two pieces of damp sponge. Since fish have no eyelids, they are extremely photophobic. As fish are lifted out of the water, an attempt should be made to protect their eyes. Frequently, it is apparent that if a fish is "blinkered," stress responses are minimized (Fig. 6–2). Light and vibrational stimuli, including sound, should be reduced to a minimum during the examination.

In some countries (Finland/Norway), when a salmon broodfish is taken from a pond in winter it is placed in snow for 5 to 10 minutes. The sudden drop in temperature lowers the basal metabolic rate of the fish and enables the fish farmer to hand strip it without the fish damaging its skin when attempting to escape. The physiological consequences of such a sudden drop in water temperature are potentially lethal, and it is generally used only in circumstances in which anesthesia is unavailable or not permitted to be used by law.

GENERAL PRINCIPLES OF IMMOBILIZATION, ANALGESIA, AND TRANQUILIZATION

Stressors should be removed from the environment before a fish is anesthetized. Food should be withheld for up to 24 hours and the fish should not be disturbed prior to anesthesia. Anesthetic tanks for immersion anesthesia and recovery tanks should be prepared ahead of time for smooth induction and

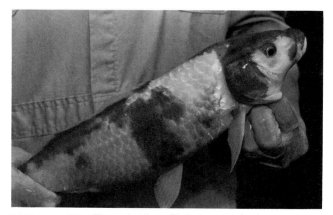

FIGURE 6–1. Handling a koi broodfish for transfer from one pond to another. The fish is held under the pectoral fins in the palm of the hand, with the other hand holding the tail. The latex gloves help the handler maintain a grasp without damaging the fish's skin.

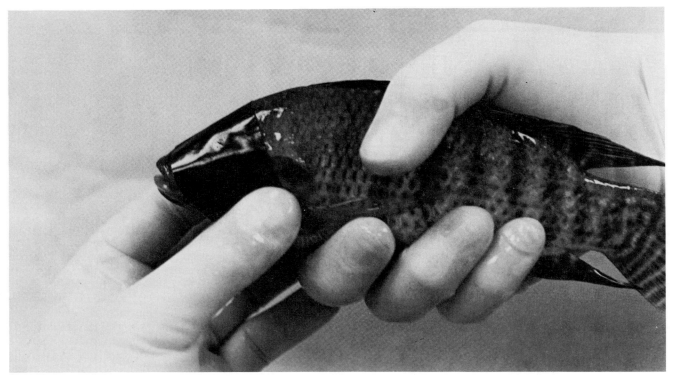

FIGURE 6–2. "Blinkering" a fish to reduce photophobic responses when bright lights are being used in the examination.

recovery. Anesthetic solutions should be properly buffered, and careful calculation of the anesthetic agent is important.

Anesthetized fish should be handled carefully to avoid damage to the delicate epidermis. The hands of the operator should always be wet. For long procedures, a recirculation system may be used to deliver anesthetic for maintenance (Brown, 1987).

Several stages of anesthesia have been attributed to fish (McFarland, 1959; Stoskopf, 1985). Generally, most species go through these phases of anesthesia; however, variation occurs in individual fish, from agent to agent, and related to the induction dose. Some stages are completely omitted in the process of anesthesia in certain fish. Table 6–1 shows a classification of anesthesia planes useful in fish.

When anesthetizing a group of fish of a new species, a small number should always be anesthetized first and their recovery carefully monitored. This allows the dose and anesthetic agent to be assessed for suitability before all fish are involved. After anesthesia, constantly monitor the fish for up to 24 hours to make sure that no long-term side effects of the anesthetic agent occur. Anesthetic solutions should be aerated constantly. When fish are under stress they remove more oxygen from the water, and this must be taken into account during anesthetic procedures.

ROUTES AND METHODS OF DELIVERY

Fish anesthesia can be administered by chemical and nonchemical methods. Nonchemical methods include lowering body temperature either by snow or crushed ice, electrical stimuli, or even mechanical methods such as a blow to the head.

The preferred methods of fish anesthesia are in the chemical category and involve the use of an anesthetic agent. Anesthesia may be administered by immersion, placing the fish either in an anesthetic solution or in a position where the anesthetic agent can pass over the gills. Most anesthetic agents for fish are administered in this way. Other routes include parenteral intramuscular or intraperitoneal injection and oral ingestion.

Topical Administration of Anesthesia in Water

In immersion anesthesia, the fish is placed in a container of water that has been taken from its own aquarium, and the anesthetic is gradually added to the solution as the fish is monitored for changes in behavior. The fish is removed from the water when the required depth of anesthesia has been reached. Generally, procedures are performed on fish out of water. A recovery container of water from the aquarium should always be on hand so that the fish can be placed in this container for recovery if there has been an error in administration of the anesthetic agent. Both anesthesia and recovery containers should always be aerated. This method is very good for procedures requiring only a short duration of anesthesia and procedures in which individual fish need to be operated on out of water.

TABLE 6–1. Stages of Anesthesia in Fishes

Stage	Plane	Category	Behavioral Response of Fish
0		Normal	Swimming actively Reactive to external stimuli Equilibrium normal Muscle tone normal
I	1	Light sedation	Voluntary swimming continues Slight loss of reactivity to visual and tactile stimuli Respiratory rate normal Equilibrium normal Muscle tone normal
I	2	Deep sedation	Voluntary swimming stopped Total loss of reactivity to visual and tactile stimuli Slight decrease in respiratory rate Equilibrium normal Muscle tone slightly decreased Still responds to positional changes
II	1	Light narcosis	Excitement phase may precede increase in respiratory rate Loss of equilibrium Efforts to right itself Muscle tone decreased Still responds to positional changes weakly
II	2	Deep narcosis	Ceases to respond to positional changes Decrease in respiratory rate to approximately normal Total loss of equilibrium No efforts to right itself Muscle tone decreased Some reactivity to strong tactile and vibrational stimuli Suitable for external sampling, fin biopsies, gill biopsies
III	1	Light anesthesia	Total loss of muscle tone Responds to deep pressure Further decrease in respiratory rate Suitable for minor surgical procedures
III	2	Surgical anesthesia	Total loss of reactivity Respiratory rate very low Heart rate slow
IV		Medullary collapse	Total loss of gill movement followed in several minutes by cardiac arrest

Adapted from Stoskopf, M. K. (1985) Manual for the Aquatic Workshop. American Association for Laboratory Animal Science, National Capital Area Branch, Washington, D.C.

Although a fish can survive for periods of several minutes in air and recover in water well, it causes stress to the fish. If long operations are to be performed, constant recirculation systems must be used and the fish must be given access to oxygenated water at all times.

Administration of Anesthesia by Injection

The sites for intramuscular and intraperitoneal injections are shown in Figure 6–3. An 18- to 23-gauge, 2- to 4-cm needle is recommended for larger fish, although a 25- to 28-gauge needle is favored for smaller fish. Obviously, the viscosity of the anesthetic agent will also have a bearing on the gauge of the needle to be used. Intramuscular injections are not an ideal route of anesthetic administration in fish, since swimming movements after injection force some of the drug out of the body, and the dosage is then difficult to quantify. In addition, depending on the volume of the agent injected, necrotic lesions can occur at the site of the injection with some agents. Intraperitoneal injections are usually made on the ventral midline with the needle pointing in a rostro-dorsal direction away from the spleen. For small ornamental fishes, a short needle (0.25 to 0.50 inch) is especially important for this route because of the proximity of the spleen to the point of injection.

Administration of Anesthesia Per Os

Chemical agents have been administered orally to fish either by gavage, using a capsule, or in food. Pellets containing diazepam fed to American shad resulted in a slow induction of anesthesia as the drug was absorbed via the gut (Murae et al., 1979).

MONITORING ANESTHESIA

Tranquilization or anesthesia should be constantly monitored throughout any procedure. Once fish are anesthetized their gill covers move, albeit at a slower rate. When placed in air, opercular movement may be reduced or even stop altogether. If procedures do not take too long (1 to 2 minutes), then no action need be taken, and the fish will probably make an uneventful recovery.

However, for longer periods of time, opercular movement should be accurately observed. If the fish is returned to fresh water and does not appear to move the opercula, then forced recovery procedures may be employed. This involves holding the fish and pushing it through the water head first so that water enters the mouth and then passes back over the gills.

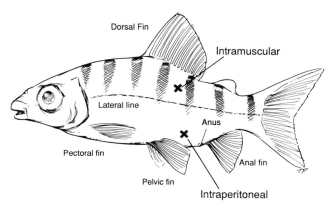

FIGURE 6–3. Routine sites for intraperitoneal and intramuscular injections in fish.

After one motion in this manner, the fish should be raised from the water and placed back at the starting point before repeating the procedure. It is important to stress that water should not be forced through the mouth at too great a velocity. This will only cause gross capillary damage to the lamellar area, making passage of oxygen across the gills even harder.

For smaller fish it is possible to place a tube into the fish's mouth through which fresh water is directed until recovery is observed. Recovery for many species of fish is seen as a "cough" reflex. The fish suddenly opens and closes its opercula and makes a jerky movement backward.

ANESTHETIC AGENTS

In discussing the pharmacology of anesthetic agents, references from mammalian literature have been given where necessary. This is because there is very little information available on the pharmacology of these agents in fish.

In order for a chemical to be a good anesthetic agent it should have rapid and smooth induction and recovery. Anesthesia should be achieved in doses that are much lower than any concentration calculated to produce toxic effects either to the fish or the operator. Finally, the anesthetic agent should be soluble in water.

Anesthesia is a triad of narcosis, analgesia, and skeletal muscle relaxation. These phenomena are produced by sensory nerve block, motor nerve block, and reflex activity reduction. For major procedures, total loss of sensory, motor, and reflex activity is required. However, for tranquilization only, sensory and motor loss sufficient to block activity is required. Anesthetic agents vary as to the degree of anesthesia that can be administered either because of the molecule itself or because of different concentrations used. The pH of an anesthetic agent can alter the efficacy of the agent, perhaps by affecting the ratio of charged to uncharged molecules. Occasionally, different effects are noted in sea water versus fresh water. Solubility and stability of agents affect the efficacy of anesthesia for various drugs. Finally, variation between species and from individual fish to fish occurs. Information on the most frequently used anesthetic agents in fish is given below (Martindale's Pharmacopoeia, 1977). Table 6–2 lists other agents that have been reported in the literature as useful for fish anesthesia.

PAIN AND FISH

Equating pain in animals with that of humans is very subjective. It is suggested that three stages of suffering should be recognized in animals: discomfort, stress, and pain. Discomfort may be characterized by such negative signs as poor condition, torpor, and diminished appetite. Stress is defined as a condition of tension or anxiety predictable or readily

TABLE 6–2. Other Anesthetic Agents for Fishes

Agent	Common Name	Dosage	Reference*
Chlorbutanol	Salmonids	2.8–3.5 mM	Nelson (1953)
Ethanol in H_2O	Killifish	Anesthesia not controllable	
Ether	Goldfish		
Lidocaine	Tilapia, carp	0–50 ml/L	Carrasco et al. (1984)
Lidocaine HCO_3		Dosage very variable between species	
		Better in adults than lidocaine, use as a combination of lidocaine, 250–350 mg/L and $NaHCO_3$	
Methylparafynol	California killifish	1.5–3.5 ml	
Methlpentynol		0.5–0.9 ml/L	
Pentobarbitone	Tench, roach	2 mg/100 gm IM	Shelton and Randall (1962)
2-Phenoxyethanol	Pacific salmon	0.1–0.5 ml/L	Klontz and Smith (1968)
Procaine			
Propanidid	Carp	4 ml/L ip	Jeney et al. (1986)
Propoxate	Goldfish	1–4 mg/L	Jolly et al. (1972)
Quinaldine sulfate	Tropical marines warmwater spp.	200 mg/L	
		15–70 mg/L, 2.5–2.0 mg/L	
Salt	Rainbow trout	Questionable	Dixon and Milton (1978)
Sodium amytal	California killifish	Freshwater: 0.05–0.08 g/L	Barton and Peter (1982)
		Saltwater: 0.4–0.65 g/gal	Brooke et al. (1978)
Sodium bicarbonate	Carp	642 g/L, pH = 6.5	
4-Styrylpyridine		20–50 mg/L	McFarland and Klontz (1969)
Tertiary-amyl alcohol	California killifish	1.0–1.75 ml/L	
		0.5–1.1 ml/L	
Urethane†	Goldfish	0.3 g/L	Anders and Ostrow (1986)
Etorphine/Acepromazine (Immobilon)		8–10 mg/kg	
		(Recover with Revivon)	

*All references cited by Brown (1988).
†Potential carcinogen.

explicable from environmental causes, including physical causes. Finally, pain itself is recognized by more positive signs such as struggling, screaming or squealing, convulsions, or severe palpitations. These definitions will be assumed when referring to pain, stress, and discomfort in this chapter.

Attempts to assess pain in animals are made more difficult by adaptive responses. It is well known that the fight and flight mechanism can override pain perception. Individual differences exist between various species in their ability to tolerate or react to pain. One theory for the perception of pain in higher animals involves the modulation of sensory cues that are normally controlled by specific cells in the spinal cord operating a gating mechanism. The sensory input is relayed to central receptors by fast myelinated and slow unmyelinated fibers up the spinothalamic tract. An imbalance of input between these two sets of fibers is thought to be the cause of pain. There is a wealth of evidence that interruption of this tract, either by injury or disease, results in a loss of the ability to feel pain. A British Veterinary Association Fish Sub-Committee meeting in 1984 concluded that although the scientific evidence shows that fish do not have a spinothalamic pathway, there seems to be no way of showing whether or not another part of the brain has adapted to take over the function of the thalamus (Brown, 1985). In man, parts of the nonspecific or association cortex have been shown to be concerned with nociceptive input. There are marked differences in cortical development between mammals, birds, reptiles, amphibia, and cartilaginous fishes, the simplest of which have no recognizable cerebral cortex, but there is a paucity of information available on centrally mediated reception of sensory cues in fish.

Fish physiologists (Lagler et al., 1977) argue that pain is probably not experienced as a strong sensation by fishes, though forceful or noxious physical or chemical stimuli evoke violent reactions. This contention still does not relieve us of the responsibility of giving animals the benefit of the doubt concerning pain. The main sensory cues to which fish respond in the aquatic environment are chemical, hydrodynamic, acoustic, thermal, electrical, light, and mechanical. The receptor sites for these stimuli vary from species to species. Physical changes in heat flow or touch are recognized by skin receptors, and visual cues are observed as changes in light intensity and/or quality. The inner ear and lateral line receive acoustic input, whereas chemical reception occurs in smell and taste organs located all over the body. No authorities so far appear able to identify the presence of nociceptors in fish.

To summarize, we are not able to say if fish perceive pain. Sensory receptors are present for external environmental cues. The central reception of these sensory inputs is unclear in fish. Clinical signs of acute and chronic stress can be observed in fish, and we are able to determine physiological stress by assaying serum cortisol. Fish act in a reflex manner by removing themselves from an adverse stimulus.

We may, therefore, postulate that fish need to be cognizant of their surroundings to react to stressors in their environment. In any event, we should give fish the benefit of the doubt in situations that might be considered either stressful or painful.

MOST FREQUENTLY USED ANESTHETICS

Tricaine Methane Sulfonate

Synonyms. 3-Aminobenzonic acid ethyl ester; ethyl m-aminobenzoate; tricaine; MS222; Finquel; methane sulfonate; TS-222 Sandoz; TS-222; tricaine—Sandoz; metacaine; metacaine methanesulfonate; TMS.

Tricaine methane sulfonate, or tricaine, was discovered by accident when research workers were looking for a reliable synthetic substitute for cocaine. It is the only anesthetic fully licensed for use in fish and is one of the most widely used anesthetic agents for poikilotherms world wide. It is a derivative of benzocaine, which has an additional sulfonate radical, rendering it more water soluble and more acidic than its parent compound (Fig. 6–4).

Chemical Attributes

Tricaine (MW = 261.31), $C_{10}H_{15}NO_5S$ is a fine white crystalline powder. It is soluble to 11%, where it forms a clear colorless acid solution.

Stability

The melting point of tricaine is 145°C. It leaves only minimum traces of ash and is free from chlorides, sulfates, alkaloids, and heavy metals. It loses less than 0.5% of its weight upon heating to 103°C.

Physiological Impact

Tricaine has no effect on ciliary action, but its effect on muscular activity is rapid. Recovery is also rapid. In weak solutions, no long-term toxic effects have been reported in fish, so it is used for transporting fish long distances. Tricaine is a very popular anesthetic agent because of its solubility in water. However, since tricaine is acid in aqueous solution, it should be buffered with imidazole, sodium hydro-

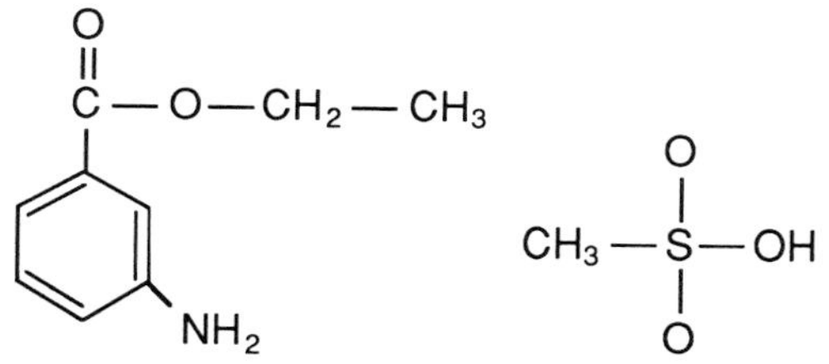

FIGURE 6–4. The structure of tricaine methane sulfonate.

gen phosphate, or sodium hydroxide. Tricaine administration also reduces the blood pH of freshwater fish (Soivio et al., 1977). When fish are anesthetized with unbuffered tricaine solutions, there is an increase in blood urea nitrogen concentrations, hypercholinesteremia, and increased ACTH production (Wedemeyer, 1970).

Tricaine has been noted by many authors to be an hypoxic agent. During stage III plane 2 of anesthesia, it is noted that there is insufficient water flow over the gills due to depression of the medullary respiratory center. This is associated with several physiological changes, including bradycardia (possibly induced by the hypoxic water in the area of the gills), an increase in the resistance to blood flow through the gill lamellae, and erythrocyte swelling that impedes blood passage through the gills (Fromm et al., 1971; Holeton and Randal, 1967; Garey and Rahn, 1970). Further physiological effects due to hypoxia during tricaine anesthesia can include:

1. Increased concentrations of blood glucose, lactate, potassium, magnesium, hemoglobin, and hematocrit.
2. Increased urinary output and electrolyte loss. These changes are reported to occur immediately following anesthesia and may persist up to 4 to 7 days after anesthesia.

Dose (Table 6–3)

In general, a 1:10,000 solution of tricaine can be used for surgical anesthesia, whereas 1:20,000 to 1:30,000 solutions are used for tranquilization and transport. Tricaine has also been administered in sharks as a solution sprayed onto the gills at a strength of about 1 ppt. Table 6–2 shows doses of tricaine recommended for a variety of species; however, since individual variation from fish to fish can be very wide with this agent, the table should be used with extreme caution.

TABLE 6–3. Tricaine Dosages

Variety of Fish	Concentration	Anesthesia Time
Tropicals at 24 to 27°C		
Live bearers	0.32 g/U.S. gal (approx. 1:12,000)	To 12 hours uncrowded
Egg layers	0.24 g/U.S. gal (approx. 1:15,000)	To 12 hours uncrowded
For uncrowded shipment of pugnacious species without oxygen:		
Bettas, Piranhas, etc.	0.25 g/U.S. gal (approx. 1:15,000)	To 48 hours
Goldfish, with oxygen	0.14 g/U.S. gal (approx. 1:24,000)	

From Bove, F. J. (date unknown) MS. 222 Sandoz. The Anaesthetic and Tranquilizer for Fish, Frogs and Other Cold-Blooded Organisms. Sandoz Technical Bulletin, Sandoz Ltd. Basle, Switzerland.

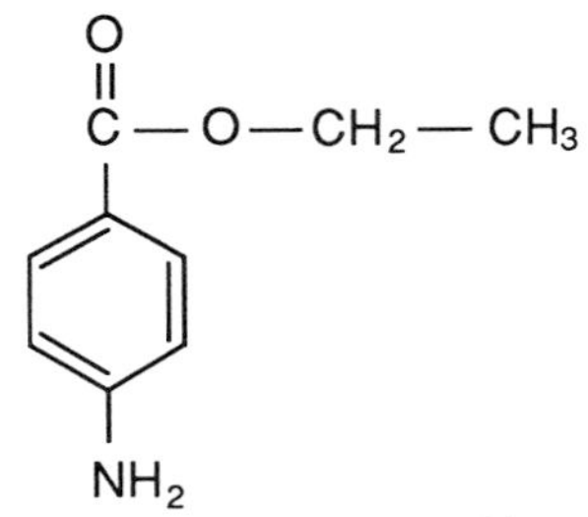

FIGURE 6–5. The structure of benzocaine.

Benzocaine

*Synonyms.** (BP, EurP.) benzocainum; ethyllis aminobenzoas (IP); ethyl aminobenzoate; anaesthesinum (RusP); Ethoforme; ethyl p-aminobenzoate.

Benzocaine is as popular an anesthetic agent in fish as is its derivative tricaine (Fig. 6–5). It is, however, much less expensive and so tends to be used on a routine basis. Its insolubility in water is usually countered by the preparation of a stock solution in ethanol, methanol, or acetone.

Chemical Attributes

A colorless crystal or white odorless crystalline powder with a slightly bitter numbing taste, benzocaine (MW = 165.2), $C_9H_{11}NO_2$, is mainly insoluble in water (1:2500); 1:8 alcohol, 1:2 in chloroform, 1:4 in ether, and 1:50 in fixed oils. It is soluble in liquid paraffin and dilute acids. In solution, benzocaine is neutral and is said to cause a less stressful reaction than tricaine.

Stability

The melting point of benzocaine is 89 to 92°C. Benzocaine should be stored in air-tight containers and protected from light. When stored in an alcohol-based solution, it should be kept in dark glass bottles and held at room temperature.

Mechanism of Action

Benzocaine in humans is a surface anesthetic of the ester type. It is comparatively nonirritant and has a low systemic toxicity. Since benzocaine is not very soluble in water, it must first be dissolved in ethanol or acetone (0.5 g in 5 ml) before use in fish.

Physiological Impact

In humans, benzocaine is hydrolyzed in the body to p-aminobenzoic acid and should not, therefore, be used in patients being treated with sulfonamides. Benzocaine tends to suppress stress effects

---

*Abbreviations: BP, *British Pharmacopoeia*, EurP., *European Pharmacopoeia*; IP, *International Pharmacopoeia*; RusP, *Russian Pharmacopoeia*.

in stages I and II of anesthesia. The side effects noted with benzocaine are as for tricaine and are associated with hypoxic changes. Since benzocaine is fat soluble, the duration of anesthesia may be prolonged (with extended recovery times) in large older fish or gravid females.

Dose

A stock solution of benzocaine (100 g benzocaine in 1 L of ethanol or acetone) is prepared and stored in a dark glass bottle (Ross and Ross, 1984). This stock solution is added to the water intended for anesthetic use drop-wise and mixed thoroughly. A small batch of fish are first anesthetized and allowed to recover in a recovery tank to ensure that the concentration of benzocaine used is adequate. Higher doses of both benzocaine and tricaine are required at higher temperatures (Ross and Ross, 1984).

Etomidate

Synonyms. Etomidate (sulfate) R. 26490; R 16659 (base); R-(+)-ethyl 1-(α-methylbenzyl)imidazole-5 carboxylate (sulfate).

Etomidate sulfate is used parenterally in humans for the induction of anesthesia (Fig. 6–6). Dosage is generally expressed in terms of the base. Toxic effects in the human include pain on injection, involuntary muscle movement, and hypotension.

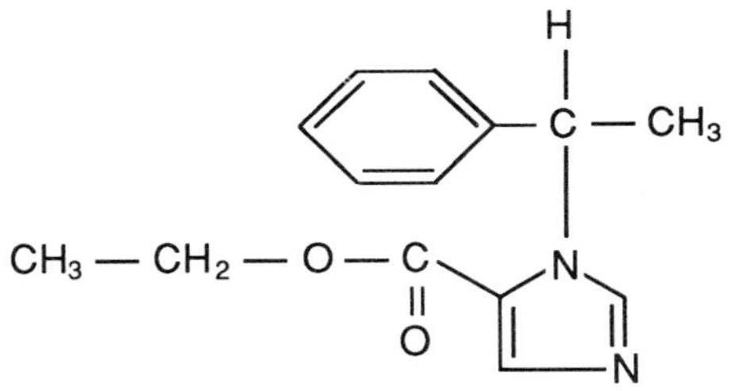

Chemical Attributes

Etomidate (MW = 342.4), $C_{14}H_{16}N_2O_2H_2SO_4$, is a white crystalline powder. It is very soluble in water, alcohol, methyl alcohol, and propylene glycol and also is freely soluble in chloroform and macrogols 200, 400, and 600. However, it is sparingly soluble in acetone and practically insoluble in ether.

NOTE: 140 mg etomidate sulfate is approximately equivalent to 100 mg etomidate base.

Stability

The melting point of etomidate is about 115°C. Etomidate should be stored in air-tight containers and protected from light.

Mechanism of Action

Etomidate is an imidazole-based nonbarbiturate hypnotic agent. It has no analgesic properties in humans and should never be used as an anesthetic agent for surgical procedures on fish, assuming that a similar mechanism of action occurs for both species. The specific mechanism of action of etomidate is as yet unclear. Etomidate induction in human anesthesia is associated with an increase in adrenocorticotrophic hormone (Stoskopf and Arnold, 1985). Low cortisol levels would thus be expected to exert a

FIGURE 6–6. The structure of etomidate.

negative feedback effect on the pituitary gland, causing an elevation of ACTH.

Physiological Impact

In humans, etomidate selectively suppresses the production of cortisol through inhibition of 11-β hydroxylation of cholesterol. It is thought that a similar phenomenon may occur in fish, causing a frequently observed reduction in plasma cortisol and plasma glucose. This is thought to be detrimental to the long-term survival of the fish, owing to a suppression of the inflammatory response, decreased concentration of circulating leukocytes, and suppressed leukocyte migration and phagocytic activity (Wedemeyer, 1970).

Dose

Etomidate is thought to be a tranquilizing agent only. Sedation of striped bass at a dose of 0.1 mg/L etomidate has been reported (Davis et al., 1982). It has been used to suppress physiological changes when research workers investigated stress mechanisms.

Metomidate

Synonyms. (+)Methyl-1-(alpha-methylbenzyl)-5-imidazole-carboxylate hydrochloride (R 7315, Janssen); Marinil.

Metomidate is an analogue of etomidate (Fig. 6–7). It is an imidazole-based nonbarbiturate hypnotic agent that has no analgesic properties in humans (Godefroi et al., 1965).

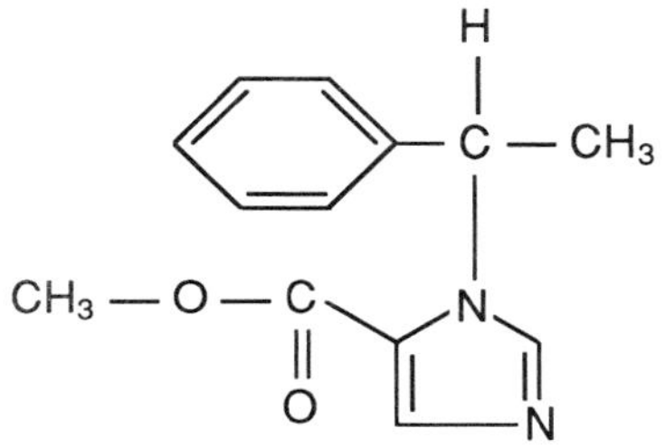

FIGURE 6–7. The structure of metomidate.

Chemical Attributes

Metomidate (MW = 266.73), $C_{13}H_{14}N_2O_2$:HCl, has chemical attributes similar to those of etomidate.

Stability

The melting point of metomidate is about 115°C. Metomidate should be stored in well-closed opaque containers.

Mechanism of Action

Metomidate is classed as a hypnotic and is thought to have a similar mechanism of action as for etomidate.

Physiological Impact

Metomidate has been found to be effective in subduing fish so they can be handled. Long recovery times have been seen with this drug. Metomidate is known to reduce plasma cortisol and glucose concentrations; however, the cortisol reduction is possibly due to a suppression of 11β-hydroxylation of cholesterol as for etomidate (Allolio et al., 1984). Etomidate does not increase plasma histamine (Sebel et al., 1983). An increase in fish pigmentation, presumably due to the increased production of melanocyte-stimulating hormone on the same primary protein as ACTH, has been noted for metomidate (Stoskopf and Arnold, 1985).

Dose

In rainbow trout, small adults may be tranquilized with 5 mg/L of metomidate. At these doses, total loss of reflexes does not occur. Channel catfish fingerlings can be tranquilized at 5 mg/L (Brown et al., 1986), although the authors think that this dose may have been too high. Tranquilization occurs in 10 min after administration. Catfish tranquilized at this dose show no reaction to handling for up to 24 hours. Muscle fasciculation is a common occurrence with the use of this drug, precluding it from being effective for detailed procedures on fish. Dosages generally used in freshwater and marine tropical species of fish vary from 2.5 to 5 mg/L. Doses reported for tropical marine fishes for tranquilization or transportation are in the range of 0.06 to 0.20 ppm.

Doses for metomidate anesthesia have been cited by Wildlife Laboratories Inc. (Fort Collins, Colorado) as 6 to 10 mg/L for rainbow trout and channel catfish. As a tranquilizer for sunfish (Centrarchidae), a dose of 0.5 to 1 mg/L is effective. For anesthesia, 5 to 10 mg/L is considered effective.

Diazepam

Synonyms. (BP) diazepam; LA111; Ro 5-2807; Wy 3467; 7-chloro-2,3-dihydro-1-methyl-5-phenyl-1H-1,

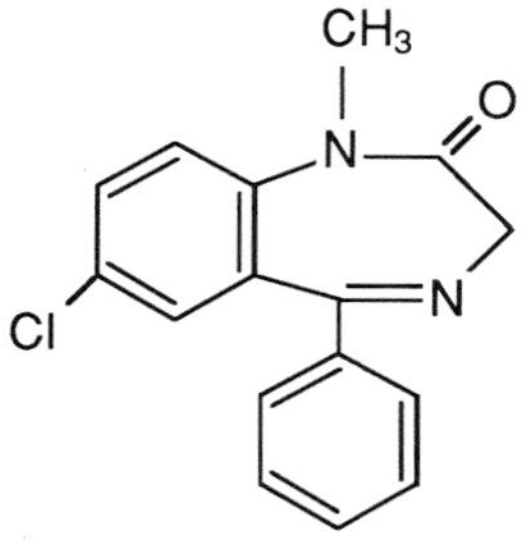

FIGURE 6–8. The structure of diazepam.

4-benzodiazepin-2-one; Valium; Apozepam; Stesolid; E-Pam; Paxel; Serenack; Vivol; Relanium.

Diazepam is a benzodiazepine tranquilizer and, as well as being used for the treatment of anxiety and tension states in humans, it also has the effect of controlling muscle spasm (Fig. 6–8).

Chemical Attributes

Diazepam (MW = 284.7), $C_{16}H_{13}C_1N_{20}$, is a white or almost white, odorless or almost odorless, crystalline powder, tasteless at first with a bitter aftertaste.

Stability

The melting point of diazepam is 130 to 134°C. It is very slightly soluble in water; soluble 1:25 in alcohol, 1:2 in chloroform, and 1:30 in ether. Diazepam should be stored in airtight containers and protected from light.

Mechanism of Action

Diazepam is rapidly absorbed from the gastrointestinal tract of most mammals. While blood concentrations tend to be variable, it is usually eliminated in a biphasic manner. This is because it is initially distributed and subsequently converted to active metabolites. In man, the major metabolites are desmethyl diazepam and temazepam. In mammals, up to 75% of a dose has been reported to be excreted in the urine, mainly as conjugated oxazepam. In man, 10% is excreted in the feces. The mechanism of action in fish is unclear but may mimic the mammalian mechanism of action.

Physiological Impact

Diazepam has anticonvulsant, sedative, muscle relaxant, and amnesic properties. It has been used in humans to control anxiety and tension states as a sedative and as a premedication agent.

Dose

Diazepam has been given in feed to American shad at 9.94 mg/kg (Murae et al., 1979). Problems encountered were connected with reliable incorpo-

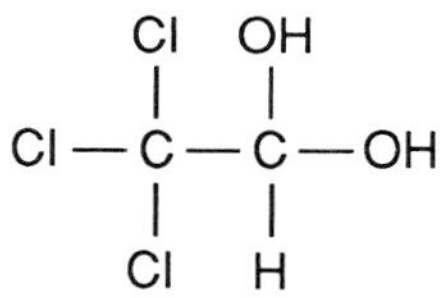

Cl   OH
| |
Cl — C — C — OH
| |
Cl   H

FIGURE 6–9. The structure of chloral hydrate.

ration in the diet and the unwillingness of fish to eat the food. Both of these factors give concern about actual dose available to each fish. The drug has been administered to green moray eels intramuscularly and intravenously at doses of 0.1 to 0.5 mg/kg with variable effect (Stoskopf, 1990).

Chloral Hydrate

Synonyms. (BP, EurP) chloral Hydr; (IP) chlorali hydras; chloral; 2,2,2-trichloroethane-1,1-diol.

Chloral hydrate is a sedative and hypnotic with properties similar to those of the barbiturates (Fig. 6–9). In humans, chloral hydrate has a rubifacient action and was formerly employed as an anodyne and counterirritant.

Chemical Attributes

Chloral hydrate (MW = 165.42), $C_2H_3Cl_3O_2$, is a colorless crystal with a pungent but not acrid odor and a pungent bitter caustic taste. It volatilizes slowly on exposure to air and liquefies between 50 and 58°C.

Stability

Chloral hydrate is soluble at 1:0.3 in water; 1:0.2 in alcohol; 1:3 in chloroform, 1:>1 in ether; 1:0.5 in glycerol and in fixed and volatile oils. A 10% solution of chloral hydrate in water has a pH of 3.5:4.4. Unfortunately, it is incompatible with many alkaline compounds. It should be stored in a cool place in airtight containers and protected from light.

Mechanism of Action

Chloral hydrate is rapidly absorbed from the stomach in man and starts to act within 30 minutes. It is widely distributed throughout the body and is metabolized to trichloroethanol and trichloroacetic acid in the blood, liver, and other tissues. In the urine, it is excreted slowly as trichloroethanol and its glucuronide (urochloralic acid) and as trichloroacetic acid.

Physiological Impacts

Because chloral hydrate decomposes rapidly when exposed to UV light, reliable maintenance of anesthesia when used in fish is difficult. As it decomposes, it forms hydrochloric acid, trichloroacetic acid, and formic acid. In humans, chloral hydrate is corrosive to skin and mucus membranes unless well

diluted. Thus chloral hydrate should not be considered an agent of choice.

Dose

In killifish, a dose of 0.8 to 0.9 gm/L has been used for handling and transport (McFarland, 1960). It is not used very often in fish anesthesia, since so many other agents are available that are less toxic, more predictable, and more efficacious.

Carbon Dioxide

Synonyms. (BP, EurP) carbon dioxide; carbon diox; (IP) carbonei dioxydum; carbonei dioxidum; carbonic anhydride; carbonic acid gas.

Gaseous anesthesia as strictly defined is impossible with fish. Gill lamellar collapse occurs out of water, which decreases exchange area for absorption of a gas across the lamellar membrane.

Chemical Attributes

Carbon dioxide (MW = 44.01), CO_2, is a colorless odorless gas that does not support combustion (Fig. 6–10). It is about 1.5 times as heavy as air. As a solution in water, it has weakly acidic properties. Carbon dioxide can be liquefied by pressure at 31°C or lower; at 31°C, a pressure of 72 atmospheres is required. It is soluble in water at a dilution of 1:1.2 by volume at normal temperature and pressure. It is also available as a liquid and as a solid (dry ice).

Mechanism of Action

In humans, above a concentration of 7%, carbon dioxide gives rise to headache, dizziness, mental confusion, palpitations, hypertension, and dyspnea, and eventually, at a concentration of 10% or more, to unconsciousness. Carbon dioxide is important for regulating the acid-base balance of the body. In humans, CO_2 given per os in solution promotes the absorption of liquids by the mucous membranes. Such a factor in fish would severely debilitate the osmotic balance and would also tend to produce a metabolic alkalosis. Since too much CO_2 in the blood can have a depressive effect on respiratory drive, it is important that sufficient aeration is added to the water to allow the fish to maintain correct pO_2 levels.

Dose

In fish, carbon dioxide is noted to be an effective anesthetic, but it has only been used occasionally as

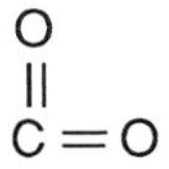

O
‖
C = O

FIGURE 6–10. The structure of carbon dioxide.

a sedative for transportation. The gas is bubbled through the water. The final concentration of CO_2 in the water is very difficult to control by this method. Takeda and Itazawa (1983) felt that this method was impractical, since pO_2 must be maintained at a very high level when pCO_2 is high.

Ketamine

Synonyms. (USNF*) ketamine hydrochloride; CI 581; CL 369; 2-O-chlorophenyl-2-methyl aminocyclohexanone hydrochlande. Proprietary names include Ketalar, Ketaject, and Ketanest.

In humans, ketamine is a short-acting general anesthetic, producing dissociative anesthesia (Fig. 6–11).

Chemical Attributes

Ketamine (MW = 274.2), $C_{13}H_{16}ClNO$:HCl, is a white crystalline powder with a slight characteristic odor. Ketamine hydrochloride, 1.15 mg, is approximately equivalent to 1 mg of ketamine base.

Stability

The melting point of ketamine is about 259°C. It is freely soluble in water and methyl alcohol, soluble in alcohol, and sparingly soluble in chloroform. A 10% solution has a pH of 3.5:4.1.

Physiological Impact

In humans, emergence reactions are common during recovery from ketamine anesthesia and include vivid and often unpleasant dreams, confusion, hallucinations, irrational behavior, and increased muscle tone. These actions may be controlled by tranquilizers. In doses above 45 mg/Kg given intramuscularly to fish, deleterious effects occur (Williams et al., 1988). Verbal and tactile stimuli should be kept to a minimum during recovery in an attempt to reduce the risk of emergence reactions.

Dose

A dose of 14 to 18 mg/Kg by the intramuscular route has been used in a variety of temperate water fishes for anesthesia (Williams et al., 1988).

---

*Abbreviation: USNF, *U.S. National Formulary.*

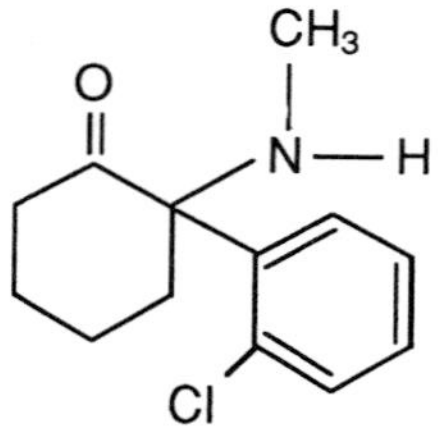

FIGURE 6–11. The structure of ketamine hydrochloride.

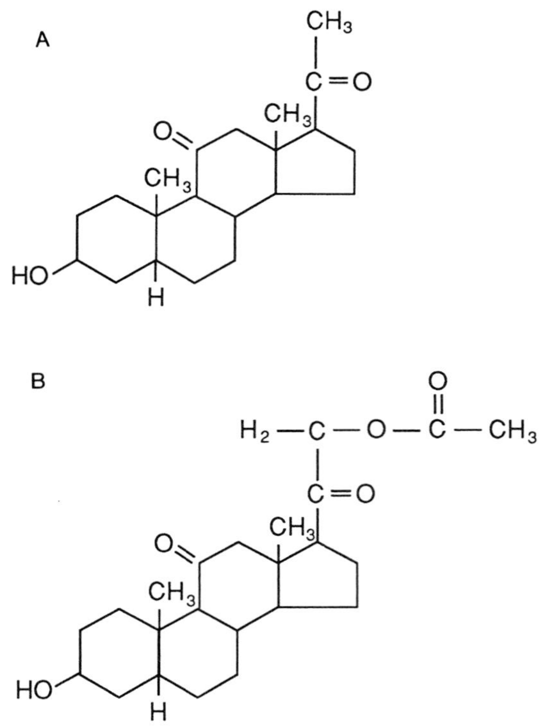

FIGURE 6–12. The structures of alphaxalone (A) and alphadolone acetate (B).

Saffan

Synonyms. Saffan (CT 1341 and alphadione) is a combination of alphaxalone and alphadolone. Other proprietary names include Athesin and Alfathesin (Fig. 6–12).

Alphadolone acetate is GR 2/1574; 21-acetoxy-3-α-hydroxy-5-α-pregnane-11,20-dione.

Alphaxalone is GR2/234; 3-α-hydroxy-5-α-pregnane-11,20-dione.

Alphadolone (MW = 390.5), $C_{23}H_{34}O_5$, is a white or almost white, odorless, crystalline powder. Its melting point is 175 to 181°C. It is insoluble in water but freely soluble in acetone and chloroform.

Alphaxalone (MW = 332.5), $C_{21}H_{32}O_3$, is a white or almost white, odorless, crystalline powder. Its melting point is 165 to 171°C, and it is practically insoluble in water but freely soluble in acetone and chloroform.

CT1341 and alphadione describe an aqueous solution of alphadolone acetate 0.3% and alphaxalone 0.9% with sodium chloride 0.25% and 20% of polyoxyethylated castor oil (Cremephor E.L.). Alphadolone is used to enhance the solubility of alphaxalone. It possesses some anesthetic properties and is considered to be about half as potent as alphaxalone.

Mechanism of Action

Both alphaxalone and alphadolone acetate are rapidly and widely distributed following injection. In the human, they are metabolized in the liver and excreted in the urine. In animals, some excretion in the feces has been noted. There is evidence of enterohepatic recirculation. Up to 50% of alphaxalone may be bound to plasma proteins.

Physiological Impact

In humans, this combination may produce involuntary muscle movements, which may be common with high doses. Alphaxalone is thought to lack many of the side effects of barbiturates or other steroid hormones. The gills appear bright red and engorged, in contrast to the dull purplish color associated with tricaine or benzocaine. The ECG shows a normal QRS complex. In humans, the preparation has little analgesic effect.

Dose

When the dose is low, fish lose equilibrium and muscle tone. Respiration and circulation are maintained at approximately the basal level (Tytler and Hawkins, 1981). At high doses, it is advisable to irrigate the gills for the fish, since respiration tends to be reciprocative (Tytler and Hawkins, 1981).

Quinaldine

Synonyms. 2-Methylquinoline.

Quinaldine is a quinoline compound that is insoluble in water (Fig. 6–13). Supplied by Eastman Kodak Co., it has been used to good effect by many fish workers. Unfortunately, there are an equal number of workers in the literature who report adverse effects on fish physiology with the use of this compound.

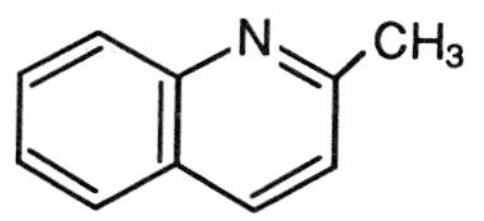

Chemical Attributes

Quinaldine (MW = 143.18), $C_{10}H_9N$, is an oily liquid, which must be dissolved in acetone or ethanol in order to make it miscible with water. Quinaldine sulfate, however, is readily soluble in water, but owing to its acidic nature, it should be buffered with sodium bicarbonate (0.45 gm $NaHCO_3$/1 gm quinaldine sulfate).

Stability

At pH 5 or less, quinaldine is ineffective. The higher the water pH, the more potent quinaldine becomes. It is oxidized on exposure to air.

Mechanism of Action

Quinaldine sulfate is not easily available commercially. Although it is an effective anesthetic, it is an irritant and is insoluble. Corneal damage has been reported following its use with salmonids.

Physiological Impact

Quinaldine has been reported to be irritant to gills and cause increased bronchial mucus secretion.

FIGURE 6–13. The structure of quinaldine.

Although it produces a loss of equilibrium and depression of medullary centers in stage III of anesthesia, fish do not lose all reflex response, thus precluding its use for delicate surgery (Tytler and Hawkins, 1981). The required solvents produce a noxious vapor that is harmful to the eyes of operators.

Dose

Analgesia with quinaldine is thought to be minimal (Tytler and Hawkins, 1981). Anesthesia with quinaldine is considered to be good by some workers, and it has become a popular agent for use when collecting fish from tidal pools and small lagoons. In tropical marine fishes, a dose of 200 mg/L is recommended (Blasiola, 1976). For warm-water species, generally 15 to 70 mg/L is used. The dose required to reach stage III anesthesia in many fish species is 16 mg/L. Doses of 50 to 1000 mg/L have been used in tilapia (Sado, 1985). Induction and recovery times of 2 to 6 minutes were recorded (Tytler and Hawkins, 1981).

Halothane

Synonyms. (BP, EurP) halothanum: alotano; phthorothanum; 2-bromo-2-chloro-1,1, 1-trifluoroethane.

Halothane is widely used as an inhalation anesthetic in animals after being vaporized (Fig. 6–14).

Chemical Attributes

Halothane (MW = 197.4), $CHBrClCF_3$, is a colorless, mobile, heavy, noninflammable liquid with a characteristic chloroformlike odor and a sweet burning taste. It contains 0.01% w/w of thymol as a preservative. It weighs 1.867 to 1.872 g/ml.

Stability

The distillation range of halothane is 49 to 51°C. It is soluble at 1:400 in water and miscible with dehydrated alcohol, chloroform, ether, trichloroethylene, and fixed and volatile oils. Halothane is soluble in rubber. In the presence of moisture, it reacts

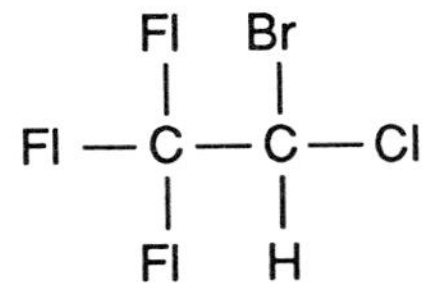

FIGURE 6–14. The structure of halothane.

with many metals. Halothane should be stored at a temperature not exceeding 25°C in airtight containers and protected from light. On prolonged exposure to ultraviolet radiation, halothane decomposes with the formation of halogens and halogen acids.

Mechanism of Action

Halothane reduces muscle tone. In humans, halothane is absorbed on inhalation. It has a relatively low solubility in blood. It is more soluble in neutral fats of adipose tissue than in the phospholipids of brain cells. Halothane is excreted unchanged through the lungs, and a variable amount is metabolized by the liver. Urinary metabolites in the human include trifluoroacetic acid and bromide and chloride salts.

Physiological Impact

When passing halothane into water for fish, there is great danger of generating "hot-spots" in the solution where high concentrations may be toxic to the fish in the system.

Dose

Dose levels of 0.5 to 2.0 ml/L of halothane produce anesthesia. Halothane may also be vaporized and dissolved to effect. Induction is dose related and rapid with excellent maintenance and rapid recovery (2 to 5 minutes). However, the technique is difficult to control (Ross and Ross, 1984). It is relatively little used these days and is not a preferred anesthetic agent.

Other anesthetic agents not included in this section are listed, together with dosages and references for use, in Table 6–2.

LITERATURE CITED

Allolio, B., Stuttman, R., Fisher, L., and Winklemann, W. (1984) Adrenocortical suppression by a single dose of etomidate. Klin. Wochenschr. 62:1014–1017.

Anders, J.J., and Ostrow, M.E. (1986) Goldfish in research: Use and maintenance. Lab. Anim. 15:33–41.

Barton, V.A., and Peter, R.E. (1982) Plasma cortisol stress response in fingerling rainbow trout, Salmo gairdneri Richardson, to various transport conditions, anaesthesia, and cold shock. J. Fish Biol. 20:39–51.

Blasiola, G.C. (1976) Quinaldine sulphate, a new anesthetic formulation for tropical marine fish. J. Fish Biol. 10:113–120.

Booke, H.E., Hollender, B., and Lutterbie, G. (1978) Sodium bicarbonate, an inexpensive fish anesthetic for field use. Progressive Fish Culturist 40:11–13.

Bove, F.J. (date unknown) MS222 Sandoz. The Anaesthetic and Tranquilizer for Fish, Frogs and Other Cold-Blooded Organisms. Sandoz Technical Bulletin, Sandoz Ltd., Switzerland.

Brown, L.A. (1985) Pain in fish. In: Pain in Animals. British Veterinary Association, Animal Welfare Foundation Symposium, London.

Brown, L.A. (1987) Recirculation anesthesia for laboratory fish. Lab. Anim. 21:210–215.

Brown, L.A. (1988) Anesthesia in fish. Small animal practice. Tropical fish medicine (M. Stoskopf, ed.). Vet. Clin. North Am. 18(2):317–330.

Brown, L.A., Ainsworth, J.A., Beleau, M.H., Bentinck-Smith, J., Francis-Floyd, R., Waterstrat, P.R., and Freund, J.A. (1986) The effects of tricaine methane sulphonate, flunixin meglumide and metomidate on serum cortisol in channel catfish (Ictaluris punctatus Rafinesque). Conference Proceedings. 17th International Association for Aquatic Animal Medicine conference and workshop, Biloxi, Mississippi.

Carrasco, S., Sumano, H., and Navarro-Fierro, R. (1984) The use of lidocaine-sodium bicarbonate as anaesthetic in fish. Aquaculture 41:395–398.

Davis, K.B., Parker, N.C., and Suttle, M.A. (1982) Plasma corticosteroids and chlorides in striped bass exposed to tricaine methanesulfonate, quinaldine, etomidate and salt. Progressive Fish Culturist 44(4):205–207.

Dixon, R.N., and Milton, P. (1978) The effects of the anesthetic quinaldine on oxygen consumption in an intertidal teleost, Blennius pholis (L). J. Fish Biol. 12:359–369.

Fromm, P.O., Richards, B.D., and Hunter, R.C. (1971) Effects of some insecticides and MS222 on isolated perfused gills of trout. Progressive Fish Culturist 33:138–305.

Garey, W.F., and Rahn, H. (1970) Normal arterial gas tensions and pH and breathing frequency of the electric eel. Resp. Physiol. 9:141–150.

Godefroi, E.F., Janssen, P.A.J., Van der Eycken, C.A.M., Van Heertum, H.M.T., and Niemeyeers, C.J.E. (1965) DL-1-(1-arylalkyl) imidazole-5-carboxylate esters. A novel type of hypnotic agent. J. Med. Chem. 9:220–223.

Holeton, G.F., and Randall, D.J. (1967) Changes in blood pressure in the rainbow trout during hypoxia. J. Exp. Biol. 46:297–305.

Jeney, Z., Jeney, G., and Olah, J. (1986) Propanidid, a new anaesthetic for use in fish propagation. Aquaculture 54:149–156.

Jolly, D.W., Mawdesley-Thomas, L.E., and Bucke, D. (1972) Anesthesia of fish. Vet. Rec. 91:424–426.

Klontz, G.W., and Smith, L.S. (1968) Methods of using fish as biological research subjects. In: Methods of Animal Experimentation. Vol. 3. Academic Press, New York.

Lagler, K.F., Bardach, J.E., Miller, R.E., and Passino, D.R.M. (1977) Ichthyology. 2nd ed. John Wiley & Sons, New York.

Martindale (1977) The Extra Pharmacopoeia. 27th ed (Wade, A., ed.). The Pharmaceutical Press, London.

McFarland, W.N. (1960) The use of anesthetics for the handling and the transport of fishes. Calif. Fish Game 46:407–431.

McFarland, W.N., and Klontz, G.W. (1959) Anesthesia in fishes. Fed. Proc. 28:1535–1540.

Murae, T., Andrews, J.W., and Muller, J.W. (1979) Fingerling American shad: Effect of Valium, MS-22 and sodium chloride on handling mortality. Progressive Fish Culturist 15(2):74.

Nelson, P.R. (1953) Use of three anesthetics on juvenile salmon and trout. Progressive Fish Culturist 15(2):74.

Pickering, A.D. (1981) Stress and Fish. Academic Press, London, pp. 1–9.

Ross, L.G., and Ross, B. (1984) Anaesthetic and sedative techniques for fish. Institute of Aquaculture. University of Stirling, Scotland.

Sado, E.K. (1985) Influence of the anaesthetic quinaldine on some tilapias. Aquaculture 10:55–62.

Sebel, P.S., Verghese, C., and Makin, H.L.J. (1983) Effect of plasma cortisol concentrations on a single induction dose of etomidate or thiopentone. Lancet 2(8350):625.

Shelton, G., and Randall, D.J. (1962) The relationship between heart beat and respiration in teleost fish. Comp. Bichem. Physiol. 7:237–250.

Soivio, A., Nyholm, K., and Huhti, M. (1977) Effects of anesthesia with MS 222, neutralized MS-22 and benzocaine on the blood constituents of rainbow trout, Salmo gaidneri. J. Fish. Biol. 10:91–101.

Stoskopf, M.K. (1990) Personal communication.

Stoskopf, M.K. (1985) Manual for the Aquatic Animal Workshop. American Association for Laboratory Animal Science National Capital Area Branch, Washington, D.C.

Stoskopf, M.K., and Arnold, J. (1985) Metomidate anesthesia of ornamental freshwater fish (Proc. International Association for Aquatic Animal Medicine. Also Data on File: Wildlife Laboratories Inc.

Takeda, T., and Itazawa, Y. (1983) Examination of the possibility in applying anesthesia by carbon dioxide in the transportation of live fish. Bull. Jpn. Soc. Sci. Fish. 49(5):725–732.

Tytler, P., and Hawkins, A.D. (1981) Vivisection, anaesthetics and minor surgery. In: Aquarium systems (Hawkins, A.D., ed.). Academic Press, London, pp. 247–278.

Wedemeyer, G. (1970) Stress of anesthesia with MS222 and benzocaine in rainbow trout. J. Fish. Res. Bd. Canad. 27:909–914.

Williams, T.D., Christiansen, J., and Nygren, S. (1988) A comparison of intramuscular anesthetics in teleosts and elasmobranchs. IAAAM Proc. 19:148.

Chapter 7

SURGERY

MICHAEL K. STOSKOPF

Fish are generally excellent surgical patients. At first glance, this might appear an absurd statement, but a wide variety of complex surgical procedures have been performed successfully on fish, using relatively primitive techniques. The advent of better surgical practices with fish can only be expected to improve the therapeutic value of fish surgery. This chapter reviews several techniques developed primarily for research purposes and discusses clinical surgical applications in the hopes of bringing veterinary surgeons into the future advancement of fish surgery.

PREOPERATIVE CONSIDERATIONS

Most surgical texts open with a discussion of preoperative preparations and positioning considerations. This chapter will not be an exception. Preparation of the surgical area on fish is quite controversial. The desire for sterile operating fields seems intuitively important, but fish skin is easily damaged, and the constant mucus production makes any form of sterilization transient at best. Disinfectants can damage fish skin to the point that surgical wounds will not heal, and skin preparation with standard disinfecting protocols is not feasible. Fish skin is easily damaged by alcohols and surgical scrub solutions, and the exuberant response of the mucus-producing glands to that damage far exceeds any potential benefits derived from using them.

Alcohol should not be used on fish. Dilute povidone-iodine solutions have been used without harm to some fish species, but they chemically burn the skin of other species. The problem of maintaining a sterile field in fish surgery is further complicated by the need to keep the patient moist at all times and provide high-quality water for the animal to breathe. Surgical preparation for fish is usually limited to a gentle sponging of most of the mucus from the immediate surgical area. Surgical infections do not seem to be a serious problem when skin preparation is handled this way, as long as good sterile techniques are practiced in the surgery. It is possible to sew a drape to the wound edges in larger fish. This seems appropriate and useful when the animal is large enough to allow it to be done efficiently.

Underwater Surgery

One of the first approaches to fish surgery that comes to mind is to perform the surgery under water. At first thought, this seems the logical solution to maintaining respiration and skin protection for the animal. It has been used on occasion, but this method has usually been abandoned early in the careers of budding fish surgeons. Aside from the expected drawbacks of wound contamination and osmotic tissue damage, the altruistic basis of the approach wears thin with some of the difficulties the surgeon faces. Not the least of these is the difficulty in viewing the field when the water surface is constantly disturbed by the surgeon's hand motions. The rippling water makes it nearly impossible to focus on the surgical site. This has been solved by placing the operating field under a glass-bottomed viewing box; however, the solution is not elegant. If the viewing bucket is large, the surgeon must move his arms and hands around the viewing aid to reach the surgical site. The problem of refraction bending the light and making the surgical site appear in a position different from expected is less of a problem than expected. Most surgeons acclimate to this correction nearly automatically after just a few minutes working. The problem is exacerbated by deeper water, and it is best to keep the fish patient in a shallow container. When doing microsurgery, the problem essentially disappears unless the surgeon has the bad habit of looking around the microscope.

What does cause a great deal of aggravation when operating under water is the loosely floating suture material. Controlling suture material under water is a quite different skill from working in air. Under water, the suture material does not tend to make it to rest before it is time to manipulate it again, and the capture of free-floating suture with needle holders is akin to catching flies with chopsticks. It is possible with practice, but it is not an instinctive art.

Surgery Out of Water

Many fish surgeries are performed with the fish out of water, laying flat on a surface that will either absorb water or allow it to run off without running into the surgeon's lap. This has obvious advantages for the surgeon, who can work in the surgical site in much the same way as in any other animal. There are, however, important disadvantages for the fish patient and the anesthesiologist. Delivery of adequate oxygenated water to the fish to maintain respiration is very difficult. The relatively low oxygen capacity of water makes it necessary to move considerable volumes of water past the gills to keep a fish surgical patient oxygenated. The amount of water involved exceeds the absorbance capacity of most materials for any procedure longer than a few minutes. Even troughs designed to carry the water away from where the surgeon is working are generally inadequate to handle the necessary water volumes. A few designs for fish surgical tables have been published (Reinecker and Ruddell, 1974). One design that works reasonably well has a mesh screen in the head region of the fish to allow water to fall through to a bucket. A second relatively successful design simply uses a perforated plastic board under the entire fish.

Even with a functioning water-removal system, the fact that large amounts of water are being passed over the gills to exit out the opercular openings can

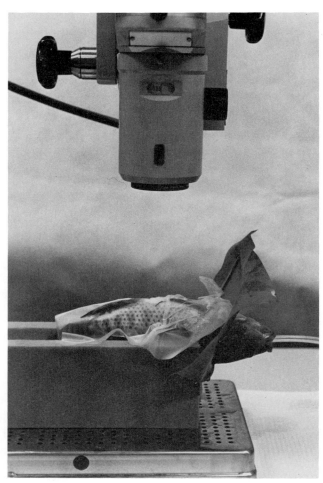

FIGURE 7–2. Fish prepared for surgery with a rubber dental dam in place to prevent flooding of the surgical site.

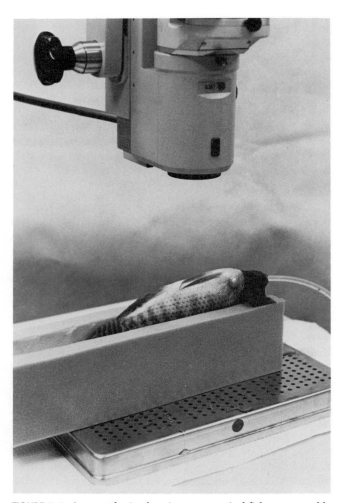

FIGURE 7–1. An anesthetized patient on a typical fish surgery table with the area under the head perforated.

cause difficulties in any abdominal surgery. An innovative approach to keeping the surgical site free of water coming from the opercula is to use a rubber dental dam placed around the fish just anterior to the incision site (Fig. 7–2). The dam can be restrained by a normal dental dam frame, or some surgeons have made their own frames. In the absence of a dental dam rubber, the palms of latex rubber gloves have been used successfully, although a dental dam is more reliable.

The hole in the dam is made close to one edge of the frame and the fish is pushed head first through the dam until the gills and opercula are not obstructed. With this apparatus in place, water coming out of the opercula hits the dam and flows down through the table to the reservoir.

An extension of the dental dam method has been used in a variety of forms that I call "diving helmet" systems. In these systems, the fish patient's head is enclosed in a water-filled container with a rubber membrane fitted behind the opercula. Anesthetic and water is circulated through the chamber, and the remainder of the fish's body is available for surgery. For longer, more complex procedures, this approach is useful; however, commercial helmets are not available, and each fish surgeon has to make his own. Also, depending on the design of the helmet, calibrating flows to keep the helmet full without blowing out the rubber gasket can be tricky.

Even if all water is kept out of the surgical sites by a well-functioning dam device, the skin and fins of the patient must still be kept moist. The mucus production of the skin will also make picking up sutures from the body surface very difficult. The use of drapes has not yet been established in fish surgery. The arguments against them center around the ease with which the cuticle of fish skin can be damaged, and the fact that cloth or paper drapes invariably become wet anyway and, therefore, pose no barrier to bacteria. Proponents of the use of drape materials generally argue that their purpose is entirely to aid the surgeon in working with suture materials, and the failure to serve as a barrier to bacteria is not an issue, since if they are not used, there is no barrier anyway. Using light-weight, absorbent drape materials has several potential advantages. They keep mucus produced by the fish from getting on instruments and suture material. They can be moistened and serve to keep the body and fins of the fish from drying during the surgery with much less interference than constantly spraying the body with water. The material used to drape the fish should be soft and absorbent enough to hold considerable water. A plastic drape may be placed around the surgical site and over any cloth or porous drape used.

Keeping a drape in place is an interesting problem in fish surgery. Even pediatric towel forceps are much too large for use on most fish, and frankly, they do not work very well, even on large patients. Some investigators glue the edges of their drapes down around the incision using methacrylate glue. I have not found this particularly useful and have observed that some species of fish develop quite dramatic allergic reactions to methacrylate glues placed on their skin. Other approaches that are used include applying a thin bead of Vaseline around the surgical site with a syringe and pressing the drape into it (Fig. 7–3). Other materials could probably also be used in this manner. This approach does not hold as well as glue, but it has the advantage of being much easier to remove. As mentioned, some surgeons sew a drape to the edge of surgical incisions in larger specimens. This technique works very well.

Positioning

For operations on fins, or the lateral body, positioning is easy with most fusiform fishes. They are relatively stable when placed in lateral recumbency. Stability and positioning can be improved with the use of water-soaked foam pads in various shapes. Small wedges of loose-celled foam are very helpful.

The majority of invasive clinical surgeries in fishes, including laparotomies, are usually performed through a ventral midline incision with the fish in dorsal recumbency. For fusiform fishes, this presents a greater challenge than the positioning for a lateral approach. A number of fish-positioning devices have been illustrated in the research literature, and frankly most of them are not particularly applicable to clinical surgery. They often consist of complex clamps and rods, with or without pads, that hold the fish in position (Goetz et al., 1977). They can be no more than a vice with foam-padded jaws (Tytler and

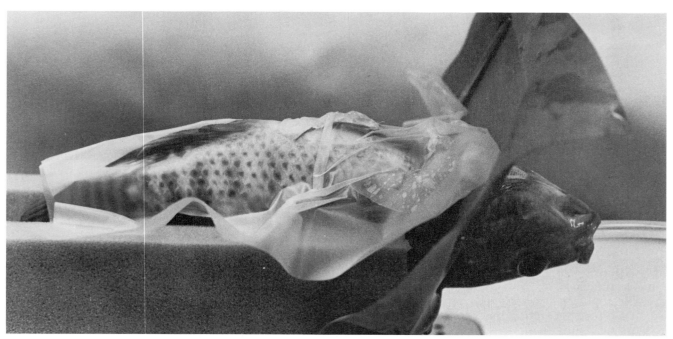

FIGURE 7–3. Plastic drape being held in place with Vaseline.

Hawkins, 1981). The fish can be held in an appropriate position with foam troughs or by foam wedges, although the latter tend to slip out at inopportune moments. Another technique is to strap the fish to a padded plastic board with padded elastic bands, and then clamp the board vertically in a vice. This works reasonably well but does not give the surgeon much support and restricts one side of the fish. A cut out in the edge of the board helps, but I prefer to use a foam trough. Hopefully, future innovation by clinical surgeons will improve the options available for positioning fish for laparotomy.

MICROSURGERY TECHNIQUES

A good portion of fish surgery qualifies as microsurgery. Most fish patients are relatively small and freshwater tropical ornamental species are often extremely small. It behooves anyone interested in clinical surgery of fishes to develop microsurgical skills and equip their facility with appropriate instruments. Good courses in microsurgery are available, but consistent practice of the skills is critical to developing a good microsurgeon. It is important to have a quiet environment free of interruption and other activity in your clinical facility for performing microsurgery. The surgical table should be a comfortable height (usually 30 to 33 inches) and allow relaxed work from a sitting position with the forearms and wrists supported on the table surface. The surgeon should avoid strenuous activity or manual labor for at least 24 hours prior to operating to minimize normal physiologic tremor. Avoidance of caffeine and nicotine is also advisable on the same grounds. Try to exercise your surgical skills on practice situations at least once a week if clinical surgical cases are not plentiful.

Microscope Selection and Use

Much of the microsurgery performed in fish can be accomplished using optical loupes (Fig. 7–4). These are available as separate binoculars or as insets to your own prescription glasses. You get what you pay for in these important instruments. It is worthwhile to order custom-fitted loupes. Less expensive loupes with plastic lenses or mounted on plastic headbands are available, but excellent custom loupes can be obtained for less than $600, and they offer many advantages. Custom loupes are adjusted specifically to your own interpupillary distance and are constructed with a focal length based upon your own arm length and body posture during surgery. They decrease fatigue and greatly improve operative control. For fish surgery, a magnification of 2 to 3.5 times is sufficient.

The next step-up in microscope equipment is an expensive one. Operating microscopes are considerably more costly than operating loupes but offer significant advantages if frequent surgical procedures

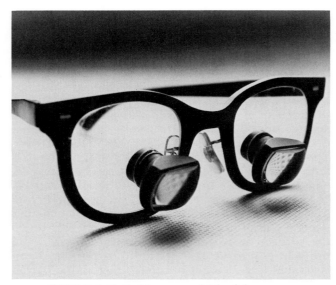

FIGURE 7–4. Optical loupes useful for fish surgery.

are performed (Fig. 7–5). Major advantages include adjustable magnifications, the ability to have dual observation of the surgical field, allowing an assistant to participate in the procedure, and in more expensive units, the ability to photograph the procedure. Disadvantages of the operating microscope include the capital investment cost and the lack of portability.

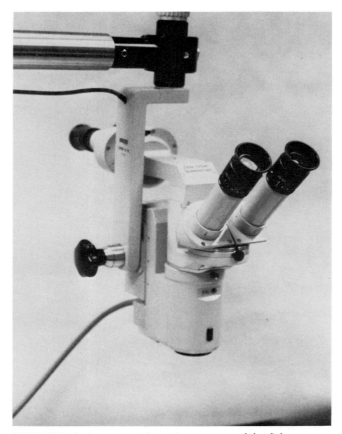

FIGURE 7–5. A stereo operating microscope used for fish surgery.

Instrument Selection and Use

Microsurgical instruments are expensive, delicate, and come in a wide variety of designs. Fish surgeons may want to design their own specialized instruments. Microsurgical instruments should have dull nonreflective surfaces to avoid glare, and when spring handles are employed, should close with gentle tension to avoid finger fatigue (Serafin and Georgiade, 1986).

The essential components of a microsurgical instrument kit are a pair of microscissors with curved iris tips, a needle holder with curved, tapered jaws, a Downing-Bonn 1 X 2 tooth forceps, a Downing-Harms tying forceps, and two number 4 jeweler's forceps (Fig. 7–6). If the surgeon intends to accomplish vessel reanastomosis, two atraumatic microvessel clamps, a microvessel approximating clamp, and an angled clamp applicator should be included in the kit (Serafin and Georgiade, 1986). Additions to the kit may also include retractors, microsuction tips, and fine hot-wire cautery devices. A wide variety of forceps is available, but all are extremely fragile and must be handled carefully. Prior to surgery, the tips of all forceps to be used should have been examined under the loupes or the microscope for bent tips or burred, rough edges. Jeweler's forceps make a good substitution for more expensive specialized needle holders; however, the surgeon must avoid grasping the needle so that it twists or slips during the manipulation.

Suture Materials

A broad range of suture materials can be obtained for microsurgical uses. Most commonly used are 8/0 (45 μ diameter) to 11/0 (14 μ diameter) monofilament nylon sutures with swedged-on needles. Other materials commonly used include polypropylene, polyglactin 910, and polydioxanone. All appear suitable for use in fish. Needles are available with tapered, reverse cutting or cutting tips as 3/8 circle, 1/2 circle, 1/4 circle, or straight shapes. Needle shape is very often a preference of the individual surgeon. A small needle-to-suture diameter ratio is a benefit in most situations. Tapered needle tips are valuable for repair of friable fascial tissues. Needles with a slight cutting tip are advantageous for working with skin.

Other Microsurgical Techniques

Plasma suturing is a technique that may have broad application in fish surgery. In this method, small amounts of fish plasma are directed to the area requiring stabilization, and then the plasma is encouraged to clot with the addition of tiny quantities of a calcium-containing solution. The technique has not been adequately tested in fish surgery but bears consideration and development.

Blunt dissection techniques are critical to fish surgery. They avoid rupturing vessels and minimize difficulties due to blood loss. After initial skin incisions are made, the bulk of all surgical approaches to fish rely on blunt dissection with forceps or scissors. The closed jaws of the instrument are pushed into connective tissues and then gently opened, separating tissues to create exposure. Hemostasis is critical in the surgical field. This is perhaps best achieved in fish surgery with a small fine-wired heat-cautery unit that uses electrical resistance in small wires to achieve finely directed cauterization. Bipolar coagulators that allow current to flow only between the forceps tips can also be used. Systems that require electrical current to dissipate throughout tissues such as standard Bovie units should not be used with fish. Electrocoagulation in small fish patients can be excessively damaging to adjacent tissues, so great care must be taken to carefully direct its application.

Suction can be used in larger patients to maintain a clear surgical field. It can also be used, especially in smaller patients for surgical ablation and even organ biopsy. Suction tips used for neurosurgery are available and can be adapted to fish surgery, or customized instruments can be made by drawing out and shaping glass Pasteur pipettes commonly found in the laboratory. In small fish, these suction devices are best manipulated using small rubber squeeze bulbs, rather than attaching them to vacuum or suction lines. This allows finer control and avoids excessive tissue removal.

SPECIFIC SURGICAL PROCEDURES

Too few clinically relevant surgical procedures have been adequately described in the literature to

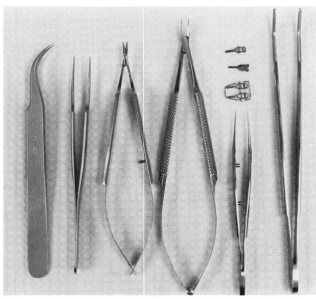

FIGURE 7–6. A typical microsurgical instrument pack.

establish a compendium of approaches and procedures in this chapter. Hopefully, this unfortunate situation will be remedied in the future as more clinicians lend their talents to the field. When in doubt, the surgical principles and techniques that have been established in mammals serve very well in fish surgery.

Laparoscopy

Laparoscopy can be performed in medium- to large-sized fish without difficulty. The approach has been used infrequently but bears more consideration in the future. Laparoscopic examination and guided biopsy are useful tools in fish diagnostics. The approach has been worked out in sharks (Fig. 7–7). The anesthetized shark is placed in left lateral recumbency. An insufflation cannula can be placed in the abdomen in the region of the ventral midline. A 2-mm skin incision made by inserting a number 15 blade is necessary to insert the cannula. The abdomen is insufflated with room air. A second incision is made just above the dorsal base of the right pelvic fin, between the major muscle bundles. Then the shark is tilted head down at about a 35-degree angle to help pull the abdominal organs, including the large liver, forward, away from the trocar insertion site. The laparoscopic trocar is inserted and the shark is returned to a horizontal position. From the insertion point, the liver, spiral valve, rectal gland, and, with difficulty, the caudal kidney can be visualized and biopsied. The liver lobes must be repositioned with a Veres needle to see the other organs. After

the procedure, it is important to remove the excess air from the abdomen before releasing the fish. The entry incision for larger laparoscopes can be closed with simple interrupted resorbable sutures in the skin. Smaller incisions for the insufflation needle and Veres needle can be closed with methacrylate adhesive. The adhesive does not seem to cause contact allergies in the sharks.

Catheter Implantation

The best known procedure in fish surgery is probably the implantation of an arterial cannula in the dorsal aorta of salmon and trout (Smith and Bell, 1964, 1967) (Fig. 7–8). The technique involves implantation of a protective flanged polyethylene tube through the roof of the mouth, exiting just cranial to the nostrils, and anchored in the nasal bone. A smaller polyethylene tube is run through the protective tube, and in the original technique, a hubless needle is attached. The needle is then inserted through the roof of the mouth into the confluence of the efferent branchial arteries as they join the dorsal aorta. The needle and tube can be anchored in various ways, including an oral suture around the needle. This type of cannula is useful for repetitive blood sampling, and for administration of some drugs into the blood. The cannula must be kept heparinized.

In sharks, it is possible to catheterize the dorsal cutaneous vein which runs along dorsal midline just below the surface of the skin. It is easiest to find just cranial or caudal to the first dorsal fin. This vein is

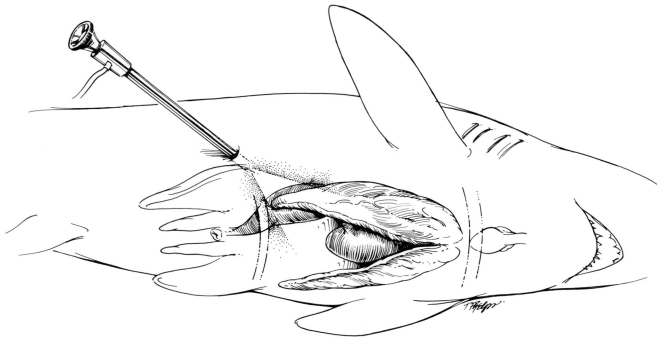

FIGURE 7–7. Laparoscopic examination of the abdominal cavity of the shark.

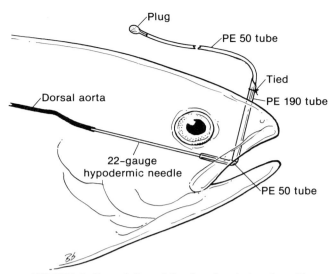

Plug

PE 50 tube

Tied

PE 190 tube

Dorsal aorta

22-gauge
hypodermic needle

PE 50 tube

FIGURE 7–8. Cannulation of the dorsal aorta in salmonids.

small but can be cannulated in larger animals (greater than 20 lbs). This site is preferable for cannulation to the larger ventral caudal vein commonly used for blood sampling, because it is not subject to the movement of the tail and allows the catheter to exit dorsal to the shark rather than ventral.

Laparotomy

The abdominal exploratory procedure in fish is normally performed through a ventral midline incision. The fish is positioned in dorsal recumbency and an incision is made from just anterior to the anal opening, extending forward to the level required for visualization. In scaled fishes, the incision is facilitated by removing a row of scales, but many surgeons do not feel this is necessary. The ventral midline incision provides reasonable visualization of the liver and bowel. With manipulation the stomach and spleen can be located and usually exteriorized. It is difficult in most fish to adequately visualize the swim bladder or the kidneys through this approach. Clinical surgical approaches to the swim bladder have not been worked out but would be of great value.

An exception to the routine ventral midline approach for a routine laparotomy would be the sturgeon. The heavy armored plates of this fish make a

ventral lateral incision more appropriate. It is possible that this approach would also be of value in other fishes. The anus and the pectoral girdle apparatus are used as landmarks for locating the incision over the organs of interest. The ventral midline laparotomy is also impractical in the flounder and presumably in other flatfishes. The preferred approach to abdominal surgery in the flounder is a ventral approach, which is actually a lateral approach because of the unusual development and posture of these fishes.

CLOSURE

Closure in fish surgery is an issue that has not been well studied. It is possible to use absorbable sutures successfully. Polyglycolic acid is frequently employed. Great care must be taken to adequately knot the individual sutures as there is a tendency for polyglycolic acid sutures to untie in sea water. The main advantage of these sutures is there is no need to handle the fish twice to remove sutures. Surgical steel has been used successfully in skin sutures in sharks. It must be removed. Other sutures which have been used successfully in skin incisions in fish include propylene, nylon, and Dacron.

As mentioned earlier in the chapter, specific procedures for approaching various abdominal organs in fish have not been worked out. Surgeons operating on fish are unfortunately required to invent approaches as they go along, based upon their knowledge of mammalian or avian surgery. Hopefully, more of these approaches will be published in the future as more veterinarians explore surgery of fish.

LITERATURE CITED

Goetz, F.W., Hoffman, R.A., and Pancoe, W.L. (1977) A surgical apparatus for fish and its use in the pinealectomy of salmonids. J. Fish Biol. 10:287–290.

Reinecker, R.H., and Ruddell, M.O. (1974) An easily fabricated operating table for fish surgery. Progressive Fish Culturist 36:111–112.

Serafin, D., and Georgiade, N.G. (1986) A Laboratory Manual of Microsurgery. Duke University Medical Center, Durham, North Carolina.

Smith, L.S., and Bell, G.R. (1964) A technique for prolonged blood sampling in free swimming salmon. J. Fish. Res. Bd. Can. 21:711–717.

Smith, L.S., and Bell, G.R. (1967) Anaesthetic and surgical techniques for Pacific salmon. J. Fish. Res. Bd. Can. 24:1579–1588.

Tytler, P., and Hawkins, A.D. (1981) Vivisection, anaesthetics and minor surgery. In Aquarium Systems (Hawkins, A.D., ed.). Academic Press, New York, pp. 247–278.

Chapter 8

HOSPITALIZATION

MICHAEL K. STOSKOPF

Hospitalization of ill fish is still in its infancy. It is being pioneered by large public aquaria and progressive veterinarians developing practices treating large numbers of pet fish. Currently, most clinical fish practices are based on ambulatory visits to obtain diagnostic samples or outpatient clinic visits. This will change as innovative veterinarians develop improved methods for housing patients in the hospital setting. The same advantages and disadvantages accrue to the hospitalized fish patient that are recognized in treating other types of patients. Hospitalized patients can be afforded more intensive treatment and observation by trained medical staff. At the same time, hospitalized animals are subjected to the stresses of being placed in an unfamiliar environment. The advantages and disadvantages must be weighed in each individual case.

This chapter deals with the current state of small aquarium fish housing as it applies to hospitalization. Information on keeping fish is available in a variety of books on aquaculture and mariculture. Although this chapter is focused on criteria for selecting equipment and deploying it, every practitioner considering hospitalization of fish should realize that dedicated staff, trained and experienced in keeping healthy fish, are the most important asset to fish wards. High-technology filtration and monitoring systems can never substitute for individuals experienced in good animal husbandry.

GENERAL CONSIDERATIONS

Properly designed hospital facilities should provide an even better environment for the patient than it experiences in its exhibit or home tank. This, of course, is a difficult goal to achieve, but all aspects of a fish's husbandry needs must be considered in designing a successful hospital tank. First and foremost, the water must be of the highest quality and stable. This is complicated in a hospital system because the need to disinfect often limits the choices of filtration available, as will be discussed later in this chapter. On the other hand, the proper design of a hospital system should provide tremendous flexibility in water manipulation, making it easier to respond to an individual's water needs.

It is critical that the hospital tank design provide easy observation and access to the patient. The viewing areas of the tank should allow observation of all corners of the tank. It should be possible to capture a patient calmly and without undue effort to allow close examination or delivery of medication. A well-designed hospital tank should provide appropriate light cycles and substrates to allow a fish to be comfortable, and it must facilitate environmental manipulation, including adjustment of temperature, modifications of salinity, and execution of water changes. In addition, a hospital tank must be more easily cleaned, broken down, disinfected, and restarted than a home or display aquarium.

SYSTEM DESIGNS

An integral decision in system design for a fish hospital is the size and shape of the tanks to be used. Perhaps the first decision is to determine how many tanks are going to be required, and how large or small they should be. Small tanks offer great flexibility for keeping large numbers of patients from different sources in a relatively small space. They are also economical if expensive drugs are going to be used as water treatments. Unfortunately, small tanks are also inherently more volatile and must be watched much more carefully to avoid environmental problems that can be detrimental to a fish patient.

Large tanks offer a greater latitude with water quality and are less confining to the patient. Unfortunately, besides taking up space, large tanks take much more time to drain and refill for disinfection, etc., and medications delivered in the water can become prohibitively expensive. The decision of what size and how many tanks to set up depends upon your practice expectations. However, in most cases, it is a good idea to have a mix of tank sizes. Even if you expect your practice will be exclusively small tropical freshwater species, it is inevitable that with time you will be called upon to treat older, larger specimens, and the option to hospitalize them will be dependent upon the availability of a suitable, large hospital tank. A good starting mix of tanks for a pet fish practice would include three or four 15-gal tanks, three or four 30-gal tanks, at least one 50-gal tank, and perhaps a 100-gal tank (Fig. 8–1). This would vary, of course, if your clientele has a predilection for large carnivorous fishes. If you have clients that maintain large systems, you may want to consider hospital tanks that hold 300 gals.

In general, it is a good idea to avoid tanks smaller than 15 gal unless you expect to have a large Siamese fighting fish practice. These fish will tear up their

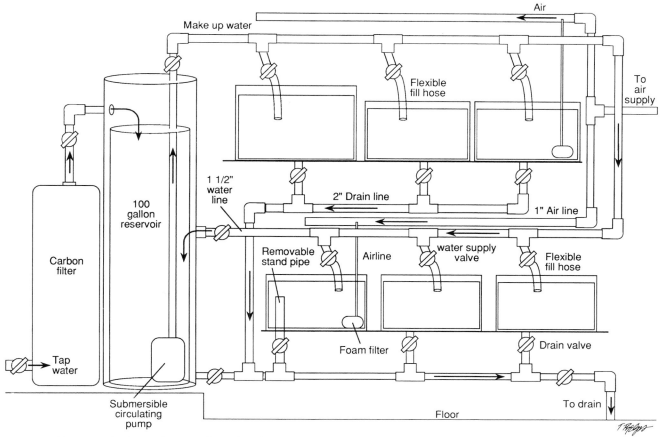

FIGURE 8–1. Diagram of a hospital system for a clinic beginning to see pet fish patients. Three 15-gallon, two 30-gallon, and a 50-gallon tank are arranged on two shelves with enough room for twice the height of the tanks plus room for the pipes. Tap water is filtered through a carbon filter using tap pressure to remove chlorine. Dechlorinated water is stored in a 100-gallon reservoir and circulated through the make-up water loop with a magnetic drive submersible pump. Each tank has a bulkhead fitting in the bottom connected to a drain through a valve to allow easy draining of the tank. Standpipes are used only as an extra security measure to avoid accidental draining from leaky valves. Each tank has a fill hose and valve above it connected to the make-up water loop. Air is supplied through a manifold system from a remote air pump. The system is designed for frequent (daily) water changes and tank disinfections. Foam filters can be used if desired.

fins if placed in too large a tank. Otherwise, it is usually much easier to place a fish in an oversized tank than to try and keep it alive in a tank that is too small. In addition, it costs about the same to buy filters, lights, tops, etc., for 15-gal tanks as it does for smaller tanks.

Most small aquaria are square or rectangular. This offers the advantage of being able to place a maximum number of tanks in a given space. On the other hand, corners can present some disconcerting problems in water circulation and fish management. These will not usually be a problem working with smaller species, but if you have clients who maintain sharks or other rapidly swimming fish, you may need to consider round tanks. Round tanks allow continuous swimming patterns in pelagic species and can be manipulated to direct water flow around the periphery of the tank, minimizing incidences of fish colliding with tank walls or rubbing in corners of the tank.

If you choose rectangular tanks, remember, not all rectangles are created equal. The depth of the

tank and the width-to-length ratio will be important. A hospitalized fish must be able to turn around freely in its tank. It must also be able to make its normal vertical movements within the water column. From a husbandry standpoint, it is always best to have a working depth that allows the aquarist to reach the bottom of the tank with ease. Certainly, the issue of surface area for air exchange is important, but even more important in a hospital system, tanks should not require the veterinarian to get his sleeve and armpit wet to reach the bottom and corral a patient. It simply is not conducive to good medical care to have a tank that makes it very difficult to catch the patient.

HUMAN ERGONOMICS

Woe to the veterinarian who fails to consider the ergonomics of maintaining and working with a fish hospital tank. There is no quicker way to convince yourself and your staff that aquatic medicine is not for you or them than to have a labor-intensive fish ward. Certainly, one of the largest problems is provision of adequate overhead clearance. It is very tempting to try and pack as many tanks as possible into a vertical space. Not only is this a bad idea because of the disease transmission problems discussed later, but it makes it very difficult to operate the tanks.

Remember that to be used conveniently, a net should reach the bottom of a tank with enough of the handle exposed to allow easy manipulation. That means the minimum overhead clearance for any tank should exceed the depth of the tank if nets are going to be used without impediment. Certainly, it is possible to catch a fish by slipping a net in sideways and carefully maneuvering the fish to a place in the tank where it can be carefully lifted out, but considerable time and irritation can be saved by making the access to the top of a tank complete. Net access to tanks can be enhanced by having tops that are completely removable, and lighting systems that are also easily moved to allow open access to the tank. If you are putting in large systems, do not forget that the distance from the top of the water to the ceiling should be at least as great as the depth of the tank.

Make the controls and monitors for the environmental systems of the tanks easily accessible. This makes it much more likely that they will be examined regularly and adjusted when necessary. If you or your technician must squat down and peer under a dark shelf to examine a pump's bearings, chances are it will not happen.

Also, spare no effort to provide good visibility into the tanks from a comfortable position. Tanks made entirely of glass provide excellent visibility, but it is common for larger tanks, built with opaque materials, to have large blind spots that can only be seen by major contortions of the viewer, if they can be seen at all. Do not attempt to save money on the viewing ports of your tanks.

Finally, no matter how difficult it is, be sure to design your systems so they can be drained completely without having to resort to baling buckets, mops, or sponges (Fig. 8–2). Unfortunately, many bulkhead systems for installing bottom drains have a significant lip, which results in not being able to passively drain a tank completely dry. Consider building up the bottoms of these tanks to minimize the amount of moping and sponging required, or use a tank design that does not require a bulkhead fitting. It will repay you many times over with saved labor.

PISCEAN ERGONOMICS

Of course, the consideration of your fish patient's comfort is also important in hospital tank design. Unfortunately, the wide variety of fish patients, with their often very specialized needs, makes

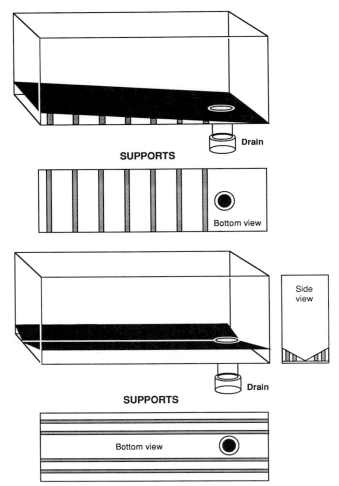

FIGURE 8–2. Alternative ways of building up the bottom of a tank to make it drain more easily.

an exhaustive treatment of this subject impossible in this chapter. It must suffice to say that the hospital tank system you design should be flexible and allow provision of appropriate light cycles, thermoregulation, space, and cover for your patient. Light cycles are often neglected in fish management, and they should not be. It may even be valuable to be able to have certain patients on partially reversed day/night cycles. This certainly aids in the observation of nocturnal feeders, allowing them to be fed and watched during normal practice hours.

Likewise, cover and substrates must allow a fish to be comfortable in the tank but, at the same time, not hinder capture or observation of the patient. Plastic piping can often be used to provide hiding places for fish (Figs. 8–4 and 8–5). Clear piping is often accepted by a fish just as well as opaque piping, especially if tank lighting is kept subdued except during observation. Animals that need to burrow in sand can be easily observed through clear glass gravel placed in patches, in removable containers, or covering the entire bottom of the tank.

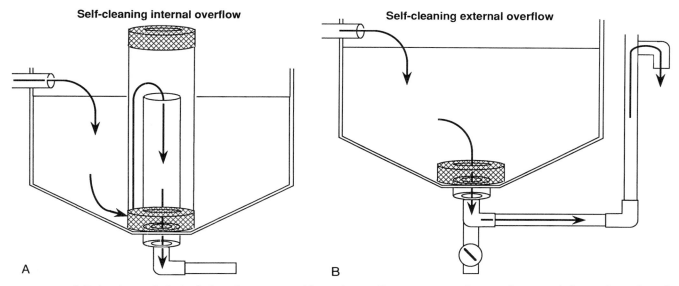

FIGURE 8–3. Self-cleaning tank drain designs for systems with continuous-flow or automated water changers. *A.* Internal overflow. *B,* External overflow.

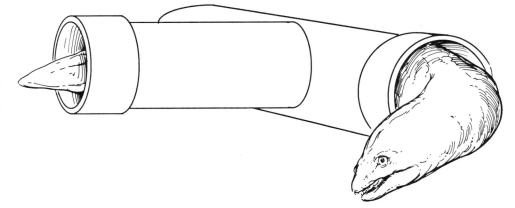

FIGURE 8–4. Plastic piping can be used to provide easily disinfectable hiding places for fish in a hospital tank.

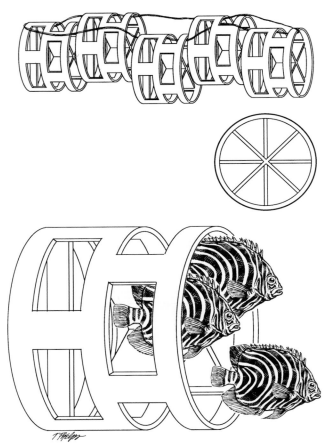

FIGURE 8–5. Smaller fish use large floating plastic bio-rings for cover. The rings can be strung together to make structures that will float just under the surface of the water.

SAFETY

The issue of safety in hospital tank design affects both patients and your staff. The major safety hazard of hospital aquaria is electrocution. It is very important to design your facility to minimize the chance of an electrical accident. Use ground fault breakers in the receptacles that provide power to the room. Make sure all grounds are properly wired. Train your employees in the safe use of electricity near water. Make sure the floors and drains of the facility do not add to the hazard by retaining standing water. Use nets with nonconducting handles. Avoid any form of exposed wiring.

Equally devastating for your patients would be an accidental loss of power or equipment failure which resulted in the draining of the water from the hospital tank (Figs. 8–6 and 8–7). It is possible to design your plumbing approach so that if the system should stop running adequate water remains in the tank to allow the patient to survive. Generally, this means that in normal operation, you want the process of removing water from the tank limited by a standpipe or another device that protects the tank water level. If a pump fails, no siphons should allow the tank to continue to drain without return flow.

Finally, good tops on your tanks are important to your staff and to your patients. They can prevent fish from jumping out of tanks unobserved and dying on the floor of your facility. A good top can also stop dropped objects from accidentally finding their way into your tanks.

PLUMBING

The limitations on hospital tank filtration methods make their plumbing rather straightforward. Most small tanks made of glass simply have their filters attached through tubes run over the side of the tank like a typical home aquarium. However, if several small systems are being installed, consider the plumbing rules for larger systems, which minimize the labor required to clean and change water and decrease the potential for accidental tank drainings.

The general rule in plumbing a larger system is to use gravity as much as possible. Minimize the use of power pumps and make sure it is impossible for tanks to drain if a pump fails, power is interrupted, or water circulation stops for any reason (see Figs. 8–6 and 8–7). At the same time, ensure that it is

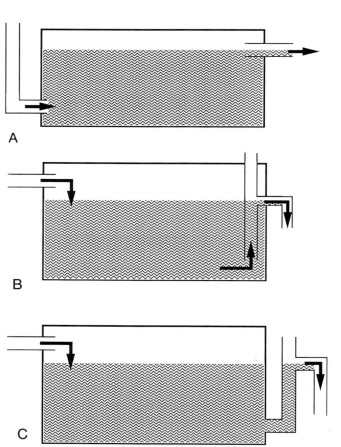

FIGURE 8–6. Three designs that allow water to circulate into and out of a tank continuously without risk of the tank draining if a pump or the electrical supply fails. *A.* Top level effluent method. *B.* Internal open siphon method. *C.* External open siphon method.

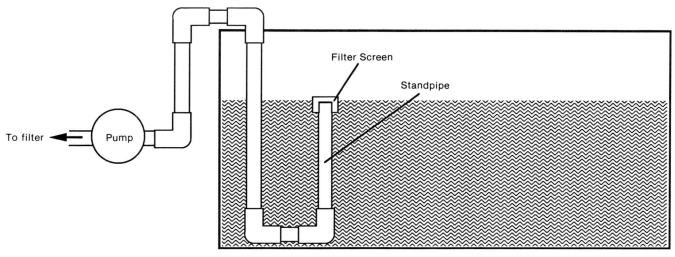

FIGURE 8–7. A way of retrofitting a tank that cannot be drilled for an internal standpipe system, which will not drain the tank in case of a power failure.

possible to completely drain the enclosures. Accomplishing these feats is usually simpler in hospital systems than in those that use complex filters and biological filtration. The need to be able to adequately disinfect the entire hospital system limits the complexity of the plumbing problem. Bottom drains can be fitted with standpipes to prevent accidental draining. Return water can be sprayed onto the water surface of the tank to increase aeration (Fig. 8–8) or delivered beneath the surface to minimize aerosolization (Fig. 8–9). Circulation can be provided by standing free-standing airlifts.

The need for frequent water changes in the hospital systems means consideration of reserve water sources must have high priority in fish hospital design. Reserve water systems should be thermally tempered and preferably designed to allow delivery of water of appropriate pH and hardness to every hospital tank in the wards (Fig. 8–10). The reserve should minimally allow an immediate 50% water change of the entire ward volume in cases of emergency (Fig. 8–11).

MATERIALS SELECTION

Aquaria can be constructed of anything that will retain water. Whether a fish will survive in the tank is another question. Only a few materials and designs are suitable for hospital tanks, but your clients may be using a wider variety of materials. These are also discussed, if only to make sure their use is avoided in hospital tank construction.

Glass

For small hospital systems, all-glass tanks are probably an ideal choice. They afford excellent visibility and are relatively chemically inert. Glass has certain advantages over plastic. It is harder and less easily scratched during maintenance than acrylic plastics (although plastic-coated safety plate is also readily scratched). Plastics require solvent sealing and cannot be properly sealed with silicone sealants, making construction and repair more difficult. Glass is also less expensive than high-quality, clear acrylics.

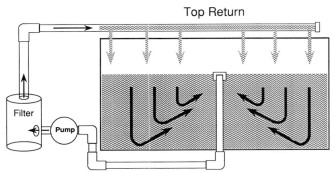

FIGURE 8–8. Top withdrawal with surface return. Turbulence will be least near the bottom, and debris will accumulate around the standpipe base.

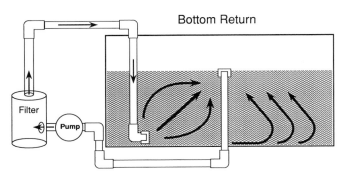

FIGURE 8–9. Top withdrawal with bottom return. Turbulence will be least at the surface around the perimeter. Debris will accumulate in the far bottom corners and behind the influent pipe.

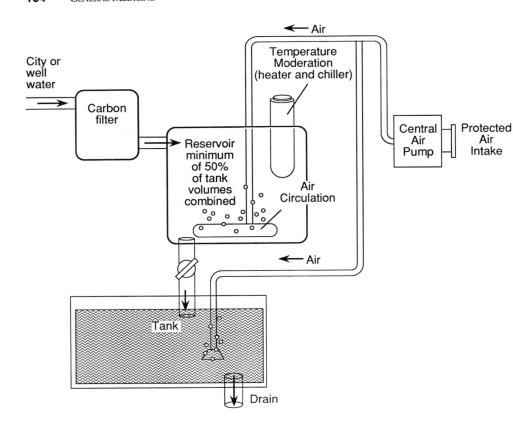

FIGURE 8–10. Diagram of a freshwater recirculating system with carbon prefiltration, and a minimum of 50% reserve reservoir of tempered and aerated water for emergency water changes.

FIGURE 8–11. Schematic of a marine reservoir system that requires a brine reservoir and optimally a marine water make-up reservoir in addition to the freshwater reservoir.

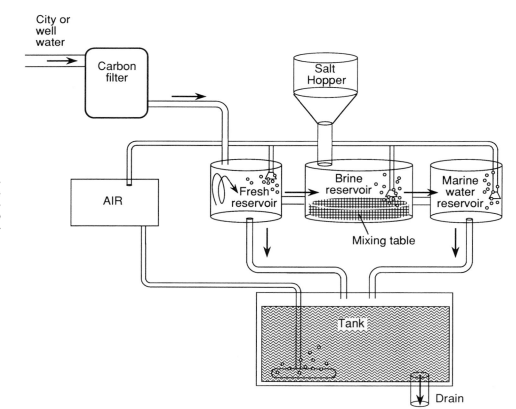

On the negative side, glass is infinitely more breakable than most plastics and difficult to drill for some plumbing applications. If you construct or repair your own all-glass tanks, remember to use only high-grade silicone. Low-grade, inexpensive silicone caulks contain heavy metals, cyanide, and organic toxins, which can kill fish. Systems larger than 200 L require extremely thick glass. Complex plumbing is also more common in these systems, making plastic construction a major benefit.

Plastics

Plastics cover a wide range of materials with quite diverse properties. Do not accept plastic construction materials without careful consideration of the type of plastic. Clear plastics used as glass substitutes are usually highly specialized acrylics. They are expensive, relatively soft, and susceptible to scratching. Acrylics have the advantage over glass that they can be molded in panes to fill very large spans (Hawkins and Lloyd, 1981). They are not subject to shattering with the same forces that affect glass but can be broken. Acrylic panes are subject to melting from the heat of photographic lights and can catch fire. Little is known about their interaction with chemicals and drugs used in the treatment of fish.

Opaque plastics are also used as structural components of tanks. Many plastics have been used for this purpose. New or unknown materials should be tested for toxicity with a bioassay before they are used with a client's fish. Materials graded as acceptable for foodstuffs are usually acceptable for aquarium systems. Recycled plastics should be avoided.

Fiber glass has the highest tension-loading capacity of the plastics (Wheaton, 1977a). It is relatively inexpensive, and probably the most commonly used structural plastic in aquarium construction (Hawkins and Lloyd, 1981). It is not suitable for construction of toxicological evaluation facilities because of the variability of toxin leaching from the hardening resins. Newly constructed tanks incorporating fiber glass should be treated carefully to rid the system of polymerizing agent and trapped metals in the fiber glass resin. This can be accomplished by alternately running the filled system for a day with fresh water of pH 3.0 or lower, followed by fresh water of pH 11 or higher, and finally fresh water at pH 3.0, discarding the water after each pH shift. A final leeching with salt water for an additional day is desirable if the tank is destined to be a marine aquarium. The entire treatment process is facilitated by the use of warm water (37 to 40°C). A bioassay is still advisable before using such a system for patients.

Vinyl is a flexible plastic used in swimming pool liners, which is used in the manufacture of inexpensive makeshift holding facilities. It is not durable, easily damaged, and can have tremendous residuals of toxic plasticizer and heavy metals trapped in the polymerization process. These leach out into the water. Dioctyl phthalate is a common contaminant,

and although 10 days of soaking and etching is recommended for its removal (Carmignani and Bennett, 1976), it makes vinyl a poor choice in any fish system.

High-density linear polyethylene and polypropylene tanks are relatively inert and can be stripped with the same protocol described for fiber glass, making them essentially free of heavy metal and plasticizer contaminants. Such tanks are expensive. They are opaque and quite suited for use in fish systems.

Polyvinyl chloride generally is not used in tank construction, but it is used in the construction of the plumbing systems that operate tanks. Polyvinyl chloride is basically inert to salt water, however, it comes in several types or schedules. These have different properties. High-impact or unplasticized polyvinyl chloride is most commonly used for plumbing applications but can contain trace amounts of metals, particularly lead, which can be leached in acid water systems (Hawkins and Lloyd, 1981). Acrylonitrile butadiene styrene pipes are less likely to cause subtle toxicity problems and are recommended in construction of hospital systems.

Concrete

Concrete is widely used for very large systems because of its durability, low cost, and formability. It is a consideration when constructing a facility for large fish and may be used by aquaculture or display aquarium clients.

Concrete has a strong resistance to compression but lacks tensile strength and shear resistance, which must be provided by metal reinforcement buried in the concrete. Concrete is very alkaline because of free lime produced by hydration of the surface of the cement. It also contains small amounts of foreign materials, including chromates, which can leach out slowly over a long period after tank construction. In seawater, the alkalinization effect of concrete is buffered by the carbonate system. Nevertheless, concrete structures should be thoroughly washed or leached with dilute muriatic acid, and coated with several layers of sodium silicate or other sealant before being used for fish. A soaking period of several weeks, adjusting pH and discarding water, is recommended.

Generally, concrete is very durable, even in seawater, although it can be made more durable by the exclusion of tricalcium aluminate and substitution of tetracalcium aluminoferrite to inhibit sulfate attack. To minimize salt penetration to reinforcing bars, a layer of 50 to 75 mm of compacted concrete must separate the metal from the exposure surface (Hawkins and Lloyd, 1981). When concrete does fail in an aquarium, it is usually due to the failure of the reinforcing steel being oxidized by seawater. The steel is passivated by the concrete, but exposure to seawater and oxygen will destroy this protection, allowing corrosion. Protection of the structural steel is of tantamount importance in concrete tank maintenance. Quick-setting, high alumina cement should not be used in aquaria because of the tendency to crumble with prolonged exposure to moisture (Hawkins and Lloyd, 1981; Wheaton, 1977a).

Wood

You may have clients that use wood construction. It is a useful material. Your clients should use well-dried, seasoned heartwood, preferably of teak or afrormosia, which are most resistant to decay (Hawkins and Lloyd, 1981). Mahogany, oak, and Western red cedar are also useful (Hawkins and Lloyd, 1981). Plywoods must be marine ply. You should keep in mind that many wood preservatives are toxic (Radeleff, 1970).

Metal

Metals and water are not compatible. Unfortunately, in many instances, metals are required for the completion of a system where no other material will serve. The major problem with metals and water, particularly seawater, is corrosion. Corroded metals lose structural integrity and strength, and the metal being lost through corrosion is toxic to fish. Stainless steel is considered the most resistant metal to seawater corrosion, but its resistance is only relative. The most available stainless steel, AISI type 316, is a high molybdenum alloy resistant to pitting and crevice corrosion. It is not a high-strength steel, and it will corrode (Hawkins and Lloyd, 1981). Where strength and maximal corrosion resistance are needed, titanium is preferred over stainless steel.

Other Metals

Other common metals used in tank construction include galvanized fittings and brass or copper. Unfortunately, the galvanized coat placed on iron contains considerable zinc. Enough zinc can dissolve from galvanized fittings to be lethal to fish within very short periods, even when calcium protection is in effect in seawater. Bronze can be a fatal source of zinc and copper. In hospital design, it is important to avoid the sublethal and lethal effects of heavy metals on fish behavior and physiology.

WATER FILTRATION SYSTEMS

Filtration is the removal of unwanted materials from the water. In basic aquatic design, there are three major types of filtration: mechanical, biological, and chemical, each with its own purpose and application. In hospital systems, biological filters are rarely used because of the need to disinfect between patients. Hospital tank filtration relies heavily on mechanical and chemical filtration. The practicing veterinarian dealing with pet fish must, however, be well-versed in biological filters because they are the most commonly used filter in home aquaria.

Mechanical Filtration

Mechanical filtration, sometimes referred to as primary filtration, removes suspended particles from water by passing it through a fine medium, which obstructs the particles. The mesh of the medium used depends on the size of the particulates to be removed and the amount of resistance that can be placed on the pump. More pumping effort is required to move water through finer meshed filters. When the physical limits of flow are reached in a pumping system, reduced through-put results in longer turnover times and reduced impact of the filter. Another limiting factor on the mesh size of filters is the occlusion rate. Very fine meshed filters, by their nature, occlude more quickly than coarser mesh filters. When occlusion occurs, or the head differential across the filter becomes too great, the filter must be backwashed to avoid cracking the filter medium or damaging the pumps. Mechanical filter design involves compromises between the size of particles cleared (degree of polishing) and the need to achieve reasonable turnover times, in proportion to particulate loading of the system while keeping backwash labor at reasonable limits.

In hospital systems, clogging is usually less of a problem. Only a very small bioload is being maintained in most hospital tanks, often a single fish. Also, water changes are routinely performed frequently to compensate for the lack of biological fixation, and to dilute out medications and free-swimming forms of parasites. This allows finer meshed media to be used than is generally practical in production or home systems. A uniform medium with an effective size of 0.3 mm will remove about 95% of particles down to 6 μ in diameter (Wheaton, 1977b). A coarser medium, 0.45 mm in diameter, will retain 15-μ particles (Wheaton, 1977b). For complete retention of all bacteria, a mechanical filter must exclude particles down to 0.2 μ in diameter. This is impractical in most systems because the cost of operating a filter large enough to provide reasonable turnover time is prohibitive.

Mechanical filters, with easily changeable media, are ideal for hospital tank systems. It is particularly beneficial if the media can be disinfected and reused. Canister filters with high-quality paper media are often used in systems up to about 1500 L. A variety of polymer filters are also available, but these are somewhat more expensive.

Chemical Filtration

Chemical filtration covers a wide range of methodology for removing molecular contaminants from water. These include ion exchange, both specific (resins) and nonspecific (activated carbon), and oxidative systems (ozone). Foam fractionation by protein modification and ultraviolet filtration can also be considered methods of chemical filtration, since they rely on basic modifications of chemical structure to remove contaminants.

Activated carbon filters are the most commonly applied form of chemical filtration. This is sometimes described as absorption filtration, but it is actually a relatively nonspecific exchange situation. A finite number of binding sites are available on the carbon, depending upon the surface area of the carbon particles (Fig. 8–12). These are capable of binding cations and anions with binding strengths that vary with the ion being bound. These ions undergo constant exchange with ions in the water at a rate inversely proportional to their binding strength to the carbon sites. Ions with strong binding affinity are effectively removed from the water. This works well until all of the binding sites are saturated and competitive binding between the more toxic compounds reaches a point where not all toxic ions can be bound simultaneously. At this point, some ions must be released by mass action (Spotte, 1979). The filter also fails

when a very strongly binding ion is introduced into the system that displaces more weakly bound toxic compounds from the binding sites (Beleau, 1988). In either of these cases, the filter designed to remove toxic compounds becomes a source of the toxin.

In a hospital system, individual filtration systems are the best plan, and this can make some chemical filtration methods difficult to implement on a small scale. For removal of waste products, disposable cartridges or polymer pads in external canister filters are probably the best route. Disinfection of the complex surface areas involved in these types of media is a false economy. The potential for transmitting disease from one patient to the next through incompletely disinfected chemical filtration media is high. For larger facilities, it may be practical to build a contact chamber for delivery of ozone or ultraviolet filtration to various hospital tanks in series. If you intend to invest in this technology, it is best to arrange for a knowledgeable consultant. It will be critical that the contact chamber provide complete disinfection before returning the water to the hospital tanks, or disease transmission will be a major problem. Systems adequate to kill bacteria may not be adequate to kill protozoa or fungi.

Biological Filtration

Biological filtration in aquaria refers to the biological fixation of nitrogenous wastes into less toxic compounds by bacteria (Fig. 8–13). Other forms of biological filtration, including the concentration of metals and certain toxic organics in algal scrubbers, are also employed. A biological filter must maintain enough heterotrophic bacterial colonies to process the solid nitrogenous wastes of fish into soluble wastes such as ammonia. The ammonia from this process and that directly excreted by the fish is then converted by autotrophic bacteria to nitrite (by *Nitrosomonas* spp.) and then to nitrate (by *Nitrobacter* spp.). The surface area for bacterial growth is usually the limiting factor in biological filters, along with the ability to circulate the waste-laden water into contact with the bacteria responsible for nitrogen fixation. This is the principle behind so-called "undergravel filters."

Numerous augmenting systems to increase the efficiency of waste fixation have been developed, primarily to provide additional surface area for bacterial growth and easier water contact. These include plastic-fluted spheres and cylinders that maximize surface area while minimizing flow impedance. Biofilter dynamics can be very important to fish health. They need to provide adequate turnover of the tank water to avoid accumulation of toxic wastes, but at the same time they must provide enough contact time with waste-laden water to allow effective waste metabolism by the bacteria. An imbalance results in an ineffective biofilter.

In a hospital system, where frequent disinfection is required, some types of filters are better than

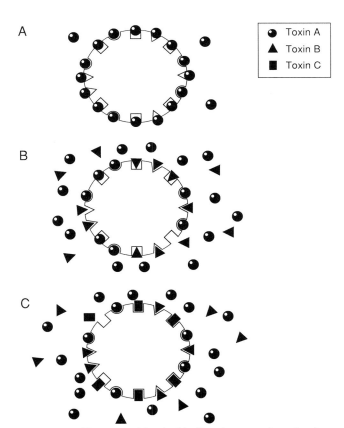

FIGURE 8–12. The competition for binding sites on activated carbon. *A.* An activated carbon particle is saturated with toxin, A, which has occupied all available sites, some with stronger binding than other less-suitable sites. *B.* A second toxin (B) is introduced into the system that fits some binding sites better than toxin A. As toxin B binds preferentially to those sites, toxin A levels in the water increase dramatically. *C.* A third toxin (C) serves to release even more toxin A and toxin B into the water by better competing for specific binding sites on the carbon particle.

Toxin A
Toxin B
Toxin C

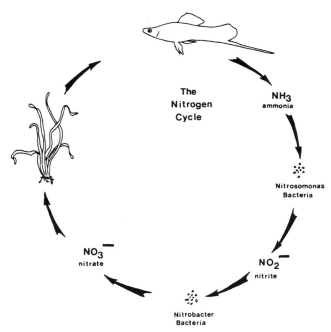

FIGURE 8–13. The nitrogen fixation cycle of biological filtration. (With permission from Stoskopf, M.K. [1988] Tropical fish medicine. Taking the history. Vet. Clin. North Am., Small Anim. Pract. 18[2]:283–291.)

others. In general, biological filters are not useful. They cannot be disinfected easily by their very nature, and to do so makes them completely ineffective. It takes about 6 weeks to restart a disinfected biofilter and to have it working at full capacity. This is much too long for any practical hospital system to be down. One way to avoid the problem of downtime is to have portable biofilters that are growing in a reserve system designed to keep the filters healthy. Strings of biorings or other plastic support media suspended in the water are a common approach. In the hospital tank, the strings of plastic afford cover for the patient and also accomplish some nitrogen fixation. They are not as efficient as if they were deployed in a spray chamber to maximize contact time and flow past their surfaces, but they are easier to remove and replace when a tank changes patients.

Remember two things when using a portable biofilter system in a hospital setting. First, your disinfection must be excellent. The high surface area of the biofilter makes it difficult to get complete disinfection, and unless you do, you will be introducing pathogens into your reserve system and contaminating all of your hospital tanks that receive biofilters. Dilute formalin or chlorine soaks for 24 to 48 hours are used for this purpose. Biofilters are rinsed thoroughly after disinfection and soaked again for a day in untreated water before being returned to the reserve system for reseeding.

In a well-established reserve system, reseeding may require no more than placing the biofilter into the system. It may be beneficial to keep the disinfected biofilter downstream of and in close contact with well-seeded biofilters. It will take a minimum of 3 weeks to reseed the disinfected biofilter to a level that will be of any value in your hospital tank. This can be hastened somewhat by keeping your biofilter reserve system warmer; however, it is difficult to say whether this is a long-term benefit or not. The bacteria working on the biofilters are very susceptible to environmental changes, and a large drop in fixation efficiency can occur with just the careful transfer of a biofilter from the reserve system to a tank. This loss is greater if the environmental conditions, including the water temperature, of the hospital tank and reserve system are widely disparate.

It is important to feed your biofilters while they are in the reserve system. This can be accomplished in a number of ways. Some aquarists maintain fish or invertebrates in the reserve system to provide waste material to feed the bacteria. This minimizes the work involved in operating the reserve system but has the obvious disadvantage of having potential reservoirs of infection in the reserve system itself. Another approach is to introduce ammonia into the system on a periodic or continuous basis. In marine systems, this is often done with ammonium chloride solutions.

AIR SYSTEMS

Do not overlook the importance of a safe air delivery system when designing a fish hospital ward. If you install several hospital tanks, a central air system is often cost effective and energy efficient and should be considered. Any air system should have a backup, and this includes central systems. This can be a box full of small individual pumps stored in the pharmacy for deployment in case of a mechanical failure or a second central pump. Mechanical breakdowns happen, and according to Murphy's law, they will happen at the most inopportune time, when your hospital is full of critically ill patients. If your hospital has an emergency power generator, your air system should be wired to it.

Another important issue in air system design is the location of the air intake. Remember, the air being brought into your air pump will be exchanged as it is bubbled through your hospital tanks. Locating your air intake in a garage or near a parking lot where exhaust fumes accumulate can result in mysterious toxicity problems in the hospital tanks. Also, be aware of painting, pesticide spraying, or the use of cleaning solutions in the vicinity of the air intake for your air pumps.

Take precautions to prevent accidental exposure of fish to infectious disease through the air system. Wherever possible, use plastic airstones, which are easily disinfected for reuse. Design your delivery system with intermediate connectors for relatively short tubing leaders to the tanks themselves. This minimizes the cost of discarding contaminated air tubing after an infectious patient. It is a good idea to periodically replace your leaders, even when you have not had particularly serious infectious problems in your patients. This avoids microbial colonization of the tubing and contamination of your central system or pump.

TEMPERATURE CONTROL

Many fish hospital and holding facilities are designed to control temperature through regulation of the room air temperature. This design is energy efficient but requires careful attention to the dynamics of the heating and cooling system of the building. The human comfort range shifts seasonally with changes in our dress. In the winter, we wear heavier clothes and tend to heat buildings to lower temperatures than we find comfortable in summer, when we run our air conditioning systems. While this change is not very large, and usually not noticed by us, it does occur on the edge of the temperature tolerance ranges of a large number of tropical fish species. The difference between 20 and 23°C (68 to 73.4°F) can be life threatening to a critically ill tropical fish. Many tropical fish need temperatures in the range of 24 to 26°C (77 to 78.8°F), and temperatures of 27°C (80.6°F) are sometimes used when treating protozoal infections. Facilities using air heating should be maintained at room temperatures in the 24 to 25°C (75.2 to 77.0°F) range. Supplemental heaters should be available to boost temperatures in specific tanks. Glass-encased heaters are safer than metal-enclosed heaters, particularly in marine systems. Take extreme precaution with any electrical wiring in a fish hospital facility. All connections and wires should be well insulated. Ground fault circuit breakers should be used for all outlets.

Selection of heater wattage is based on the volume of water that must be heated. It is not particularly critical. A small heater in a large volume will be on a greater proportion of the time. A rule of thumb is 50 to 100 watts of heater for every 40 L (10 gals) of water in the system. For larger tanks, fused silica heaters may be required. Longer-barreled heaters have lower surface temperatures than shorter heaters of the same wattage and are, therefore, less liable to cause burns to fish caught up against them. Protective, guard fences can be placed around heaters to keep fish away. Placing the heater horizontally near the bottom of the tank improves the convection dynamics of the heater but requires a sealed, submersible heater (Fig. 8–14). Submersible heaters are easier to disinfect and may be preferable in hospital situations. If a facility has a large number of tanks, a heater calibration bucket is a worthwhile investment. This is a bucket or tank of water maintained at a desired temperature by a thermostatic heater. Other heaters can be placed in the tank and rapidly calibrated to roughly the temperature of the bucket before being placed in a tank with fish.

The other side of temperature control is cooling water to maintain hospitalized temperate or cold-water species. Refrigeration systems are expensive.

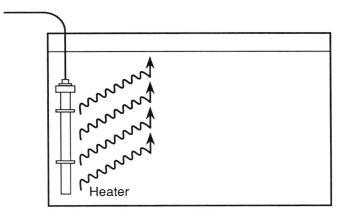

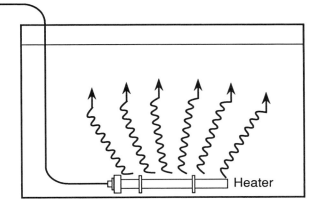

FIGURE 8–14. Placing a submersible heater horizontally has the advantage of more even distribution of temperature over a vertically placed heater.

It is common for a hospital facility to own one or two assembled on movable carts so they can be deployed in different tanks as the need arises. They are a necessity if you are going to hospitalize cold-water fish. The most common refrigeration systems are heat exchangers driven by a compressible refrigerant such as Freon. Heat exchangers constructed of a variety of materials are available. Most plastics are poor conductors of heat, making them relatively useless in exchangers. Titanium is the only metal proven suitable for heat exchangers used in marine systems. Coatings on coils of other metals are susceptible to scratching and other damage, resulting in toxicity problems from leached metals and serious corrosion problems in the chiller. These chillers can be used with some impunity in freshwater systems but are too dangerous for marine systems. Graphite exchange blocks are available and may prove useful in marine systems.

Frequently, an intermediate-stage refrigerant is used to give a more stable temperature than is achieved with compressible gases such as Freon. Liquid phases (usually calcium chloride brine), which are less toxic than refrigerant gases, are circulated, releasing heat to a compressed gaseous coolant away from the tank system, and accepting heat from the water in the tank. This type of system is preferable to exchangers, which place Freon circulating coils in direct contact with the aquarium water.

An inexpensive system can be constructed using a freezer compartment of a standard refrigerator, plastic airline tubing, and a peristaltic pump. In home aquaria, the pump is usually used to move aquarium water through the tubing, which is coiled in the freezer section of the refrigerator. The temperature of the returning water and the tank being cooled is regulated by the length of tubing coiled in the freezer and the rate at which the water is pumped. This type of system is not suitable for a hospital situation because calibration of the system is tedious and time consuming and disinfection is nearly impossible.

An alternate system that uses the same low capital investment parts can be adapted for hospital use (Fig. 8–15). Rather than circulating the water from the tank through the tubing, the principle of using a secondary refrigerant can be employed. Coils of tubing are placed in the freezer section of a refrigerator, with both ends of the line extending through holes drilled in the freezer wall. These are then connected to three-way stopcock valves that can serve as connectors for a length of tubing that will connect the loop outside the refrigerator. This length of tubing will be in contact with the hospital tank being chilled. It can be removed for disinfection. When a new tank needs to be chilled, the completed plastic tubing loop is filled with either calcium chloride solution or water, using the three-way stopcocks and bleeding out any air in the tubing. The peristaltic pump is attached to the tubing on the outside of the refrigerator, and coils of plastic tubing are placed in the tank. Temperature can be regulated by increasing or decreasing the number of loops of tubing placed in the hospital tank, and by changing the speed of the peristaltic pump. When it is time to change tanks

or patients, the tubing in the tank can be detached and carefully disinfected or discarded.

MONITORING TANKS

Fish hospital systems can be designed to minimize most catastrophic events, but a program of careful environmental monitoring is necessary in any aquarium system. Three critical factors should be monitored essentially continuously: temperature, water level, and power failure. Other aspects such as pH and nitrate monitoring are discussed in Chapter 13.

Water temperature can rise catastrophically when a heater thermostat fails. More subtle changes that have a negative impact on fish patients may occur gradually. Temperature can be monitored with a simple thermometer. In hospital tanks, liquid crystal thermometers applied to the outside of the tanks reduce disinfection problems. Place these away from the heater near the top of the water. External thermometers usually read a degree or so under what a thermometer inside a tank would read because of the insulating properties of the tank wall. This differential varies with different tank materials, but it will be consistent for any given tank. The outside thermometer can be calibrated to a floating thermometer and the temperature readings adjusted in use.

A variety of accidents can cause the water level in a tank to rise or fall. The most obvious problem is a ruptured tank, but failed water pumps, loose hoses, or errant siphons can all result in a fish being left out of water. It is important to recognize this type of problem immediately.

Power failure can affect your hospital tanks in several ways. In improperly designed systems, power failure can result in draining a tank when

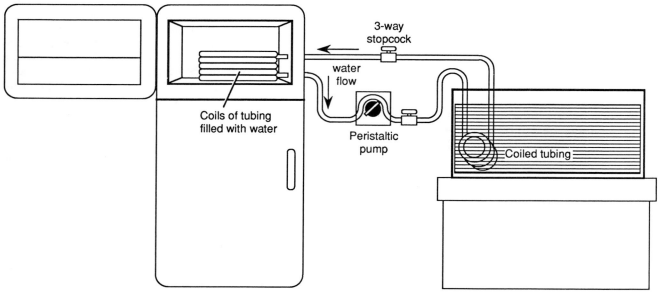

FIGURE 8–15. A low-cost refrigeration system suitable for hospital use.

electric pumps malfunction. Usually, the most critical concern is the loss of the air system and circulation that maintain dissolved oxygen levels. Certainly, loss of electric heaters or chillers can result in problems with temperature.

Electronic tank monitoring systems capable of measuring temperature, water level, and interruption in electrical supply are available commercially. Systems designed for monitoring incubators and laboratory equipment can be adapted to use in fish tanks. They can also be built from parts available in most electronics stores carrying burglar or fire alarm components. These systems can be programmed to call a prescribed telephone number and notify whoever answers that a problem exists. Many can even communicate what the problem is. These systems are extremely valuable security in lieu of staffing a fish hospital 24 hours a day.

INFECTIOUS DISEASE CONTROL

Once the basic issue of life support for your fish patients is settled through the selection of tanks, filters, substrates, and accessories, the very real problem of infectious disease control must be considered. The fact that fish are subject to all forms of infectious agents common in other animals is well established throughout this book. Here the issue becomes how to prevent one patient from infecting others hospitalized in the same facility. This is not as trivial an issue as it might seem. It is important in fish medicine to consider each vector route for disease transmission established in terrestrial veterinary medicine.

Spread of infection through direct contact occurs in fish. Fish suspected to have bacterial, viral, fungal, or protozoal diseases should not be placed in the same hospital tank as other otherwise unexposed fish. Many fish diseases are also readily spread through the water, so for general purposes of fish ward design, the term "tank" should include the filtration system. Each hospital tank should have its own separate filtration and water management system. Ideally, each system or tank would also be housed in its own room. This is never practical, but is the most effective way to eliminate a third, very important mode of transmission of disease between fish, aerosolization. The fine bubbles coming to the surface of tanks from airstones and airlifts cast millions of small aerosol droplets into the air. Anyone who has maintained a marine aquarium is aware of how far these droplets carry because they hold small amounts of salt, which result in the white salt crusting of everything in the vicinity of the aquarium. These droplets also carry bacteria, viruses, and fungal spores. The entire process might be considered analogous to a terrestrial animal's sneeze. All hospital tanks should have tops, and, preferably, tops that minimize the chances for direct aerosolization into the room. If possible, tanks should be placed far enough apart to prevent the aerosolized droplets of one tank from settling on another. This distance is dependent upon the type of top employed, the location of holes in the top, and the degree of aeration and spray used in the tank system. It is never a good idea to place a tank for infectious patients above another tank, but because of space considerations, it is often a necessity. When this occurs, every precaution should be taken to avoid splash or spill contamination of the lower tanks. If you have tiered tank systems, patients with highly infectious problems should be kept in lower aquaria, not in top aquaria.

Fomite transmission of disease in fish is a very real problem, particularly in a hospital setting. Each tank should have its own set of implements (nets, feeding sticks, tongs, etc.), which are used only on the fish in that system. Although disinfection of implements may seem a more economical approach initially, in the actual day-to-day rush of caring for the sick animals in your wards, disinfection becomes impractical. Implements do not remain in contact with disinfectants long enough to be effective. In addition, hurried rinsing of "disinfected" implements can lead to complications from exposing your patients to the disinfectant. The individualized nets and implements can be thoroughly disinfected each night, minimizing the risk of fomite transmission of disease. Practitioners treating pet fish may want to give the thoroughly disinfected net and feeding tongs, used with a hospitalized fish, to the owner when the fish goes home. Many pet fish owners do not own proper nets and find the feeding tong useful.

Implements are best disinfected by first rinsing the net or object in running water to remove slime and debris and then submerging the tool in a container of disinfectant. Selecting a disinfectant is controversial. Chlorine solutions are popular. They are inexpensive and can be monitored with simple swimming pool test kits or amperometric titrators to assure that they remain active. Implements disinfected in chlorine are often rinsed in a vat of dilute sodium thiosulfate to reduce any residual chlorine. The major drawback to this method is that prolonged exposure to chlorine weakens and destroys nets. This is, of course, true to some extent of any oxidizing disinfectant. Some facilities prefer the use of dilute formalin as a disinfectant, although the potential human health risk of this procedure makes it questionable. A variety of quaternary ammonium compounds have been used to disinfect nets and tools. Many of these contain dyes and perfumes, which make it easy to establish that an implement has been placed in the disinfectant. These same dyes also make it easy to detect inadequate rinsing, a common error in fish husbandry.

A major consideration in maintaining a fish hospital is the disinfection and decontamination of the tanks and filter systems themselves between patients. This can be the major labor involved in maintaining a fish hospital, and the problem of disinfecting filters has been considered earlier in the chapter. Each time a hospital tank and filter is recycled for a new patient, they should be disinfected. This is no more or less important than cleaning out a dog or cat kennel before placing a new patient inside. The water should be drained from the tank. A variety of tank disinfection schemes have been invented. There still needs to be study as to their efficacy.

Currently, there are three levels of effort being employed in fish hospitals for cleaning or disinfecting tanks. Most commonly, the water in a hospital tank is drained and replaced, perhaps after cleaning any visible dirt from the tank sides. This is certainly an improvement over simply putting a new patient in the same water as a previous patient, but it provides minimal disease control, if any at all. Proponents of this approach argue that it saves time, presents less risk of accidental poisoning with disinfectants, and is cost effective.

Spraying the walls of the tank with 70% ethanol or isopropyl alcohol and allowing the alcohol to evaporate, or spraying and rinsing with dilute chlorine or formalin solutions, is another level of disinfection that has been used successfully in fish hospital situations. The use of formalin has potential health risks to operators and should probably be avoided. Spraying tank walls will disinfect the tank and is definitely superior to merely draining the system and refilling it. However, this approach will not disinfect the plumbing or filtration systems. If disposable filters are being used, this may not be a major problem, but safer disinfection is accomplished by circulating disinfectant throughout the tank system.

Usually, chlorine is the disinfectant of choice when the entire system is disinfected between patients. This process is time consuming and is usually reserved for systems that have held fish with highly infectious problems. The tank and system should be drained and cleaned of visible debris. Then the tank is refilled with a dilute chlorine or quaternary ammonium solution and circulated for an hour or more. The tank is drained and the system rinsed. A major concern is to be sure all disinfectant is removed from the system before it goes back on line. Using removable or disposable filtration systems greatly aids in this process as disinfection, and removal of disinfectant from the complex surfaces of filters takes a great deal of time. If chlorine was used, the water can be tested for residual chlorine or thiosulfate added after the tank is refilled. Dilute vinegar solutions have also served as disinfectants of hospital and home aquarium systems. Considerable disinfection can be accomplished through merely altering the pH of the water running through the system and then discarding the water.

LITERATURE CITED

Beleau, S. (1988) Water quality. Vet. Clin. North Am., Small Anim. Pract. 18:291–304.

Carmignani, G.M., and Bennett, J.P. (1976) Leaching of plastics used in closed aquaculture systems. Aquaculture 7:89–91.

Ford, D. (1981) Small aquaria. In: Aquarium Systems (Hawkins, A.D., ed.). Academic Press, New York, pp. 149–170.

Hawkins, A.D., and Anthony, P:.D. (1981) Aquarium design and construction. In: Aquarium Systems. (Hawkins, A.D., ed.). Academic Press, New York, pp. 1–46.

Hawkins, A.D., and Lloyd, R. (1981) Materials for the aquarium. In: Aquarium Systems (Hawkins, A.D., ed.). Academic Press, New York, pp. 171–222.

Radeleff, R.D. (1970) Veterinary Toxicology. 2nd ed. Lea & Febiger, Philadelphia, pp. 312–313.

Schreck, C.B. (1981) Stress and compensation in teleostean fishes: Responses to social and physical factors. In: Stress and Fish (Pickering, A.D., ed.). Academic Press, New York, pp. 295–321.

Spotte, S. (1979) Seawater Aquariums, The Captive Environment. John Wiley & Sons, New York.

Wheaton, F.W. (1977a) Ponds, Tanks and Other Impounding Structures in Aquacultural Engineering. John Wiley & Sons, New York, pp. 414–462.

Wheaton, F.W. (1977b) Energy in Aquatic Systems in Aquacultural Engineering. John Wiley & Sons, New York, pp. 64–113.

Chapter 9

CLINICAL PATHOLOGY

MICHAEL K. STOSKOPF

Clinicians tend to equate clinical pathology with hematology and perhaps serology. These are important elements of the discipline, but they are not the "whole kettle of fish." In any practice, but particularly in the practice of fish medicine, clinicians must be competent with a wide range of clinical pathological examinations, including hematology, serology, cytology, immunology, and scatology. This chapter focuses on the methods and general interpretation of the first three subdisciplines. Immunology and scatological techniques and interpretation are similar to those used in mammals. Points salient to fish medicine are covered in Chapters 10 and 11.

HEMATOLOGY

Despite popular dogma to the contrary, fish hematology is a valuable tool in disease diagnosis and prognostication. Although it is enjoying a period of rapid advances, the study of fish blood has only recently begun to evolve consistent rules of nomenclature and procedures along the lines of mammalian hematology. This does not mean it is a young science. The foundations for fish hematology were well established by the late 1800s. Scientists examining the basic functional properties of blood studied fish models. By the turn of the twentieth century, several studies of peripheral fish blood were available, including Meinertz's exhaustive studies of the white cell staining characteristics of reptile, fish, and invertebrate blood. This work is illustrated with 177 color illustrations of leukocytes, each with a different name (Meinertz, 1902).

The nomenclature of fish blood cells remains confusing, but the introduction of the term *heterophil* for any granulocyte other than an eosinophil or basophil, regardless of shape or staining characteristics, greatly simplified communication (Kyes, 1929). This term was adopted by Jordan in a chapter in Downey's *Handbook of Hematology*, which first established the nomenclature of fish hematology in its modern form, sanctioning the heterophil and the monocyte as accepted cell types (Jordan, 1938). Unfortunately, fish hematology has never been as organized since. Individual investigators have invented new names for cells, paying little or no attention to consistency in methods. Without standardized criteria for naming cells and standardized techniques for quantitating hematological values, fish hematology

is not clinically useful. That is why this chapter spends much of its effort presenting the details of standardized methods and nomenclature which should be used as a basis for clinical fish hematology.

SAMPLING TECHNIQUES

The method used to draw a blood sample can affect the values obtained when it is analyzed. Until recently fish hematology was considered a postmortem technique performed on fish sacrificed for the purpose. This remains the case for extremely small specimens or in some production animals. In these fish, the size of the sample taken is limited only by the blood volume of the fish and the efficiency of the method used to collect it. However, for fish 200 g or larger, it is not necessary to sacrifice the animal to obtain suitable quantities of blood for analysis. Fish easily tolerate blood samples proportionate in volume to those drawn from similar-sized mammals (0.08 to 0.1% of body weight). In vivo blood sampling techniques are covered in Chapter 5.

ANTICOAGULANTS

A controversy yet to be resolved is the selection of an anticoagulant for fish blood samples destined for formed element analysis. No perfect anticoagulant has been found, so when selecting one, it is important to consider the eventual use of the blood sample, particularly for chemistry determinations. Early studies with unspecified heparin salts (heparin), dipotassium ethylenediamine tetraacetic acid (EDTA), disodium oxalate (oxalate), and trisodium citrate (citrate) demonstrated that heparin used in appropriate concentrations has the least effect on blood pH, divalent cation concentration, and hematocrit. EDTA acidifies blood, whereas oxalate and citrate raise blood pH to a smaller extent. The chelating activity of EDTA lowers calcium and other divalent ion concentrations, while obviously the salt selected for any of these anticoagulants determines their impact on specific monovalent cation determinations. The proper selection of volume and concentration of anticoagulant should minimize these changes.

To complicate things, however, recent work with avian erythrocytes implicates heparin in increased nuclear permeability to chromatin, resulting in artifactual formation of swollen nuclei and cytoplasmically displaced chromatin (Freidlin, 1985). Heparin can also cause erythrocyte clumping, and particularly important, it can be extremely variable from vial to vial, even between vials from a single manufacturing lot (Freidlin, 1985). This suggests the need for caution in storing and handling heparin.

ERYTHROCYTES

Erythrocyte Morphology

Mature fish erythrocytes are oval, nucleated cells with abundant pale eosinophilic cytoplasm (Fig. 9–1). The nucleus is usually oval with its long axis matching that of the cell, but in some species the nucleus can be nearly round. The nuclear chromatin is dense and stains darkly. Some anisocytosis and polychromasia is normal (Fig. 9–2). Occasionally, mitotic activity will be seen in fish peripheral blood. Erythropoiesis can occur normally in the circulation in fishes (Stokes and Firkin, 1971). Ultrastructurally the cytoplasm of fish erythrocytes is finely granular with no inclusions and few mitochondria (Hyder et al., 1983). There may be prominent cytoplasmic vacuoles believed to be autophagic vacuoles derived from degenerating mitochondria (Stokes and Firkin, 1971).

Methods for Examining Erythrocytes

TOTAL ERYTHROCYTE COUNT. Many methods are available for determining total erythrocyte counts.

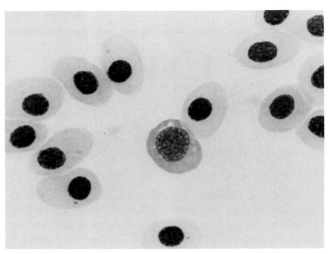

FIGURE 9–2. Polychromasia in a peripheral blood smear from a spiny dogfish (Giemsa, 1000×).

Each has advantages and disadvantages. Automated techniques give reasonable estimates, although fish erythrocytes are quite large compared to mammalian erythrocytes and are larger than small lymphocytes and the nucleated thrombocytes of fish. These white cells will be included in a total erythrocyte count unless very careful adjustments of the lower exclusion limits are made for each individual sample.

Manual methods for counting erythrocytes are performed at the same time as the total leukocyte count, since differential staining methods are needed to distinguish fish leukocytes from nucleated erythrocytes. These methods will be discussed in more detail later under the leukocytes. A specific dilution of the blood is made with a staining solution and a standard Neubauer cell counting chamber flooded (Fig. 9–3). A total erythrocyte count (cells per microliter) is obtained by counting the erythrocytes in the four small corner boxes and the center box of the center square of the apparatus. This number is multiplied by a factor dependent upon the dilution used. The same mathematics is used as for mammalian samples.

The total area of the central primary square on the counting surface is 1 mm² and the area of each of the five secondary squares actually counted is 0.2 mm². The depth under the coverslip is 0.1 mm, making the fluid volume for the five counted secondary squares 0.02 μl. For the common dilution of 1/100 (20 μl of blood in 1980 μl of diluent), the number obtained in the count is multiplied by 5000 to obtain the total erythrocyte count.

HEMOGLOBIN. Several methods for determining the hemoglobin content of fish erythrocytes are available. Each method gives somewhat different values for the same sample, so standardization of methodology is quite important if comparisons are to be made between data from different laboratories. The cyanmethemoglobin method has been adopted internationally as the reference method for hemoglobin determination in mammals and is generally accepted

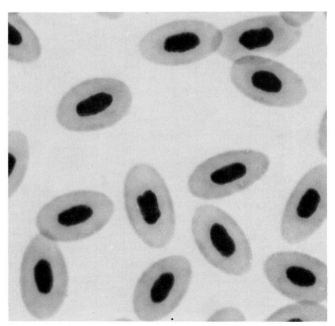

FIGURE 9–1. Normal erythrocytes from a peripheral blood smear from a goldfish (Giemsa, 1000×).

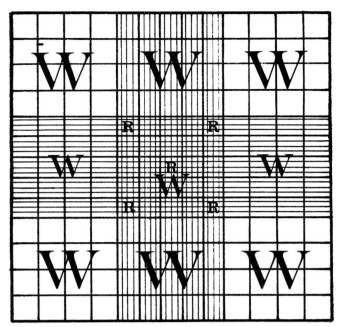

FIGURE 9–3. Counting patterns on the standard Neubauer cell counting chamber for total leukocyte counts (W) and total erythrocyte counts (R).

as such for fish. It is rapid and precise and measures all hemoglobin derivatives.

The cyanmethemoglobin method converts all hemoglobin derivatives to methemoglobin using ferricyanide and cyanide ions. Methemoglobin is a stable red compound that can be measured spectrophotometrically, reading optical density at 540 nm. Whole blood is mixed with Drabkin's solution (Table 9–1) to achieve a 1:251 ratio of blood to reagent. After mixing, 10 minutes is allowed for the reaction to be completed and then the optical density of the mixture is read. A standard curve is made from serial dilutions of a cyanmethemoglobin standard or a standard sample is run with the sample to allow calculation of hemoglobin concentration.

TABLE 9–1. Cyanmethemoglobin Method

1. Transfer 5 ml Drabkin solution to a clean dry cuvette.
2. Add 20 μl whole blood (1:251 blood-to-reagent ratio).
3. Mix well and allow to stand for 10 minutes.
4. Read optical density (OD) at 540 nm using Drabkin solution as a blank.
5. Calculate hemoglobin concentration from a standard curve made from readings taken from a hemoglobin standard at various dilutions or from a simultaneously run standard.

$$\text{hemoglobin (g/dl)} = \frac{\text{OD blood}}{\text{OD standard}} \times \text{hemoglobin conc. of standard}$$

Reagent:
Drabkin Solution:
   Put 500 ml distilled water in a 1 L volumetric flask.
   Add 1 g sodium bicarbonate ($NaHCO_3$).
   Add 0.05 g potassium cyanide (KCN).
   Add 0.02 g potassium ferricyanide ($K_3Fe(CN)_6$).
   Dissolve the contents.
   Add distilled water to bring the volume to 1 L.

Unfortunately, interference from red cell nuclei affects the optical density measured in the cyanmethemoglobin method, causing inaccurately high values for hemoglobin. This effect can be eliminated by centrifuging the lysed blood (1000 G for 2 minutes) to precipitate nuclear debris before the hemoglobin determination is made. This requires additional handling steps and is rarely done. The various fractions of hemoglobin in fish erythrocytes may also cause some of the observed differences between methods of determinations. Usually the cyanmethemoglobin method gives a higher reading than the acid or alkaline hematin methods.

Other hemoglobin determination methods have been used in fish. The oxyhemoglobin methods give comparatively lower values than the cyanmethemoglobin method. Automated systems such as the Coulter hemoglobinometer give artificially high readings, also because of the interference of the nuclear debris in fish blood.

HEMATOCRIT. The packed cell volume or hematocrit in fish is usually determined by the microhematocrit method. Small capillary tubes are filled approximately two-thirds full with anticoagulated blood, sealed on one end with clay, and centrifuged for 5 minutes at 14,000 G. The percentage of packed cells to total volume is determined by direct measurement. This parameter is stable for approximately 24 hours after a heparinized blood sample has been taken. It is considered less stable if EDTA is used as an anticoagulant (Fourie, 1977), but this is probably due to osmotic problems with certain preparations of EDTA.

MORPHOLOGICAL EVALUATION OF ERYTHROCYTES. The differential smear made for the examination of leukocytes is also used for evaluating erythrocyte morphology. Fish normally exhibit some degree of polychromasia, and some mitogenic activity is frequently seen in the peripheral erythrocytes. However, a large number of immature erythrocytic cells is indicative of a regenerative anemia. Nuclear abnormalities and high numbers of erythrocytes without nuclei are seen in toxicities and nutritional deficiencies such as folic acid deficiency, which often results in amitosis, and irregular nuclear fragmentation that can be observed in the stained differential smear (Hibiya, 1985). Eels in polluted estuaries show nuclear fragmentation of erythrocytes (Eiras, 1983), and fatty liver syndrome in fish due to feeding on rancid oils or to low levels of vitamin E can result in increased fragmentation and breakdown of erythrocytes as well as arrested maturation (Ferguson, 1989). Hypersenescent erythrocytes in a fish blood smear may accompany an anemic condition associated with hypersensitivity. Hypersensitivity occurs in fish but the mechanism is somewhat distinct from the mechanism of hypersensitivity reactions seen in mammals (Ellis, 1984) (see Chapter 11). Careful evaluation of erythrocyte morphology can be a valuable adjunct to clinical diagnosis.

WINTROBE ERYTHROCYTE INDICES. The Wintrobe erythrocyte indices—mean corpuscular volume

(MCV), mean corpuscular hemoglobin (MCH), and mean corpuscular hemoglobin concentration (MCHC)—are frequently used in fish hematology. They are determined by the same formulas used for mammals (Table 9–2). Their usefulness is directly related to the accuracy of the data used in their calculations.

EVALUATION OF ANEMIA. Using the Wintrobe indices, it is possible to classify and evaluate fish anemias in much the same manner as in mammals. This can be particularly important in fish, since clinical signs of anemia are often masked until quite late in the pathogenesis of the disease. For example, rainbow trout can compensate for a 70% reduction in hematocrit while maintaining resting oxygen levels to all tissues. This is accomplished by increased cardiac output due to an increased stroke volume. So fish with significant anemias may show few clinical signs other than branchial pallor unless they are forced to exercise (Ferguson, 1989).

A large number of immature erythrocytes or major polychromasia observed on the blood smear is indicative of a regenerative anemia. Unless a large number of blast forms are present, the MCV will be smaller than normal. This is just the opposite of what occurs in mammals. In fish the younger erythrocytes are somewhat smaller than mature erythrocytes (Ferguson, 1989). Microcytic anemias of fish include hemorrhagic and hemolytic anemias. Hemorrhagic anemias are seen after stripping of eggs from broodfish that have been handled too roughly, after other forms of trauma, or after surgery. They can also be seen in heavy infestations of external parasites such as leeches, lampreys, or blood-sucking copepods. Microcytic anemias with increased polychromasia are also seen in fish infected with the viral hemorrhagic septicemia virus owing to a loss of vascular integrity that facilitates hemorrhagic blood loss. It is also seen in vitamin K–deficient fish (Ferguson, 1989).

Hemolytic anemias in fish result from exposure to bacterial hemolysins (*Vibrio* spp.). They also occur with heavy hematozoa infections of *Trypanosoma*, *Cryptobia*, or *Haemogregarina*. Viral infections such as the erythrocytic necrosis virus also cause erythrocyte lysis and hemolytic anemia. Toxic situations can result in hemolysis. Massive erythrocyte destruction and methemoglobin formation occurs with chlorine exposure (Ferguson, 1989). Methemoglobin formation with or without red cell destruction can be seen in nitrite, aniline, and nitrobenzene toxicities (Ferguson, 1989).

Microcytic normochromic anemia is seen associated with high population density stress (Murray and Burton, 1979). Microcytic hypochromic anemia with elongated erythrocytes is seen in trouts fed diets containing yeasts, and is the result of peroxides produced by the yeast (Sanchez-Muiz et al., 1982). Other oxidative stressors can also cause significant anemias in fish.

Hypoplastic anemias in fish are seen in folic acid deficiency and in vitamin B_{12} deficiency. In folic acid deficiency, the anemia is normochromic and macrocytic. The anemia seen in vitamin B_{12} deficiencies is hypochromic. Other nutritionally related anemias have been produced experimentally with induced niacin, pyridoxine, inositol, riboflavin, vitamin C, and iron deficiencies (Ferguson, 1989).

OTHER TESTS. A variety of other tests are used in mammalian clinical pathology to evaluate erythrocytes. Erythrocyte sedimentation rate (ESR), erythrocyte osmotic fragility testing, and a variety of immunologic tests such as the Coombs test have proved useful in various diagnostic efforts in mammals. In fish hematology, these methods have not been widely employed and little is known about their diagnostic value.

LEUKOCYTES

The leukocytes are the most morphologically and functionally diverse of the three major groups of formed elements in fish blood. Erythrocytes and thrombocytes are essentially monotypic groups. Fish leukocytes include at least five distinct subgroups on the basis of morphology and function, each of which must be considered separately.

Heterophils

The fish heterophil is generally a round cell with a multilobed nucleus and prominent spindle-shaped or bar-shaped cytoplasmic bodies in Wright-Giemsa–stained smears of peripheral blood. These cells appear relatively uniform in size within a given species and are usually round. The nucleus is usually eccentric and may be segmented into two or three lobes (Fig. 9–4). Less mature cells have round or reniform nuclei. The occurrence of hypersegmented nuclei with five or more nuclear lobes is relatively rare in fish (Fig. 9–5).

The cytoplasm of heterophils stained with Romanowsky stains is usually pale and gray, with numerous small granules which stain variably depending on the species of the fish and the maturity

TABLE 9–2. Wintrobe Erythrocyte Indices

$$MVC\ (fl) = \frac{Hct\ (ml/dl)}{RBC\ (million/\mu l)} \times 10$$

$$MCH\ (pg) = \frac{Hb\ (g/dl)}{RBC\ (million/\mu l)} \times 10$$

$$MCHC\ (g/dl) = \frac{Hb\ (gm/dl)}{Hct\ (ml/dl)} \times 100$$

Hb: Hemoglobin
Hct: Hematocrit
MCH: Mean corpuscular hemoglobin
MCHC: Mean corpuscular hemoglobin concentration
MCV: Mean corpuscular volume
RBC: Total erythrocyte count
fl (femtoliter): 10^{-15} L
pg (picogram): 10^{-12} g

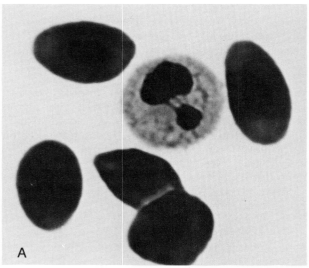

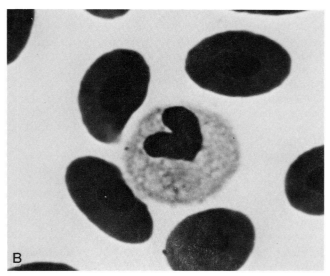

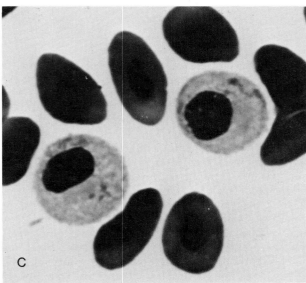

FIGURE 9–4. Circulating heterophils can have a variable nuclear morphology. The three plates show heterophils from a tilapia peripheral blood smear. *A.* Heterophil with a classic bilobed nucleus. *B.* Heterophil with a typical indented nucleus. *C.* Two heterophils with nearly round nuclei (Giemsa, 1000×).

FIGURE 9–5. A rarely seen hypersegmented heterophil from a peripheral blood smear of a sandtiger shark (Giemsa, 1000×).

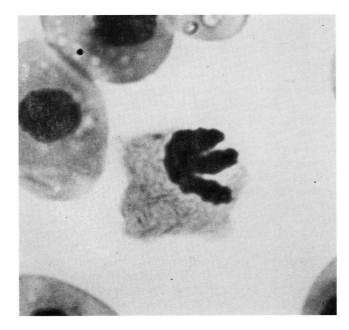

of the cell. These granules are usually rod-shaped and can be gray or pale blue to pale red. They are often distinctly eosinophilic and frequently obscure nuclear detail. For this reason, they are termed heterophils rather than neutrophils, although they appear analogous to mammalian neutrophils.

The staining characteristics of fish heterophils are quite variable with different fish species. This also occurs among mammalian species and should not be that surprising in fish (Sierecki, 1955). Heterophilic granules in fish are usually peroxidase positive, although heterophilic granules from tench and river bleak are reported to be negative for the benzidine peroxidase test (Kelényi and Németh, 1969). Otherwise, positive peroxidase staining is considered an identification criterion for fish heterophils (Weinreb, 1963). Heterophilic granules of plaice, brown trout, roach, and Atlantic salmon are all peroxidase positive. The granules of heterophils from brown trout, Spanish mackerel, and plaice are also Sudan black B positive (Campbell, 1988; Ellis, 1977) as well as PAS positive. Plaice heterophils are acid and alkaline phosphatase positive (Ellis, 1977).

Ultrastructurally, two types of heterophilic granules are described in fish, small homogeneous granules and large oval granules with axial crystalloids (Kelényi and Németh, 1969). The smaller homogeneous granule is composed of a dense matrix of alternating light and dark bands with approximately 100 Å periodicity when stained with phosphotungstic acid. The larger granules vary in size. Their axial electron-dense crystalloids are similar to those found in eosinophils. The crystalloids are not found in all fish species (Ferguson, 1976).

The major granulopoietic organ of fish is the kidney, but the spleen may play a minor role in the production of fish heterophils (Ellis, 1977). In sharks the majority of heterophil production seems to occur in the lymphoid tissues of the esophagus (Fange, 1968). Blast cells similar to mammalian granuloblasts found in bone marrow are seen in these tissues. The maturation sequences and nomenclature of granulocytes remain to be well established in fish, but adoption of the granuloblast system of nomenclature seems most appropriate.

The functional activity of fish heterophils remains a topic of study. For example, the phagocytic nature of the fish heterophil remains in question. Studies in plaice and rainbow trout have indicated that the heterophil is not phagocytic for carbon particles (Ellis et al., 1976; Klontz, 1972). On the other hand, studies examining heterophilic activity in bacterial infections have shown a high phagocytic response in rainbow trout (Finn and Nielson, 1971) and goldfish (Watson et al., 1963). Goldfish heterophils are also highly phagocytic for thorium dioxide (Thorotrast), a radiographic contrast agent (Weinreb and Weinreb, 1969). Also, chemotaxis has not been well demonstrated experimentally in fish heterophils. However, fish heterophils infiltrate injured tissues early in the inflammatory response (Thorpe and Roberts, 1972; Joy and Jones, 1973) and observations strongly suggest chemotaxic stimuli are involved.

The range of heterophil numbers in fish blood is quite wide, but they are usually not the predominate leukocyte in peripheral circulation. Infectious disease and stressful conditions elevate the number of heterophils in fish blood (Ellsaesser et al., 1985). The heterophilia seen in response to infection with bacteria or protozoa is a relatively rapid response in fish (within 24 hours) and appears to be independent of temperature. An increase in young heterophils, called a shift to the left of the Arneth scale (Schilling shift), does occur in response to acute inflammations in fish. Increased numbers of cells with hypersegmented nuclei (right shift) are also observed in long-standing chronic conditions. In fish, a heterophilia is most frequently associated with a lymphopenia (Slicher, 1961). This is particularly true of heterophilia due to stress responses, such as cold shock, or to responses to iatrogenic injection of cortisone or adrenocorticotropic hormone (ACTH).

Eosinophils

The piscean eosinophil is roughly the same size as or a bit smaller than the heterophil. It is usually 4.5 to 10.0 μ in diameter and is round in fixed and stained smears. Its nucleus is lobate, although, as in the heterophil, the nucleus may be obscured by the presence of numerous large cytoplasmic bodies. The opinion that the nucleus of fish eosinophils is less heavily lobated than that of the heterophil has not been carefully examined, but seems to hold true. The denser staining characteristics of the spherical cytoplasmic bodies in eosinophils may obscure this feature (Fig. 9–6). Nevertheless, the round bodies are distinct from the rod-shaped bodies of the heterophil and serve as a good identifying characteristic.

Ultrastructurally, the eosinophil granules of fish consist of dense material enclosing one or more rod- or disc-shaped inclusions (Weinreb, 1963). Smaller

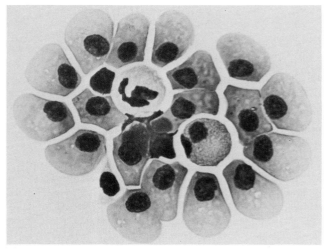

FIGURE 9–6. A heterophil of a sandtiger shark has larger, spindle-shaped cytoplasmic granules that do not stain (left), whereas an eosinophil has smaller, round cytoplasmic granules that stain dark pink (right) (Giemsa, 1000×).

granules lack crystalloids. The crystalloids are not a good differentiating feature between eosinophils and heterophils in fish blood, since both cell types may or may not exhibit them.

Eosinophils are formed in the granulocytic series similar to the heterophil. They become differentiable at the level of the progranulocyte. They are involved in hypersensitivity reactions and although they are more prevalent than basophils, they are still relatively rare. Eosinophils account for only 2 to 3% of normal total leukocyte counts in those species where they are recorded to occur. Occasionally reports of counts above 10% of the total leukocyte count are seen.

Eosinophils can phagocytize bacteria and other foreign substances, but probably not with the efficiency of the heterophil. There is little doubt that eosinophils play a roll in the control of metazoan parasite infection and that they are involved in immune responses to a variety of antigens. Considerably more work needs to be done on the biochemistry of fish eosinophils. It is a reasonable assumption that the anaerobic glycolysis pathway (the hexose monophosphate shunt) is important to eosinophils, since they contain abundant, large mitochondria and do phagocytize. The level of this importance remains to be studied. Similarly, although mammalian eosinophil granules are known to contain many lysosomal enzymes, including peroxidase, β-glucuronidase, phospholipase, and arylsulfatase as well as many characterized cationic proteins, the cytoplasmic bodies from fish eosinophils have not been as well studied.

Basophils

The fish basophil is not well studied. It is a granulocyte and apparently develops from the same series of precursor cells as the heterophil and eosinophil. It is distinct in blood smears stained with Romanowsky stains for light microscopy by the presence of several deeply basophilic cytoplasmic bodies approximately 0.8 μ in diameter with no clearly defined internal structure (Fig. 9–7). These usually appear round and are often fewer in number than the cytoplasmic bodies of heterophils and eosinophils. In Spanish mackerel these basophilic granules are PAS positive (Pitombeira and Martins, 1970). The nucleus of the fish basophil is eccentric and lobated, although often not as extensively as the nucleus of heterophils. The chromatin is homogeneous.

Ultrastructurally, the cytoplasmic bodies of basophils are large oval electron-dense areas enclosed in a membrane in the region of the rough endoplasmic reticulum. These cells contain histamine and are target cells in acute inflammations and hypersensitivity reactions. Their number varies among species of fish and there is some question about whether they occur in all species, but they have been reported in a wide range of fishes. Basophils have been reported in fairly high numbers in some studies in carp (Lowenthal, 1930), but they seldom constitute more than 1% of the total leukocyte count of fish.

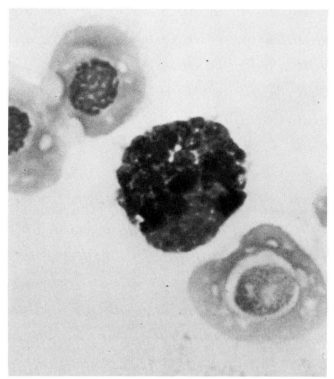

FIGURE 9–7. A basophil from a spiny dogfish peripheral blood smear showing large round dark-staining cytoplasmic granules (Giemsa, 1000×).

The function of basophils has not been established. They resemble mast cells, but the relationship is not clear. Basophils are affected by hormones from the adrenals and are seen in allergic and stress situations. Anomalous basophils and monocytes are seen along with anemia in chronic cadmium toxicity (Gill and Pant, 1985).

Monocytes

A clear-cut morphologic distinction between the lymphocytic series and monocytes is not present in most fish blood. This distinction is usually based on size and the regularity of the nucleus (Fig. 9–8). Monocytes are large, usually with more abundant cytoplasm than large lymphocytes, and often, but not always, have more irregular nuclear shapes. The nucleus of a monocyte usually occupies less than half the cell volume, and has coarsely granular chromatin, which does not show the peripheral clumping of dense chromatin seen in the nuclei of lymphocytes. The cytoplasm of monocytes is usually blue to blue-gray and may appear vacuolated. Occasionally, fine PAS- and acid phosphatase–positive granules may be present in the cytoplasm. Sometimes pseudopodia are seen.

Fish monocytes are only present in large numbers in the blood and anterior kidney. They may be formed from stem cells in the anterior kidney, although more complete studies are needed. Fish

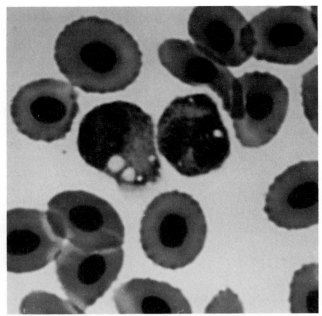

FIGURE 9–8. The distinction between large lymphocytes and monocytes is not clear-cut in fish hematology. The two leukocytes from peripheral blood of a channel catfish shown here are larger, with more cytoplasm than is common in large lymphocytes, and are most likely monocytes. The nucleus of the one cell is deeply indented, uncommon in lymphocytes (Giemsa, 1000×).

monocytes are phagocytic and take up colloidal carbon (Ellis et al., 1976) and Thorotrast (Weinreb and Weinreb, 1969). The term monocyte/macrophage is sometimes used for fish monocytes because cells resembling transitional forms are often seen in fish peripheral blood (Campbell, 1988). This usage is misleading and adds to confusion. It is recommended that the term *monocyte* be used for circulating cells and *macrophage* be reserved for differentiated cells in the connective tissues of fish.

Lymphocytes

Piscean lymphocytes are usually the most abundant leukocyte in the peripheral blood of fish. They are mononuclear cells with a round, or occasionally, a slightly indented nucleus, and they resemble the lymphocytes found in other vertebrates. They have a high nucleus-to-cytoplasm ratio and the nuclear chromatin pattern is generally distinct from that of thrombocytes, monocytes, and blast cells in a given sample. The lymphocytes are commonly divided into two or three groups on the basis of size.

SMALL LYMPHOCYTES. Small lymphocytes are round on stained smears and have very little deep to pale blue cytoplasm. They are about one-half to one-third the size of the erythrocytes, and they must be differentiated from the thrombocytes in some species of fish. Usually the small lymphocytes are slightly larger than thrombocytes (Fig. 9–9). Lymphocytes may conform to adjacent cells, causing an irregular outline, but they are usually round. Also

lymphocytes can have azurophilic granules that can lead to their being confused with thrombocytic granules. When this occurs similar granules in the cytoplasm of larger lymphocytes often alert the hematologist to the problem.

MEDIUM-SIZED LYMPHOCYTES. Medium-sized lymphocytes form a size continuum between the small lymphocytes and the large lymphocytes. They have a slightly increased amount of cytoplasm, which may appear to bleb out from the otherwise round border of the cell membrane. Ultrastructurally this cytoplasm contains more mitochondria than that of the small lymphocytes. The nuclear morphology of the medium-sized lymphocyte is consistent with the small and large lymphocytes and presents little trouble in differentiation. The chromatin is more open than that of the small lymphocyte but still represents a similar pattern. These are often the easiest lymphocytes to unequivocally identify. They may exhibit small round azurophilic granules, as mentioned earlier, which are sometimes considered an indication of activation.

LARGE LYMPHOCYTES. Large lymphocytes approach the size of monocytes and blast cells but are rarely as large. Their differentiation can be quite difficult for the novice, and, in some cases, trying for the expert. The fact that large lymphocytes represent a member of a size continuum with the smaller lymphocytes can help to differentiate them from monocytes. Their nuclei are more regular and the chromatin pattern is distinct from that of monocytes in any given sample. These young lymphocytic cells have more cytoplasm than the more mature, smaller lymphocytes, and their cytoplasm is filled with abundant mitochondria. The differentiation between large

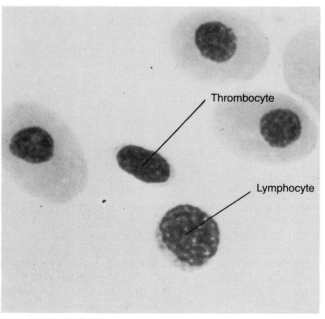

FIGURE 9–9. A small lymphocyte (lower) and a thrombocyte (above) from a brown shark peripheral blood smear (Giemsa, 1000×).

lymphocytes and lymphoblasts at the level of light microscopy can be a relatively academic exercise.

Numbers of circulating lymphocytes can be affected by disease and physiological states. Fish with infectious disease or exposed to stress may have low lymphocyte counts (Campbell, 1988), and lymphopenia is commonly associated with the heterophilia seen in bacterial septicemias (Brenden and Huizinga, 1986). Administration of exogenous cortisol or dexamethasone to salmon results in a reduction of the number of circulating lymphocytes in the blood (McLeay, 1973) and a lymphopenia is a well-established stress reaction in fish.

Plasma Cells

Plasma cells morphologically similar to those found in mammals occur in fish and are found occasionally in the peripheral blood. These cells are characterized by an eccentrically positioned nucleus that is intensely stained, showing a wheel-spoke pattern of chromatin and prominent nucleoli. A conspicuous Golgi area appears as a pale perinuclear halo in the otherwise deep blue cytoplasm.

Methods of Evaluating Leukocytes

Most controversies in fish hematologic methodology center around leukocyte counts. Numerous methods for obtaining total leukocyte counts (cells per microliter) have been proposed and used by different workers, providing ample evidence that the optimal method is not yet at hand. Historically, when all quantification was done manually by counting cells in known volumes of blood under a microscope, this issue was not nearly as controversial. The development of lysis techniques to facilitate counting mammalian samples by removing enucleated erythrocytes inaugurated the distinction between mammalian and fish hematology. Fish samples cannot be accurately counted with some new methods because of the interference of erythrocyte nuclei. Differential stains are still needed and leukocytes must be discerned from the much more numerous erythrocytes.

The introduction of automated cell counting on the basis of cell size accented the disparity between fish and mammalian cell counting techniques and fueled the controversy over the value of fish leukocyte counts. Attempts to apply cell size counter technology to fish samples are plagued by the overlap in sizes between the very small lymphocytes and the relatively large nucleated erythrocytes of fish. Although the rapid analysis possible with automated techniques allows investigators to examine and report on larger numbers of fish and more varied species, these reports do not agree with the literature based on hand counting. Very fine adjustments in the size exclusion parameters have a very major impact on automated total leukocyte counts, causing totally unacceptable variation and poor reproducibility.

Unfortunately this variability and lack of consistency leads to the erroneous conclusion that fish leukocyte counts are not useful tools for differential diagnosis. In reality, inappropriate methods adopted to speed the counting procedure, including some indirect methods that would never be acceptable for mammalian samples, are responsible for the lack of consistency.

Indirect leukocyte counts from differential smears are extremely dependent upon uniform distribution of white and red cells in the smear and the absence of cell lysis in the sample. Methods that count white cells in a predetermined number of high-powered fields and then multiply that number by a factor to obtain a count are not reliable and should not be used. Estimated leukocyte counts using an actual erythrocyte count and a ratio of leukocytes to erythrocytes taken from a smear are somewhat better, but depend heavily on the methods used to obtain the erythrocyte count and the cell type ratio. The difficulties in distinguishing early erythrocytic precursors from leukocytes on fish blood smears can also result in very bizarre and clinically unusable data when these methods are employed.

Another indirect method currently seeing considerable use because it requires little skill discerning cellular morphology is vital staining a portion of the leukocytes in a sample for counting in a chamber. The total leukocyte count is determined mathematically using a ratio determined from the differential smear. Here accuracy depends not only on the quality of the differential smear and its evaluation, but on the precision and selectivity with which the vital stain shows a given cell type. For example, the commonly used Eosinophil Unopette (Becton-Dickinson, Franklin Lakes, New Jersey) actually stains both eosinophils and heterophils in practice, a situation that must be accounted for in the mathematics of determining the total leukocyte count (Zinkl, 1986). This technique is relatively accurate if heterophils and eosinophils make up the majority of leukocytes in the sample. Its accuracy and precision suffer as the percentage of lymphocytes in the total white count increases. It is more suitable where lymphocytes make up less than half of the total leukocytes, a rare situation in fish.

Direct counting of leukocytes on a Neubauer chamber is the preferred method of determining fish total leukocyte counts (see Fig. 9–3). It is relatively consistent and reliable if performed by an experienced hematologist, and it can be performed on the same preparation used for the erythrocyte count. Its major drawback is the need for the hematologist to be competent in the differentiation of thrombocytes from small lymphocytes when counting the chamber. Several differential staining diluents have been developed for use on fish blood to assist in this differentiation. The most useful is Natt-Herrick solution (Natt and Herrick, 1952). The recipe for this diluent is given in Table 9–3. Twenty microliters of blood is added to 1980 μl of Natt-Herrick solution to achieve a 1 to 100 dilution.

TABLE 9–3. Natt-Herrick Diluent

1. Add 500 ml distilled water to a 1 L volumetric flask.
2. Dissolve 3.88 g NaCl.
3. Dissolve 2.50 g Na_2SO_4.
4. Dissolve 2.91 g Na_2HPO_4 •12 H_2O.
5. Dissolve 0.25 g KH_2PO_4.
6. Add 7.5 ml 37% formaldehyde.
7. Dissolve 0.10 g methylviolet 2B.
8. Bring the flask volume to 1 L with distilled water.
9. After allowing the solution to stand overnight, filter the solution through Whatman no. 2 filter paper.

In the direct, complete fish total leukocyte count, white cells in all nine primary squares on the Neubauer chamber are counted. In other words, all white cells on the entire counting surface or the equivalent of the cells contained in 0.9 µl of the diluted sample are tallied. Ten percent of this count is then added to the count to represent the number of cells expected in a full microliter of diluted sample. Finally, this number is multiplied by the dilution factor to obtain the number of leukocytes in 1 µl of undiluted blood. For the common dilution of 20 µl of blood in 1980 µl of staining diluent, the dilution factor is 100. The cells counted in nine primary squares is increased by 10% and multiplied by 100.

DIFFERENTIAL CELL COUNTS. The morphological characteristics of fish blood cells have been well documented since before the turn of the century, yet no aspect of fish hematology is fraught with more uncertainty than the differential leukocyte count. Most of this timidity is unwarranted. With a modicum of experience most people can differentiate fish cells readily and accurately. Difficulties involved in discerning immature erythrocytic series cells from leukocytic cells are one source of confusion. The basophilic cytoplasm of young red cells can be confused for that of a lymphocyte if nuclear morphology is ignored. This problem can be avoided by initially examining the blood smear to identify characteristic cells in the erythrocytic series and comparing them against well-defined lymphocytes prior to beginning the differential count.

Another source of confusion in fish differentials is the presence of discernible eosinophilic cytoplasmic granules in granulocytes otherwise analogous to mammalian neutrophils. The morphological distinction in the shape of the granules, round for eosinophils and spindle shaped or elongated in heterophils, is useful. This differentiation may be augmented by sometimes subtle differences in staining. The granules in eosinophils are usually more intensely stained than those in heterophils, but these differences are not always consistent or reliable. The nuclei of heterophils also tend to be more segmented than the nuclei in eosinophils, giving another distinguishing characteristic.

The usefulness of the differential count depends heavily on the proper preparation of the blood smear to be counted. Differential smears are best made from fresh blood immediately after it is drawn. They can also be made from anticoagulant-treated samples, but the quality of smear may not be as good. If anticoagulated samples are used, it is important that the sample be adequately mixed prior to making the smear to assure a representative sample. One to 2 minutes of carefully rotating the sample vial is usually adequate.

Two techniques predominate the preparation of thin smears for differential counting, the slide method and the coverslip method. The slide method of blood smear preparation is identical to the method commonly used in mammalian hematology (Fig. 9–10). It is prepared by placing a slide on a flat level surface and then placing a small drop of blood near one end. The blood is then spread with the edge of another slide held at about a 30-degree angle to the slide being prepared. Preparing this type of slide properly requires considerable practice. A good smear should have a smooth appearance and long straight borders that end in a feathered edge. Erythrocytes should be well distributed in a single cell layer over a reasonable portion of the smear. Inexperienced preparers tend to use too large a drop of blood, resulting in thick smears which overrun the sides of the slide. Wavy films with varying thickness are caused by an unsteady and uneven motion of the spreader slide when the smear is prepared. Holes and streaks in the smear occur if the preparation slide is dirty or if the spreader slide is chipped or dirty. Any of these conditions result in a suboptimal preparation.

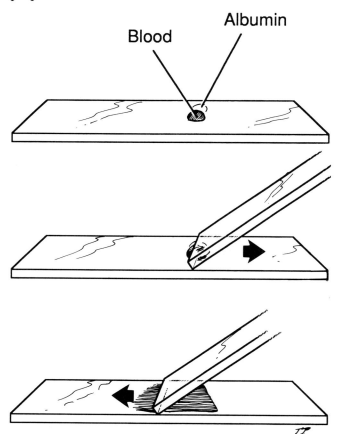

FIGURE 9–10. The two-slide method for making a blood smear for differential cell counting.

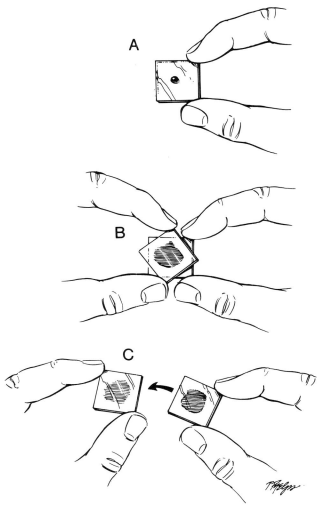

FIGURE 9–11. The coverslip method for differential blood smear preparation.

The coverslip method uses two coverslips (Fig. 9–11). A drop of blood is placed on one coverslip and the second coverslip is dropped on the first at a 45-degree offset. This spreads the blood uniformly across the coverslips. The coverslips are gently separated and the blood film allowed to dry before fixation and staining.

Proper staining of the blood smears made by either technique may be more critical for fish samples than it is for mammalian samples. Commonly the Romanowsky-type stains are used. The selection of a stain is based considerably on personal preference, but different stains do provide different advantages. Wright's stain tends to show the azurophilic granules of monocytes well and preserve the cytoplasmic bodies of heterophils better than May-Grunwald Giemsa stain. The May-Grunwald Giemsa stain is a more intense stain which improves the differentiation of immature cells. The Wright-Giemsa stain seems to combine the benefits of both parent stains and is very good for preparation of slides destined to be photographed. More important than the stain se-

lected is perhaps the consistent application of the stain to produce uniform staining from slide to slide. This will greatly influence the slide reader's ability to produce consistent and meaningful differential counts. Many find it beneficial to coverslip blood smears before they are counted, although this may not be practical in a busy clinical laboratory. When the coverslip method is used, the stained coverslip is usually mounted on a slide.

When approaching a differential count, the stained blood film should always be examined initially at low power (100 to 200×) to survey the slide for areas with good cell distribution in a monolayer. Next, high dry magnification (400×) should be used to appraise the staining characteristics of the different cell types seen on the slide. During this phase of the differential count, cells distinctly characteristic of the various leukocytes are sought out and used as standards for the eventual decisions that will be necessary to classify ambiguous cells. Experienced hematologists may then proceed to a well-distributed area of the smear to perform the actual differential count under high dry magnification (400×). Others may prefer to use oil emersion (1000×) to perform the differential.

Several methods of counting cells have been examined for their ability to provide consistent and representative results. This is particularly necessary with thin smears prepared on slides because heterophils tend to marginate and lymphocytes tend to remain in the body of the smear. The selection of the area to count and the method for counting can significantly affect the picture presented by a differential count. The battlement method of counting along the edges of the smear is accepted as the most representative (MacGregor et al., 1940) (Fig. 9–12). In the battlement method, a count is made in three fields in the horizontal direction along the length of the slide followed by counting two fields toward the center of the slide. Then two horizontal fields are counted in the same direction as before, followed by two fields toward the edge of the slide. This returns the slide reader to the initial level along the edge of the slide, advanced five fields. The procedure is repeated until the desired number of leukocytes have been categorized and counted.

The question of how many cells should be

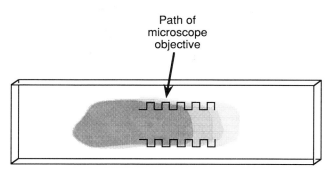

FIGURE 9–12. The battlement approach to examining a differential blood smear.

counted in a fish differential blood leukocyte count has not been resolved. The differential count is subject to considerable error because a small number of leukocytes are sampled in relation to the total sample in even the most aggressive counts. The distribution of cells on the smear and in the area counted has a profound impact on the final results obtained, and obviously the more cells counted, the better the chances of achieving a true representation of the percentages of leukocyte cell types present. On the other hand, the differential count is one of the most time-consuming procedures in fish hematology, and counting large numbers of cells can severely limit the number of samples which can be counted in a day. Even when 400 cells are counted, the error in a given cell type due to chance may be as much as 7.5% of the total count (Barnett, 1933). Optimally 200 cells should be counted in a routine differential count. An exception would be in certain fish and in cases of viral infections where the lack of leukocytes in the smear makes the differential count much more time consuming. In these cases every effort should be made to count 100 cells.

THROMBOCYTES

Fish thrombocytes are small, spindle-shaped or elongated oval cells with a single round-to-ovoid, dense nucleus and a scant cytoplasm, which stains blue to blue-gray with Romanowsky stains (Fig. 9–13). Cytoplasmic granules are often present and can be deeply basophilic or lightly eosinophilic. Granules are not always present. A single PAS-positive cytoplasmic granule has been reported near the nucleus of plaice thrombocytes (Ellis, 1976). Thrombocytes are routinely negative for Sudan black B and benzidine-peroxidase stains (Yuki, 1957) and may appear PAS negative in some species (Blaxhall and Daisley, 1973).

Fish thrombocytes are morphologically distinct from small lymphocytes at the electron microscopy level, having a distinctly ribbed chromatin and many cytoplasmic vesicles similar to the surface-connecting system of platelets in mammals (Ferguson, 1976). At the light microscopy level the distinction between these two cell types causes considerable difficulty in some samples. Classic thrombocytes should have a distinctly elongate shape. The nuclear patterns are generally more dense. Cytoplasmic granules are extremely rare in small lymphocytes.

The origins of fish thrombocytes are not clear. Early workers felt fish thrombocytes were formed from small lymphocytes (Jordan, 1926; Gardener and Yevich, 1969), whereas other workers have felt fish thrombocytes may develop from the same stem cell as the lymphocytes (Catton, 1951; Klontz, 1972). This is considered highly unlikely, but some evidence exists for thrombocyte development occurring in the fish spleen (Ellis, 1977).

Thrombocytes of fish respond to disease situations in much the same manner as is seen with platelets in mammals. Administration of cortisol or dexamethasone can lead to an increased clotting time in fish through a reduction in thrombocyte count (McLeay, 1973). Thrombocytopenia is also seen along with a lymphocytosis and mild heteropenia in chronic cadmium toxicity (Gill and Pant, 1985).

Methods for Evaluating Thrombocytes

Usually, evaluation of the thrombocytes in fish centers around a total count. Actual counts can be made using a counting chamber and stained dilutions of blood such as Natt-Herrick solution. The most common counting method uses the same standard 1/200 dilution used in the erythrocyte and leukocyte counts. All of the small squares in the large center square of an improved Neubauer hemocytometer are counted (see Fig. 9–3). This number is multiplied by 2000 to obtain the total thrombocyte count. To improve the accuracy of the count, many clinical pathologists count two or more chambers and average the number of thrombocytes counted.

More frequently, in fish hematology thrombocyte counts are estimated from the stained thin smear. There are two methods used to accomplish this, both of which are heavily dependent upon a well-distributed, properly made blood smear. The tendency for thrombocytes to clump contributes considerable opportunity for error in these estimates and they should be evaluated with care.

The more accepted method of estimation is to count the number of thrombocytes seen while counting 100 leukocytes. This is reported as thrombocytes per 100 leukocytes but can be converted to an estimated absolute value by multiplying the number of thrombocytes counted by the total leukocyte count divided by 100. The reporting style remains a matter of personal preference. An alternative estimation technique that is even more subject to the vagaries of cell distribution on the thin smear is to count the number of thrombocytes per high-powered (1000×) field for 10 or more fields and report the average as

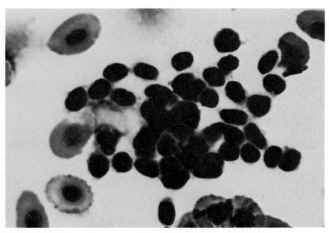

FIGURE 9–13. A raft of thrombocytes from a peripheral blood smear from a channel catfish (Giemsa, 1000×).

thrombocytes per high-powered field. If the reported value is greater than 3, the platelet count is assumed to be normal.

CYTOLOGY

Surface Smears

There is a reasonable argument that cytology is the most useful of the clinical pathology techniques applied to fish. Certainly the most commonly performed procedure in fish clinical practice is the body surface smear for identification of protozoan parasites. A description of taking these smears can be found in Chapter 5. A major advantage of the technique is that it can be applied to fish of any size without harming them. Indications for taking a surface smear include any externally visible lesion, excessive mucus production, or behavioral signs of irritation such as flashing or rubbing.

Surface or skin smears of fish are usually examined as unstained wet mounts to facilitate the observation of moving parasites. With practice, it is possible to identify fish cell types in this type of preparation. This is facilitated by using a microscope equipped with phase contrast. It is also possible, and useful, to stain surface smears after the initial wet mount examination. This helps identify suspected pathogens and facilitates evaluation of the response of the fish to the condition affecting it. If the clinician suspects that more than one stain may be needed for a complete examination, several smears should be made when the fish is handled. Although some stains can be decolorized and restained with another process, it is much simpler and more reliable to have multiple slides available.

New methylene blue stain is often used as a general stain to allow better visualization of formed elements in the smear. It is quick and similar enough to Wright-Giemsa stains to allow easy interpretation. The Gram stain is used to identify bacteria and the acid-fast stain for detecting mycobacteria. Rapid Wright's stains (Diff-Quik, Harleco, Gibbstown, New Jersey) are used extensively in veterinary practices and work well to stain the formed elements in a fish surface smear. Most clinicians are adept at interpreting blood smears stained with these stains, which makes it easier to interpret cytologic smears stained the same way. Lactophenol cotton blue stain is used to selectively stain fungal elements. All of these stains can be purchased as commercial kits, or they can be made using the formulas provided in Tables 9–4 to 9–7. They are all quick and require little in the way of special apparatus.

Fish skin is commonly noncornified stratified squamous epithelium, and specimens obtained from scraping the skin usually have numerous squamous epithelial cells and scales (Fig. 9–14). Epithelial cells are large flat polygonal cells with abundant cytoplasm and, typically, very round nuclei with uniform chromatin density. They may be found in sheets, but

TABLE 9–4. New Methylene Blue Staining Procedure

1. Air-dry slide.
2. Add small drop of methylene blue stain.
3. Coverslip.

Reagent:
New methylene blue: Dissolve 0.5 g new methylene blue in 99 ml 0.85% saline. Add 1 ml 37% formaldehyde, filter, and store in a brown bottle.

in smears from fish, they are more often seen as individual cells. Fish scales come in a variety of shapes, sizes, and structures. Their morphology is discussed in Chapter 1. Commonly, the small scales seen on surface smears of most fish have a fingerprint appearance. They have no nucleus and are easily distinguished from cellular components.

The other prominent feature of most skin smears is the mucus produced by the goblet cells. This appears as background strands or amorphous patches of transparent material, often containing cells. When stained with Romanowsky stains or new methylene blue, mucus protein stains pale blue to purple.

Occasionally goblet cells may be seen in a smear. They are tall columnar epithelial cells with a basal nucleus and abundant cytoplasm. Their cytoplasm contains several clear vacuoles, and when they are stained fine eosinophilic granules are visible in the basophilic cytoplasm. Also seen on occasion are melanophores and iridiophores, which may exfoliate with the epithelial tissues. These cells can have an intricate stellate appearance. The pseudopodia of these pigment-bearing ameboid cells can take on intricate and elaborate shapes. They usually contain yellow, red, or black pigment and are quite prominent when they occur in a smear. In fresh smears they may be actively moving pigment and appear in motion. They should not be mistaken for an unusual pathogenic organism.

Abnormal epithelial cells may also be identified on cytological examination. These include the grossly enlarged cells infected with the lymphocystis virus

TABLE 9–5. Harleco Diff-Quik Staining Technique

1. Air-dry the slide, and then dip into fixative for five 1-second dips. Drain off any excess fixative.
2. Dip the slide in solution I five times for 1 second each, and then drain off any excess stain.
3. Dip the slide into solution II five times for 1 second each, and drain off any excess stain.
4. Rinse the slide in distilled water and allow it to air-dry.

Reagents:
Fixative: A methanol-based fixative solution.
Solution I: Buffered eosin Y.
Solution II: Buffered methylene blue and azure A dye.

The procedure results in a stain similar to Wright-Giemsa. Increasing or decreasing the staining intensity can be accomplished by altering the number of dips into solutions I and II. Overstained specimens can be destained with acid alcohol and restained.

TABLE 9–6. Gram Stain Technique

1. Prepare slide, air-dry, heat-fix gently, and allow to cool.
2. Cover slide 1.5 to 2 minutes with gentian violet solution.
3. Wash with tap water.
4. Cover slide with Gram's iodine solution for 1 minute.
5. Wash with tap water.
6. Decolorize with alcohol for a few seconds.
7. Wash with tap water.
8. Counterstain with safranin for 0.5 to 1 minute.
9. Wash with tap water, blot dry, and examine.

Reagents:
Gentian violet: Dissolve 4.0 g crystal violet (85% dye content) in 20 ml ethanol (95%), then dilute 1:10 with distilled water. Dissolve 0.8 g ammonium oxalate in 80 ml distilled water. Make a 1:4 mixture (crystal violet:ammonium oxalate) (v/v).

Gram iodine: Dissolve 1 g iodine and 2 g potassium iodide in 300 ml distilled water. (Make fresh every 2–3 weeks.)

Safranin: Make a 2.5% (w/v) solution of safranin in 95% ethanol, then dilute 1:10 (vv) with distilled water.

Decolorizing alcohol: Use either 95% ethanol or 1:1 (v/v) acetone and 95% ethanol.

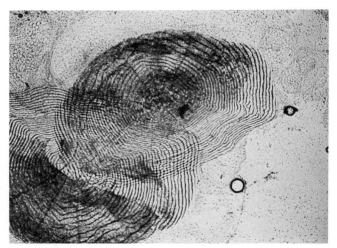

FIGURE 9–14. Squamous epithelial cells and scales are commonly seen in skin impression smears.

(Fig. 9–15). These can be seen in smears of typical lymphocystis lesions but are more commonly identified in skin biopsy preparations where a small part of the exuberant tumor is excised and prepared in a squash smear.

Other cells that may be identified in a surface smear from a fish include spindle-shaped fibroblasts and large adipocytes, which contain a single large vacuole. These connective tissue cell types are usually only encountered in smears from areas where the epithelial layers are not intact. They do not exfoliate as readily as epithelial cells and are less frequently seen.

Inflammatory responses on the skin of fish are similar to other animals. The leukocytic hemocytes are involved. The predominate leukocyte type seen in fish surface smears resembles macrophages or monocytes. Heterophils, eosinophils, and even basophils can be seen in surface smears, as can lymphocytes and occasional thrombocytes. The astute clinician can judge the condition of the leukocytes in the smear. In severe sepsis, toxic or lytic leukocytes are seen. Toxic cells have increased cytoplasmic vacuolization, atypical granulation, and some degree of karyorrhexis of their nuclei.

Of course, it is also possible to observe parasites, including bacteria, in the mucus smear. Protozoan parasites are usually easier to identify while still living and moving in a freshly prepared smear. They can be identified by their specific morphological features as well as distinctive movement patterns. Helminth parasites are relatively easy to find in surface smears and are identified by their characteristic morphology. Bacteria in large colonies are identifiable as such in a fresh smear but are more easily studied in stained preparations.

Fluid Aspirates

The other major use of clinical cytology in fish practice is the examination of fluids aspirated from various organs or the body cavity. Common sources of specimens include aspirations from the swim bladder or of ascitic fluid in the body cavity. The same staining techniques are used with these specimens as are used with surface smear preparations.

Swim bladder taps usually yield only gas in healthy fish. Even small amounts of fluid obtained from taps of the swim bladder are worth examining. Large numbers of mononuclear leukocytes or immature heterophils in such specimens suggest infectious processes and are indicative of a septic swim bladder. The presence of intracellular bacteria in leukocytes from swim bladder taps is essentially diagnostic for bacterial sepsis. The prognosis for such cases is fair in the absence of systemic disease with proper antibiotic therapy.

When swim bladder taps yield large amounts of fluid that is essentially acellular, it is suggestive of

TABLE 9–7. Acid-Fast Staining Procedure

1. Prepare smear, air-dry, and gently heat-fix.
2. Cover the smear with Ziehl-Nielsen carbolfuchsin and steam gently for 5 minutes.
3. Wash with tap water.
4. Decolorize with acid alcohol until the film is colorless.
5. Wash with tap water.
6. Counterstain with methylene blue for 5 to 20 seconds.
7. Wash with tap water and dry.

Reagents:
Ziehl-Nielsen carbolfuchsin: Dissolve 3 g basic fuchsin in 100 ml 95% ethanol. Dissolve 5 g phenol in 100 ml distilled water. Mix 1 part of the carbolfuchsin solution with 9 parts of the phenol solution (v/v), let stand 24 hours, and filter.

Acid alcohol: Combine 98 ml 95% ethanol with 2 ml concentrated hydrochloric acid.

Methylene blue: Take 30 ml saturated methylene blue (1.5 g methylene blue powder in 100 ml 95% ethanol) and add to 100 ml distilled water and 0.1 ml 10% potassium hydroxide solution. Filter and dilute 1:20 (v/v) with distilled water.

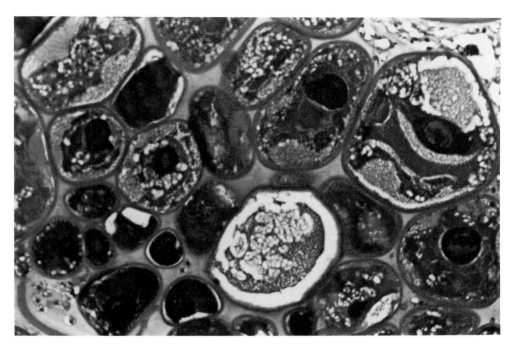

FIGURE 9–15. *Lymphocystis*-infected fibroblasts seen in a stained 7 μm-histologic section. The large cells are also prominent in fresh squash preparations (H & E, 100×). (Courtesy of L. Khoo.)

chromic inflammatory occlusion of the pneumatic ducts. The prognosis for a fish with this condition is poor.

Gas-forming enteritis can mimic diseases of the swim bladder. In addition to the development of abnormal swimming postures, bulges from gas-filled bowel can cause the clinician to misidentify the bowel as the swim bladder. The presence of ciliated columnar epithelial cells along with considerable debris indicates an intestinal tap.

Abdominal taps of ascitic fluid can also accidentally result in an intestinal tap. These are readily identified by the presence of food debris. Leukocytes will not be seen in any large numbers in contrast to the relatively rare event of an intestinal or gastric rupture spilling bowel contents into the coelom, resulting in peritonitis.

Ascites accumulations in fish are often dominated by mononuclear cells. The cellular content of ascitic fluids is often very low and centrifugation of the sample to sediment cellular elements is a useful technique to facilitate cytologic examination. It shortens reading time by reducing the slide coverage required to encounter cells. The technique can make interpretation a bit more difficult, since cell numbers cannot be estimated without volume measurements made before and after the centrifugation step. Also, centrifugation often distorts the cells, making them more difficult to identify.

SERUM CHEMISTRY

Serum chemistry studies of healthy fish are relatively scarce and well-designed studies of fish with specific diseases are almost nonexistent. This makes interpretation of fish serum chemistries from clinical patients very difficult. Much more work is needed in this area, both in the establishment of baseline parameters and in studying well-defined cohorts with specifically diagnosed diseases.

As in any aspect of veterinary practice, the methods used to obtain samples and the handling of those samples can be of paramount importance to the reliability of the information obtained from analysis of the sample. Serum is the preferred sample for chemistry analysis, although plasma is often used because of the difficulty of obtaining two samples from one patient. The yield of plasma from a sample is also greater than the yield of serum. If plasma is used, it is important to consider the anticoagulant involved when interpreting the results. Obviously, sodium or potassium salts of EDTA or heparin will affect serum sodium or potassium levels. In addition, the calcium-binding activity of EDTA will modify the serum calcium reading obtained from an EDTA-treated plasma sample. When plasma samples are destined to be examined for enzymatic activities and electrolytes, ammonium heparin or lithium heparin are the anticoagulants of choice.

As in mammalian samples, glucose determinations are most useful when performed on serum separated from cellular elements shortly after sampling. If more than 30 minutes to an hour is required to get whole blood samples back to the laboratory and processed, fluoride anticoagulant needs to be used to slow glycolysis in the whole blood. Unfortunately fluoride inhibits not only glycolysis, but also other enzymatic processes in the serum and in test reagents used in automatic serum analyzers. It should only be used when glucose levels are of particular interest to the clinician and rapid processing of the sample is not practical.

Improper specimen handling is the number one

cause of analytic inaccuracies in serum chemistry evaluations. Blood should ideally be processed within 1 hour of sampling. Clot formation requires approximately 15 to 30 minutes at room temperature. At this time, the clot can be rimmed and the specimen centrifuged for 5 to 10 minutes at a relative centrifugal force (RFG) of 1000 (3000 rpm in a 10-cm radius centrifuge). Better yield is obtained using serum separator devices. These may require more relative centrifugal force to be effective.

Hemolysis is a large source of inaccuracy in serum chemistry analysis. Hemolysis increases serum lactate dehydrogenase (LDH), aspartate aminotransferase (AST) (formerly SGOT), and potassium levels in many fish species. If there is enough hemolysis to interfere with colorimetric assays, other values can be inaccurate from automated processors. Hemolysis can be minimized in most cases by avoiding exposure of the blood to moisture or water, careful transfer of the blood, and avoiding rapidly emptying of blood through needles. Tubes of blood should be handled gently, avoiding excessive shaking, extreme clot rimming, or overcentrifugation.

NITROGENOUS WASTE PRODUCTS

Blood Urea Nitrogen

The evaluation of nitrogenous compounds in fish serum is particularly complex, since it becomes necessary to distinguish saltwater and freshwater species as well as a host of very specialized fishes. With the exception of the elasmobranchs (sharks and rays), coelocanth, and lungfishes, the first two enzymes of the urea cycle, carbamoyl phosphate synthetase and ornithine transcarbamoylase, do not seem to occur in fish. Nevertheless, urea appears in all fish, thought to be derived from both exogenous and endogenous arginine, purine nucleotides, and the purine precursor amino acids, glutamine, serine, and glycine, rather than being formed from ammonia via the Krebs-Henseleit cycle. Most urea in fish is produced by the liver, but urea passes rapidly through most internal membranes and is consequently found in all fish tissues. It is excreted in small quantity in relation to total nitrogen excretion, primarily by the gills. Accordingly, in bony fishes, an elevated blood urea nitrogen (BUN) is not necessarily indicative of renal disease, but is more likely associated with gill or liver disease. Species differences occur, although most healthy freshwater fish seem to have a low BUN of around 10 mg/dl, whereas marine teleosts normally have BUN levels of about 5.0 mg/dl. In teleost fishes, a falling BUN can reflect liver disease or starvation.

In contrast, elasmobranchs have much higher normal BUN concentrations and use these levels to maintain osmotic balance with salt water. In elasmobranchs, urea is actually resorbed by kidney tubules from the urine, probably with simultaneous reabsorption of sodium. The coelocanth is similar to elasmobranchs in this regard. Though elasmobranchs maintain high urea concentrations, they are not more tolerant of urea toxicity. None of their enzymes are enhanced by urea and the enzymes of oxidative processes and glycolysis are definitely inhibited by urea. Nor do sharks appear to use control of urea concentration in their bodies to extend their external salinity tolerance range. In elasmobranchs and coelacanths, then, BUN may serve as an indicator of renal disease, particularly if it is falling.

Creatinine and Creatine

In fish, creatine predominates over creatinine. Creatine is excreted through the kidneys, not the gills, and forms more than half of the urinary nitrogen of most fish. Creatinine is found in fish, formed by spontaneous, nonenzymatic cyclization of creatine. The levels found in muscle do not appear to correlate with levels of creatine, and once formed, creatinine is not metabolized further, but excreted unchanged. Blood levels of creatinine in teleost fishes usually are on the order of 0.5 to 2 mg/dl, being higher in marine species.

Uric Acid

Uric acid is formed by fish from exogenous and endogenous purine nucleotides and by catabolism of proteins via purines. It is converted in the liver, and to a lesser extent in the kidney, to urea for excretion by the gills.

Ammonia

Ammonia is the main excretory product of fish. It is derived from the deamination of amino acids and the breakdown of purines and pyrimidines and is excreted primarily across the gills by passive diffusion and in an exchange mechanism for sodium as ammonia or ammonium ion. The rate of excretion of ammonia increases after feeding, whereas urea excretion does not. It also increases during periods of physical activity. In fish blood, ammonia is buffered by glutamic acid and the activities of glutaminase and glutamine synthetase. Teleost serum ammonia nitrogen ranges between 0.3 and 5.5 mg/dl. Significant spikes in serum ammonia are normal about 4 hours after eating.

SERUM ELECTROLYTES

Although fish kidneys make a negligible contribution to the excretion of nitrogenous waste, they are concerned with water excretion in freshwater fishes or divalent cation (magnesium and sulphate) elimination in marine fishes. Freshwater fishes have numerous glomeruli and clear about 30% of their body weight in free water every day, resorbing sodium and chloride in the distal tubules of the kidney and producing a very dilute urine. In contrast, marine fishes have a reduced number of smaller glomeruli and must compensate for diffusional water loss through their gills by drinking seawater. This creates a major salt burden to be eliminated. Sodium and chloride are excreted primarily by chloride cells in the gills, but magnesium and sulfate loads are handled by the kidney of marine fishes.

In freshwater fishes, a decrease in the glomerular filtration rate for any reason results in an acutely oliguric fish which mimics a normal marine fish. Sodium reabsorption is decreased to facilitate water removal and magnesium reabsorption is shifted to magnesium secretion. Serum sodium and magnesium levels fall and serum sulfate levels should also be expected to fall. In marine fishes, impairment of the renal tubular function reduces magnesium and sulfate secretion and should cause increased serum sulfate and magnesium levels.

Apart from renal involvement, in freshwater fishes, sodium and chloride usually fall in generalized infections, suggesting impairment of gill function. Baseline electrolyte values vary by species and environment but sodium levels around 150 mEq/L and chloride levels around 130 mEq/L are expected in most fishes. Potassium and calcium levels also fall in generalized infections, from expected baselines of about 3.2 mEq/L and about 5 mEq/L, respectively. In marine fishes, calcium baselines are nearer 6.5 mEq/L and egg-laden females from either marine or freshwater environments have higher calcium levels. The difficulty of interpreting simultaneous declines in multiple electrolytes in fish has led some workers to propose a potassium-to-sodium ratio of 0.02 as a better index of health than absolute electrolyte levels. This system has yet to be proven in sound clinical trials.

Electrolyte levels can be indicators of external influences from the environment. Excessively acid fresh water, for example, results in decreases in serum sodium and chloride that may or may not be related to concomitant rises in serum cortisol (Scherer et al., 1986). Calcium levels are also decreased under acidic conditions, contributing to an overall serum osmolality decrease.

Because of the complexity of evaluating the various electrolyte components of serum in fish, total osmolality is frequently assessed. A major portion of serum osmolality is due to sodium, chloride, and serum protein. This parameter is accordingly more easily affected by gill disease than by renal dysfunction and does not readily reflect changes in minor serum electrolytes such as magnesium, calcium, or potassium. Caution must be exercised when evaluating serum osmolality, since it may be maintained near normal limits even in the face of precipitous decreases in serum sodium, potassium, chloride, calcium, and even total protein. This is not well understood but may be accomplished through the contribution of amino acids liberated during the breakdown of proteins. Serum osmolality is generally around 295 mOsm/L in freshwater fishes and about 300 to 305 mOsm/L in marine fishes.

SERUM PROTEINS

Lowered serum protein levels often attributed to renal involvement do not necessarily follow increases in urine protein levels and should be interpreted with caution. Alternate causes of low total proteins include decreased intake through starvation, decreased synthesis due to hepatic dysfunction, increased capillary permeability for plasma proteins, or degradation of proteins by proteolytic enzymes released from endothelial cells destroyed by viruses or bacteria. Serum albumin levels fall with liver disease (Casillas et al., 1986). Serum calcium levels fall along with falling serum albumin levels owing to liver disease. This is probably a result of albumin acting as a ligand carrier for serum calcium (Wortsman and Traycoff, 1980). Total protein levels also fall in septicemic *Aeromonas* infections owing to decreased circulating immunoglobulins (Evenberg et al., 1986).

SERUM ENZYMES

The enzymes alanine aminotransferase (ALT) (formerly SGPT) and aspartate aminotransferase (AST) (formerly SGOT) occur in fish. They are concentrated in hepatic tissues. Serum AST and ALT levels are increased in severe acute necrotic hepatic disease of fish due to exposure to hepatotoxins such as carbon tetrachloride (Casillas et al., 1982). Levels of these enzymes are not reliably elevated in chronic liver disease (Casillas et al., 1986).

Severe septicemic infections, particularly with *Aeromonas* spp., have been shown to be associated with elevations in serum AST and decreases in serum ALT. Such severe infections also result in initially elevated serum glucose levels that subsequently fall, and anemia with lowered hemoglobin, total erythrocyte counts, and hematocrits (Brenden and Huizinga, 1986).

The method of sampling can have a major effect on serum enzyme determinations. Alanine aminotransferase, lactate dehydrogenase, creatinine, and phosphorus are all significantly higher in sera collected from a severed tail peduncle than in sera collected from heart puncture (Ikeda and Ozaki, 1981). Total serum protein, albumin, glucose, urea nitrogen, cholesterol, magnesium, creatinine, ALT, alkaline phosphatase, amylase, and acetylcholine esterase do not appear to be affected by tissue contamination associated with tail severing (Ikeda and Ozaki, 1981).

OTHER SERUM PARAMETERS

Glucose is probably the most studied of the nonenzymatic and nonprotein components of fish serum. Glucose elevates in severe bacterial infections for 24 hours but then falls precipitously (Brenden and Huizinga, 1986). Glucose values tend to increase with increased age in fish (Das, 1964). Fish are also alloxan sensitive and can be rendered temporarily diabetic with repeated intraperitoneal injections of the drug at 200 to 300 mg/kg body weight. This results in major increases in serum glucose that return to normal in 3 to 4 days (Young and Chavin, 1963).

Other serum parameters besides glucose shift with age. Serum amylase, chloride, creatinine, total protein, and total blood hemoglobin all increase with age in fish (Das, 1964). Serum calcium and alkaline phosphatase decrease with increasing age, and serum total cholesterol, uric acid, and urea nitrogen show a hyperbolic function with age, first decreasing, then increasing with age (Das, 1964).

ESTABLISHING BASELINE VALUES

The lack of good baseline values for most fish species means clinicians will need to be involved in this process for the next many years. Although clinicians are trained to use baseline values, the methods for determining them are not often readily available. The veterinary literature is replete with papers purporting to provide baseline information, but all too often, too few samples have been examined and often not with the rigor needed to provide truly useful reference values.

The first step in establishing the normal range of a parameter in fish blood is to find the mean and standard deviation (SD) of the distribution for a value using a random sampling design from a population of normal animals. One way to achieve a random sampling is to identify all animals in a healthy population with unique numbers. Then numbers are selected from a random numbers table or a random number generator, and the corresponding animals are entered into the study group. Numbers appearing more than once from the random number source are ignored after the first use.

The number of animals required to accomplish a decent baseline range determination depends on the amount of variation seen in the values of the parameter being studied and how much difference you will accept in the mean your experiment obtains from the true mean of the population. With the assumption of a gaussian distribution of the data, the required number of samples or replications to achieve a mean value with 95% confidence can be calculated from the following formula:

$$N = \frac{3.8416 \cdot (SD)^2}{(Distance)^2}$$

As an example, consider that you want to determine the baseline values for a serum enzyme. You have done a few determinations and have calculated a standard deviation of 4 units. You would like to

achieve a mean value within 1 unit of the true mean of the population. From the formula you would need to have 61.5 (rounded to 66) samples in your study. However, if you could accept a mean value from your experiment that might be as far as 2 units from the true mean, you would only need 15.4 (rounded to 15) samples.

Usually the convention of two times the standard deviation is used to establish the boundaries of values which would be considered "normal." This convention means that only 2.5% of all normal animals would be expected to have a value above the range and 2.5% below the range established. This results in some "normal" animals being considered abnormal, but it is a reasonable trade-off for not accepting too many abnormal animals as normal. This method does not consider the distribution of abnormal animals. There are many types of abnormalities and there may be many different distributions of these abnormalities, many of which may not be gaussian. The assumption applied when using the convention of two times the standard deviation to establish a baseline range is that an abnormal animal's value for the parameter will be enough above or below the center of the distribution to be outside the range for normal animals.

Not all serum chemistry values show a gaussian distribution. They can be quite asymmetric. This is called skewed data (Fig. 9–16). In these cases the mean (average value) and the mode (most frequent value) will not agree. If the skewedness is enough, it can result in values from the sample "normal" population falling outside of the 2 standard deviation range. When skewed data are obtained, they can sometimes be given a more gaussian distribution with a transformation such as taking the logarithm or square root value of each data point. An alternative method is to use percentiles. The normal range would be set at the 2.5 and 97.5 percentiles of all normal data. This technique will misclassify 5% of the normal animals as abnormal, an error called a Type 1 error. Calling a diseased animal normal is considered a Type 2 error. Changing the reference values to minimize one type of error increases the probability of the other type of error. Using a differ-

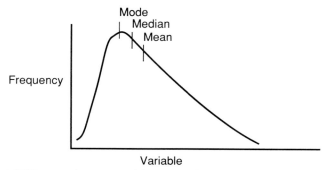

FIGURE 9–16. A nonnormal frequency distribution of data skewed to the right. The mean and mode are not the same. This can result in normal values falling outside of a 2-SD range.

ent percentile cut-off other than 2.5 and 97.5% is advisable only if an aspect of the disease or parameter being studied demands a different ratio of Type 1 and Type 2 errors.

LITERATURE CITED

Bailey, R.E. (1957) The effect of estradiol on serum calcium, phosphorus and protein of goldfish. J. Exp. Zool. 136(3):455–469.

Barnett, C.W. (1933) The unavoidable error in the differential count of the leukocytes of the blood. J. Clin. Invest. 12:77.

Blaxhall, P.C., and Daisley, K.W. (1973) Routine hematological methods for use with fish blood. J. Fish Biol. 5:771–782.

Brenden, R.A., and Huizinga, H.W. (1986) Pathophysiology of experimental Aeromonas hydrophila infection in goldfish, Carassius auratus (L.). J. Fish Dis. 9:163–167.

Campbell, T.W. (1988) Tropical fish medicine. Fish cytology and hematology. Vet. Clin. North Am. [Small Anim. Pract.] 18(2):347–364.

Casillas, E., Sundqvist, J., and Ames, W.E. (1982) Optimization of assay conditions for, and selected tissue distribution of alanine aminotransferase and aspartate aminotransferase of, English sole (Parophrys vetulus girard). J. Fish Biol. 21:197–204.

Casillas, E., Myers, M.S., Rhodes, L.D., and McCain, B.B. (1986) Serum chemistry of diseased English sole, Parophrys vetulus Girard, from polluted areas of Puget Sound, Washington. J. Fish Dis. 8:437–449.

Catton, W.T. (1951) Blood cell formation in certain teleost fishes. Blood 6:39–60.

Das, B.C. (1964) Age-related trends in the blood chemistry and hematology of the Indian carp (Catla catla). Gerontologia 10:47–64.

Eiras, J.C. (1983) Erythrocyte degeneration in the European eel, Anguilla anguilla. Bull. Eur. Assoc. Fish Pathol. 3:8–10.

Ellis, A.E. (1976) Leucocytes and related cells in the plaice, Pleuronectes platessa. J. Fish Biol. 8:143–156.

Ellis, A.E. (1977) The leucocytes of fish: A review. J. Fish Biol. 11:453–491.

Ellis, A.E. (1984) Bizarre forms of erythrocytes in a specimen of plaice, Pleuronectes platessa L. J. Fish Dis. 7:411–414.

Ellis, A.E., Munro, A.L.S., and Roberts, R.J. (1976) Defence mechanisms in fish. I. A study of the phagocytic system and the fate of intraperitoneally injected particulate material in the plaice (Pleuronectes platessa). J. Fish Biol. 8:67–78.

Ellsaesser, C.F., Miller, N.W., and Cuchens, M.A. (1985) Analysis of channel catfish peripheral blood leukocytes by bright-field microscopy and flow cytometry. Trans. Am. Fish. Soc. 114:279–285.

Evenberg, D., de Graaff, P., Fleuren, W., and Van Muiswinkel, W.B. (1986) Blood changes in carp (Cyprinus carpio) induced by ulcerative Aeromonas salmonicida infections. Vet. Immunol. Immunopathol. 12:321–330.

Fange, R. (1968) The formation of eosinophilic granulocytes in the eosophageal lymphomyeloid tissue in the elasmobranchs. Acta Zool. (Stockh.) 49:155–161.

Ferguson, H.W. (1976) The ultrastructure of plaice leucocytes. J. Fish Biol. 8:139–142.

Ferguson, H.W. (1989) Systemic Pathology of Fish. Iowa State University Press, Ames, Iowa.

Finn, J.P., and Nielson, N.O. (1971) Effect of temperature on inflammatory response in rainbow trout. J. Pathol. Bacteriol. 105:257–268.

Fourie, F. (1977) Effects of anticoagulants on the haematocrit, osmolarity and pH of avian blood. Poultry Sci. 56:1842–1846.

Freidlin, P.J. (1985) Destructive effect of heparin on avian erythrocytes. Avian Pathol. 14:531–536.

Gardener, G.R., and Yevich, P.P. (1969) Studies on the blood morphology of three estuarine cyprinodontiform fishes. J. Fish. Res. Bd. Can. 2:433–447.

Gill, T.S., and Pant, J.C. (1985) Erythrocytic and leukocytic responses to

cadmium poisoning in a freshwater fish, Puntius conchonius Ham. Environ. Res. 36(2):327–337.

Hibiya, T. (ed.) (1985) An Atlas of Fish Histology. Normal and Pathological Features. Kodansha, Tokyo.

Hyder, S.L., Cayer, M.L., and Pettey, C.L. (1983) Cell types in peripheral blood of the nurse shark: An approach to structure and function. Tissue Cell 15(3):437–455.

Ikeda, Y., and Ozaki, H. (1981) The examination of tail peduncle severing blood sampling method from aspect of observed serum constituent levels in carp. Bull. Jpn. Soc. Sci. Fish. 47(11):1447–1453.

Jordan, H.E. (1926) On the nature of the basophilic granulocytes of the blood and tissues. Anat. Rec. 33:89–106.

Jordan, H.E. (1938) Comparative Hematology. In: Handbook of Hematology. Vol. 2. (Downey, H., ed.). Paul B. Hoeber, New York, pp. 703–862.

Joy, J.E., and Jones, L.P. (1973) Observations on the inflammatory response within the dermis of a white bass, Morone chrysops, infected with Lernea cruciata. J. Fish Biol. 5:21–23.

Klontz, G.W. (1972) Haematological techniques and the immune response in rainbow trout. In: Diseases of Fish (Mawdesley-Thomas, L.E., ed.). Symp. Zool. Soc. London No. 30. Academic Press, London, pp 89–99.

Kyes, P. (1929) Normal leucocyte content of birds' blood. Anat. Rec. 43:197.

Lowenthal, N. (1930) Nouvelles observations sur les globules blancs du sang chez animaux vertebres. Arch. Anat. Histol. Embryol. 8:223–309.

MacGregor, R.G.S., et al. (1940) The differential leukocyte count. J. Pathogen. Bacteriol. 51:337.

McLeay, D.J. (1973) Effects of cortisol and dexamethasone on the pituitary-interrenal axis and abundance of white blood cell types in juvenile Coho salmon, Oncorhynchus kisutch. Gen. Comp. Endocrinol. 21:441–450.

Meinertz, J. (1902) Beitrage zur vergleichenden Morphologie der farblosen Blutzellen. Arch. Pathol. Anat. Klin. Med. 168:353–398.

Murray, S.A., and Burton, C.B. (1979) Effects of density on goldfish blood. II. Cell morphology. Comp. Biochem. Physiol. 62A:559–562.

Natt, M.P., and Herrick, C.A. (1952) A new blood diluent for counting the erythrocytes and leucocytes of the chicken. Poultry Sci. 31:735–738.

Pitombeira, M., and Martins, J.M. (1970) Haematology of the Spanish mackerel. Copeia 1:182–186.

Sanchez-Muiz, F.J., Higuera, M. De La, and Varela, G. (1982) Alterations of erythrocytes of the rainbow trout, Salmo gairdneri, by the use of Hansenula anomola yeast as sole protein source. Comp. Biochem. Physiol. 72A:693–696.

Scherer, E., Harrison, S.E., and Brown, S.B. (1986) Locomotor activity and blood plasma parameters of acid-exposed lake whitefish, Coregonus clupeaformis. Can. J. Fish. Aquatic Sci. 43:1556–1561.

Sieracki, J.C. (1955) The neutrophil. Ann. N.Y. Acad. Sci. 59:690–705.

Slicher, A.M. (1961) Endocrinological and haematological studies in Fundulus heteroclitus (Linn.). Bull. Birmingham Oceanographic Coll. 17:3–55.

Stokes, E.E., and Firkin, B.G. (1971) Studies of the peripheral blood of the Port Jackson shark (Heterodontus porusjacksoni) with particular reference to the thrombocyte. Br. J. Hematol. 20:427–435.

Thorpe, J.E., and Roberts, R.J. (1972) An aeromonad epidemic in the brown trout (Salmo trutta L.). J. Fish Biol. 4:441–452.

Watson, L.J., Shechmeister, I.L., and Jackson, L.L. (1963) The haematology of goldfish (Carassius auratus). Cytologia 28:118–130.

Weinreb, E.L. (1963) Studies on the fine structure of teleost blood cells. Anat. Rec. 147:219–238.

Weinreb, E.L., and Weinreb, S. (1969) A study of experimentally induced endocytosis in a teleost. I. Light microscopy of peripheral blood cell response. Zool. N.Y. 54:25–34.

Wortsman, J., and Traycoff, R.B. (1980) Biological activity of protein-bound calcium in serum. Am. J. Physiol. 238:E104–E107.

Young, J.E., and Chavin, W. (1963) Serum glucose levels and pancreatic islet cytology in the normal and alloxan diabetic goldfish, Carassius auratus L. Am. Soc. Zool. 3(4):510.

Yuki, R. (1957) Blood cell constituents in fish. I. Peroxidase staining of leucocytes in rainbow trout. Bull. Fac. Fish. Hokkaido Univ. 8:36–44.

Zinkl, J.G. (1986) Avian hematology. In: Schalm's Veterinary Hematology. 4th ed. (Jain, N.C., ed.) Lea & Febiger, Philadelphia, pp. 256–273.

Chapter 10

GENERAL PARASITOLOGY

STEPHEN A. SMITH   EDWARD NOGA

Fish can serve in the life cycle of parasites as definitive, intermediate, or paratenic hosts. Both adult and larval parasites can be found in almost every tissue of the host fish. Larval parasites, often observed in the musculature of the fish, are unsightly and cause economic hardships for fishermen, aquaculturists, and fish processors.

Most parasites cause little pathology under normal conditions, and wild fish may harbor a variety of parasites without any associated morbidity or mortality. However, parasites of fish can cause decreased weight gains and emaciation. Some parasites decrease host fecundity, or indirectly jeopardize their host's survival, causing susceptibility to predation owing to blindness or abnormal behavior. Parasite attachment sites can also provide a portal of entry for secondary bacterial or fungal infections. Parasites can also act as vectors of bacteria, viruses, or parasitic protozoa (Cusack and Cone, 1986).

In culture, where large numbers of fish are concentrated under sometimes stressful environmental conditions, parasites can cause serious disease, often resulting in mass epidemics. Identification of fish parasites and an understanding of parasite life cycles are prerequisites to the prevention or management of a parasitic disease outbreak.

Some parasites of fish also pose a threat to public health, particularly when humans eat the larval parasites in raw or undercooked fish. A number of genera of digenetic trematodes, such as *Clonorchis*, *Opisthorchis*, and *Heterophyes*, include species that can infect humans (Healy, 1970; Rim, 1982; Velasquez, 1982). Several species of the cestode genus *Diphyllobothrium* infect humans who eat the larval plerocercoid stage found in the muscles of freshwater and marine fishes (Bauer, 1961; Meyer, 1970). A number of larval nematodes that occur in fish also infect humans. Species in the genera *Anisakis*, *Contracaecum*, and *Porrocaecum* can cause serious acute abdominal pain in man (Smith and Wootten, 1978; Rohde, 1984). In addition, nematodes of the genera *Dioctophyma*, *Phocanema*, and *Gnathostoma* infect humans (Myers, 1970). Fortunately, most fish parasites with zoonotic potential can be eliminated by thorough cooking of the fish.

This chapter provides an introduction to methods of collection, preservation, and identification of parasites. The morphology, general life cycle, and typical pathology associated with the major groups of parasites is described, and a partial morphological key to some of the more common fish parasites is included (Table 10–1).

SPECIMEN COLLECTION

The smaller the parasite, the more fragile it is, and the more care is required for diagnostically useful preservation. For example, ciliates and flagellates may die rapidly after their host dies, making identification difficult. These parasites are best identified from wet mounts of live preparations. Metazoan parasites are generally recognizable for longer periods. Some parasites, especially ectoparasites, leave a dead host, whereas others (e.g., larval nematodes) migrate to aberrant locations. The rapid autolysis of fish tissues can also make identification of parasites difficult. Therefore, it is always best to examine a live or recently euthanatized host.

Before examining a clinical case for parasites, always determine if the fish can be euthanatized. Intentionally killing a fish that a client desires to be returned alive can be embarrassing. If necessary, live fish can be maintained in an aquarium for several days before they are examined. However, some parasites may leave their host, whereas others (e.g., ectoparasites) may multiply rapidly and infect other individuals in the aquarium. If holding facilities are not available, or if a fish cannot be kept alive until examination, it can be euthanatized and refrigerated or stored on ice for up to 24 hours. However, small parasites may be unidentifiable after refrigeration.

Fish can also be preserved in fixative (10% neutral buffered formalin or 70% ethanol). This allows collection and archiving of a large number of samples, but it is not recommended for routine parasitologic examination.

Freezing is the least desirable method of sample preservation and may make some parasites impossible to identify. Many parasites, especially protozoa and small metazoans, lyse during freezing and thawing of the host. In large fish, endoparasites may undergo degradation and autolyze before the tissue has completely frozen.

THE PARASITOLOGIC EXAMINATION

Keep all parasites collected from different anatomical sites separate, along with accurate records.

TABLE 10–1. Artificial Key to the Common Parasites of Fish

The following key is for the identification of protozoan and metazoan parasite groups that commonly infect fish. This key is designed to facilitate identification of the major taxa based upon selected major morphological features. It does not include all of the major criteria that define each taxa, nor does it include all possible clinical presentations of the parasite. Refer to the previously cited literature sources for detailed taxonomic criteria of the specific groups.

I. Unicellular Organism (Protozoa) . . . . . Kingdom Protista
  1a. Flagella or cilia present in trophozoite (2)
   b. No flagella or cilia present in trophozoite (3)
  2a. Cilia present, which may be restricted to certain parts of the body. At least 2 nuclei present, a larger macronucleus and a smaller micronucleus. Present mainly on skin or gills . . . . . Phylum Ciliophora
   b. Flagella present. Present mainly on skin or gills, or in bloodstream . . . . . Phylum Sarcomastigophora, Subphylum Mastigophora
  3a. Spores with polar capsules . . . . . Phylum Myxozoa
   b. Spores without polar capsules, stain gram positive . . . . . Phylum Microspora
   c. Trophozoite ameboid; no spores present that are gram positive or have polar capsules. Present mainly on gills . . . . . Phylum Sarcomastigophora, Subphylum Sarcodina
   d. Trophozoite intracellular, apical complex present. Present mainly in the viscera . . . . . Phylum Apicomplexa
   e. Trophozoite with tentacles. Present on gills . . . . . Phylum Ciliophora, Subclass Suctoria
II. Multicellular Organism (Metazoa) . . . . . Kingdom Animalia
  1a. Without a backbone (invertebrate) (2)
   b. With a backbone (vertebrate) . . . . . Phylum Chordata, Subphylum Vertebrata, Class Cyclostomata (lampreys)
  2a. Digestive system absent or primitive, no developed respiratory or circulatory system (3)
   b. Complete digestive system, with developed respiratory and circulatory systems (8)
  3a. Body dorsoventrally compressed, usually displaying bilateral symmetry, with pseudocoelum filled with connective tissue or parenchyma (acoelomate). Organ of attachment in the form of suckers, hooks, clamps, or scolices . . . . . Phylum Platyhelminthes (flatworms) (4)
   b. Body cylindrical, unsegmented, with fluid-filled pseudocoelum (7)
  4a. Digestive system primitive, usually in the form of blindly ending ceca, organ of attachment in the form of suckers, hooks, and/or clamps . . . . . Class Trematoda (flukes) (5)
   b. Digestive system absent, body generally segmented, organ of attachment usually in the form of scolex . . . . . Class Cestoda (tapeworms) (6)
  5a. Organ of attachment, or holdfast organ, in form of a prohaptor at anterior end of body and opisthaptor at posterior end of body, which may contain anchors, hooks, clamps, and/or suckers. Adults usually ectoparasitic on fishes, only occasionally endoparasitic in fishes . . . . . Subclass Monogenea
   b. Holdfast organ in form of a large disc occupying almost entire ventral surface, which may contain septa and loculi, transverse rugae, or a linear series of ventral suckers. Adults usually endoparasitic in fishes . . . . . Subclass Aspidogastrea
   c. Holdfast organs in form of oral and ventral suckers. Adults endoparasitic in fishes . . . . . Subclass Digenea
  6a. Without a scolex, without internal or external segmentation, and contains only one set of reproductive organs . . . . . Subclass Cestodaria
   b. Scolex present, internal and external segmentation generally present, usually contain one or more sets of reproductive organs per segment . . . . . Subclass Eucestoda
  7a. Intestine present, usually with complete primitive digestive system . . . . . Phylum Aschelminthes, Class Nematoda (roundworms)
   b. Intestine absent, with incomplete or closed primitive digestive system, anterior end with retractile proboscis armed with hooks . . . . . Phylum Acanthocephala (thorny-headed worms)
  8a. Without limbs (9)
   b. With limbs, body consisting of unequal segments grouped in three sections (head, thorax, and abdomen), segments may be partially or completely fused, entire body covered with chitinous cuticle (exoskeleton) . . . . . Phylum Arthropoda, Class Crustacea (10)
  9a. Body laterally compressed, covered by a thin bivalve shell with small hooks or teeth lining the anterior edge of each valve . . . . . Phylum Mollusca, Class Bivalvia
   b. Body flat, occasionally cylindrical, divided into segments and often differentiated into a distinct head, neck, and trunk, well-developed anterior and posterior suckers, and body generally lacking setae . . . . . Phylum Annelida, Class Hirudinea (leeches)
  10a. Compound eyes absent, egg sacs present . . . . . Subclass Copepoda
   b. Compound eyes present (11)
  11a. Body elongated, usually dorsoventrally flattened, segmented into distinct thorax and abdomen, no carapace present, female with ventral brood pouch . . . . . Subclass Isopoda
   b. Body oval to round, compressed ventrally, cephalothorax almost completely covered with carapace, pair of ventral suctorial discs present . . . . . Subclass Branachiura

Make a thorough, methodical examination of the fins, body, buccal cavity, and gills. Carefully remove large ectoparasites and place them in a small container of the water used to submit the fish for later identification and/or preservation. Skin samples should be taken from several areas, including lesions, before excessive handling of the fish causes a loss of smaller, fragile ectoparasites. The use of anesthetics may also cause some parasites to detach from their host. A blood sample can be collected for preparation of both wet and air-dried smears.

With euthanatized or otherwise dead fish, follow the routine necropsy procedure presented in Chapter 12. Several gill arches can be excised, placed in water, and gently shaken to dislodge small monogeneans, which can be found in the sediment. These are removed with a Pasteur pipette and placed in physiological saline for later fixation. Arthropods collected from the sediment can be placed directly in 70% ethanol, since they do not contract at death like many of the softer parasites.

Examine the internal organs. The abdominal cavity may contain larval digeneans, nematodes, cestodes, or acanthocephalans. Larval helminths may be encysted in the viscera, and pseudocysts of microsporidians and myxozoans may be found in various organs. Squash preparations of liver, gallbladder, spleen, urinary bladder, swim bladder, kidney, gonads, and heart can be made. The gastrointestinal tract should be examined by opening the viscera with a pair of fine scissors and making wet mounts of representative areas to look for adult worms and protozoa, such as *Hexamita*. An incision should also be made in the muscles to look for encysted parasites. The eyes should be examined carefully for larval digeneans in the lens and vitreous humor. Finally, the brain should be removed and squashes made. It is often advisable to also fix representative tissues for histopathology.

FIXATION

The purpose of these procedures is to preserve the parasite in a state that will allow the examination of the morphological features needed for taxonomic identification. Only the most commonly used procedures are described. The reader should refer to Pritchard and Kruse (1982) for details on other methods.

Protozoa

The parasitic protozoa are best identified using live preparations. However, in fixed tissues, most flagellates and ciliates can be readily identified from routinely processed material that is stained with hematoxylin and eosin (H&E). Giemsa stain is especially good for identifying myxozoan spores, since the polar capsules stain intensely. Microsporidia are the only protozoal cysts or spores that are gram positive. Periodic acid–Schiff reveals a distinct, purple-red granule, the polar cap, at the anterior end of the spore (Canning and Lom, 1986). The spores are also birefringent (Tiner, 1988). Hemoprotozoa are generally identified from Giemsa-stained blood smears.

Metazoa

The first step in the preservation of most helminths is often a relaxation procedure that prevents the parasite from contracting after being placed into fixative. This may include placing the parasite (acanthocephalans and trematodes) into water or saline for several hours or placing it (leeches) in an anesthetic for several minutes (Table 10–2).

Following relaxation, parasites are immediately placed in a fixative, most commonly alcohol–formalin–acetic acid (AFA), 70% ethanol, or 10% neutral buffered formalin. AFA is the best fixative for most parasites, providing rapid killing and preservation, and parasites can be stored in it for a long time. Formalin is a general-purpose fixative that is often used if histological sections are to be made (Pritchard and Kruse, 1982). Except when preserving arthropods, which have a rigid cuticle, fixatives should be used hot (50°C) to kill rapidly and prevent contraction of the parasite. Hot fixatives emit toxic fumes and should be used under a fume hood. Gently flattening large cestodes and trematodes during initial fixation using a coverslip or microscope slide often increases the ability to observe morphologic details.

Arthropods that are embedded in host tissue (e.g., many copepods) may be excised along with a piece of host tissue and the entire mass fixed in 70% ethanol. After 24 hours, the parasite can be carefully dissected out of the host tissue.

Prepared samples can be sent to a reference laboratory for identification or be stained, cleared, and mounted. Unless a large number of specimens are to be collected, it is often better to have staining and mounting done by the reference laboratory.

STAINING

Staining enhances visualization of taxonomically important internal structures. Routine stains are either alcohol based such as Semichon's acetocarmine or Mayer's acid carmine stains, or water based like Mayer's hematoxylin or Van Cleave's combination hematoxylin stains. Depending upon the stain base, specimens must be either hydrated or dehydrated by using a series of increasing or decreasing alcohol concentrations. The choice of stain generally depends on the investigator's personal preference, and often specimens will be stained several ways for comparison.

Specimens for staining are washed for 12 to 24 hours to remove any residual fixative. Specimens from AFA or 70% ethanol are washed in 70% ethanol and specimens from 10% formalin are washed in distilled water (Fig. 10–1). Depending upon the stain to be used, specimens are either hydrated or dehydrated in a series of alcohol concentrations for 10 to 30 minutes at each concentration. For example, a parasite fixed and stored in AFA to be stained with carmine should be washed in 70% ethanol for 12 to 24 hours, placed in fresh 70% ethanol for 15 minutes, and then placed in the alcohol-based stain. Conversely, a specimen fixed and stored in 10% formalin should be washed in distilled water for 12 to 24 hours, passed through an alcohol dehydration series of 15 minutes at each concentration, and then placed in the alcohol-based stain. Specimens can be moved between solutions with a camel hair brush or forceps, or by removing the fluid from the container with a Pasteur pipette and immediately replacing it with the next solution. Whichever method is used, keep an

TABLE 10–2. Recommended Methods of Preserving Metazoan Parasites for Identification

Parasite Group	Relaxation Procedure	"Relaxed" Parasite	Fixation	Storage	Final Preparation for Identification
Trematodes*	None usually needed for small worms Gently flatten under a coverslip and flood slide with fixative for 5 min	Not contracted Allows some expulsion of eggs from uterus	Hot (55–65°C) AFA or hot NBF	AFA or ETOH	Stained and permanently mounted in mounting medium
Cestodes*	Cold (4–8°C) water or saline for 1–12 hr Gently flatten under a coverslip and flood slide with fixative for 5 min	Not contracted Allows some expulsion of eggs from uterus	Hot AFA or hot NBF or hot ETOH	AFA or ETOH	Stained and permanently mounted in mounting medium
Nematodes	None usually needed for small worms Stretch large worms by holding at both ends with forceps and add fixative for 5 min	Completely uncoiled	Hot AFA or hot ETOH	AFA or ETOH or glycerol:ETOH	Small nematodes can be cleared in glycerol:ETOH and mounted permanently in glycerol jelly. Large nematodes are cleared and temporarily mounted in glycerol:ETOH
Acanthocephalans	Cold (4–8°C) water or saline for 1–12 hr	Proboscis fully extruded	Hot AFA or hot NBF or hot ETOH (puncture cuticle)	AFA or ETOH	Small: stained and mounted Large: unstained and mounted in glycerol:ETOH
Hirudineans	Tricaine methane sulfonate Pentobarbitol sodium	Not contracted	Hot ETOH	ETOH	Small: stained and mounted Large: glycerol:ETOH
Arthropods	Not required	Not required	Cold (4–8°C) ETOH	ETOH	Unstained and cleared in 10% KOH or Hoyer mounting medium

Abbreviations: AFA, alcohol–formalin–acetic acid; NBF, 10% neutral buffered formalin; ETOH, 70% ethanol; glycerol:ETOH, glycerol: 70% ethanol.

*Before beginning preservation procedures, encapsulated larvae should be manually dissected out of the capsule or the capsule should be digested with 0.2% pepsin in 0.1 M HCl.

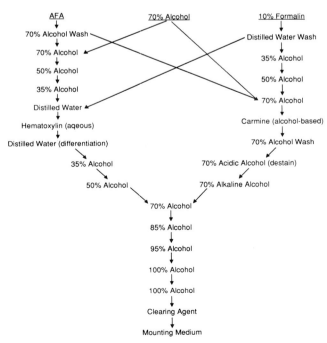

FIGURE 10–1. Methods for preparing permanent whole mounts of trematodes, cestodes, and small acanthocephalans.

identification label with the specimens so that the parasites can be correctly identified at any time.

Staining can be progressive, where specimens are gradually stained until the desired color intensity is obtained, or regressive, where specimens are intentionally overstained and then the stain is partially removed. In regressive staining, specimens are stained for 12 to 24 hours until internal organs maximally absorb the stain. The stain is then removed by washing the specimen or destaining it until the outer cortical tissue of the parasite is relatively free of stain, whereas the internal organs retain enough stain to be readily distinguished.

To permanently mount specimens on glass slides, a mounting medium, such as Canada balsam, synthetic piccolyte, or Permount, is used. Both of the latter mounting media work well and are relatively inexpensive; however, for archival material Canada balsam is minimally affected by environmental changes (Pritchard and Kruse, 1982). Place a drop of mounting medium onto a clean glass slide and put the parasite into the drop. Be careful not to expose the specimen to air. This would cause the formation of air bubbles in the preparation. Elongated trematodes and short cestodes can be mounted whole on a single slide, with the trematode ventral side up. For most cestodes, sections of the parasite must be arranged in parallel rows on the slide. Representative cestode specimens should contain the scolex, neck, and mature and gravid proglottids.

Touch the edge of a coverglass to one side of the mounting medium and carefully lower it over the parasite. Use the smallest coverglass possible to minimize the amount of mounting medium required. Air bubbles trapped under the coverglass will usually migrate to the edges during the hardening process. Large or thick specimens often need small pieces of broken coverglass or capillary tubing permanently placed under the edges of the coverglass to help support it. Add additional mounting medium to the margins of the coverglass as medium recedes during the hardening process to prevent the specimen from being exposed to the air. Hardening may take several weeks at room temperature, or it can be accelerated using a slide-warming tray or a drying oven between 40 and 50°C. Keep the slides level. When the mounting medium is hard remove excess with a razor blade and clean the slide with a lint-free cloth moistened with 95% ethanol.

Small monogenetic trematodes can be permanently mounted unstained in glycerol jelly, which partially clears the parasite. Heat glycerol jelly in a water bath until it liquifies and place a drop on a clean glass slide. Carefully transfer the trematode from 70% ethanol directly into the glycerol jelly and position it. Place a coverglass over the specimen and allow it to harden at room temperature. Remove any excess glycerol jelly with a razor blade and seal the edges of the coverglass with a double layer of fingernail polish.

Nematodes are best examined after being cleared in a mixture of glycerine:alcohol (Fig. 10–2). The glycerine concentration is increased over time by leaving the container with the parasite open and allowing the alcohol to gradually evaporate. Additional glycerine may have to be added to prevent exposing the specimens to the air and dessication. Nematodes are not usually mounted permanently, but are examined in temporary preparations of glycerol jelly or glycerine to allow manipulation of the parasite to observe taxonomically important structures. Small nematodes can also be permanently mounted in glycerol jelly, like the monogenetic trematodes (Pritchard and Kruse, 1982).

Acanthocephalans and small leeches can be stained with either carmine or hematoxylin, cleared, and permanently mounted on glass slides. The cuticle of acanthocephalans should be punctured several times to allow more rapid fluid exchange. Specimens too large to mount on glass slides are usually not stained but cleared in glycerine:alcohol like nematodes.

Copepods and isopods can be examined untreated or cleared in 10% KOH solution. Smaller specimens can be cleared in 10% KOH and mounted permanently in mounting medium, or mounted directly in Hoyer mounting medium, which clears the specimen and hardens for a permanent preparation.

Mounted slides should be stored at a constant temperature away from light and dust in a level horizontal position to prevent drifting of the specimen in the mounting medium. Nematodes not mounted on slides should be permanently stored in sealed containers of glycerine:alcohol. All unmounted material should be stored in 70% ethanol.

Parasites on slides to be shipped to individuals for identification or to museum collections for deposit should be individually wrapped in cloth or tissue paper and packed in postal service–approved slide mailers. Specimens in fixative must be sealed to prevent leakage. Before sending any specimens, always contact the destination and ask their preferred methods for submission of material.

Holotype material, from which original taxonomic descriptions are made, should be deposited in a national depository such as the U.S. National Helminth Collection (c/o Animal Parasitology Institute, B.A.R.C. East, Building 1180, Beltsville, Maryland 20705). Paratype material and voucher specimens should be deposited in a public collection or institution where the specimens may be loaned and studied further.

The permanent collection record should include (1) an individual identification number; (2) the common and scientific names of the host; (3) specific host

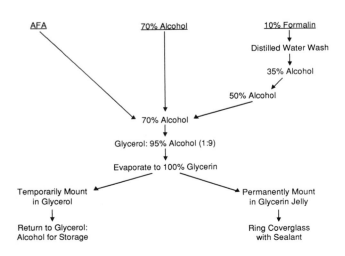

FIGURE 10–2. Methods for preparing nematodes for examination.

information, such as age, size, and sex; (4) the date the host was collected; (5) the location where the host was collected, including the nearest town, state, river, lake, or geographic coordinates; (6) the method of collection; and (7) the collector's name. Also include: (1) the general type of parasite, such as trematode or cestode; (2) the specific identification if known; (3) the number of parasites collected; (4) the location in the host; (5) the method of fixation; and (6) the person who specifically identified the parasite.

GENERAL MORPHOLOGY, LIFE CYCLES, AND PATHOLOGY

Protozoa

Not all protozoa associated with fish produce overt clinical disease. Some are harmless commensals, whereas others may cause clinical signs of disease only in large numbers or when the host is stressed. However, protozoa cause more disease in cultured fish than any other parasite group (Hoffman, 1970), and in intensive aquaculture systems they can cause serious morbidity and mortality. Important fish pathogens include members of the phyla Sarcomastigophora, Ciliophora, Apicomplexa, Microspora, and Myxozoa. Detailed taxonomic descriptions of specific protozoa are available (Hoffman, 1970; Bykhovskaya-Pavlovskaya et al., 1964; Lee et al., 1985) as well as reviews of taxonomic groups such as the flagellates (Becker, 1977), ciliates (Hoffman, 1978), and amebae (Noble and Noble, 1966).

Sarcomastigophoran Protozoa

The phylum Sarcomastigophora includes a diverse assemblage of protozoa with either flagella and/or pseudopodia. Members of the subphylum Mastigophora have one to many flagella, typically present in the trophozoite stage. Asexual reproduction is by intrakinetal (symmetrogenic) binary fission. The subphylum Mastigophora is further subdivided into Phytomastigophorea, which includes dinoflagellates (*Amyloodinium*) and other algal groups, and Zoomastigophorea, or heterotrophic flagellates.

Most of the important zoomastigophorean parasites of fish are members of the order Kinetoplastida, which are characterized by the presence of a kinetoplast, a Fuelgen-positive mass of extranuclear deoxyribonucleic acid (DNA) that is typically associated with the large, single, looped mitochondrion of this group. The life cycle may be direct (*Ichtyoboda*) or indirect (*Trypanosoma*). These parasites commonly inhabit mucosal surfaces (skin, gills, intestinal tract) or blood.

Other zoomastigophorean parasites include members of the orders Retortamonadida, Diplomonadida, and Trichomonadida. Most are considered to be relatively harmless ectocommensals. They are differentiated based on the number and position of flagella, number of nuclei, and other morphologic features.

The subphylum Sarcodina includes protozoa that form pseudopodia or are mobile by locomotive protoplasmic flow. Flagella, if present, are restricted to developmental stages and are not present in trophozoites. Asexual reproduction is by fission. This is probably a polyphyletic group that includes amebae of unrelated origins, but which have been included together because of a lack of taxonomic relationships between some groups. Fish pathogens are relatively uncommon in this group and include *Thecamoeba* and *Paramoeba*.

Ciliated Protozoans

The Ciliophora are taxonomically distinguished by the presence of two or more nuclei, including one or more larger macronuclei, which regulate cell metabolism, and a smaller micronucleus, which is primarily involved in genetics and sexual recombination. Most ciliates ingest nutrients through a cytostome-cytopharynx that may be surrounded by rows of cilia. Patterns of ciliature, which may be restricted to certain parts of the cell, are often used to distinguish certain groups. Ciliate reproduction is usually by binary fission, but may occur by multiple fission. Ciliates inhabiting fish range from ectocommensals to obligate parasites.

The subclass Peritrichia includes two major groups. The order Mobilida (*Trichodina*) are free-swimming parasites with a characteristic denticulate ring. They attach to hosts using a scopula or holdfast disc (Fig. 10–3). The order Sessilida (*Ambiphrya*) at-

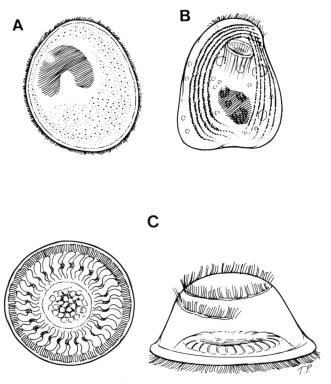

FIGURE 10–3. Common ciliate parasites of fishes. *A. Ichthyophthirius multifiliis. B. Chilodonella* sp. *C. Trichodina* sp.

tach to the host as a trophozoite. They have one or more bands of cilia around each organism and feed on suspended particles. Many are colonial. Reproduction is by a mobile stage (telotroch). Peritrichs are usually weak pathogens.

Other important ciliate parasites are members of the subclass Hymenostomatia (*Ichthyophthirius, Tetrahymena, Uronema*). These are holotrichous ciliates often having multiple stages in a direct life cycle. The subclass Phylophararyngea includes two important pathogens, *Chilodonella* and *Brooklynella*, which have cilia present mainly on their ventrum (see Fig. 10–3). The subclass Suctoria (*Trichophrya*) are sessile with one or more tentacles for ingesting prey; cilia are present only in the mobile infective stage.

Apicomplexa

The Apicomplexa was formerly a part of the obsolete phylum Sporozoa; this was a misnomer because many apicomplexans do not form spores. However, all members possess an apical complex used to penetrate the host cell. Most of the apical complex structure is visible only by electron microscopy. All apicomplexans are parasitic, and most fish pathogens in this group are intracellular parasites.

Two subclasses infect fish: the Coccidiasina (*Eimeria, Hemogregarina*) and the Piroplasmasina. The most important apicomplexan group infecting fish is the family Eimeriidae, where the infective stage (sporozoite) is formed within an oocyst. In the host cell, the coccidian parasite forms a meront, which produces many merozoites by asexual reproduction (merogony). The merozoites then sexually differentiate into flagellated microgametes and oocytelike macrogametes, which mate, producing a zygote (gamogony). The zygote then forms an oocyst, containing sporocysts with the sporozoites (sporogony).

Eimeriids are very common fish parasites, and the prevalence of these agents is probably underestimated. Intestinal infections are usually asymptomatic, but extraintestinal parasites can cause severe morbidity and mortality. Common extraintestinal infection sites include the reproductive organs, liver, and swim bladder. Transmission is per os and almost always direct, although there is evidence for an intermediate or paratenic host in a few species. Diagnosis of fish coccidia is based on spore morphology. Oocysts are characteristically thin walled compared to those of coccidia infecting mammals and are usually sporulated when shed. All species infecting fish have oocysts with four sporocysts, each with two sporozoites.

The family Hemogregarinidae includes several poorly studied blood parasites having a life cycle that is believed to include merogony in the circulatory system of the fish host and gamogony and sporogony in a blood-sucking invertebrate vector such as a leech or parasitic crustacean. Most infections have been described from feral fishes. The piroplasmids (e.g., *Babesiosoma*) are uncommon fish hemoparasites that are believed to require an invertebrate vector. Identification of hemoparasites is based on their morphology in blood smears.

Microspora

Classification of the Microspora is based upon the life cycle, type of sporogony, and spore morphology. Fish are infected by several members of the order Microsporida. Microsporidians form a thick-walled spore that contains a sporoplasm. When a host ingests the spore, the sporoplasm is discharged through the channel of a tubular polar filament that is stored coiled within the spore. The sporoplasm then migrates to the target organ and starts a proliferative phase, producing a large number of cells (meronts) by binary or multiple fission or plasmotomy. In the final stage of development, meronts give rise to sporonts, which undergo sporogony.

There are two suborders of microsporidia. In the suborder Pansporoblastina (*Glugea, Pleistophora, Loma*), spores develop in membrane-bound packets known as sporophorous vesicles (pansporoblast membranes), which may be seen in wet mounts of lesions. The number of spores per sporophorous vesicle is diagnostic. In the suborder Apansporoblastina (*Ichthyosporidium, Spraguea*), spores are free within the host cell cytoplasm.

Some species induce the formation of a tremendously hypertrophied host cell, which together with the parasite forms a xenoma, or xenoparasitic complex. Xenomas are whitish, cystlike structures up to several millimeters in diameter. Some species (*Ichthyosporidium giganteum*) may form very large (up to 2 cm or larger) pseudotumors consisting of many individual xenomas.

Depending on the parasite species and its tissue predilection, infections can be widely disseminated throughout various organs. How infections spread within a host is unknown. Possibilities include migration of meronts and autoinfection, where spores hatch in the individual and begin another propagation cycle. Clinical signs depend on the organ infected and range from being asymptomatic to causing the death of the host. While mild infections may be innocuous, mechanical displacement and tissue disruption caused by parasite growth can lead to serious organ dysfunction (intestinal blockage, parasitic castration, muscle loss) with severe morbidity and/or mortality. Mature spores may be released from lesions on body surfaces (e.g., skin, gills, intestine) or after death of the host. Spores are typically very resistant to environmental conditions and are very small, usually 7 μm or less. Important pathogens include *Glugea* and *Pleistophora*.

Myxozoa

Myxozoa are restricted to invertebrates (mostly annelids) and poikilothermic vertebrates. The Myxozoa that infect fish are all members of the class Myxosporea (Fig. 10–4). The vast majority infect fishes. They are obligate parasites of tissues and

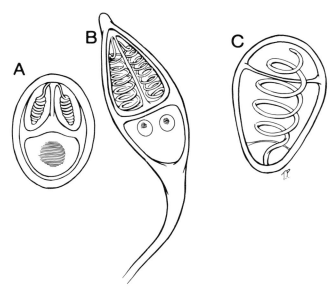

FIGURE 10–4. Myxozoan spores. *A. Myxobolus* sp. *B. Henneguya* sp. *C.* Typical microsporidian spore.

organ cavities. Key characteristics include the development of a multicellular spore, the presence of polar capsules in the spores, and endogenous cell cleavage in both the trophozoite and sporogony stages. One of the most important characteristics of myxosporeans is the development of multinucleated forms that have primary cells containing enveloped secondary cells.

Myxosporidian spores have one binucleate or two uninucleate sporoplasms, one to six (usually two) polar capsules, which are refractile in live spores and have a polar filament, and a shell with two to six valves. When a host ingests a spore, it triggers the rapid release of the coiled polar filaments. This probably facilitates the adherence of the spore to the intestinal mucosa. The spore valves separate, releasing the infective sporoplasm. Upon hatching, fusion of the two uninucleate sporoplasms or the nuclei of the binucleate sporoplasm produces the only uninucleate stage in the parasite's life cycle. This zygote or synkaryon then migrates to the target tissue. In some species *(Sphaerospora),* there is evidence that there may also be a separate proliferative phase in organs other than the final target tissue.

In the final target tissue, the trophozoite may reproduce in one of two ways. In some, the nucleus divides to produce a massive plasmodium containing generative cells and many vegetative nuclei. In others, a large number of very small plasmodia, each with only one vegetative nucleus, divide to produce many parasites prior to sporogony, each giving rise to one or two spores.

The method of transmission for virtually all myxozoans is unknown, but there is evidence that some may have an indirect life cycle that involves an invertebrate intermediate host. What is astounding is that this may require completion of two different life cycles involving a vertebrate (fish) and an invertebrate (annelid) host, each life cycle having its own asexual and sexual stages (Wolf et al., 1986). Such an alternation of life cycles has not been documented in other parasites.

Most myxosporean infections of fish are relatively innocuous, inciting only moderate host reactions. Heavy infections can cause serious, mechanical damage from the pseudocysts or tissue necrosis and inflammation from trophozoite feeding. Young fish are usually most seriously affected by myxozoan infections.

The early stages of the life cycle usually incite little host reaction, but plasmodia with mature spores often induce considerable inflammation. Interestingly, in many cases, tissue damage is greatest after the death of the host, when enzymes released by the parasites are believed to cause massive muscle liquefaction (tapioca disease). Muscle lysis can cause serious reduction in carcass value.

The taxonomy of the Myxosporea is based solely on spore structure, including spore size and shape, the number and position of polar capsules, and the characteristics of the polar filaments. Spores range from about 8 to 25 μm, which is considerably larger than the typical microsporidian spore. The order Bivalvulida *(Myxobolus)* has spore walls with two valves. The order Multivalvulida *(Kudoa)* has spore walls with three to six valves; most live intracellularly in myocytes *(Kudoa).* Spores may have projections of various sorts that facilitate their maintenance in the water column or passive attachment to food of potential hosts. The pseudocysts induced by many species can look similar to lesions induced by microsporidians, but they are easily differentiated by examining spores.

Metazoa

Monogenetic Trematodes

The majority of the monogenetic trematodes of fish are ectoparasites on the body, fins, gills, and/or oral cavity, where they feed on the host's mucus, epithelium, or blood. Notable exceptions are several *Dactylogyrus* species, which occur in the nasal cavities (Strelkov and Ki, 1964), intestine (Gusev and Fernando, 1973), and ovipositor (Yukhimenko and Danilov, 1977); *Acolopenteron* species, which occur in the ureters and urinary bladder (Fischthal and Allison, 1940); and a single *Enterogyrus* species that occurs in the intestine (Paperna, 1963).

Most species of monogenetic trematodes are highly host specific and site specific on the body of the host. Monogeneans have a direct life cycle and complete their entire development on a single host (Fig. 10–5). Most are oviparous, producing a small number of large eggs that are released into the water, which embryonate and release a ciliated oncomiracidium. These free-swimming larvae must locate and infect a suitable host where maturation is completed. Conversely, gyrodactylids are viviparous, producing larvae which usually remain on the same individual

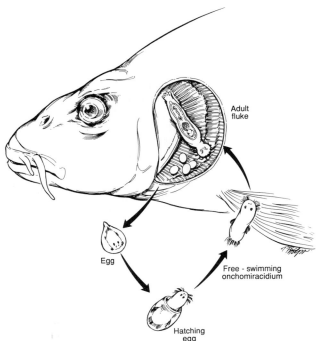

FIGURE 10–5. Representative life cycles of monogenetic trematodes of the genus *Dactylogyrus*.

host as the adult parasite. Spread of gyrodactylids from fish to fish probably occurs during physical contact of the hosts.

The monogeneans are divided into two major groups based upon the morphology of the posterior attachment organ, or opisthaptor (Fig. 10–6). In the Monopisthocotyle, the opisthaptor is a single distinct unit composed of several large centrally located anchors (hooks) and small marginal hooklets. In the Polyopisthocotyle, the posterior attachment organ consists of muscular adhesive suckers or clamps supported by cuticular sclerites. Other anatomic structures diagnostic in these parasites include one or more oral suckers, prohaptors, and distinct glandular areas in the anterior end, and pigmented eye spots may be present or absent. The digestive system may be simple or branched with numerous blind pouches, called ceca. The morphology of the testes, which may be single, paired, or multiple, and the ovaries, which may be oval or branched, may also be of taxonomic importance. Excellent taxonomic reviews of the monogenetic trematodes are available (Sproston, 1946; Bychowsky, 1957; Yamaguti, 1963a; Bykhovskaya-Pavlovskaya et al., 1964; Dawes, 1968; Schell, 1985; Hargis and Thoney, 1983).

Adults of many monogenean species appear to remain permanently attached to a single site on the host, whereas others move about on the skin and/or gills. Morbidity and mortality caused by epidemics of these parasites in cultured fish are generally a result of stressful environmental conditions due to poor husbandry or poor water quality. Disease outbreaks have rarely been reported in wild fish populations.

The most economically important monogeneans

in cultured fish are in the families Dactylogyridae and Gyrodactylidae (Needham and Wootten, 1978). Dactylogyrids are primarily gill parasites of freshwater fishes, and gyrodactylids are skin and gill parasites of both freshwater and marine fishes. Lesions caused by both groups of monogeneans appear to be due to the feeding activity of the parasites as well as to the mechanical damage produced by the anchors and hooklets of the opisthaptor. These parasites cause little, if any, harmful effects to the host, but this is dependent upon the number of parasites present, the condition and age of the host, and the involvement of any secondary pathogens. Large numbers of monogeneans on the gills of young stressed fish can cause severe pathologic effects in a short period of time. These include hemorrhage and hyperplasia of the gill tissue, fusion and clubbing of the gill lamellae, and secondary bacterial and protozoal infections of gill lesions. Skin infestations are usually less pathogenic than gill infestations owing to the rapid regenerative ability of fish skin (Kearn, 1963).

Digenetic Trematodes

The digenetic trematodes are a very large group of endoparasites that have indirect and often complex life cycles (Fig. 10–7). All digeneans of fish are

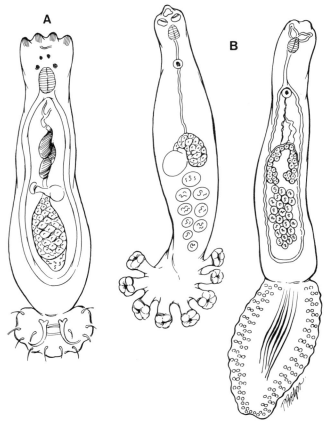

FIGURE 10–6. Representative morphology of monogenetic trematodes from fishes. *A.* Monopithocotyle. *B.* Polyopisthocotyle. (Adapted from Schell, S.C. [1985] Handbook of Trematodes of North America North of Mexico. University Press of Idaho, Moscow.)

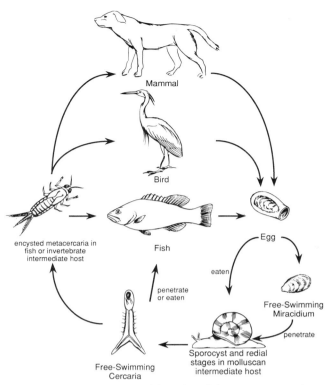

FIGURE 10–7. Representative life cycles of digenetic trematodes.

monecious and oviparous. A large, usually operculated egg is passed in the feces of the definitive host. A ciliated, free-swimming larva (miracidium) hatches, infects a mollusc intermediate host, and undergoes asexual reproduction. The resulting cercaria is released into the water, after which it penetrates or is ingested by a second host, which may be the definitive host in which the adult digenetic trematode matures, or a second intermediate host in which a metacercaria develops. Metacercariae may be found encapsulated in numerous sites throughout the body of the second intermediate host. The life cycle of digeneans with a second intermediate host is completed when the metacercaria-infected tissues are ingested by the definitive host. Adult digenetic trematodes are generally found in the stomach, pyloric ceca, and intestine of fish, but some are found in the swim bladder, ovary, and body cavity (*Acetodextra* sp. and *Nematobothrium* sp.), the urinary bladder (*Phyllodistomum* sp.), and the circulatory system (*Sanguinicola* sp. and *Cardicola* sp.). Larval digeneans can be found in almost any fish tissue and may as adults parasitize a wide variety of carnivorous vertebrate hosts, including fish, mammals, and birds.

Adult digeneans usually have an anterior muscular oral sucker and a ventral holdfast organ, although the suckers may be vestigial or completely absent in some species (*Sanguinicola* spp.). Other diagnostic features include the presence of cephalic structures around the oral cavity; the size and location of the ventral sucker; the number, position, and shape of the testes and ovary; the location of the genital pore; the distribution of the vitellaria; and the morphology of the ceca. Taxonomic keys and bibliographies to the adult trematodes exist (Yamaguti, 1958, 1971; Bykhovskaya-Pavlovskaya et al., 1964; Skrjarbin, 1964; Dawes, 1968; Hoffman, 1970; Schell, 1985).

Metacercariae often display many of the taxonomic characteristics of the adult trematode, but they usually lack fully developed reproductive organs. Metacercariae that produce a cyst secrete the membranous material from cystogenous glands. The host may also produce a cellular response to the larval stage, resulting in the formation of a connective tissue capsule around the parasite that may or may not be pigmented. Illustrations and keys to the known species of North American larval trematodes are available (Hoffman, 1960, 1970).

Three types of metacercariae commonly occur in fish. A larval digenean of the *Diplostomulum* spp., called a diplostomulum, have well-developed muscular pseudosuckers (cotylae) on each side of the anterior oral sucker. Found in the eyes, coelom, and central nervous system of fish, these metacercariae are usually not encysted, but they may be contained in a connective tissue capsule of host origin. Metacercariae of *Tetracotyle* spp., called tetracotyles, also have a well-developed cotyle and are usually encysted in a thick, tight-fitting, transparent membrane of parasite origin. The neascus type of metacercariae belong to the genus *Neascus,* and do not have cotylae. These immature trematodes are encysted in a thin, loose-fitting membrane of parasite origin and are commonly called "white grubs," or when surrounded by pigment from the host are commonly known as "black spot" or "black spot disease."

Adult digeneans generally cause very little pathology in the gastrointestinal tract of fish, though heavy infections of *Crepidostomum* spp. have been reported to cause inflammation of the gut (Hoffman, 1975). Adult trematodes of the circulatory system, called blood flukes, can cause considerable damage to the blood vessels of the gills of freshwater fishes, including carp in Europe and the U.S.S.R. and salmonids in North America (Needham and Wootten, 1978). However, larval digenetic trematodes are often found in large numbers in the abdominal cavity and viscera where they can cause considerable damage. Blindness due to diplostomulum metacercariae in the eyes of salmonids may cause them difficulty in feeding as well as make them more susceptible to predation. Large numbers of metacercariae in the musculature often make fillets unacceptable to the consumer.

Cestodes

Tapeworms may occur in fish as sexually mature adults that are found in the intestine and pyloric ceca or as larval forms (plerocercoids) in the abdominal cavity, visceral organs, and/or musculature. Cestodes are divided into the subclasses Cestodaria and Eucestoda. In the more primitive Cestodaria, the adult cestode is without a scolex, without internal or external segmentation, and contains only one set of reproductive organs (monozoic). The embryo (lycophora) in the egg of these oviparous parasites contains 10 hooklets. Additional information about their life cycle is not known. These cestodes are mostly parasites of sturgeons, silurids, and the primitive chimaerids.

The Eucestoda usually have a scolex, internal and external segmentation, and, with the exception of the orders Caryophyllidea and Spathebothriidea, one or more sets of reproductive organs per segment (polyzoic). The embryo (oncosphere) in the egg of these cestodes contains only six hooklets. Eleven of the 13 orders within the subclass Eucestoda have species that are parasitic in freshwater or marine fishes, with six of these orders being exclusively parasites of elasmobranchs. The general life cycle of these parasites may include one or two intermediate hosts, with a fish acting as an intermediate host, a definitive host, or both.

The general morphology of the Eucestoda usually consists of an organ of attachment and locomotion (scolex), followed by an undifferentiated area (neck), and a chain of segments (proglottids) with one or more sets of reproductive organs. The scolex may be provided with suckers, grooves, hooks, spines, or combinations of these or may lack any specializations. Classification of adult cestodes in species depends on the characteristics of the scolex and the organ systems of the mature proglottid, whereas immature cestodes can often be classified in an order only on the basis of morphology. A detailed account of the reproductive anatomy and other internal organ systems of cestodes (Schmidt, 1986; Yamaguti, 1959), excellent keys to the adult and larval cestodes of North American freshwater fishes (Hoffman, 1970), and discussions of many of the adult and larval cestodes of marine species of fishes (Overstreet, 1978) have been published.

The Eucestoda, like the Cestodaria, are oviparous, passing eggs into the water in the feces of the definitive host (Fig. 10–8). Either the egg or a free-swimming larval stage (coracidium) released from the egg is eaten by an intermediate host, usually a copepod. Whether the immature cestode is ingested as a coracidium or as an egg that hatches in the gut, the larval cestode penetrates through the gut wall into the hemocoel of the intermediate host and develops into either a procercoid or a plerocercoid. If a procercoid develops, then a second intermediate host, which may be a fish, is required in the life cycle. In the fish intermediate host, the parasite again penetrates the gut wall, then encysts in the coelom, viscera, or musculature where it develops into a plerocercoid. These immature cestodes may grow considerably in length and occasionally show signs of external segmentation. After being ingested by a carnivorous fish, bird, or mammal, the plerocercoids develop into adult cestodes in the intestinal tract of the definitive host.

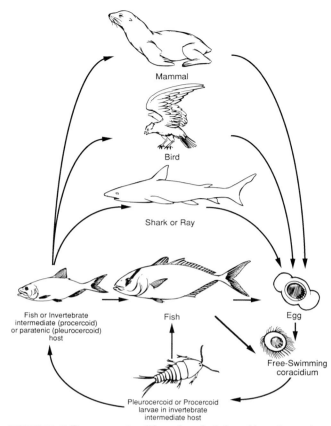

FIGURE 10–8. Representative life cycles of adult and larval cestodes.

Adult cestodes are common in the digestive tracts of both freshwater and marine fishes. These parasites generally cause minimal pathology, although heavy infestations may retard the growth rate in catfishes (Hoffman, 1970) and salmon (Smith, 1973), and cause hemorrhagic enteritis in carp (Bauer et al., 1973). Larval cestodes are probably the most harmful of all the parasites of the body cavity and can severely decrease both the sporting and commercial value of fish. Migrating plerocercoids can cause extensive damage to the liver, spleen, and kidney of fish, while also causing adhesions and compression of the viscera. Death, if not caused directly from the migrating parasites, can be caused indirectly by affecting the swimming ability of the fish, thus making it more susceptible to predation. Reduced reproductive potential and sterility have also been attributed to massive numbers of plerocercoids in the gonadal tissue. In addition, plerocercoids decrease the market value of fillets when the parasite occurs in the musculature and are in general esthetically undesirable.

Nematodes

The class Nematoda consists of bilaterally symmetrical organisms that have a pseudocoelom and a gut. Nematodes are cylindrical and possess a complete digestive tract with an esophagus, intestine, and anus. They commonly occur in both larval and adult forms in freshwater and marine fishes. Most adult nematodes occur in the stomach and intestine of fish, though a number of species do occur in other organs. Some nematodes that use extraintestinal sites as adults are species of *Philonema* and *Philometra*, parasites of the body cavity, gonads, and musculature of freshwater and marine fishes, *Cystidicola* in the swim bladder of freshwater fishes, and *Pancreatonema* in the pancreatic ducts of skates. Larval nematodes, like the metacercariae of digenetic trematodes, can occur in almost any fish tissue. Species of the genera *Philonema, Spiroxys, Eustrongylides, Contracaecum,* and *Anisakis* can cause considerable damage to the visceral organs and other tissues during migration through the fish host.

Identification of nematodes is based on external and internal anatomic structures. External characteristics may include modifications of the cuticle at the anterior end, alae, cervical or caudal papillae, location of the vulva, and the presence of a copulatory bursa in male nematodes. Internally, the digestive, reproductive, and excretory systems display a wide variety of forms. In the digestive system, the shape of the buccal cavity and the presence of lips and teeth may have taxonomic value, while the length and morphology of the esophagus may vary. In a number of genera, the male reproductive system has a pair of chitinized spicules used during copulation that may vary between the species in shape, size, and length. In addition, the shape, size, and internal contents of the egg may also be of diagnostic value. For a review of the nematodes affecting fish the reader is referred to Hoffman (1970) for freshwater species and to Margolis (1970) and Rohde (1984) for marine species. Taxonomic accounts of the various groups of parasitic nematodes have been presented by Yamaguti (1961), Bykhovskaya-Pavlovskaya et al. (1964), Skrjabin (1968), Chaubard (1974, 1975a,b, 1978), Hartwich (1974), Petter and Quentin (1976), Anderson (1978), Lichtenfels (1980a,b), and Anderson and Bain (1976, 1982).

The sexes of nematodes are separate, and most nematodes parasitizing fishes are oviparous, passing eggs into the water that release a free-swimming larva (Fig. 10–9). Exceptions to this are females in the genera *Camallanus* and *Philometra*, which are viviparous and release larvae directly into the water. In either case, the larvae are ingested by an arthropod intermediate host where development of the parasite continues. When the intermediate host is ingested by a fish, the immature nematode either completes development to the adult stage or becomes encysted as a larval form in the tissues or body cavity of the fish. The fish in which larvae encyst may serve as a second intermediate host or a paratenic (transport) host. The life cycle of these parasites is completed when the fish host is ingested by another carnivorous fish, a bird, or a mammal.

Very little pathology has been associated with the presence of adult nematodes in the gastroin-

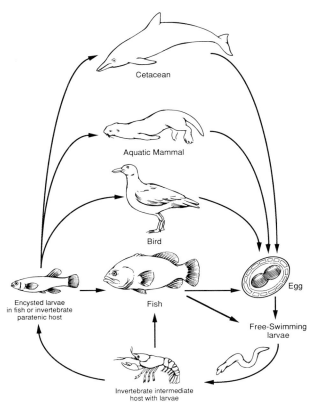

FIGURE 10–9. Representative life cycles of adult and larval nematodes. (Modified from Overstreet, R.M. [1978] Marine Maladies? Worms, Germs, and Other Symbionts from the Northern Gulf of Mexico. Blossman Printing, Ocean Springs, Mississippi; and Olsen, O.W. [1974] Animal Parasites: Their Life Cycles and Ecology. 3rd ed. University Park Press, Baltimore.)

tinal tract of fish. Inflammation and ulceration of the gut of fish and emaciation in aquarium fish due to *Capillaria* have been reported (Hoffman, 1970; Amalacher, 1970). Like the cestodes, the majority of the pathology occurring in fish due to nematodes is caused by the migrating larval forms. Larvae of *Philonema* can cause severe visceral adhesions in salmon, trout, and striped bass, while larval ascarids, such as *Porrocaecum, Contracaecum,* and *Anisakis*, can cause serious damage to the liver and mesenteric tissues of freshwater fishes. Anisakid larvae may also occur throughout the musculature and visceral organs of marine fishes and produce significant pathology in the liver (Smith and Wootten, 1978).

Acanthocephalans

The so-called "thorny-headed worms," like the nematodes, are bilaterally symmetric, cylindrical, and dioecious. However, they have no digestive tract and have an anterior, retractile proboscis armed with chitinoid hooks. Acanthocephalan life cycles require at least one intermediate host.

Most adult acanthocephalans in fish inhabit the intestine or sometimes the pyloric ceca. A few also use fish as a second intermediate or paratenic host, where the immature acanthocephalan (cystacanth) is encysted in the mesenteries and/or liver. Many acanthocephalan species use marine fishes as hosts, and encysted larval stages of acanthocephalans are more commonly observed in marine fishes than in freshwater fishes.

Identification of adult acanthocephalans depends upon the characteristics of the proboscis and its associated structures, presoma, as well as various internal structures of the body. The hooks of the proboscis are very important in the classification of these parasites. These vary in number, shape, conformation, and location, and may occur in rows, spirals, or randomly along the proboscis (Fig. 10–10). Additional structures used in the specific identification are the copulatory organs of the male, cement glands found in males and used to seal the genital pore of the female after fertilization, and the paired lemnisci used in the evagination and invagination of the proboscis. Taxonomic keys to the known species of acanthocephalans have been published (Yamaguti, 1963b; Petrochenko, 1971).

The life cycle of these parasites starts with an egg containing a larva, called an acanthor, which is passed into the water in the feces of the definitive host (Fig. 10–11). The egg is ingested by an invertebrate host, usually an arthropod. The acanthor is

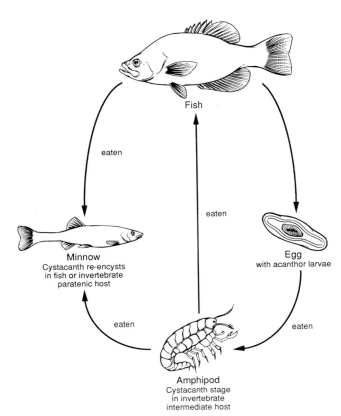

FIGURE 10–11. Life cycles of acanthocephalans of fishes.

released in the gut of the intermediate host and penetrates into the hemocoel, where development to a second immature form, called a cystacanth, occurs. When the intermediate host is ingested by a fish, the immature acanthocephalan cystacanth either completes development to the adult stage or becomes encysted as a larval form in the tissues of the fish. A fish with encysted cystacanths, like one infected with immature encysted nematodes, may serve as a second intermediate host or a paratenic host for the parasite. The life cycle of the acanthocephalan is completed by the ingestion of the cystacanth-infected tissues by other fishes, birds, or mammals.

The acanthocephalans rarely cause mortality in either freshwater or marine fishes, and therefore are not generally considered to be serious pathogens of fishes. However, acanthocephalans can cause severe local damage at the site of attachment in the intestine where the proboscis may be deeply embedded in the mucosa. This may also be accompanied by an intense inflammatory response by the host. Necrotic hemorrhagic ulcers in trout infected with acanthocephalans has been reported (Bullock, 1963), and large numbers of the parasites can completely obstruct the gastrointestinal tract and may ultimately cause the death of fish (Reichenbach-Klinke, 1973).

Molluscs

Most freshwater bivalve molluscs, particularly members of the family Unionidae, have an obligatory

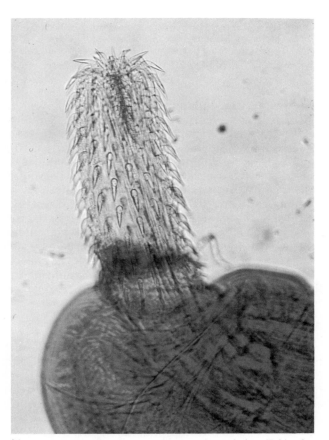

FIGURE 10–10. The proboscis of an acanthocephalan (*Echinorhynchus salmonis*) from a largemouth bass. Note the numerous recurved spines used for attachment of the parasite to the intestine of the host fish.

parasitic larval phase. These glochidia consist of a small, thin bivalve shell with small hooks on the inner edges, and are usually encysted in the gills or skin epithelium of the fish. Glochidia are nonmotile and are dispersed by water currents after being released from the adult clam. Attachment of the glochidium to the surface of the fish appears to stimulate the epidermis of the fish to proliferate around the larval clam. After metamorphosis on the host fish, juvenile clams are shed into the water and develop into adult clams. Although rarely a problem, heavy glochidial infections of the gills have been reported to cause mortalities of salmonids (Davis, 1953).

Leeches

Leeches are occasionally parasites of freshwater and marine fishes (Fig. 10–12). They have a segmented body with a coelom largely filled with connective tissue, and have distinct anterior and posterior suckers. Leeches resemble large digenetic trematodes in body form, but unlike the trematodes, they have a complete digestive system with a mouth located in the anterior sucker and an anus located in the posterior sucker. They have a direct life cycle. Juvenile leeches hatch from cocoons produced by hermaphroditic adults. Both immature and adult leeches may periodically attach to fish where they ingest blood. The pathology produced by leeches on fish depends on the number of leeches, the amount of blood loss, and the development of secondary bacterial or fungal infections at the site of attachment. Some leeches infest a wide range of hosts, while others have some degree of host specificity. The freshwater leech, *Piscicola geometra*, reaches epidemic proportions in cultured rainbow trout and cyprinids (Needham and Wootten, 1978). The marine leech, *Hemibdella* sp., has been a problem for cultured Dover sole and turbot (Needham and Wootten, 1978). *Myzobdella lugubris* has been associated with skin lesions on gulf mullet (Paperna and Overstreet, 1981). Leeches also serve as vectors for several protozoan parasites, including trypanosomes, *Cryptobia* spp., and possibly haemogregarines (Mann, 1962). Keys to the freshwater species have been published (Meyer, 1940, 1946; Hoffman, 1970).

Crustaceans

Parasitic crustaceans often exhibit extreme anatomic modifications to a parasitic mode of life. They have a complete digestive system and are usually dioecious, with females generally larger than males.

Classification of the parasitic crustaceans depends on body form, segmentation, the number and structure of the limbs, the form of the attachment organ, and the morphology of the egg sac or brood pouch. The biology, life history, and pathology of some of the more important parasitic crustaceans of fishes have been reviewed (Kabata, 1970, 1981, 1984; Mann, 1970; Smith, 1975; Schmidt and Roberts, 1989). The taxonomy of the known parasitic species of this group has also been extensively reviewed (Cressey, 1972; Kabata, 1970; Yamaguti, 1963c; Bykhovskaya-Pavlovskaya et al., 1964).

Copepods

Copepods are important both as parasites of fish and as intermediate hosts for other fish parasites. Most copepods have two main body divisions; the cephalothorax, consisting of the head and thorax, and the abdomen (Fig. 10–13). The cephalic region is generally greatly modified and possesses specialized mouth parts for piercing or sucking. These parasites typically possess two pairs of antennae, of which the second pair may be modified into a prehensile organ. The thoracic appendages are often reduced and usually consist of four pairs of swimming appendages. There are many families in this subclass that contain members that are ectoparasitic on freshwater and marine fishes, and even one family with members that are exclusively endoparasitic in the subdermal ducts and canals of teleosts and elasmobranchs (Kabata, 1970). Members of the family

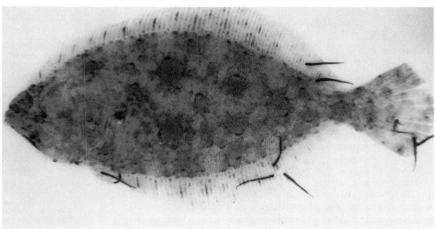

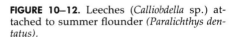

FIGURE 10–12. Leeches (*Calliobdella* sp.) attached to summer flounder (*Paralichthys dentatus*).

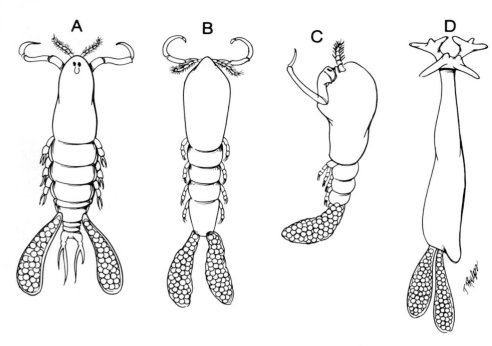

FIGURE 10–13. Representative morphology of copepods. *A–C.* Adult female ergasilids. *D.* Adult female lernaeid. (Adapted from Wootten, R. [1989] Fish Pathology. 2nd ed. [R.J. Roberts, ed.]. Bailliere Tindall/W.B. Saunders, Paris and Philadelphia; and Kabata, Z. [1970] Diseases of Fishes. Book 1. Crustacea as Enemies of Fishes [S.F. Sniezko and H.R. Axelrod, eds.]. T.F.H. Publications, Jersey City, New Jersey.)

Ergasilidae are probably the most common parasitic crustaceans of fish. This family includes the cosmopolitan genus *Ergasilus*, members of which have the typical copepod body form. In general, these are parasites of the gills or buccal cavity. As with most parasitic copepods, only the mature female is parasitic, whereas the immature developing female is free living. The males of parasitic species are free living throughout their life.

Members of the family Lernaeidae, most of which belong to the genus *Lernaea*, have species where adult females exhibit extreme modification of the cephalothorax. The mouth parts of the adult female are severely reduced, the body is elongate and vermiform, and the head is modified into large, anchor-shaped, cephalic horns (see Fig. 10–13). Thus, these ectoparasites have commonly been called "anchor worms." The horns are used for attachment to the host and are buried beneath the epidermis. As with the ergasilids, only the adult female lernaeids are parasitic, whereas the males and immature forms of both sexes are free living. Most of the members of this family occur on freshwater teleosts.

Members of the family Lernaeopoidae are parasites of both freshwater and marine species of fish, and include the genus *Salmincola*, which are parasitic on salmonids. Members of the family Lernaeoceridae are primarily parasites of marine fish.

In low numbers, parasitic copepods cause little damage to fish. They may cause localized inflammation and ulceration at the area of attachment and allow the entrance of secondary bacterial and fungal infections. Individuals of the genus *Lernaea* can also cause a localized hemorrhagic lesion and tissue proliferation at the attachment site. However, owing to the rapid reproductive potential of these parasites, massive numbers of parasitic copepods can cause serious pathology in fish under crowded culture conditions.

Branchiura

These "fish lice" are obligate ectoparasites of the skin and rarely the buccal cavity of freshwater and marine fishes. Most belong to the genus *Argulus*. They have a dorsoventrally flattened body covered with a carapace that extends laterally and posteriorly from the head, forming a shell over the thoracic and abdominal segments (Fig. 10–14). They have a retractile preoral sting or stylet, a proboscislike mouth, and four pairs of jointed swimming appendages. In

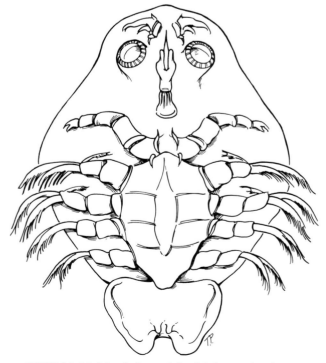

FIGURE 10–14. Morphology of the fish louse, *Argulus* sp.

addition, the first pair of maxillae are modified into a pair of large sucking discs used in the attachment of the parasite to the host. These parasitic crustacea are periodic parasites of fish and exhibit very little host specificity. Unlike the parasitic copepods, which undergo several metamorphic changes in becoming an adult, the branchiurans have a relatively simple development. Juveniles, which are similar in morphology to the adult, hatch from eggs and eventually develop into sexually mature individuals. The damage produced in the fish host by these parasites is a result of repeated piercing of the skin by the preoral sting, which injects a toxic substance into the underlying epidermis.

Isopods

Most isopods infest marine and brackish water fishes, but some are also parasitic on elasmobranchs and freshwater teleosts. They are usually attached to the gills or within the buccal or opercular cavity. Rarely, they may also be found embedded beneath the scales of the fish. Isopods are usually larger than the other parasitic crustacea and have chitinous plates over the dorsum of each body segment and a pair of appendages associated with each body segment (Fig. 10–15). The biting and sucking mouth parts of many species are highly modified for parasitism. Many are parasitic as both juveniles and adults, although some species of parasitic isopods are only parasitic as juveniles (pranizae).

Lampreys

Lampreys (cyclostomes) are eel-like, jawless fishes. The adults of these mostly freshwater or anadromous fishes are ectoparasitic on a number of commercially important freshwater and marine spe-cies of fishes. Cyclostomes have a circular suctorial mouth with a number of sharp, horny teeth. Once a lamprey attaches to a fish, the teeth rasp the skin, producing characteristic circular ulcers at the site of attachment (King and Edsall, 1979). Lampreys spawn in the spring in fresh water. Each fertilized egg hatches into a small, wormlike larva (ammocoete). The larvae are structurally and biologically different from the adult, being toothless, nonparasitic, and filter feeders. After spending several years buried in the mud, the larvae metamorphose into adult lampreys, which depending on the species may migrate to the ocean or remain in fresh water.

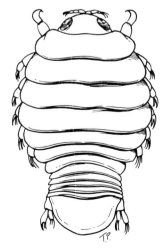

FIGURE 10–15. Representative morphology of an isopod. (Adapted from Kabata, Z. [1970] Diseases of Fishes. Book 1. Crustacea as Enemies of Fishes [S.F. Sniezko and H.R. Axelrod, eds.]. T.F.H. Publications, Jersey City, New Jersey.)

LITERATURE CITED

Amlacher, E. (1970) Textbook of Fish Diseases. T.F.H. Publishers, Neptune, New Jersey.

Anderson, R.C. (1978) CIH Keys to the Nematode Parasites of Vertebrates, No. 5. (Anderson, R.C., Chabaud, A.G., and Willmott, S., eds.). Commonwealth Agricultural Bureaux, Farnham Royal, Bucks, England.

Anderson, R.C., and Bain, O. (1976) CIH Keys to the Nematode Parasites of Vertebrates, No. 3, Part 3. (Anderson, R.C., Chabaud, A.G., and Willmott, S., eds.). Commonwealth Agricultural Bureaux, Farnham Royal, Bucks, England.

Anderson, R.C., and Bain, O. (1982) CIH Keys to the Nematode Parasites of Vertebrates, No. 9. (Anderson, R.C., Chabaud, A.G., and Willmott, S., eds.). Commonwealth Agricultural Bureaux, Farnham Royal, Bucks, England.

Bauer, O.N. (1961) Fish as carriers of human helminthosis. In: Parasitology of Fishes (Dogil, V.A., Petrushevski, G.K., and Polyanski, Y.I., eds.). Oliver and Boyd, Edinburgh, Scotland, pp. 320–334.

Bauer, O.N., Musselius, V.A., and Strelkov, Y.A. (1973) Diseases of Pond Fishes. Israel Programme for Scientific Translations, Jerusalem.

Becker, C.D. (1977) Flagellate parasites of fishes. In: Parasitic Protozoa. Vol. 1 (Kreier, J.P., ed.). Academic Press, New York, pp. 357–416.

Bullock, W. (1963) Intestinal histology of some salmonid fishes with particular reference to the histopathology of acanthocephalan infections. J. Morphol. 112:23–44.

Bychowsky, B.E. (1957) Monogenetic Trematodes. Their Systematics and Phylogeny. (Hargis, W.J., ed.). American Institute of Biological Sciences, Washington, D.C.

Bykhovskaya-Pavlovskaya, E.I., et al. (1964) Key to Parasites of Freshwater Fish of the U.S.S.R. Israel Program for Scientific Translations, National Science Foundation, Washington, D.C.

Canning, E.U., and Lom, J. (1986) The Microsporidia of Vertebrates. Academic Press, Orlando, Florida.

Chabaud, A.G. (1974) CIH Keys to the Nematode Parasites of Vertebrates, No. 1. (Anderson, R.C., Chabaud, A.G., and Willmott, S., eds.). Commonwealth Agricultural Bureaux, Farnham Royal, Bucks, England.

Chabaud, A.G. (1975a) CIH Keys to the Nematode Parasites of Vertebrates, No. 3, Part 1. (Anderson, R.C., Chabaud, A.G., and Willmott, S., eds.). Commonwealth Agricultural Bureaux, Farnham Royal, Bucks, England.

Chabaud, A.G. (1975b) CIH Keys to the Nematode Parasites of Vertebrates, No. 3, Part 2. (Anderson, R.C., Chabaud, A.G., and Willmott, S., eds.). Commonwealth Agricultural Bureaux, Farnham Royal, Bucks, England.

Chabaud, A.G. (1978) CIH Keys to the Animal Parasites of Vertebrates, No. 6. (Anderson, R.C., Chabaud, A.G., and Willmott, S., eds.). Commonwealth Agricultural Bureaux, Farnham Royal, Bucks, England.

Cressey, R.F. (1972) The genus Argulus (Crustacea: Branchiura) of the United States. Identification Manual, No. 2, United States Government Printing Office, Washington, D.C.

Cusack, R., and Cone, D.K. (1986) A review of parasites as vectors of viral and bacterial diseases of fish. J. Fish Dis. 9:169–171.

Davis, H.S. (1953) Culture and Diseases of Game Fishes. University of California Press, Berkeley.

Dawes, B. (1968) The Trematoda. Cambridge University Press, Cambridge, England.

Fischthal, J.H., and Allison, L.N. (1940) Acolpenteron ureteroecetes n.g., n. sp., a monogenetic trematode from the ureters of black basses. J. Parasitol. 26:34–35.

Gusev, A.V., and Fernando, C.H. (1973) Dactylogyridae (Monogenoidea) from the stomach of fishes. Folia Parasitol. 20:207–212.

Hargis, W.J., and Thoney, D.A. (1983) Bibliography of the Monogenea. Virginia Institute of Marine Science, Gloucester Point.

Hartwich, G. (1974) CIH Keys to the Animal Parasites of Vertebrates, No. 2. (Anderson, R.C., Chabaud, A.G., and Willmott, S., eds.). Commonwealth Agricultural Bureaux, Farnham Royal, Bucks, England.

Healy, G.R. (1970) Trematodes transmitted to man by fish, frogs and crustacea. J. Wildlife Dis. 6:255–261.

Hoffman, G.L. (1960) Synopsis of Strigeoidea (Trematoda) of fishes and their life cycles. U.S. Fish and Wildlife Service, Fishery Bulletin 175, 60:439–469.

Hoffman, G.L. (1970) Parasites of North American Freshwater Fishes. University of California Press, Berkeley.

Hoffman, G.L. (1975) Lesions due to internal helminths of freshwater fishes. In: The Pathology of Fishes (Ribelin, W.E., and Migaki, G., eds.). University of Wisconsin Press, Madison, pp. 151–186.

Hoffman, G.L. (1978) Ciliates of freshwater fishes. In: Parasitic Protozoa. Vol. 2 (Kreier, J.P., ed.). Academic Press, New York, pp. 583–632.

Kabata, Z. (1970) Diseases of fishes. In: Book 1. Crustacea as Enemies of Fishes. (Snieszko, S.F., and Axelrod, H.R., eds.). T.F.H. Publications, Jersey City, New Jersey.

Kabata, Z. (1981) Copepoda (Crustacea) parasitic on fishes: Problems and perspectives. Adv. Parasitol. 19:1–74.

Kabata, Z. (1984) Diseases caused by Metazoans: Crustaceans. In: Diseases of Marine Animals (Kinne, O., ed.). Biologische Anstalt Helgoland, Hamburg, pp. 321–399.

Kearn, G.C. (1963) The life cycle of the monogenean Entobdella soleae, a skin parasite of the common sole. Parasitology 53:253–263.

King, E.L., and Edsall, T.A. (1979) Illustrated Field Guide for the Classification of Sea Lamprey Attack Marks on Great Lakes Lake Trout. Special Publication 79-1, Great Lakes Fishery Commission, Ann Arbor, Michigan.

Lee, J.J., Small, E.B., Lynn, D.H., and Bovee, E.C. (1985) Some techniques for collecting, cultivating and observing protozoa. In: An Illustrated Guide to the Protozoa (Lee, J.J., Hunter, S.H., and Bovee, E.C., eds.). Society of Protozoologists, Lawrence, Kansas, pp. 1–7.

Lichtenfels, J.R. (1980a) CIH Keys to the Animal Parasites of Vertebrates, No. 7. (Anderson, R.C., Chabaud, A.G., and Willmott, S., eds.). Commonwealth Agricultural Bureaux, Farnham Royal, Bucks, England.

Lichtenfels, J.R. (1980b) CIH Keys to the Animal Parasites of Vertebrates, No. 8. (Anderson, R.C., Chabaud, A.G., and Willmott, S., eds.). Commonwealth Agricultural Bureaux, Farnham Royal, Bucks, England.

Mann, K.H. (1962) Leeches (Hirudinea): Their Structure, Physiology, Ecology and Embryology. Pergamon Press, New York.

Mann, H. (1970) Copepoda and Isopoda as parasites of marine fishes. In: A Symposium on Diseases of Fishes and Shellfishes (Snieszko, S.F., ed.). American Fisheries Society, Washington, D.C., pp. 177–189.

Margolis, L. (1970) Nematode diseases of marine fishes. In: A Symposium on Diseases of Fishes and Shellfishes (Snieszko, S.F., ed.). American Fisheries Society, Washington, D.C., pp. 190–208.

Meyer, M.C. (1940) A revision of the leeches (Piscicolidae) living on freshwater fishes of North America. Trans. Am. Microscope Soc. 59:354–376.

Meyer, M.C. (1946) Further notes on the leeches (Piscicolodae) living on freshwater fishes of North America. Trans. Am. Microscope Soc. 65:237–249.

Meyer, M.C. (1970) Cestode zoonoses of aquatic animals. J. Wildlife Dis. 6:249–254.

Myers, B.J. (1970) Nematodes transmitted to man by fish and aquatic mammals. J. Wildlife Dis. 6:266–271.

Needham, T., and Wootten, R. (1978) Parasitology of teleosts. In: Fish Pathology (Roberts, R.J., ed.). Macmillan, New York, pp. 144–182.

Noble, E.R., and Noble, G.A. (1966) Amebic parasites of fishes. J. Protozool. 13:478–480.

Overstreet, R.M. (1978) Marine Maladies? Worms, Germs, and Other Symbionts from the Northern Gulf of Mexico. Blossman Printing, Ocean Springs, Mississippi.

Paperna, I. (1963) Enterogyrus cichlidarum n. gen., n. sp., a monogenetic trematode parasite in the intestine of a fish. Bull. Res. Council Isr. 4:183–187.

Paperna, I., and Overstreet, R.M. (1981) Parasites and diseases of mullets (Mugilidae). In: Aquaculture of Grey Mullets (Oren, O.H., ed.). Cambridge University Press, Cambridge, England, pp. 411–493.

Petrochenko, V.I. (1971) Acanthocephala of Domestic and Wild Animals (Skrjabin, K.I., ed.). Israel Program for Scientific Translations, Ltd., National Science Foundation, Washington, D.C.

Petter, A.J., and Quentin, J. (1976) CIH Keys to the Animal Parasites of Vertebrates, No. 4. (Anderson, R.C., Chabaud, A.G., and Willmott, S., eds.). Commonwealth Agricultural Bureaux, Farnham Royal, Bucks, England.

Pritchard, M.H., and Kruse, G.O.W. (1982) The Collection and Preservation of Animal Parasites. University of Nebraska Press, Lincoln.

Reichenbach-Klinke, H. (1973) Fish Pathology. T.F.H. Publications, Neptune, New Jersey.

Rim, H. (1982) Clonorchiasis. In: CRC Handbook Series in Zoonoses, Section C: Parasitic Zoonoses (Steele, J.H., ed.). CRC Press, Boca Raton, Florida, pp. 17–32.

Rohde, K. (1972) The Aspidogastrea, especially Multicotyle purvisi Daws, 1941. In: Advances in Parasitology, Vol. 10 (Dawes, B., ed.). Academic Press, New York, pp. 78–152.

Rohde, K. (1984) Diseases caused by Metazoans: Helminths. In: Diseases of Marine Animals (Kinne, O., ed.). Biologische Anstalt Helgoland, Hamburg, pp. 193–320.

Schell, S.C. (1985) Handbook of Trematodes of North America North of Mexico. University Press of Idaho, Moscow.

Schmidt, G.D. (1986) CRC Handbook of Tapeworm Identification. CRC Press, Boca Raton, Florida.

Schmidt, G.D., and Roberts, L.S. (1989) Parasitic crustaceans. In: Foundations of Parasitology (Schmidt, G.D., and Robert, L.S., eds.). C.V. Mosby, St. Louis, pp. 560–585.

Skrjabin, K.I. (1964) Keys to the Trematodes of Animals and Man (Arai, H.P., ed.). University of Illinois Press, Urbana.

Skrjabin, K.I. (1968) Keys to Parasitic Nematodes. Vols. 1–3. National Science Foundation, Washington, D.C.

Smith, F.G. (1975) Crustacean parasites of marine fishes. In: The Pathology of Fishes (Ribelin, W.E., and Migaki, G., eds.). University of Wisconsin Press, Madison, pp. 189–203.

Smith, H.D. (1973) Observations on the cestode Eubothrium salvelini in juvenile sockeye salmon (Oncorhynchus nerka) at Babine Lake, British Columbia. J. Fish Res. Bd. Can. 30:947–964.

Smith, I.W., and Wootten, R. (1978) Anisakis and Anisakiasis. In: Advances in Parasitology. Vol. 16 (Lumsden, W.H.R., Muller, R., and Baker, J.R., eds.). Academic Press, New York, pp. 93–163.

Sproston, N.G. (1946) A synopsis of the monogenetic trematodes. Trans. Zool. Soc. Lond. 25:185–600.

Strelkov, U.A., and Ki K. (1964) A new case of unusual localization of a monogenetic trematode of the genus Dactylogyrus in the nasal cavities of fishes. Zool. Zhurn. 43:1236–1238.

Tiner, J.D. (1988) Birefringent spores differentiate Encephalitozoon and other Microsporidia from Coccidia. J. Vet. Pathol. 25:227–230.

Velasquez, C.C. (1982) Heterophyidiasis. In: CRC Handbook Series in Zoonoses, Section C: Parasitic Zoonoses (Steele, J.H., ed.). CRC Press, Boca Raton, Florida, pp. 99–107.

Wolf, K., Markiw, M.E., and Hiltunen, J.K. (1986) Salmonid whirling disease: Tubifex tubifex (Muller) identified as the essential oligochaete in the protozoan life cycle. J. Fish Dis. 9:83–85.

Yamaguti, S. (1958) Systema Helminthum. Vol. 1. The Digenetic Trematodes of Vertebrates, Parts 1 and 2. Interscience Publishers, New York, pp. 1575.

Yamaguti, S. (1959) Systema Helminthum. Vol. 2. The Cestodes of Vertebrates. Interscience Publishers, New York, pp. 860.

Yamaguti, S. (1961) Systema Helminthum. Vol. 3. The Nematodes of Vertebrates. Interscience Publishers, New York, pp. 1261.

Yamaguti, S. (1963a) Systema Helminthum. Vol. 4. Monogenea and Aspidocotylea. Interscience Publishers, New York, pp. 699.

Yamaguti, S. (1963b) Systema Helminthum. Vol. 5. Acanthocephala. Interscience Publishers, New York, pp. 423.

Yamaguti, S. (1963c) Parasitic Copepoda and Branchiura of Fishes. Interscience Publishers, New York, pp. 1104.

Yamaguti, S. (1971) Synopsis of Digenetic Trematodes of Vertebrates, Vols. 1 and 2. Keigaku Publishing, Tokyo.

Yukhimenko, S.S., and Danilov, V.A. (1977) A New Case of Transition to Endoparasitism in Monogeneans. In: Investigation of Monogeneans in the U.S.S.R. (Skarlato, O.A., ed.). Oxonian Press, New Delhi, pp. 75–76.

Chapter 11

IMMUNOLOGY

SUZANNE KENNEDY-STOSKOPF

Knowledge of the fish immune system has been accumulated following two lines of investigation. The first is comparative immunology. As the most primitive vertebrates, fish are an important link between invertebrates and the higher vertebrates. Fish possess the phagocytic mechanisms associated with granulocytic and mononuclear phagocytic cells of invertebrates and are the first species to exhibit both the humoral and the cell-mediated immunity most commonly associated with mammals. They have both B and T lymphocytes capable of responding to foreign antigens by antibody production and various effector mechanisms, respectively. Studying piscine immune systems has provided valuable insight into the evolution of antigen-specific responses. Comparative studies, in turn, provide the framework for the second line of investigation designed to determine how fish respond to pathogens.

THE IMMUNE SYSTEM

Lymphoid and Myeloid Tissue

All fish lack bone marrow, the source of myeloid cells in anurans and higher vertebrates. They also lack lymph nodes. Lymphoid and myeloid tissues are more intermingled in fish, commonly associated with the kidney of teleosts and sturgeons and the liver of hagfishes and elasmobranchs. The spiral valve of sharks and other cartilaginous fishes is also rich in lymphomyeloid tissue (Fig. 11–1). In addition, sharks have lymphomyeloid tissue associated with the epigonal and Leydig organs. Sturgeons have additional lymphomyeloid tissue associated with the meninges and pericardium (Fange, 1986). Fish possess a well-developed thymus and spleen except for the hagfishes, which do not have a true thymus and only a rudimentary spleen (Horton and Lackie, 1989). In fishes, the thymus develops the earliest of all lymphoid tissues. Lymphocytes are the predominant cell population, although they are not organized into a distinct cortex and medulla as occurs in mammals (Chilmonczyk, 1985; Fange and Pulsford, 1985). The spleen is divided into red and white pulp as in mammals but lacks germinal centers.

A unique feature of piscine lymphomyeloid tissue is the presence of melanomacrophage centers in the liver, spleen, and kidney (Fig. 11–2). These melanomacrophage centers may be the forerunners of the germinal centers present in the spleen and lymph nodes of birds and mammals (Agius, 1985). Both germinal and melanomacrophage centers are aggregates of reticular cells, lymphocytes, macrophages, and plasma cells. Germinal centers develop in response to antigen trapping within lymphoid tissue and are believed to be necessary to establish immunological memory. Although fish exhibit anamnestic responses, this function has not been conclusively linked with melanomacrophage centers.

Instead, the melanomacrophage centers are repositories of pigment. The pigments include lipofuscin, melanin, and hemosiderin. All three pigments may occur in the same macrophage. Lipofuscin, formed in part by the oxidation of unsaturated tissue lipids, is the most abundant pigment. Melanin is

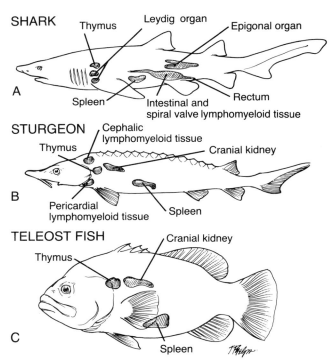

FIGURE 11–1. The locations of lymphopoietic tissues in sharks, sturgeons, and most teleost fishes. A. The shark has lymphopoietic tissues in the thymus, Leydig organs, spleen, and epigonal organ and in the walls of the intestine and spiral valve. B. The sturgeon has lymphopoietic tissues in the thymus, spleen, and cranial kidney as well as in special pericardial and cephalic lymphomyeloid tissues. C. The majority of teleosts have lymphopoietic tissues in the thymus, cranial kidney, and spleen.

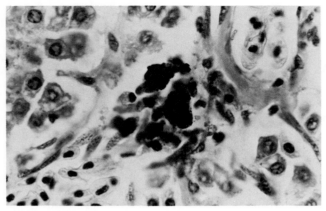

FIGURE 11–2. Melanomacrophage centers in the liver of an American eel (1000×).

commonly present at variable levels but is quite abundant in the kidneys of salmonid species. Hemosiderin, a by-product of hemoglobin degradation, consists of the protein apoferritin and ferric iron. Hemosiderin is abundant in the fish spleen under conditions of starvation and disease (Agius, 1985). This pigment has not been seen in the shark spleen. Occasionally ceroid, a lipid pigment, is observed in pathological conditions in fish.

The high lipofuscin content of melanomacrophages is attributed to the peroxidation of unsaturated fatty acids, which are abundant in fish in order to allow them to maintain membrane fluidity at low temperatures. Melanin is capable of neutralizing the free radicals and cation activity associated with oxidizing conditions. This would explain its close association with lipofuscin in macrophages and its increased accumulation during infections and injuries. The ferric iron associated with hemosiderin is believed to be recycled for metabolic processes as in mammals, but the process is unknown.

The role of melanomacrophage centers for modulating infections is speculative. The pigments may have a direct bactericidal effect (Edelstein, 1971) or may simply accumulate as a result of tissue damage at the sites of infection, thereby enlarging the melanomacrophage centers.

Phagocytosis

Phagocytosis is the most primordial defense mechanism. Primarily a nutritive function in lower life forms, phagocytosis has evolved solely to a protective function in vertebrates. Phagocytosis involves recognition and attachment of a foreign particle, engulfment, and digestion. Signals for recognition and attachment are largely unknown in fish. In bony fishes, the kidney and spleen are the major sites of antigen localization by phagocytic cells. There are two kinds of phagocytic cells common to all vertebrates: monocyte-macrophages and granular leukocytes.

MONOCYTES AND MACROPHAGES. Monocytes are

restricted to the peripheral circulation, whereas macrophages are located in the tissues. These mononuclear cells are actively phagocytic. Until recently, opsonization, or enhancement of phagocytosis via antigen-antibody complexes, was considered doubtful because fish macrophages could not be shown to possess Fc receptors for binding antibody (Wrathmell and Parish, 1980). Fc receptors have been demonstrated in the nurse shark by using cytochalasin D to inhibit nonspecific phagocytosis (Haynes et al., 1988). The authors speculate that specific binding via an Fc receptor could not be distinguished from nonspecific phagocytic activity that is quite high in shark leukocytes.

GRANULAR LEUKOCYTES. Granular leukocytes include heterophils, eosinophils, and basophils. This is a mammalian classification scheme based on the staining characteristics of granules that has been adopted for fish even though the morphology and perhaps function of piscine granular leukocytes are not identical to those of mammals (Mainwaring and Rowley, 1985).

Heterophils are the predominant granulocyte in fish blood. The preponderance of evidence supports a phagocytic function for these cells, although they are not as actively phagocytic as fish monocytes and macrophages or mammalian neutrophils. Ellis (1981) speculates that fish heterophils kill extracellularly through the discharge of their hydrolytic and oxidizing enzymes rather than intracellularly via phagosome-lysosome fusion as occurs in mammals. This would explain why bacterial infections in fish are associated with hemorrhagic liquefaction instead of the suppuration seen in mammals. This would also substantiate the role of melanomacrophage centers as modulators of superoxide radicals.

Eosinophils are also believed to be phagocytic (Mainwaring and Rowley, 1985). Additional phagocytic cells include thrombocytes in plaice (Ferguson, 1976a) and coho salmon (Lester and Budd, 1979), endothelial cells lining the blood sinuses and gill pillar cells in rainbow trout (Chilmonczyk and Monge, 1980), ventricular endothelial cells in the Amazon molly (Woodhead, 1981), and atrial endocardial macrophages in plaice (Ferguson, 1975).

Humoral Immunity

Through the complex interactions of antigen-presenting cells, activated helper T lymphocytes, and soluble cell factors known as interleukins, B lymphocytes are stimulated to produce immunoglobulins (Fig. 11–3). Macrophages are the primary antigen-presenting cells in fish. Conflicting reports exist regarding the presence in fish of dendritic cells, which are antigen-presenting cells in mammals (Ellis, 1980; Ferguson, 1976b; Stuart, 1970). The presence of helper T lymphocytes is inferred by lymphoproliferative responses to mitogens. Recognition of different subsets of T lymphocytes using monoclonal antibodies is just beginning to be developed (Miller et al.,

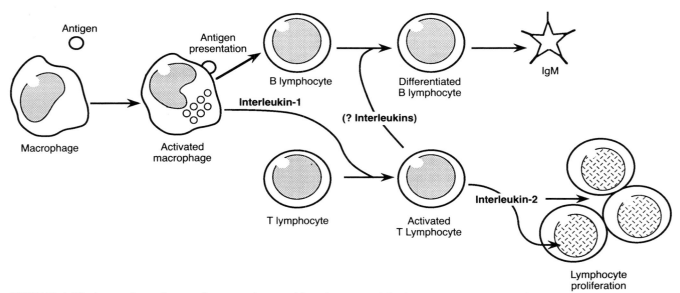

FIGURE 11–3. The interactions of macrophages, antigen, and lymphocytes in fish. Antigen activates macrophages, which serve as antigen-presenting cells to B lymphocytes. Activated macrophages also produce interleukin-1, which activates T lymphocytes. T lymphocytes in turn produce unidentified interleukins, which activate B lymphocytes that have been presented with antigen by activated macrophages to produce IgM. Activated T lymphocytes also produce interleukin-2, which induces lymphoblast proliferation.

1987). Likewise, the existence of interleukinlike molecules in fish is primarily by inference. Interleukin-1 (IL-1), which is produced by macrophages after exposure to antigen, activates helper T lymphocytes in mammals. Human IL-1 combined with suboptimal concentrations of mitogen enhances the lymphoproliferative responses of catfishes. Supernatants from cultured carp epithelial cells have IL-1–like properties (Sigel et al., 1986). Activated helper T lymphocytes, in turn, produce interleukin-2 (IL-2), which supports proliferation of lymphoblastic cells. Supernatants of mitogen- and alloantigen-stimulated carp peripheral blood leukocytes promote the growth of carp T lymphocytes, suggesting the presence of an IL-2–like molecule (Caspi and Avtalion, 1984). Activated helper T lymphocytes then stimulate B lymphocytes to produce immunoglobulins.

Fish synthesize only one class of immunoglobulin equivalent to mammalian immunoglobulin M (IgM) (Fig. 11–4). Serum IgM in teleosts is tetrameric, and in cartilaginous fishes it is pentameric, although monomeric IgM is found in sharks and rays (Ambrosius et al., 1982). Epitopes on piscine μ chains are highly conserved and shared with μ chains of other vertebrates (Litman and Marchalonis, 1982). Immunoglobulin M is the major immunoglobulin isotype produced in a primary immune response in mammals. IgM is produced in secondary immune responses, but the presence of IgM is obscured by the predominance of IgG (Tizard, 1987). IgG is the most abundant serum immunoglobulin in mammals and consequently plays a prominent role in antibody-mediated defense mechanisms. Despite the absence of IgG in fish, protective humoral responses occur. In general, IgM is more efficient than IgG in comple-

ment activation, opsonization, neutralization of viruses, and agglutination (Tizard, 1987).

Secretory immunity, as opposed to systemic immunity, refers to the localized production of antibodies at mucosal surfaces and is associated with the IgA isotype in mammals. The primary role of IgA is the prevention of adherence of microorganisms rather than activation of the complement and opsonization that IgM facilitates. In teleosts, antigen-spe-

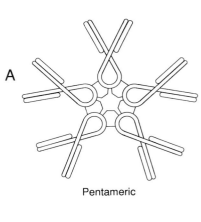

A

Pentameric

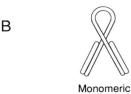

B

Monomeric

FIGURE 11–4. Diagram of the structure of pentameric (A) and monomeric (B) IgM of fishes.

cific antibodies occur in the mucus as IgM (St. Louis-Cormier et al., 1984; Lobb, 1987).

Cell-Mediated Immunity

T lymphocytes, which originate from the thymus, mediate cellular immunity. Different subsets regulate different functions. Helper T cells enhance, whereas suppressor T cells downregulate, the responses of other T and B lymphocytes. Cytotoxic T cells destroy foreign and abnormal cells. Another subset of T lymphocytes mediates delayed-type hypersensitivity reactions. Bony fishes presumably have heterogenic T lymphocytes because the described cellular immune responses are demonstrable either in vitro or in vivo, although no functional markers distinguish the various subsets (Fig. 11–5).

Bony fishes have acute allograft rejections in vivo (≤14 days) and strong mixed lymphocyte reactions in vitro (Jurd, 1985). These two tests demonstrate functional disparity between two individuals, and thus support the existence of a major histocompatibility complex (MHC) in teleosts. Acute allograft rejections imply the presence of class I MHC antigens and strong mixed lymphocyte reactions suggest class II MHC antigens. Like functional markers for T lymphocytes, the piscine MHC has not been characterized.

Hagfishes, sharks, skates, rays, and sturgeons exhibit chronic or subacute rejection (≥30 days) of skin and scale allografts, suggesting that these fishes lack an MHC and reject foreign antigens nonspecifically (Jurd, 1985). Sharks and sturgeons also have weak mixed lymphocyte reaction (MLR), but hagfishes (class Agnatha) have a strong MLR (Horton and Lackie, 1989). The significance of this is not known.

Nonspecific Mediators of Immunity

Host defense mechanisms that do not involve specific recognition of antigen as occurs in humoral and cell-mediated immunity are considered to be nonspecific. The term *nonspecific* is somewhat misleading, since some of these defense mechanisms are triggered in the presence of specific molecular configurations that are common in nature. Because the recognition sites are not restricted to a particular microorganism, the term *nonspecific* is used to describe mechanisms that function to limit the spread or remove the cause of host-tissue damage. Phagocytosis, which has already been discussed, is an example of a nonspecific immune response.

The skin, which is a physical barrier to invading microorganisms, is often overlooked as an important nonspecific defense mechanism. Unlike the skin of higher vertebrates, fish epidermis is composed of nonkeratinized living cells (Roberts and Bullock, 1980). Wound healing is much more rapid in fish

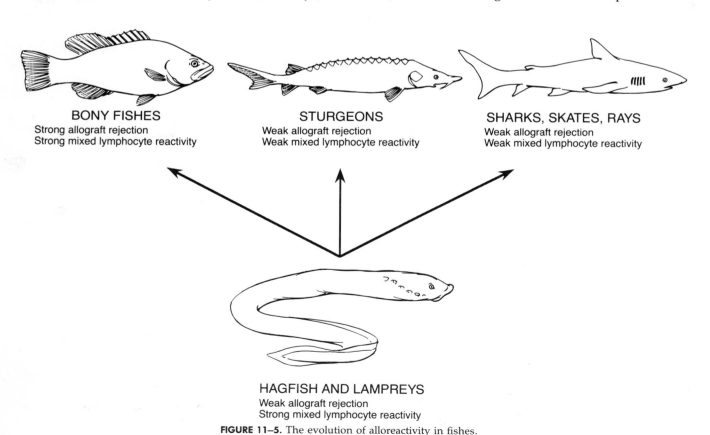

BONY FISHES
Strong allograft rejection
Strong mixed lymphocyte reactivity

STURGEONS
Weak allograft rejection
Weak mixed lymphocyte reactivity

SHARKS, SKATES, RAYS
Weak allograft rejection
Weak mixed lymphocyte reactivity

HAGFISH AND LAMPREYS
Weak allograft rejection
Strong mixed lymphocyte reactivity

FIGURE 11–5. The evolution of alloreactivity in fishes.

than in mammals. This is viewed as an adaptive advantage to an aquatic environment in order for fish to maintain their osmolarity (Ellis, 1981).

Mucus is an additional external barrier shared by fish that is absent on the skin of other vertebrates. Mucus inhibits the colonization of microorganisms on the integument as well as on the gills and gastrointestinal mucosa. Fish mucus has been found to contain natural antibodies, lysozyme, and bacteriolysins (Diconza, 1970; Fletcher and White, 1973; Ourth, 1980). Natural antibodies are not the result of a previous exposure to a specific epitope on a foreign antigen but represent exposure to related epitopes, which commonly occur in nature. These related epitopes are usually carbohydrate constituents of cell walls. Agglutination of xenotropic erythrocytes is a function of natural antibodies and has been demonstrated in teleost mucus (Suzuki and Kaneko, 1986). Lysozyme is an enzyme produced by phagocytic cells that recognizes carbohydrate moieties of cell walls, in particular, bacterial mucopolysaccharides. The nature of the bacteriolysin reported in the skin mucus of channel catfish is not known (Ourth, 1980). Natural antibodies, lysozyme, and lysins are also found in the serum. The exact contribution of these nonspecific factors to piscine defense mechanisms is not known.

Complement is also present in mucus and serum. The complement system involves a series of carefully regulated, interlinking enzyme reactions. The end result of this cascade mechanism is disruption of cell membranes. The complement system may be activated by three distinct pathways. Hagfishes are thought to possess only the terminal complement components, the so-called third pathway (Horton and Lackie, 1989). This is not a true cascade reaction, but a series of aggregations by which a membrane-damaging complex is formed from the activated third component. The other two complement pathways are alternate routes for the activation of the third complement component (C3). The classic complement pathway, so named because it has been recognized longer than the alternate pathway, is activated by antigen-antibody interactions. The alternate pathway provides the host with a mechanism for eliminating invading pathogens without the presence of antibody. Most fish have classic and alternate complement pathways analogous to those of mammals (Koppenheffer, 1987).

C-reactive protein that can activate complement is present in the normal serum of plaice (Pepys et al., 1978), dogfishes (Robey et al., 1983), lumpsucker (Fletcher et al., 1977), and rainbow trout (Winkelhake and Chang, 1982). Flounder, which are closely related to plaice, apparently do not have C-reactive protein (Fletcher and Baldo, 1976). In plaice and rainbow trout, C-reactive protein is elevated following inoculation with bacterial lipopolysaccharide and *Vibrio anguillarum*, respectively, and thus acts as an acute phase protein (White et al., 1981; Murai et al., 1990). C-reactive protein in mammals enhances

phagocytosis and may function similarly in fish, although it has not been demonstrated.

α-Antiprotease found in normal rainbow trout serum (Ellis et al., 1981) is analogous to mammalian α_2-macroglobulin, another acute phase protein. α-Antiprotease neutralizes the proteolytic activity of *Aeromonas salmonicida* exotoxin in vitro and in vivo. Ellis (1981) suggests that α-antiprotease, like α_2-macroglobulin, may also stabilize macrophage lysosomes and thus explains the relative resistance of salmonids to endotoxin shock.

Nonspecific cytotoxic leukocytes have been described in fish (Hinuma et al., 1980; Graves et al., 1984; Moody et al., 1985). Analogous to mammalian natural killer cells, these cells in carp, channel catfish, and salmonids lyse a variety of mammalian cell lines and teleost cell lines in the case of salmonids (Moody et al., 1985). Viral infections and interferon stimulate mammalian natural killer cell activity above normal levels. Infecting teleost cells with infectious pancreatic necrosis virus enhances the killing function of salmonid "natural killer" cells. Interferon has been described in fish (Ingram, 1980), but its effect on nonspecific cytotoxicity has not been documented.

Certain teleost species exhibit behavioral reactions compatible with type I hypersensitivity, or anaphylaxis (Goven et al., 1980; Ellis et al., 1981). Controversy exists as to whether fish can truly experience anaphylaxis, since they do not have the IgE and mast cells that interact in mammals to release histamine, thereby triggering type I hypersensitivity. Fish do have eosinophilic granular cells widely distributed in connective tissue. Intraperitoneal injection of *Aeromonas salmonicida* extracellular products in rainbow trout causes rapid degranulation of eosinophilic granular cells with a concomitant increase in serum histamine and a decrease in gut-associated histamine levels (Ellis et al., 1985). Ultrastructure and cytochemical studies suggest that tissue eosinophils are mast cell–like (Ezeasor and Stokoe, 1980). Interestingly, antihistamines inhibit eosinophilic granular cells but not mast cell degranulation (Vallejo and Ellis, 1989). Clearly, some teleost fishes have a mechanism, yet to be fully elucidated, which mediates piscine type I hypersensitivity.

Type II and type III hypersensitivity reactions have not been documented in fish but probably occur. Type II hypersensitivity reactions are caused by the release of biologically active cell breakdown products following antibody-dependent cell cytotoxicity or complement-mediated lysis. Reaction from an incompatible blood transfusion is an example of type II hypersensitivity. Blood groups in fish appear to exist phylogenetically between orders (Sakai et al., 1987). Normal serum from salmonid fishes (rainbow trout, masu salmon, and sockeye salmon) lyse erythrocytes of nonsalmonid fishes (goldfish and carp). Heat inactivation of the serum abolishes the lytic activity, implying complement mediation and possibly a type II hypersensitivity reaction. Salmonid erythrocytes also survive less than 1 day in nonsalmonid fishes. Intraspecific erythrocyte rejection and hemolysis with serum from different species of fish within the same taxonomic group does not occur.

Type III hypersensitivity is mediated by deposition of complement-activating immune complexes in tissue. Although not specifically documented in fish, all the necessary components of type III hypersensitivity are present and could cause immune complex–mediated pathologic changes like glomerulonephritis and skin ulcerations (Ellis, 1981).

MODULATION OF THE IMMUNE RESPONSE

Temperature

The physiological processes of poikilotherms are influenced by temperature. Numerous studies have demonstrated that low temperatures depress nonspecific, humoral, and cell-mediated defense mechanisms in fish. Helper T-lymphocyte functions and allograft rejections are temperature dependent, and primary antibody responses develop faster at optimal temperatures. Although the kinetics of primary antibody response is slower at suboptimal temperatures, the magnitude and duration of the response is not significantly different from the response that develops more quickly at higher temperatures (Stolen et al., 1984). Phagocytosis does not seem to be impaired by low temperatures, but the intracellular killing of ingested organisms is.

Fluctuations in water temperature are natural seasonal phenomena. Likewise, mortalities from infectious agents have a seasonal incidence. Bacteria and parasites are associated with spring die-offs, and some viruses cause epizootic diseases in the fall. Bisset (1946) hypothesized that the seasonal incidence of infectious diseases was related to temperature-dependent immunocompetency. Infections acquired during the cooler months would persist as immune functions were depressed, then as temperatures increased, the infections would overwhelm the ectothermic host before its defense mechanisms could compensate. This is probably an oversimplification. Studies in carp and channel catfish have shown that antibodies develop at cool temperatures if fish are first exposed to the antigen at optimal temperatures (Avtalion, 1969; Plumb et al., 1986). In fact, the antibody responses of channel catfish immunized against *Edwardsiella ictaluri* are greater if they are exposed to cooler temperatures following antigen inoculation at optimal temperatures than if they are just maintained at optimal temperatures (Plumb et al., 1986). This suggests that the fish immune system has adapted to seasonal temperature fluctuations, and that other mitigating factors besides temperature alone contribute to seasonal mortalities.

By selecting a higher environmental temperature, fish show a febrile response. Bluegill and largemouth bass injected with *Aeromonas hydrophila* prefer an environmental temperature 2 to 3°C higher than before infection (Reynolds et al., 1976). The mechanism for this behavioral febrile response is unknown. Acetaminophen, however, diminishes the febrile response in bluegills (Reynolds, 1977), as it does in higher vertebrates, so perhaps piscine and mammalian physiological responses to pyrogens share similar features.

Neuroendocrine Functions

The interactions between the hypothalamus and pituitary gland on such target organs as the adrenals and gonads is well established. Increasing awareness is developing that neuroendocrine functions impact on immunocompetence. This has fostered a whole new area of investigation called neuroendocrinimmunology. The cornerstone of these studies is the effect of stress on immune functions.

Any number of stimuli may be perceived by the hypothalamus as stressful, which activates the release of adrenocorticotropin (ACTH) from the pituitary and the subsequent production of corticosteroids by the interrenal cells. The major corticosteroid in fish is cortisol. Corticosteroids can affect leukocyte circulation, lymphocyte effector mechanisms, and inflammation in a negative fashion. All these effects have been reported in fish. When plaice are either environmentally stressed or given exogenous cortisol, they have fewer leukocytes in the peritoneal cavity following glycogen injection (MacArthur et al., 1984). This is attributed to cortisol-related inhibition of leukocyte migration. Cortisol is also believed to inhibit interleukin production. Cultures of splenic- and pronephric-derived lymphocytes from coho salmon exposed to physiological concentrations of cortisol have dose-dependent, decreased antibody responses to a hapten conjugated *Escherichia coli* lipopolysaccharide (Tripp et al., 1987). This suppression can be abrogated by adding supernatants from antigen-stimulated lymphocytes that would have interleukin activity.

Heavy Metals, Pollutants, and Drugs

Anemia is a widely recognized toxic effect of the exposure to heavy metals in fish. Cadmium, lead, mercury, and zinc at concentrations of 10 μg/L for 1 to 2 months have caused some degree of anemia in teleosts (Heath, 1987). The effects of heavy metals on leukocytes is more variable. Cadmium causes a dose-dependent lymphopenia in cunners (Newman and MacLean, 1974), and a lymphocytosis in perch from a cadmium-polluted river has been reported (Larsson et al., 1985). The significance of decreased or increased numbers of lymphocytes to function is not known. Interspecies variability to cadmium exposure apparently exists in fish, however. Sublethal concentrations of cadmium enhance antibody responses against *Bacillus cereus* in striped bass and inhibit the response in cunners (Robohm, 1986).

The effects of heavy metals on nonspecific immunity is also variable. Cadmium (12 ppm) increases phagocytosis in cunners, but intracellular killing is decreased (Robohm and Nitkowski, 1974). Copper severely depresses phagocytic activity and aluminum less so (Elsasser et al., 1986). Mercuric chloride (0.3 ppm) causes a steady decline in serum lysozyme of plaice over 7 days exposure (Fletcher, 1986).

Dioxin (2,3,7,8-tetrachlorodibenzo-p-dioxin, TCDD), a by-product of the production of the herbicides (2,4,5-trichlorophenoxy)acetic acid, 2,4,5-T, and 2,4-D, is being detected in many freshwater and marine fishes. It is exceedingly immunosuppressive in mice at doses lower than those that cause histopathology and liver microsomal enzyme induction. The reverse appears to be true in fish. Intraperitoneal injection of TCDD at doses ranging from 0.1 to 10 μg/kg had no significant effect on phagocytosis and humoral and cellular immunity of rainbow trout (Spitsbergen et al., 1986). A dose of 10 μg/kg, however, caused hypophagia, fin necrosis, ascites, and suppressed hematopoiesis.

Petroleum distillates contain varying amounts of saturated and unsaturated aliphatic and aromatic hydrocarbons. Macrophage chemotactic and phagocytic activities were depressed in spot and hogchokers collected in a river with high concentrations of polycyclic aromatic hydrocarbons (Weeks and Warinner, 1986).

Not only are environmental contaminants potentially detrimental to the piscine immune system, but therapeutic agents may also be immunosuppressive. Certain antibiotics are known to immunosuppress vertebrates. The immunomodulating effects of oxytetracycline are the best documented in teleost fish (Grondel and Boeston, 1982; van Muiswinkel et al., 1985). A single intraperitoneal injection of oxytetracycline 24 hours prior to antigen administration delays primary antibody responses 2 to 4 days (Grondel et al., 1987). The rate of development of plaque-forming cells (PFCs) is not altered, but their number is decreased. Their numbers are also decreased if oxytetracycline is administered following inoculation of antigen.

Nutrition

Although there is general agreement that a well-balanced diet is essential to adequate host defense mechanisms, very little has been done to study the effects of specific nutrients on immune functions in fish. As dietary levels of ascorbic acid increase, mortality rates of catfish fingerlings infected with *Edwardsiella tarda* and *E. ictaluri* decrease (Durve and Lovell, 1982; Li and Lovell, 1985). Circulating antibody titers to *E. ictaluri* and phagocytic indices were lower in channel catfish fed diets with no ascorbic acid (Li and Lovell, 1985). Humoral immunity and phagocytosis are not impaired in mammals with severe vitamin C deficiencies (Beisel, 1982).

Species Variability

Intraspecies differences in disease susceptibility exist in fish and have formed the basis of selective breeding programs. Different strains of rainbow trout exhibit varying degrees of resistance to furunculosis that is associated with the magnitude of the serum neutralization titers against *Aeromonas salmonicida* (Cipriano, 1982). Different strains of salmon have varying resistance to vibriosis (Gjedrum and Aulstad, 1974). Susceptibility of coho salmon to bacterial kidney disease is related to their different transferrin genotypes (Suzumoto et al., 1977; Winter et al., 1980).

Pathogens

Many organisms are successful pathogens because they can modulate the host immune response. The observed effects of infection with *Aeromonas salmonicida* suggest that the bacteria is immunosuppressive and possibly even evades the immune system (Evenberg et al., 1986). Affected fish have concurrent opportunistic infections and immunoglobulin concentrations are decreased. Immunological memory does not develop following sublethal infections.

Viruses and parasites can also be immunosuppressive. Persistent infection of Atlantic salmon with the infectious pancreatic necrosis virus suppresses phytohemagglutinin blastogenesis (Knott and Munro, 1986). The microsporidian *Glugea stephani* causes a decline in serum immunoglobulins of experimentally infected winter flounder and suppresses antibody responses to unrelated antigens (Laudan et al., 1986). When indomethacin is given twice weekly following inoculation of spores, there is no decrease in immunoglobulins. This suggests that prostaglandins mediate the observed immunosuppression.

VACCINES

An ideal vaccine should be relatively inexpensive to produce, easy to administer, safe, and effective. Often these features are mutually exclusive. The principles for making vaccines are quite old. Microorganisms, either killed or attenuated, are administered by appropriate routes, at appropriate intervals, and in appropriate vehicles to trigger a protective host response. Historically, vaccine development has focused on these variables to achieve success. Basically, vaccines were a matter of luck. The vaccinated host was protected, but the mechanism of this protection was not fully appreciated. Antigenic determinants of the microorganism that were the most immunogenic and the nature of the protective host response (cell-mediated versus humoral immunity) were often unknown.

Since 1976, only three licensed vaccines have been marketed commercially for fish. The first was against enteric-redmouth (ERM) followed by vaccines against vibriosis and furunculosis. All three vaccines are formalin-inactivated whole cell preparations. The ERM and vibriosis vaccines are highly efficacious, whereas the vaccines for furunculosis offer merely low levels of protection that are thought to be mediated by stimulation of nonspecific defense mechanisms (Ellis, 1988). Considerable effort is being made to develop effective, safe, economical vaccines for numerous bacterial and viral diseases. Success depends on identifying the antigenic determinants that elicit a protective host response, establishing the nature of that protective response (humoral versus cell-mediated versus nonspecific), amplifying the protective response by the use of adjuvants, and packaging all this so that it is economical and easy to use. This is no small task and explains why so few vaccines are commercially available.

Types of Vaccines

Organisms in killed vaccines are inactivated by numerous chemical and physical treatments. Commercial vaccines used to control bacterial fish diseases rely on formalin (Austin, 1984). Formalin acts on amino and amide groups in proteins and on non–hydrogen-bonded amino groups in the purine and pyrimidine bases of nucleic acids to form cross-links, which preserve the structural integrity of immunogenic, antigenic determinants. Formalin (0.3% v/v) has been used to kill *Aeromonas hydrophila, Edwardsiella ictaluri, Pasteurella piscicida, Pseudomonas anguilliseptica, Vibrio anguillarum,* and *V. ordalii* to produce immunogenic vaccines (Austin, 1984). Other chemicals used to kill organisms with lipids in their outer membranes (most bacteria and enveloped viruses) are chloroform and phenol. Physical disruption by sonication and lysis with sodium hydroxide at pH 9.5 or the detergent sodium dodecyl sulfate has been used to inactivate bacteria for experimental vaccines of fish. Killing organisms by heat denatures protein and oxidizes lipids, often destroying crucial antigenic sites important for the development of protective immunity. Despite this, fish vaccinated with heat-killed *V. anguillarum* and *V. ordalli* are protected to the same levels as those vaccinated with formalin-treated preparations of the same bacteria (Austin, 1984).

Attenuated vaccines are not used commercially, although viable *Aeromonas salmonicida* microorganisms have been detected in formalin-treated vaccines (Rogers and Austin, 1985). Exposing organisms to sublethal concentrations of chemicals or gentle heat treatment are in fact old methods for reducing the virulence of bacteria. More commonly used methods of bacterial attenuation include culturing in unfavorable media or at an unfavorable temperature. Viruses are attenuated by prolonged passage in tissue culture or adaptation in an aberrant host. Attenuated vaccines require fewer inoculating doses than killed vaccines and often elicit higher antibody titers. This makes them quite attractive for treating the large numbers of individuals in fish farms, yet concern

over reversion of attenuated organisms to a virulent state has hindered commercial development of modified live vaccines.

Alternative strategies include subunit vaccines and synthetic peptides. Both techniques require that antigens that elicit a protective response from a host be known. In the former, deoxyribonucleic acid (DNA) coding for the antigen of interest is placed in a bacterium, yeast, or other cell and allowed to code for that protein. In the latter, if the sequence of protective epitopes within a protein is known, then these peptides can be synthesized. In both instances, the expressed proteins and synthesized peptides can be incorporated into vaccines.

Knowledge of protective antigenic determinants for fish pathogens is just emerging. The protective antigens in *Vibrio* and enteric-redmouth vaccines are the lipopolysaccharides, though the specific epitopes are unknown (Evelyn, 1984; Amend et al., 1983). For *Aeromonas salmonicida,* the etiologic agent of furunculosis, the protective antigen appears to be the extracellular protease (Ellis et al., 1988). Using monoclonal antibodies to each of six antigens expressed by the Egtved virus, the rhabdovirus responsible for viral hemorrhagic septicemia, the protective antigen as demonstrated by passive immunization experiments is the membrane glycoprotein protein G (Lorenzen et al., 1987).

Methods of Vaccine Administration

Most vaccines used in vertebrates are injected. Intraperitoneal injections of fish vaccines have produced high antibody titers to numerous bacterial and viral pathogens (Austin, 1984; Wolf, 1988) but are not feasible with large numbers of fish. Alternative routes of administration include orally via food or by anal intubation. In general, oral vaccines against bacteria have proved disappointing presumably because protective antigenic determinants are destroyed in the gastrointestinal tract (Austin and Austin, 1987).

Anal intubation has been suggested as a method that would avoid the potential degradation of an orally administered vaccine in the stomach and intestine, but as it requires individual manipulation of fish, it offers no significant advantage over intraperitoneal injections.

For vaccinating large numbers of fish, immersion and bath techniques are favored. With a bath, the vaccine is diluted and fish spend several hours in the preparation. Immersion is quicker, requiring a 30- to 120-second exposure to a vaccine solution. Protection is greater with immersion vaccines against *Edwardsiella ictaluri, Vibrio anguillarum,* and *V. ordalii* than with injectable vaccines (Austin, 1984). In an effort to get more vaccine into a fish during immersion, the fish is first exposed to a strong salt solution, 3 to 8% (w/v) sodium chloride, for 30 to 60 seconds. This technique, called hyperosmotic infiltration, is not universally used as it can be very stressful to the fish (Austin and Austin, 1987).

An alternative to immersion and bathing is spraying or showering the vaccine onto the fish (Gould et al., 1978). This method has provided superior protection over injection with *Vibrio* vaccines (Austin, 1984).

Enhancement of Vaccines

Adjuvants are substances that when combined with antigen enhance specific immune responses in addition to nonspecific defense responses. The mechanism of enhancement is not always understood. In general, adjuvants slow the rate of antigen elimination, thereby prolonging antigen contact with macrophages and lymphocytes and augmenting a specific immune response. Freund's complete adjuvant is a potent adjuvant composed of mineral oil, emulsifier, and killed mycobacteria. The mineral oil creates a local inflammatory response while antigen is slowly leached from the emulsifier. The mycobacteria stimulate polyclonal activation of lymphocytes and activate macrophages. This represents the nonspecific augmentation of the immune response. Freund's complete adjuvant has been used in experimental fish vaccines to augment antibody responses successfully. However, its widespread use in fish vaccines is impractical and undesirable because it is designed for use with injectable preparations and it causes severe tissue damage at the site of inoculation.

Alternative adjuvants are being considered for use with immersion and oral vaccines. Aluminum potassium sulfate (alum) is an insoluble salt that can be used as a colloidal suspension with antigenic material absorbed to it. It has been used to improve the efficacy of oral *Vibrio* vaccine (Agius et al., 1983) and enhances antigen uptake in *Vibrio* immersion vaccines (Tatner and Horne, 1983). Dimethyl sulfoxide increases antibody production in rainbow trout when combined with enteric-redmouth immersion vaccine (Anderson et al., 1984). When added to immersion vaccines, BCG, the live, attenuated vaccine strain of *Mycobacterium bovis*, and Quilaja saponin fail to enhance antibody responses to enteric-redmouth disease (Grayson et al., 1987). Bacterial clearing, however, is improved and represents enhancement of a nonspecific defense mechanism.

ASSESSMENT OF IMMUNE FUNCTION

Assays used to evaluate immune functions in mammals have been readily adapted to fish. Care must be exercised that assays which utilize cells are conducted at constant, optimal temperatures. Consideration must also be given to the ambient temperatures experimental fish encounter. Suboptimal environmental temperatures may result in less than optimal test responses, even if the in vitro experiment is conducted at optimal temperatures.

Humoral immunity equates with antibody production. Plaque assays are used to quantitate the number of B lymphocytes producing antibody, usually to sheep red blood cells. Antibody-producing cells collected from the pronephros or spleen of a fish previously inoculated with sheep erythrocytes are incubated in media containing sheep red blood cells and a source of complement. If the B lymphocytes have been activated to produce antibody, then the erythrocytes migrate to these cells, where they become coated with immunoglobulin and are then lysed by complement. As a result, a clear zone or plaque forms around the antibody-producing cells. This assay is a good experimental technique for determining if the cellular components responsible for humoral immunity are intact. Plaque assays, however, have little use clinically.

Numerous assays exist for the measurement of antibody in serum. Primary binding tests that include enzyme-linked immunosorbent assays, immunofluorescence assays, and radioimmunoassays are the most sensitive methods. These tests directly measure the binding of antibodies to antigen. The biggest problem in developing these assays to detect antibodies in fish against specific pathogens is purification and concentration of the immunogenic component of a disease organism.

Secondary binding tests, although less sensitive than primary binding tests, are easier to perform. These tests measure the consequences of antibody interacting with antigen in vitro. Examples of such interactions include precipitation of soluble antigens, agglutination of particulate antigens, and complement activation. The Ouchterlony technique, or double diffusion test, depends on the precipitation of antigen with antibody in agar gel. A positive reaction with fish serum, however, may not be antigen specific because of the high incidence of so-called natural antibodies. Even C-reactive protein can form precipitates with a variety of microorganisms (Baldo and Fletcher, 1973), although this can be circumvented by the addition of chelating agents to bind calcium ions. Furthermore, not all species of fish produce good precipitating antibodies (Ellis, 1982).

Tertiary binding tests measure the ability of antibody to protect either an individual or cell culture from the harmful effects of a pathogen. Neutralization assays are in vitro tertiary binding tests, and passive transfer of immune serum followed by a challenge is an example of an in vivo test. Passive transfer of immune serum and challenge is an excellent way to determine if antibodies specific to a particular organism are truly protective. The presence of antibodies is not necessarily indicative of protection following vaccination or elimination of an organism following natural infection. Similarly, the failure to produce antibodies does not necessarily imply generalized immunosuppression, since many pathogens can successfully evade the immune system.

Among the more commonly performed tests used to evaluate cellular immunity are lymphoproliferative assays. Cells dividing in response to antigen have increased DNA synthesis, which can be detected by the incorporation of radiolabeled thymidine. Antigens used in lymphoproliferative assays include intraspecies lymphocytes (mixed lymphocyte culture), purified preparations of infectious organisms, and mitogens. Mixed lymphocyte tests evaluate T-lymphocyte immunocompetence as do most specific antigen preparations. Mitogens include plant lectins and other substances that nonspecifically stimulate lymphocytes to proliferate. Different mitogens stimulate different populations of lymphocytes in humans and mice. The assumption is generally made that they function similarly in fish. The lectins, phytohemagglutinin and concanavalin A, stimulate T lymphocytes to proliferate. In humans, phytohemagglutinin appears to preferentially stimulate helper T cells, and concanavalin A seems to primarily stimulate proliferation of cytotoxic/suppressor T cells. No evidence exists to support this differential stimulation of T lymphocytes in fish. Pokeweed mitogen, *Staphylococcus* protein A, and bacterial lipopolysaccharides are B-cell mitogens.

During the past decade, chemiluminescence has been used extensively to evaluate the phagocytic abilities of piscine granulocytes and macrophages. This test requires all steps prior to actual killing to be intact. Phagocytic cells emit small amounts of electromagnetic radiation following ingestion of microorganisms that can be detected as light by sensitive photomultiplier tubes such as those in liquid scintillation counters.

Literature Cited

Agius, C. (1985) The melano-macrophage centres of fish. In: Fish Immunology (Manning, M.J., and Tatner, M.F., eds.). Academic Press, London, pp. 85–105.

Agius, C., Horne, M.T., and Ward, P.D. (1983) Immunization of rainbow trout, *Salmo gairdneri* Richardson, against vibriosis: Comparison of an extract antigen with whole cell bacterins by oral and intraperitoneal routes. J. Fish Dis. 6:129–134.

Ambrosius, H., Fiebig, H., and Scherbaum, I. (1982) Phylogenetic aspects of fish immunoglobulins and lymphocyte receptors. Dev. Comp. Immunol. Suppl. 2:3–13.

Amend, D.F., Johnson, K.A., Croy, T.R., and McCarthy, D.H. (1983) Some factors affecting the potency of *Yersinia ruckeri* bacterins. J. Fish Dis. 6:337–344.

Anderson, D.P., van Muiswinkel, W.B., and Roberson, B.S. (1984) Effects of chemically induced immune modulation on infectious diseases of fish. In: Chemical Regulation of Immunity in Veterinary Medicine (Kende, M., Gainer, J., and Chirigos, M., eds.). Alan L. Liss, New York, pp. 182–211.

Austin, B. (1984) The future of bacterial fish vaccines. Vaccine 2:249–254.

Austin, B., and Austin, D.A. (1987) Bacterial Fish Pathogens: Disease in Farmed and Wild Fish. Ellis Horwood, Chichester, England.

Avtalion, R.R. (1969) Temperature effect on antibody production and immunological memory in carp (Cyprinus carpio) immunized against bovine serum albumin (BSA). Immunology 17:927–931.

Baldo, B.A., and Fletcher, T.C. (1973) C-reactive protein-like precipitins in plaice. Nature 246:145–147.

Beisel, W.R. (1982) Single nutrients and immunity. Am. J. Clin. Nutr. 35S:417–468.

Bisset, K.A. (1946) The effect of temperature on non-specific infections of fish. J. Pathol. Bacteriol. 58:251–258.

Caspi, R.R., and Avtalion, R.R. (1984) Evidence for the existence of an IL-2 like lymphocyte growth promoting factor in a bony fish, *Cyprinus carpio*. Dev. Comp. Immunol. 8:51–60.

Chilmonczyk, S. (1985) Evolution of the thymus in rainbow trout. In: Fish Immunology (Manning, M.J., and Tatner, M.F., eds.). Academic Press, London, pp. 285–292.

Chilmonczyk, S., and Monge, D. (1980) Rainbow trout gill pillar cells: Demonstration of inert particle phagocytosis and involvement in viral infection. J. Reticuloendothel. Soc. 28:327–332.

Cipriano, R.C. (1982) Resistance of salmonids to *Aeromonas salmonicida*: Relation between agglutinins and neutralizing activities. Transactions of the Am. Fish. Soc. 112:95–99.

Diconza, J.J. (1970) Some characteristics of natural haemagglutinins found in serum and mucus of catfish, *Tachysurus australis*. Aust. J. Exp. Biol. Med. Sci. 48:515–523.

Durve, V.S., and Lovell, R.T. (1982) Vitamin C and disease resistance in channel catfish (Ictalurus punctatus). Can. J. Fish. Aquat. Sci. 39:948–951.

Edelstein, L.M. (1971) Melanin: A unique polymer. In: Pathobiology Annual (Ioachim, H.L., ed.). Appleton-Century-Crofts, New York, p. 309.

Ellis, A.E. (1980) Antigen trapping in the spleen and kidney of the plaice (Pleuronectes platessa L.). J. Fish Dis. 3:413–426.

Ellis, A.E. (1981) Non-specific defense mechanisms in fish and their role in disease processes. Dev. Biol. Stand. 49:337–352.

Ellis, A.E. (1982) Differences between the immune mechanisms of fish and higher vertebrates. In: Microbial Diseases of Fish (Roberts, R.J., ed.). Academic Press, London, pp. 1–29.

Ellis, A.E. (1985) Eosinophilic granular cells (EGC) and histamine responses to *Aeromonas salmonicida* toxins in rainbow trout. Dev. Comp. Immunol. 9:251–260.

Ellis, A.E. (1988) Current aspects of fish vaccination. Dis. Aquat. Org. 4:159–164.

Ellis, A.E., Burrows, A.S., Hastings, T.S., and Stapleton, K.J. (1988) Identification of *Aeromonas salmonicida* extracellular protease as a protective antigen against furunculosis by passive immunization. Aquaculture 70:207–218.

Elsasser, M.S., Roberson, B.S., and Hetrick, F.M. (1986) Effects of metals on the chemiluminescent response of rainbow trout (Salmo gairdineri) phagocytes. In: Fish Immunology (Stolen, J.S., Anderson, D.P., and van Muiswinkel, W.B., eds.). Elsevier, Amsterdam, pp. 243–250.

Evelyn, T.P.T. (1984) Immunization against pathogenic vibriosis. In: Symposium on Fish Vaccination (de Kinkelin, P., ed.). O.I.E., Paris, pp. 121–150.

Evenberg, D., de Graaf, P., Fleuren, W., and van Muiswinkel, W.B. (1986) Blood changes in carp (Cyprinus carpio) induced by ulcerative *Aeromonas salmonicida* infections. In: Fish Immunology (Stolen, J.S., Anderson, D.P., and van Muiswinkel, W.B., eds.). Elsevier, Amsterdam, p. 321.

Ezeasor, D.N., and Stokoe, W.M. (1980) A cytochemical, light and electron microscope study of eosinophilic granule cells in the gut of rainbow trout *Salmo gairdneri* Richardson. J. Fish Biol. 17:619–634.

Fange, R. (1986) Lymphoid organs in sturgeons. In: Fish Immunology (Stolen, J.S., Anderson, D.P., and van Muiswinkel, W.B., eds.). Elsevier, Amsterdam, pp. 153–161.

Fange, R., and Pulsford, A. (1985) The thymus of the angler fish [Lophius piscatorius (Pisces:Teleostei)]: A light and electron microscopic study. In: Fish Immunology (Manning, M.J., and Tatner, M.F., eds.). Academic Press, London, pp. 293–311.

Ferguson, H.W. (1975) Phagocytosis by the endocardial lining cells of the atrium of plaice (Pleuronectes platessa). J. Comp. Pathol. 85:561–569.

Ferguson, H.W. (1976a) The ultrastructure of plaice (Pleuronectes platessa) leucocytes. J. Fish Biol. 8:139–142.

Ferguson, H.W. (1976b) The relationship between ellipsoids and melano-macrophage centres in the spleen of turbot (Scophthalmus maximus). J. Comp. Pathol. 86:377–380.

Fletcher, T. C. (1986) Modulation of nonspecific host defenses in fish. In: Fish Immunology (Stolen, J. S., Anderson, D. P., and van Muiswinkel, W.B., eds.). Elsevier, Amsterdam, pp. 59–67.

Fletcher, T.C., and Baldo, B.A. (1976) C-reactive protein-like precipitins in lumpsucker (Cyclopterus lumpus L.) gametes. Experientia 32:1199–1200.

Fletcher, T.C., and White, A. (1973) Lysozyme activity in the plaice (Pleuronectes platessa). Experientia 29:1283–1285.

Fletcher, T.C., White, A., and Baldo, B.A. (1977) C-reactive protein-like precipitin and lysozyme in the lumpsucker Cyclopterus lumpus L. during the breeding season. Comp. Biochem. Physiol. 57:353–357.

Gjedrum, T., and Aulstad, D. (1974) Selection experiments with salmon. I. Differences in resistance to vibrio disease of salmon parr (Salmo salar). Aquaculture 3:51–59.

Gould, R.W., O'Leary, P.J., Garrison, R.L., Rohovec, J.S., and Fryer, J.L. (1978) Spray vaccination: A method for the immunization of fish. J. Fish Pathol. 13:63–68.

Goven, B.A., Dawe, D.L., and Gratzek, J.B. (1980) In vivo and in vitro anaphylactic type reactions in fish. Dev. Comp. Immunol. 4:55–64.

Graves, S.S., Evans, D.L., Cobb, D., and Dawe, D.L. (1984). Nonspecific cytotoxic cells in fish (Ictalurus punctatus) I. Optimum requirements for target cell lysis. Dev. Comp. Immunol. 8:293–302.

Grayson, T.H., Williams, R.J., Wrathmell, A.B., Munn, C.B., and Harris, J.E. (1987) Effects of immunopotentiating agents in the immune response of rainbow trout, *Salmo gairdneri* Richardson, to ERM vaccine. J. Fish Biol. 31(Suppl. A):195–202.

Grondel, J.L., and Boeston, J.A.M. (1982) The influence of antibiotics on the immune system 1. Inhibition of the mitogenic leukocyte response in vitro by oxytetracycline. Dev. Comp. Immunol. 2S:211–216.

Grondel, J.L., Nouws, J.F.M., and van Muiswinkel, W.B. (1987) The influence of antibiotics on the immune system: Immuno-pharmokinetic investigations on the primary anti-SRBC response in carp, *Cyprinus carpio* L., after oxytetracycline injection. J. Fish Dis. 10:35–43.

Haynes, L., Fuller, L., and McKinney, E.C. (1988) Fc receptor for shark IgM. Dev. Comp. Immunol. 12:561–571.

Heath, A.G. (1987) Water Pollution and Fish Physiology. CRC Press, Boca Raton, Florida.

Hinuma, S., Abo, T., Kumagi, K., and Hata, M. (1980) The potent activity of freshwater fish kidney cells in cell-killing I. Characterization and species-distribution of cytotoxicity. Dev. Comp. Immunol. 4:653–666.

Horton, J., and Lackie, A. (1989) Evolution of immunity. In: Immunology (Roitt, I.M., Brostoff, J., and Male, D.K., eds.). C.V. Mosby, St. Louis, pp. 15.1–15.16.

Ingram, G.A. (1980) Substances involved in the natural resistance of fish to infection—A review. J. Fish Biol. 16:23–60.

Jurd, R.D. (1985) Specialization in the teleost and anuran immune response: A comparative critique. In: Fish Immunology (Manning, M.J., and Tatner, M.F., eds.). Academic Press, London, pp. 9–28.

Knott, R.M., and Munro, A.L.S. (1986) The persistence of infectious pancreatic necrosis virus in Atlantic salmon. In: Fish Immunology (Stolen, J.S., Anderson, D.P., and van Muiswinkel, W.B., eds.). Elsevier, Amsterdam, pp. 359–364.

Koppenheffer, T.L. (1987) Serum complement systems of ectothermic vertebrates. Dev. Comp. Immunol. 11:279–286.

Larsson, A., Haux, C., and Sjobeck, M. (1985) Fish physiology and metal pollution: results and experiences from laboratory and field studies. Ecotoxicol. Environ. Saf. 9:250–281.

Laudan, R., Stolen, J.S., and Cali, A. (1986) The immune response of marine teleost, *Pseudopleuronectes americanus* (winter flounder) to the protozoan parasite *Glugea stephani*. In: Fish Immunology (Stolen, J.S., Anderson, D.P., and van Muiswinkel, W.B., eds.). Elsevier, Amsterdam, pp. 403–412.

Lester, R.J.G., and Budd, J. (1979) Some changes in the blood cells of diseased coho salmon. Can. J. Zool. 57:1458–1464.

Li, Y., and Lovell, R.T. (1985) Elevated levels of dietary ascorbic acid increase immune responses in channel catfish. J. Nutr. 115:123–131.

Litman, G.W., and Marchalonis, J.J. (1982) Evolution of antibodies. In: Immune Regulation—Evolutionary and Biological Significance (Ruben, L.N., and Gershwin, M.E., eds.). Marcel Dekker, New York, p. 29.

Lobb, C.J. (1987) Secretory immunity induced in catfish, *Ictalurus punctatus*, following bath immunization. Dev. Comp. Immunol. 11:727–738.

Lorenzen, N., Vestergard Jorgensen, P., and Oleson, N.J. (1987) Passive protection of rainbow trout *(Salmo gairdneri)* against Egtved virus with monoclonal antibodies. Abstracts of Fish Immunology Symposium, Plymouth Polytechnic, Plymouth, England.

MacArthur, J.I., Fletcher, T.C., Pirie, B.J.S., Davidson, R.J.L., and Thomson, A.W. (1984) Peritoneal inflammatory cells in plaice, *Pleuronectes platessa* L.: Effects of stress and endotoxin. J. Fish Biol. 25:69–81.

Mainwaring, G., and Rowley, A.F. (1985) Studies on granulocytic heterogeneity in elasmobranchs. In: Fish Immunology (Manning, M.J., and Tatner, M.F., eds.). Academic Press, London, pp. 57–69.

Miller, N.W., Bly, J.E., van Ginkel, F., Ellsaesser, C.F., and Clem, L.W. (1987) Phylogeny of lymphocyte heterogeneity: Identification and separation of functionally distinct subpopulations of channel catfish lymphocytes with monoclonal antibodies. Dev. Comp. Immunol. 11:739.

Moody, C.E., Serreze, D.V., and Reno, P.W. (1985) Non-specific cytotoxic activity of teleost leukocytes. Dev. Comp. Immunol. 9:51–64.

Murai, T., Kodama, H., Naiki, M., Mikami, T., and Izawa, H. (1990) Isolation and characterization of rainbow trout C-reactive protein. Dev. Comp. Immunol. 14:49–58.

Newman, M.W., and MacLean, S.A. (1974) Physiological response of the cunner, *Tautogolabrus adspersus*, to cadmium. VI. Histopathology. NOAA Tech. Rep. NMFS SSRF-681:27–33.

Ourth, D.D. (1980) Secretory IgM, lysozyme and lymphocytes in the skin mucus of the channel catfish, *Ictalurus punctatus*. Dev. Comp. Immunol. 4:65–74.

Pepys, M.B., Dash, A.C., Fletcher, T.C., Richardson, N., Munn, E.A., and Feinstein, A. (1978) Analogues in other mammals and in fish of human plasma proteins, C-reactive protein, and amyloid P component. Nature 273:168–170.

Plumb, J.A., Wise, M.L., and Rogers, W.A. (1986) Modulatory effects of temperature on antibody response and specific resistance to challenge of channel catfish, *Ictalurus punctatus*, immunized against *Edwardsiella ictaluri*. In: Fish Immunology (Stolen, J.S., Anderson, D.P., and van Muiswinkel, W.B., eds.). Elsevier, Amsterdam, pp. 297–304.

Reynolds, W.M. (1977) Fever and anti-pyresis in the bluegill sunfish, Lepomis macrochirus. Comp. Biochem. Physiol. 57:165–167.

Reynolds, W.M., Casterlin, M.E., and Convert, J.B. (1976) Behavioural fever in teleost fish. Nature 259:41–42.

Roberts, R.J., and Bullock, A.M. (1980) The skin surface ecosystem of teleost fishes. Proceedings of the Royal Society of Edinburgh 79B:87–91.

Robey, F.A., Tanaka, T., and Liu, T.-Y. (1983) Isolation and characterization of two major serum proteins from the dogfish, *Mustelas canis*, C-reactive protein and amyloid P component. J. Biol. Chem. 258:3889–3894.

Robohm, R.A. (1986) Paradoxical effects of cadmium exposure on antibacterial antibody responses in two fish species: inhibition in cunners *(Tautogolabrus adspersus)* and enhancement in striped bass *(Morone saxatilis)*. In: Fish Immunology (Stolen, J.S., Anderson, D.P., and van Muiswinkel, W.B., eds.). Elsevier, Amsterdam, pp. 251–262.

Robohm, R.A., and Nitkowski, M.F. (1974) Physiological response of the cunner, *Tautogolabarus adspersus* to cadmium. IV. Effects on the immune system. NOAA Tech. Rep. NMFS SSRF-681:15–20.

Rodgers, C.J., and Austin, B. (1985) Oral immunization against furunculosis: An evaluation of two field trials. In: Fish Immunology (Manning, M.J., and Tatner, M.F., eds.). Academic Press, London, pp. 185–194.

St. Louis-Cormier, E.A., Osterland, C.K., and Anderson, P.D. (1984) Evidence for a cutaneous secretory immune system in rainbow trout *(Salmo gairdneri)*. Dev. Comp. Immunol. 8:71–80.

Sakai, D.K., Okada, H., Koide, N., and Tamiya, Y. (1987) Blood type compatibility of lower vertebrates: Phylogenetic diversity in blood transfusion between fish species. Dev. Comp. Immunol. 11:105–115.

Sigel, M.M., Hamby, B.A., and Huggins, E.M. (1986) Phylogenetic studies on lymphokines. Fish lymphocytes respond to human IL-1 and epithelial cells produce an IL-1 like factor. In: Fish Immunology (Stolen, J.S., Anderson, D.P., and van Muiswinkel, W.B., eds.). Elsevier, Amsterdam, pp. 47–58.

Spitsbergen, J.M., Schat, K.A., Kleeman, J.M., and Peterson, R.E. (1986) Interactions of 2,3,7,8-tetrachlorodibenzo-p-dioxin (TCDD) with immune responses of rainbow trout. In: Fish Immunology (Stolen, J.S., Anderson, D.P., and van Muiswinkel, W.B., eds.). Elsevier, Amsterdam, pp. 263–280.

Stolen, J.S., Gahn, T., Kaspar, V., and Nagle, J.J. (1984) The effect of environmental temperature on the immune response of a marine teleost *(Paralichthys dentatus)*. Dev. Comp. Immunol. 8:89–98.

Stuart, A.E. (1970) The Reticulo-Endothelial System. Livingstone, Edinburgh.

Suzuki, Y., and Kaneko, T. (1986) Demonstration of the mucous hemagglutinin in the club cells of eel skin. Dev. Comp. Immunol. 10:509–518.

Suzumoto, B.K., Schreck, C.B., and McIntyre, J.D. (1977) Relative resistance of three transferrin genotypes of coho salmon *(Oncorhynchus kisutch)* and their hematological responses to bacterial kidney disease. J. Fish. Res. Bd. Can. 34:1–8.

Tatner, M.F., and Horne, H.T. (1983) Factors influencing the uptake of ^{14}C-labelled *Vibrio anguillarum* vaccine in direct immersion experiments with rainbow trout, *Salmo gairdneri* Richardson. J. Fish Biol. 22:585.

Tizard, I. (1987) Veterinary Immunology. W.B. Saunders, Philadelphia.

Tripp, R.A., Maule, A.G., Schreck, C.B., and Kaattari, S.L. (1987) Cortisol mediated suppression of salmonid lymphocyte responses in vitro. Dev. Comp. Immunol. 11:565–576.

Vallejo, A.N., and Ellis, A.E. (1989) Ultrastructural study of the response of eosinophil granule cells to *Aeromonas salmonicida* extracellular products and histamine liberators in rainbow trout *Salmo gairdneri* Richardson. Dev. Comp. Immunol. 13:133–148.

van Muiswinkel, W.B., Anderson, D.P., Lamers, C.H.J., Egberts, E., van Loon, J.J.A., and Ijssel, J.P. (1985) Fish immunology and fish health. In: Fish Immunology (Manning, M.J., and Tatner, M.F., eds.). Academic Press, London, pp. 1–8.

Weeks, B.A., and Warinner, J.E. (1986) Functional evaluation of macrophages in fish from a polluted estuary. In: Fish Immunology (Stolen, J.S., Anderson, D.P., and van Muiswinkel, W.B., eds.). Elsevier, Amsterdam, pp. 313–320.

White, A., Fletcher, T.C., Pepys, M.B., and Baldo, B.A. (1981) The effect of inflammatory agents on C-reactive protein and serum amyloid P-component levels in plaice (*Pleuronectes platessa* L.) serum. Comp. Biochem. Physiol. 69c:325–329.

Winkelhake, J.L., and Chang, R.J. (1982) Acute phase (C-reactive) protein-like macromolecules from rainbow trout *(Salmo gairdneri)*. Dev. Comp. Immunol. 6:481–489.

Winter, G.W., Schreck, C.B., and McIntyre, J.D. (1980) Resistance of different stocks and transferrin genotypes of coho salmon, *Onchorhynchus kisutch*, and steelhead trout, *Salmo gairdneri*, to bacterial kidney disease and vibriosis. Fish. Bull. 77:795–802.

Wolf, K. (1988) Fish Viruses and Fish Viral Diseases. Cornell University Press, Ithaca.

Woodhead, A.D. (1981) Penetration and distribution of carbon particles in a teleost fish, *Poecilia formosa* (Girard), the Amazon molly. J. Fish Biol. 19:237–242.

Wrathmell, A.B., and Parish, N.M. (1980) Cell surface receptors in the immune response in fish. In: Phylogeny of Immunological Memory (Manning, M.J., ed.). Elsevier/North Holland, Amsterdam, p. 143.

Chapter 12

POSTMORTEM EXAMINATION

RENATE REIMSCHUESSEL

The postmortem examination is an important tool for diagnosing diseases of fish (Reimschuessel, 1988). Unfortunately, most pathology services do not provide fish necropsies, so it is especially important that clinicians know the basics of this procedure. Before embarking on a necropsy, the clinician should obtain a detailed history and make a clinical assessment. The history should include a description of the holding facilities or capture site, the number of fish affected, the total number of mortalities, the number of mortalities per day, the color, behavior, and age of the affected fish, and any current or prophylactic treatments. This information may determine what type of samples to take (bacterial cultures, tissues for viral or parasite isolation, and tissues critical for histologic or toxicologic evaluation). Interpretation of any postmortem finding depends on an understanding of the entire case, not just the physical lesions and laboratory analyses. This chapter describes the procedure for postmortem examination of fish and provides a step-by-step outline (Table 12–1) of the systems to evaluate and sample for histology.

PREPARATION

If possible, first examine the affected fish in their normal surroundings, noting any behavioral signs (see Chap. 5). You will obtain the best results if you use a live fish exhibiting signs of disease for the necropsy. The fish may be narcotized prior to sacrifice (see Chap. 6) and blood samples can be collected at this point (see Chap. 5). To euthanatize the narcotized fish, sever the spinal cord caudal to the brain case, using the caudal margin of the operculum as a guide for the location of the incision.

When a dead fish is submitted for necropsy, it should be wrapped in moist paper to prevent drying, and refrigerated or placed on ice. It should not be kept floating in water or frozen. Freezing renders the tissues unsuitable for many diagnostic laboratory procedures. Fish that are found dead are often autolyzed, but a gross necropsy examination can occasionally yield information even in these specimens. Fish that have been floating at room temperature for 6 to 8 hours usually are unsuitable for histopathology. Specimens refrigerated soon after death, however, can be held for about 12 hours. In either case, the longer the delay before necropsy and fixation of the tissues, the more decomposition occurs.

Select sterile instruments appropriate for the size of the fish. Usually a scalpel, a pair of forceps, and two pairs of scissors (one pair of heavy dissecting scissors and one of fine tissue scissors) are all that is needed (see Fig. 12–1). Bone cutters may be needed when examining larger fish. For very small fish, a dissecting microscope and fine ophthalmic instruments are very useful. The instruments should be sterilized after use and preferably be dedicated for postmortem examinations only.

Have glass slides, culture materials, and fixatives at hand. For histology, fixatives such as Bouin's or 10% neutral buffered formalin are routinely used (Luna, 1968). Samples for viral studies can be rapidly frozen in liquid nitrogen or on dry ice. Methods of collecting various samples are discussed in some detail in Chapter 5. If you do have a diagnostic laboratory, you should find out how they prefer specimens to be prepared and submitted for virology, parasitology, microbiology, toxicology, and histology.

THE POSTMORTEM

Each postmortem examination should be done in a systematic and consistent sequence. The protocol in Table 12–1 is recommended for most fish. It ensures that all organs are examined and appropriate samples taken. For small ornamental fish, modifications are required, and a good dissecting scope is essential. Rapid techniques, such as preparing direct squash preparations of various organs, can also be extremely useful when examining small fishes or when a quick diagnosis is critical.

External Examination

General Condition

If you are unfamiliar with the anatomy of the fish you are preparing to necropsy, you should review Chapter 1. External variations in shape may be marked. The external anatomy of the eel with its serpentine shape is quite different from that of fishes like the angelfishes or the flounder. Examine all external surfaces, noting loss of scales, ulcers, areas of discoloration, masses, or other abnormalities. The location of all lesions is important and must be noted. Look at the body form and palpate to determine if

TABLE 12–1. Protocol Postmortem Examination

External Examination
1. General condition
2. Fins
3. Skin scraping
4. Weight and length
5. Eyes and nares
6. Oral cavity
7. Anus

Internal Examination
1. Disinfect
2. Remove the eye
3. Remove the operculum with the pseudobranch
4. Remove the second and third gill arches
5. Open the body cavities
6. Remove the heart
7. Remove the abdominal body block
8. Dissect out the liver
9. Dissect out the spleen
10. Remove the gonads
11. Remove the swim bladder
12. Remove cranial and caudal wedges of kidney, vertebrae, spinal cord, and muscle
13. Sample the skin, including the lateral line and nares
14. Remove the brain
15. Open and sample the stomach and intestines

From Reimschuessel, R., May, E.B., Bennett, R.O., and Lipsky, M.M. (1988) Necropsy examination of fish. Vet. Clin. North Am. 18(2):427–433.

there is any change suggesting muscle atrophy, ascites, or skeletal deformity. Radiographs can be useful in demonstrating and documenting skeletal deformities such as scoliosis, lordosis, brachycephaly, vertebral fusions, accessory processes, or hyperossification (Sindermann, 1978). Reversed laterality in flatfishes should also be noted.

Fins

Fins vary in shape and size with different species of fishes. Some have an adipose fin located between the dorsal and caudal fins. Others have fused fins, and others are missing some fins entirely. Examine all of the fins for fraying, erosion, necrosis, or small discolored spots that may be parasites. Check for bent or broken fin rays. Because fins are so thin, they can easily be examined microscopically.

Skin Scraping

Prepare a skin scraping with a clean scalpel, evaluating both normal skin and the margins of any lesions. Because time and subsequent procedures will reduce the quality of the preparations, this should be done during the examination of external surfaces. The scraping should be deep enough to remove a few scales in addition to the mucus layer. Examine the fresh scraping for bacteria, fungi, or parasites as you would a biopsy specimen. Because parasites often leave the host shortly after death, and bacteria proliferate, the time of death is important. Use sterile technique to take microbiologic cultures from ulcerative lesions (see Chap. 5). Note any excess mucus and save the scales for aging the fish.

Weight and Length

Record the weight. Ornamental tropical fishes can weigh less than 1 g and large species can weigh hundreds of kilograms. The length is taken either from the snout to the tail fork (fork length) or from the snout to the caudal fin margin (total length). The fork length is less susceptible to error caused by eroded fins.

Eyes and Nares

Examine the eyes for corneal opacity or exophthalmia. Also examine the anterior chamber for the presence of blood or exudates. Note the lenses; they should be transparent. The nares can be examined by pressing behind the external orifices. Culture any exudates expressed by this procedure.

Oral Cavity

Open the mouth and view the oral cavity. Note any raised or discolored areas or macroscopic parasites. Dentition varies with the species. Note any missing teeth or gingivitis.

Anus

Examine the anus for swelling, redness, or ulcerations. If fecal material protrudes, examine it now (see Chap. 10).

Internal Examination

Disinfecting

After the external examination, disinfect the surface of the fish with 70% alcohol. Place the fish in

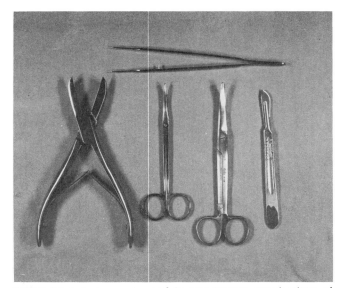

FIGURE 12–1. Instruments used in postmortem examinations of fish. (Courtesy of R. Reimschuessel.)

left lateral recumbancy on a nonslip surface such as wood, a sponge, or a disposable drape. An approach through the right side gives better access to the spleen (May, 1985). The internal anatomy varies with the shape, age, and species of the specimen. Although the organs retain their positions with respect to each other, they may be pushed craniad as in the flatfishes or surrounded by thick fibrous connective tissue as in the eel.

Removing the Eye

With a forceps, grasp the eye by the conjunctiva and gently free it from the surrounding skin with a pair of fine scissors (Fig. 12–2A). Pull gently on the globe and cut the underlying muscles. Examine the orbit for exudates, hemorrhage, or masses. At least one eye should be included with the tissues submitted for histology. The other eye can be opened to evaluate the lens closely. Parasites, such as the trem-atode *Diplostomum spathaceum*, can be located in the lens, sometimes causing "herniation" of the lens. If any lesions are noted in the eyes, submit both eyes. Bouin's fixative penetrates unopened eyes well. Eyes fixed in formalin can be incised through the sclerae to allow better penetration of fixative. Very large eyes can be injected with fixative.

Removing the Operculum with the Pseudobranch

The pseudobranch, a gill-like structure present in some fish, is located on the medial-cranial surface of the operculum (see Fig. 12–2B). It normally has a striated appearance and is bright red. It should be included with tissues submitted for histology.

Removing the Second and Third Gill Arches

The gills should be bright red in fresh specimens. Animals submitted for necropsy longer than 8 hours

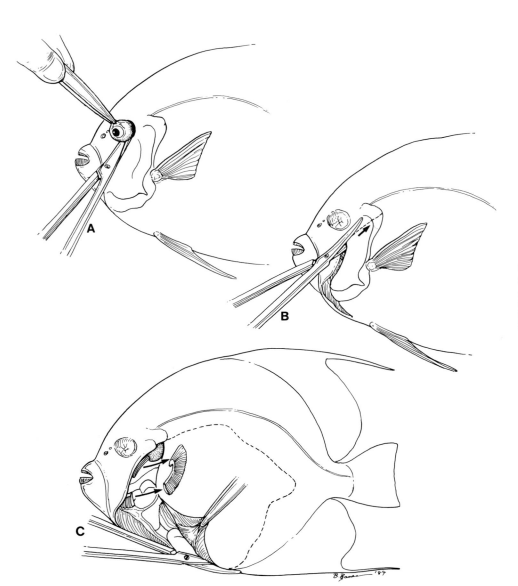

FIGURE 12–2. Standard fish post-mortem examination procedure. *A*. Removal of the eye with curved scissors. *B*. Removal of the operculum. *C*. Opening the body cavity.

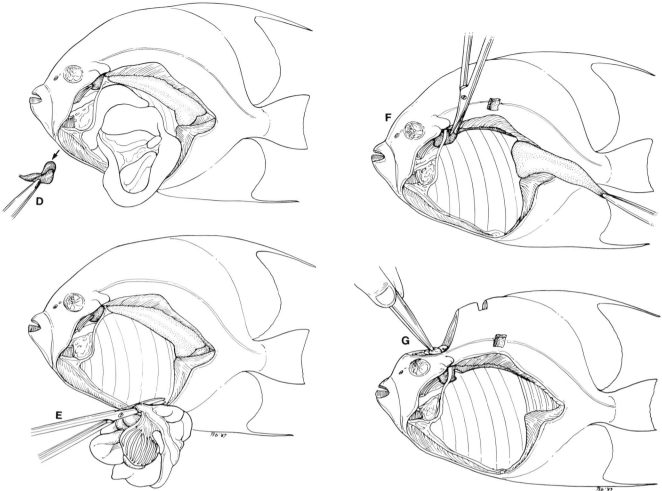

FIGURE 12–2 *Continued D.* Removal of the heart from the pericardial cavity. *E.* Removal of the abdominal body block. *F.* Sampling lateral line, cranial kidney, showing swim bladder reflected. Caudal kidney should also be sampled. *G.* Samples taken of dorsal musculature and skin; approach to the brain.

after death often have very pale or white gills and are unsuitable for histology owing to autolysis. Fresh animals with pale gills may be anemic or have serious fluid imbalances. Look for any abrasions, hemorrhages, excess mucus, or parasites. Remove a gill arch and place it between two slides. If the arches are large, remove the cartilage. Press the slides together, spreading the lamellae apart. Examine this wet mount of gill microscopically for parasites. Handle gills gently, grasping and cutting them at each end of the cartilaginous arch. A section of the second and third arches usually provides an adequate sample for histopathologic examination.

Opening the Body Cavities

Using sterile technique, make an incision starting at the operculum (Fig. 12–2C). Cut through the pelvic girdle, and extend the incision dorsally to the spine. Cut through the pectoral girdle. Continue the incision caudally along the spine, then follow the curve of the abdominal cavity in a ventrocaudal direction to the anus. Finally, extend the incision from the operculum along the ventral midline to the anus, and remove the body wall. Watch for adhesions from any organs to the body wall.

Once the contents of the pericardial cavity and the abdomen are exposed, culture any fluid in the body cavities and record its volume, color, and consistency. Note the size, color, and consistency of each organ in situ and how much adipose tissue is located between the organs. Before disturbing any organ, culture any tissue that appears abnormal. If the abdomen has been contaminated during entry, first sear the surface of the organ to be cultured. A heated scalpel works well. Then, remove the organs for closer examination and collection of histologic specimens, impression smears, or squash preparations. With very small fish, if the situation is not acute, it may be best to place the entire fish in fixative for histologic examination while the organs are still in situ. If the operculum and one body wall have been removed, the tissues should be adequately preserved. Be sure to open the skull dorsal to the operculum to allow fixative to penetrate the brain. In acute situations, squash smears may be more useful. It is best to remove organs from fish larger than 8 cm long.

Removing the Heart

The heart is found between and just caudal to the gills (Fig. 12–3). The elastic, whitish bulbus arteriosis is attached to the ventricle and usually is easy to see even in small fish. Grasp the cranial border of the bulbus arteriosus, pull caudally gently, and sever the connection to the ventral aorta (see Fig. 12–2D). Then pull the heart far enough out of the body to expose and sever the sinus venosus. Examine the surface of the heart for any raised or discolored lesions. A large heart can be cut open to examine the endocardial surface and valves. Place fine scissors into the bulbus, cutting through the ventricle longitudinally. Then cut through the sinus venosus and atrium in the same manner. Finally, extend this incision from the atrium into the ventricle. Look for any adhesions or raised nodules on the valves or walls.

Removing the Abdominal Body Block

Remove the abdominal body block by transecting the esophagus (see Fig. 12–2E). Then grasp the esophagus and lift it out of the body while gently pulling caudally. Transect the intestine at the anus. The stomach, intestines, liver, spleen, and possibly the swim bladder and gonads will be removed by this procedure.

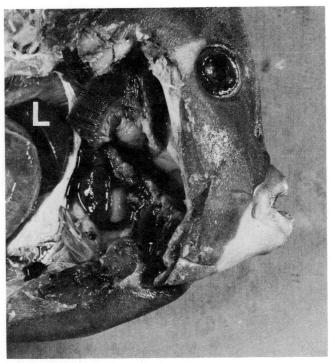

FIGURE 12–3. Dissection of a marine angelfish showing the heart in situ under the gills (L marks liver). (Courtesy of R. Reimschuessel.)

Dissecting Out the Liver

Free the liver from the surrounding tissue. Examine the edges, which should be sharp. Note the color. The liver is usually a reddish tan, but it can show marked variations in color, becoming quite yellow in fish raised on some hatchery diets. Make several slices into the parenchyma, and examine the color and texture of the cut surface. Note any discolored or raised foci. Parasites, such as cestode plerocercoids, appear as small linear white foci. If you see lesions, take a section to examine as a wet mount, and save some of the foci for histopathology.

Gallbladder

The gallbladder is usually located between the liver lobes and may be quite distended if the fish has not been eating. Note the color of the bile, which may vary from dark green to straw-colored yellow. Bile can be sampled using a Vacutainer or syringe and frozen for toxicologic evaluation.

Dissecting Out the Spleen

The spleen is usually a flat, triangular, dark red organ located adjacent to the left dorsal aspect of the stomach. In some species, the spleen is embedded in fat and is difficult to see on gross examination. Unlike the mammal, the white pulp of a fish spleen is not prominent unless active. As with the liver, examine the edges and a cut surface. If the spleen is swollen and round, it should be cultured. If the spleen has been contaminated during the necropsy procedure, sear the surface before culturing.

Removing the Gonads

The gonads are usually located in the caudal abdomen and may not be grossly visible in sexually inactive animals. If the gonads are visible, note their size, color, and consistency. Make several incisions into the glands, and evaluate the cut surface. Note the stage of development (inactive, developing, mature). Mature ova are different colors in different species, but they are often yellowish. Immature but developing ova are often a greenish color. Mature testes are large and white. In fresh samples, sperm can be examined microscopically for viability and progressive motility.

Removing the Swim Bladder

The swim bladder, if present, is a white or clear hollow organ located dorsally along the spinal column. It is usually easily identified if it has not been ruptured. The number of chambers varies, as can the prominence of the red gas-forming organ. If the swim bladder is present, gently open it, watching for any exudates or hemorrhagic areas. Be ready to take cultures if this is the case. The swim bladder can fail to develop or to inflate in some hatchery-reared species (Bennett, 1987; Weppe and Bonami, 1981). This may be associated with skeletal deformities (Kitajima et al., 1981; Paperna, 1978). Overinflation also occurs (Yamashita, 1966). Include part of the swim bladder in samples for histology. If it is not inflated, include its remnant in the wedge described below.

Removing a Cranial and Caudal Wedge of Kidney, Vertebrae, Spinal Cord, and Muscle

Examine the kidneys next. The kidneys of fish are retroperitoneal, lying next to the spinal column, dorsal to the swim bladder. They are dark reddish brown and may be distinctly lobed or intimately embedded along the vertebrae (Hickman and Trump, 1969). The cranial kidney may be separate or fused with the caudal kidney. A urinary "bladder," formed by fusion of the mesonephric ducts, may be present near the anus. If samples are being taken for histology, be sure to include tissues from the cranial and caudal portions of the organ (see Fig. 12–2F). Sections of tissues containing kidney, spinal cord, and muscle can be obtained by cutting a wedge from the abdomen through the dorsal body of the fish. If septicemia is suspected, culture the kidney because bacteria tend to localize within this organ (Roberts, 1989).

Sampling the Skin, Including the Lateral Line and Nares

Take samples of skin for histologic analysis. The sections should include normal skin at the margins of lesions. Fix samples of the lateral line and the nares. Make several large cuts into the muscles after sampling the skin. Look for parasites and small dark foci that could be metacercaria embedded in the musculature. Note the color and texture of the muscles.

Removing the Brain

The brain should be examined by opening the skull just dorsal to the eyes. If it is difficult to find the brain, remove both eyes and follow the optic nerves caudad. Remove enough of the bone to fully expose the brain (see Fig. 12–2G). It is normally white and fairly firm. Note any hemorrhage or discoloration of the cerebrospinal fluid or the brain itself. Then transect at the spinal cord and gently tease the brain away from its neural connections. Brain rapidly undergoes autolysis and liquefaction; therefore, if any histologic work is to be done, it is important that the specimen be very fresh.

Opening and Sampling the Stomach and Intestines

Examine the stomach and intestinal tract. Variations in the length and shape of the intestines occur

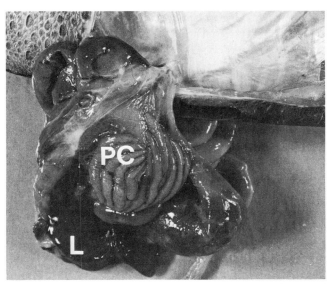

FIGURE 12–4. Dissection of a marine angelfish with abdominal body block reflected to show the pyloric ceca (PC) and liver (L).

in different species. Some fish have multiple pyloric ceca (Fig. 12–4), others may have a spiral intestine, and others may have a short, relatively straight gut. Note any raised or hemorrhagic areas on the serosal surface. Cut open the lumen and examine the contents of the entire tract. If undigested material is in the stomach, try to identify what the fish was eating. Note any irregularities in the mucosal surface. Scrapings can be evaluated for microscopic parasites (see Chap. 10). Include sections of the stomach, intestine, and colon for histology.

LITERATURE CITED

Bennett, R.O., Kraeuter, J.N., Woods III, L.C., Lipsky, M.M., and May, E.B. (1987) Histological evaluation of swim bladder noninflation in striped bass larvae Morone saxatilis. Dis. Aquat. Organ. 3:91–95.

Hickman, C.P., Jr., and Trump, B.F. (1969) The kidney. In: Fish Physiology. Vol. 1 (Hoar, W.S., and Randall, D.J., eds.). Academic Press, New York.

Kitajima, C., Tsukashima, Y., Fujita, S., Watanabe, T., and Yone, Y. (1981) Bull. Jpn. Soc. Sci. Fish. 47:1289–1294.

Luna, L.G. (1968) Manual of Histologic Staining Methods of the Armed Forces Institute of Pathology. 3rd ed. McGraw-Hill, New York.

May, E.B. (1985) Workshop, "The Aquatic Animal," held at the National Aquarium in Baltimore, January 16–17.

Paperna, I. (1978) Swimbladder and skeletal deformations in hatchery bred Sparus aurata. J. Fish Biol. 12:109–114.

Reimschuessel, R., May, E.B., Bennett, R.O., and Lipsky, M.M. (1988) Necropsy examination of fish. Vet. Clin. North Am. 18(2):427–433.

Roberts, R.J. (1989) Fish Pathology. 2nd ed. Bailliere Tindall, London.

Sindermann, C.J., Ziskowski, J.J., and Anderson, V.T., Jr. (1978) A guide for the recognition of some disease conditions and abnormalities in marine fish. National Marine Fisheries Service, U.S. Dept. of Commerce, Technical Series Report No. 14.

Weppe, M., and Bonami, J.R. (1981) Non-inflation of the swimbladder in hatchery-reared sea bass and sea bream: a significant problem in marine aquaculture. Bull. Eur. Assoc. Fish Pathol. 3:59–60.

Yamashita, K. (1966) Fundamental studies for the culture of Chrysophrys major—VI. On disease of larval and young fish (2). Abnormal expansion of the swimbladder. Bull. Jpn. Soc. Sci. Fish. 32:1006–1014.

Chapter 13

WATER ANALYSIS

CRAIG S. TUCKER

The aquatic environment is a complex system subject to constant physical and chemical changes. These changes result from natural processes, such as the variation in salinity of an estuary with tidal flow, or from man's activities, such as the effects of pollution. Fish have evolved by natural selection to live in an optimal range of environmental conditions. When fish are exposed to conditions outside this range, they are stressed.

Stress involves a series of physiological and behavioral reactions to help fish adapt. When stress is severe or prolonged, the capacity of fish to adjust can be exceeded. The ultimate result may include reduced growth, decreased reproductive performance, impaired immune function, or death (Pickering, 1981). The physiological responses of fish to environmental stressors are complex, and hematological or histological tests alone are rarely sufficient to assess the cause or impact. Therefore, evaluation of environmental conditions is central to any fish health investigation.

DESIGNING WATER-ASSESSMENT PROGRAMS

Most environmental analyses conducted in connection with fish health investigations are done (1) to assess the suitability of water for holding or rearing fish, (2) to monitor environmental conditions to ensure fish health, or (3) to investigate causes of fish health problems. In any of these situations, the design of a suitable water-assessment program depends on knowledge of complex chemical and biological relationships because hundreds of water-quality variables impact fish health, and the concentrations of these variables are not constant in space or time.

Obviously, it is impossible to sample constantly from all possible locations or analyze for all possible deleterious substances. We must choose those variables that will hopefully alert us to potentially stressful conditions or provide insight into the cause of fish health problems. We must then design a sampling program to assure valid data. No single measurement program applies to all situations; the variables to be measured and the sampling procedures depend on the problem at hand (Hunt and Wilson, 1986; Keith, 1988).

TYPES OF WATER-ASSESSMENT PROGRAMS

Assessing Water Supplies

The suitability of a water supply for holding or rearing fish is determined primarily by the environmental requirements of the fish. Specific environmental requirements for certain fishes are given in the appropriate chapters in Part II. The unique characteristics of the source of water and the type of system used to hold or grow fish must also be considered when assessing a water source for fish culture.

Sources of water for fish culture facilities include ground water and surface water, either of which may be of various salinities. Small-scale systems, such as home aquaria or small research facilities, sometimes use tap water from the public water supply. Each source has unique characteristics that affect its suitability as a supply for fish culture.

Ground water is generally considered the best source of water for fish culture. It is usually free of suspended matter, fish disease organisms, and is less easily polluted than surface water. The temperature and composition are relatively constant and the supply is usually dependable. However, some ground water has objectionable characteristics that make it unsuitable for use unless the water is treated; for example, much ground water is devoid of dissolved oxygen and must be aerated before use. The composition of ground water varies with the location and depth of the well used to obtain the water. Chemical and physical analyses can be obtained from local water-well drilling companies or from analysis of a small test well. The quality of most ground water is fairly constant with time and a single analysis will suffice initially. The water should be reanalyzed at least annually to document long-term changes in quality.

Surface water supplies include streams, rivers, ponds, lakes, reservoirs, estuaries, and oceans. Evaluate surface water carefully before use because it is subject to contamination or pollution, and the quality varies with time. Even the quality of near-shore ocean water varies significantly with time, especially near the mouths of large rivers. Another major drawback to using a surface water supply for fish culture is the potential for contamination of the system with wild fish, fish disease organisms, or waterborne predators. Surface water, particularly estuarine and marine water, also contains fouling organisms which can enter the water system and clog supply lines.

The quality of the water from public supplies depends on the original source of the water and how it is treated before distribution. Of particular concern is the chlorine that is added to most public water supplies for disinfection. Chlorine and chloramines are toxic to fish and must be removed before the water is used.

The suitability of a water supply must also be assessed relative to the type of facility used to hold or culture fish. Most of the systems used to rear fish can be placed into one of four categories: (1) flow-through systems, (2) closed water-recirculating systems, (3) ponds or lakes, and (4) net-cages placed in open water.

Flow-Through Water Systems

The water in flow-through systems passes through each culture chamber once and ultimately exits into a receiving body of water. Metabolic wastes are removed by dilution. This type of system is common in hatcheries and requires an abundant supply of water. Fish in flow-through systems are exposed to water that is nearly identical to the original source unless the water is treated before it enters the system. The quality of the water supply must therefore meet all the environmental requirements of the fish or be treated to render it suitable before use.

Closed Water-Recirculating Systems and Ponds or Lakes

Closed water-recirculating systems consist of a culture chamber and a series of water-treatment systems such as mechanical filters to remove particulate matter and biological filters to convert the toxic metabolic waste, ammonia, to a less toxic product, nitrate. In the closed system, water is added initially and subsequent additions are made only to replace losses such as evaporation. A home aquarium with a simple mechanical and biological filter is an example of this type of system.

A pond or lake is really just a variation of the closed water-recirculating system. The basic difference is the nature of the impoundment and the lack of formal filtration. Water quality changes rapidly when it is used in closed water-recirculating systems or ponds. The temperature increases or decreases with local air temperature, and diffusion alters the concentrations of gases. Water quality in closed systems is altered by the addition of feed or fertilizers to a greater extent than water in flow-through systems. Water in ponds is also affected by interactions with bottom muds. The most important initial quality considerations for water to be used in closed systems or ponds are salinity, total alkalinity and hardness, and the absence of toxic substances.

Net-Cages

Net-cages are placed in lakes, estuaries, or sheltered marine water. The wastes generated by the captive fish are diluted into the water around the cages, aided by wind-generated or tidal currents. Surface water can vary greatly in quality with time and some indication of the range of temperature, salinity, and dissolved oxygen must be obtained before selecting a site for net-cage fish culture. Water in the area must not be polluted by municipal, agricultural, or industrial wastes, and the site should not be subject to blooms of potentially toxic phytoplankton (Beveridge, 1987).

Monitoring Environmental Conditions

Routine water-quality monitoring is necessary in systems used to hold high densities of fish. If the initial quality of the water is adequate, only a few variables need to be monitored routinely once the system is in use. The critical variables are usually those affected by biological processes because they change rapidly. The recommendations in Table 13–1 are examples of monitoring programs appropriate for various fish culture systems. These are only guidelines. Design your monitoring programs considering the species being cultured and the specific characteristics of the culture environment. Another important consideration in the design of a monitoring program is the value of the fish in the system. An intensive, diligent monitoring program, perhaps involving continuous automatic monitoring of key variables, is appropriate for systems containing rare or important fish, or in commercial culture systems containing a large biomass of fish.

Fish Disease Investigations

Consider adverse environmental conditions in any fish disease investigation, but be aware that the unequivocal diagnosis of poor water quality as a cause of disease is difficult. The lesions that result from environmental stressors are often generalized or subtle. Lesions also vary with the species of fish, the duration of exposure, and interactions with other environmental variables. Diagnosis must be based on observations of behavior, histopathological changes, and analysis of the water. A historical record of environmental conditions is invaluable in such investigations. Unfortunately, often no information is available about environmental conditions before the disease outbreak. Collect water samples as soon as possible because conditions can change rapidly in an aquatic environment and analysis of samples collected after some delay may fail to identify the stressor, or worse, provide misleading information. If possible, collect water samples from a comparable but unaffected area. Comparison of environmental conditions in the two areas may provide insight into the cause of the disease.

TABLE 13–1. Examples of Sampling Programs for Monitoring Environmental Conditions in Various Fish Culture Systems

Type of System	Sampling Frequency			Comments
	Twice Daily	Daily	Weekly	
Flow-through				
Low density		DO, NH₃, pH		Check DO twice daily if load changes
High density	DO	NH₃, pH, CO₂		Check twice daily if load changes, check DO before and after feeding
Closed				
Newly loaded	DO, NH₃, NO₂, pH, CO₂		salinity NO₃	Check more often if concentrations are rapidly changing
Established		DO	NH₃, NO₂, pH CO₂, salinity NO₃	Check DO and NH₃ more frequently in high-density systems, or if load changes
Freshwater Ponds				
Low density		DO	NH₃, pH	
High density	DO		NH₃, NO₂, pH	Monitor DO at nighttime during warm weather
Saltwater Ponds				
Low density		DO	NH₃, pH salinity	
High density	DO		NH₃, pH salinity	Monitor DO at nighttime during warm weather
Freshwater Cages	DO		NH₃, NO₂, pH	
Saltwater Cages		DO	salinity	Check more often during unusual tide or weather conditions

Abbreviations: DO, dissolved oxygen; NH₃, un-ionized ammonia; NO₂, nitrite; NO₃, nitrate; CO₂, carbon dioxide.

Interpretation of water-quality data is difficult because there are few absolute values for toxic or stressful water-quality variables. The effect of a stressor depends on other physical and chemical factors as well as the fish species involved, the stage of development, nutritional status, degree of acclimation, and other factors. These interactions and modifying factors must be considered when interpreting environmental analyses as part of a diagnostic procedure (Rand and Petrocelli, 1985; Heath, 1987).

VARIABILITY OF WATER QUALITY

The objective of water sampling is to collect a representative portion of water small enough to transport conveniently without introducing significant changes in composition before analysis. An appropriate sampling method and accurate analysis allows inference of the quality of the whole body of water from the sample. However, be cautious no matter how accurate; sample analysis results represent only a few values from an array of values that vary with time and location. Be aware of potential variation in environmental conditions and design measurement programs, and interpret their results accordingly. The following factors should always be considered.

Variation with Time

Many water-quality variables show cyclic changes in magnitude over time (Fig. 13–1). Diurnal fluctuations are particularly evident for variables that are affected by photosynthesis and respiration. Concentrations of dissolved oxygen, carbon dioxide, and pH vary during a 24-hour period in natural waters (Fig. 13–2). Variations in environmental pH are caused by changes in carbon dioxide concentrations; the diurnal changes in pH then affect pH-dependent equilibria (such as the ammonia-ammonium system) and cause these to exhibit daily cyclic changes.

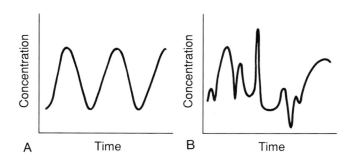

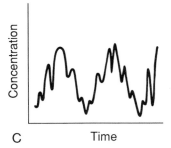

FIGURE 13–1. Variation in water quality with time. *A.* Periodic, cyclic variation. *B.* Aperiodic, irregular variation. *C.* Long-term periodic variation with short-term irregular variation.

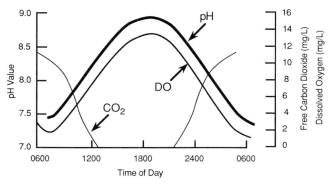

FIGURE 13–2. Diurnal changes in dissolved oxygen (DO), carbon dioxide (CO_2), and pH in a eutrophic fish culture pond. The amplitude of the variation would be much less in most surface waters.

Systematic changes in water quality also occur in aquaria or other fish-holding facilities where fish are fed on a regular schedule. Concentrations of dissolved oxygen will be highest and carbon dioxide lowest shortly before fish are fed (see Fig. 13–2). Feeding activity and the metabolic demands of digestion increase oxygen uptake and carbon dioxide production. Deamination of feed proteins and excretion of ammonia also cause environmental ammonia concentrations to vary with feeding schedule.

Not all cyclic variations are driven by biological processes. Diurnal wind cycles, increasing during the day and abating at dusk, cause mixing of water and may affect the concentration of certain constituents. For example, wind-induced turbulence increases diffusion of gases into or out of water and may affect concentrations of dissolved oxygen. Wind can also cause upwelling of the cool, oxygen-deficient bottom water of ponds, lakes, or estuaries. This water mixes with the surface water and decreases the surface water temperature and dissolved oxygen content and may bring reduced substances such as hydrogen sulfide to the surface. The effect will be most noticeable along the windward shore where upwelling occurs. Seasonal changes in temperature and wind velocity are responsible for the annual mixing-stratification cycle in deep lakes in the temperate zone, and this cycle is associated with predictable changes in water quality (Wetzel, 1975).

Tides affect water quality in estuaries on a predictable, periodic cycle by mixing water from different sources. Temperature, salinity, ionic composition, and pH may fluctuate regularly with tidal flow depending on the location within the estuary. Estuarine water quality is also affected by seasonal changes in the inflow of fresh water. Salinity, for example, is lowest during periods of high river discharge.

Cyclic variations in water quality also occur unrelated to natural environmental cycles. The concentration of a toxicant cycles daily in a river as the volume of effluent from a point source of pollution varies with the operating schedule of the plant or factory producing the waste.

Irregular or aperiodic variations occur when concentrations vary in a complex manner (see Fig. 13–1B). In natural water, the concentrations of few substances vary strictly irregularly. Substances unaffected by biological activity often vary with climatic factors, such as rainfall and temperature. Most changes in water quality, particularly over a long term, have a cyclic component with shorter-term irregular variations (see Fig. 13–1C).

Short-term cyclic variations may incorrectly appear to be irregular because of an inappropriate sampling program. For example, if only a few measurements of dissolved oxygen concentrations in a lake are made over several days, concentrations may appear to vary without pattern. In fact, the variation may be cyclic. More frequent sampling would make this evident. Failure to recognize extraneous sources of error may also make variation incorrectly appear to be irregular. This occurs when large random errors are introduced during sampling, sample handling, or analysis.

Sample Timing

The ideal water-sampling procedure would obtain a continuous record of the magnitude of the variable of interest. Except for a few variables such as temperature or dissolved oxygen this is impractical, and we must rely on discrete samples collected and analyzed at intervals. How rapidly and how much a variable changes dictate the timing and frequency of sampling. The nature of variation with time may also dictate the optimal times to sample to ensure fish health. It may also influence the interpretation of data collected as part of a diagnostic procedure.

A historical record is a valuable tool for designing a sampling program. If insufficient past data are available, you should sample as frequently as possible. Let the information gained in the early stages of the program be a guide to subsequent sampling frequencies and times. The sampling procedure should not be fixed. Be guided by trends and changes in sources of variability. If the concentration of a substance suddenly changes, sample more frequently to document the critical concentrations.

When cyclic variations are present, choose a particular method and location of sampling and collect samples at a constant time interval. The data of interest dictate the timing and frequency of sampling. If the magnitude and duration of the cycle is of interest, three samples on each side of the inflection points should be collected throughout three or four cycles. If the period of the cycle is known and only the highest or lowest value is of interest, samples can be collected at the appropriate time during the cycle. For example, in natural waters, dissolved oxygen concentrations are lowest at dawn and highest in the late afternoon. Measurements at these times will document critical concentrations. When a single sample is analyzed as part of a fish disease investigation, it is important to know when the sample was collected and how this relates to the periodicity of the variable.

When irregular variation dominates the period of interest, determine the average concentration of the variable by sampling at a constant time interval. The frequency of sampling is dictated by the level of uncertainty tolerable for the variable or the margin of safety of the variable. If the objective is to document critical concentrations, pick a sampling frequency to minimize the probability of missing critical episodes. Samples collected as part of a diagnostic procedure can be difficult or impossible to interpret when the concentration of the variable of interest varies irregularly. If a historical record is not available, there may be no way to even estimate the magnitude of the variable when the actual damage was done.

Statistical methods are available for determining optimal sampling frequencies and times. Spectral analysis (United States Environmental Protection Agency, 1982) is a powerful method for determining the periods and amplitudes of complex cyclic variations, and the sampling frequencies necessary to characterize the variation. Spectral analysis requires a computer and a comprehensive set of historical data. Techniques are also available for determining sampling frequencies necessary to document critical concentrations of substances that vary irregularly (Kateman and Pijpers, 1981). These techniques are complex and also require a comprehensive past record of the concentrations of the variable to be measured. Often, statistically based sampling plans require more samples than can feasibly be collected and the sampling program must be down-scaled based on simplifying assumptions. Clinicians or analysts involved in detailed water-assessment programs, particularly if part of a regulatory process, should seek the advice of a statistician before undertaking the sampling program. Fortunately, most sampling programs for routine fish health investigations can be established intuitively from a general knowledge of the variability of the substance of interest and the type of environment sampled.

Variation with Depth and Location

The composition of water varies with depth. This is usually caused by incomplete mixing of the strata of different composition or heterogeneous distribution of substances affected by biological activity. The first situation is common in thermally stratified lakes and reservoirs. It also occurs in estuaries where salt and fresh water stratify. Density differences prevent mixing, and stratification may persist for long periods.

Biological processes cause the composition of water to vary with depth, even in otherwise homogeneous bodies of water. Photosynthesis proceeds most rapidly in the upper layers of water where light intensity is greatest. This causes the concentrations of dissolved oxygen and carbon dioxide and pH to vary with depth. Biological uptake, excretion, and biodegradation also cause the concentration of bio-

logically active substances to vary with depth. Concentrations of ammonia, nitrite, hydrogen sulfide, carbon dioxide, and other products of decomposition and anaerobic metabolism tend to increase with depth. Less metabolically active substances like sodium, potassium, calcium, and magnesium and aggregate properties like salinity and total alkalinity tend to be uniform with depth unless water from different sources is in the process of mixing.

Samples taken from the same depth but at different locations within a body of water may also vary in composition. Variation with location is also caused by incomplete mixing or differences in biological activity, but variation with location is generally less predictable than that with depth. Site-to-site variation is common in situations where two bodies of water are in the process of mixing, such as in estuaries or in rivers receiving an effluent or flow from a tributary. Variation in composition of large bodies of water is often related to temporary wind-induced upwelling of the deeper strata of water.

Heterogeneity may be present even in apparently well-mixed systems like aquaria, tanks, or raceways. Variations in these systems can be caused by "dead-spots" or poor mixing. Water quality gradients in these systems may also be caused by localized areas of high biological activity. Water in raceways often shows a horizontal gradient in dissolved oxygen, carbon dioxide, and ammonia concentrations because fish tend to gather in the upper section of the raceway.

Heterogeneous bodies of water require multiple samples to characterize, and in some programs samples from specific locations are needed. Each situation is different, and it is not possible to generalize when selecting sampling locations. Local knowledge of the body of water to be sampled is indispensable. Otherwise, set up a preliminary sampling program to assess the degree of heterogeneity. Collect samples from relevant locations and depths and analyze for the substance of interest. Samples should be collected at the same time to minimize the effects of short-term temporal variations. Results of the analyses can be used to determine the number of samples necessary to characterize the water from constraints put on either the allowable variability or desired precision of estimates of the mean at a given confidence level (United States Environmental Protection Agency, 1982). The degree and pattern of heterogeneity often changes with time, so occasionally recheck the variability and change the sampling program if required.

The results of preliminary or ongoing tests for heterogeneity can also be used to choose specific sampling locations to monitor critical (high or low) concentrations of a substance within a system. Samples obtained near the inflow and discharge of raceways or tanks can be used to document the range of water quality in these systems. Dissolved oxygen concentrations and pH will be highest and carbon dioxide and total ammonia concentrations lowest in the upper end of the system, with the situation reversed in the lower end. If tanks or raceways are in a series, water quality also changes from tank-to-tank within the series. As a minimum, sample ponds and larger bodies of water near the windward and lee shores because of the effects of wind-induced turbulence. Obtain samples from 0.5 to 1 m deep in shallow waters less than 2 m deep. Analysis of samples obtained from near the surface and near the bottom of deeper bodies of water will usually document the extreme values for substances affected by biological activity. Do not assume that the pattern or degree of heterogeneity will be similar for apparently identical fish culture systems or natural waters. Subtle differences in water flow or microbial activity can cause large differences in water quality.

SAMPLING DEVICES

A water-sampling device obtains a portion of water from the whole for analysis. Sampling devices can be as simple as a bottle held by hand, or much more complex. Automated, microprocessor-controlled sampling systems exist for the collection of samples at predetermined locations and times within a body of water. No one sampling device is ideal for all purposes. The choice of sampling device depends on the objectives of the specific sampling program. The device should (1) be appropriate for the variable to be measured, (2) provide a sample of adequate volume, (3) be chemically inert and not contaminate the sample nor absorb constituents from the water, and (4) should be simple to use (United States Environmental Protection Agency, 1982; Hunt and Wilson, 1986). A variety of sampling devices are available from commercial sources, but equally suitable devices can sometimes be constructed from commonly available, inexpensive materials.

For routine, periodic analysis of dissolved ionic constituents in surface water, aquaria, or well-mixed bodies of water, samples can be dipped with an open container or taken in a wide-mouthed bottle held beneath the surface. Avoid contaminating the sample during the sampling procedure. When sampling streams or rivers, the container opening should be held upstream from the sampling position so that the sample is not contaminated with material stirred up during the sampling activity.

Subsurface samples can be collected using a simple weighted bottle sampler (Fig. 13–3). When the device reaches the desired depth, the stopper is removed by jerking the line. The bottle is hauled to the surface when bubbles stop rising to the surface. There is some contamination of the sample with water from shallower depths as the device is brought to the surface, but the degree of contamination is negligible for most purposes. Contamination with surface water can be minimized by using a device which removes and replaces the bottle cap while the sample bottle is submerged. Such a device, called a "grab sampler," is available from many scientific supply companies.

Sampling devices into which water simply bubbles or flows without overflow are not suitable for

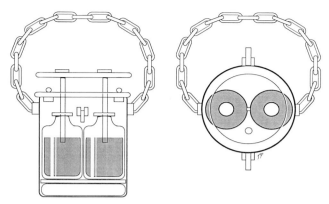

FIGURE 13–3. A weighted bottle sampler.

the collection of samples for measuring dissolved gases because the water entering the sampler contacts the air it replaces and gases are exchanged by diffusion. The "sewage sampler" or "BOD" sampler is a simple device for obtaining water for dissolved gas analysis. The sample bottle is usually a special 300-ml glass BOD bottle (Fig. 13–4) and is filled from the bottom and overflows several times while the inside of the sampler fills. The bottle is then removed and stoppered. The final sample volume does not contact air or require transfer to another container for transport or storage. Collect larger samples for dissolved gas analysis in Van Dorn or Kemmerer samplers (Figs. 13–5 and 13–6). These consist of an open cylinder which is continually flushed as it is lowered through the water. When the sampler reaches the desired depth, it is closed by a "messenger" dropped down the suspension line. The sampler is brought to the surface and drained into a sample bottle through a valved tube. Insert the tube in the bottom of the sample bottle and allow the bottle to overflow at least two bottle-volumes before stoppering. Kemmerer and Van Dorn samplers are available in capacities of 1 to 10 or more liters.

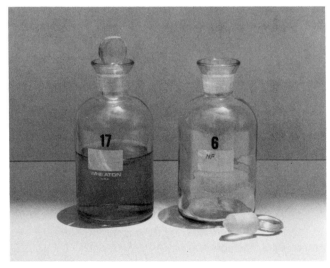

FIGURE 13–4. BOD (biochemical oxygen demand) bottles.

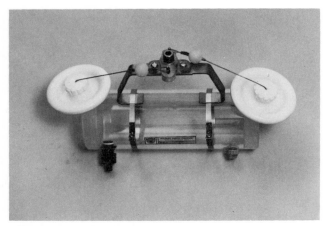

FIGURE 13–5. Van Dorn water sampler (Wildlife Supply Co., Saginaw, Michigan).

Automated sampling systems are attractive alternatives to traditional sampling programs in applications where frequent or semicontinuous monitoring is required. Automated sampling systems collect discrete samples at set time intervals and sometimes from different locations. The samples can be pooled

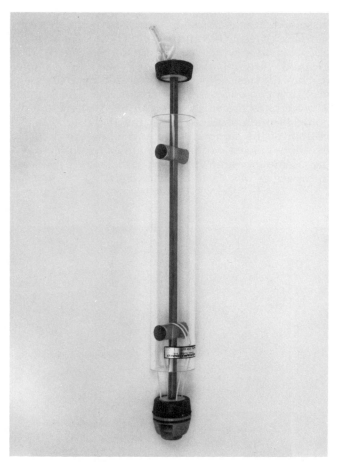

FIGURE 13–6. Kemmerer water sampler (Wildlife Supply Co., Saginaw, Michigan).

as time-composite or location-composite samples, or maintained as discrete, individual samples. The samples are periodically transferred to the laboratory for analysis by standard methods. Careful attention to adequate sample preservation and upkeep of the sampling system is necessary to obtain valid samples for analysis (United States Environmental Protection Agency, 1982). The use of automated sampling systems is usually limited to the collection of samples for measurement of water quality variables that are fairly stable in storage, such as salinity, alkalinity, and hardness.

SAMPLE STORAGE

A water-sample collection container can serve as a storage container. A surface water sample dipped from the water in an appropriate glass or plastic bottle does not usually need to be transferred before analysis. However, some sampling devices require the sample to be transferred to a bottle for transport and storage. The type of container to use depends on the variable to be measured.

Use borosilicate glass, polyethylene, or polypropylene bottles for routine sampling for major ionic constituents. Use borosilicate glass when trace organic compounds such as pesticides are to be measured. For trace metal analysis, use conventional polyethylene. Stoppers should be glass or plastic; avoid rubber or cork. Before each use, wash containers thoroughly and rinse with tap water, followed by distilled water. Wash the sample bottle several times with portions of the water to be sampled before actually taking a sample (United States Environmental Protection Agency, 1982).

Chemical changes begin to occur in samples immediately after collection. Whenever possible, conduct the analysis immediately after sample collection. If immediate analysis is not possible, techniques to retard the rate of change are available, but complete stabilization of a sample is impossible.

Methods of preserving samples for storage inhibit biological activity, slow the rate of chemical reactions, prevent precipitation, or prevent adsorption of substances onto container walls. Preservation methods include freezing, refrigeration, pH control, or chemical addition.

Freezing the sample immediately after collection and storing the frozen sample at -10 to $-20°C$ is an acceptable method of preserving samples for analysis of major ionic constituents. Freezing is never acceptable for samples for dissolved gases, pH, or trace metals (Hunt and Wilson, 1986). Frozen samples must be completely thawed and thoroughly mixed before withdrawing an aliquot for analysis.

Refrigeration or storage of samples on ice is the best way to temporarily preserve samples for most analyses. Refrigeration is also the best precaution when the stability of a particular variable is not known. The sample should be thoroughly mixed before analysis.

TABLE 13–2. Summary of Methods for Preserving Water Samples

Variable	Preservation	Recommended Maximum Storage Period
Alkalinity, total	Cool, 4°C	14 days
Carbon dioxide	Analyze immediately	—
Chloride	None required	1 month
Chlorine, residual	Analyze immediately	1 hr
Conductivity	Cool, 4°C	1 month
Hardness	Cool, 4°C	14 days
Nitrogen		
Ammonia	Add H_2SO_4 to pH < 2	7 days
	Cool, 4°C	24 hr
Nitrate	Add H_2SO_4 to pH < 2	7 days
	Cool, 4°C	24 hr
Nitrite	Cool, 4°C	24 hr
Oxygen		
Electrode	Analyze immediately	—
Winkler	Fixation (see method)	6 hr
pH	Analyze immediately	2 hr
Salinity	None required	6 months
Sulfide	Precipitation as ZnS	6 hr
Temperature	Analyze immediately	—
Total gas pressure	Analyze immediately	—

Acidification stabilizes samples by inhibiting biological activity and preventing precipitation or adsorption of metals. A concentrated mineral acid, usually nitric or sulfuric acid, is added in amounts to decrease the pH to less than 2. Acidification of samples cannot be used in trace metal analysis if speciation is of interest because lowering the pH may dissolve solid species or desorb metals from particulate matter. Before using acidification to preserve samples, the investigator should know the analytical method to be used because the addition of acid affects procedures if the reaction involved is pH dependent. For example, measurement of total ammonia requires adding a base to raise the sample pH to over 10. If acid is used to preserve the sample, it will neutralize some of the base and may interfere with the analysis.

The most common chemical, other than acids, used to preserve samples is mercuric chloride, $HgCl_2$, a strong biocide. Mercury interferes with some analyses, such as the gas-sensing electrode method for ammonia and the cadmium-reduction method for nitrate, and should not be used as a general preservative.

Recommendations for water-sample preservation are summarized in Table 13–2. Additional information regarding sampling and storage is also presented with analytical procedures.

SHIPPING SAMPLES

It is often necessary to ship water samples to laboratories for analysis. Contact the laboratory before collecting samples to avoid problems that may invalidate the results of the analysis. Tell the laboratory your objectives and specific analytical requirements (preferably in writing) so the laboratory director can determine whether the information can be provided with the resources available. Be quantitative and precise. Define the type of water to be sampled and the variables to be measured. State the accuracy and limits of detection you require. The frequency of sampling and the total number of samples to be collected as well as the frequency with which samples will be shipped to the laboratory should be discussed, including the estimated dates of shipment. Discuss the preferred method of sample preservation and data-handling requirements, such as turnaround time for receiving analytical results. Request a price schedule and cost estimate. Chemical analyses of water are expensive, and you might be forced to reevaluate the measurement program if the cost of the analyses is too high.

After consultation with the laboratory, follow the plan throughout the program to avoid introducing extraneous sources of bias. Identify each sample container by attaching a tag or label inscribed with waterproof ink. Provide the sample identification number, name of the sample collector, date, time, and location of sample collection, the preservation method, and any other sample pretreatment procedures, such as filtration. Pack sample containers carefully to avoid loss or contamination. Leave an air space of about 1% of the sample volume in the sample container to allow for thermal expansion of the sample during shipment. Samples preserved by freezing or refrigeration should be packed with dry ice or reusable refrigerant packs in well-insulated containers. Avoid packing in ice because of leakage as the ice melts. A description of the samples should be included with the shipping container, preferably attached outside. The method of shipment depends on the size of package, distance, and speed with which delivery must be made. If possible, register the package with return receipt requested. Samples shipped for regulatory compliance monitoring or samples collected as evidence during enforcement investigations must conform to precisely defined procedures regarding sample handling, shipment, and chain-of-custody documentation (United States Environmental Protection Agency, 1982).

ANALYTICAL METHODS

It is important that fish disease specialists be familiar with the methods used to obtain water-quality data, not only because they may be called upon to perform the analysis, but also because such an understanding is critical to interpretation of the results. Detailed descriptions of analytical methods for the measurement of environmental variables of interest in routine fish health investigations are described in the remainder of this chapter. These descriptions assume a working knowledge of basic laboratory techniques and rudimentary quantitative analysis. Reviews of laboratory techniques and analytical chemistry are provided by Boyd (1979), Snoeyink and Jenkins (1980), and Shugar et al. (1981).

The procedures described in this chapter are

adapted from "standard" or "recommended" methods commonly used in the analysis of waste water and natural fresh water (United States Environmental Protection Agency, 1979; American Public Health Association et al., 1989; Fresenius et al., 1988), water used in aquaculture (Boyd, 1979; Stirling, 1985) and aquaria (Spotte, 1979), and seawater (Strickland and Parsons, 1972; Grasshof et al., 1983; Parsons et al., 1984). When these methods are used properly, they can provide results that are sufficiently reliable and of adequate detection limits and accuracy to be of use in virtually any fish health investigation. These methods generally require an investment in laboratory equipment (mainly a spectrophotometer and analytical balance) and are most conveniently used where only a moderate number of discrete samples are to be analyzed at any one time. Where facilities are limited and the requirements for accuracy, precision, and limits of detection are less stringent, inexpensive portable test kits can be used to approximate most of these analyses. The use of test kits is discussed after the standard analytical procedures.

Salinity

Salinity is the salt content of water and is expressed as grams per kilogram (g/kg) or parts per thousand (ppt). The salinity of natural water ranges from essentially zero to over 40 ppt. The salinity of fresh water is usually less than 0.5 ppt; seawater generally varies from 33 to 37 ppt. The salinity of estuarine water is usually intermediate and depends on the relative amounts of fresh river water and seawater that are mixed together. Salinity thus varies with both time and location within an estuary. The salinity of some estuaries is also strongly influenced by the rate of evaporation relative to freshwater input, and during periods of drought estuary salinities may be higher than seawater.

Each fish species is best adapted to a particular range of salinities. The optimum salinity for the growth and reproduction of most freshwater fish species is in the range of 0.01 to 1 ppt, although many species can tolerate salinities much greater than this. Some euryhaline fishes such as red drum, *Sciaenops ocellatus*, and various salmonids may tolerate salinities from less than 1 to over 35 ppt. However, even fishes that can survive in waters over a wide range of salinities will not tolerate sudden, drastic changes in salinity.

Direct measurement of salinity is difficult, and salinity is usually calculated after determination of some related quantity such as chlorinity, conductivity, refractive index, or specific gravity. Chlorinity is determined by titrating a sample of water with silver nitrate, using potassium chromate as an indicator. This method is often used for precise salinity determinations, and salinity was until recently operationally defined in terms of chlorinity. However, salinity is now defined in terms of electrical conductance (Grasshof et al., 1983). Portable conductivity meters

with direct readout in parts per thousand salinity are available from commercial sources. These meters are convenient for rapid in situ estimates of salinity. Salinity can also be estimated from refractive index, and hand-held refractometers are useful for quick, semiquantitative estimates. Hand-held refractometers with direct readings in parts per thousand salinity are available from most scientific equipment supply companies. The hydrometric method of determining salinity is based on the determination of the specific gravity of a water sample with a hydrometer (American Public Health Association, 1989). Although this method is simple and fast, it has been supplanted by the use of refractometers in most applications.

pH Value

pH expresses the intensity of the acidic or basic character of a solution. It is effectively the negative logarithm of the hydrogen ion concentration. The pH scale is usually represented as ranging from 0 to 14. Conditions become more acidic as pH values decrease and more basic as pH values increase. At 25°C, pH 7.0 is the neutral point and the activities of the hydrogen ions and hydroxyl ions are equal (each at 10^{-7} mol/L).

Most ground water contains dissolved carbon dioxide, bicarbonate, and carbonate and has pH values between 5 and 8. In general, ground water in contact with silicate minerals is poorly buffered, has a higher carbon dioxide content, and, consequently, has a lower pH than water from carbonate rock deposits. High pH values (>8.5) are usually associated with ground water with a high sodium carbonate content. Very low pH values (<4) occur in acid mine water as a result of the microbial oxidation of sulfides to sulfuric acid.

The pH of surface water ranges from less than 4 to over 12 but usually falls in the range of 6 to 9. Surface water pH may vary diurnally because photosynthesis affects the concentration of dissolved carbon dioxide. Very high pH values (>9) are common in lakes in arid regions, where the water has a high sodium carbonate content. Low pH values (<4) are caused by the presence of mineral acids and are typical of streams and lakes in coal-mining areas or volcanic regions. Sulfuric acid causes low pH in water in contact with a certain type of soil developed from marine sediments. This soil, called cat's clay, contains large amounts of sulfide produced under anaerobic conditions by sulfate-reducing bacteria. When the soil is drained and exposed to oxygen, sulfide is oxidized to sulfuric acid and it is then called acid-sulfate soil. Water in fish ponds built on acid-sulfate soil may have a pH of less than 4 (Boyd, 1979). Low pH values are also found in water that is rich in organic acids produced by decaying vegetation. Poorly buffered water, such as that occurring in the mountainous regions of eastern North America, may have low pH values as a result of "acid precipitation." Usually precipitation is acidic because it contains carbon dioxide, but in areas where the atmosphere is polluted by industrial emissions of sulfur dioxide or nitrogen oxides, the pH of rain or snowfall is further decreased as these oxides form strong acids in the atmosphere. Acid precipitation can have a pH less than 5.

Seawater is buffered by the bicarbonate-borate system and indirectly by the formation of magnesium carbonate ion pairs. It has a relatively stable pH between 8.0 and 8.5. High rates of biological activity in nutrient-rich marine water may result in higher or lower pH values, but the pH is seldom lower than 7.5 or greater than 9.0.

The pH of water in fish culture systems changes with time. As water flows through a raceway or series of raceways, pH decreases as carbon dioxide is added by fish respiration. The pH of water in closed water-recirculating systems decreases with time as acid is produced during nitrification of ammonia to nitrate. In poorly buffered systems, pH may decrease to 6 or less. In pond culture, the amplitude of diurnal fluctuations in pH generally increases with time as the density of phytoplankton increases through the growing season.

Measurement of pH is fundamental when assessing a potential water supply for fish culture, or when evaluating fish health problems that are environment related because extremes of pH are detrimental to fish health. Most freshwater fishes are stressed, grow slowly, and are prone to infectious diseases when the pH falls outside a range of about pH 6 to 9. Saltwater fishes have a narrower range of pH tolerance, from about pH 7.5 to 8.5. The pH of water may also affect the likelihood or severity of other water-quality problems. For example, toxicity from zinc, copper, or aluminum is more common in acidic water because they are more soluble in acid conditions. pH is also measured as part of the analytical method for other variables such as un-ionized ammonia, hydrogen sulfide, and alkalinity.

Colorimetric Determination of pH

Colorimetric measurement of pH of water uses weak organic acids and bases whose color changes with pH. The more commonly used indicators show a distinct change in color over a pH range of about 1 pH unit. With the use of six to eight indicators, either alone or in various combinations with one another, it is possible to determine pH to an accuracy of about 0.2 units in colorless, turbidity-free samples of well-buffered water (Haines et al., 1983). Reliability under other conditions is poor, and even under optimum conditions, best results are achieved if the sample pH is near the midpoint of the pH color change range for the indicator. Colorimetric pH measurement is used in some portable water-analysis kits. The reliability of these test kits is adequate for some applications, but the general availability of low-cost, portable pH meters has largely supplanted the use of colorimetric measurement of pH, even for field use.

Potentiometric Determination of pH

Potentiometric pH measurements of water usually use a glass electrode with a bulb of special glass containing a fixed concentration of hydrogen ion into which is immersed an internal reference electrode. Glass separates the internal solution of constant hydrogen ion activity from the sample of variable hydrogen ion activity. A potential, proportional to the hydrogen ion concentration of the solution, develops because of the different amounts of hydrogen ion adsorbed by the two sides of the glass. The potential is measured by completing the electrochemical circuit with a calomel or silver:silver chloride reference electrode through a high-impedance millivoltmeter. The electromotive force developed varies linearly with pH. The relationship between electromotive force and pH is determined by calibrating the system with buffers of known pH.

pH meters available from commercial supply houses range from inexpensive, portable, battery-operated units to elaborate multifunction meters incorporating a microprocessor. Lower-cost instruments are suitable for routine analyses related to fish health investigations, but the system should minimally be accurate and reproducible to 0.1 pH unit. A plastic-bodied, general-purpose combination electrode, incorporating a glass and a reference electrode into a single probe, is less expensive and more convenient than separate reference and glass probes.

Sampling, Storage, and Preparation

Water samples for pH determination should be obtained with as little contact with the atmosphere as practical and the sample container should be filled to exclude all air. Store the sample in the dark at low temperature for no more than 2 hr before analysis. Samples and standard buffers should be brought to about the same temperature for analysis.

Calibration buffers can be prepared from ACS-grade chemicals (Table 13–3) or purchased as tablets, powders, or liquids from scientific supply houses.

TABLE 13–3. Preparation and pH Values of Primary Standard Buffer Solutions

Temperature (°C)	Potassium Hydrogen Phthalate[1] (0.05 M)	Phosphate[2] (about 0.04 M)	Borate[3] (0.01 M)
10	3.996	7.472	9.331
15	3.996	7.449	9.276
20	3.999	7.430	9.227
25	4.004	7.415	9.183
30	4.011	7.403	9.143

[1]Dissolve 10.12 g $KHC_8H_4O_4$ (dried at 105°C) in distilled water and dilute to 1,000 ml.
[2]Dissolve 1.179 g of KH_2PO_4 and 4.303 g Na_2HPO_4 (dry both at 130°C) in distilled water and dilute to 1,000 ml.
[3]Dissolve 3.80 g $Na_2B_4O_7\cdot10H_2O$ in distilled water and dilute to 1000 ml.

From Standard Methods for the Examination of Water and Wastewater. 17th ed. Copyright 1989 by the American Public Health Association, the American Water Works Association, and the Water Pollution Control Federation. Reprinted with permission.

Prepackaged commercial buffers are most convenient for routine use. Buffers should be prepared from freshly boiled (to expel CO_2) and cooled distilled water. They can be stored at 4°C for up to a month in stoppered polyethylene bottles.

Procedure

The operating instructions for pH meters vary widely. Consult the instruction manual and follow the manufacturer's instructions for maintenance of electrodes.

Electrode response is affected by temperature, and the temperature of calibration buffers and samples should not differ by more than about 3°C. To calibrate, remove the electrode from the storage solution (a pH 4 buffer is a good storage solution), rinse with distilled water, and blot dry with a soft tissue. Place the probe in gently stirred buffer of about pH 7. After the reading has stabilized, set the meter to the buffer pH value for the temperature at which the measurement is taken. Wash the electrode and immerse it in a second buffer to bracket the expected sample pH. After the reading has stabilized, set the meter to read the second buffer pH value correct for the measurement temperature. Depending on the particular pH meter, the control for the adjustment of the second buffer pH may be labeled "slope," "temperature," or "offset." On microprocessor-controlled meters the correct second buffer pH is simply entered into the microprocessor. The instrument should be calibrated before each series of water samples.

To measure the sample pH, wash the probe with distilled water and blot it dry before immersing the probe into the gently stirring sample. Wait about 30 seconds before taking the reading. The measured pH of the sample is correct only for the temperature at which the measurement is made. The pH of water buffered by the bicarbonate system declines by about 0.01 unit for each 1°C increase in temperature. Samples collected from cold water and allowed to warm to room temperature may have a measured pH 0.2 units lower than the actual in situ pH. The in situ pH can be calculated from:

In Situ pH = Measured pH + 0.0114 × (Measuring Temperature − In Situ Temperature)

The temperature coefficient, 0.0114, is useful for general purposes. The actual temperature coefficient depends on the buffer intensity, salinity, and temperature range. For more accurate temperature corrections, consult Strickland and Parsons (1972) or Grasshof et al. (1983).

ALKALINITY

Alkalinity measures the capacity of water to neutralize strong acid. It is an aggregate property and cannot be precisely interpreted unless the composition of the water is known. The usefulness of the value stems from the fact that for most natural waters, alkalinity is primarily attributable to the presence of bicarbonate (HCO_3^-) and carbonate (CO_3^{2-}), and it is often interpreted as a measure of these. This interpretation is sometimes erroneous because other bases such as hydroxide, silicates, borates, phosphates, or organic bases also contribute to alkalinity.

Alkalinity is expressed either as milligrams per liter (mg/L) as $CaCO_3$ or as milliequivalents per liter (mEq/L). Expression of alkalinity in the latter way is common in oceanography and limnology. This expression is unambiguous and clearly shows the meaning of alkalinity as the aggregate acid-neutralizing capacity of water. Expression of alkalinity as mg/L as $CaCO_3$ is traditional in civil and sanitary engineering and fishery biology. The term is somewhat misleading because it implies only carbonate contribution to alkalinity as well as a stoichiometric relationship with calcium, which may not be true. Alkalinity expressed as mg/L as $CaCO_3$ can be divided by 50 to convert to mEq/L.

The alkalinity of natural waters ranges from less than 0.2 to over 10 mEq/L. The composition of inland water depends on the geology of the aquifer or watershed. Water in contact with carbonate-bearing minerals such as limestone has relatively high alkalinities compared to water from areas dominated by silicate minerals or acidic topsoils. The alkalinity of estuarine water is determined by the composition of the river inflow and the degree of mixing with seawater. Seawater has an alkalinity of about 2.5 mEq/L. About 5% of the alkalinity of seawater is attributable to borate.

Measurement of alkalinity is useful for assessing the general suitability of a water for the culture of fish. Water of low alkalinity (<0.2 meq/L) is poorly buffered and pH fluctuates drastically with relatively small additions of acid or base. Dissolved metals such as copper, zinc, and aluminum are more toxic to fish in water of low alkalinity. In water with ample alkalinity, metals form relatively nontoxic hydroxide and carbonate precipitates and dissolved carbonate and bicarbonate complexes. Adequate alkalinity is also essential for the proper function of aquaria and other recycled-water fish culture systems that use nitrification biofilters to convert ammonia to nitrate. The nitrification process produces acid and unless the system is adequately buffered, the environmental pH may fall below 6.0 (Wheaton, 1977).

Determination of Total Alkalinity

A known volume of water is titrated with a standard solution of sulfuric acid to a pH between 4 and 5. The endpoint of the titration is detected with a pH meter or color change of an indicator, usually bromocresol green. The true endpoint of the titration corresponds to the pH of the solution when the bases hydroxide, carbonate, and bicarbonate have been neutralized to water and carbonic acid. This pH depends on the amount of carbon dioxide formed as the bases are neutralized. The true endpoint will thus be lower for samples of high alkalinity than for samples of low alkalinity. The following endpoint pH values for corresponding alkalinity concentrations are recommended: alkalinity = 0.6 mEq/L as $CaCO_3$, pH 4.9; alkalinity 3 mEq/L, pH 4.6; alkalinity 10 mEq/L, pH 4.3 (American Public Health Association et al., 1989). For routine analysis, titrate to pH 4.5 or use a color indicator that gives a sharp color change at a pH of around 4.5.

Sampling, Storage, and Preparation

No special precautions are needed during sampling for total alkalinity and samples can be held at room temperature for 24 hours before analysis. Samples can be refrigerated and held for up to 2 weeks. Do not filter, dilute, or concentrate the sample.

Standard sulfuric acid titrant (approximately 0.02N) is made by diluting 2.8 ml concentrated H_2SO_4 to 1000 ml to prepare an approximately 0.1N solution. Dilute 200 ml of the 0.1N H_2SO_4 solution to 1000 ml to prepare an approximately 0.02N solution. Standardize this solution against a 0.0200N sodium carbonate, Na_2CO_3, solution by pipetting 10 ml of the Na_2CO_3 solution into a 250-ml beaker. Add 90 ml of distilled water and 5 drops of bromocresol green indicator. Place the beaker on a magnetic stirrer under a buret. While gently stirring, titrate with acid to the endpoint where 1 drop of acid will change the color of the solution from yellow to blue. Alternatively, titrate to pH 4.5 using a glass electrode and pH meter. Calculate the normality of the sulfuric acid solution by dividing 0.2 by the volume of acid in milliliters used in the titration.

The standard Na_2CO_3 solution (0.0200N) is made by dissolving 1.0600 g of oven-dried (140°C) Na_2CO_3 and diluting to 1000 ml in boiled (to expel CO_2) and cooled distilled water. Use within a few hours of preparation. The bromocresol green indicator is made by dissolving 100 mg bromocresol green (sodium salt) in 100 ml of distilled water.

Procedure

Add 5 drops bromocresol green indicator to 100 ml of sample and titrate with the standard sulfuric acid until the color changes from yellow to blue. The titration can be carried out potentiometrically by omitting the indicator and titrating to pH 4.5 or the appropriate endpoint based on the approximate alkalinity. Total alkalinity is calculated as follows:

$$\text{Total Alkalinity (mEq/L)} = \frac{(\text{ml Titrant}) (N) (1000)}{(\text{Sample Volume in ml})}$$

where ml Titrant is milliliters of standard sulfuric acid required to titrate the sample to the endpoint, and N is the normality of the standard sulfuric acid.

TOTAL HARDNESS AND CALCIUM

Total hardness is the sum of the concentrations of calcium and magnesium expressed as equivalent $CaCO_3$. Other divalent cations contribute to hardness, but their concentration in natural water is usually low. The concentration of calcium alone in water is unambiguously expressed in milligrams per liter. Calcium concentrations sometimes are expressed as equivalent $CaCO_3$, but this method of expression is more properly termed calcium hardness. Calcium concentrations in milligrams per liter can be multiplied by 2.5 to give calcium hardness as $CaCO_3$.

The total hardness of natural water ranges from near 0 to over 10,000 mg/L as $CaCO_3$. The proportion of hardness contributed by calcium also varies widely and depends on the geology of the watershed. Most fresh water has hardness values less than 200 mg/L as $CaCO_3$; seawater has a hardness of about 6500 mg/L as $CaCO_3$. Seawater contains about 400 mg/kg calcium (an approximately calcium hardness of 1000 mg/L) and about 1350 mg/kg of magnesium (an approximate magnesium hardness of 5500 mg/L as $CaCO_3$).

Most freshwater fishes grow well over a wide range of hardness values, but they may be more susceptible to other adverse water-quality conditions when hardness values (in particular, calcium concentrations) are low. For example, increased environmental calcium concentrations decrease the toxicity of ammonia (Tomasso et al., 1980) and low pH (McWilliams, 1982) to freshwater fishes, probably by decreasing plasma sodium efflux at the gills. This reduces the osmoregulatory stress imposed on fish in acid water or environments with high un-ionized ammonia concentrations. Increasing the hardness of water also decreases the toxicity of dissolved metals such as copper and zinc because calcium and magnesium compete with the metals for branchial adsorption sites, decreasing the rate of metal uptake. Adequate hardness is also desirable because environmental calcium deficiencies in water may cause poor survival, decreased growth, or poor disease resistance in fry (Piper et al., 1982). In general, the calcium content of fresh water should be greater than about 5 mg/L (calcium hardness of 12.5 mg/L as $CaCO_3$) for raising freshwater fishes. Calcium and magnesium are abundant in natural seawater and do not limit normal life function of marine fishes.

EDTA Titrimetric Method for Total Hardness

Calcium and magnesium ions are titrated with the complexing agent ethylenediaminetetraacetic acid disodium salt (EDTA) to form chelated soluble complexes. The titration is performed at pH 10, and the endpoint is marked by the dye Calmagite (1-[1-hydroxy-4-methyl-2-phenylazo]-2-naphthol-sulfonic acid), which changes color from wine-red to blue when all the calcium and magnesium in solution have been complexed.

Sampling, Storage, and Preparation

No special precautions are required during sampling for total hardness. Samples can be stored at room temperature for several days before analysis or cooled to 4°C and held for at least 2 weeks.

To perform total hardness assays, prepare an ammonium chloride buffer solution by dissolving 16.9 g ammonium chloride (NH_4Cl) in 143 ml concentrated ammonium hydroxide (NH_4OH) and diluting it to 250 ml. Store this buffer in a tightly capped polyethylene bottle for no more than a month.

Calmagite indicator is made by dissolving 0.10 g Calmagite in 100 ml distilled water. This indicator is stable for many months.

Standard calcium solution (0.010 M) is prepared by transferring 1 g anhydrous calcium carbonate, $CaCO_3$, to a 500 ml Erlenmeyer flask. Add 1:1 HCl slowly until the $CaCO_3$ just dissolves, then dilute with about 200 ml distilled water. Boil this solution for a few minutes to expel CO_2 and then cool. Adjust the pH to 7 with 3N ammonium hydroxide, NH_4OH. Transfer this to a 1000-ml volumetric flask and dilute to volume with distilled water.

Standard EDTA titrant is made by dissolving 4.0 g disodium ethylenediaminetetraacetic acid and 100 mg $MgCl_2 \cdot 6\ H_2O$ in distilled water and diluting to 1000 ml. Standardize this solution against the standard calcium solution. Pipette 10.0 ml of the standard calcium solution into a 250-ml Erlenmeyer flask and add 90 ml of distilled water. Add 2.0 ml of ammonium chloride buffer solution and mix. Add 2 ml of Calmagite indicator solution and titrate with the EDTA solution. At the endpoint the solution will change from wine-red to blue. Calculate the molarity of the EDTA solution by dividing 0.1 by the volume in milliliters of EDTA solution required to see the color change.

Procedure

To perform the assay, measure 100 ml of water sample into a 250-ml Erlenmeyer flask and mix it with 2.0 ml of ammonium chloride buffer. Add 2.0 ml Calmagite indicator and titrate with the EDTA solution until the color changes from wine-red to blue. If less than 100 ml of sample is used, dilute to 100 ml with distilled water before titrating. If more than 100 ml of sample is used, add proportionately more buffer and indicator before titrating.

$$\text{Total Hardness (mg/L as } CaCO_3) = \frac{(\text{ml Titrant}) (M) (100,100)}{(\text{Sample Volume in ml})}$$

where ml Titrant is milliliters of standard EDTA solution required to titrate the sample to the endpoint, and M is the molarity of the standard EDTA solution.

EDTA Titrimetric Method for Calcium

Calcium is determined by complexation with EDTA after precipitating magnesium as its hydroxide at pH 12 to 13. Murexide (ammonium purpurate) indicator is used, which is more or less specific for calcium. Concentrations of calcium less than 10 mg/L can be determined more accurately by atomic absorption spectrometry, but such sensitivity is seldom required in routine environmental analyses.

Sample Storage and Preparation

Samples can be stored at room temperature for several days or refrigerated for 2 weeks before analysis.

Murexide indicator is made by mixing 200 mg of murexide with 100 g of NaCl. Grind this thoroughly with a mortar and pestle and store in an opaque bottle.

A 1N sodium hydroxide solution is prepared by dissolving 40 g NaOH and diluting it to 1000 ml with distilled water. Store this solution in a tightly stoppered polyethylene bottle.

The standard EDTA titrant is prepared as described in the section on measuring total hardness.

Procedure

Measure 100 ml of water sample into a 250-ml Erlenmeyer flask and add 4.0 ml of the 1N NaOH and mix. Next add 0.2 g of murexide (which can be measured with a calibrated scoop) and titrate with the standard EDTA solution. The color change from pink to orchid-purple is not abrupt; add titrant until a single drop of EDTA causes no further intensification of the color. Subtract the volume of this last drop from the buret reading.

$$\text{Calcium (mg/L)} = \frac{(\text{ml Titrant}) (M) (40,100)}{(\text{Sample Volume in ml})}$$

where ml titrant is milliliters of standard EDTA solution required to titrate sample to the end point, and M is the molarity of the standard EDTA solution. This can be converted to calcium hardness (mg/L as $CaCO_3$) by multiplying by 2.5.

DISSOLVED OXYGEN

Oxygen is a major component of the atmosphere, comprising about 21% of dry air by volume. However, oxygen is only sparingly soluble in water and the concentration of oxygen at equilibrium (saturation) for water in contact with moist air at 760 mm Hg ranges from about 6 to 15 mg/L at temperatures and salinities normally encountered in water holding fish (Table 13–4). The solubility of oxygen in water decreases as water temperature and salinity

TABLE 13–4. Saturation Concentrations of Dissolved Oxygen (mg/L) for Water in Contact with Moist Air at 760 mm Hg

Temp (°C)	Salinity (ppt)								
	0	5	10	15	20	25	30	35	40
0	14.60	14.11	13.64	13.18	12.74	12.31	11.90	11.50	11.11
1	14.20	13.72	13.27	12.82	12.40	11.98	11.58	11.20	10.82
2	13.81	13.36	12.91	12.49	12.07	11.67	11.29	10.92	10.55
3	13.44	13.00	12.58	12.16	11.76	11.38	11.00	10.64	10.29
4	13.09	12.67	12.25	11.85	11.47	11.09	10.73	10.38	10.04
5	12.76	12.34	11.94	11.56	11.18	10.82	10.47	10.13	9.80
6	12.44	12.04	11.65	11.27	10.91	10.56	10.22	9.89	9.57
7	12.13	11.74	11.36	11.00	10.65	10.31	9.98	9.66	9.35
8	11.83	11.46	11.09	10.74	10.40	10.07	9.75	9.44	9.15
9	11.55	11.18	10.83	10.47	10.16	9.84	9.53	9.23	8.94
10	11.28	10.92	10.58	10.24	9.93	9.62	9.32	9.03	8.75
11	11.02	10.67	10.34	10.02	9.71	9.41	9.12	8.83	8.56
12	10.77	10.43	10.11	9.80	9.50	9.21	8.92	8.65	8.38
13	10.52	10.20	9.89	9.59	9.29	9.01	8.73	8.47	8.21
14	10.29	9.98	9.68	9.38	9.10	8.82	8.55	8.29	8.04
15	10.07	9.77	9.47	9.19	8.91	8.64	8.38	8.13	7.88
16	9.86	9.56	9.28	9.00	8.73	8.47	8.21	7.97	7.73
17	9.65	9.36	9.09	8.82	8.55	8.30	8.05	7.81	7.58
18	9.45	9.17	8.90	8.64	8.38	8.14	7.90	7.66	7.44
19	9.26	8.99	8.73	8.47	8.22	7.98	7.75	7.52	7.30
20	9.08	8.81	8.56	8.31	8.06	7.83	7.60	7.38	7.17
21	8.90	8.64	8.39	8.15	7.91	7.68	7.46	7.25	7.04
22	8.75	8.48	8.23	8.00	7.77	7.54	7.33	7.12	6.91
23	8.56	8.32	8.08	7.85	7.63	7.41	7.20	6.99	6.79
24	8.40	8.16	7.93	7.71	7.49	7.28	7.07	6.87	6.68
25	8.24	8.01	7.79	7.57	7.36	7.15	6.95	6.75	6.56
26	8.09	7.87	7.65	7.44	7.23	7.03	6.83	6.64	6.46
27	7.95	7.73	7.51	7.31	7.10	6.91	6.72	6.53	6.35
28	7.81	7.59	7.38	7.18	6.98	6.79	6.61	6.42	6.25
29	7.67	7.46	7.26	7.06	6.87	6.68	6.50	6.32	6.15
30	7.54	7.33	7.14	6.94	6.75	6.57	6.39	6.22	6.05
31	7.41	7.21	7.02	6.83	6.64	6.47	6.29	6.12	5.96
32	7.29	7.09	6.90	6.72	6.54	6.36	6.19	6.03	5.87
33	7.17	6.98	6.79	6.61	6.43	6.26	6.10	5.94	5.78
34	7.05	6.86	6.68	6.51	6.33	6.17	6.01	5.85	5.69
35	6.93	6.75	6.58	6.40	6.24	6.07	5.91	5.76	5.61

increase. Barometric and hydrostatic pressure also influence the solubility of oxygen. The major factor influencing barometric pressure is elevation above sea level. When calculating the effect of high altitude, the standard saturation concentration is multiplied by the ratio of the actual barometric pressure in millimeters of mercury to 760. The effects of hydrostatic pressure can be important for deep-water fishes. Effectively the saturation concentration of oxygen in water is increased by multiplying the appropriate value in Table 13–4 by the number of atmospheres of pressure involved at depth.

The concentration of dissolved oxygen in natural water is influenced by the relative rates of diffusion to and from the atmosphere, photosynthesis by aquatic plants, and respiration by the entire aquatic biological community. Ground water usually contains little or no dissolved oxygen because biological processes in the aquifer recharge zone remove oxygen as the water percolates through the ground. Likewise, unless mixed with surface water, deep lake water may be oxygen deficient as biological activity consumes oxygen and the water is deprived of reaeration. Dissolved oxygen concentrations are usually near saturation in surface water of unpolluted rivers,

lakes, estuaries, and oceans because of turbulent mixing and low rates of respiration. If phytoplankton or other aquatic plants are abundant, dissolved oxygen concentrations may vary significantly during the day, being highest in late afternoon and lowest at sunrise. Oxygen is produced by photosynthesizing plants during the day. At night, photosynthesis ceases, and oxygen-consuming respiration continues. In water with excessive plant and animal life, high rates of respiration may deplete dissolved oxygen. This occurs in high-density fish culture facilities, polluted bodies of water, and during phytoplankton blooms in lakes, estuaries, or near-shore ocean water.

The availability of oxygen is the most common limiting factor to fish life. This is particularly true for marine fishes and fishes living in warm water because of the decreased solubility of oxygen in warm water and the higher rate of basal metabolism in poikilothermic animals living in warm water. The respiratory and circulatory systems of fish function effectively over a range of environmental dissolved oxygen concentrations, but fish perform best and are healthiest when dissolved oxygen concentrations are near saturation. As dissolved oxygen concentrations decrease, fish are stressed and immune function may

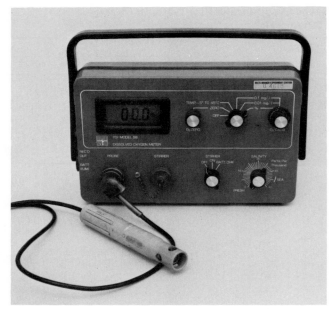

FIGURE 13–7. Dissolved oxygen meter and polarographic membrane electrode (Yellow Springs Instrument Co., Yellow Springs, Ohio).

be compromised. Below the critical environmental oxygen concentration, fish die from tissue hypoxia. The critical oxygen concentration depends on species, acclimation, activity, size, temperature, and other environmental conditions. Generally, warmwater species survive for long periods at dissolved oxygen concentrations as low as 2 or 3 mg/L. Many cold-water fishes tolerate 4 or 5 mg/L indefinitely. The United States Environmental Protection Agency (1976) sets a minimum of 5 mg/L as the criterion for maintaining a good fish population. The embryonic and larval stages of fish are particularly intolerant of low dissolved oxygen concentrations because their respiratory and circulatory systems may not be fully developed. The early life stages of fish also have a limited ability to enviroregulate by moving away from areas of low oxygen.

Dissolved oxygen measurements can be made either with one of the modifications of the classic "Winkler" iodometric procedure or by using a membrane electrode and meter. The iodometric procedure offers a reliable and relatively inexpensive method for dissolved oxygen measurements, but it is laborious if many measurements must be made and the results are not available instantly. The method is also subject to serious errors resulting from poor sampling technique. Dissolved oxygen measurements with a membrane electrode and meter (Fig. 13–7) are usually not as accurate or precise as properly conducted iodometric measurements, and accuracy and precision can be especially suspect in water supersaturated with dissolved oxygen or in water with very low dissolved oxygen concentrations. However, accuracy and precision are adequate for most purposes, and membrane electrodes are less subject to interfering substances. Membrane electrodes are portable,

easy to use, and give practically instantaneous readings. Their construction makes them particularly suited for field use and for continuous monitoring of fish culture systems.

Winkler Iodometric Determination of Dissolved Oxygen

Manganous sulfate, potassium iodide, and sodium hydroxide are added to a sample of water. Under the alkaline conditions, any oxygen present oxidizes manganous ion to manganic oxide, a brown precipitate. Acidification dissolves the precipitate, freeing manganic ion to react with iodide to produce iodine. The amount of iodine produced is proportional to the amount of dissolved oxygen originally present. The amount of iodine is determined by titration with a reducing agent, usually sodium thiosulfate.

Oxidizing or reducing agents present in the sample also react with iodide or iodine causing errors. Nitrite is the most common interfering substance in water holding fish. Interference from nitrite is overcome by adding sodium azide to reduce nitrite to dinitrogen oxide and nitrogen gas.

Samples for the iodometric determination of dissolved oxygen should be collected in 300-ml glass-stoppered BOD bottles, avoiding contact with air during and after sampling. Bottles must not contain any bubbles. If possible, determine the dissolved oxygen concentration immediately. Samples may be stored in the dark for a few hours after adding the manganous sulfate solution, alkali-iodide-azide solution, and sulfuric acid solution. (Clinicians interested in applying this method should consult American Public Health Association et al., 1989.)

Membrane Electrode Method for Dissolved Oxygen

Most of the commercially available oxygen electrodes, often called probes, are of the polarographic type. The working part of the probe (Fig. 13–8)

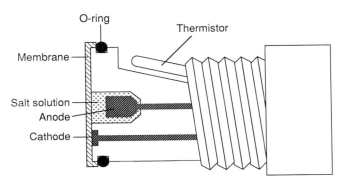

FIGURE 13–8. Cross-section of a polarographic membrane electrode.

consists of a pair of electrodes bathed in a salt solution. The electrodes and salt solution are separated from the sample by a thin fluorocarbon membrane. The membrane is essentially impermeable to dissolved ions, but it is permeable to most gases. An electrical potential is applied across the two electrodes by an external voltage source to polarize the electrodes. Molecular oxygen diffusing across the membrane is reduced to hydroxide at the cathode. Hydroxide ions migrate to the anode and react with the electrode to form a metallic oxide or hydroxide. This completes the circuit, allowing a current to flow. The current is measured with a sensitive ammeter. The current produced is proportional to the overall reaction rate. Since the oxygen concentration beneath the membrane is kept low (virtually zero) because oxygen is rapidly consumed in the cathodic reaction, the rate of reaction is controlled by the rate at which oxygen diffuses across the membrane from the sample. The partial pressure of oxygen in the sample is the driving force behind oxygen diffusion; thus the measured electrode current is proportional to oxygen partial pressure. Automatic or manual compensation for temperature, pressure, and salinity allows the readings to be conveniently read in concentration units after appropriate calibration.

Several brands and models of oxygen-sensitive membrane electrodes and meters are available commercially. Use a system capable of an accuracy of at least ± 0.2 mg/L at the calibration temperature. Preferred are probes that incorporate a thermistor together with an appropriate meter with a temperature readout. For convenience, the meter should incorporate a system to compensate for changes in sample temperature. A manual system for salinity compensation is also convenient.

The probe and meter electronics are designed to provide a linear response to partial pressure of oxygen. The meter response is calibrated against the partial pressure of oxygen in moist air or against a water sample of known dissolved oxygen concentration. Calibration against oxygen in air is most convenient and sufficiently accurate for most purposes. Electrode response is highly temperature dependent. Most commercial probe-meter systems incorporate manual or automatic temperature compensation, but the exact temperature coefficient varies depending on the condition of the membrane and electrodes. For highest accuracy, calibration should be conducted at a temperature near the measurement temperature following the manufacturer's instructions closely. Calibration is quite stable on most modern probe-meter systems and frequent calibration is not necessary. Calibration before each series of measurements is generally sufficient. The instrument should be left on between successive measurements to avoid depolarizing the probe unless the instrument will not be used for an hour or longer. Then it should be turned off and recalibrated when next needed to extend the life of the electrodes and batteries.

Water must flow across the membrane surface of polarographic probes to obtain an accurate, stable measurement of dissolved oxygen. Otherwise, a zone of oxygen-deficient water will develop at the membrane surface, causing erroneous low readings. Polarographic probes do not give a spontaneous reading. From 5 seconds to over 1 minute may be required for the probe-meter system to indicate within 10% of actual dissolved oxygen concentrations. Probe response time is longer in cold water or as oxygen concentrations deviate from saturation values. Thin, high sensitivity membranes improve response time but are less durable than standard membranes.

CARBON DIOXIDE

Carbon dioxide (CO_2) is highly soluble in water, but equilibrium concentrations are very low because carbon dioxide is a minor constituent of the atmosphere. Carbon dioxide is produced by organisms during respiration and consumed during photosynthesis. The amount of free carbon dioxide* in water is usually determined by the relative rates of respiration and photosynthesis, and the rate of diffusion to and from the atmosphere. Free carbon dioxide concentrations in surface water are usually less than 10 mg/L and vary diurnally; highest concentrations occur after daybreak and lowest concentrations in midafternoon. High concentrations of free carbon dioxide are encountered in surface water polluted with organic wastes and in high-density fish culture systems where rates of respiration are high. The ground water and bottom water of deep lakes or reservoirs can be considerably enriched with carbon dioxide produced in the decomposition of organic matter. Free carbon dioxide concentrations greater than 100 mg/L are found in some ground water.

An increase in free carbon dioxide concentration in water reduces the concentration gradient necessary for diffusion of carbon dioxide from blood through the gills. This causes an increase in blood carbon dioxide levels and a decrease in blood pH. These conditions decrease the affinity of hemoglobin for oxygen and reduce oxygen uptake by blood even when normally sufficient dissolved oxygen is present in the water. The quantitative relationship between free carbon dioxide in the environment and the oxygen-combining capability of hemoglobin varies greatly among fish species and with other environmental conditions. Free carbon dioxide concentrations less than 10 mg/L are usually well tolerated by fish if dissolved oxygen concentrations are near saturation.

Prolonged exposure of fish to free carbon dioxide concentrations greater than 10 to 20 mg/L has been implicated as causing mineral deposits within kidney tubules, collecting ducts, and ureters. This condition, known as nephrocalcinosis, rarely results in high

---

*Free carbon dioxide refers to the concentration of dissolved carbon dioxide plus carbonic acid, H_2CO_3. Carbonic acid constitutes less than 1% of the total.

mortality unless other environmental conditions are marginal (Landolt, 1975). The mechanisms responsible for the development of this condition are not fully understood.

Two methods are commonly used to estimate free carbon dioxide concentrations in fresh water (American Public Health Association et al., 1989). The nomograph method is based upon mathematical relationships among free carbon dioxide concentration and the pH, alkalinity, temperature, and dissolved solids content of the water. The nomograph method provides highly accurate results but requires very accurate pH determinations and analysis for total dissolved solids. It is also limited to use in dilute fresh water.

The other commonly used method is titrimetric. It is easy to perform and reasonably accurate. In the variation given below, sodium carbonate is substituted for the usual titrant, sodium hydroxide, to eliminate a standardization step. Titration with prestandardized sodium hydroxide is the basis for most portable test kit methods.

Titrimetric Method for Free Carbon Dioxide

A known volume of water sample is carefully titrated with standard sodium carbonate. Free carbon dioxide reacts with sodium carbonate to form sodium bicarbonate. The reaction is complete at about pH 8.3. The endpoint of the titration is marked by phenolphthalein indicator which changes from colorless to pink as the pH is increased through pH 8.3.

Sampling, Storage, and Preparation

Samples must be collected without contact with air to avoid gain or loss of carbon dioxide. Sample bottles should be filled completely and kept at a temperature lower than that at which the water was collected. Analysis should be conducted as soon as possible, and not more than 2 hours, after sample collection. Do not filter or dilute the sample.

To prepare the phenolphthalein indicator solution, dissolve 0.5 g phenolphthalein in 50 ml of 95% ethyl alcohol and add 50 ml distilled water. Remove carbon dioxide from the indicator by adding 0.0454N sodium carbonate dropwise until a faint pink color appears.

Standard 0.0454N sodium carbonate is prepared by transferring 2.407 g of dried Na_2CO_3 (140°C, 2 hours) to a 1000-ml volumetric flask and diluting to volume with boiled and cooled distilled water. This solution should be prepared fresh every few days and stored tightly stoppered in a plastic bottle.

Procedure

Siphon the water sample into a 100-ml graduated cylinder, allowing about 100 ml to overflow. Remove excess sample from the cylinder, leaving 100 ml. The 100-ml sample volume can be changed so that a convenient volume of sodium carbonate will be used in the titration. Add 4 drops of phenolphthalein indicator and gently stir with a glass rod. If the sample turns pink, the pH is above 8.3 and free carbon dioxide is not present. If the sample remains colorless, titrate rapidly with 0.0454N Na_2CO_3 while gently stirring with the glass rod. The endpoint is marked by a persistent faint pink color.

$$\text{Free CO}_2 \text{ (mg/L)} = \frac{(\text{ml Na}_2\text{CO}_3 \text{ Titrant}) (1000)}{(\text{Sample Volume in ml})}$$

AMMONIA

Ammonia* in water establishes an equilibrium that can be written as:

$$NH_3 + H_2O = NH_4^+ + OH^-$$

The relative proportions of NH_3 and NH_4^+ depend primarily on pH and temperature, and, to a lesser degree, salinity. For a given concentration of total ammonia, the concentration of un-ionized ammonia proportionately increases as temperatures and pH values increase, and decreases as salinities increase.

Total ammonia-nitrogen concentrations are usually less than 1 mg/L in natural water. At common environmental pH values and temperatures, this results in un-ionized ammonia-nitrogen concentrations much less than 0.1 mg/L. Locally high total ammonia-nitrogen concentrations are sometimes found in oil-field brines, ground water in volcanic areas, and ground and surface water polluted by industrial wastes, sewage, or runoff from agricultural areas. Ammonia frequently accumulates in high-density fish culture systems because ammonia is the major end product of nitrogen catabolism excreted by most fish. Some aquatic animals produce urea in significant quantities, but it is rapidly hydrolyzed to ammonia and carbon dioxide.

Ammonia can be toxic to fish, and un-ionized ammonia is much more toxic than the ionized form. Un-ionized ammonia freely diffuses across the gill membranes, the major route of ammonia excretion. As the concentration of environmental un-ionized ammonia increases, the concentration gradient between blood and environment decreases and the rate of ammonia excretion decreases. This results in increased blood and tissue ammonia levels that can have serious physiological consequences (Colt and Armstrong, 1981).

Suggested criteria for environmental ammonia are usually based on the concentration of un-ionized ammonia, and range from less than 0.01 to more than 0.2 mg/L NH_3-N (Meade, 1985). A maximum

---

*The following convention will be used in this section: NH_3 will be referred to as un-ionized ammonia; NH_4^+ will be referred to as ionized ammonia; and the sum $NH_3 + NH_4^+$ will be referred to as total ammonia or, simply, ammonia. All concentrations will be expressed on a nitrogen basis.

concentration of 0.0125 mg/L NH_3-N has been suggested for optimum health in salmonids under continuous exposure (Smith and Piper, 1975). However, 0.04 mg/L NH_3-N is considered "reasonably safe" for production of rainbow trout in raceway systems (Meade, 1985). Warm-water fish are somewhat more tolerant to ammonia than cold-water fish (Arthur et al., 1987), but insufficient data are available on which to base recommendations for "safe" concentrations. The criterion set by the United States Environmental Protection Agency (1976) as "safe" for freshwater aquatic life under continuous exposure is 0.02 mg/L un-ionized ammonia-nitrogen.

No convenient method exists for directly measuring un-ionized ammonia concentrations. Determination of the un-ionized ammonia concentration initially involves analytical measurement of the total ammonia concentration. The un-ionized ammonia concentration is then calculated using formulas or tables. Four methods for the determination of total ammonia in water are commonly used. Method selection depends primarily upon the sensitivity and precision required, and the possible presence of interfering substances.

Direct nesslerization is a rapid and convenient method applicable to waters with ammonia concentrations greater than about 0.1 mg/L total ammonia-nitrogen. The nessler reagent is stable for a year or more, and direct nesslerization is the method used in most portable water analysis kits. Direct nesslerization is often used for routine monitoring of ammonia concentrations because of the simplicity of the method and the stability of the reagents. The direct nesslerization procedure, however, lacks precision and reliability. The nessler reagent yields an unstable colloidal product that absorbs light over a wide range of wavelengths that causes nonlinearity of calibration curves and poor reproducibility, as well as an increased probability of interference from colored substances in water. This method is described by the American Public Health Association et al. (1989).

The indophenol method is less subject to interference than direct nesslerization and is more reproducible, particularly when ammonia concentrations are low. The indophenol method is useful in fresh water and seawater with total ammonia-nitrogen concentrations of 0.02 mg/L or greater. The reagents used in the indophenol method are not stable and the intensity of the blue color that develops is affected by the age of the reagents. This necessitates carrying a blank and standards through the procedure with each set of samples.

The salicylate method is a variation of the indophenol method, but the reagents are more stable. The method is more sensitive and reproducible than direct nesslerization and is useful in both fresh and salt water. Despite these advantages, the salicylate method is not widely used. This method is described by Krom (1980).

The use of the ammonia-selective electrode method is increasing because of its value as a rapid diagnostic technique. This method is not subject to

as many interferences as the nessler, indophenol, or salicylate method and is useful over a wide range of ammonia concentrations. It obviates preliminary sample treatment such as distillation and dilution and is best suited for rapid screening of environmental ammonia as an aid in the diagnostic procedure, particularly if ammonia concentrations vary over a wide range. However, the response of the electrode is slow, and the accuracy and precision of the method are suspect at low ammonia concentrations.

Sampling, Storage, and Preparation

No special precautions are needed during sampling if only total ammonia is to be measured. Samples for total ammonia analysis can be stored temporarily in glass or polyethylene bottles, but analysis should not be delayed for more than 2 hours. Samples can be cooled to 4°C and stored for up to 24 hours. Addition of sulfuric acid (1 ml concentrated H_2SO_4/L) or mercuric chloride (40 mg $HgCl_2$/L), with refrigeration, allows sample storage for up to 7 days. If sulfuric acid is used as preservative, the sample should be neutralized with 1N NaOH prior to analysis. Mercuric chloride should not be used as a preservative if the ammonia-selective electrode method is to be used. Samples to be used in the indophenol method should be filtered through Whatman 42, or equivalent, filter paper. Do not filter under vacuum as some NH_3 may be lost. No filtration is necessary for the electrode method. If un-ionized ammonia concentrations are to be calculated, in situ measurement of temperature and appropriate sampling procedures for subsequent measurement of pH are required.

Indophenol Method for Total Ammonia

Phenol, hypochlorite, and un-ionized ammonia react under strongly alkaline conditions to form indophenol, an intensely blue compound. The reaction is catalyzed by sodium nitroprusside. The intensity of the blue color is measured spectrophotometrically. Turbidity due to precipitation of calcium and magnesium hydroxide under alkaline conditions is avoided by using sodium citrate as a complexing agent. The indophenol method is suitable for use in most natural water with total ammonia-nitrogen concentrations above 0.02 mg/L. For use in fresh water, a simpler, but less sensitive variation of this method is available (American Public Health Association et al., 1989).

Procedure

All reagents and standards are prepared with ammonia-free distilled water. This is made by passing distilled water through a column containing a strongly acidic cation exchange resin, such as Dowex 50W-X8.

Phenol solution is made by dissolving 10 g

phenol in 100 ml 95% ethyl alcohol. This reagent is stable for several weeks.

To make sodium nitroprusside solution, dissolve 0.5 g $Na_2[Fe(CN)_5NO] \cdot 2H_2O$) in 100 ml distilled water. This reagent is stable for at least a month if stored in a dark glass bottle.

Alkaline-citrate solution is made by dissolving 100 g sodium citrate and 5 g sodium hydroxide in 500 ml of distilled water. It is stable indefinitely.

The oxidizing solution is prepared by mixing 100 ml of alkaline-citrate solution and 25 ml of fresh household bleach (about 5% sodium hypochlorite). The oxidizing solution should be prepared fresh every day.

A stock ammonia-nitrogen solution, 1000 mg/L, is prepared by dissolving 1.9079 g NH_4Cl and diluting to 500 ml with ammonia-free distilled water. This solution can be stored refrigerated for a month. Dilute 5 ml of the 1000-mg/L stock solution to 500 ml with ammonia-free water to give a 10.0-mg/L solution of total ammonia-nitrogen. Dilute 2.0 ml of the 10-mg/L solution to 100 ml with ammonia-free water to give a 0.20-mg/L standard ammonia-nitrogen solution. The standard should be prepared fresh daily.

To run the test, add 2 ml phenol solution to 50 ml of filtered water sample in a 125-ml Erlenmeyer flask and swirl to mix. Next add 2 ml sodium nitroprusside solution and 5 ml of oxidizing solution, mixing after each addition. Cover or stopper the flask and allow 1 hour for full color development. The color is stable for 24 hours. Carry 50 ml of ammonia-free distilled water (reagent blank) and 50 ml of the standard 0.20-mg/L ammonia-nitrogen solution through the procedure with each set of samples. Measure the absorbance with a spectrophotometer at 640 nm. Use the reagent blank of ammonia-free distilled water to set the instrument at 0 absorbance. Total ammonia nitrogen (mg/L) = 0.2(A1/A2), where A1 is the absorbance of the sample and A2 is the absorbance of the standard.

Ammonia-Selective Electrode Method for Total Ammonia

The ammonia-selective electrode is a pH electrode immersed in an ammonium chloride solution that is separated from the sample by a gas-permeable membrane. Ammonia in the sample is converted to un-ionized ammonia by raising the pH of the sample above 11 with a strong base. Un-ionized ammonia diffuses across the membrane and changes the pH of the internal ammonium chloride solution. The change in pH is sensed by the pH electrode. Potentiometric measurements are made with either a pH meter having an expanded millivolt scale, or, more conveniently, with a specific ion meter.

The electrode will respond to total ammonia-nitrogen over the range of about 0.2 to 1400 mg/L, and is subject to few interferences. However, measurements of ammonia-nitrogen below 1 mg/L should be considered semiquantitative. Standards and samples should have the same temperature and about the same level of dissolved ions. The addition of 10 N NaOH serves as an ionic strength adjustment buffer as well as the base to raise sample pH above 11. The sodium hydroxide solution is prepared by dissolving 400 g NaOH in 800 ml water, allowing the solution to cool, and bringing the total volume to 1000 mL with water.

The general procedure is to place 100 ml of each standard solution in a 125 ml Erlenmeyer flask. Immerse the electrode into the standard at an angle so bubbles will not accumulate on the membrane and add 1 ml of 10 N NaOH while stirring. Keep the electrode in the solution until a stable reading is obtained. Repeat the procedure for each standard, proceeding from the lowest to highest concentrations. Use standards of 0.1, 1.0, 10.0, and 100.0 mg/L ammonia-nitrogen. The results of the calibration can be recorded in the memory of some specific ion meters, but they must be recorded manually when using most pH millivolt meters. Plot the ammonia-nitrogen concentration of the standards versus the electrode potentials to construct a calibration curve. The total ammonia-nitrogen concentrations in water samples are then obtained from the calibration curve (American Public Health Association et al., 1989).

Calculation of Un-ionized Ammonia

The un-ionized ammonia-nitrogen concentration can be computed from the following formula derived from the equilibrium expression:

$$(NH_3\text{-}N) = (Ammonia\text{-}N)/[1 + antilog\ (pK_a\text{-}pH\ of\ the\ solution)]$$

where (Ammonia-N) is the measured total ammonia-nitrogen concentration and pK_a is the negative logarithm of the ionization constant for the reaction. The pK_a value is a function of temperature and salinity (Whitfield, 1974; Emerson et al., 1975). Tabular lists of percent un-ionized ammonia in water are useful when there is only an occasional need to compute un-ionized ammonia concentrations. Table 13–5 lists the percent of total ammonia in the un-ionized form as a function of pH and temperature for dilute fresh water or seawater. Tabular lists are available for percent un-ionized ammonia in more concentrated fresh water (Messer et al., 1984) and seawater of lower salinities (Bower and Bidwell, 1978).

NITRITE

Nitrite (NO_2^-) is an intermediate product in two bacteria-mediated processes involving transformations of nitrogen in soil and water. In the first process, called nitrification, two groups of highly aerobic, autotrophic bacteria (mainly *Nitrosomonas* spp. and *Nitrobacter* spp.) oxidize ammonia to nitrite and then to nitrate. Nitrite is also an intermediate in the process of denitrification. In this process, a number of species of common facultative anaerobic bac-

TABLE 13–5. Percentage Un-ionized Ammonia in Dilute Freshwater (salinity <0.5 ppt) or Seawater (salinity of 32–40 ppt) at Different pH Values and Temperatures

	Freshwater Temperature (°C)							
pH	4	8	12	16	20	24	28	32
6.0						0.1	0.1	0.1
6.2					0.1	0.1	0.1	0.1
6.4			0.1	0.1	0.1	0.1	0.2	0.2
6.6		0.1	0.1	0.1	0.2	0.2	0.3	0.4
6.8	0.1	0.1	0.1	0.2	0.2	0.3	0.4	0.6
7.0	0.1	0.2	0.2	0.3	0.4	0.5	0.7	0.9
7.2	0.2	0.3	0.3	0.5	0.6	0.8	1.1	1.4
7.4	0.3	0.4	0.5	0.7	1.0	1.3	1.7	2.3
7.6	0.5	0.6	0.9	1.2	1.7	2.1	2.7	3.5
7.8	0.7	1.0	1.4	1.8	2.4	3.2	4.2	5.5
8.0	1.2	1.6	2.1	2.9	3.8	5.0	6.5	8.4
8.2	1.8	2.5	3.3	4.5	5.9	7.7	10.0	12.7
8.4	2.8	3.8	5.2	6.9	9.0	11.7	15.0	18.8
8.6	4.4	5.9	7.9	10.5	13.6	17.4	21.8	26.8
8.8	6.8	9.1	12.0	15.7	20.0	25.0	30.6	36.7
9.0	10.3	13.7	17.8	22.7	28.4	34.6	41.2	47.9
9.2	15.5	20.1	25.6	31.8	38.6	45.6	52.6	59.3
9.4	22.4	28.5	35.3	42.5	49.9	57.0	63.7	69.8
9.6	31.4	38.7	46.3	53.9	61.2	67.8	73.6	78.6
9.8	42.0	50.0	57.8	65.0	71.4	76.9	81.5	85.3
10.0	53.4	61.3	68.4	74.6	79.8	84.1	87.5	90.2
10.2	64.5	71.5	77.5	82.3	86.3	89.3	91.7	93.6

	Seawater Temperature (°C)							
pH	4	8	12	16	20	24	28	32
7.4	0.2	0.3	0.4	0.5	0.7	1.0	1.4	1.9
7.6	0.4	0.5	0.7	0.7	1.2	1.6	2.1	2.9
7.8	0.6	0.8	1.1	1.4	1.9	2.6	3.4	4.6
8.0	0.9	1.2	1.7	2.2	3.0	4.0	5.3	7.1
8.2	1.5	2.0	2.6	3.5	4.7	6.2	8.2	10.7
8.4	2.3	3.1	4.1	5.4	7.2	9.4	12.4	16.0
8.6	3.5	4.8	6.3	8.4	10.9	14.2	18.3	23.2
8.8	5.5	7.4	9.7	12.6	16.3	20.8	26.2	32.4
9.0	8.5	11.2	14.5	18.6	23.6	29.4	36.0	43.1
9.2	12.9	16.6	21.2	26.6	32.9	39.8	47.1	54.6

teria use nitrate as an exogenous terminal electron acceptor during the oxidation of organic compounds under anaerobic conditions. In most natural bodies of water, the intermediate product of these reactions, nitrite, does not accumulate, and concentrations of nitrite-nitrogen are usually much less than 0.1 mg/L. Nitrite is sometimes found at higher concentrations in surface water polluted with nitrogen-containing wastes, such as sewage or runoff from agricultural lands.

Nitrite is occasionally detected in some high-density fish culture systems. This is usually the result of a breakdown in the nitrification process in systems with high nitrogen loading rates in the form of feed protein. In closed water-recirculating fish culture systems, biofilters, or nitrification filters, are used to convert ammonia to nitrate. The process is used to prevent the accumulation of a potentially toxic compound (un-ionized ammonia) by converting it to relatively nontoxic nitrate. In properly designed and operating recirculating systems, nitrite does not accumulate because it is converted to nitrate as quickly as it is produced. Nitrite may accumulate when systems using biofilters are operated without proper acclimation of the filter. This is the result of faster initial colonization of the filter by the ammonia-oxidizing *Nitrosomonas* group of bacteria than the nitrite-oxidizing *Nitrobacter* group. A similar situation occurs when bactericidal chemicals are introduced into the system to treat certain fish diseases. The chemical may kill nitrifying bacteria and the filter will be recolonized initially by *Nitrosomonas* spp. The *Nitrobacter* group is also more sensitive to certain environmental aberrations such as sudden temperature changes. Thus, a decrease in water temperature may result in the accumulation of nitrite in the system. Nitrite also accumulates in some fish culture ponds. In temperate climates, the incidence of nitrite in ponds is seasonal, occurring most frequently in the fall and spring. It appears that this is related to the differential effect of temperature on the relative rates of ammonia and nitrite oxidation.

Environmental nitrite can be toxic to some fish species at relatively low concentrations. Waterborne nitrite enters the fish circulatory system through the gills. Uptake may be either active or passive depending on the fish species and environmental pH. Nitrite in the blood oxidizes the ferrous iron (Fe^{2+}) in the hemoglobin molecule to the ferric (Fe^{3+}) state. The resulting product, called methemoglobin, is incapable of reversibly combining with oxygen. Thus, methemoglobinemia may cause considerable respiratory distress because of the impairment of oxygen transport by the blood. Methemoglobin has a characteristic brown color that becomes grossly noticeable when the methemoglobin concentration of the blood exceeds 20 to 30% of the total hemoglobin.

The concentration of methemoglobin formed in the blood of fish is related to the rate nitrite enters the bloodstream and the rate the resultant methemoglobin is reduced to hemoglobin either spontaneously or by NADH-dependent methemoglobin reductase. There is considerable variation among fish species in the rates and mechanism of nitrite uptake and in methemoglobin reductase activity. Furthermore, rates of nitrite uptake are influenced by environmental factors such as temperature, pH, and environmental chloride concentration. These modifying factors make defining a "safe" nitrite concentration difficult, even for an individual species. Generally, freshwater-inhabiting species of the Salmonidae, Ictaluridae, Cichlidae, and Cyprinidae are quite susceptible to nitrite toxicosis, and nitrite-nitrogen concentrations less than 0.5 mg/L may cause acute methemoglobinemia if environmental chloride concentrations are low. Species of the Percidae, Esocidae, and Centrarchidae are more tolerant, and saltwater fish are generally at the lowest risk to nitrite toxicosis because of the inhibiting effect of environmental chloride on nitrite uptake. The toxicology of nitrite is reviewed by Freeman et al. (1983), Tomasso (1986), Lewis and Morris (1986), and Williams and Eddy (1986).

Diazotization Method for Nitrite

Under acid conditions, nitrite (as nitrous acid) reacts with a diazotizing reagent to form a diazonium salt. The diazonium salt is coupled with an aromatic compound to form highly colored pinkish red azo dyes. In the method given here, sulfanilamide is the diazotizing reagent and N-(1-napthyl)-ethylenediamine dihydrochloride is the coupling reagent. Spectrophotometric measurements can be made without dilution in the range of 0.01 to 0.2 mg/L nitrite-nitrogen with a 1-cm light path length. Modifications of this method, often substituting chromotropic acid as the coupling agent, are used in test kit methods for nitrite.

Chemical interferences are unlikely because nitrite and interfering compounds seldom coexist. The presence of color in the sample can cause positive interference but can be compensated for photometrically by adding only the sulfanilamide reagent to a separate sample and using this as a blank.

Sample, Storage, and Preparation

Samples should be analyzed within 1 to 2 hours after collection to prevent bacterial conversion of nitrite to nitrate or ammonia. Filtered samples can be stored refrigerated for 24 hours, or for up to 2 days by either freezing or adding 40 mg $HgCl_2$/L and refrigerating. Do not use acid to preserve samples for nitrite analysis. Samples should be filtered through Whatman 42 or equivalent filter paper or vacuum filtered through Whatman GF-C, or equivalent, glass-fiber filters. Filter about 75 ml, discarding the first 20 ml of filtrate.

Diazotizing reagent is prepared by diluting 50 ml concentrated HCl to about 300 ml with distilled water. Dissolve 5 g sulfanilamide and dilute to 500 ml. This solution is stable for several months.

The coupling reagent is made by dissolving 500 mg of N-(1-napthyl)-ethylenediamine dihydrochloride in 500 ml distilled water. This reagent should be replaced when it turns dark brown.

The standard nitrite-nitrogen solution (1.0 mg/L) is made by dissolving 0.4925 g sodium nitrite, $NaNO_2$, in 1000 ml distilled water to give a 100-mg/L NO_2^--N solution. Dilute 10.0 ml of the 100-mg/L solution to 1000 ml with distilled water to give 1.0 mg/L NO_2^--N. These solutions deteriorate rapidly and must be prepared fresh.

Procedure

Measure 50 ml of filtered sample into a 125-ml Erlenmeyer flask. Add 1.0 ml diazotizing reagent and swirl to mix allowing 2 to 4 minutes for a complete reaction. Add 1.0 ml of coupling reagent and mix. Let the solution stand at least 10 minutes, but not more than 2 hours, to form the azo compound. Measure the absorbance of the lavender color spectrophotometrically at 543 nm in a 1-cm cuvette. Use a reagent blank to set the spectrophotometer at 0.00 absorbance. Obtain the nitrite-nitrogen concentration from a calibration graph generated from running nitrite standards made as shown in Table 13–6 through the same procedure. Redetermine the calibration curve for each new batch of reagents.

TABLE 13–6. Preparation of Nitrite-Nitrogen Standards for Use in a 1-cm Cuvette

Nitrite-Nitrogen (mg/L)	ml of 1 mg/L Nitrite-Nitrogen Standard Diluted to 100 ml
0.00	0.00
0.02	2.00
0.04	4.00
0.06	6.00
0.08	8.00
0.10	10.00
0.15	15.00
0.20	20.00

NITRATE

The nitrate (NO_3^-) content of most ground and surface water rarely exceeds 5 mg/L NO_3^--N. Higher concentrations are found in some ground water as the result of pollution in the aquifer recharge zone. Nitrate can accumulate in aquaria and other closed water-recirculating fish culture systems because nitrate is the final product in the nitrification of ammonia entering the water in fish excretory products. Nitrate is the least toxic of the inorganic nitrogen compounds to aquatic animals, and 96-hour LC_{50} values invariably exceed 1000 mg/L NO_3^--N (Colt and Armstrong, 1981). Acute lethal $NaNO_3$ concentrations for freshwater fish are comparable to lethal NaCl concentrations, indicating that toxicity of nitrate is related to effects on osmoregulation at high solute concentrations. However, little is known of the effects of fish of long-term exposure to lower concentrations of nitrate. Measurements of environmental nitrate are important when conditioning biological nitrification filters in recycled systems to ensure that ammonia is being oxidized to nitrate. Analysis for nitrate can also be used indirectly to assess the suitability of ground water as a supply for large-scale fish culture. Concentrations of nitrate-nitrogen over 10 mg/L may indicate pollution of the ground water with industrial or agricultural wastes and the water may contain toxic substances, even though the nitrate itself is harmless.

Cadmium Reduction Method for Nitrate

Nitrate in a filtered sample of water is reduced almost quantitatively to nitrite after passing through a column containing cadmium granules loosely coated with metallic copper. The nitrite thus produced as well as any nitrite initially present are determined by diazotizing with sulfanilamide and coupling with N-(1-napthyl)-ethylenediamine to form a highly colored dye, as described in the procedures for determining nitrite. A separate determination is made of any nitrite initially present in the sample and subtracted from that found after cadmium reduction to obtain the nitrate-nitrogen concentration. Concentrations of nitrate plus nitrite-nitrogen in the range 0.01 to 0.2 mg/L can be determined, without dilution, using a 1-cm light path length.

The cadmium reduction method is the most sensitive and reliable method available for routine determination of nitrate. This method is also the basis for most portable test kit determinations of nitrate but is usually simplified for field testing by adding cadmium directly to the sample rather than using the more reliable reduction column technique.

Chemical interferences (other than by nitrite) with the cadmium reduction method are unlikely in samples from natural water or fish culture systems. Background color in the sample causes false high absorbances, but this can be photometrically com-

pensated for by adding only sulfanilamide to a separate reduced sample and using this as a blank.

Sample Storage and Preparation

Samples should be analyzed within 1 to 2 hours after collection. Filtered samples can be refrigerated and stored for a day or two; frozen samples are stable for weeks. Do not use cellulosic membrane filters unless they are thoroughly washed because they may contaminate the samples with traces of nitrate. Avoid using $HgCl_2$ as a preservative because the mercuric ion deactivates the cadmium reduction column over time.

A reduction column can be constructed from common laboratory glassware, but it is more convenient to purchase a column specially constructed for nitrate analysis (Fig. 13–9). The column must then be filled with copper-coated cadmium granules. Pre-

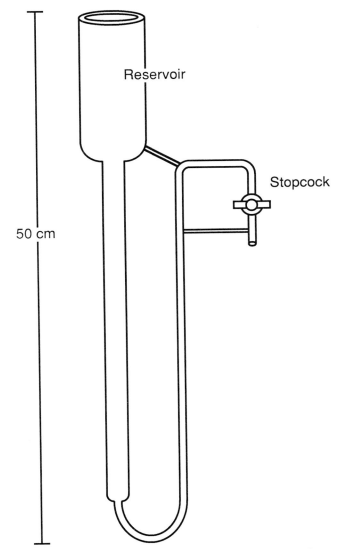

FIGURE 13–9. Glass column used in nitrate analysis (Anderson Glass Co., Fitzwilliams, New Hampshire).

pare the Cu-Cd granules by washing 50 g of cadmium granules (40- to 60-mesh) with 6N HCl and then rinsing copiously with distilled water. Add 250 ml of a 2% solution of copper sulfate pentahydrate, $CuSO_4 \cdot 5H_2O$, and swirl until the blue color fades. Wash the Cu-Cd granules at least 10 times with distilled water. Plug the bottom of the reduction column with very fine copper turnings or glass wool and fill the column with water. Add Cu-Cd granules to produce a column about 30 cm long. Add a small plug of copper or glass wool at the top of the column. Wash the column thoroughly by passing through several 100-mL portions of dilute ammonium chloride solution (6.25 g NH_4Cl/L of distilled water) at a flow of 7 to 10 ml/minute. Activate the column by passing through at least five washes of 100 ml of 0.20 mg/L nitrate-nitrogen standard to which has been added 2 ml of concentrated ammonium chloride solution (250 g NH_4Cl/L of distilled water).

The 0.20 mg/L nitrate-nitrogen standard is prepared fresh daily from a 100-mg/L stock nitrate-nitrogen solution. Make the stock solution by dissolving 0.6072 sodium nitrate, $NaNO_3$, in distilled water and diluting to 1000 ml. This solution can be stored refrigerated for several months. Prepare the standard by diluting 10.0 ml of the 100 mg/L NO_3^--N stock solution to 100 ml with distilled water to give a 10-mg/L NO_3^--N solution. Dilute 10 ml of this solution to 500 ml to give the 0.20-mg/L NO_3^--N standard.

Procedure

Measure 100 ml of filtered sample into a 125-ml Erlenmeyer flask and mix in 2 ml of concentrated ammonium chloride solution. Pour about 5 ml of the sample onto the top of the column and let it pass through. Add the remainder of sample and collect at a rate of 7 to 10 ml/minute. Discard the first 30 to 40 ml, and collect 50 ml of sample in the original sample flask. The procedure from this point is identical to the diazotization method for nitrite. Carry 100 ml of 0.20-mg/L NO_3^--N standard through the procedure with each set of samples. Reduction efficiency varies among columns, so if more than one column is to be used, carry a standard for each column and use it to calculate nitrate concentrations for that particular column: nitrate + nitrite-nitrogen (mg/L) = 0.20 (A_1/A_2), where A_1 is the absorbance of the sample and A_2 is the absorbance of the standard. Nitrate-nitrogen is calculated by measuring the nitrite-nitrogen concentration in a part of the sample not run through the column and subtracting this value from the combined nitrate and nitrite-nitrogen value obtained from the sample run through the cadmium column.

There is no need to wash the column between samples, but if columns are not to be used for several hours, wash with 50 ml dilute ammonium chloride. Store columns in this solution and never allow the Cu-Cd granules to dry. The column becomes deactivated with continual use, leading to poor reduction efficiency. Verify reduction efficiency every 10 to 20

samples by comparing a nitrite standard to a reduced nitrate standard of the same concentration. If reduction efficiency is below 75%, reactivate columns by stripping the copper with acid and recoating the cadmium granules (Strickland and Parsons, 1972; American Public Health Association, 1989).

CHLORIDE

Chloride (Cl^-) is usually the major anion in water of high salinity, and as a contributor to salinity it is important in the culture of brackish water or marine species. However, chloride influences the survival and growth of some euryhaline fish species in fresh water, and this effect is somewhat independent of the general contribution of chloride to salinity. For instance, when juvenile red drum are cultured in water of low salinity, survival is maximized when environmental chloride concentrations are greater than about 125 mg/L, regardless of the salinity (Miranda and Sonski, 1986). In fresh water, the concentration of environmental chloride usually is of minor concern as a factor in fish health. However, concentrations of chloride greater than about 20 mg/L are desirable in intensive freshwater fish culture systems and aquaria because chloride counteracts nitrite toxicosis in some fish (Lewis and Morris, 1986).

Measurement of chloride concentration alone is seldom required in seawater analyses and is difficult because bromide and iodide interfere with most analytical methods. However, a related quantity, chlorinity, is often measured and used to calculate salinity. The procedure for determination of chlorinity is similar to the silver nitrate titrimetric method for the determination of chloride in fresh water, but it also includes bromide and iodide, both reported as chloride. Procedures for measurement of chlorinity are described by Strickland and Parsons (1972) and the American Public Health Association et al. (1989).

Three methods are routinely used to measure the chloride concentration of fresh water: the silver nitrate method, the mercuric nitrate method, and the potentiometric method (American Public Health Association et al., 1989). Potentiometric titration probably is the most accurate and reliable method, but it requires a special silver billet indicating electrode. The silver nitrate and mercuric nitrate titration procedures are similar in sensitivity and accuracy, and selection is a matter of personal preference, although the endpoint of the mercuric nitrate procedure is easier to detect. Both procedures are used in portable test kit methods.

Mercuric Nitrate Method for Chloride

Mercuric ion reacts with chloride to form slightly dissociated mercuric chloride. The endpoint of the titration is indicated by diphenylcarbazone, which changes color in the presence of excess mercuric ion. The sharpness of the endpoint is highly pH dependent, so the sample is acidified to pH 2.3 to 2.8 with nitric acid, HNO_3. Xylene cyanol FF is added to the indicator solution as an endpoint enhancer and pH indicator.

Sampling, Storage, and Preparation

No special precautions are needed during sampling and samples can be stored for at least a month before analysis. Samples with high chloride concentrations can be diluted with distilled water to reduce the titrant used to a convenient volume.

To prepare the indicator solution, dissolve, in the order named, 250 mg of s-diphenylcarbazone, 4.0 ml of concentrated nitric acid, and 30 mg of xylene cyanol FF in 100 ml of 95% ethyl alcohol. Store this in a dark bottle and discard it when the color changes from blue-green to brown.

The standard sodium chloride solution, 0.0141 N, is made by dissolving 0.8241 g of dried NaCl (190°C, 2 hours) in distilled water and diluting to 1000 ml.

Standard mercuric nitrate titrant is made by dissolving 2.3 g $Hg(NO_3)_2$ in about 100 ml of distilled water in a 1000-ml volumetric flask. Add 0.25 ml of concentrated nitric acid and dilute to volume. Standardize this solution against the 0.0141N NaCl solution by pipetting 10.0 ml of the NaCl solution into a 250-ml Erlenmeyer flask. Dilute to about 100 ml with distilled water and add 10 mg sodium bicarbonate, $NaHCO_3$. Add 1.0 ml of indicator and titrate with the standard mercuric nitrate until the solution turns from green-blue to blue. Slowly continue the titration to a definite purple end point. Titrate a reagent blank containing 100 ml of distilled water, 10 mg $NaHCO_3$, and 1 ml of indicator solution. The normality of the standard mercuric nitrate solution is equal to 0.141 divided by the volume in milliliters of mercuric nitrate used to titrate the NaCl solution minus the volume in milliliters of mercuric nitrate used to titrate the blank.

Procedure

Measure 100 ml of water sample into a 250-ml Erlenmeyer flask and add 1.0 ml of indicator. For most fresh water, the pH of the solution at this point will be in the proper range of 2.3 to 2.8 and the color will be green-blue. A light green color indicates that the pH is too low; a pure blue color indicates that the pH is too high. The pH should be adjusted to be within the proper range with 0.1 N HNO_3 or 0.1 N NaOH. The pH of the solution can also be checked with the appropriate narrow range pH test paper and adjusted accordingly. Titrate to a definite purple color with the mercuric nitrate titrant. Also titrate a reagent blank containing 100 ml of distilled water, 10 mg $NaHCO_3$, and 1.0 ml of indicator solution.

$$\text{Chloride Concentration (mg/L)} = \frac{(Vs - Vb)\ (N)\ (35,450)}{(\text{Sample Volume in ml})}$$

where Vs = the sample titration in ml
Vb = the blank titration in ml
N = the normality of the mercuric nitrate titrant

CHLORINE

Chlorine is added to public water supplies and waste water as an oxidizing agent and a disinfectant. Chlorine is applied as a gas (Cl_2) or as salts of hypochlorous acid (HOCl), such as sodium hypochlorite, NaOCl, or calcium hypochlorite, $Ca(OCl)_2$, also called HTH or high-test hypochlorite. The salts dissociate to yield hypochlorite ion, for example:

$$Ca(OCl)_2 + H_2O = Ca^{2+} + H_2O + 2OCl^-$$

Chlorine gas reacts with water to form hypochlorous and hydrochloric acid:

$$Cl_2 + H_2O = HOCl + H^+ + Cl^-$$

The end result, whether chlorine is added as a gas or salt, is similar because hypochlorous acid and hypochlorite establish a pH- and temperature-dependent equilibrium:

$$HOCl = OCl^- + H^+$$

Hypochlorous acid is the dominant species below pH 7.5 at 25°C; hypochlorite predominates above pH 7.5. Hypochlorous acid has far more disinfecting ability and is more toxic to fish than hypochlorite. The sum of the concentrations of Cl_2, HOCl, and OCl^-, expressed in milligrams per liter as Cl_2, is referred to as free chlorine or free residual chlorine.

Hypochlorous acid or chlorine react with ammonia to form chloramines:

$$NH_3 + HOCl = NH_2Cl + H_2O \text{ (monochloramine)}$$
$$NH_3 + 2HOCl = NHCl_2 + 2H_2O \text{ (dichloramine)}$$
$$NH_3 + 3HOCl = NCl_3 + 3H_2O \text{ (trichloramine)}$$

The amount of each chloramine formed depends on pH and the relative amounts of chlorine and ammonia. Mono- and dichloramine have disinfecting power and are also toxic to fish. The sum of the concentrations of mono-, di-, and trichloramine, expressed in milligrams per liter as Cl_2, is referred to as combined chlorine or combined residual chlorine. Total chlorine, or total residual chlorine, is the sum of free chlorine and combined chlorine.

Fish are exposed to chlorine when incompletely dechlorinated municipal water supplies are used to hold them, or when chlorinated effluents are added to natural waters. The most common forms of chlorine found in natural water are HOCl, OCl^-, NH_2Cl, and $NHCl_2$. Generally, HOCl and $NHCl_2$ are the most toxic forms to fish, followed by NH_2Cl and OCl^- (Brooks and Bartos, 1984). Toxicity also varies with fish species, duration of exposure, temperature, and other water-quality conditions. Analysis for each form of chlorine is too laborious for routine environmental monitoring. For these reasons, water-quality criteria are often based on total residual chlorine.

The United States Environmental Protection Agency (1976) recommends that maximum total residual chlorine concentration for long-term exposure not exceed 0.002 mg/L for salmonids and 0.01 mg/L for other aquatic organisms.

Eight methods are described by the American Public Health Association et al. (1989) for the determination of free, combined, and total residual chlorine. The DPD colorimetric method for total residual chlorine described below is the most widely used method. Most portable test kit methods are also based on the DPD method.

DPD Method for Total Residual Chlorine

Hypochlorous acid and hypochlorite oxidize N,N-diethyl-p-phenylenediamine (DPD) to produce a magenta color. The reaction is pH dependent and the solution must be buffered in the range of 6.2 to 6.5 for accurate, repeatable results. Total residual chlorine is determined by adding iodide to the reaction mixture. Iodide is oxidized to iodine by chloramines; the iodine liberated then reacts with DPD to form the magenta color. Absorbance at 515 nm is measured, and the concentration of total residual chlorine is then determined from a calibration curve prepared by reacting DPD with potassium permanganate standards of known chlorine equivalence.

Sampling, Storage, and Preparation

No special precautions are needed during sampling, but chlorine in an aqueous solution is not stable and measurements must be made immediately after sampling. Exposure to strong light or agitation will accelerate the reduction of chlorine. Samples should not be filtered before analysis; turbidity and background color are compensated by incorporating a turbidity or color blank into the procedure.

Prepare the phosphate buffer solution required for this assay by dissolving 24 g anhydrous Na_2HPO_4 and 46 g anhydrous KH_2PO_4 in 500 ml distilled water in a 1000-ml volumetric flask. Dissolve 0.8 g disodium ethylenediaminetetraacetic acid (EDTA) in about 100 ml distilled water and add it to the 1000-ml volumetric flask. Add 20 mg mercuric chloride, $HgCl_2$, to the contents of the flask to inhibit mold growth, then dilute the contents to 1000 ml with distilled water. This buffer is stable for months.

N,N-Diethyl-p-phenylenediamine (DPD) solution for this assay is made by dissolving 1 g DPD oxalate in 100 ml of distilled water in a 1000-ml volumetric flask. Add 8 ml of a solution prepared from 1 part concentrated H_2SO_4 and 3 parts distilled water. Then add 200 mg disodium EDTA and dilute contents to 1000 ml. Store in the dark and discard when solution becomes discolored.

Procedure

Add 5 ml of the phosphate buffer solution and 5 ml DPD solution to a 250-ml Erlenmeyer flask. Add 100 ml of sample and mix. Immediately add about 1 g of potassium iodide, KI, crystals from a calibrated scoop and mix to dissolve the crystals. Let stand about 2 minutes and transfer to a 1-cm cuvette or cell and measure the absorbance spectrophotometrically at 515 nm. Use a distilled water reagent blank or a corresponding color or turbidity blank to set the spectrophotometer at 0.00 absorbance. Obtain the total residual chlorine concentration from the calibration graph.

The standards used to prepare the calibration graph are prepared by diluting aliquots of a potassium permanganate stock solution to obtain a series of chlorine-equivalent concentrations (Table 13–7). The stock solution is made by dissolving 0.891 g $KMnO_4$ in distilled water in a 1000-ml volumetric flask and diluting to volume. Pipet 10.0 ml of this solution into a 100-ml volumetric flask and dilute to volume. This solution must be made immediately before preparing the calibration standards. Measure 100-ml portions of each calibration standard and develop the color as described above. Use the 0.00 mg/L chlorine-equivalent solution to set the spectrophotometer at 0.00 absorbance. Plot absorbance versus chlorine equivalent concentrations (in milligrams per liter as Cl_2) to obtain the calibration graph.

HYDROGEN SULFIDE

Hydrogen sulfide (H_2S) is a soluble gas that smells like rotten eggs. It is produced under anoxic conditions by anaerobic bacteria, chiefly species of *Desulfovibrio*. Sulfides are readily oxidized to sulfate in the presence of oxygen, and sulfide is rarely detected in aerobic surface water. However, total dissolved sulfide-sulfur concentrations may exceed 10 mg/L in the anaerobic bottom water of lakes and reservoirs. If this water is discharged into rivers, sulfide may be detectable for miles downstream. Sulfide can also be present in rivers and streams as a waste product from industries such as paper mills, chemical plants, and oil refineries. Ground water often contains hydrogen sulfide, and hot springs, deep seawater aquifers, and oil-field brines may have unusually high total sulfide-sulfur concentrations, some over 100 mg/L.

TABLE 13–7. Preparation of Potassium Permanganate, $KMnO_4$, Standards for Calibration of DPD Method for Total Residual Chlorine*

Chlorine Equivalence (mg Cl_2/L)	ml of $KMnO_4$ Stock Solution Diluted to 500 ml
0.00	0.00
0.05	0.25
0.10	0.50
0.20	1.00
0.50	2.50
1.00	5.00
2.00	10.00

*These standards are suitable for use in a 1-cm cuvette.

Hydrogen sulfide is very toxic to fish. Fry apparently are the most sensitive life stage of fish to hydrogen sulfide toxicosis (Bonn and Follis, 1967; Smith et al., 1976). Because of the extremely toxic nature of hydrogen sulfide, hydrogen sulfide-sulfur concentrations for hatchery water supplies should not exceed 0.1 µg/L for optimum growth and survival of most fish species (Piper et al., 1982). The United States Environmental Protection Agency (1976) suggests that exposure to concentrations of hydrogen sulfide-sulfur greater than 2 µg/L constitutes a long-term health hazard for fish.

Hydrogen sulfide-sulfur concentrations are calculated from concentrations of total dissolved sulfide-sulfur and measurements of pH and temperature. Hydrogen sulfide is in a pH- and temperature-dependent equilibrium with HS^- and S^{2-}. Both HS^- and S^{2-} are relatively nontoxic to fish. The proportion of total dissolved sulfide present as H_2S increases as pH and temperature decrease.

Two methods are available for routine measurements of total dissolved sulfide. The iodometric titration method (American Public Health Association et al., 1989) is simple but lacks the sensitivity required to measure the low concentrations of sulfide of interest in fish health investigations. The methylene blue colorimetric method (Strickland and Parsons, 1972) is more sensitive and accurate. Calibration of the method is involved, but subsequent measurements of sulfide are fairly simple. Variations of the methylene blue method also are used in portable test kit procedures for sulfide measurement.

Methylene Blue Method for Total Sulfide

The total dissolved sulfide-sulfur concentration is determined by acidifying the sample to convert all sulfide to hydrogen sulfide. Hydrogen sulfide reacts with N,N-dimethyl-p-phenylenediamine and ferric chloride to form the dye methylene blue. Ammonium phosphate is added after color development to remove the ferric chloride color. The amount of methylene blue formed is proportional to the total sulfide concentration in the original sample and is measured spectrophotometrically. Measurements can be made in the range of 0.10 to 2.0 mg/L sulfide-sulfur using a 1-cm light path length. Sensitivity is improved by incorporating a preconcentration step where sulfide is precipitated under alkaline conditions as zinc sulfide. This step is also useful for short-term sample preservation before analysis. Hydrogen sulfide is calculated from total sulfide, pH, and temperature.

Sampling, Storage, and Preparation

Sulfide is rapidly oxidized in the presence of dissolved oxygen and samples must be collected to minimize contact with the atmosphere. Samples collected in a Kemmerer or Van Dorn sampler should be transferred to a 300-ml BOD bottle by inserting the drain tube to the bottom of the BOD bottle, filling the bottle, and allowing two bottle-volumes to over-

flow before stoppering. Samples should be analyzed within an hour of collection or preserved with zinc acetate. Preserved samples should be analyzed within 6 hours of collection.

The following reagents are required for sample pretreatment, a zinc acetate solution of 22 g $Zn(C_2H_3O_2)_2 \cdot 2H_2O$ dissolved in 87 ml of distilled water and a sodium hydroxide solution of 24 g NaOH dissolved in distilled water and diluted to 100 ml. Pipet 0.5 ml of zinc acetate solution beneath the surface of the sample in the BOD bottle. Restopper with no air bubbles and mix by inverting the bottle several times. Pipet 0.3 ml of sodium hydroxide solution again beneath the surface, restopper, and mix. A white precipitate will form and the sample is then stable for several hours. If the sulfide concentration is high enough to be measured without concentrating the sample, let the precipitate settle for at least 30 minutes, decant as much of the supernatant as possible, and refill the bottle with distilled water. Resuspend the precipitate and withdraw a sample for analysis.

Very low sulfide levels require the sample to be concentrated. Decant the supernatant and quantitatively transfer the precipitate to a 100-ml graduated glass cylinder. Rinse the BOD bottle with three small volumes of distilled water from a wash bottle and add the rinses to the cylinder. Record the volume in the cylinder. Resuspend the precipitate, withdraw a sample, and proceed with the analysis. Multiply the result by the ratio of final volume to initial volume. For routine analysis, it is assumed that a BOD bottle has an initial volume of 300 ml. The actual volume of these bottles is usually within a few percent points of 300 ml, and this error, and the slight error introduced by adding 0.8 ml of zinc acetate plus sodium hydroxide, are not significant.

Procedure

You will need the following reagents to perform a sulfide analysis:

1. Sulfuric acid solution, 1 + 1: Cautiously add 500 ml concentrated H_2SO_4 to 500 ml distilled water with continuous mixing. Allow to cool before using.

2. Amine-sulfuric acid stock reagent: Dissolve 27 g N,N-dimethyl-p-phenylenediamine oxalate in a cold mixture of 50 ml concentrated sulfuric acid and 20 ml distilled water. Cool and dilute to 100 ml with distilled water. Store in a dark glass bottle.

3. Amine-sulfuric acid reagent: Dilute 25 ml amine-sulfuric acid stock solution with 975 ml 1 + 1 H_2SO_4.

4. Ferric chloride solution: Dissolve 100 g $FeCl_3 \cdot 6H_2O$ in 40 ml distilled water.

5. Diammonium hydrogen phosphate solution: Dissolve 40 g $(NH_4)_2HPO_4$ in 80 ml of distilled water.

Transfer 7.5 ml of the sample to each of two 10-ml mixing cylinders or two test tubes using a wide-mouth pipet. To the first cylinder add 0.5 ml amine-sulfuric acid reagent and 3 drops of ferric chloride solution. Immediately stopper and mix by slowly inverting the cylinder once. To the second cylinder add 0.5 ml 1 + 1 H_2SO_4 and 3 drops of ferric chloride solution and mix. If sulfide is present, a blue color will develop in the first cylinder. After 5 minutes add 1.6 ml of diammonium hydrogen phosphate solution to each cylinder. After 3 minutes, but before 15 minutes, transfer the contents of the second cylinder to a 1-cm cell or cuvette and zero the absorbance of the color in a spectrophotometer at 664 nm. Then measure the absorbance of the blue color in the first cylinder. Refer to the calibration graph to obtain the total sulfide-sulfur concentration.

Preparation of the Calibration Graph

The following reagents are required to prepare the calibration graph:

1. Stock sulfide-sulfur solution, 1 g/L: Dissolve 7.5 g $Na_2S \cdot 9H_2O$ in boiled, cooled distilled water. Dilute to 1000 ml in a volumetric flask. Prepare fresh before using.

2. Standard sulfide-sulfur solution, approximately 20 mg/L: Dilute 20 ml stock sulfide solution to 1000 ml with boiled, cooled distilled water.

3. Starch indicator: Add 2 g soluble starch to 100 ml of distilled water in a 250-ml beaker. Heat slowly on a hot plate until transparent and add 0.5 ml formalin as a preservative.

4. Standard sodium thiosulfate titrant, approximately 0.025N: Dissolve 6.21 g $Na_2S_2O_3 \cdot 5H_2O$ in distilled water. Add 0.4 g NaOH and dilute to 1000 ml.

5. Standard potassium dichromate solution, 0.025N: Dissolve 1.226 g $K_2Cr_2O_7$ in distilled water, dilute to 1000 ml.

6. Iodine solution, approximately 0.025N: Dissolve 20 to 25 g potassium iodide (KI) in a little distilled water and add 3.13 g iodine. After the iodine has dissolved, dilute to 1000 ml.

First the 0.025N thiosulfate titrant is standardized by dissolving 2 g KI in a 250-ml Erlenmeyer flask with 100 ml distilled water. Add 10 ml of a solution of 1 part concentrated H_2SO_4 and 9 parts distilled water. Then add 20 ml standard 0.025N dichromate solution and place in the dark for 5 minutes. Dilute to 200 ml and titrate with 0.025N thiosulfate solution until a pale straw color is reached. Add 8 drops of starch indicator and titrate until the blue color of the indicator suddenly disappears. Calculate the normality of the thiosulfate titrant by dividing 0.5 by the volume of thiosulfate in milliliters used in the titration.

Next standardize the approximately 20 mg/L sulfide-sulfur solution by pipetting 100 ml of the standard sulfide solution into a 250-ml Erlenmeyer flask. Immediately add 10.0 ml of the approximately 0.025N iodine solution and 2 drops concentrated HCl. Titrate the residual iodine with the standardized thiosulfate titrant using starch indicator as described above. Record the volume used in the titration. Prepare a blank by combining 100 ml of distilled water, 10.0 ml of the approximately 0.025N iodine

solution, and 2 drops of concentrated HCl and titrate again. Calculate the exact concentration (mg/L) of sulfide-sulfur in the solution:

$$\text{sulfide-sulfur (mg/L)} = 160N(B-A),$$

where N is the normality of thiosulfate titrant previously determined, B is the ml of thiosulfate used in the blank titration, and A is the milliliters of thiosulfate used in the sulfide titration.

Aliquots of the standardized sulfide solution diluted to 100 ml with boiled and cooled distilled water are used to obtain a series of sulfide-sulfur concentrations from 0.0 to 2.0 mg/L sulfide-sulfur. Pipet 7.5 ml of each standard into a 10-ml mixing cylinder and add 0.5 ml amine-sulfuric acid reagent and 3 drops of ferric acetate solution. Stopper and slowly invert once to mix. After 5 minutes, add 1.6 ml of diammonium hydrogen phosphate to each cylinder. After 3 minutes, but before 15 minutes, measure the absorbance at 664 nm. Zero the spectrophotometer with the 0 mg/L solution. Plot absorbance versus sulfide-sulfur concentration.

Calculation of Hydrogen Sulfide

The percentages of un-ionized hydrogen sulfide (H_2S) in fresh water or seawater (Table 13–8) at different pH values and temperatures were calculated from the equilibrium expression for the reaction,

$$H_2S = HS^- + H^+$$

using equilibrium constants as a function of temperature and conductivity (American Public Health Association et al., 1989).

To calculate hydrogen sulfide-sulfur concentration, measure the total dissolved sulfide-sulfur concentration and the pH and temperature of the water at the time of sample collection. Find the percentage

TABLE 13–8. Percentage Hydrogen Sulfide in Freshwater (salinity <0.5 ppt) or Seawater (salinity 33–37 ppt) at Different pH Values and Temperatures

| | Freshwater Temperature (°C) | | | |
pH	15	20	25	30
5.0	99.3	99.2	99.1	98.9
5.5	99.7	97.4	97.0	96.5
6.0	93.5	92.3	91.1	89.7
6.5	81.7	79.2	76.4	73.4
7.0	58.5	54.6	50.6	46.6
7.5	30.8	27.5	24.4	21.6
8.0	12.4	10.7	9.3	8.0
8.5	4.4	3.7	3.1	2.7
9.0	1.4	1.2	1.0	0.9
	Seawater Temperature (°C)			
pH	15	20	25	30
7.0	51.2	47.1	43.1	39.2
7.5	24.9	22.0	19.3	17.0
8.0	9.5	8.2	7.1	6.1
8.5	3.2	2.7	2.3	2.0
9.0	1.0	0.9	0.8	0.6

hydrogen sulfide on the table from pH and temperature data and divide this number by 100. Multiply the resulting factor by the total dissolved sulfide-sulfur concentration to obtain the hydrogen sulfide-sulfur concentration.

TOTAL GAS PRESSURE

All atmospheric gases are dissolved to some extent in water. Total gas pressure is the sum of the partial pressures of all gases in solution. Equilibrium conditions occur when total gas pressure is equal to local barometric pressure ($\Delta P = O$). When total gas pressure is greater than barometric pressure ($\Delta P > O$), the water is supersaturated and gases tend to come out of solution. When total gas pressure is less than barometric pressure ($\Delta P < O$), the water is undersaturated and gases tend to enter the water from the atmosphere. Gas saturation is sometimes reported as a percentage of local barometric pressure (BP):

$$\% \text{ Total Gas Pressure} = \frac{BP + \Delta P}{BP} \times 100$$

For example, assume the local barometric pressure is 760 mm Hg and the ΔP is 38 mm Hg. The total gas pressure is 105% of saturation.

Gas bubble trauma (also called gas bubble disease) occurs in fish living in supersaturated waters. Supersaturation is an unstable condition, and as gases come out of solution they form bubbles. If the gases in solution diffuse across the gills of fish before coming out of solution, emboli will be formed in the vascular system and other tissues. Acute gas bubble trauma occurs at high levels of supersaturation, usually at ΔP values greater than 76 mm Hg (about 110% saturation at sea level). Acute gas bubble trauma is caused by vascular emboli that restrict blood flow, resulting in tissue anoxia. Mortality may be high over short (a few days) exposure. Chronic gas bubble trauma may occur after long-term exposure to positive ΔP values less than 76 mm Hg. Chronic gas bubble trauma is associated with hyperinflation of the swim bladder and extravascular emboli in the gut and buccal cavity. Mortality is usually less than 5% over extended time periods and may be related to secondary, stress-related infections.

The actual development of acute or chronic gas bubble trauma varies with a number of biological and physical factors (Weitkamp and Katz, 1980; Colt, 1986). Tolerance to gas supersaturation varies with fish species and developmental stage. Warm-water fish are generally more tolerant than cold-water fish; eggs of most species are very tolerant to supersaturation and juveniles are usually least tolerant. The development of gas bubble trauma is also related to the composition of the gases in solution. Gas bubble trauma is more likely as the partial pressure ratio of (nitrogen + argon):oxygen increases because the contribution of oxygen partial pressure to ΔP is somewhat moderated by the biological uptake of oxygen within the fish.

One of the most important factors affecting the development of gas bubble trauma is the depth at which the fish is positioned in the water column. The deeper the fish, the less actual ΔP the fish experiences because of the hydrostatic pressure of the overlying water. In fresh water at 20°C, ΔP is reduced by 74 mm Hg for every meter beneath the surface (Colt, 1984). This explains why animals confined to shallow water, such as fishes in hatcheries, are particularly susceptible to gas bubble trauma. These fishes cannot increase their depth, so that hydrostatic pressure can reduce the effect of a high ΔP.

Gas supersaturation can be caused by a variety of processes. Much ground water is supersaturated because the water in the aquifer is under considerable hydrostatic pressure and atmospheric gases in the recharge zone are driven into solution. The ΔP of ground water ranges from negative values to over 500 mm Hg. Surface water becomes supersaturated when water passes over a dam or through penstocks and is carried to depth in a plunge basin. At depth, the increased hydrostatic pressure increases the solubility of atmospheric gases and the air goes into solution. Supersaturated conditions also develop when a water source is rapidly heated in a closed system such as occurs in cooling waters for steam electrical generating plants. Gas solubility decreases with increasing temperature, but the volume of gas dissolved in the water remains the same, since these systems are closed to the atmosphere. Supersaturation can also occur if there is an air leak on the low pressure side of a pump in the supply line for an aquaculture facility. The air is drawn in through the leak and mixed with the water. The water is then pressurized after moving through the pump and some of the air is passed into solution. Colt (1986) has reviewed these and numerous other causes and occurrences of gas supersaturation in water.

Membrane-diffusion instruments, or "saturometers" (Fig. 13–10), are convenient and widely used to measure total dissolved gas pressure. The saturometer is simple to use, but 10 to 20 minutes may be required for a single measurement. Other methods, such as volumetric gasometry (Van Slyke and Neill, 1924) and quantitative gas chromatography (Swinnerton et al., 1962), have been used for dissolved gas analysis, but they are time-consuming and require expensive equipment. These methods also require transport of samples from the field for laboratory analysis. Measurements of total gas pressure should be made in situ because diffusion of gases during sampling and transport causes serious errors.

Saturometer Method for Total Gas Pressure

The saturometer is a long length of small-diameter, gas-permeable, dimethyl silicone tubing wound around a frame and connected to a low-volume pressure gauge. Dissolved gases diffuse between the interior of the tubing and the water. Equilibrium is reached between the gas pressure inside and outside

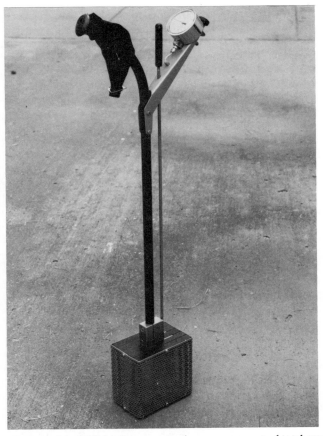

FIGURE 13–10. A Weiss Saturometer for measurement of total gas pressure in water (ECO-Enterprises, Seattle, Washington).

solved oxygen depletions occur most frequently at night when photosynthesis stops and oxygen is rapidly consumed in respiration by the great phytoplankton biomass. Oxygen depletions can also occur during daylight hours when conditions for photosynthesis are poor, such as during extended periods of cloudy weather. Sudden die-offs of dense phytoplankton blooms and subsequent decomposition can also cause oxygen depletion. Bloom die-offs may occur naturally or can be triggered by herbicides applied to the water. Natural die-offs are common in dense blooms dominated by blue-green algae. Die-offs can be recognized by the change in the color of the water from green or green-brown to a gray-brown and the noxious odor of decomposing algae.

Estimates of phytoplankton abundance are of limited usefulness in assessing potential environmental problems. The impact of phytoplankton on the environment is related not only to abundance, but also to the community species composition and physiological state, water temperature, and physical processes such as reaeration and mixing of the water. The effect of phytoplankton on water quality is best assessed by frequent measurements of dissolved oxygen concentrations.

Certain species of marine and freshwater algae produce toxins that can kill fish. Although many species (Table 13–9) have been implicated in fish kills, only a few have been proven directly responsible for natural intoxications. In many instances, fish kills are caused by dissolved oxygen depletion associated with bloom conditions but are mistakenly attributed to algal toxins by the coincident occurrence of suspected toxin-producing algae.

the tubing, and this change in pressure is read on the pressure gauge, relative to local atmospheric pressure, in millimeters of mercury.

Step-by-step instructions for operation of the saturometer provided with the instrument must be followed carefully to ensure accurate measurements. The dimethyl silicone tubing is fragile and the instrument should be frequently tested for pressure leaks.

PHYTOPLANKTON COMMUNITIES

Phytoplankton are minute, autotrophic, chlorophyll-bearing organisms suspended in water. Phytoplankton include certain photosynthetic bacteria (cyanobacteria or blue-green algae) and plants (algae). Phytoplankton are the base of the food chain in most natural waters and are important in oxygenating waters and cycling nutrients. Fish health can be affected when phytoplankton become overabundant, or when the phytoplankton community comprises certain undesirable species.

An overabundance of phytoplankton can indirectly stress or kill fish by depleting the water of dissolved oxygen. Dense phytoplankton blooms often develop in warm, nutrient-rich waters such as fish ponds and polluted lakes and estuaries. Dis-

TABLE 13–9. Algal Species Known or Suspected to Have Caused Toxicosis in Fishes

Pyrrophyta (Dinoflagellates)*	Chrysophyta (Yellow-Green Algae)
Protogonyaulax tamarensis	
Protogonyaulax acatenella	*Prymnesium parvum*
Protogonyaulax catanella	*Ochromonas malhamensis*
Gonyaulax spinifera	(FW)
Gonyaulax polyedra	*Ochromonas danicum* (FW)
Gonyaulax polygramma	*Ochromonas minuta* (FW)
Gessnerium monilatum	
Pyrodinium bahamense	Chlorophyta (Green Algae)
Noctiluca miliaris	*Chaetomorpha minima*
Prorocentrum concavum	
Peridinium polonicum (FW)	Cyanobacteriales (Blue-Green Algae)
Ptychodiscus brevis	
Gymnodinium venificum	*Microcystis aeruginosa* (FW)
Gyrodinium aureolum	*Anabaena flos-aquae* (FW)
Amphidinium klebsii	*Aphanizomenon flos-aquae* (FW)
Amphidinium rhynocephalum	(FW)
Amphidinium carterae	*Oscillatoria agardhii* (FW)
	Oscillatoria rubescens (FW)
	Schizothrix calcicola

Abbreviation: FW = freshwater species; all other are marine or brackish-water species.

*Taxonomy of the dinoflagellates has been in a state of flux for years. The disposition used here is based upon the review by Taylor (1984).

Data from Collins, 1978; Steidinger, 1979; Carmichael and Mahood, 1984; Taylor, 1984; White, 1984.

Certain marine dinoflagellates (most notably species of *Protogonyaulax* and *Pyrodinium*) produce potent neurotoxins, collectively called paralytic shellfish toxins. These organisms occur worldwide and in certain areas populations dramatically increase and cause "red tides." Paralytic shellfish toxins are relatively nontoxic to most invertebrates, but certain vertebrates, including fish, are poisoned when they eat shellfish or crustaceans that have concentrated the toxins while feeding on the toxin-producing dinoflagellates (White, 1984). Fish kills can also result when phytoplanktonivorous fish such as menhaden feed directly on the toxic dinoflagellates. A fish intoxicated by paralytic shellfish toxins swims irregularly and loses equilibrium, followed by immobilization with occasional bursts of hyperactivity. Fish that do not ingest a lethal dose recover within hours with no apparent consequence (White, 1984).

Red tides comprising *Ptychodiscus brevis* cause extensive fish kills in the Gulf of Mexico and perhaps elsewhere. *Ptychodiscus brevis* produces at least two potent neurotoxins (brevetoxins) that are released into the water upon cell lysis (Baden et al., 1984). The mode of action and chemical structures of neurotoxins produced by *P. brevis* differ from paralytic shellfish toxins, but the symptoms of intoxication in fish are similar. Fish become intoxicated after exposure to the toxin or after feeding on *P. brevis* cells during red tides. A related species, *Gyrodinium aureolum*, has been implicated in fish kills, including cage-cultured salmonids, in waters of the north Atlantic (Jones et al., 1982).

The trophont stage of the dinoflagellate *Amyloodinium ocellatum* is parasitic on marine fishes. *Amyloodinium ocellatum* invades primarily the gills, causing inflammation, hemorrhage, and necrosis. The disease is called oodiniasis or velvet disease. It can cause great losses of aquarium fish or fish held in high-density culture systems (Lauckner, 1984). Toxin production by *A. ocellatum* has not been verified. A related freshwater dinoflagellate, *Oodinium* sp., is parasitic on some freshwater fishes (Hoffman, 1970).

Prymnesium parvum is a flagellated, marine alga associated with fish kills in Europe and the Middle East. Waterborne toxins produced by *P. parvum* cause reversible loss of the selective permeability of the gill epithelium, resulting in the uptake of toxins (Shilo, 1981) and osmoregulatory dysfunction. *Prymnesium parvum* occurs in water with salinities of 1.2 to 50.0 ppt; maximum toxin production is found at salinities of about 20 ppt (Padilla, 1970). Blooms of *P. parvum* have caused the large-scale loss of fish in brackish water fish culture ponds in Israel, but losses can be controlled by monitoring toxin levels in ponds and applying aqueous ammonia, which lyses *P. parvum* cells (Shilo, 1981).

Dense blooms of the marine diatom *Chaetoceros* sp. have been associated with the death of Pacific salmon cultured in net-cages (Kennedy, 1978). This diatom does not produce toxins but causes physical damage to gill epithelium. Death of fish follows massive blood loss or secondary infection.

Several species of cyanobacteria (blue-green algae) produce compounds that are extremely toxic to warm-blooded animals (Carmichael and Mahmood, 1984), but documentation of the direct toxicity of blue-green algal blooms to fish is lacking. The toxin of one cyanobacterium, *Microcystis aeruginosa*, is toxic to rainbow trout after intraperitoneal injection, but immersion of fish in cultures of toxin-producing *M. aeruginosa* resulted in no deleterious pathological changes (Phillips et al., 1985).

Sample Collection

Collect samples for the quantification or identification of phytoplankton using any of the common samplers and techniques used to obtain water samples for chemical analysis. Communities of bloom-forming dinoflagellates and blue-green algae tend to be patchy, and many samples may be required to describe their distribution. Steidinger (1979) and the American Public Health Association et al. (1989) discuss sampling plankton communities.

Cell Counts

The abundance of phytoplankton can be estimated by direct cell counts using an appropriate counting chamber under a microscope (American Public Health Association et al., 1989). Direct counts do not adequately represent biomass because algal cells vary greatly in size. Cell counts can be converted to cell volume by measuring the dimensions of the cell and calculating volume using geometric formulas. The resulting data are expressed on a volume to volume basis (such as cubic millimeters per liter) for individual species or summed for all species in the sample to estimate total phytoplankton volume. Cell volume determinations are extremely tedious, and indirect methods are more commonly used to estimate total algal biomass. Chlorophyll A constitutes, on average, about 1.5% of the ash-free dry weight of phytoplankton. Chlorophyll A is determined by extracting the pigments into an organic solvent (usually acetone) and measuring the absorbance of the extract with a spectrophotometer. The chlorophyll A concentration is then calculated using standard formulas (American Public Health Association et al., 1985). The phytoplankton biomass can then be roughly estimated by multiplying the chlorophyll A concentration by 67.

Identification of Algae

Identification of algae is based primarily on morphological characteristics. Identification even to the genus level is difficult, particularly for dinoflagellates. Samples collected as part of fish health investigations must be examined by a competent taxonomist for a meaningful identification. Store samples temporarily in the dark at ambient temperature in

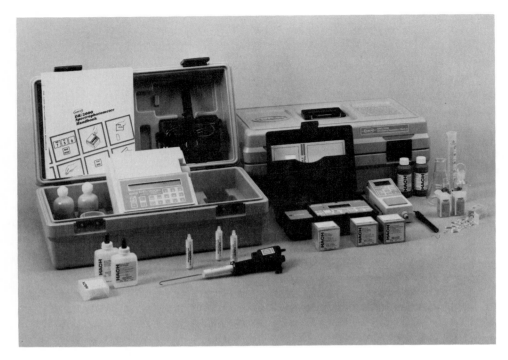

FIGURE 13–11. A portable water quality test kit with reagents and apparatus for 29 different tests (DREL/2000, Hach Company, Loveland, Colorado).

partially filled glass or plastic bottles. Do not refrigerate or ice the samples, and handle carefully because some species, such as *Ptychodiscus brevis*, are delicate and lyse under extremes of temperature. Have the sample examined as soon after collection as possible. If examination is not possible within 24 hours, preserve seawater samples with 5 ml of 50% gluteraldehyde to 100 ml of sample or with 0.5 ml buffered formalin to 100 ml of sample. Buffered formalin is prepared by supersaturating formalin with sodium tetraborate, $Na_2B_4O_7 \cdot 10H_2O$. Freshwater samples can be preserved with 0.3 ml Lugol's solution to 100 ml of sample. Lugol's solution is prepared by dissolving 20 g potassium iodide and 10 g iodine crystals in 200 ml of distilled water containing 20 ml of glacial acetic acid.

WATER-ANALYSIS KITS

Portable water-analysis kits use prepackaged reagents and simple analytical equipment so balances and other expensive apparatus are not required. Test kits generally sacrifice some accuracy, precision, detection limits, and sensitivity for convenience, portability, rapidity of analysis, and expense. However, the overall performance of some kits is quite good and the results of their use are adequate for many practical purposes. The advantages of portable kits include the availability of results without delay, allowing immediate remedial action. Field testing is also desirable when samples would have to be stored for long periods before laboratory analysis. Laboratory analysis might not accurately represent the composition of the stored water samples because of changes during storage.

Test kit methods are usually modifications of "standard" methods. Sophisticated kits are capable of performance near that of "standard" laboratory methods. With these kits, colorimetric analyses are usually conducted with a simple spectrophotometer, which may operate on line voltage or a battery. Titrations are conducted with hand-held, precisely calibrated syringes or small burets. Multiple parameter kits (Fig. 13–11) may contain equipment and reagents for analysis of over 20 different variables, including pH and conductivity. In general, these kits are capable of estimates within 20% of values obtained with standard laboratory procedures (Boyd, 1976, 1977, 1980, 1981; Boyd and Hollerman, 1984; Boyd and Daniels, 1988). Actual performance depends on the particular kit used, the variable being measured, and the concentration range of interest.

Less sophisticated kits are also available for rapid approximations of water quality. These kits often use subjective "color-comparators" where visual estimates of color intensity are made. Titrations are performed by counting drops or by delivering the titrant from calibrated syringes. Estimates of pH are made colorimetrically with pH indicators. The performance of these kits varies widely, and results should be regarded as useful only for rapid screening of large numbers of samples to identify those with exceptional concentrations. Before using any kit, it is important to determine if it is sufficiently reliable for the particular use. The manufacturer's directions must then be followed carefully to obtain the desired degree of accuracy.

LITERATURE CITED

American Public Health Association, American Water Works Association, and Water Pollution Control Federation (1989) Standard Methods for the Examination of Water and Wastewater. 17th ed. American Public Health Association, Washington, D.C.

Arthur, J.W., West, C.W., Allen, K.N., and Redtke, S.F. (1987) Seasonal toxicity of ammonia to three fish and nine invertebrate species. Bull. Environ. Cont. Toxicol. 38:324–331.

Baden, G.G., Mende, T.J., Poli, M.A., and Block, R.E. (1984) Toxins from Florida's red tide dinoflagellate *Ptychodiscus brevis*. In: Seafood Toxins (Ragelis, E.P., ed.). American Chemical Society, Washington, D.C., pp. 359–367.

Beveridge, M.C.M. (1987) Cage Aquaculture. Fishing News Books, Farnham, England.

Bonn, E.W., and Follis, B.J. (1967) Effects of hydrogen sulfide on channel catfish, *Ictalurus punctatus*. Trans. Am. Fish. Soc. 96:31–36.

Bower, C.E., and Bidwell, J.P. (1978) Ionization of ammonia in seawater: Effects of temperature, pH, and salinity. J. Fish. Res. Bd. Can. 35:1012.

Boyd, C.E. (1976) An evaluation of a water analysis kit. Auburn University Agricultural Experiment Station Leaflet 92, Auburn, Alabama.

Boyd, C.E. (1977) Evaluation of a water analysis kit. J. Environ. Qual. 6:381–384.

Boyd, C.E. (1979) Water Quality in Warmwater Fish Ponds. Auburn University Agricultural Experiment Station, Auburn, Alabama.

Boyd, C.E. (1980) Reliability of water analysis kits. Trans. Am. Fish. Soc. 109:239–243.

Boyd, C.E. (1981) Comparisons of water analysis kits. Proc. Annu. Conf. S.E. Assoc. Fish Wildlife Agencies 34:39–48.

Boyd, C.E., and Daniels, H.V. (1988) Evaluation of Hach Fish Farmer's Water Quality Test Kits for saline water. J. World Aquacult. Soc. 19:21.

Boyd, C.E., and Hollerman, W.D. (1984) Performance of a Water Analysis Kit. Auburn University Agricultural Experiment Station Circular 274. Auburn, Alabama.

Brooks, A.S., and Bartos, J.M. (1984) Effects of free and combined chlorine and exposure duration on rainbow trout, channel catfish, and emerald shiners. Trans. Am. Fish. Soc. 113:786–793.

Carmichael, W.W., and Mahmood, N.A. (1984) Toxins from freshwater cyanobacteria. In: Seafood Toxins (Ragelis, E.P., ed.). American Chemical Society, Washington, D.C., pp. 377–389.

Collins, M. (1978) Algal toxins. Microbiol. Rev. 42:725–746.

Colt, J. (1984) Computation of dissolved gas concentrations in water as functions of temperature, salinity, and pressure. Special Publication No. 14. American Fisheries Society, Bethesda, Maryland.

Colt, J. (1986) The impact of gas supersaturation on the design and operation of aquatic culture systems. Aquacult. Eng. 5:49–86.

Colt, J., and Armstrong, D.A. (1981) Nitrogen toxicity to crustaceans, fish, and molluscs. In: Bio-engineering Symposium for Fish Culture (Allen, L.J., and Kinney, E.C., eds.). American Fisheries Society, Bethesda, Maryland, pp. 34–47.

Emerson, K., Russo, R.C., Lund, R.E., and Thurston, R.V. (1975) Aqueous ammonia equilibrium calculations: Effect of pH and temperature. J. Fish. Res. Bd. Can. 32:2379–2383.

Freeman, L., Beitinger, T.L., and Huey, D.W. (1983) Methemoglobin reductase activity in phylogenetically diverse piscine species. Comp. Biochem. Physiol. 75B:27–30.

Fresenius, W., Quentin, K.E., and Schneider, W. (eds.) (1988) Water Analysis. Springer-Verlag, New York.

Grasshof, K., Ehrhardt, M., and Kremling, K. (eds.) (1983) Methods of Seawater Analysis. Verlay Chemie, Weinheim, Germany.

Haines, T.A., Akielaszek, J.J., Norton, S.A., and Davis, R.B. (1983) Errors in pH measurements with colorimetric indicators in low alkalinity waters. Hydrobiologia 107:57–61.

Heath, A.G. (1987) Water Pollution and Fish Physiology. CRC Press, Boca Raton, Florida.

Hoffman, G.L. (1970) Parasites of North American Freshwater Fishes. University of California Press, Berkeley.

Hunt, D.T.E., and Wilson, A.L. (1986) The Chemical Analysis of Water: General Principles and Techniques. Alden Press, Oxford, England.

Jones, K.J., Ayres, P., Bullock, A.M., Roberts, R.J., and Tett, P. (1982) A red tide of *Gyrodinium aureolum* in sea lochs of the Firth of Clyde and associated mortality of pond-reared salmon. J. Mar. Biol. Assoc. U.K. 62:771–782.

Kateman, G., and Pijpers, F.W. (1981) Quality Control in Analytical Chemistry. John Wiley & Sons, New York.

Keith, L.H. (ed.) (1988) Principles of Environmental Sampling. American Chemical Society, Washington, D.C.

Kennedy, W.A. (1978) A handbook on rearing pan-sized Pacific salmon using floating seapens. Fisheries and Marine Services Independent Report 107. Department of Fisheries and Environment Canada, Ottawa.

Krom, M.D. (1980) Spectrophotometric determination of ammonia: A study of a modified Berthelot reaction using salicylate and dichloroisocyanurate. Analyst 105:305–316.

Landolt, M.L. (1975) Visceral granuloma and nephrocalcinosis of trout. In: The Pathology of Fishes (Ribelin, W.E., and Migaki, G., eds.). The University of Wisconsin Press, Madison, pp. 793–799.

Lauckner, G. (1984) Diseases caused by protophytans (algae). In: Diseases of Marine Animals. Vol. VI, Part 1 (Kinne, O., ed.). Biologische Anstalt Helgoland, Hamburg, pp. 169–179.

Lewis, W.M., and Morris, D.P. (1986) Toxicity of nitrite to fish: A review. Trans. Am. Fish. Soc. 115:183–195.

McWilliams, P.G. (1982) The effects of calcium on sodium fluxes in the brown trout, Salmo trutta, in neutral and acid water. J. Exp. Biol. 96:439–442.

Meade, J.W. (1985) Allowable ammonia for fish culture. Progressive Fish Culturist 47:135–145.

Messer, J.J., Ho, J., and Grenney, W.J. (1984) Ionic strength correction for extent of ammonia ionization in freshwater. Can. J. Fish. Aquat. Sci. 41:811–815.

Miranda, L.E., and Sonski, A.J. (1986) Survival of red drum fingerlings in fresh water: Dissolved solids and thermal minima. S.E. Assoc. Fish Wildlife Agencies.

Padilla, G. (1970) Growth and toxigenesis of the chrysomonad *Prymnesium parvum* as a function of salinity. J. Protozool. 17:456–462.

Parsons, T.R., Maita, Y., and Lalli, C.M. (1984) A Manual of Chemical and Biological Methods for Seawater Analysis. Pergamon Press, Oxford, England.

Phillips, M.J., Roberts, R.J., Stewart, J.A., and Codd, G.A. (1985) The toxicity of the cyanobacterium *Microcystis aeruginosa* to rainbow trout, *Salmo gairdneri* Richardson. J. Fish. Dis. 8:339–344.

Pickering, A.D. (1981) Introduction: The concept of biological stress. In: Stress and Fish (Pickering, A.D., ed.). Academic Press, London, pp. 1–9.

Piper, R.G., McElwain, J.B., Orne, L.E., McCraren, J.P., Fowler, L.G., and Leonard, J.R. (1982) Fish Hatchery Management. United States Department of Interior, Fish and Wildlife Service, Washington, D.C.

Rand, G.M., and Petrocelli, S.R., Eds. (1985) Fundamentals of Aquatic Toxicology. Hemisphere, Washington, D.C.

Shilo, M. (1981) The toxic principles of *Prymnesium parvum*. In: The Water Environment: Algal Toxins and Health (Carmichael, W.W., ed.). Plenum Press, New York, pp. 27–47.

Shugar, G.J., Shugar, R.A., Bauman, L., and Bauman, R.S. (1981) Chemical Technicians Ready Reference Handbook. McGraw-Hill, New York.

Smith, C.E., and Piper, R.G. (1975) Lesions associated with chronic exposure to ammonia. In: The Pathology of Fishes (Ribelin, W.E., and Migaki, G., eds.). Univ. Wisconsin Press, Madison, pp. 497–514.

Smith, L.L., Oseid, P.M., Kimball, L.L., and El-Kandelgy, S.M. (1976) Toxicity of hydrogen sulfide to various life history stages of bluegill (*Lepomis macrochirus*). Trans. Am. Fish. Soc. 105:442–449.

Snoeyink, V.L., and Jenkins, D. (1980) Water Chemistry. John Wiley & Sons, New York.

Spotte, S. (1979) Seawater Aquariums. John Wiley & Sons, New York.

Steidinger, K.A. (1979) Collection, enumeration and identification of free-living marine dinoflagellates. In: Toxic Dinoflagellate Blooms (Taylor, D.L., and Seliger, H.H., eds.). Elsevier, Amsterdam, pp. 435–442.

Stirling, H.P. (Ed.) (1985) Chemical and Biological Methods of Water Analysis for Aquaculturists. Institute of Aquaculture, Stirling, Scotland.

Strickland, J.D.H., and Parsons, T.R. (1972) A Practical Handbook of Seawater Analysis. Fisheries Research Board of Canada, Ottawa.

Swinnerton, J., Linnebonn, V.J., and Cheek, C.H. (1962) Determination of dissolved gases in aqueous solutions by gas chromatography. Anal. Chem. 34:483–485.

Taylor, F.J.R. (1984) Toxic dinoflagellates: Taxonomic and biogeographic aspects with emphasis on *Protogonyaulax*. In: Seafood Toxins (Ragelis, E.P., ed.). American Chemical Society, Washington, D.C., pp. 77–97.

Tomasso, J.R. (1986) Comparative toxicity of nitrite to freshwater fishes. Aquat. Toxicol. 8:129–137.

Tomasso, J.R., Goudie, C.A., Simco, B.A., and Davis, K.B. (1980) Effects of environmental pH and calcium on ammonia toxicity in channel catfish. Trans. Am. Fish. Soc. 109:229–234.

U.S. EPA (1976) Quality Criteria for Water. EPA-440/9-76-023. United States Environmental Protection Agency, Washington, D.C.

U.S. EPA (1979) Methods for Chemical Analysis of Water and Wastes. EPA-600/4-79-020. Office of Research and Development, United States Environmental Protection Agency, Cincinnati, Ohio.

U.S. EPA (1982) Handbook for Sampling, and Sample Preservation of Water and Wastewater. EPA-600/4-82-029. Environmental Monitoring and Support Laboratory. United States Environmental Protection Agency, Cincinnati, Ohio.

Van Slyke, D.D., and Neill, J.M. (1924) The determination of gas in blood and other solutions by vacuum extraction and manometric measurement. J. Biol. Chem. 61:523–574.

Weitkamp, D.E., and Katz, M. (1980) A review of dissolved gas supersaturation literature. Trans. Am. Fish. Soc. 109:659–702.

Wetzel, R.G. (1975) Limnology. W.B. Saunders, Philadelphia.

Wheaton, F.W. (1977) Aquacultural Engineering. Wiley-Interscience, New York.

White, A.W. (1984) Paralytic shellfish toxins and finfish. In: Seafood Toxins (Ragelis, E.P., ed.). American Chemical Society, Washington, D.C., pp. 171–180.

Whitfield, M. (1974) The hydrolysis of ammonia ions in seawater—A theoretical study. J. Mar. Biol. Assoc. U.K. 54:565–580.

Williams, E.M., and Eddy, F. B. (1986) Chloride uptake in freshwater teleosts and its relationship to nitrite uptake and toxicity. J. Comp. Physiol. B 156:867–872.

Chapter 14

SOIL AND SUBSTRATE ANALYSIS

MICHAEL K. STOSKOPF

Very few clinicians working with terrestrial species give much thought to the composition or makeup of soils, although most are at least cognizant of several ways soils can affect health, including their impact on feeds grown in nutrient-deficient or over-abundant soils. Practitioners involved with health management of pond-reared fish have long appreciated that the nature and composition of the soils making up ponds is a primary factor in fish productivity and health dynamics (Durum and Hem, 1972). Soil provides major components of water-nutrient composition, including supplying nitrogen, phosphorus, potassium, selenium, copper, iodine, and cobalt. The importance of soil composition in fish culture may be less apparent to practitioners dealing with marine or aquarium fish, but the impact of solid substrates used to construct fish facilities or marine sediments can be every bit as important to the long-term health of fish as the factors of water quality. This chapter will concentrate on natural soils.

Aquatic clinicians are only rarely involved in pond site selection, construction materials selection, or watershed development planning, but they should be conscious of the impact of these factors on fish health. They must be particularly aware of the remedial measures that can be employed to correct problems created by these factors. Clinically effective aquatic medicine, therefore, requires a basic working knowledge of soils and their health interactions, including an understanding of the impact of soils on water stabilization, nutrient provision, and toxic leaching.

TYPES OF SOILS

Soil Composition

Soil is a term that covers a variety of substances with widely differing properties. The major components of soil are clay, sand, and silt or humus, which give soil its properties. The major properties of soils that are important to fish health include color, bulk density, texture, and content.

Properties of Soil

The most readily observable property of soil is its color, which often delineates the natural drainage conditions of the area. Soil has primarily two color agents. Organic matter is responsible for the darkness or blackness of soil, and iron content can give soil a red, yellow, or gray color. The color imparted by iron is related directly to the oxidation state and hydration of the soil. Red soil is oxidized and not hydrated. Yellow soil is hydrated but not oxidized, and gray soil is chemically reduced owing to wetness and lack of oxygen. Examination of soil color gives a clinician insight into the natural percolation and drainage features of a pond site. While yellow soils are indicative of good hydration and available water, gray soils point to anaerobic conditions and potential problems.

Another basic property of soil is the bulk density. This is the relative weight per volume of soil. The bulk density of a soil is inversely related to its permeability. Heavy dense soils tend to be relatively impermeable to water whereas light soils of low bulk density percolate readily. The implications for water retention are obvious. Less obvious perhaps is the impact of percolation through low-density soils, increasing leaching from soils remote from a pond, stream, or lake. The topology of the area, combined with the bulk density of the soils, greatly affects the impact of agricultural chemicals, natural deposits of minerals, or industrial by-products on the health of fish.

Most ways to express soil texture rely on definitions that refer to content. For example, soil with harsh or coarse grains of sand visible is called "sandy" soil. Moist but nonsticky soil is referred to as "silty" soil, and soil that is sticky and can be rolled into a ribbon is called "clay" soil. Other texture definition systems delineate between coarse earths and fine earths. Coarse earths are usually defined as consisting primarily of particles 2 mm in diameter or larger, whereas fine earths have particles ranging from 0.5 to 2 mm in diameter. Although soil texture does not particularly affect fish management directly, it is a good tool for rapid on-site estimation of soil properties through an appreciation of the probable ratios of the soil components.

Soil Components

Soils are usually composites or mixtures of soil separates. These mixtures are referred to as loams. The three soil separates or components are clay, sand, and silt, or humus. The properties of a soil are due to the properties and ratios of the soil separates, which make up the soil proper. An average loam, for example, might consist of 40% sand, 40% silt, and 20% clay. A loam with 50% sand, 20% silt, and 30% clay would be considered a sandy clay loam. The relationship between sand, silt, and clay content and texture is summarized in the textural triangle shown in Fig. 14–1.

Clays

There are several types of clays, each with slightly different properties. Clays play a major role in the interactions between water and soils. In general, clays have very large surface areas per unit weight. For example, 5 g of an average clay can have a surface area equal to an American football field. Clays swell or shrink with wetting and drying, a property important in water retention. Clays affect the stabilization of soils by their abilities to hold water. They also vary in their tendency to hold and release nutrients and toxicants.

Clays are classified on the basis of their structure, content, and properties. Structurally there are two major types of clays: 2:1 clays and 1:1 clays (Fig. 14–2). The 2:1 clays have a sandwichlike arrangement, usually with two layers of silica around a single layer of alumina. Examples of this type of clay include the montmorillonite and hydrous mica clays. The 1:1 clays are the pottery clays. These have a single layer of silica fastened to a layer of alumina in an open-

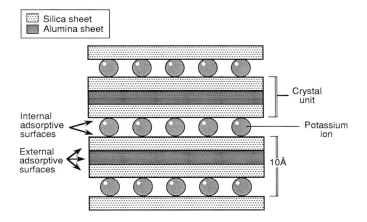

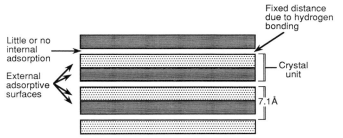

FIGURE 14–2. Diagram of the differences between a 2:1 clay (top) and a 1:1 clay (bottom). (Modified from Harpstead, M.I., and Hole, F.D. [1980] Soil Science Simplified. Iowa State University Press, Ames.)

faced sandwich. An example of a 1:1 clay familiar to veterinarians would be the kaolinite clays used to treat diarrhea.

On the basis of content, clays are usually divided into the silicate clays and the oxide clays. Oxide clays are found most often in tropical and subtropical areas where weathering has removed much or all of the silica, leaving a clay with little crystallinity and poor nutrient-holding capacity. Silicate clays provide the properties more generally associated with clay.

A common silicate clay that is not particularly beneficial in pond construction is montmorillonite, a 2:1 clay with a high capacity to hold nutrients. Unfortunately, it also has a high capacity for swelling and shrinking depending on its degree of wetting or drying. Soils containing this type of clay are very troublesome because when they are wet, their layers slip past each other, giving them a very low bearing strength. These soils are often very sticky and difficult to navigate when wet. Silicate clay is common in grassland areas, or in soil formed from shale or basic rocks.

Hydrous mica clays are another type of 2:1 clay in which the lattice layers are held together by potassium ions. This slight structural change minimizes shrinking and swelling and gives the clay a good bearing strength with less stickiness. Unfortunately, it also reduces the clay's capacity to hold nutrients. This type of clay is found in soils in cool climates where reasonable precipitation has removed soluble salts from the soil.

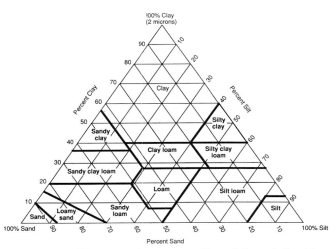

FIGURE 14–1. Diagrammatic representation of the relationships between soil types and soil components. (Modified from Harpstead, M.I., and Hole, F.D. [1980] Soil Science Simplified. Iowa State University Press, Ames.)

The kaolinite clays are 1:1 clays with considerable hydrogen bonding of the alumina layer to the oxygen in the silica layer. As a result they are less sticky and have a greater bearing strength than other silicate clays. Kaolinite clays also have a very low nutrient holding capacity and are slow to adsorb water.

Sands

While sand has a major effect on the texture of soils, and indirectly affects water retention, the various types of sands have not been well studied for their contributions to the health of fish through the contribution or abstraction of various trace minerals and metals. Two basic types of sands are generally discussed in soils texts, volcanic and silica sands. However, as a soil component, sand is usually defined on the basis of coarseness and rapid settling (density). In this definition, gravels of various sizes must be considered, and these may be derived from any rocks with widely varying trace mineral and metal contents. While examining gravels, it is only a small step to consideration of soil generating rock in the area. Sands (including gravels) should always be suspected when trace metal or mineral problems are implicated in a diagnosis.

While silica sands are considered relatively inert, the trace element compositions of a given sand may have more impact on water properties than is generally recognized. Fluorine is found primarily in silicates. Micas are silicon compounds with high potassium and magnesium contents. They also contain strontium, lead, and barium. Quartz is silicon dioxide, but it can also contain high levels of phosphorus, molybdenum, calcium, and magnesium.

Granites are acid rocks. They often are composed of orthoclase, a potassium-rich compound. They also commonly contain considerable lithium, beryllium, and boron. They can contain enough molybdenum to contribute to molybdenum toxicity in some areas. Acidic granites are poor sources of cobalt, as are most sandy soils. Cobalt is generally associated with clay.

Sands from basic rocks contain essential micronutrient metals, including iron, cobalt, manganese, copper, and zinc (Beeson, 1976). Calcium silicates, including the hornblends, pyroxenes, and plagioclases, also occur more often in basic rocks (Beeson, 1976). Hornblends can have excessive levels of zinc. In general, in low-pH soils, iodine and fluorine solubility is enhanced, and leaching of these compounds can become a problem.

Limestones contain carbonates of biological origin and alkaline earths, boron, sulfur, manganese, and iodine. Limestone sands are low in cobalt, although weathering of limestone soils removes calcium carbonate and concentrates other nutrients, correcting deficiencies to some extent. Glacial till containing fragments of limestone usually has a higher concentration of nutrient elements than a till composed of silica sandstone. In recent volcanic rocks, mineral levels are high, although selenium levels are very low.

Knowledge of regional trends in rock or sand structures can be useful. For example, the highland rim of Tennessee is low in phosphates (Beeson, 1976), as are the fine sand soils of Georgia and the lower and middle Atlantic coastal plain. The metamorphic rocks of the Eastern states are low in selenium. On the other hand, selenium concentrations in South Dakota, Nebraska, and Wyoming can be toxic to fish.

Humus

Humus, or silt, is the third component of a soil. It is made up of the organic matter in the soil. In temperate humid regions, most surface soils will consist of 2 to 6% humus by weight. It is derived from the decay of plant and animal matter and generally holds soil loosely to allow air and water to percolate. Soils that become dense and cloddy when tilled are low in humus. Humus greatly affects the availability of nutrients in the soil both by releasing them during decomposition and by binding cations, including metals. This latter property of humus is highly dependent upon the soil pH. Humus retains a greater negative charge in slightly acid, or alkaline, soil, binding more cationic nutrients than when the soil is extremely acidic. This in turn affects the stability of the soil. For example, sodium binding causes the humus and the soil to disperse rather than to cluster in colloids suitable for flocculation, reducing stability. Humus also interacts with many organic contaminants, including pesticides and herbicides. The humus, or silt, component of the soil can be important when investigating this type of problem in a fish facility or natural stream. Copper and molybdenum problems usually occur in poorly drained humus soils with high organic content, such as the peats, in which these metals form stable complexes. For example, molybdenum toxicosis is common in wet parts of alluvial fans.

POND SITE SELECTION

An aquaculturist examining a site for its potential as a pond evaluates the soil for two major factors, nutrient content and water retention. In the United States, the Federal Soil Conservation Service will give advice on these aspects free of charge, and the veterinary clinician will rarely be involved. If a species is to be reared on the natural production of the pond, then nutrient-rich soils are a major benefit, and even supplemental fertilization will be employed. On the other hand, if fish are to be fed from external sources (catfishes or eels), an extremely nutrient-rich pond soil is unnecessary and may contribute to water problems due to secondary production. The issue of water stabilization is more universal. High water retention and low percolation are generally beneficial, reducing overall water requirements and usually costs.

WATER STABILIZATION

Soil has impact on water stabilization in two distinct ways, physical retention and chemical equilibration. Water retention by soils is of universal importance in aquacultural construction. Leaky ponds can be repaired, but the expense can be devastating. Opinions as to what soil composition provides the optimal retention of water differ, but either high clay content soils or soils with 70% sand and 25% clay and just enough silt to fill in spaces are best for water retention. The type of clay and the treatment of the pond bottom and levees during construction will also greatly affect the water retention of the soil.

When a pond has been constructed in soils with poor water retention, it may be necessary to repair the situation with sealants to achieve an economically viable pond. Bentonite clay can be used to seal earth ponds. Its major drawbacks are the relatively huge quantities of material that must be applied to the pond and the requirement that the clay be applied to a dry pond bottom. Generally 0.5 to 1.5 kg of bentonite clay must be applied for every square meter of pond containment surface depending on the laboratory analysis of the preexisting soil. This type of treatment will be effective on sandy or silty soils but will not affect percolation due to leaks from cracking of swelling clay soils.

Leaking in fine-grained soils will also occur when clay particles are not adequately dispersed. This is often due to low salt content of the soil. As a rule of thumb, when more than half the soil consists of particles under a millimeter in diameter and the soluble salt content of the soil is less than 0.5%, adding salts to the soil will help improve water retention. A variety of salts will work as sealants, including sodium chloride and the sodium polyphosphates, such as tetrasodium pyrophosphate (TSPP) and sodium tripolyphosphate (STPP). Sodium chloride is generally applied to the soil at the rate of 0.04 to 0.17 kg/m^2 to correct this type of problem. Polysphosphates are administered at 0.01 to 0.02 kg/m^2.

SOIL NUTRIENT MANAGEMENT

An important aspect of pond management is chemical stabilization of pond soils (Bardarch et al., 1972). Fertilization is one way this is accomplished. For example, since sandy soils are often poor in potassium, supplementation is beneficial. This is often applied at the same time as phosphate fertilizers (Bennett, 1962). The results of fertilization vary tremendously from pond to pond, and the timing of fertilization can be critical to whether it is beneficial or detrimental to the fish population of a pond. Fertilizer falling onto fish eggs in the spring kills embryos. In the summer, excessive fertilization leads to algal blooms, which in turn deplete oxygen and result in fish mortality; fertilization in the winter increases winter kill by suffocation if the pond freezes

over. By default, fall seems to be the most opportune time for fertilization with phosphates.

Liming a pond is the application of calcium oxide (quicklime) to buffer sulfate-induced acidity, precipitate iron, and make potassium and phosphate more readily available. Quicklime is applied at least 2 to 3 weeks before fish are to be stocked in the pond and not into ponds already full of fish. It should never be applied at the same time as the application of phosphate fertilizer.

Of course, soil compositions are not static. Several factors contribute to constantly changing soil dynamics, including the tilling and turnover of soils by benthic invertebrates. Their activity increases soil-to-water exchange, increasing nutrient or toxicant release from the soil. On the other hand, mass blooms of benthic invertebrates can result in nutrient depletions as they utilize soil nutrients to sustain their own cycles. They also increase leaching efficiency.

SOIL SAMPLE COLLECTION AND HANDLING

An important decision is where to take your soil samples. At a pond construction site, roadcuts and ditch banks are tempting but are not satisfactory sampling sites unless they are freshly made. The exposure these sites get to wet-dry cycles and oxidation affect many tests of interest. Usually soil samples for a pond should be taken from a sampling pit. The pit should be dug in the region of interest, into an area representative of the most common topography of the area. It may be advisable to sample from several sampling pits depending on the homogeneity of the area being studied. When investigating established ponds, the mineral composition of the water is roughly similar to the mineral composition of the soils of the bottom and surrounding basin. It is not often useful to drain a pond or lake for the purpose of soil testing (Bennett, 1962).

Sampling for Pesticides in Soil

Sampling for soil pesticides can be very important when investigating a die-off, or when locating a site for a new pond. It is particularly important in areas where cotton has been grown. These areas typically are treated heavily with chlorinated hydrocarbons and soil levels can have deleterious effects on subsequent fish production. When sampling for pesticides, the depth of the sample required is determined by the behavior of the pesticide of interest. For example, many herbicides are absorbed in the surface layer and sampling greater than 50 to 75 mm dilutes the sample with uncontaminated material, making detection harder, rather than easier. Unfortunately, the depth of sampling is not always easy to determine. When sampling for pesticides suspected of recently being applied to the surface, take a sample 12 in. deep. It is optimal to divide the sample into a deep and a surface aliquot for analysis

(Eagle et al., 1983). The major special transport precaution for a soil sample being submitted for pesticide analysis is to avoid contamination with pesticides. Polyethylene bags (Rourke et al., 1977) and cloth bags (Levi and Nowicki, 1972) may release interfering substances into the sample, making analysis worthless; paper sacks are often used. Samples should be stored on the basis of the stability of the suspected pesticide. Many pesticides are very stable when deep frozen. Diazinon, malathion, parathion, and dichlorvos are exceptions (Kawar et al., 1973). It is usually wise to get the sample analyzed immediately rather than storing it.

SOIL NOMENCLATURE

The nomenclature involved in classifying soils in soil maps and reports you receive from testing laboratories can seem like a foreign language to the uninitiated. In fact, it can seem like many foreign languages, since there is a plethora of soil classification terms that have survived in common usage despite the evolution of soil taxonomy. Also, in various parts of the world, different supplanted soil classification schemes remain extant, further complicating the issue (Harpstead and Hole, 1980). Consequently, soil analysis reports provide little or no information to the average biologist or veterinarian unfamiliar with the subject or its jargon. Luckily, a solid background in biology is excellent preparation for a short foray into soil taxonomy, which follows the same basic principles of classification used in zoology or botany.

A short explanation of the U.S. Comprehensive Soil Classification System, which is now in use in the United States and can be considered the most modern of the classification systems, is justified if only to allow the clinician to get some idea of what basic soil properties are implied by the various classifications. The strength of the U.S. system lies in the definition of taxa using differentiating characteristics that are properties of the soils.

The U.S. Comprehensive Soil Classification System

There are technically six levels of classification of soils in the U.S. system, from order to series. There are 10 orders, each differentiated from the other on the basis of soil-forming processes and the presence or absence of various layers called diagnostic horizons. There are a total of 47 suborders, subdividing the orders on the basis of wetness, parent material, and vegetation effects. These are in turn divided into about 230 great groups on the basis of temperature and the presence or absence of diagnostic layers of mineral types. The lowest level of division, the "series," is equivalent to "species" in biological classification. There are over 12,000 distinct soil species separated on color, texture, and chemical reactions (Buol et al., 1980).

The Ten Orders of Soils

HISTOSOLS. The histosols form the only order of the "organic soils." These soils contain more than 25% humus overall or more than 30% humus to a depth of 40 cm. They cover only a small portion of the total land area and form wherever organic matter production exceeds mineralization. These are usually conditions of continuous previous or current water saturation. Histosols are commonly formed at seepage sites or in depressions that go below the water table, especially in cool areas where anaerobic conditions are prominent. The peat bogs of the Irish and Scottish highlands are histosols. The degree of decomposition is particularly important to the hydraulic properties of the histosols. Well-decomposed histosols have very high water-holding capacity, and their hydraulic conductivity can be lower than clay sediments (Boelter, 1974). On the other hand, slightly decomposed histosols can have very high water movement. While low hydraulic conductivity can be a problem in trying to drain land with high water tables, it can be used to advantage in efforts to retain water. A major feature of histosols, however, is their changeability, particularly when drained. Settling, or compaction, usually termed "subsidence," can be very dramatic, affecting any structures built on histosols. They have very low bearing capacity.

OXISOLS. The oxisols are highly weathered soils found in tropical regions. They are not generally found in geographic areas that would be developed for aquaculture, with the possible exception of limited areas of the Amazon basin and the area between Brasilia and São Paulo. They are not suited to aquaculture. Oxisols are mineral soils with very low nutrient reserve, and particularly low water-holding capacity. These infertile soils are actively acidic, and although exchangeability of minerals is variable depending on the vegetation breaking up the soil, they generally have low exchangeable aluminum, high permeability, and low erodibility.

SPODOSOLS. The spodosols are the white earths. They are acid, ashy gray sands over sandy loams, often found in conifer hardwood forests. Spodosols have a subsurface rich in organic matter and iron. They are generally cobalt deficient. Spodosols are often found overlying sand plains or northern slopes in the temperate and arctic zones. They are also extensive in the southeastern United States. There are four suborders of spodosols based primarily on the degree of wetness.

MOLLISOLS. The mollisols are thick, black topsoils with a clay-enriched subsurface. They are prominent in short-grass grasslands, steppes, plains, and prairies, including the American Midwest. There are seven suborders of mollisols based on moisture content and climate temperature.

ALFISOLS. The alfisols have the same clay-enriched subsurface of the mollisols, but a thinner layer of topsoil. They are generated over a fertile parent layer in temperate, subtropical, and tropical regions. Alfisols have a high cation-exchange capability, and although they exchange aluminum to some extent, aluminum toxicity is not a problem.

ULTISOLS. The ultisols are essentially alfisols overlying an infertile parent layer. They are found in hardwood pine forests between the tropics and more temperate latitudes. Ultisols are geologically old compared to glaciated areas, and all are formed in areas of relatively high precipitation. These are weathered soils that are subject to agricultural overuse, which exposes clay layers with low water-infiltration characteristics.

INCEPTISOLS. The inceptisols are less weathered immature soils with a thin subsoil under the topsoil. They are usually moist and are considered embryonic. Inceptisols are often volcanic soils and can be strong sulfate fixers. Phosphate is also often strongly fixed in these soils. There are six suborders of inceptisols based on moisture and organic material content.

ARIDISOLS. The aridisols are dry soils of the general construction of inceptisols. They are low in nitrogen and high in potassium and other nutrients. Aridisols are generally alkaline. They are rarely encountered in aquaculture construction because of the lack of available water.

ENTISOLS. The entisols consist of topsoil directly over a parent substance that is not dominated by swelling clay. They are usually young soils such as those found in the sand hills of Nebraska, salt flats, and the barrier islands off Long Island, New York.

VERTISOLS. The vertisols are entisols which are dominated by swelling clay. In the United States, they are common in Texas, particularly in the Houston area, and other Western states. They are desirable for retention of surface water, and yet pose several engineering problems because of their propensity to swell and contract as hydration changes. Vertisols are particularly prone to give misleading percolation tests that are falsely high in the dry season. To test retention or percolation in these soils they should be fully saturated with water at the beginning of the test. Vertisols are usually alkaline soils.

Additional Soil Vocabulary

ALKALIZATION. Alkalization is the accumulation of sodium ions in clay. Calcium and magnesium precipitate from solution first, leaving high sodium content in solution available for binding to clay.

DECALCIFICATION. Decalcification refers specifically to the loss of carbonates in soil. This is common in humid areas.

DESILICATION. Desilication occurs in high-temperature regions with extreme leaching. It is usually accompanied by accumulation of iron or fertilization due to immobilization of ferric oxide in oxidizing conditions.

GLEIZATION. Gleization is the reduction of iron in poorly drained soils due to segregation or leaching. It results in the formation of iron sulfide. When areas undergoing this process are drained, they become acidic and sulfuric acid is formed with exposure to oxygen.

PALUDIZATION. Paludization is an accumulation of a thicker mass of organic materials in a poorly drained site due to preservation under anaerobic conditions.

SALINIZATION. Salinization is the salt accumulation in depressional soils with a high clay content and low permeability. Sulfates and chlorides are the predominant salts involved. Nitrates and borates occur rarely.

LITERATURE CITED

Bardach, J.E., Ryther, J.H., and MacLarney, W.O. (1972) Aquaculture, The Farming and Husbandry of Freshwater and Marine Organisms. Wiley-Interscience, New York.

Beeson, K.C. (1976) The Soil Factor in Nutrition. Marcel Dekker, New York.

Bennett, G.W. (1962) Management of Artificial Lakes and Ponds. Reinhold, New York.

Boelter, D.H. (1974) The hydrologic characteristics of undrained organic soils in the lakestates. In: Histosols: Their Characteristics, Classification, and Use (Aandahl, A.R., et al., eds.). Soil Science Society of America Special Publication No. 6, Madison, Wisconsin, pp. 33–46.

Buol, S.W., Hole, F.D., and McCracken, R.J. (1980) Soil Genesis and Classification. (2nd ed.) Iowa State University Press, Ames.

Durum, W.H., and Hem, J.D. (1972) Geochemical Environment in Relation to Health and Disease. Ann. N.Y. Acad. Sci. 199:26–34.

Eagle, D.J., Jones, J.L.O., and Jewell, E.J. (1983) Determination of pesticides by gas chromatography and high pressure liquid chromatography. In: Soil Analysis (Smith, K.A., ed.). Marcell Dekker, New York. pp. 455–511.

Harpstead, M.I., and Hole, F.D. (1980) Soil Science Simplified. Iowa State University Press, Ames.

Kawar, N.S., de Batista, G.C., and Gunther, F.A. (1973). Pesticide stability in cold-stored plant parts, soils, and dairy products, and in cold-stored extractives solutions. Residue Rev. 48:45.

Levi, I., and Nowicki, T.W. (1972) Spurious GLC peaks in cereal grains stored in cloth bags. Bull. Environ. Contam. Toxicol. 7:133.

Rourke, D.R., Mueller, W.F., and Yang, S.H. (1977) J. Assoc. Off. Anal. Chem. 60:233.

Chapter 15

Specific Ion and Toxicologic Analysis

Joseph V. Kitzman

Technological advances have produced more effective and useful chemicals to benefit all phases of our lives, but they have also increased the risk of toxicity to fish and other aquatic wildlife from accidental or illegal dumping of potentially dangerous pollutants into water sources.

Pollutants vary in their toxic potential, so qualitative and quantitative determinations are needed to assess the toxic risk to the environment of each individual pollutant. For example, nitrate fertilizers applied in proper quantities are beneficial to agricultural crops as well as to plant life in streams and ponds. However, nitrates can become pollutants if runoff situations produce accumulations in water sources, with resulting algal blooms. On the other hand, heavy metal pollutants including lead, mercury, and tin are toxicants at all concentrations, becoming more of a serious problem with increasing concentrations. This chapter will focus on several toxicants that often bioaccumulate in the tissues of the fish and plants of water systems. Chapter 13, which deals with the analysis of water quality and samples, should be reviewed. The important goal here will be to identify which tissue samples should be submitted for laboratory analysis, how they should be collected, and a brief overview of the appropriate analytical methodology needed to detect the presence and concentration of the pollutants in fish tissues.

TRACE METALS

Many heavy metals are micronutrients in the diet of fish and mammals. Although the specific dietary requirements of copper, iron, zinc, cobalt, manganese, tin, nickel, selenium, iodine, and molybdenum are largely unknown in fish, minor concentration changes of these elements have been shown to cause depressed health and growth states (Awadallah et al., 1985; Hilmy et al., 1986). Marked changes in the concentration of one or more of these elements can cause rapid death. Lead, cadmium, and mercury are commonly found in natural water and soils and are not known to be required micronutrients (Jorgensen and Heisinger, 1987; Sherman et al.,

1987). They are widespread and are a potential health hazard to fish and mammals. Therefore, the United States Environmental Protection Agency (EPA) closely monitors water and surrounding soil concentrations for these three metals, along with nickel, chromium, tin, copper, zinc, and aluminum, as a priority monitoring program (United States EPA, 1980a–d; Segner, 1987; National Research Council of Canada, 1982). Reference material is available concerning the chemistry of trace metals in water, and the toxicological and homeostatic responses of aquatic vertebrates and invertebrates to trace metal contamination. For more details on the subject, several good reviews are available (Moore and Ramarmoorthy, 1984; Leland and Kuwabara, 1985).

Sample Analysis

The gill is most often the organ of absorption for the metals. If it is impractical to submit one or more whole fish for analysis, a sample of gill tissue should be included with other organ specimens whenever trace metal intoxication is suspected. Specific target organ samples should also be collected, if the trace metal causing the water contamination is known (Table 15–1). However, when collecting fish samples from a body of water of unconfirmed or unknown trace metal content, collect at least 25-g samples of the gill, liver, kidney, and muscle. The muscle sample should have the skin attached and should be taken from the dorsum of the fish. Dorsal sampling

TABLE 15–1. Fish Tissues to Submit for Determination of Heavy Metals

Metal	Tissues
Lead	Kidney, gills, liver, muscle
Mercury	Liver, gills, kidney, muscle
Cadmium	Liver, kidney, gills
Nickel	Liver, gills, kidney, muscle
Chromium	Liver, kidney, gills, muscle
Tin	Liver, brain, muscle
Copper	Gills, liver
Zinc	Liver, gills, kidney
Aluminum	Gills, liver

reduces error caused by the contact contamination of bottom swimming fishes (Schmitt and Finger, 1987). If possible, also collect whole fish, representative samples of the gastrointestinal tract, and serum in case further analysis is needed.

When collecting samples from fish, erroneously high concentrations of trace metals may occur if the samples come in contact with polluted water or soil during collection. When sampling in the field, whole fish should be doubled bagged in plastic containers, and transported to the laboratory on ice whenever possible. In the lab, the tissues must be handled for subsampling with acid-cleaned instruments under ultraclean conditions. Marked differences occur in trace metal concentrations when samples are collected in the field using standard techniques, as opposed to sampling done under laboratory conditions using ultraclean techniques (Schmitt and Finger, 1987).

Detection and Quantitation Techniques

Graphite furnace atomic absorption spectrometry is one of the most useful and sensitive techniques available for trace metal quantitation. The technique has become even more sensitive and reliable in recent years by the use of an alternating magnetic field at the furnace atomizer to avoid spectral interferences (Zeeman background correction). With suitable preparation, plant, animal, water, and soil samples can be assayed for one or more of the trace metals (Welz et al., 1986). Other analytical methods are used to identify and quantitate specific metals. Gas liquid chromatography with electron capture detection can be used to detect mercury (Kai et al., 1986). Selenium can be quantitated by fluorometry (Kai et al., 1986).

Iron can be detected in several body tissues with inductively coupled plasma-atomic emission spectroscopy (Sargent and Youson, 1986). Cadmium, copper, and zinc in liver-soluble fractions can be determined by high-performance liquid chromatography with inductively coupled argon plasma-atomic emission spectrometry (Suzuki et al., 1987). Several metals, including tin, manganese, iron, nickel, copper, zinc, and selenium, can be determined in fish and shrimp samples by particle-induced x-ray emission (PIXE) (Khan et al., 1987). Finally, a novel approach to detect aluminum on gill epithelial cells uses transmission electron microscopy and electron probe x-ray microanalysis (Youson and Neville, 1987).

PESTICIDES

Modern effective pest control began with the development of DDT as an insecticide in the mid–1940s. Extensively used in the United States until 1962, DDT proved to be a highly successful, but extremely persistent, compound (Virtanen, 1986) (Fig. 15–1). Because the molecule of DDT is very stable and resists chemical change in the soil, significant concentrations of DDT and two of its major metabolites, DDD and DDE, can be found in the soil in and around streams, lakes, and rivers throughout the world today.

Insecticides in current use are often divided into categories based on their chemical structure and properties. These include the organochlorine insecticides (chlorinated hydrocarbons), organophosphate insecticides, carbamates, and pyrethrins, or botanical insecticides. Table 15–2 lists several examples of each class.

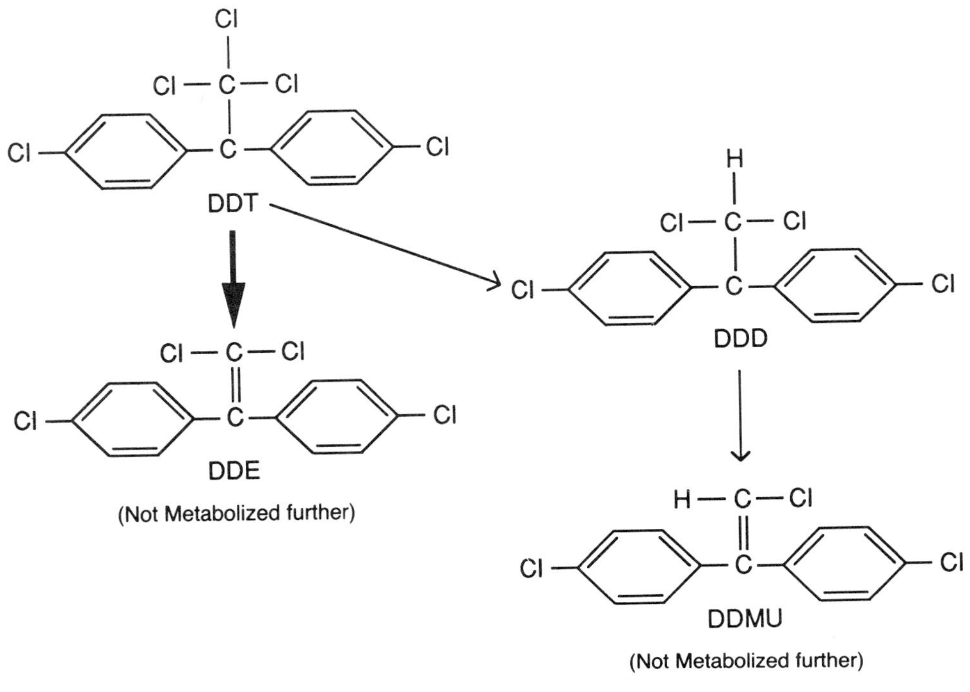

FIGURE 15–1. The metabolic pathways of DDT in fishes.

TABLE 15–2. Insecticide Groups and Examples

Organochlorine	**Carbamate**
(Chlorinated Hydrocarbon)	Aldicarb
DDT	Carbaryl
Dieldrin	Carbofuran
Endosulfan	Diallate
Endrin	Ethiofencarb
Heptachlor	Methomyl
Lindane	**Pyrethrins (Botanicals)**
Methoxychlor	Allethrin
Mirex	Cyclethrin
Organophosphate	Permethrin
Amiton	Pyrethrin
Coroxon	
Demeton	
Fensulfothion	
Parathion	
Trichlorfon	

Herbicides are also pesticides and have a major impact on fish health. Synthetic organic herbicides available today permit selective weed control for farmers and are commonly used to control nuisance aquatic vegetation around lakes and reservoirs, increasing the possibility of toxicity to fish. Examples of commonly used herbicides include linuron, trifluralin (Fig. 15–2), glyphosate, atrazine, molinate, and endothall (Benedeczky et al., 1986; Nemcsok et al., 1987; Kawatsu, 1977; Berry, 1984).

Sample Analysis

When pesticide pollution is suspected, whole fish or tissue samples should be submitted along with accompanying water samples. Since many organic pesticides are highly lipid soluble, tissues with high lipid content, such as the brain and the body fat, should be submitted in addition to gill, liver, and kidney samples. Because detection of a few parts per billion (micrograms per liter) of organic toxicants is possible using currently available methodology, it is critical to avoid specimen contamination during collection and preparation. Knives and scalpel blades used to open the abdomen must not be used to

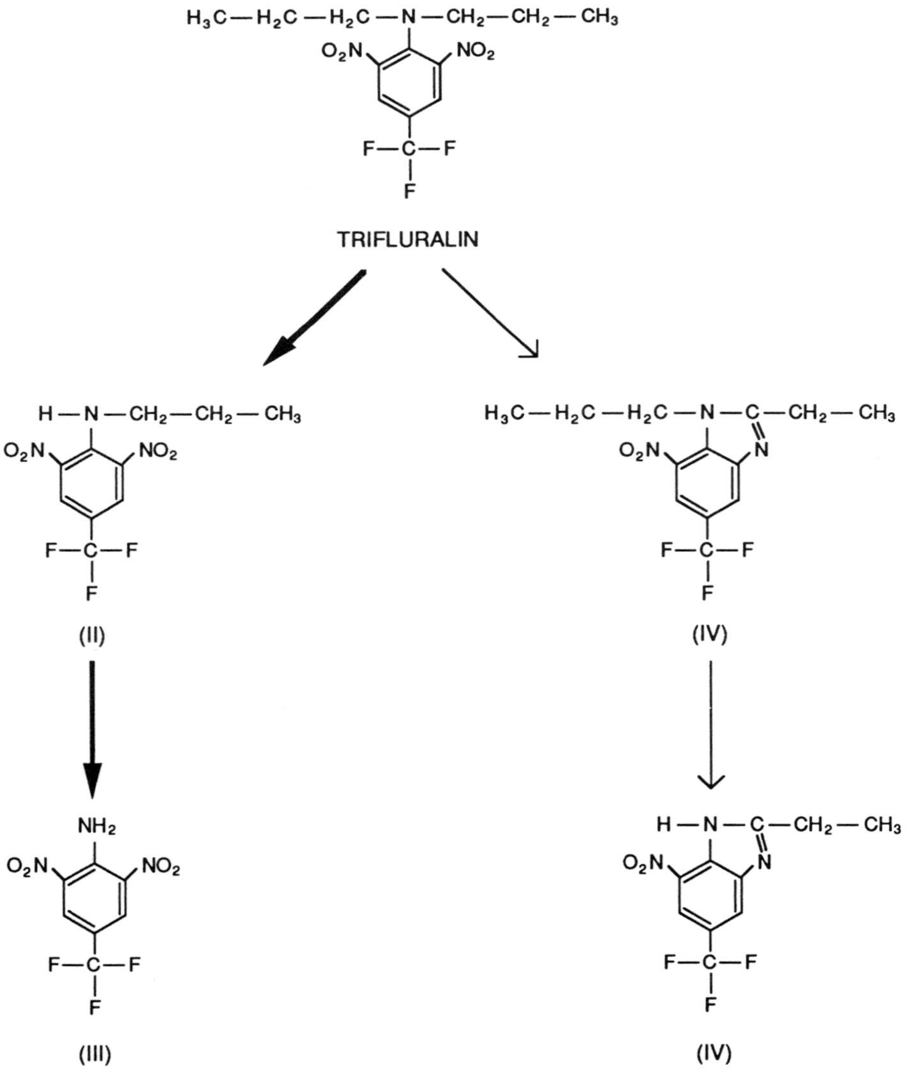

FIGURE 15–2. The metabolic pathways of trifluralin in soil and water.

remove internal organs for submission. Also, collection equipment should be thoroughly cleaned and rinsed between fish. Tissue samples for pesticide analysis should be frozen immediately, preferably at ultralow temperatures (–70°C), and should be analyzed within 7 days of collection. Water samples should be stored, refrigerated but not frozen (4°C), in glass containers and should be analyzed as soon as possible after collection.

Detection and Quantitation

Detection and quantitation of pesticides are performed primarily using gas chromatography, or occasionally by liquid chromatography (Villeneuve et al., 1987; Price et al., 1986; Phipps and Holcombe, 1985). Samples for chromatographic analysis are first prepared for extraction and then usually purified and concentrated before being injected into the gas chromatograph. The gas chromatograph heats the sample to volatilization and then separates the gas phase sample on a column. Compounds may be detected by flame ionization detection, nitrogen-phosphorus flame ionization detection, and/or electron capture detection. Although these methods provide relatively good quantitation of how much compound is present, they provide little direct evidence of the structure and identity of the compound other than comparison of retention times with standards. Gas chromatography linked to mass spectrometry can be particularly useful for positive identification of an unknown chemical in water or fish tissue (Camanzo et al., 1987; Lay et al., 1979). High-performance liquid

chromatography (HPLC) is used to separate organic compounds in aqueous samples. Pesticides are most frequently detected in HPLC systems by changes in ultraviolet light absorption, changes in refractive index, or by direct electrochemical detection. The decision to use gas chromatography or HPLC to detect a particular compound is based on the chemical properties of the substance, type of sample (water, soil, tissue), and the sensitivity of detection needed. Gas chromatography has the greater sensitivity and is most often the method of choice for detecting pesticides in water or tissues.

INDUSTRIAL TOXICANTS

Polycyclic Aromatic Hydrocarbons

Polycyclic aromatic hydrocarbons are a class of organic pollutants formed by fusing two or more benzene rings. Common examples are naphthalene, anthracene, and derivatives of pyrene such as benzo[a]pyrene (see Fig. 15–3). Polycyclic aromatic hydrocarbons in the environment come from three primary sources: high-temperature combustion of fossil fuels, transformation of organic material into oil and natural gas, and direct synthesis by bacteria and some plants. The predominant source is the burning of fossil fuels. If fossil fuels are incompletely burned, saturated and unsaturated aromatic compounds fuse to form polycyclic aromatic hydrocarbons of 100 to 300 molecular weight units. Automobile exhaust, smoke produced by burning coal, cigarette smoke, wood-burning fireplaces, and petro-

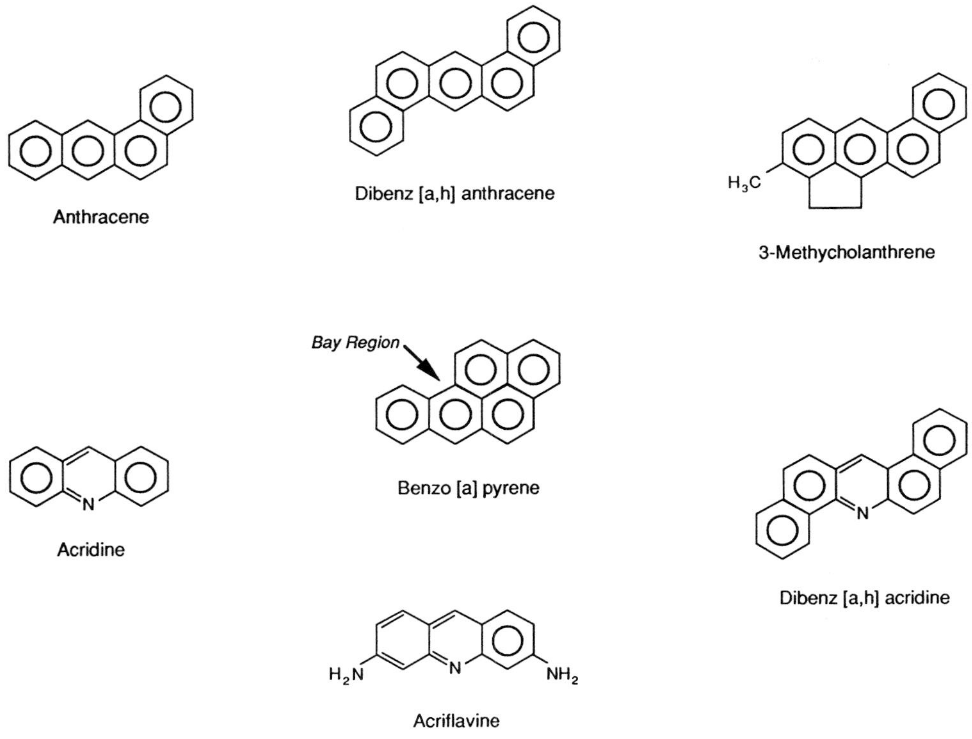

FIGURE 15–3. The structures of important polycyclic hydrocarbons including benzo(a)pyrene and the popular fish treatment agent acriflavine.

leum refining are sources of polycyclic aromatic hydrocarbon pollution.

Low-temperature conversion of organic material into fossil fuels also produces small amounts of these toxins; however, because this conversion generally occurs underground in anaerobic environments, the release of polycyclic aromatic hydrocarbons from this source into air, water, or surface soil is rare. Natural formation of hydrocarbons also occurs as the result of the metabolic activity of some bacteria, fungi, and plants, and this must be considered a minor contributing source of pollution (Bossert and Bartha, 1986).

Polycyclic aromatic hydrocarbons reach the aquatic environment by runoff from contaminated land, airborne contamination, and oil spills. Their concentrations in an aquatic environment usually reflect the degree of human and industrial activity within and surrounding the water and its sources. Because of their hydrophobicity, polycyclic aromatic hydrocarbons in water generally adsorb onto particulate matter. This may result in their settling to the bottom of ponds or streams. Once settled on the bottom, these compounds can concentrate significantly (Butler and Sibbald, 1986; DouAbdul et al., 1987; Broman et al., 1987). This is of particular importance to bottom-feeding fish that will have contact with the high polycyclic aromatic hydrocarbon concentrations in sediment.

Sample Analysis

Polycyclic aromatic hydrocarbons are metabolized primarily by mixed function oxidase activity in the liver. Therefore, samples to be submitted to determine concentrations should include liver, kidney, intestine, muscle, fat, and whole fish, if possible.

Detection and Quantitation Technique

Detection and quantitation of polycyclic aromatic hydrocarbons is primarily performed using gas chromatography or gas chromatography–mass spectrometry.

Polychlorinated Biphenyls

Polychlorinated biphenyls are a group of nonflammable, chemically stable oils used in transformers, condensers, and some closed heat-transfer systems. The basic chemical structure of these compounds is shown in Figure 15–4. Chlorine atoms are found at one or more of the sites marked (X). Although closely related chemically and toxicologically to many pesticides used today, polychlorinated biphenyls were not initially considered significant environmental pollutants owing to their "closed-system" uses as nonflammable lubricants and fluids in electrical transformers, pumps, and compressors.

Polychlorinated biphenyl production peaked at about 75 million pounds per year in the United States

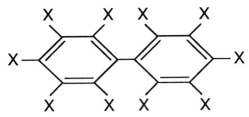

FIGURE 15–4. The general structure of polychlorinated biphenyls. X marks possible chlorination sites.

in 1970. Calculations based on the number of transformers and condensers taken out of service and discarded each year indicate that about 290 million pounds of polychlorinated biphenyls were discarded in landfills or dumps (Nimmo, 1985) and must be considered as a source of land and water pollution. In fact, contaminated municipal sewage sludge and runoff from landfills are principal sources of polychlorinated biphenyl accumulation in streams (Shaw and Connell, 1987; Wren et al., 1987; Crossland, et al., 1987; Greig and Sennefelder, 1985).

Sample Analysis

If exposure to polychlorinated biphenyls is suspected, samples of body fat, liver, and brain from affected fish should be submitted along with soil samples from in and around the stream.

Detection and Quantitation Technique

Detection and quantitation of polychlorinated biphenyls are usually performed by gas chromatography or gas chromatography-mass spectrometry.

LITERATURE CITED

Awadallah, R.M., Mohamed, A.E., and Gabr, S.A. (1985) Determination of trace elements in fish by instrumental neutron activation analysis. J. Radioanal. Nucl. Chem. 95:145–151.

Benedeczky, I., Nemcsok, J., and Halasy, K.J. (1986) Electronmicroscopic analysis of the cytopathological effect of pesticides in the liver, kidney, and gill tissues of carp. Acta Biol. Szeged. 32:69–91.

Berry, C.R. (1984) Toxicity of the herbicides diquat and endothall to goldfish. Environ. Poll. 34:251–258.

Bossert, I.D., and Bartha, R. (1986) Structure-biodegradability relationships of polycyclic aromatic hydrocarbons in soil. Bull. Environ. Contam. Toxicol. 37:490–495.

Broman, D., Colmsjo, A., and Naf, C. (1987) Characterization of the PAC profile in settling particulates from the urban waters of Stockholm. Bull. Environ. Contam. Toxicol. 38:1020–1028.

Butler, A.C., and Sibbald, R.R. (1986) Isolation and gas-chromatographic determination of saturated and polycyclic aromatic hydrocarbons in mussels. Bull. Environ. Contam. Toxicol. 37:570–578.

Camanzo, J., Rice, C.P., Jude, D.J., and Rossmann, R. (1987) Organic priority pollutants in nearshore fish from 14 Lake Michigan tributaries and embayments, 1983. J. Great Lakes Res. 13:296–309.

Crossland, N.O., Bennett, D., and Wolff, C.J.M. (1987) Fate of 2,5,4'-trichlorobiphenyl in outdoor ponds and its uptake via the food chain compared with direct uptake via the gills in grass carp and rainbow trout. Ecotoxicol. Environ. Safety 13:225–238.

DouAbdul, A.A.Z., Abaychi, J.K., Al-Edanee, T.E., and Ghani, A.A., Al-Saad, H.T. (1987) Polynuclear aromatic hydrocarbons (PAHs) in fish from the Arabian Gulf. Bull. Environ. Contam. Toxicol. 38:546–552.

Greig, R.A., and Sennefelder, G. (1985) Metals and PCB concentrations in mussels from Long Island Sound. Bull. Environ. Contam. Toxicol. 35:331–334.

Hilmy, A.M., el-Domiaty, N.A., Daabees, A.Y., and Abdel Latife, H.A. (1986) Toxicity in Tilapia zilli and Clarias lazera (Pisces) induced by zinc, seasonally. Comp. Biochem. Physiol. [C] 87(1):181–186.

Jorgensen, D. and Heisinger, J.F. (1987) The effects of selenium on the distribution of mercury in the organs of the black bullhead (Ictalurus melas). Comp. Biochem. Physiol. [C] 87(1):181–186.

Kai, N., Ueda, T., Takeda, M., Takeda, Y., and Kataoka, K.A. (1986) The levels of mercury and selenium in gonad of yellow fin and albacore. Jpn. Soc. Sci. Fish. 52(6):1049–1053.

Kawatsu, H. (1979) Studies on the anemia of fish—VIII. Hemorrhagic anemia of carp caused by a herbicide, molinate. Bull. Jpn. Soc. Sci. Fish. 43:905–912.

Khan, A.H., Ali, M., Biaswas, S.K., and Hadi, D.A. (1987) Trace elements in marine fish from the Bay of Bengal. Sci. Total Environ. 61:121–130.

Lay, M-M., Niland, A.M., Debaun, J.R., and Menn, J.J. (1979) Metabolism of the thiocarbamate herbicide molinate (Ordram) in Japanese carp, in pesticide and xenobiotic metabolism in aquatic organisms. Am. Chem. Soc. Symp. Series 99:95–120.

Leland, H.V., and Kuwabara, J.S. (1985) Trace metals. In: Fundamentals of Aquatic Toxicology (Rand, G.M., and Petrocelli, S.R., eds.). Hemisphere, Washington, D.C.

Moore, J.W. and Ramarmoorthy, W. (1984) Heavy metals in natural waters: Applied monitoring and impact assessment. Springer-Verlag, New York.

National Research Council of Canada (1982): Thermal effects upon fishes, NRCC 18566. Ottowa, Canada.

Nemcsok, J., Orban, L., Asztalos, B., and Vig, E. (1987) Accumulation of pesticides in the organs of carp, Cyprinus carpio L., at 4°C and 20°C. Bull. Environ. Contam. Toxicol. 39:370–378.

Nimmo, D.R. (1985) Pesticides. In: Fundamentals of Aquatic Toxicology. (Rand, G.M., and Petrocelli, S.R., eds.). Hemisphere, Washington, D.C.

Phipps, G.L., and Holcombe, G.W. (1985) A method for aquatic multiple species toxicant testing: Acute toxicity of 10 chemicals to 5 vertebrates and 2 invertebrates. Environ. Poll. 38:141–157.

Price, H.A., Welch, R.L., Schell, R.H., and Warren, L.A. (1986) Modified multiresidue method for chlordane, toxaphene, and polychlorinated biphenyls in fish. Bull. Environ. Contam. Toxicol. 37:1–9.

Sargent, P.A., and Youson, J.H. (1986) Quantification of iron deposits in several body tissues of lampreys (Petromyzon marinus L.) throughout the life cycle. Comp. Biochem. Physiol. 83A(3):573–577.

Schmitt, C.J., and Finger, S.E. (1987) The effects of sample preparation on measured concentrations of eight elements in edible tissue of fish from streams contaminated by lead mining. Arch. Environ. Contam. Toxicol. 16:185–207.

Segner, H. (1987) Response of fed and starved roach, Rutilus rutilus, to sublethal copper contamination. J. Fish Biol. 30:423–437.

Shaw, G.R., and Connell, D.W. (1987) Comparative kinetics for bioaccumulation of polychlorinated biphenyls by the polychaete (Capitella capitata) and fish (Mugil cephalus). Ecotoxicol. Environ. Safety 13:84–91.

Sherman, R.E., Gloss, S.P., and Lion, L.W. (1987) A comparison of toxicity tests conducted in the laboratory and in experimental ponds using cadmium and the fathead minnow (Pimephales promelas). Water Res. 21:317–323.

Suzuki, K.T., Sunaga, H., Kobayashi, E., and Hatakeyama, S. (1987) Environmental and injected cadmium are sequestered by two major isoforms of basal copper, zinc-metallothionein in gibel (Carassius auratus Langsdorfi) liver. Comp. Biochem. Physiol. 87C(1):87–93.

United States Environmental Protection Agency (1980a) Ambient water quality criteria for copper. EPA 440/5–80–036. Washington, D.C.

United States Environmental Protection Agency (1980b) Ambient water quality criteria for zinc. EPA 440/5–80–079. Washington, D.C.

United States Environmental Protection Agency (1980c) Ambient water quality criteria for lead. EPA 440/5–80–057. Washington, D.C.

United States Environmental Protection Agency (1980d) Ambient water quality criteria for mercury. EPA 440/5–80–058. Washington, D.C.

Villeneuve, J.P., Fowler, S.W., and Anderlini, V.C. (1987) Organochlorine levels in edible marine organisms from Kuwaiti coastal waters. Bull. Environ. Contam. Toxicol. 38:266–270.

Virtanen, M.T. (1986) Histopathological and ultrastructural changes in the gills of Poecilia reticulatus induced by an organochlorine pesticide. J. Environ. Pathol. Toxicol. Oncol. 7:73–86.

Welz, B., Schlemmer, G., and Voellkopf, U. (1986) Trace element determination in biological materials using stabilized temperature platform furnace AAS and Zeeman-effect background correction. Acta Pharmacol. Toxicol. Suppl. 59(7):589–592.

Wren, C.D., Hunter, D.B., Leatherland, J.F., and Stokes, P.M. (1987) The effects of polychlorinated biphenyls and methylmercury, singly and in combination on mink. II: Reproduction and kit development. Arch. Environ. Contam. Toxicol. 16:449–454.

Youson, J.H., and Neville, C.M. (1987) Deposition of aluminum in the gill epithelium of rainbow trout (Salmo gairdneri Richardson) subjected to sublethal concentrations of the metal. Can. J. Zool. 65:547–656.

Chapter 16

Epidemiology

G. W. KLONTZ

Epidemiology is the branch of medicine describing the occurrence, distribution, and types of diseases in populations of animals (Austin and Werner, 1974, Kleinbaum et al., 1982). Traditionally, the term *epidemiology* has been associated with disease episodes or epidemics in human populations, and the term *epizootiology* has been used to indicate similar issues associated with disease episodes in populations of domestic and free-living mammals, birds, reptiles, amphibians, and fish. However, during the past two decades the term *epizootiology* has been dropped from common usage in favor of the term *epidemiology*. This application has given rise to a more inclusive definition of epidemiology as the medical aspects of ecology (Schwabe, 1969). Epidemiological principles have a role in fish health management, although published reports where they have been rigorously applied to fish populations are few (Klontz, 1984). The task before the worldwide fish health management community today is to adopt and adapt these principles to increase our understanding of the nature of diseases in confined and free-living populations of fish.

DESCRIPTIVE MEASUREMENTS OF DISEASE

One of the chief impediments to applying epidemiologic principles to disease episodes in populations of animals is the lack of uniform nomenclature. Many terms currently used are actually misused by the uninformed, resulting in considerable confusion. For example, the term *disease* is often used to allude to the causal agent or pathogen. For example, there are many instances where "diseases" are said to be transmitted. It would be more technically correct to state that the pathogenic organism is transmitted. Disease, then, is the result of the transmission, but it is not transmitted.

MEASURES OF DISEASE OCCURRENCE

The usual method of quantifying disease episodes is to establish ratios and rates. The data used to establish these are of two types, discrete and continuous. Discrete, or categorical, data are easily placed into distinct categories. For example, data collected on whether animals in a population are dead or alive are a form of discrete data. There is no intermediary position or continuum to consider. This type of data is essentially qualitative. On the other hand, continuous data, which are sometimes referred to as numeric data, do not offer convenient discrete categories for data division. They are quantitative data. An example of continuous, or numeric, data would be the body weight of animals in a population. It is reasonable to expect that a fish's weight can be any number or fraction of kilograms, grams, and milligrams.

Ratios

Ratios are a fractional relationship between two numeric quantities. The data used to determine a ratio can be continuous or discrete. In a ratio, data or animals in the numerator are not represented in the denominator. This is in distinct contrast to a proportion. For example, in a ratio, the number of dead animals (A) compared to the number of live animals (B) at a single time point can be expressed as the ratio A/B.

Proportions

Proportions are a fractional value ranging between 0 and 1 that are often represented as a percentage. In contrast to ratios, individuals or data in the numerator of a proportion are included in the denominator. For example, the proportion or percentage of rainbow trout with proliferative kidney disease in a raceway population would be equal to the number of affected fish (A) divided by the total fish population of the raceway (T), which includes both affected and unaffected fish.

Fatality Proportion

Another example of a proportion is a fatality proportion (sometimes inappropriately called a fatality rate). This calculation gives information about the lethality of a condition. The numerator is the number of deaths due to a specific disease. The denominator is the number of cases of the disease identified in the population being examined. The statistic is a proportion because the fatal cases are included in the total number of cases being used in the denominator.

Prevalence

Prevalence is essentially a proportion that specifically looks at the number of affected individuals within a population at a specified time. The numerator is the number of individuals in the population affected. The denominator is the total number of individuals in the population at risk at the time point of interest. For example, if 1000 plaice caught in a specific locality were examined for the presence of a fungal infection, such as *Ichthyophonus hoferi*, and 355 of the fish examined had the disease, a proportion of affected animals to the entire population examined (the population at risk) would be 35.5%. This would be the prevalence of the disease in the population, and it is a useful description of disease data.

Rates

Rates are dynamic measurements that describe the occurrence of events within a given time period rather than at a point in time. The numerator of a rate consists of events, and the denominator is the population in which the events occurred over a period of time. For example, a mortality rate would describe the number of deaths expected within a specified time period. The numerator would be the number of deaths, and the denominator would be the population in which the deaths occurred. If 36 fish out of a population of 1000 died over a year, the mortality rate for the population would be 3.6%/year.

Incidence Rate

An incidence rate represents the rate of development of new cases occurring as a result of a specific cause during a specified time. Often the standard time period used is 1 year. It is similar to other rates and is generated by using the number of new cases due to a specific cause as the numerator and dividing by a denominator representing the estimated population at risk over time. For example, if 20 new cases of infectious pancreatic necrosis virus infection are detected in 1 month in a population of brown trout that includes 2000 fish, the incidence of pancreatic necrosis in that population is 1%/month.

INVESTIGATION OF DISEASE OUTBREAKS

Morbidity/Mortality Curves

The measures of disease occurrence described above are used to depict morbidity and mortality in populations. Patterns of disease occurrence can also be depicted graphically, and the shape of the curves generated often helps identify temporal trends that reflect the cause of the outbreak (Russell, 1977). If the number of events or the percent representation

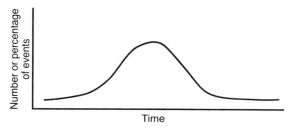

FIGURE 16–1. An epidemiform propagative event curve. The bell-shaped distribution of this curve suggests that an infectious agent or toxic substance has moved through a population and is no longer affecting the number of events in the population.

of a ratio or proportion is plotted versus time, characteristic curves can be seen. Of course, these curves can become quite complex when multiple factors are affecting the transmission of disease agents and the development of disease within the population being studied.

Propagative Source Curves

A propagative source curve is a curve that is either epidemiform (Fig. 16–1) or sigmoidal (Fig. 16–2). In an epidemiform curve, the number of events is initially a very low number, but over time the number of events builds to a peak, which then falls off to return to the initial low number. This bell-shaped, epidemiform curve suggests that an infectious agent or toxic substance has moved through a population or the population's environment and at the end of the time scale is no longer affecting the number of events in the population. It is indicative of a direct horizontal transmission of the causal agent, and the breadth of the curve is related to the incubation time and the period of communicability of the disease agent as well as to the efficiency of the surveillance system.

Deviations from bell-shaped to sigmoidal-shaped curves are related to latent periods or periods during the course of the disease in which the agent is not communicable or is less communicable.

Point Source Curves

A very abruptly spiked curve (Fig. 16–3) is sometimes referred to as a point source curve. Its shape,

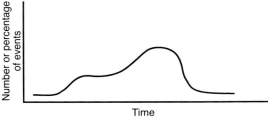

FIGURE 16–2. A sigmoid propagative event curve. The deviations from the bell shape are related to latent periods or periods of less communicability.

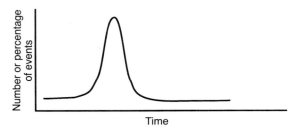

FIGURE 16–3. A point source event curve. This very sharp curve suggests a single time point exposure.

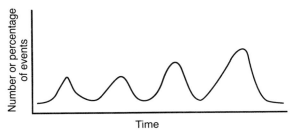

FIGURE 16–5. A broad, multiple-source event curve. This type of curve suggests multiple independent exposures to a disease agent.

rising rapidly to a peak and falling away rapidly to baseline levels, suggests the population at risk was exposed to the disease agent at a single time point, and that all susceptible members of the population were affected within a very brief time span. This type of curve can be seen in infectious disease situations with highly virulent organisms exposed to a completely susceptible population. Typically, it suggests the potential association of environmental toxicants or the presence of an inanimate vehicle that serves as a source of infectious agent.

Broad Source Curves

The opposite extreme of a point source curve is a broad source curve. It can be a plateau-shaped curve (Fig. 16–4), which is indicative of exposure to an agent over a long period of time or a slow incubation or transmission rate. It also can consist of multiple spiked curves (Fig. 16–5), which result from frequent intermittent exposure to the disease agent. Often the difference between which of these types of curves is generated will be a function of the data collection cycle. If data are collected very infrequently, the individual spikes of an multipeak curve will be lost and blended into a plateau appearance.

Investigative Approaches

Disease outbreak investigation requires the skills of individuals from a variety of disciplines, including microbiology, pathology, physiology, toxicology, limnology, ecology, and epidemiology. Epidemiological disease investigations focus on the identification of environment-, host-, and agent-related factors

associated with disease outbreaks. Fish in confined and free-living conditions are subject to many biotic and abiotic factors potentially associated with episodes of noninfectious and infectious diseases (Klontz, 1979).

Retrospective Studies

Retrospective studies are used to look backward in time after a disease problem has been identified. Investigators utilize data collected by a variety of often unrelated sources during the time of the outbreak and attempt to describe the "who, what, when, where, and how" of an episode in their efforts to explain an unusual increase in occurrence of a disease. There are several fundamental steps to the process.

1. Confirm the nature of the problem. An important first step is to establish a definitive diagnosis of the disease entity being studied based on clinical signs or laboratory tests. Although this may seem like an obvious first step, it can all too often be the root of serious embarrassment. Establish a definitive diagnosis or diagnostic criteria for the entity you are studying.

2. Characterize the events. In this step you must document the historical aspects of the events you wish to study. This means collect data on the clinical, environmental, social, and other factors that precede or are concomitant with the events.

3. Identify the population at risk. The investigator must identify the total number of individuals that the events under study had the opportunity to affect. This requires the investigator to catalog the age, size, and year-class of affected and unaffected individuals, when the cases occurred, and where they were observed.

4. Establish proportions, rates, and ratios of events. The prevalence, incidence, and other proportions, ratios, and rates related to the disease outbreak in the population under study are calculated.

5. Identify the suspected associated causal factors. This is accomplished by comparing the derived rates. A skilled investigator can identify and characterize the factors potentially associated with the disease episode from examination of the mathematical or graphic data generated in step 4.

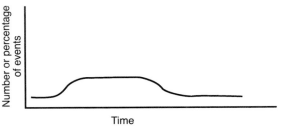

FIGURE 16–4. A broad, single-source event curve. This type of curve may indicate a slow incubation period or transmission rate.

6. Formulate and test hypotheses. Having identified suspected associated causal factors, it should be possible to form hypotheses about the cause of the outbreak, and question the roles of each associated factor. This process involves asking questions of the data already in hand that would either tend to confirm or challenge the hypotheses.

7. Presentation of recommendations. No study would be complete without careful preparation of a report of the investigation, preferably subjected to peer review.

8. Experimental testing. Although the retrospective study may be considered completed with the presentation of recommendations, it may be warranted to experimentally examine the validity of the associations identified in the retrospective study. At this point, the retrospective approach becomes a prospective approach.

Prospective epidemiology is essentially experimental epidemiology. It seeks to monitor a population or, more frequently, multiple populations over a time period in the future to examine the impact of associated and causal factors. Prospective epidemiology is often based upon the foundations of retrospective studies that have provided support to particular hypotheses, which can be tested prospectively.

LITERATURE CITED

Austin, D.F., and Werner, S.B. (1974) Epidemiology for the Health Sciences. Charles C. Thomas, Springfield, Illinois.

Kleinbaum, D.G., Kupper, L.L., and Morgenstern, H. (1982) Epidemiologic Research: Principles and Quantitative Methods. Van Nostrand Reinhold, New York, pp. 56–57,97.

Klontz, G.W. (1979) Fish Health Management. Vol. II: Concepts and Methods of Fish Disease Epidemiology. Office of Continuing Education, University of Idaho, Moscow.

Klontz, G.W. (1984) Epidemiology of diseases in wild fish populations. In: Contaminant Effects on Fisheries (Cairns, V.W., Hodson, P.W., and Nriagu, J.O., Eds.). John Wiley & Sons, New York, pp. 9–18.

Russell, L.H. (1977) A Syllabus: The Principles of Epidemiology. Texas A&M University, College Station.

Schwabe, C.W. (1969) Veterinary Medicine and Human Health. 2nd ed. Williams & Wilkins, Baltimore.

Chapter 17

ZOONOTIC DISEASES

THOMAS G. NEMETZ   EMMETT B. SHOTTS, JR.

Zoonoses involving transmission of disease-producing agents from fish to man have been reviewed previously (Shotts, 1980, 1987; Eastaugh and Shepherd, 1989). Examination of recent literature pertaining to fishborne zoonotic diseases reveals three salient points. First, the number of reported outbreaks of fish-related diseases in the United States is increasing. Factors responsible include the increased awareness of disease symptoms; the increased rates of exposure to contaminated or infected fish via consumption or recreational activities; the increased contamination of marine, estuarine, and freshwater environments by chemical and biological pollutants; and the increased susceptibility to disease as a result of immunocompromising diseases such as acquired immunodeficiency syndrome (AIDS). Second, the overall incidence of fish-related diseases in the United States remains relatively low. Third, disease episodes in immunocompetent hosts are often self-limited bouts of gastroenteritis; however, patients may suffer serious disease and subsequent mortality if their conditions are improperly diagnosed, or if they have a preexisting disease that compromises their immune system. The purpose of this chapter is to review and summarize recently published information concerning known and potential fishborne zoonoses that occur in the United States.

BACTERIA

Bacterial diseases of fish are described in Part II of this book and in other texts (Frerichs and Roberts, 1989). The major bacterial diseases of fish in incidence and severity are caused primarily by gram-negative rods. A few of these organisms, and a small number of gram-positive species, also cause disease in humans. An important feature of many of bacterial organisms is their opportunistic nature. The development of disease in the human host often requires a preexisting state that compromises the immune system. In general, humans contract fishborne bacterial disease through ingestion of contaminated fish tissue or water, or by injection of the organisms into puncture wounds or abrasions. Exposures often result in inapparent or mild episodes of gastroenteritis or in localized infections of the skin and underlying tissue. However, a few bacteria are highly pathogenic and may produce high rates of mortality.

Gram-Positive Organisms

STREPTOCOCCUS. Members of the genus *Streptococcus* have been found to produce disease outbreaks among freshwater and saltwater fishes in the southern United States and Japan (Frerichs and Roberts, 1989). Many fish isolates are of the Lancefield group B and D serotypes (Shotts and Teska, 1989). Although no transmission from fish to man has been documented, the potential for human infection does exist among individuals who handle diseased fish.

STAPHYLOCOCCUS. Members of the genus *Staphylococcus* occasionally produce disease in fish (Shotts and Teska, 1989). *Staphylococcus* sp. has been isolated from aquarium water and has been found in aquaculture pond water in Africa (Ogbondeminu and Okaeme, 1986). The greatest potential for staphylococcal fishborne disease is probably by means of enterotoxin synthesis during improper food handling, rather than by infection with intact organisms.

CLOSTRIDIUM. Members of the genus *Clostridium* are found as commensal organisms in the intestinal tract of many marine and freshwater fishes. In fish, the bacteria rarely produce disease; however, isolated outbreaks of fish mortality have been described in salmonids (Frerichs and Roberts, 1989).

Clostridium species can cause serious and potentially fatal disease in humans who consume fish tissues in which the vegetative form has proliferated and produced heat-labile toxins. Two species (*C. perfringens* and *C. botulinum*) have produced disease outbreaks as a result of consumption of contaminated fish (Bean and Griffin, 1990). *Clostridium perfringens* causes clinical signs of gastroenteritis, which often resolve within 24 hours with minimal or no treatment. In contrast, *C. botulinum* produces five different forms of a neurotoxin that causes presynaptic blockage of acetylcholine release and consequent signs of diffuse lower motor neuron disease (e.g., generalized muscle dystonia, difficulty in swallowing or speaking, and ptosis). Death in affected individuals is usually caused by respiratory paralysis.

In fish tissues, type E toxin is produced almost exclusively (Telzak et al., 1990), although one disease outbreak involving contaminated fish was attributed to type A toxin (Rigau-Perez et al., 1982). Ingestion of uneviscerated whitefish (kapchunka) was determined to be the source of two outbreaks of type E food poisoning in the United States (Centers for Disease Control, 1987a; Telzak et al., 1990). The reasons why type E toxin is preferentially produced in fish are unknown, but it is believed to be a function of the fishes' intestinal microflora and tissue composition (Smith and Turner, 1989).

ERYSIPELOTHRIX. The genus *Erysipelothrix* has only one member, *E. rhusiopathiae* (formerly *E. insidiosa*). It is a facultative anaerobic rod with worldwide distribution. The organism appears to cause no disease in fish and is thought to be present in the external mucus of many freshwater and marine species (Wood, 1975).

Erysipelothrix rhusiopathiae does cause disease in humans, swine, sheep, avian, and other species. The clinical syndrome in man has recently been reviewed (Reboli and Farrar, 1989). Infections with *E. rhusiopathiae* are considered to be an occupational disease of individuals who handle animal tissues containing the organism. Butchers, abattoir workers, veterinarians, and cooks, both home and professional, have a higher risk of infection than the general population. The disease is considered to be particularly prevalent among persons handling fish. Three forms of the disease have been described in humans: a localized skin infection (erysipeloid, or "fish rose") often involving the fingers or hands, a diffuse cutaneous form in which a localized infection spreads to adjacent tissues, and a septicemic form.

The literature concerning *E. rhusiopathiae* septicemia has recently been summarized (Gorby and Peacock, 1988). Only 49 cases have been reported in the United States since 1912; however, the syndrome produced a 38% mortality rate among affected individuals. Endocarditis was the most common and serious sequela, occurring in 90% of patients. Fish or shellfish were believed to be the source of infection in 22% of reported cases. A history of alcohol abuse was found to be a predisposing factor to septicemia (33% incidence).

MYCOBACTERIUM. Organisms in the genus *Mycobacterium* are nonmotile acid-fast rods. Three species are recognized as pathogens of fish (Frerichs and Roberts, 1989). *Mycobacterium fortuitum* produces disease in a variety of fish found in tropical and temperate climates. *Mycobacterium chelonei* has been isolated primarily from salmonids. *Mycobacterium marinum* is a pathogen of tropical species of freshwater and saltwater fishes. Of interest is the fact that *M. fortuitum* grows at 30° and 37°C, whereas the other two species grow only at 30°C (Frerichs and Roberts, 1989). *Mycobacterium chelonei* and *M. marinum* may not be detected in some instances because the incubation of human isolates is commonly done at 37°C.

The advent of AIDS has spurred considerable interest in these and other mycobacteria other than tuberculosis (MOTT) species. Mycobacterial infections are common sequelae to AIDS, and MOTT species (primarily *M. avium* complex, formerly *M. avium-intracellulare*) are currently isolated at a higher frequency than *M. tuberculosis* in human immunodeficiency virus (HIV)–infected individuals (Centers for Disease Control, 1987b). The increased number of mycobacterial infections is of concern because the rates of infection have also risen in nonimmunocompromised individuals (Prince et al., 1989), and because inadequate diagnosis and treatment may result in excessive morbidity and mortality (Iseman, 1989).

In contrast to *M. avium*, only a low number of human infections with the three fish pathogens has been reported. Clinical data regarding these and other MOTT species have been reviewed (Woods and Washington, 1987). Persons infected with *M. fortuitum* and *M. chelonei* demonstrate a variety of clinical presentations that are correlated with the presence or absence of immunocompromising diseases such as AIDS. Typically, HIV-positive individuals show signs of disseminated or respiratory disease, whereas immunocompetent patients are more likely to exhibit circumscribed cutaneous lesions acquired through penetrating wounds. No cases of infection in the reported survey resulted from exposure to fish. However, *M. fortuitum* has been reported to produce cutaneous lesions on the hands of individuals handling contaminated aquaria (Shotts, 1987; Frerichs and Roberts, 1989).

Case histories of human infections with *M. marinum* have been reported (Donta et al., 1986; Gray et al., 1990). This organism is the agent of swimming pool and fish tank granuloma in humans and tuberculosis of fish. Humans are infected with *M. marinum* by contamination of lacerated or abraded skin during activities such as swimming or cleaning tropical fish aquaria. Two clinical syndromes are observed (Woods and Washington, 1987). A single granulomatous nodule may form at the site of infection, most commonly on the hands or fingers (Fig. 17–1). This lesion often resolves over a period of weeks to months without antibiotic treatment. The customary lack of dissemination to adjacent tissues is believed to be a reflection of the organism's inability to grow at 37°C (Brown and Sanders, 1987).

A "sporotrichoid" form of infection with *M. marinum* is sometimes seen. Localized infection is followed by spread to nearby lymph nodes, resulting in the appearance of nodules at the original site of infection and in regional lymphatic tissues. The bacterium has also been observed to occasionally spread deeper into adjacent tissues and produce arthritis, osteomyelitis, and tenosynovitis. Such infections may be the result of T-cell unresponsiveness to specific mycobacterial antigens in immunoincompetent patients (Dattwyler et al., 1987). More disseminated forms of the disease are likely in patients infected with HIV, and those individuals are advised

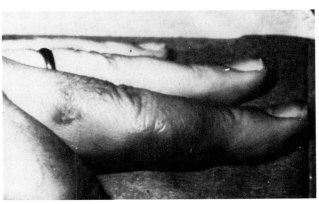

FIGURE 17–1. Human infection with *Mycobacterium marinum.*

to avoid cleaning tropical fish aquaria (Ries et al., 1990).

NOCARDIA. *Nocardia asteroides* and *N. kampachi* have been isolated at very low frequencies from tuberculoid lesions of both fish and man (Shotts, 1980, 1987; Frerichs and Roberts, 1989). Infections with these organisms may be misdiagnosed as mycobacterial disease because of the similarity of clinical signs and the positive reaction to acid-fast staining.

Gram-Negative Organisms

VIBRIO *SPP.* Members of the genus *Vibrio* are facultatively anaerobic, pleiomorphic rods that are commonly isolated from marine and estuarine waters; however, some species are also found in fresh water. They are considered to be the most significant bacterial pathogens of marine fish (Frerichs and Roberts, 1989). Nine species have been associated with foodborne diseases in humans, the most important species of which are *V. cholerae* 0 group 1, *V. cholerae* non-01, *V. parahemolyticus,* and *V. vulnificus* (Eastaugh and Shepherd, 1989).

Foodborne infections with *Vibrio* spp. in the United States are most often associated with consumption of raw or inadequately cooked shellfish. Clinical signs include vomiting and diarrhea that vary in severity according to the bacterial species causing the disease. In general, *V. cholerae* 0 group 1 causes the most severe signs. *Vibrio cholerae* non-01 infections are seen less frequently and are less debilitating. *Vibrio parahemolyticus* infections are frequently inapparent (Morris et al., 1981; Lowry et al., 1989). The apparent ubiquity of this organism in marine water gives credence to the idea that ingestion of improperly cooked fish may also be a source of human infection. In Japan, *V. cholerae* non-01 has been isolated at relatively high frequencies from market fish (Murase et al., 1988). One case of septicemia caused by ingestion of catfish contaminated with *Vibrio hollisae* has been reported in the United States (Lowry et al., 1986).

Human infections with *V. vulnificus* have been the object of some scrutiny (Johnston et al., 1985; Klontz et al., 1988; Hoffmann et al., 1988; Vartian and Septimus, 1990). The disease is one of low incidence and high mortality. Two clinical syndromes have been described. The first is a primary septicemia and is most often associated with consumption of raw oysters. Signs of infection include fever, changes in mental status, ecchymotic hemorrhages, bulla formation, and pain in the lower extremities. The mortality rate among affected individuals is approximately 50%, even with prompt diagnosis and treatment. A prominent predisposing factor is preexisting liver disease, especially cirrhosis, which is believed to adversely affect leukocyte migration (Morris, 1988).

The second clinical syndrome produced by *V. vulnificus* is one of wound infections and is characterized by cellulitis, edema, hemorrhages, bulla formation, and extensive tissue necrosis. Despite prompt and aggressive treatment, the mortality rate ranges from 25 to 30% among affected individuals. In most cases, infection is acquired by introduction of contaminated seawater into skin wounds.

PLESIOMONAS SHIGELLOIDES. The taxonomy of the genus *Plesiomonas* is uncertain, but at present it is considered to be a member of the family Vibrionaceae. *Plesiomonas shigelloides* is a facultatively anaerobic rod that causes septicemia in various species of fishes (Shotts and Teska, 1989). The organism is found in fresh water and salt water and has been isolated from the intestinal tract of tropical freshwater fishes (Centers for Disease Control, 1989).

Human infections with *P. shigelloides* are acquired through ingestion of contaminated water or uncooked fish and shellfish. Two clinical syndromes have been described (Brenden et al., 1988). The first and most common syndrome is one of gastroenteritis, which is characterized by fever, abdominal pain, vomiting, and diarrhea. The low incidence of positive cultures among asymptomatic individuals is believed to reflect the absence of a carrier state in humans. A majority (70%) of patients with this disease have either a preexisting debilitating disease such as cancer or cirrhosis or a risk factor such as recent foreign travel or seafood consumption. Contaminated water from a tropical aquarium has been implicated as the source in one case (CDC, 1989).

The second clinical syndrome caused by *P. shigelloides* is one of extraintestinal disease and is rarely encountered. Affected individuals may demonstrate meningitis, sepsis, and cellulitis. A recent clinical report described treatment of a pancreatic abscess from which *P. shigelloides* was cultured (Kennedy et al., 1990).

AEROMONAS. Aeromonad organisms are members of the family Vibrionaceae and are facultatively anaerobic rods. *Aeromonas salmonicida* is the agent of furunculosis in salmonids and is not considered to be a human pathogen. Five other species (*A. hydrophila, A. sobria, A. caviae, A. schubertii,* and *A. veronii*) are currently considered to be members of the motile aeromonas complex (Shotts and Teska, 1989). These organisms can produce septicemia in infected fishes and are routinely found in the aquatic environment. The species most commonly isolated is *A. hydrophila*. It is found worldwide in tropical and temperate fresh water and is considered to be part of the normal intestinal microflora of healthy fish (Frerichs and Roberts, 1989). *Aeromonas* spp. have been found in nearly 100% of freshwater tropical aquaria in a survey of English pet shops (Sanyal et al., 1987).

Despite the ubiquity of *Aeromonas* spp., available data suggest that motile aeromonads produce a low number of human infections. California reported a 1-year disease rate of 0.7/million population (Centers for Disease Control, 1990). Individuals infected with *Aeromonas* may show a variety of clinical signs, but the two most common syndromes are gastroenteritis and localized wound infection. Aeromonad gastroenteritis is produced by ingestion of contaminated water and is characterized by diarrheic states that range from acute and self-limiting to chronic and unresolving (George et al., 1985). Wound infections due to aeromonads are sporadically reported and result from introduction of the organism via laceration or puncture wound. Such infections may be superficial or may progress to cellulitis, deep muscle necrosis, or septicemia. Although such infections have occasionally been documented in the nonimmunocompromised host (Heckerling et al., 1983; Karam et al., 1983), the primary concern from a public health standpoint is with individuals who have an immune deficiency as a result of AIDS or other chronic diseases and who acquire an aeromonad infection as a result of wound contamination (Flynn and Knepp, 1987).

PSEUDOMONAS. The genus *Pseudomonas* is a member of the family Pseudomonadaceae. Pseudomonads are motile aerobic rods that are commonly found in soil and water. *Pseudomonas fluorescens* infrequently produces a septicemic disease in pond, aquarium, and marine fish that is similar to the one seen with *Aeromonas* (Frerichs and Roberts, 1989). Although the potential exists for this organism to produce infections in humans with preexisting immunocompromising disease, no documented cases related to fish exposure have been reported.

THE ENTEROBACTERIACEAE. Members of the genera *Escherichia*, *Salmonella*, *Klebsiella*, *Edwardsiella*, and *Yersinia* are included in the family Enterbacteriaceae, which occur as facultatively anaerobic rods. Enteropathogenic *Escherichia coli* has been isolated from fish but apparently does not produce disease (Shotts, 1987). *Salmonella* spp. have been isolated from freshwater aquaria, and fish are apparent carriers of the organism (Shotts, 1987; Sanyal et al., 1987). Similarly, *Salmonella* spp. have been isolated from numerous marine species, including fishes, shellfishes, cetaceans, and pinnipeds (Minette, 1986). At present, the primary risk of infection with *E. coli* and *Salmonella* appears to be through the ingestion of improperly prepared contaminated fish food products. Isolated instances of such food poisonings have been reported (Bean and Griffin, 1990; Bean et al., 1990). *Klebsiella* spp. are found in aquatic environments, and one case of *K. pneumoniae* septicemia has been reported as a consequence of handling contaminated fish (Reagan et al., 1990).

Two species of *Edwardsiella* are known pathogens of fish. *Edwardsiella ictaluri* is the agent of enteric septicemia in channel catfish. No instance of human infection with this bacterium has been reported. *Edwardsiella tarda* is the agent of emphysematous putrefactive disease in catfish and is found in the intestinal microflora of rats, birds, amphibians, fish, and other species (Frerichs and Roberts, 1989). *Edwardsiella tarda* infections in humans have recently been reviewed (Wilson et al., 1989). Infection with this organism is by ingestion or a penetrating wound. Infected fish and contaminated water are sources of infection. A variety of disease states may develop, including gastroenteritis (the most common symptom), localized infection, an asymptomatic carrier state, or septicemia. Documented infections are rare. Persons with serious preexisting illnesses are predisposed to infection with *E. tarda,* and as a consequence the mortality rate is high (44%).

Yersinia ruckeri is the agent of enteric red-mouth disease in salmonids and is considered to be highly pathogenic to infected fish. In contrast, only one case of human infection with this organism has been reported (Farmer et al., 1985).

LEPTOSPIROSIS. Three cases of *Leptospira icterohaemorrhagica* infection among fish farmers in England in 1981 caused concern that fish and other aquatic species could harbor *Leptospira* and transmit the disease to humans. An epidemiologic survey concluded that English fish farmers were at increased risk of developing *leptospirosis* (Gill et al., 1985). However, the authors were unable to identify any factors or husbandry practices that predisposed to development of the disease.

Definitive data are lacking concerning the existence of *Leptospira* infections in fish and the possible role of fish in disease transmission. An early report (Maestrone and Benjaminson, 1962) stated that *Leptospira* could be isolated from goldfish tissues up to 17 days after experimental infection. Since that time, little has been published concerning the possible role of fish in the etiology of human disease. Studies of leptospirosis in aquatic species have concluded that fish can harbor the organism. However, more field and experimental data are needed to accurately determine the risk of human infection (Minette, 1983).

TOXINS

A large number of marine organisms produce toxic substances that can cause illness and death in man. In most instances, however, poisonings caused by marine species occur as isolated events. The toxicology and clinical syndromes produced by these agents have been comprehensively reviewed (Halstead, 1988). Ciguatera and scombroid food poisonings are worthy of discussion because they are frequently implicated as causes of foodborne intoxications in the United States and other countries. Statistics compiled by the Centers for Disease Control showed that chemical poisonings accounted for 26% of foodborne disease outbreaks and 2% of all clinical cases from 1983 to 1987 (Bean et al., 1990). Fish poisonings resulting from ingestion of ciguatoxin and scombrotoxin accounted for 73% of these outbreaks.

Ciguatera Poisoning

The term *ciguatera* is believed to be derived from *cigua,* the common name for a Cuban gastropod that produces similar clinical signs when ingested (Lee, 1980). The intoxication is highly endemic in tropical regions (Morris et al., 1982). However, modern transportation of fish and man has made ciguatera a condition of worldwide occurrence (Lawrence et al., 1980; Halstead, 1988).

Ciguatera poisoning is caused by ingestion of the meat of carnivorous reef fishes such as grouper, snapper, kingfish, and barracuda. Ciguatoxin is probably produced by the dinoflagellate *Gambierdiscus toxicus*. The dinoflagellate adheres to the surfaces of reef plants, which are consumed by herbivorous fishes. These fishes are in turn consumed by predatory species. Ciguatoxin accumulates in the liver, intestines, reproductive organs, and muscles, and affected fish may demonstrate clinical signs of neurotoxicity (Halstead, 1988). Factors resulting in increased rates of dinoflagellate growth (storms, rains, chemical and organic pollutants) also produce increased levels of ciguatoxin in fish meat (Lee, 1980).

Ciguatera poisoning in man is primarily a syndrome of high morbidity, although deaths have been reported (Bagnis et al., 1979). The clinical syndrome has recently been reviewed (Frenette et al., 1988). Frequently affected individuals develop signs of gastroenteritis (nausea, vomiting, and diarrhea) within 5 to 6 hours of ingestion. These symptoms usually resolve within 1 to 2 days, although diarrhea may persist for longer periods.

A second phase of the intoxication usually starts 18 to 24 hours after ingestion of contaminated food. It is characterized by neurologic signs such as paresthesias of the mouth and extremities, pruritus, myalgia and arthralgia, headaches, and weakness. Cold sensitivity of the mouth and extremities is highly characteristic of the condition. Patients often report a paradoxical burning sensation upon exposure to cold food or objects. Bradycardia, shock, and coma may develop in cases of severe toxicity. These neurological signs may in part be attributable to cerebral edema. This could account for the dramatic clinical improvement seen in some patients after intravenous administration of mannitol (Palafox et al., 1988).

The biphasic clinical syndrome may be related to the presence of more than one toxin in contaminated fish (Halstead, 1988). Ciguatoxin has been characterized as a lipid-soluble polyether. It is believed to produce neurological symptoms by acting on the sodium channels of nerve cells and effecting changes in their permeability and electrical potential (Palafox et al., 1988). The lipid nature of ciguatoxin may render it soluble in body fluids. In two recently described cases of ciguatera poisoning, the sources of exposure were believed to be sexual contact and breast feeding (Lange et al., 1989; Blythe and de Sylva, 1990).

Diagnosis of ciguatera poisoning is based on the clinical signs and a history of recent ingestion of carnivorous marine fish. Although the toxin is currently not detectable in human samples, an enzyme immunoassay system can screen for its presence in fish tissues (Hokama, 1985). Treatment of the toxicity is largely symptomatic. In addition to mannitol, other recently tested drugs include the sodium channel blocker amitryptiline and the calcium channel blocker nifedipine (Calvert et al., 1987). Prevention is hampered by the fact that ciguatoxin is heat and cold stable and does not impart an odor or taste to contaminated meat.

Scombroid Poisoning

Scombroid toxicity derives its name from the fact that most cases are seen after ingestion of marine fishes of the family Scombroidae. Representative species implicated in food poisonings include tuna, mackerel, bonito, and skipjack. Other nonscombroid species (bluefish, mahi-mahi, herring, and sardines) have also been identified as vectors in outbreaks (Taylor et al., 1989). Although the reported incidence of scombroid poisoning is less than that of ciguatera, it is believed to be underreported and often misdiagnosed as food allergy (Eastaugh and Shepherd, 1989).

The exact mechanism of scombroid food poisoning is not completely understood (Halstead, 1988). Surface contamination of fish with bacteria such as *Proteus* and *Klebsiella* spp. results in the accumulation of histamine. Tissues of scombroid fish contain high levels of histidine, and the bacteria convert this amino acid to histamine via the enzyme histidine decarboxylase. Histamine may accumulate to toxic levels if contaminated fishes are left unrefrigerated for as little as 3 to 4 hours (Kow-Tong and Malison, 1987).

Ingestion of histamine has previously been believed to produce the clinical signs of scombroid food poisoning. These include a rapid onset of nausea, vomiting, diarrhea, a burning sensation of the mouth, hives, pruritus, flushing, and skin rash (Taylor et al., 1989). Levels of histamine in fish tissue are positively correlated with the occurrence and severity of clinical signs and are used to diagnose cases of scombroid poisoning. However, histamine is degraded during ingestion and does not produce signs of food poisoning when administered orally (Halstead, 1988; Eastaugh and Shepherd, 1989). It has been suggested that scombrotoxin is not histamine per se, but rather a potentiator of histamine activity (Taylor et al., 1984).

The diagnosis of scombroid poisoning is based on clinical signs and a history of recent ingestion of fish. Treatment is symptomatic and consists of supportive therapy (including antihistamines). The disease is best prevented by refrigeration of fish during all stages of handling (Bartholomew et al., 1987).

PARASITES

In the United States, the incidence of parasitic zoonoses attributable to fish is quite small. This is in contrast to other countries and geographic regions (e.g., Japan, Russia, the Far East) where rates of infection reach significant levels (Wootten, 1989). In the United States, most reported cases involve consumption of fish, which are intermediate hosts for intestinal parasites of fish predators. The incidence of fishborne parasitism has recently increased, and this is thought to be the result of dietary changes; i.e., greater consumption of raw or undercooked dishes such as sushi or sashimi (McKerrow et al., 1988; Wittner, et al., 1989).

Nematodes

ANASAKIASIS. Anasakiasis is a rare but increasingly observed clinical disease in the United States. Only 50 cases have been reported since 1958, but 70% of these have occurred since 1980 (McKerrow et al., 1988). Humans are infected by eating fish meat containing third-stage larvae of *Anasakis simplex* and *Pseudoterranova* (formerly *Phocanema*) *decipiens*. These nematodes normally parasitize marine mammals that consume infected fish. Many cases of anasakiasis occur in the western United States, and this is believed to reflect the geographical location of marine mammals and intermediate hosts such as salmon, herring, and Pacific cod (Kliks, 1986).

In many instances, human infection with anasakid parasites produces no ill effects. Larvae are often regurgitated 1 to 2 days after ingestion. However, larvae may burrow into the walls of the stomach or intestines and produce acute illness that may be clinically indistinguishable from gastric ulceration or appendicitis. Laparotomy often reveals the presence of inflamed portions of the gastrointestinal tract and the parasite. Anaskiasis is prevented by cooking or freezing fish meat.

EUSTRONGYLOIDES. Human infections with other nematode parasites have been described. *Eustrongyloides* causes an anasakiasislike syndrome of acute abdominal pain. Infection has been reported to occur after ingestion of live bait minnows and sushi (Centers for Disease Control, 1982; Wittner et al., 1989). An unusual case involved the migration of a dracunculoid nematode (*Philometra* sp.) into an open hand wound (Deardorff et al., 1986).

CESTODES. Human infections with cestode parasites such as *Diphyllobothrium latum* have been noted (Wootten, 1989; Eastaugh and Shepherd, 1989). In contrast to other fishborne parasites, most cases involve ingestion of freshwater fishes such as pike or walleye. Typical clinical signs include mild intestinal upset (cramps, loose stools). Megaloblastic anemia is occasionally found during diagnostic evaluation. Diagnosis is by demonstration of ova in feces.

TREMATODES. Trematode infections in humans are rare in the United States. One case report documented infection with *Heterophyes heterophyes* as a consequence of eating sushi (Adams et al., 1986). A number of human infections with *Nanophyetus salmincola* have recently been diagnosed (Fritsche et al., 1989; Harrell and Deardorff, 1990). This intestinal fluke is of interest to veterinarians because it is the biological vector for *Neorickettsia helminthoeca*, the agent of salmon poisoning in dogs. Human infection with *Nanophyetus* is caused by the ingestion of raw or partially cooked salmon. Clinical signs may include abdominal pain and diarrhea, but patients are often asymptomatic. Diagnosis is by demonstration of ova through fecal flotation.

PROTOZOA. Human infection with fishborne protozoans are very rare. The coccidial organism *Cryptosporidium* is known to have a wide range of hosts, including man and fish (O'Donoghue, 1985). Humans are predisposed to infection by congenital or acquired immunodeficiency diseases. Although no cases involving transmission from fish to man have been reported, it is possible that these may occur. One outbreak of giardiasis has been attributed to fecal contamination of canned salmon (Osterholm et al., 1983).

VIRUSES AND FUNGI

No human infections with fish viruses have been reported (Wolf, 1988). However, San Miguel sea lion virus, a calicivirus known to produce vesicular disease in both marine mammals and pigs, has been shown to elicit antibody production in humans and vesicular lesions in primates. The virus is believed to be transmitted by various marine fishes, and it has been suggested that humans may become infected during handling of fish vectors (Barlough et al., 1986a, 1986b). The practice of integrated fish farming may contribute to the development of human influenza pandemics (Scholtissek and Naylor, 1988). New strains of human influenza virus are thought to be produced by genetic reassortment of human and avian influenza viruses, and this reassortment is believed to occur in pigs. The proximity of humans, pigs, and birds is most notably seen in polyculture systems in Asia, where duck and/or pig feces are used to fertilize aquaculture ponds. These ponds may be fertile areas for the growth of both fish and new strains of human influenza (Scholtissek and Naylor, 1988).

No incidence of human fungal infection with fish pathogens has been described (Roberts, 1989). However, *Candida albicans* has been cultured from skin lesions of mullet (Macri et al., 1984).

LITERATURE CITED

Adams, K., Jungkind, D., Bergquist, E., and Wirts, C. (1986) Intestinal fluke infection as a result of eating sushi. Am. J. Clin. Pathol. 86:688–689.

Bagnis, R., Kuberski, T., and Laugier, S. (1979) Clinical observations on 3,009 cases of ciguatera (fish poisoning) in the South Pacific. Am. J. Trop. Med. Hyg. 28:1067–1073.

Barlough, J., Berry, E., Skilling, D., and Smith, A. (1986a). The marine calicivirus story—Part I. Compend. Contin. Ed. Pract. Vet. 8:F5–F14.

Barlough, J., Berry, E., Skilling, D., and Smith, A. (1986b) The marine calicivirus story—Part II. Compend. Contin. Ed. Pract. Vet. 8:F75–F82.

Bartholomew, B., Berry, P., Rodhouse, J., and Gilbert, R. (1987) Scombrotoxic fish poisoning in Britain: Features of over 250 suspected incidents from 1976 to 1986. Epidemiol. Infect. 99:775–782.

Bean, N., and Griffin, P. (1990) Foodborne disease outbreaks in the United States, 1973–1987: Pathogens, vehicles, and trends. J. Food Protect. 53:804–817.

Bean, N., Griffin, P., Goulding, J., and Ivey, C. (1990) Foodborne disease outbreaks, 5-year summary, 1983–1987. J. Food Protect. 53:711–728.

Blythe, D., and de Sylva, D. (1990) Mother's milk turns toxic following fish feast. J.A.M.A. 264:2074.

Brenden, R., Miller, M., and Janda, J. (1988) Clinical disease spectrum and pathogenic factors associated with *Plesiomonas shigelloides* infections in humans. Rev. Infect. Dis. 10:303–316.

Brown, J., and Sanders, C. (1987) *Mycobacterium marinum* infections: A problem of recognition, not therapy? Arch. Intern. Med. 147:817–818.

Calvert, G., Hryhorczuk, D., and Leikin, J. (1987) Treatment of ciguatera poisoning with amitryptiline and nifedipine. Clin. Toxicol. 25:423–428.

Centers for Disease Control. (1982) Intestinal perforation caused by larval *Eustrongyloides*. M.M.W.R. 31:383–384.

Centers for Disease Control (1987a) Botulism associated with commercially distributed kapchunka—New York City. M.M.W.R. 34:546–547.

Centers for Disease Control (1987b) Diagnosis and management of mycobacterial infection and disease in persons with human immunodeficiency virus infection. Ann. Intern. Med. 106:254–256.

Centers for Disease Control (1989) Aquarium-associated *Plesiomonas shigelloides* infection—Missouri. M.M.W.R. 38:617–619.

Centers for Disease Control (1990) *Aeromonas* wound infections associated with outdoor activities—California. M.M.W.R. 39:334–341.

Dattwyler, R., Thomas, J., and Hurst, L. (1987) Antigen-specific T-cell anergy in progressive *Mycobacterium marinum* infection in humans. Ann. Intern. Med. 107:675–677.

Deardorff, T., Overstreet, R., Okihiro, M., and Tam, R. (1986) Piscine adult nematode invading an open lesion in a human hand. Am. J. Trop. Med. Hyg. 35:827–830.

Donta, S., Smith, P., Levitz, R. and Quintiliani, R. (1986) Therapy of *Mycobacterium marinum* infections: Use of tetracyclines vs rifampin. Arch. Intern. Med. 146:902–904.

Eastaugh, J., and Shepherd, S. (1989) Infectious and toxic syndromes from fish and shellfish consumption: A review. Arch. Intern. Med. 149:1735.

Farmer, J. J., Davis, B. R., and Hickman-Brenner, F. C. (1985) Biochemical identification of new species and biogroups of *Enterobacteriaceae* isolated from clinical specimens. J. Clin. Microbiol. 21:46–76.

Flynn, T., and Knepp, I. (1987) Seafood shucking as an etiology for *Aeromonas hydrophila* infection. Arch. Intern. Med. 147:1816–1817.

Frenette, C., MacLean, J., and Gyorkos, T. (1988) A large common-source outbreak of ciguatera fish poisoning. J. Infect. Dis. 158:1128–1131.

Frerichs, G., and Roberts, R. (1989) The bacteriology of teleosts. In: Fish Pathology (Roberts, R., ed.). Baillière Tindall, Philadelphia, p. 289.

Fritsche, T., Eastburn, R., Wiggins, L., and Terhune, C. (1989) Praziquantel for treatment of human *Nanophyetus salmincola* (*Troglotrema salmincola*) infection. J. Infect. Dis. 160:896–899.

George, W., Nakata, M., Thompson, J., and White, M. (1985) Aeromonas-related diarrhea in adults. Arch. Intern. Med. 145:2207–2211.

Gill, O., Coghlan, J., and Calder, I. (1985) The risk of leptospirosis in United Kingdom fish farm workers: Results from a 1981 serological survey. J. Hyg. (Cambridge) 94:81–86.

Gorby, G., and Peacock, J. (1988) *Erysipelothrix rhusiopathiae* endocarditis: Microbiologic, epidemiologic, and clinical features of an occupational disease. Rev. Infect. Dis. 10:317–325.

Gray, S., Smith, R., Reynolds, N., and Williams, E. (1990) Fish tank granuloma. Br. Med. J. 300:1069–1070.

Halstead, B. (1988) Poisonous and Venomous Marine Animals of the World. Darwin Press, Princeton, New Jersey.

Harrell, L., and Deardorff, T. (1990) Human nanophyiasis: Transmission by handling naturally infected coho salmon (*Oncorhynchus kisutch*). J. Infect. Dis. 161:146–148.

Heckerling, P., Stine, T., Pottage, J., Levin, S., and Harris, A. (1983) *Aeromonas hydrophila* myonecrosis and gas gangrene in a nonimmunocompromised host. Arch. Intern. Med. 143:2005–2007.

Hoffmann, T., Nelson, B., Darouiche, R., and Rosen, T. (1988) *Vibrio vulnificus* septicemia. Arch. Intern. Med. 148:1825–1827.

Hokama, Y. (1985) A rapid, simplified enzyme immunoassay stick test for the detection of ciguatoxin and related polyethers from fish tissues. Toxicon 23:939–946.

Iseman, M. (1989) *Mycobacterium avium* complex and the normal host: The other side of the coin. N. Engl. J. Med. 321:896–898.

Johnston, J., Becker, S., and McFarland, L. (1985) *Vibrio vulnificus*: Man and the sea. J.A.M.A. 253:2850–2853.

Karam, G., Ackley, A., and Dismukes, W. (1983) Posttraumatic *Aeromonas hydrophila* osteomyelitis. Arch. Intern. Med. 143:2073–2074.

Kennedy, C., Goetz, M., and Mathisen, G. (1990) Postoperative pancreatic abscess due to *Plesiomonas shigelloides*. Rev. Infect. Dis. 12:813–816.

Kliks, M. (1986) Human anasakiasis: An update. J.A.M.A. 255:2605.

Klontz, K., Lieb, S., Schreiber, M., Janowski, H., Baldy, L., and Gunn, R. (1988) Syndromes of *Vibrio vulnificus* infections: Clinical and epidemiologic features in Florida cases, 1981–1987. Ann. Intern. Med. 109:318.

Kow-Tong, C., and Malison, M. (1987) Outbreak of scombroid fish poisoning, Taiwan. Am. J. Public Health 77:1335–1336.

Lange, W., Lipkin, K., and Yang, G. (1989) Can ciguatera be a sexually transmitted disease? Clin. Toxicol. 27:193–197.

Lawrence, D., Enriquez, M., Lumish, R., and Maceo, A. (1980) Ciguatera fish poisoning in Miami. J.A.M.A. 244:254–258.

Lee, C. (1980) Fish poisoning with particular reference to ciguatera. J. Trop. Med. Hyg. 83:93–97.

Lowry, P., McFarland, L., and Threefoot, H. (1986) *Vibrio hollisae* septicemia after consumption of catfish. J. Infect. Dis. 154:730–731.

Lowry, P., McFarland, L., Peltier, B., Roberts, N., Bradford, H., Herndon, J., Stroup, D., Mathison, J., Blake, P., and Gunn, R. (1989) *Vibrio* gastroenteritis in Louisiana: A prospective study among attendees of a scientific congress in New Orleans. J. Infect. Dis. 160:978–984.

Macri, B., Panebianco, A., Costa, A., and Midili, S. (1984) Yeast-induced disease in sea fish. II. Studies on the causal agent, the lesions and food hygiene aspects. Summa 1:89–94.

Maestrone, G., and Benjaminson, M. (1962) Leptospira infection in the gold fish. Nature 195:719–720.

McKerrow, J., Sakanari, J., and Deardorff, T. (1988) Anasakiasis: Revenge of the sushi parasite. N. Engl. J. Med. 319:1228–1229.

Minette, H. (1983) Leptospirosis in poikilothermic vertebrates: A review. Int. J. Zoon. 10:111–121.

Minette, H. (1986) Salmonellosis in the marine environment: A review and commentary. Int. J. Zoon. 13:71–75.

Morris, J. (1988) *Vibrio vulnificus*—A new monster of the deep? Ann. Intern. Med. 109:261–262.

Morris, J., Wilson, R., Davis, B., Wachsmuth, I., Riddle, C., Wathen, H., Pollard, R., and Blake, P. (1981) Non-0 group 1 *Vibrio cholerae* gastroenteritis in the United States: Clinical, epidemiologic, and laboratory characteristics of sporadic cases. Ann. Intern. Med. 94:656–658.

Morris, J., Lewin, P., Smith, C., Blake, P., and Schneider, R. (1982) Ciguatera fish poisoning: Epidemiology of the disease on St. Thomas, U.S. Virgin Islands. Am. J. Trop. Med. Hyg. 31:574–578.

Murase, M., Nakanishi, H., and Sakazaki, R. (1988) CT-like enterotoxin production of non-01 *V. cholerae* isolated from river water, fish and shrimps in Kobe City. Jpn. J. Vet. Sci. 50:363–370.

O'Donoghue, P. (1985) Cryptosporidium infections in man, animals, birds and fish. Aust. Vet. J. 62:253–258.

Ogbondeminu, F., and Okaeme, A. (1986) Bacterial flora associated with an organic manure-aquaculture system in Kainji Lake basin area, Nigeria. Int. J. Zoon. 13:54–58.

Osterholm, M., Forgang, J., Ristinen, T., Dean, A., Washburn, J., Godes, J., Rude, R., and McCullough, J. (1983) An outbreak of foodborne giardiasis. N. Engl. J. Med. 304:24–28.

Palafox, N., Jain, L., Pinano, A., Gulick, T., Williams, R., and Schatz, I. (1988) Successful treatment of ciguatera fish poisoning with intravenous mannitol. J.A.M.A. 259:2740–2742.

Prince, D., Peterson, D., Steiner, R., Gottlieb, J., Scott, R., Israel, H., Figueroa, W., and Fish, J. (1989) Infection with *Mycobacterium avium* complex in patients without predisposing conditions. N. Engl. J. Med. 321:863–868.

Reagan, D., Nafziger, D., and Wenzel, R. (1990) Handfishing-associated *Klebsiella* bloodstream infection. J. Infect. Dis. 161:155–156.

Reboli, A., and Farrar, E. (1989) *Erysipelothrix rhusiopathiae*: An occupational pathogen. Clin. Microbiol. Rev. 2:354–359.

Ries, K., White, G., and Murdock, R. (1990) Atypical mycobacterial infection caused by *Mycobacterium marinum*. N. Engl. J. Med. 322:633.

Rigau-Perez, J., Hatheway, C., and Valentin, V. (1982) Botulism from acidic food: First cases of botulinic paralysis in Puerto Rico. J. Infect. Dis. 145:783–785.

Roberts, R. (1989) The mycology of teleosts. In: Fish Pathology (Roberts, R., ed.). Baillière Tindall, Philadelphia, pp. 320–336.

Sanyal, D., Burge, S., and Hutchings, P. (1987) Enteric pathogens in tropical aquaria. Epidemiol. Infect. 99:635–640.

Scholtissek, C., and Naylor, E. (1988) Fish farming and influenza pandemics. Nature 331:215.

Shotts, E. B., Jr. (1980) Bacteria associated with fish and their relative importance. In: CRC Handbook Series in Zoonoses. Section A: Bacterial, Rickettsial and Mycotic Diseases (Steele, J., ed.). CRC Press, Boca Raton, Florida, pp. 517–525.

Shotts, E. B., Jr. (1987) Bacterial diseases of fish associated with human health. Vet. Clin. North Am. Small Animal Pract. 17(1):241–247.

Shotts, E. B., Jr., and Teska, J. J. (1989) Bacterial pathogens of aquatic vertebrates. In: Methods for the Microbiological Examination of Fish and Shellfish (Austin, B., and Austin, D., eds.). John Wiley & Sons, New York, pp. 164–186.

Smith, G., and Turner, A. (1989) The production of *Clostridium botulinum* toxin in mammalian, avian and piscine carrion. Epidemiol. Infect. 102:467–471.

Taylor, S., Hui, J., and Lyons, D. (1984) Toxicology of scombroid poisoning. In: Seafood Toxins (Ragelis, E., ed.). American Chemical Society, Washington, D.C., pp. 417–430.

Taylor, S., Stratton, J., and Nordlee, J. (1989) Histamine poisoning (scombroid fish poisoning): An allergy-like intoxication. Clin. Toxicol. 27:225.

Telzak, E., Bell, E., Kautter, D., Crowell, L., Budnick, L., Morse, D., and Schultz, S. (1990) An international outbreak of type E botulism due to uneviscerated fish. J. Infect. Dis. 161:340–342.

Vartian, C., and Septimus, E. (1990) Osteomyelitis caused by *Vibrio vulnificus*. J. Infect. Dis. 161:363.

Wilson, J., Waterer, R., Wofford, J., and Chapman, S. (1989) Serious infections with *Edwardsiella tarda*: A case report and review of the literature. Arch. Intern. Med. 149:208–210.

Wittner, M., Turner, J., Jacquette, G., Ash, L., Salgo, M., and Tanowitz, H. (1989) Eustrongylidiasis—a parasitic infection acquired by eating sushi. N. Engl. J. Med. 320:1124–1126.

Wolf, K. (1988) Fish Viruses and Fish Viral Diseases. Cornell University Press, Ithaca, New York.

Wood, R. (1975) Erysipelothrix infection. In: Diseases Transmitted from Animals to Man (Hubbert, W., McCullough, W., and Schnurrenberger, P., eds.). Charles C Thomas, Springfield, Illinois, pp. 271–281.

Woods, G., and Washington, J. (1987) Mycobacteria other than *Mycobacterium tuberculosis*: Review of microbiologic and clinical aspects. Rev. Infect. Dis. 9:275–294.

Wootten, R. (1989) Zoonoses: Fish parasites and man. In: Fish Pathology (Roberts, R., ed.). Baillière Tindall, Philadelphia, pp. 287–288.

PART II

SPECIAL MEDICINE

SECTION I

FRESHWATER TEMPERATE

FISHES

EDWARD J. NOGA, *Section Editor*

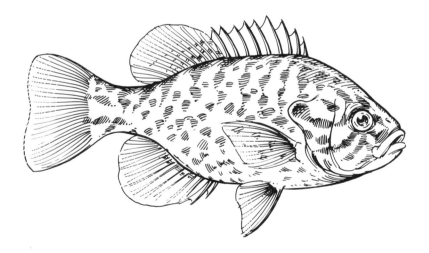

Chapter 18

Taxonomy and Natural History of Temperate Freshwater and Estuarine Fishes

LYNWOOD S. SMITH

TAXONOMY

Organizing fish species according to regional criteria, such as temperature ranges, has certain conveniences, but it has no correlation with the taxonomic groupings. Most major taxonomic groups are represented in temperate waters. One way to simplify this complexity is to divide the bony fishes (Actinopterigii) into only three major groups. The first group consists of the relict species such as sturgeon, paddlefish, bowfin, and gar, which have been mostly displaced by more specialized species. The second group is the more primal of the modern bony fishes, including the salmonids, pikes, catfishes, eels, carps, true cods, and herrings. The third group is the most recent, largest, and most diverse radiation in the evolution of the bony fishes, which consists primarily of the spiny-rayed (percomorph) fishes, including the bass, perch, pike, tunas, flatfish, sculpins, mullets, and all their relatives. These listings are incomplete and do not represent a single line of evolutionary development. The immense diversity of the bony fishes is difficult to communicate in a single chapter, so interested readers are well advised to consult an introductory ichthyology text such as Moyle and Cech (1982). Brief taxonomic comments are included with the natural history of the species of most commercial interest.

NATURAL HISTORY

The biology of temperate freshwater and estuarine fishes is as diverse as their taxonomy. In some fish families, most species inhabit similar environments. In other families, different species inhabit fresh water or sea water, or migrate.

STURGEON

Sturgeon (family Acipenseridae) are large, long-lived fish that inhabit most of the larger rivers and lakes of the cooler northern hemisphere (Binkowski and Doroshov, 1985) (Fig. 18–1). North American species have limited regional distribution. There are Atlantic coast species, Pacific coast species, species found only in the Mississippi River system or only in the Great Lakes and adjoining streams. Sturgeon were common enough at one time in the Fraser River, for example, that Indians fished for them by probing with long, forked poles. When they hit a sturgeon, they held it against the bottom until they could spear it. Commercial operations for caviar depleted most runs to noneconomic levels by the beginning of this century. Sturgeon have been cultured in Russian rivers for many years and are beginning to be cultured in the Sacramento and Columbia River systems in the United States.

Sturgeon tolerate or prefer turbid water. They feed on a variety of insects, molluscs, crustaceans, and sometimes other fishes, presumably by touch and smell. Although stereotyped as sluggish, bottom-dwelling species, the white sturgeon in the Columbia River were recently seen catching salmon smolts in midwater. Young sturgeon in tanks swim continuously. Adults spawn on sand or gravel substrate where there is a strong current. In white sturgeon on the Pacific coast, females spawn at intervals of 4 to 11 years at sizes exceeding 150 cm, and may reach a length of 365 cm and a weight of 600 kg at an estimated age of 100 years. They migrate into estuarine or near-shore ocean waters, although their marine distribution is minimally known. White sturgeon now have also become landlocked in the Columbia River where dams have blocked their passage to and from the sea.

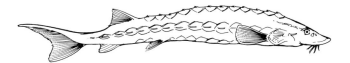

FIGURE 18–1. Green sturgeon.

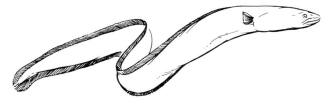

FIGURE 18–3. American eel.

PADDLEFISH

Paddlefish (family Polyodontidae) have a long snout that is half as long as the rest of their body, narrower at the base than at the tip, like a paddle (Fig. 18–2). The function of the snout, or rostrum, may be sensory, although paddlefish survive and grow normally without a snout if it is lost. The snout gives these fish a bizarre appearance, although it may be only an exaggeration of the sturgeon type of snout, some of which are also fairly long. Young paddlefish develop a rostrum and are recognizable as miniature adults only after they are about a month old.

There are only two existing species of paddlefish, one in the Mississippi River system and a second in the Yangtze River. Paddlefish grow rapidly (2.7 mm/day) during their first year, then about 5 cm/year, reaching a maximum of 150 to 190 cm total length (recent measurements are body length: anterior edge of the eye to the fork of the tail) and 23 to 40 kg at an age of 20 to 30 years. Females are generally larger than males. Because of their size, paddlefish live in large, free-flowing rivers with abundant zooplankton, their primary food (Dillard et al., 1986). Paddlefish move up and down river, sometimes hundreds of kilometers, and a few have been captured in saline waters. Some natural stocks of paddlefish have been impacted by dams without fish passage facilities and by loss of spawning habitat. Some populations have become established within reservoir systems, within which they move around vigorously.

Like sturgeon, paddlefish produce large numbers of eggs, estimated at 26,000/kg of body weight and perhaps more than 1,000,000 in one 36-kg female. Recently, paddlefish eggs have been increasingly used for caviar, increasing fishing pressure. Spawning occurs in the spring at temperatures around 12 to 14°C and over gravel bars inundated by spring freshets (overflowing streams). Hatching requires about 10 days, after which the juveniles swim mostly upward in the water column and become widely distributed downstream.

EELS

Eels are long, skinny fishes with the dorsal, caudal, and anal fins merged into a single continuous fin and with the pelvic fins absent (Fig. 18–3). Although eels belong to 22 families, most people think first of the moray eels depicted in skin-diving films or, in Asia and Europe, the anguillid eels that are widely cultured there. Since most other species are secretive or rare or both, the following deals only with the family Anguillidae.

There are only 16 species of anguillid eels. The most commonly studied are the European eel, the American eel along the Atlantic coast of North America, and the Japanese eel. Anguillid eels also occur in Southeast Asia and South Africa. Eels are catadromous, rearing in fresh water and spawning at sea (Tesch, 1977). Eels hatch as leptocephalus larvae, metamorphose into glass (unpigmented) eels that migrate onto the continental shelves, and enter rivers as pigmented elvers. They remain in fresh water for 6 to 12 years where they prey upon other fishes and are cryptically dark colored with yellow bellies. They are sometimes called yellow eels at this stage, and reach lengths of 40 to 150 cm. These eels turn silver on their bellies when they begin to mature sexually, and migrate downstream into sea water. Species in the Atlantic migrate to the Sargasso Sea. There they spawn in deep water and die. The leptocephalus larvae drift and swim for 1 to 3 years to reach their respective coast lines again.

PIKE

The pike group includes pike, pickerel, and muskellunge, all three in the genus *Esox* (family Esocidae). Pikes have elongate snouts with comparatively large teeth, forked tails, and both dorsal and anal fins placed posteriorly (Fig. 18–4). This configuration provides rapid acceleration for their lifestyle of dashing out from cover to prey on other fishes. One or more members of this family inhabit most

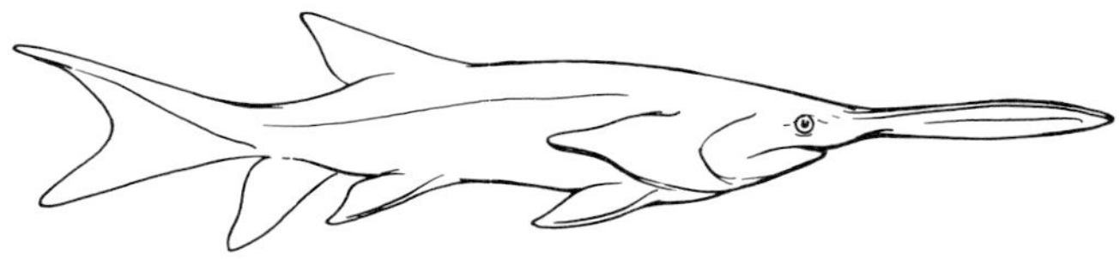

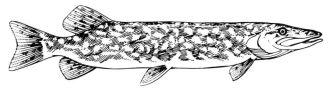

FIGURE 18–2. Paddlefish.

FIGURE 18–4. Northern pike.

temperate and northern lakes in the northern hemisphere. Although pike are considered distantly related to the salmonids because of their swim bladder and posteriorly placed pelvic fins, they have no adipose fin and no pyloric ceca. Pike require flooded vegetation for their spring spawning and adhesive eggs, as well as later growth of the young. They are negatively impacted by stabilization of lake and river levels. Hybrids are common among several species. Record sizes range from 75 to 150 cm, excepting the grass pickerel with a record size of only 38 cm, making the pike family very popular sport fishes.

PERCIFORM FISHES

In contrast to the families above, this group includes the perches, basses, and nearly 7000 fish species. The perciform fishes have similar taxonomic characteristics: fin spines; two lobes or separate parts of the dorsal fin, the anterior part being spiny; lack of an adipose fin; pectoral fins placed toward the midline on the side of the body; pelvic fins anterior and ventral or absent; and if the swim bladder is present, it is physoclistous with no pneumatic duct. White bass are widely viewed as having the archetypal body plan of this group.

Basses

There are four species of bass in the family Percichthyidae: the striped bass, the white bass, the yellow bass, and the white perch, all of which are important sport fish in North America. They can be distinguished from the sea basses by the presence of only two spines on the operculum, a tail that is usually forked, and the absence of hermaphroditism. The striped bass is anadromous, moving up rivers in spring to spawn above the tidal influence (Fig. 18–5). Landlocked stocks are known in South Carolina. Larvae feed on zooplankton. The young primarily consume invertebrates, and adults prey on other fish and larger crustaceans. Striped bass originally inhabited the Atlantic and eastern Gulf coasts of the United States, but have been widely introduced to the Mississippi River system, the Pacific coast, and Rio Grande. Adult size ranges from 46 to 198 cm. Hybrids between striped bass and white bass are becoming increasingly popular as a cultured sport fish.

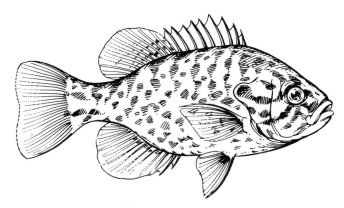

FIGURE 18–6. Sunfish.

Sunfishes

The family Centrarchidae is native to North America and includes about 30 freshwater species, some of which are commonly called bass (Fig. 18–6). They often inhabit warm-water lakes and sluggish streams, but exhibit great adaptability. Since black basses, sunfishes (includes pumpkinseed and bluegill), and crappies are very popular sport fishes, they have been widely established outside their native ranges. The largemouth bass is now established worldwide. Distinguishing features include a relatively deep body in the basses and a very deep body in the sunfishes and crappies combined with the lack of a pseudobranch.

One can stereotype this group under the name pondfishes, although the basses often prefer larger bodies of water, and often moving water. Temperature controls many aspects of bass behavior, including spawning, migration, depth preference, and growth (Stroud and Clepper, 1975). Basses survive but become torpid below 10°C and have been observed in heated effluents close to 40°C. Bass spawn in the spring and the male guards both the nest and the subsequent offspring for several weeks. This hormonally controlled behavior to prevent cannibalism includes taking prey organisms such as crayfish in their mouths and removing them from the nest area without eating them.

WALLEYE

The family Percidae, which contains mostly small darters, also includes the perches and the pike-

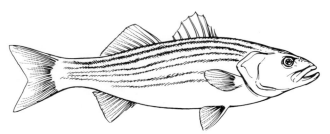

FIGURE 18–5. Striped bass.

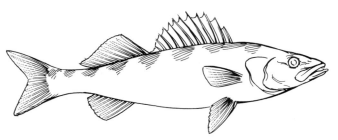

FIGURE 18–7. Walleye.

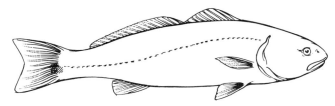

FIGURE 18–8. Red drum.

perches, both of which are highly valued food fishes (Collette et al., 1977; Craig, 1987). In North America, the largest pike-perch is the walleye (Fig. 18–7), which inhabits lakes above the thermocline and large rivers over most of the United States and southern Canada east of the Rockies, as well as a few of the larger man-made reservoirs in the west, including Roosevelt Lake of the Columbia River system. Walleye fry eat benthic invertebrates and adults prey on other fish. Walleye tolerate temperatures of 0 to 30°C. Spawning occurs on gravel or rubble (rarely sand) substrate in early spring at 3 to 16°C after an extended winter chill (less than 10°C).

The yellow perch is distributed similarly to the walleye. It is a smaller fish, with a maximum size of 30 cm total length. Perch prefer lakes with open water and a moderate amount of vegetation. Walleye are sensitive to acid rain. Yellow perch are resistant to acid rain and may become the dominant species in lakes impacted by it (Johnson, 1980). Walleye prey on young bluegill (Forsythe and Wren, 1979) and yellow perch and even on their own young when yellow perch are scarce or absent (Forney, 1974). Both species feed mostly at dusk and dawn.

Spotted Sea Trout and Drums

The family Sciaenidae includes the croakers and drums, which get their name from their ability to make noise by vibrating their multibranched swim bladder with specialized strips of muscle in the wall. Other distinguishing features include divided dorsal fins, a rounded or truncated caudal fin rather than a forked one, two anal spines rather than three, huge

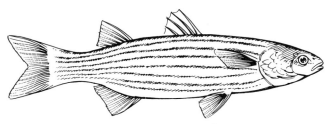

FIGURE 18–9. Gray mullet.

otoliths, and a lateral line that extends onto the caudal fin. Most species, such as the red drum (Fig. 18–8) and the spotted sea trout, inhabit warm, shallow estuaries and river mouths of the southern Atlantic and Gulf coasts of the United States. Exceptions include the freshwater drum, which is an important commercial species in the Mississippi River system.

MULLET

The family Mugilidae has about 70 species, all of which appear similar. They have round bodies, two widely separated dorsal fins with only four spines in the anterior one, forked tails, large round scales, and the pelvic fins positioned more caudally than most perciform fishes. This body plan makes them agile, fast swimmers for migration and predator avoidance. Adults feed on detritus and small algae that they scoop up from the bottom in shallow water. Mullet often ascend coastal rivers for considerable distances, but move offshore as little as 1 or 2 miles to spawn in areas where the ocean currents will bring the larvae back to shore at sizes of 2 to 3 cm. The striped mullet occurs in coastal, tropical, and subtropical waters worldwide, while other species of mullet have more limited distribution. Many of the species in the genus *Mugil* were formerly classified under the genus *Liza*. The adult size of gray mullet ranges from 23 to 36 cm (Fig. 18–9). In general, mullets are euryhaline, eurythermal, and catadromous. They also tolerate oxygen levels as low as 1 ppm.

LITERATURE CITED

Binkowski, F.P., and Doroshov, S.I. (1985) North American Sturgeons: Biology and Aquaculture Potential. Dr. W. Junk Publishers, Dordrecht/Boston/Lancaster.

Collette et al. (1977) J. Fish. Res. Bd. Canada 34:1890–1899.

Craig, J.F. (1987) The Biology of Perch and Related Fish. Freshwater Institute, Dept. of Fisheries and Oceans, Winnipeg, Manitoba, Canada.

Dillard, J.G., Graham, L.K., and Russell, T.R. (eds.) (1986) The Paddlefish: Status, Management, and Propagation. American Fisheries Society Special Publication No. 7.

Forney, J.L. (1974) Interactions between yellow perch abundance, walleye predation, and survival of alternate prey in Oneida Lake, N.Y. Trans. Am. Fish. Soc. 103(1):15–24.

Forsythe, T.D., and Wrenn, W.B. (1979) Predator-prey relationships among walleye and bluegill. In: Predator-Prey Systems in Fisheries Management (Clipper, H., ed.), pp. 475–482.

Johnson, R.E. (1982) Acid Rain/Fisheries. Proceedings of an International Symposium on Acidic Rain and Fishery Impacts on Northeastern North America. American Fisheries Society, Bethesda, Maryland.

Moyle, P.B., and Cech, Jr., J.J. (1982) Fishes: An Introduction to Ichthyology. Prentice-Hall, Englewood Cliffs, New Jersey.

Stroud, R.H., and Clepper, H. (eds.) (1975) Black Bass: Biology and Management. Sport Fishing Institute, Washington, D.C.

Tesch, F.W. (1977) The Eel: Biology and Management of Anguillid Eels. Chapman and Hall, London.

Chapter 19

Anatomy and Special Physiology of Temperate Freshwater Fishes

LYNWOOD S. SMITH

STURGEON AND PADDLEFISH

Sturgeon and paddlefish are closely related anatomically and physiologically in spite of the bizarre appearance produced by the elongated snout of the paddlefish. Both are anatomically intermediate between sharks and bony fishes. The skeletons of sturgeons and paddlefish retain considerable cartilage, and the mouth remains in a ventral position. The tail is heterocercal, meaning that the backbone extends into the upper lobe, and the intestine forms a spiral valve reminiscent of sharks. Unlike sharks, sturgeon and paddlefish gills have a single opening on each side. They have ganoid (flat, partly bone) rather than placoid (toothlike) scales. These fishes have a swim bladder, which is considered by some to be a key innovation in the evolution of the bony fishes, since a bony skeleton is too heavy for efficient swimming unless there is also a swim bladder to add compensating bouyancy. The swim bladder of the sturgeon connects to the forestomach via the pneumatic duct and has no gas secretion or absorption gland. Their anatomy is covered in more detail in Chapter 1.

Most sturgeons live in both fresh water and seawater. Although intermediate taxonomically between sharks and bony fishes, the sturgeon's osmoregulation follows the teleost pattern with no retention of urea, dilute urine in fresh water, and some increase of ion levels in both blood and urine in seawater (Potts and Rudy, 1972). This may be accompanied by an increase in muscle potassium ions (Lavrova et al., 1984). In contrast, paddlefish are considered strictly freshwater fishes whose uncommon capture in estuaries presumably has been in low-salinity areas.

Since natural spawning of paddlefish requires conditions in a large stream that would be difficult to imitate, artificial spawning methods are required for culture of paddlefish. The most successful induction of ovulation has been achieved by two intraperitoneal injections of pituitary extracts or homogenates from one or two pituitaries from other paddlefish of similar weight and degree of maturation. Induced ovulation usually causes release of less than half of the eggs (Dillard et al., 1986).

EELS

Eels have elongate, round bodies, and much of their anatomy is specially adapted to their shape. The head is wedge-shaped for poking into crevices. Gill openings are relatively far posteriorly, allowing eels to "swallow" water in the anterior portion of the mouth and pass it over the gills periodically. The esophagus is long and contributes to water and salt regulation when the eel is in seawater. Most other bony fish have a very short esophagus. Most of their other organs are longer and slimmer than in other bony fishes, including a unique, unilobular liver. Pelvic fins are absent. Tesch (1977) provided a useful summary of eel anatomy.

The physiology of anguillid eels has been extensively studied in Japan, where they are a major aquaculture species, and in Europe, but little in North America. Presumably, the physiology of the three eel species is similar. Most of the studies involve their physiology in seawater. All marine fishes drink seawater to replace the body fluids lost by passive diffusion, but control of drinking seawater has been shown only in eels. Drinking can be induced by increasing the plasma chloride levels and stopped by decreasing it (Hirano et al., 1972). Neither increased osmolality from injected sucrose nor changes in plasma sodium levels induce drinking. The long esophagus also plays a special role in processing ingested seawater. Monovalent ions are actively transported across the esophagus wall and water added to the ingested seawater, producing a fluid which is approximately isosmotic with plasma by the time it reaches the stomach.

Eels have an unusual swim bladder that possesses both a pneumatic duct and gas secretion/reabsorption capabilities. The swim bladder has a considerable blood supply, indicating some supplementary respiratory capability. Although eels can survive for long periods out of water if the temperatures are low enough (less than 7°C), they still eventually incur an oxygen debt and do so more rapidly at warmer temperatures (Tesch, 1977).

While entry of eels into seawater appears different than in salmonids, if for no other reason than the larger size and age of the individuals making the migration, eels go through many of the same physiologic changes involving chloride cells in the gills, drinking seawater, and so forth.

PIKE

Pike have a long snout, relatively long teeth, and a large mouth opening, allowing them to produce little suction for catching prey. Therefore, these fish characteristically swing their head sideways to catch prey, including fish, frogs and tadpoles, mice, and crayfish.

Fin placement in pike is characteristic of fishes adapted for rapid acceleration: The dorsal and anal fins are placed posteriorly on the body and the caudal fin is relatively large and has a high aspect ratio (span/chord). With all of these fins placed posterior to the center of gravity, the fish also is directionally stable, like an arrow. The fish dashes from cover to capture prey in a straight line (Webb, 1975).

Culture of pikes is becoming increasingly important and therefore also the need to induce ovulation artificially. Salmon gonadotropin can be used to produce viable eggs 50 degree-days after injection, although only 65% as many eggs (16,000/kg body weight) are obtained this way compared with natural spawning (25,000/kg) (Billard, 1983). Similar results are obtained with injections of carp pituitary (3 mg/kg) (Brzuska and Malczewski, 1984).

Pike responses to handling stress appear quite typical of other bony fishes. Pike held out of water three times for 30 seconds show respiratory acidosis for about 2 hours and a lactate-induced acidosis for 8 hours (Schwalme and Mackay, 1985). In salmon, which have been shown to swim to fatigue, comparable stages of recovery would be at about 1 and 4 hours, respectively.

BASSES, SPOTTED SEA TROUT, AND DRUMS

Striped and other basses are generalized spiny-rayed fishes having few distinctive features. Groman (1982) showed some aspects of their gross morphology and then provided considerable histological detail. The freshwater drum is featured in a laboratory manual by Fremling (1978).

Striped bass are an anadromous species, even though sometimes they are also described as euryhaline. Most of the physiologic information for this species relates to their culture (Parker, 1984; Parker and Geiger, 1984). Even though striped bass fingerlings may survive dissolved oxygen levels as low as 1.4 mg/L, it should not go lower than 4 mg/L and preferably should be near saturation to provide good growth. However, even slight supersaturation (102.9%) is associated with overinflation of the swim bladder. Water pH should remain between 6.8 and 10, with the most productive hatcheries being around 7.3 (mean alkalinity, 195 mg/L). Larvae and fingerlings are very fragile during the first week after hatching and require slow water velocities so they do not bump into container walls or become impinged on outflow screens. They are also very sensitive to commonly used fishery chemicals such as simazine or diesel fuel used to control aquatic insects.

Striped bass appear very sensitive to stress at all life stages. Survival during and after transport of either adults or fingerlings seems best in water with 25 mg of tricaine methsulfonate per liter and 10 g NaCl/L. Wild adults captured for broodstock are typically anesthetized and injected with human chorionic gonadotropin (250 to 300 IU/kg of body weight) at the time of capture to avoid a later reanesthetization and to minimize holding time. Attempts to hold adults for extended periods often result in all of the fish dying, one by one, within 30 days, presumably due to stress. Etomidate has also been used as an anesthetic for striped bass (Davis et al., 1982).

Water is an excellent medium for sound transmission and swim bladders are excellent resonators for enhancing hearing of underwater sounds. A few species of fish, including the drums, have gone one step further to use the swim bladder to produce sound, using strips of rapidly contracting muscle in the wall of the swim bladder. To produce a sound of a given frequency, the muscle must contract at that frequency. For example, to produce a 200-Hz sound, a sonic muscle must contract every 5 milliseconds, which is significantly faster than the usual 30 to 50 milliseconds needed for a muscle twitch. In squirrelfishes, distinct twitches up to 63 Hz, partial fusion of twitches at 112 Hz, and complete fusion above 200 Hz occur (Gainer et al., 1965). These results are probably typical of sonic muscles in many fishes.

SUNFISHES AND ALLIES

The sunfish/crappie/bluegill body plan emphasizes adaptations for maneuverability. The pectoral fins are far anterior and act as bow rudders for making sharp turns. The major portion of the spiny dorsal fin is also anterior to the center of gravity and, when erect, also enhances the turning ability by making the fish directionally unstable. The pectoral fins are near the midline to minimize changes in pitch during sudden stops and serve for slow propulsion, using flying motions like a bird's wings. The laterally compressed body minimizes sideways slippage in tight turns (Webb, 1975). The transition from larval to adult body form in these fishes follows a well-defined pattern (Meyer, 1970).

As typical pond fishes, the centrarchids, which

include sunfishes and their allies, are adapted to a greater range of temperatures than any other group of fishes. Performance polygons that cover the temperature and activity ranges for salmonids are discussed in Chapter 31. Brett (1972) compared several performance polygons for nonsalmonid species, including bass. The bass was notable for having maximum swimming performance at the upper lethal temperature in contrast to all of the other species that had showed maximum swimming performance at some intermediate temperature (Fig. 19–1).

These temperature relationships assume that fish have maximized their metabolic efficiency at a given temperature; i.e., they have become acclimated to that temperature and cannot thermoregulate. This acclimation often includes extensive molecular changes in muscle enzymes (Shaklee et al., 1977), but perhaps not in white muscle. Muscle from a wide variety of fishes, including warm-blooded ones, shows decreased muscle twitch duration of about 1 millisecond for every 1°C increase in temperature (Wardle, 1980). Temperature acclimation of muscles does not reside in the muscle ATPase, which shows no changes in activity after 4 to 6 weeks of temperature acclimation (Sidell and Johnston, 1985).

In natural waters, fish have another option for manipulating their body temperature, moving to water having a different temperature (Reynolds and Casterlin, 1980). The relationships are complex because they change for different species, different acclimation temperatures, and according to whether the temperature in question is above or below the acclimation temperature. Thermal preferences may also have intrinsic, locomotor, diel, or tidal rhythms, all of which may be different. Fish also may demonstrate behavioral fever by preferring a higher temperature when sick than when well (Covert and Reynolds, 1977).

WALLEYE AND PERCH

The walleye and perch are generalized, spiny-rayed fishes in which the first dorsal fin and first two rays of the anal fin are spiny. Chiasson (1966) presented the detailed anatomy of the yellow perch as a dissection guide for undergraduate students.

Dramatic increases in fishing pressure on walleye and perch in recent years have led to increased interest in culturing both of these species. Yellow perch have been reared experimentally, using methods similar to the rearing of bass, but the methods are still too expensive for commercial production (Heidinger and Kayes, 1986).

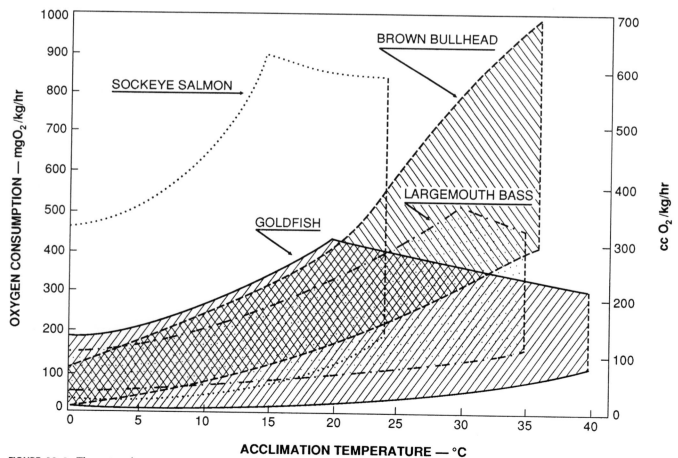

FIGURE 19–1. The rate of oxygen consumption related to temperature for four species of fish. (Adapted from Brett, J.R. [1972] The metabolic demand for oxygen in fish, particularly salmonids, and a comparison with other vertebrates. Respir. Physiol. 14:151–170.)

Several basic aspects of walleye culture have been known for over 100 years, but production methods are still not consistently dependable. After hatching, fry typically are reared in ponds where they eat zooplankton. Survival has been poor, often less than 1%, with the largest losses being due to cannibalism. Young wild walleye become piscivorous after they reach a length of about 8 cm, but both fry and fingerlings readily accept artificial food (Nickum, 1986).

MULLET

Mullets have three specialized anatomical features that relate directly to their lifestyle. Because they eat detritus and algae, which are relatively indigestible, and because they include considerable sand and mud with their food, their intestine is three to eight times their body length, depending on species. There is some indication that the mullet gut may lengthen with age and with the change from their larval diet of zooplankton to plant and algal detritus as adults. Their pyloric stomach develops as a gizzard, which is most conspicuous in species having the greatest amount of detritus and algae in their diet. They also have a pharyngobranchial organ in the roof of their mouth that, in combination with finely spaced teeth, presumably sorts out particulate organic material.

Mullets survive in salinities from zero to over 100 ppt (Ben-Yami and Grofit, 1981). Sodium-potassium ATPase is one link in the osmoregulation process carried out by the chloride cells in the gills that makes such euryhalinity possible. The activity level of this ATPase is the same in the gills of mullet adapted to 9, 24, and 40 ppt of seawater (Black, 1984), but this increases fivefold after transfer from fresh water to 45 ppt of seawater (Hossler et al., 1979). Juveniles less than 40 mm long, captured at entry into fresh water, show less than 50% survival when transferred back into 45 ppt of seawater. This suggests a developmental aspect to osmoregulatory capability. Fry survive transfer from seawater to fresh water better if the fresh water contains at least 370 ppm calcium (Auld, 1972).

Euryhalinity in mullets probably differs functionally from anadromy in salmon and catadromy in eels. In euryhaline fishes, rapid changes in sodium-potassium ATPase activity accompany changes in salinity without any changes in the quantity of enzyme present. This is probably due to changes in the catalytic rate (Towle et al., 1977), in contrast to salmonid smoltification, in which there are changes in ATPase quantity and location.

There are few data on the oxygen metabolism of mullets. The mean routine metabolic rate for a 100-g gray mullet in 18°C seawater is 84 ml of oxygen per kg per hour with a low of 44 ml/kg/hour at 15°C (Cech and Wohlschlag, 1973). The preferred temperature range of gray mullet seems to be between 12 and 25°C, although mullet have been seen feeding in a heated effluent at 40°C. Mullets have a higher metabolic rate in seawater than in brackish water.

Sexual maturation in mullets appears very sensitive to photoperiod. The thinlip gray mullet, a species which naturally spawns in December in Israel, develops mature ova only under short photoperiod (8 hours of light and 16 hours of dark) (Sagi and Abraham, 1985). Pinealectomized females were shown to develop ova only about half as large as those of intact controls when both were under short photoperiod (Sagi et al., 1983). This seems to be the difficulty in inducing ova maturation by injections of pituitary hormones in mullet when maturation is not well advanced. The decline of steroid sex hormones during normal maturation may partly explain this refractoriness (Oren and Rosenthal, 1981).

LITERATURE CITED

Auld, A.M. (1972) The effect of calcium on the osmotic tolerance of juvenile striped mullet (*Mugil cephalus* L.). In: Proceedings of the 26th Annual Conference of Southeastern Association of Game and Fish Commissioners, Knoxville, Tennessee, pp. 591–597.

Ben-Yami, M., and Grofit, E. (1981) Methods of capture of grey mullets. In: Aquaculture of Grey Mullets (Oren, O. H., ed.). Cambridge University Press, England, pp. 313–333.

Billard, R. (ed.) (1983) Efficiency of ovulation induced by gonadotropic treatment in a heterogeneous population of northern pike (*Esox lucius*); Relation to the oocyte stage, and comparison with the results of spontaneous ovulations. Coll. Hydrobiol. Aquacult. 85–95.

Black, E.W. (1984) Sodium Exchange Mechanisms in the Gill Tissue of the Striped Mullet (*Mugil Cephalus*). Ph.D. Thesis, Alabama University, Birmingham.

Brett, J.R. (1972) The metabolic demand for oxygen in fish, particularly salmonids, and a comparison with other vertebrates. Respir. Physiol. 14:151–170.

Brzuska, E., and Malczewski, B. (1984) The effect of injection of carp pituitary on oocytes maturation and ovulation in pike, *Esox lucius*. 10th International Congress on Animal Reproduction and Artificial Insemination. Congress Proceedings.

Cech, Jr., J.J., and Wohlschlag, D.E. (1973) Respiratory responses of the striped mullet, *Mugil cephalus* (L.), to hypoxic conditions. J. Fish. Biol. 5:447–455.

Chiasson, R.B. (1966) Laboratory Anatomy of the Perch. Wm. C. Brown, Dubuque, Iowa.

Covert, J.G., and Reynolds, W.W. (1977) Survival value of fever in fish. Nature 267:43–45.

Davis, K.B., Parker, N.C., and Suttle, M.A. (1982) Plasma corticosteroids and chlorides in striped bass exposed to tricaine methanesulfonate, quinaldine, etomidate, and salt. Progressive Fish Culturist 44:205–207.

Dillard, J.G., Graham, L.K., and Russell, T.R. (Eds.) (1986) The Paddlefish: Status, Management, and Propagation. American Fisheries Society Special Publication No. 7.

Fremling, C.R. (1978) Biology and Functional Anatomy of the Freshwater Drum, *Aplodinotus grunniens* Rafinesque. NASCO, Fort Atkinson, Wisconsin.

Gainer, H., Kusano, K., and Mathewson, R.F. (1965) Electro-physiological and mechanical properties of squirrel fish sound-producing muscle. Comp. Biochem. Physiol. 14:661–671.

Groman, D.B. (1982) Histology of the striped bass. American Fisheries Society Monograph No. 3.

Heidinger, R.C., and Kayes, T.B. (1986) Yellow perch. In: Culture of Nonsalmonid Freshwater Fishes (Stickney, R.R., ed.). CRC Press, Boca Raton, Florida, pp. 103–113.

Hirano, T., Satou, M., and Utida, S. (1972) Central nervous system control of osmoregulation in the eel (*Anguilla japonica*). Comp. Biochem. Physiol. 43A:537–544.

Hossler, F.E., Ruby, J.R., and McIlwain, T.D. (1979) The gill arch of mullet, *Mugil cephalus*. II. Modification in surface ultrastructure and Na+-K+ ATPase content during adaptation to various salinities. J. Exp. Zool. 208:399–406.

Lavrova, E.A., Natochin, Y.V., and Shakhmatova, E.L. (1984) Electrolytes in the tissues of sturgeon and bony fishes in fresh and salt water. J. Ichthyol. 24:156–160.

Meyer, F.A. (1970) Development of some larval centrarchids. Progressive Fish Culturist 32:130–136.

Nickum, J.G. (1986) Walleye. In: Culture of Nonsalmonid Freshwater Fishes (Stickney, R.R., ed.). CRC Press, Boca Raton, Florida, pp. 115–126.

Oren, O.H., and Rosenthal, H. (eds.) (1981) Steroid Production in the Ovary of the Greymullet (*Mugil cephalus*) During Gonadal Development. Special Publication of the European Mariculture Society, 6:221–228.

Parker, N.C. (1984) Culture requirements for striped bass. In: The Aquaculture of Striped Bass: A Proceedings (McCraren, J. P., ed.). Maryland Sea Grant Program, University of Maryland, College Park, pp. 29–43, UM-SG-MAP-84-01.

Parker, N.C., and Geiger, J.G. (1984) Production methods for striped bass. In: Third Report to the Fish Farmers: The Status of Warmwater Fish Farming and Progress in Fish Farming Research (Dupree, H.K., and Huner, J.V., eds.). U.S. Fish and Wildlife Service, Washington, D.C., pp. 106–118.

Potts, W.T.W., and Rudy, P.P. (1972) Aspects of osmotic and ionic regulation in the sturgeon. J. Exp. Biol. 56:703–715.

Reynolds, W.W., and Casterlin, M.E. (1980) The role of temperature in the environmental physiology of fishes. In: Environmental Physiology of Fishes (Ali, M. A., ed.). Plenum Press, New York, pp. 497–518.

Sagi, G., and Abraham, M. (1985) Photoperiod and ovarian activity in the grey mullet, *Liza ramada* (Pisces: Mugilidae). Isr. J. Zool. 33:1–9.

Sagi, G., Abraham, M., and Hilge, V. (1983) Pinealectomy and ovarian development in the grey mullet, *Liza ramada*. J. Fish Biol. 23:339–345.

Schwalme, K., and Mackay, W.C. (1985) The influence of exercise handling stress on blood lactate, acid-base, and plasma glucose status of northern pike (*Esox lucius* L.). Can. J. Zool. 63:1125–1129.

Shaklee, J.B., Christianse, J.A., Sidell, B.D., Prosser, C.L., and Whitt, G.S. (1977) Molecular aspects of temperature acclimation in fish: Contributions of changes in enzyme activities and isozyme patterns to metabolic reorganization in the green sunfish. J. Exp. Zool. 201:1–20.

Sidell, B.D., and Johnston, I.A. (1985) Thermal sensitivity of contractile function in chain pickerel, *Esox niger*. Can. J. Zool. 63:811–816.

Tesch, F.W. (1977) The Eel: Biology and Management of Anguillid Eels. Chapman and Hall, London.

Towle, D.W., Gilman, M.E., and Hempel, J.D. (1977) Rapid modulation of gill Na^+-K^+-dependent ATPase activity during acclimation of the killifish *Fundulus heteroclitus* to salinity change. J. Exp. Zool. 202:179–186.

Wardle, C.S. (1980) Effects of temperature on the maximum swimming speed of fishes. In: Environmental Physiology of Fishes (Ali, M. A., ed.). Plenum Press, New York, pp. 519–531.

Webb, P.W. (1975) Hydrodynamics and Energetics of Fish Propulsion. Bulletin No. 190 of the Fisheries Research Board of Canada, Ottawa.

Chapter 20

CLINICAL PATHOLOGY OF TEMPERATE FRESHWATER AND ESTUARINE FISHES

ROBERT A. BULLIS

There is a striking need for determining normal hematologic values under a wide variety of natural and experimental conditions for temperate zone fishes. Procedures and techniques are rapidly becoming standardized. Detailed investigations have established sound baseline blood values for Northern pike (Mulchay, 1990) and for killifishes (Gardner and Yevich, 1969). Work in other species remains incomplete (Tables 20–1 to 20–5).

EFFECTS OF TEMPERATURE CHANGE ON BLOOD VALUES

Few temperate freshwater fishes enjoy a stable thermal environment. Virtually all species must acclimate to large seasonal temperature fluctuations. Species occupying shallow, slow-moving, or estuarine habitats also contend with substantial diurnal temperature variation. Increases in environmental temperature impose a variety of stresses on fishes,

but erythrocyte indices have been best studied (Houston, 1980). At high temperatures, pinfishes show increased hemoglobin content and erythrocytes, but decreased hematocrit and mean corpuscular volume (Cameron, 1970). In Northern pike, sudden drops in temperature decrease both hematocrit and hemoglobin values (Kristoffersson and Brobert, 1971).

Decreases in temperature lower serum glucose in sunfish and bass, whereas the level in the closely related crappie increases (Dean and Goodnight, 1964). Killifish show dramatic differences in serum glucose between fresh water and salt water. When exposed to near-freezing temperatures, salt water–adapted fishes show only a moderate increase in serum glucose, whereas fresh water–adapted fishes increase serum glucose dramatically to the highest baseline level known for any fish (1066 mg%) (Umminger, 1971). Hyperglycemia is assumed to stabilize the blood at subzero temperatures and to increase the supply of glucose to the central nervous system

TABLE 20–1. Erythrocyte Values of Temperate Fishes

Species/Treatment/Ref.	Parameter	Values
American Eel (Altman and Dittmer, 1974)	RBC count ($\times$ 10⁶/ml) Hematocrit (%) Hemoglobin (g/dl) MCV (μ^3) MCHC (g/dl)	2.48 36.0–39.8 8.0–10.0 141–170 23.7
Bowfin (Thorson, 1961)	Hematocrit (%)	30–34
Freshwater Drum Freshwater following seine capture (Harmon and Johnson, 1980)	Hematocrit (%) Hemoglobin (g/dl) MCHC (g/dl)	20–21 4.7–5.6 22–27
Lake Sturgeon (Thorson, 1961)	Hematocrit (%)	19–29
Largemouth Bass In good body condition (Esch and Hazen, 1980)	RBC count ($\times$ 10⁶/ml) Hematocrit (%) Hemoglobin (g/dl) MCHC (g/dl)	6.5–7.1 41.7–42.3 9.1–9.3 21.9
Mummichog Freshwater 20°C Male Freshwater 20°C Female (Slicher, 1961)	RBC count ($\times$ 10⁶/ml) Hemoglobin (g/dl) RBC count ($\times$ 10⁶/ml) Hemoglobin (g/dl)	3.25–3.32 6.77–7.01 4.32–4.36 8.35–8.59
Northern Pike Freshwater 10°C Adults (Ince and Thorpe, 1976; Mulchay, 1970; Soivio and Okari, 1976)	Hematocrit (%) Hemoglobin (g/dl) MCHC (g/dl)	25–39 6.1–8.8 24–28
Brackishwater 10°C 6.2 ppt (Soivio and Okari, 1976)	Hematocrit (%) Hemoglobin (g/dl) MCHC (g/dl)	17.4–20.0 4.93–4.97 26.6–27.0
Paddlefish (Thorson, 1961)	Hematocrit (%)	24–37
Shortnose Gar (Thorson, 1961)	Hematocrit (%)	33–50
Striped Bass Freshwater 8–17°C Spawning (Westin, 1978)	RBC count ($\times$ 10⁶/ml) Hematocrit (%) Hemoglobin (g/dl) MCHC (g/dl)	3.79 47.9 9.1 19.0
White Perch (Altman and Dittmer, 1974)	RBC count ($\times$ 10⁶/ml) Hematocrit (%) Hemoglobin (g/dl) MCV (μ^3)	2.70–3.63 32.7–37.8 6.7–9.7 104–121

(Umminger, 1969). Near-freezing temperatures also apparently initiate a cyclic leukopenia and leukocytosis in killifish (Pickford et al., 1971).

EFFECTS OF STARVATION

The ability to survive for long periods without food is remarkably well developed in eels (Goran et al., 1975). They are subjected to natural starvation periods during the winter and spawning. Lowered water temperature apparently triggers cessation of eating (Goran et al., 1975). During starvation, hematocrit and mean corpuscular volumes increase first, followed by the erythrocyte count. Then hemoglobin and mean corpuscular volumes decrease

while hematocrit and erythrocyte counts remain elevated (Krajnovic-Ozretic and Ozretic, 1987).

Pike are also well adapted to periods of prolonged starvation. Forced starvation in Northern pike causes a decrease in hematocrit and serum glucose and an increase in serum cholesterol values (Ince and Thorpe, 1976). This is presumably the case for most predator species. A significant reduction in body condition has been shown to accompany exposure to thermal effluents in largemouth bass (Esch and Hazen, 1980). This deterioration can be monitored by observing a decreasing hematocrit, increasing cortisol values, and leukopenia. Increased blood iron also correlates with *Aeromonas hydrophila* infections in thermally stressed largemouth bass (Hazen et al., 1978).

CAPTURE AND HANDLING STRESS

Proper periods of acclimatization are absolutely necessary to obtain useful baseline hematologic data. Capture alone can significantly affect blood chemistry. Newly caught freshwater drum show increased plasma glucose and lactic acid, but no significant change in hematocrit or hemoglobin content compared to acclimatized fish (Harmon and Johnson, 1980). Hemolysis of blood is much more pronounced in freshly captured fish.

Following capture, the conditions of captivity can also affect blood parameters. Blood lactic acid levels increase when bass or sunfish are placed in flow-through systems and forced to swim. Peak levels occur in 1 hour and take 10 hours to return to preexercise levels (Heath and Pritchard, 1962). Subordinate individual eels exhibit a 20% reduction in serum sodium and potassium values and significant changes in gill structure compared to dominant animals in the same tank. Fish with and without bite wounds reveal no significant differences in parameters (Peters and Long, 1985). In Northern pike, serum glucose requires 2 days to return to normal following handling stress (Soivio and Okari, 1976). The serum glucose, lactic acid, sodium, magnesium, hematocrit, and hemoglobin content are all significantly higher in pike reared in fresh water versus brackish water (Soivio and Okari, 1976).

CHANGES DUE TO SPAWNING AND ESTUARINE MIGRATION

Many temperate fishes encounter changing salinities in their habitat. Hematocrits tend to be higher for a given species in fresh water (Soivio and Okari, 1976). Hematocrits and serum electrolytes are lower in individuals of the same species living in brackish water (Holmes and Donaldson, 1969; Potts and Rudy, 1972; Soivio and Okari, 1976). Dramatic differences

Text continued on page 238

TABLE 20–2. Leukocyte Counts for Freshwater and Estuarine Fishes

Species/Treatment/Ref.	Total WBC Count ($\times 10^3$)	Heterophils (%)	Lymphocytes (%)	Monocytes (%)	Eosinophils (%)	Basophils (%)	Hemocytoblasts (%)
Alligator Gar (Altman and Dittmer, 1974)	—	11	79	4	4	0	2
Longnose Gar (Altman and Dittmer, 1974)	—	0	21	2	71	4	2
American Eel (Altman and Dittmer, 1974)	—	14	38	0	46	0	2
Grass Pickerel (Altman and Dittmer, 1974)	—	0	81	2	9	4	4
Green Sunfish (Altman and Dittmer, 1974)	—	24	50	0	20	4	2
Largemouth Bass In poor flesh	2.1–2.3	0	81	3	10	0	3
In good flesh (Esch and Hazen, 1980)	2.0–3.8	0	81	4	7	0	4
Mummichog 24°C (Gardner and Yevich, 1969)	—	0	81	0	19	0	0
Freshwater 20°C Males	6.3–6.8	0	42	0	58	0	0
Freshwater 20°C Females (Slicher, 1961)	6.3–6.8	0	42	0	58	0	0
Northern Pike Adults (Mulcahy, 1970)	1.12	—	—	—	—	—	—
Pinfish (Altman and Dittmer, 1974)	—	16	59	2	21	2	0
Red Drum (Altman and Dittmer, 1974)	—	6	40	2	40	10	2
Sand Sea Trout (Altman and Dittmer, 1974)	—	8	63	0	23	4	2
Sheepshead Minnow 24°C August (Gardner and Yevich, 1969)	—	0	67	0	33	0	0
Spotted Sea Trout (Altman and Dittmer, 1974)	—	15	65	2	12	6	0
Striped Killifish 24°C (Gardner and Yevich, 1969)	—	0	59	0	41	0	0
Striped Mullet (Altman and Dittmer, 1974)	—	4	76	0	4	6	10
White Mullet (Altman and Dittmer, 1974)	—	3	75	0	19	0	3

TABLE 20–3. Serum Electrolyte Values

Species/Treatment/Ref.	Parameter (mM/L)	Values	Species/Treatment/Ref.	Parameter (mM/L)	Values
Largemouth Bass (Hazen et al., 1978)	Na K	159–166 3.7–4.6	*Plains Killifish* Freshwater (Stanley and Fleming, 1964)	Na K Ca	160 3.9 2.5
Smallmouth Bass (Shell, 1961)	Na K Ca Cl PO$_4$	128–140 8–10 10–14 111–128 6.7–9.0	*Lamprey* (Logan et al., 1980)	Na K Mg Ca Cl	122 3.2 1.1 2.4 108
Bowfin (Smith, 1929)	Na K Mg Ca Cl PO$_4$ SO$_4$ CO$_2$	133 2.0 0.4 5.3 120 4.1 2.2 4.3	*Striped Mullet* Euryhaline (Sulya et al., 1960)	Na K Cl	117 6.3 153
			White Mullet Euryhaline (Sulya et al., 1960)	Na K Cl	179 5.6 151
Red Drum Euryhaline (Sulya et al., 1960)	Na K Cl	189 8.6 160	*Mummichog* Saltwater 20°C (Umminger, 1969)	Na K Mg Ca Cl HCO$_3$	183 4.8 1.8 2.2 145 14.1
American Eel Freshwater May Silver phase (Butler et al., 1969)	Na K Mg Ca Cl	138 2.8 1.3 3.3 70	*Paddlefish* Both sexes 17°C (Grant et al., 1970)	Na K Mg Ca Cl CO$_4$	137–143 3.4–4.0 0.7–1.5 1.6–2.0 110.5–114.0 0.5–0.6
Freshwater Yellow phase (Butler et al., 1969)	Na K Mg Ca Cl	151 2.8 1.2 3.2 111	*Yellow Perch* Freshwater (Lutz, 1972)	Na K Mg Ca Cl	154 3.6 1.6 4.4 120
European Eel Freshwater Yellow phase (Chan et al., 1967)	Na K Mg Ca PO$_4$	143 2.3 3.0 2.3 1.3	*Northern Pike* Freshwater 10°C (Soivio and Okari, 1976)	Na K Mg Ca	122–128 2.0–2.2 1.3 5.0–5.6
Saltwater 5 weeks Yellow phase (Chan et al., 1967)	Na K Mg Ca PO$_4$	164 3.4 4.2 5.5 2.0	Brackishwater control (Kristoffersson et al., 1973)	Na K Ca Cl	144 3.0 3.2 117
Freshwater Silver phase (Chan et al., 1967)	Na K Mg Ca Cl PO$_4$	150 1.8 2.1 2.3 88 1.8	*Pinfish* Euryhaline (Sulya et al., 1960)	Na K Cl	183 8.3 174
Saltwater 5 weeks Silver phase (Chan et al., 1967)	Na K Mg Ca Cl PO$_4$	183 3.2 3.7 2.4 140 1.8	*Pumpkinseed* Freshwater (Grant et al., 1970)	Na K Cl	163–190 0.6–3.0 90–118
Freshwater 22°C (Peters and Long, 1985)	Na K Ca	145–155 2.2–3.0 4.9–5.1	*Spotted Sea Trout* Euryhaline (Sulya et al., 1960)	Na K Cl	195 7.8 251
Alligator Gar Low salinity (Sulya et al., 1960)	Na K Cl	153 6.2 133	*Atlantic Sturgeon* Freshwater, young fish (Holmes and Donaldson, 1969)	Na K Mg Ca Cl PO$_4$	151 2.7 0.9 1.9 113 3.1
Longnose Gar (Smith, 1929)	Na K Mg Ca Cl PO$_4$ SO$_4$ CO$_2$	140 2.7 0.3 6.1 118 3.9 2.4 9.1	*Green Sturgeon* Freshwater (Potts and Rudy, 1974)	Na K Mg Ca Cl SO$_4$	119 1.5 0.6 2.6 106 2.76
			Lake Sturgeon (Holmes and Donaldson, 1969)	Na K Mg Cl PO$_4$	143–148 3.5–4.5 0.9–1.6 104–113 2.4–2.7

Table continued on following page

TABLE 20–3. Serum Electrolyte Values *Continued*

Species/Treatment/Ref.	Parameter (mM/L)	Values	Species/Treatment/Ref.	Parameter (mM/L)	Values
White Sturgeon Saltwater males (Holmes and Donaldson, 1969)	Na	130	Pregnancy Gravid females (Urist and Van de Putte, 1967)	Na	123
	K	2.5		K	2.0
	Mg	2.1		Mg	2.2
	Ca	1.7		Ca	9.2
	Cl	115		Cl	116
	PO₄	2.9			
	SO₄	0.4	Males and nongravid females (Urist and Van de Putte, 1967)	Na	123–129
	HCO₃	5.2		K	2.0–2.7
				Mg	1.1–3.6
				Ca	1.8–4.0
				Cl	111–116
Freshwater both sexes (Holmes and Donaldson, 1969)	Na	129			
	K	2.7			
	Mg	2			
	Ca	1.8			
	Cl	111			
	PO₄	3.3			
	SO₄	0.5			
	HCO₃	6.0			

TABLE 20–4. Miscellaneous Serum Values of Freshwater Temperate Fishes

Species/Treatment/Ref.	Parameter	Values
Largemouth Bass Fresh water 5°C (Dean and Goodnight, 1964) (Hazen et al., 1978)	Glucose Lactic acid	35.0–95.0 mg/dl 11.2–98.0 mg/dl
	Iron Total iron-binding capacity Thyroxin (T₄)	72.3–161.3 mM/L 347.5–634.6 0.68–1.96
(Esch and Hazen, 1980)	Cortisol	12.0–12.8 µg/dl
Blue Gill Fresh water 20°C 3-Day fast (Hickman, 1968)	Glucose	53.0–130.0 mg/dl
Fresh water 5°C (Dean and Goodnight, 1964) (McGeachin and Debnam, 1960)	Glucose Lactic acid Amylase	32.5–85.0 mg/dl 34.7–51.2 mg/dl 290.0 U/dl
White Crappie Fresh water 5°C (Dean and Goodnight, 1964)	Glucose Lactic acid	137.5–235.0 mg/dl 59.0–125.1 mg/dl
Freshwater Drum Plasma (Harmon and Johnson, 1980)	Glucose	88–97 mg/dl
American Eel Plasma (Holmes and Donaldson, 1969)	Osmotic pressure	251.8–307.9 mOsm/L
European Eel Plasma Fresh water (Ball et al., 1971)	Cortisol	3.0 µg/dl
Plasma Fresh water 12°C Yellow phase (Lewander et al., 1976)	Cortisol	7.3–10.1 µg/dl
Plasma Fresh water 9–13°C Silver phase (Ince and Thorpe, 1977)	Insulin Amino acid nitrogen	2.4–3.8 mg/ml 3.75 mg/dl
Lamprey (Logan et al., 1980)	Osmolarity	296 mOsm

Note: Thyroxin (T_4).

TABLE 20–4. Miscellaneous Serum Values of Freshwater Temperate Fishes *Continued*

Species/Treatment/Ref.	Parameter	Values
Mummichog Serum Saltwater 10°C (Umminger, 1969)	Glucose	70.8 mg/dl
Paddlefish Males 17°C spawning (Grant et al., 1970)	Glucose Cholesterol Lactic acid Cortisol	27–36 mg/dl 437–509 mg/dl 124.3–159.5 mg/dl 22.3–29.1 µg/dl
Females 17°C spawning (Grant et al., 1970)	Glucose Cholesterol Lactic acid Cortisol	18.0–25.4 mg/dl 141.6–148.4 mg/dl 103.2–106.2 mg/dl 2.9–9.1 µg/dl
Plasma Fresh water (Thorson, 1961)	Specific gravity	1.016–1.018
Northern Pike Plasma January–June averages (Thorpe and Ince, 1974)	Glucose Cholesterol Amino acid nitrogen	25–71 mg/L 97–209 mg/dl 3.6–8.6 mg/dl
Plasma Fresh water 10°C 70% males (Ince and Thorpe, 1976) (Soivio and Okari, 1976)	Cholesterol Amino acid nitrogen	97–209 mg/dl 4.7–5.6 mg/dl
Plasma Fresh water 10–14°C (Lewander et al., 1976)	Free fatty acids	255–275 meg/L
Plasma Fresh water 15–18°C (Ince and Thorpe, 1978)	Alanine	146–180 mM/dl
Plasma Fresh water 15–18°C (Ince and Thorpe, 1978)	Valine Glycine Isoleucine Threonine Leucine Serine Proline Aspartic acid Phenylalanine Tyrosine Lysine	31–49 mM/dl 63–99 mM/dl 17–29 mM/dl 26–39 mM/dl 30–48 mM/dl 25–30 mM/dl 4–8 mM/dl 4–6 mM/dl 17–24 mM/dl 2.8–4.4 mM/dl 22–29 mM/dl
Plasma (Holmes and Donaldson, 1978)	Osmotic pressure	274 mOsm/L
Green Sturgeon Plasma Saltwater 20°C (Potts and Rudy, 1972)	Cortisol	1.4–4.0 mg/dl

TABLE 20–5. Effects of Environmental and Nutritional Factors

Species/Treatment/Ref.	Parameter	Effects Related to Controls
Largemouth Bass In poor body condition (Esch and Hazen, 1980)	RBC count Hematocrit Hemoglobin MCHC	Decrease Decrease Decrease No change
Freshwater Drum Capture stress (Harmon and Johnson, 1980)	Plasma glucose	Increase
European Eel Saltwater and 164 days starvation (Goran et al., 1975)	RBC count Hematocrit Hemoglobin MCV	Decrease Decrease No change Increase
Freshwater 22°C and stress (Peters and Long, 1985)	Na K Ca	Decrease Decrease No change
Striped Mullet Brackishwater 7°C 11 ppt (Cameron, 1970)	RBC count Hematocrit Hemoglobin MCV MCHC	Slight decrease Decrease Decrease Decrease Decrease
Mummichog Saltwater exposure 20°C (Pickford et al., 1971)	WBC count	Decrease
Freshwater exposure 11°C (Umminger, 1971)	Serum glucose	Decrease
Northern Pike Brackishwater 1 week exposure to 5 ppm phenol (Kristoffersson et al., 1973)	Na K Ca Cl	Slight decrease Increase No change Slight decrease
Pinfish Cold-water exposure 7°C (Cameron, 1970)	RBC count Hematocrit Hemoglobin MCVC MCHC	Slight decrease Slight increase Slight decrease Increase No.change
Pumpkinseed Cold-water exposure 3°C (Houston et al., 1976)	Hematocrit Hemoglobin MCHC	Increase Increase Decrease
Atlantic Sturgeon Saltwater exposure (Holmes and Donaldson, 1969)	Na K Mg Ca Cl PO₄	Increase Increase Increase No change Increase Decrease
Green Sturgeon Saltwater exposure (Potts and Rudy, 1972)	Na K Mg Ca Cl SO₄	Increase Increase Increase Increase Increase Increase

in blood chemistry values occur in anadromous or catadromous species during spawning as typified by sturgeon and eels (Butler et al., 1969; Chan et al., 1967; Potts and Rudy, 1972). Sexual dimorphism in serum nonprotein nitrogen, cholesterol, and cortisol values occurs in spawning paddlefish (Grant et al., 1970). Dimorphic changes are also reported in sturgeon (Holmes and Donaldson, 1969). The possibility

of using dimorphic serum calcium and other blood parameters to determine the sex of migrating striped bass has been investigated (Westin, 1978).

SUBLETHAL EFFECTS OF TOXINS

Measurement of plasma enzyme activity is a valuable diagnostic tool in fish toxicology, but routine methods derived from mammalian studies can lead to misinterpretation of test results. Optimal assay conditions for mullet have been described in detail (Krajnovic-Ozretic and Ozretic, 1987). Sublethal effects of phenol in mullet can be detected by increases in liver enzyme values, which correlate with changes in gross pathology and behavior (Krajnovic-Ozretic and Ozretic, 1987). Sublethal effects of phenol in pike are best determined by changes in serum amino acid concentrations (Kristoffersson et al., 1973), which can be assayed using chromatographic techniques (Ince and Thorpe, 1978). Bile is also useful in studying the elimination of biotransformed substances. An impressive compilation of bile composition for temperate freshwater fishes is available for reference (Hunn, 1976).

LITERATURE CITED

Altman, P.L., and Dittmer, D.S. (eds.) (1974) The Biology Data Book. Vol. III. Federation of American Societies for Experimental Biology, Bethesda, Maryland.

Ball, J.N., and Dittmer, D.S., (eds.) (1974) The Biology Data Book. Vol. III. Federation of the American Society for Experimental Biology, Bethesda, Maryland.

Blaxhall, R.C. (1972) The haematological assessment of the health of freshwater fish. A review of selected literature. J. Fish Biol. 4:593–604.

Butler, D.G., Clarke, W.D., Donaldson, E.M., and Langford, R.W. (1969) Surgical adrenalectomy of a teleost fish (Anguilla rostrata Lesueur): Effect on plasma cortisol and tissue electrolyte and carbohydrate concentrations. Gen. Comp. Endocrinol. 12:502–514.

Cameron, J.N. (1970) The influence of environmental variables on the hematology of pinfish (Lagodon rhomboides) and striped mullet (Mugil cephalus). Comp. Biochem. Physiol. 32:175–192.

Chan, D.D.O., Chester-Jones, I., Henderson, I.W., and Rankin, J.C. (1967) Studies on the experimental alteration of water and electrolyte composition of the eel (Anguilla L.). J. Endocrinol. 37:297–317.

Dean, M.M., and Goodnight, C.J. (1964) A comparative study of carbohydrate metabolism in fish as affected by temperature and exercise. Physiol. Zool. 37:299–380.

Esch, G.W., and Hazen, T.C. (1980) Stress and body condition in a population of largemouth bass: Implications for Red-Sore disease. Trans. Am. Fish. Soc. 109:532–536.

Gardner, G.R., and Yevich, P.O. (1969) Studies on the blood morphology of three estuarine cyprinodontiform fishes. J. Fish. Res. Bd. Can. 26:433–447.

Goran, D., Johansson-Sjobeck, M.L., Larsson, A., Lewander, K., and Lidman, U. (1975) Metabolic and hematological effects of starvation in the European eel, Anguilla anguilla L.—I. Carbohydrate, lipid, protein, and inorganic ion metabolism. Comp. Biochem. Physiol. 52A:423–430.

Grant, B.F., Mehrle, P.M., and Russell, T.R. (1970) Serum characteristics of spawning paddlefish (Polydon spathula). Comp. Biochem. Physiol. 37:321–325.

Harmon, G.J., and Johnson, D.L. (1980) Physiological responses of Lake Erie freshwater drum to capture by commercial shore seine. Trans. Am. Fish. Soc. 109:544–551.

Hazen, T.C., Esch, G.W., Glassman, A.B., and Gibbons, J.W. (1978) Relationship of season, thermal loading and Red-Sore disease with various haematological parameters in Micropterus salmoides. J. Fish Biol. 12:491–498.

Heath, A.G., and Pritchard, A.W. (1962) Changes in the metabolic rate and blood lactic acid of bluegill sunfish, Lepomis macrochirus Raf, following severe muscular activity. Physiol. Zool. 35:323–329.

Hickman, C.P., Jr. (1968) Urine composition and kidney function in Southern flounder, *Paralichthys lethostigma*, in sea water. Can. J. Zool. 46:439–455.

Holmes, W.N., and Donaldson, E.M. (1969) The body compartments and the distribution of electrolytes. In: Fish Physiology. Vol. I (Hoar, W.S., and Randall, D.J., eds.). Academic Press, New York, pp. 1–90.

Houston, A.H. (1980) Components of the hematological response of fishes to environmental temperature change: A review. In: Fish Physiology. Vol. I (Ali, M.A., ed.). Plenum Press, New York, pp. 241–298.

Houston, A.H., Mearow, K.M., and Smeda, J.A. (1976) Further observations on the hemoglobin systems of thermally-acclimated freshwater teleosts: Pumpkinseed (*Lepomis gibbosus*), white sucker (*Catostomus commersoni*), carp (*Cyprinis carpio*), goldfish (*Crassius auratus*) and carp-goldfish hybrids. Comp. Biochem. Physiol. 54A:267–273.

Hunn, J.B. (1976) Inorganic composition of gallbladder bile from freshwater fish. Copeia 3:602–604.

Ince, G.W., and Thorpe, A. (1976) The effects of starvation and force-feeding on the metabolism of the Northern pike, *Esox lucius* L. J. Fish Biol. 8:79–88.

Ince, B.W., and Thorpe, A. (1977) Glucose and amino acid-stimulated insulin release *in vivo* in the European eel (*Anguilla anguilla* L.). Gen. Comp. Endocrinol. 31:249–256.

Ince, B.W., and Thorpe, A. (1978) The effects of insulin on plasma amino acid levels in the Northern pike, *Esox lucius* L. J. Fish Biol. 12:503–506.

Krajnovic-Ozretic, M., and Ozretic, B. (1987) Estimation of the enzymes LDH, GOT, and GPT in the plasma of grey mullet *Mugil auratus* and their significance in liver intoxication. Dis. Aquat. Org. 3:187–193.

Kristoffersson, R., and Brobert, S. (1971) Effect of temperature acclimation on some blood constituents of the pike (*Esox lucius* L.). Ann. Zool. Fennici. 8:427–433.

Kristoffersson, R., Brobert, S., and Oikari, A. (1973) Physiological effects of a sublethal concentration of phenol in the pike (*Esox lucius* L.) in pure brackish water. Ann. Zool. Fennici. 10:392–397.

Lewander, K., Goran, D., Johanssen-Sjobeck, M.L., Larsson, A., and Lidman, U. (1976) Metabolic effects of insulin in the European eel, *Anguilla anguilla* L. Gen. Comp. Endocrinol. 29:455–467.

Logan, A.G., Morris, R., and Rankin, J.C. (1980) A micropuncture study of kidney function in the river lamprey, *Lampetra fluviatilis*, adapted to sea water. J. Exp. Biol. 88:239–247.

Lutz, P.L. (1972) Ionic and body compartment responses to increasing salinity in perch, *Perca fluviatilis*. Comp. Biochem. Physiol. 42:711–717.

McGeachin, R.L., and Debnam, J.W. (1960) Amylase in freshwater fish. Proc. Soc. Exptl. Biol. Med. 103:814–815.

Mulcahy, M.F. (1970) Blood values in the pike *Esox lucius* L. J. Fish Biol. 2:203–209.

Peters, G., and Long, L.Q. (1985) Gill structure and blood electrolyte levels of European eels under stress. In: Fish and Shellfish Pathology (Ellis, A.E., ed.). Academic Press, New York, pp 183–189.

Pickford, G.E., Srivastava, A.K., Slicher, A.M., and Pang, P.K.T. (1971) The stress response in the abundance of circulating leukocytes in the killifish, *Fundulus heteroclitus*. J. Exp. Zool. 177:89–96.

Potts, W.T.W., and Rudy, P.P. (1972) Aspects of osmotic and ionic regulation in the sturgeon. J. Exp. Biol. 56:703–715.

Shell, E.W. (1961) Chemical Composition of Blood of Smallmouthed Bass. U.S. Department of the Interior Fish and Wildlife Service Research Report 57:1–36.

Slicher, A.M. (1961) Endocrinological and hematological studies in *Fundulus heteroclitus* (Linn.). Bull. Bingham. Oceanog. Coll. 17(3):1–55.

Smith, A.C., and Ramos, F. (1980) Automated chemical analysis in fish health assessment. J. Fish Biol. 17:445–450.

Smith, H.W. (1929) The composition of the body fluids of the goosefish (*Lophius piscatoris*). J. Biol. Chem. 21:71–75.

Soivio, A., and Okari, A. (1976) Haemotological effects of stress on a teleost *Esox lucius* L. J. Fish Biol. 8:397–411.

Stanley, J.G., and Fleming, W.R. (1964) Excretion of hypertonic urine by a teleost. Science 14:63–64.

Sulya, L.L., Box, B.E., and Gunther, G. (1960) Distribution of some blood constituents in fish from the Gulf of Mexico. Am. J. Physiol. 199:1177–1180.

Thorpe, A., and Ince, B.W. (1974) The effects of pancreatic hormones, catecholamines, and glucose loading on blood metabolites in the Northern pike (*Esox lucius* L.). Gen. Comp. Endocrinol. 23:29–44.

Thorson, T. (1961) The partitioning of body water in osteichthyes: phylogenetic and ecological implications in aquatic vertebrates. Biol. Bull. 120:238–254.

Umminger, B.L. (1969) Physiological studies on super cooled killifish (*Fundulus heteroclitus*) II. Serum organic constituents and the problem of super cooling. J. Exp. Zool. 172:409–424.

Umminger, B.L. (1971) Osmoregulatory role of serum glucose in freshwater-adapted killifish (*Fundulus heteroclitus*) at temperatures near freezing. Comp. Biochem. Physiol. 38A:141–145.

Urist, M.R., and Van de Putte, K.A. (1967) Comparative biochemistry of the blood of fishes: Identification of fishes by the chemical composition of the serum. In: Sharks, Skates, and Rays (Mathewson, R.F., and Rall, D.P., eds.). Johns Hopkins University Press, Baltimore, Maryland.

Westin, D.T. (1978) Serum and blood from adult striped bass, *Morone saxitalis*. Estuaries 1(2):126–128.

Chapter 21

ENVIRONMENTAL REQUIREMENTS AND DISEASES OF TEMPERATE FRESHWATER AND ESTUARINE FISHES

JOSEPH R. TOMASSO, JR.

For many of the environmental diseases, definitive clinical diagnostic tests are not available. Diagnosticians must rely on their knowledge of animal behavior and environmental requirements to establish the cause of a dysfunction due to environmental problems. Diagnosis is further complicated when fish are removed from their original environment and transported to be diagnosed. In this chapter, the known environmental requirements and some environmental diseases of selected freshwater and estuarine temperate genera are presented.

TEMPERATURE

A fundamental characteristic of water that affects fish health is temperature. All fish have a specific temperature range within which they can live normally. When environmental temperatures fall outside of this range, performance is reduced, and in extreme cases survival is threatened. Table 21–1 lists some temperature ranges associated with some common freshwater temperate species.

The temperature requirements of fishes vary with several factors. Estuarine species, for example, may exhibit more or less tolerance of extreme temperatures depending on the concentration of dissolved solids in their environment. Tolerance to extreme temperatures is also dependent on the temperature to which the fish is acclimated. A given species may have differing temperature optima during different stages in their life. Finally, complex physiologic changes occurring during reproduction are very often dependent on absolute temperatures, changing temperatures, and interaction with other abiotic factors, such as photoperiod. Examples of each of these situations are given below.

Red drum are capable of surviving in water from less than 1 g/L salinity to >35 g/L. Their tolerance to cold temperatures varies in different salinities (Neill, 1987). Juvenile fish in 5 to 10 g/L salinity with >100 mg/L calcium can survive temperatures as low as 8 to 10°C provided they are brought to that temperature gradually. Decreasing the calcium concentration and either increasing or decreasing salinity increases the lower thermal limit they can survive.

Warm temperature tolerance is judged by determining a fish's critical thermal maximum. This is the temperature at which a fish dies when the water temperature is increased at a rate of 0.2°C/minute. Largemouth bass can tolerate higher water temperatures when they are acclimated for 28 days to higher temperatures. For example, if the northern subspecies is acclimated to 8°C, its critical thermal maximum is 29°C. If the same subspecies is acclimated to 32°C, then its critical thermal maximum is 41°C. This is also observed in the Florida subspecies, northern Florida hybrids, and the reciprocal hybrid bass (Fields et al., 1987).

Striped bass apparently have optimal temperatures that change during the growth of the animal (Coutant, 1985). Juvenile striped bass do well in a temperature range of 24 to 28°C, whereas suitable temperatures for adults are 18 to 25°C. In some environments, such as southeastern United States reservoirs, juveniles do well, but adults are stressed in late summer as water temperatures increase, and the deeper, cooler water becomes anoxic.

Red drum reproduction can be readily controlled by manipulating the environment (Roberts, 1987) and offers a good example of how temperature and photoperiod interact to stimulate reproduction. To initiate reproduction, red drum broodstock are accli-

TABLE 21–1. Water Temperature Ranges for Survival, Growth, and/or Reproduction of Selected Fishes

Species	Temperature (°C)	Comment	Reference
Largemouth bass	15–24	Spawning	Kramer and Smith (1960)
	25–30	Training to accept pelleted food	Nelson et al. (1974)
	27	Maximum growth	Coutant and DeAngelis (1983)
Smallmouth bass	23	Hatching	Simco et al. (1986)
	20–22	Fry growout	Simco et al. (1986)
	25–26	Maximum growth	Coutant and DeAngelis (1983)
Bluegill	21	Spawning begins	Simco et al. (1986)
	30	Maximum growth	Lemke (1977)
White crappie	18	Spawning begins	Simco et al. (1986)
	19	Egg incubation	Siefert (1968)
Muskellunge	10–14	Spawning	Westers (1986)
	9–13	Optimal incubation	Westers (1986)
Northern pike	5–10	Spawning	Westers (1986)
	9–13	Optimal incubation	Westers (1986)
Yellow perch	8–10	Spawning	Hokanson (1977)
	10–20	Fertilization to hatching	Hokanson (1977)
	24–28	Optimal growth	Hokanson (1977)
Walleye	20–23	Preferred	Ferguson (1958)
	6	Optimal hatching	Koenst and Smith (1976)
	9–12	Fertilization to yolk-sac absorption	Koenst and Smith (1976)
Striped bass	18–32	Larval rearing	Bonn et al. (1976)
	24	Good fingerling growth	Cox and Coutant (1981)
Three-spined stickleback	9–12	Preferred	Lachance et al. (1987)
Red drum	25	Optimum hatching (30 g/L salinity)	Neill (1987)
	22–25	Preferred (preliminary)	Neill (1987)
American eel	23–30	Optimum growth	Angel and Jones (1974)

mated to winter conditions of 17°C water and 9 hours/day of light. After this, the fish are brought to spring conditions of 28°C water and 14 hours/day of light over 40 days. Then the fish are taken to summer conditions of 30°C water and 16 hours/day of light in 30 days. An additional 30 days is used to bring the fish to fall conditions of 25°C water and 12 hours/day of light. Finally, 20 more days are needed to acclimate the fish to spawning conditions of 23°C water and 10 hours/day of light. Once spawning conditions are reached, spawning is stimulated by increasing the water temperature to 28°C and returning it to 23°C over 6 days. This type of complex manipulation of water temperature in concert with day lengths is not unusual when preparing temperate species for breeding.

When adjusting water temperatures or transferring fish from one vessel to another, be sure temperatures change slowly. It is best to gradually equilibrate the water temperature of the original vessel to the temperature of the receiving vessel when transferring fish. Optimal tempering rates vary among species, but generally a rate of change of 1°C or less per hour is not stressful.

DISSOLVED OXYGEN

Severe depletion of dissolved oxygen within a holding or culture system usually results in mortality. Even if some fish survive a transient oxygen depletion, they often die later of diseases activated by the stress of hypoxia (Wedemeyer, 1970; Tomasso et al., 1981).

Some species of temperate freshwater and es-

tuarine fishes are more resistant to low levels of oxygen than others; however, some generalizations are possible. A desirable dissolved oxygen concentration for warm-water pond fish is 5.0 mg/L or greater (Swingle, 1969; Boyd, 1979; Piper et al., 1982). Oxygen concentrations of 1.0 mg/L up to 5.0 mg/L allow fish to survive, but growth is inhibited in that range. A dissolved oxygen concentration below 1.0 mg/L is fatal if fish experience it for any length of time. Most fish production guidelines, including those for estuarine species, suggest maintaining dissolved oxygen concentrations of culture water above 5 mg/L (Bonn et al., 1976; Stickney, 1986; Chamberlain et al., 1987).

It is important to understand the nature of the system involved when measuring dissolved oxygen concentrations. For instance, in a warm-water fish culture pond, the dissolved oxygen concentrations fluctuate diurnally, with the lowest dissolved oxygen concentrations being present soon after sunrise, and the highest levels being present in late afternoon (Boyd, 1979). Thus, a pond with an acceptable dissolved oxygen concentration in the evening may have predictable levels that are stressful to fish by morning (Boyd, 1979).

Fish behavior can indicate inadequate dissolved oxygen levels. Feeding slows and may even stop when oxygen concentrations are below optima but are not life threatening. Several other situations can cause a similar change in feeding, including high concentrations of nitrogenous wastes, sudden changes in temperature, physical disturbances such as seining, or changes in pond or lake water levels. Fish affected by severe oxygen depletion usually swim to the surface and attempt to gulp water at the air/water interface. Oxygen depletion should be treated by immediately increasing dissolved oxygen concentrations through aeration. A prophylactic treatment for stress-induced infectious disease also may be appropriate depending on the situation.

Gas-Bubble Disease

Gas-bubble disease is a problem related to the supersaturation of gases in water. Supersaturation occurs when physical processes such as pressurized air injections are improperly applied, when rapid temperature increases occur, or when air bubbles are carried to great depths. Supersaturation refers to the total gas content of water, not just oxygen. A closed system receiving only pure oxygen can have a dissolved oxygen concentration more than double the normal saturation level of oxygen, and the water will still not be supersaturated (Schwedler et al., 1985). The excess oxygen displaces nitrogen and carbon dioxide in the water. This can have its own impact on fish physiology.

Gas-bubble disease in fish is characterized by gas emboli blocking capillaries and smaller blood vessels and interfering with the circulation, and resulting in emphysematous tissues. Fish suffering from gas-bubble disease are often exophthalmic. Emboli can often be seen in the small vessels of the fins, and subcutaneous bullae and hemorrhage occur around the opercula and fins. A diagnosis of gas-bubble disease can be confirmed by holding the affected fish under water and lancing one of the bullae. An escaping gas bubble is diagnostic. To treat gas-bubble disease, reduce the dissolved gas concentration below saturation.

"Winter Kill"

Another consideration when discussing oxygen levels is "winter kill" due to water icing over. This phenomenon causes oxygen depletion when the ice interferes with photosynthesis and mixing at the air/water interface. To prevent this problem, maintain fish at a low density during months when icing is expected. This decreases the oxygen demand on ice-covered water. Keep part of the pond surface ice-free by flowing fresh water into the pond at the surface or bubbling low-pressure air through a porous tube located on the bottom of the pond (Bennett, 1962). Also, remove snow cover from the ice. This allows more light penetration to fuel photosynthesis (Bennett, 1962).

SALINITY

Salinity is an important limiting factor in the distribution of many temperate fishes. Estuarine fishes are limited in their movements up rivers and sometimes toward the sea. Freshwater fishes are limited in their downstream movements by salinity gradients. The salinity concentration in brackish water lakes also affects the kinds of fishes found there.

Salinity requirements can vary for a particular fish species, depending on its stage of life. For example, the optimal salinity for striped bass eggs is near 1.7 g/L. Adults tolerate 35 g/L, which is full-strength seawater (Kerby, 1986). Salinity affects the temperature requirements of some species. Red drum have a higher cold tolerance in water of 5 to 10 g/L salinity with more than 100 mg/L calcium than in water with lower calcium concentrations and either higher or lower salinities (Neill, 1987).

The salinity requirements of some temperate fishes are listed in Table 21–2. Keep in mind, we do not have a comprehensive understanding of temperature-salinity interactions and the effects of changing the ionic ratios for many species. Salinity or ionic shock should be considered when transferring fish. Even if the initial and final salinities are within the tolerance range of a species, the transfer should be gradual, taking several hours to a day. Even species such as red drum, which can tolerate abrupt salinity changes, benefit from gradual change. Diadromous temperate fishes, such as the American eel and the striped bass, should also be tempered slowly, even though movements between full-strength seawater and fresh water are a part of their reproductive activities.

pH

Most temperate and freshwater estuarine fishes are tolerant of a relatively wide range of environmental pH. A pH range of 6.5 to 9.0 is a desirable range for growing warm-water fish (Swingle, 1969), and a range of 5.0 to 9.0 was considered "safe" by the European Inland Fisheries Advisory Commission (EIFAC, 1969). These ranges, however, may be too wide when considering interactions with other environmental variables or during certain stages of the life cycles of fish. For example, in water containing high levels of ammonia, a pH of 9.0 will cause a high percentage of the ammonia to exist in the toxic un-ionized form of ammonia (Emerson et al., 1975). This is a problem in poorly buffered pond water during the late afternoon hours when the natural pH rhythm peaks. Acidification of highly alkaline water can increase the free carbon dioxide concentration, resulting in CO_2 toxicity rather than pH imbalance (EIFAC, 1969). Acid water also tends to dissolve metals more readily. Aluminum concentrations, for example, are high in acid water (Haines, 1981). Mortality of fish in acid water can often be traced to the toxic interaction of the dissolved metals.

Elevating environmental calcium concentrations increases the tolerance of fishes to low pH (Haines, 1981). Calcium apparently reduces the ionic permeability of the gills. Different life stages of fishes have

TABLE 21–2. Salinity Tolerance Ranges of Some Freshwater and Estuarine Temperate Fishes

Species	Life Stage	Temperature (°C)	Salinity (g/L)		Reference
Largemouth Bass	Fry	18	0–1.8	51% survival*	Tebo and McCoy (1964)
		18	3.5	24% survival*	
		18	5.3–10.5	0% survival*	
	Fingerlings	22	0	92% survival†	
		22	12.5	33% survival†	
			15.1–22.8	0% survival†	
Bluegill	Fry	22	1.4–3.9	99–100% survival‡	Tebo and McCoy (1964)
		22	5.3–6.7	0–1% survival‡	
	Fingerlings	22	8.1	100% survival§	
			11.9–23.5	0–15% survival§	
Three-spined stickleback	Fry	20	0	78% survival§	Campeau et al. (1984)
		20	14	95% survival§	
		20	28	65% survival§	
	Fingerlings	20	0	68% survival§	
		20	14	90% survival§	
		20	21	60% survival§	
Inland silversides	Eggs	25	5–30	75% hatch	Middaugh et al. (1986)
	Larvae		5–30	45–65% survival‖	
Tidewater silversides	Eggs	25	5–15	75–85% hatch	Middaugh et al. (1986)
	Larvae		30	60% survival‖	
			5	30% survival‖	
Desert pupfish	Eggs	28	0.5	69% hatch	Gerking and Lee (1980)
		28	0.7–19.7	81–83% hatch	
		28	>31.0	0% hatch	
White perch		16	0–10	63–70% hatch	Morgan and Rasin (1982)
Red drum	Eggs	20	15	96% hatch	Holt et al. (1981)
		30	15	77% hatch	
		20	30	100% hatch	
		30	30	99% hatch	
	Larvae	20	15	97% survival¶	
		30	15	49% survival¶	
		20	30	99% survival¶	
		20	30	93% survival¶	
Spotted seatrout	Juveniles to adults	28	20	Minimum standard metabolism	Wohlschlag and Wakeman (1978)
Mullet	Eggs	22–26	30–40	optimal % hatch	Lee and Menu (1981)
Mullet	Juveniles	13–30	8.5	optimal survival	Fanta-Feofiloff, et al. (1986)
Striped bass	Eggs	18	5	80% hatch	Morgan et al. (1981)
			7.5	89% hatch	
			10.0	92% hatch	
	Larvae	18	5	80% survival¶	
		18		82% survival¶	
		18		84% survival¶	
Striped bass × white bass hybrids	Juvenile	23	0–35	good growth	Smith et al. (1986)
		23	35	poor survival	

*287-hour survival.
†70-hour survival.
‡216-hour survival.
§96-hour survival.
‖16-day survival.
¶24-hour survival.

different tolerances to low pH, with the reproductive phase being the most sensitive. Several studies have indicated that a pH of 6.5 or higher is needed for normal reproduction (Fromm, 1980).

The clinical diagnosis of pH stress is difficult. Histologic changes of the gills and changes in plasma ion concentrations due to low water pH (Haines, 1981) are inconsistent and vary by fish species. Currently, the diagnosis is best accomplished by determining the pH of the water.

AMMONIA AND NITRITE

Most work concerning the toxicity of ammonia and nitrite to fishes has been conducted on salmo-nids, cyprinids, and ictalurids (Russo, 1985; Meade, 1985; Lewis and Morris, 1986). However, some information is available on ammonia and nitrite toxicity to the fishes of interest in this chapter.

The values in Table 21–3 are presented as un-ionized ammonia (NH_3). Several studies (Russo, 1985) indicate un-ionized ammonia is the most toxic form of ammonia. Ionized ammonium (NH_4^+) contributes little to toxicity. The portion of total environmental ammonia that is un-ionized depends largely on the environmental pH and to a lesser extent on temperature (Emerson et al., 1975). Any meaningful comparison of environmental ammonia concentrations must consider pH and temperature. Ammonia toxicity is usually diagnosed by determining the

TABLE 21–3. Representative Toxicity Values of Un-ionized Ammonia and Nitrite to Several Species of Temperate Fishes

Species	Ammonia			Nitrite	
	Toxicity (mg/L NH_3-N)	Reference		Toxicity (mg/L NO_2-N)	Reference
European eel	1.1*	Sadler (1981/1982)		86.0†	Saroglia et al. (1981)
Green sunfish				160.4†	Tomasso (1986)
Bluegill	1.1†	Mayes et al. (1986)		79.9†	Tomasso (1986)
Smallmouth bass	0.7–1.8†,‡	Broderius et al. (1985)			
Largemouth bass	0.8§	Tomasso and Carmichael (1986)		137.8†	Tomasso (1986)
Guadalupe bass	0.6†	Tomasso and Carmichael (1986)		187.6†	Tomasso (1986)
Red drum	0.3‖	Holt and Arnold (1983)		100.0¶	Holt and Arnold (1983)
Walleye	1.1†	Mayes et al. (1986)			

*10-day median lethal concentration (estimated).
†96-hour median lethal concentration.
‡0.7 mg/L determined at pH 6.53; 1.8 mg/L determined at pH 8.71.
§72-hour median lethal concentration.
‖ Reduced survival of newly hatched larvae.
¶Growth not different from controls after 2 weeks.

concentration of ammonia in the suspected water. Gill epithelial hyperplasia may be present, but other environmental factors, such as residual chlorine, induce similar histologic changes (Mitchell and Cech, 1983).

"Safe" environmental ammonia concentrations are difficult to establish because of species differences and the complexity of evaluating low-level exposures. The growth of channel catfish is reduced by chronic exposure to 0.217 mg/L NH_3-N (Colt and Tchobanoglous, 1978). Most temperate fishes appear to require environments with un-ionized ammonia levels below 0.1 mg/L NH_3-N. The most effective treatment for ammonia toxicity is to move fish to ammonia-free water. If ammonia-free water is not available, lowering the pH to near neutral converts most un-ionized ammonia to the less toxic ionized form.

Toxicity values of nitrite for several species are also presented in Table 21–3. Nitrite toxicity is best diagnosed by detecting elevated methemoglobin levels in the blood (Russo, 1985). Baseline methemoglobin concentrations vary among species, but high levels may be indicative of nitrite toxicity.

Most freshwater fishes actively transport nitrite from the environment using the chloride uptake mechanism located on the chloride cell of the gills. In many species, toxicity can be prevented or treated by adding chloride as either calcium or sodium chloride to the water (Tomasso et al., 1979). Surprisingly, members of the family Centrarchidae apparently do not actively transport nitrite at the gills and thus are very resistant to nitrite toxicity (Tomasso, 1986).

CALCIUM

The main physiologic effect of environmental calcium is to reduce the permeability of the gills, decreasing water and electrolyte flux between the environment and plasma (Hunn, 1985). This occurs

in both freshwater fishes and marine fishes such as mullet (Pic and Maetz, 1981).

When working with small volumes of water, increasing the total hardness to 100 to 200 mg/L as calcium carbonate using calcium chloride is generally beneficial. Also, when working with estuarine species, it is important to use sea salt mixtures when making holding water solutions. The use of sodium chloride alone results in a calcium-poor solution.

STRESS DUE TO TRANSPORT

The physical disturbances associated with transporting fish from one location to another can result in mortality due to osmoregulatory dysfunctions or epizootic diseases induced by the stress (Wedemeyer, 1970; Carmichael et al., 1984). Transport stress in fish can be diagnosed clinically by a decrease in the plasma osmolality in freshwater fishes or an increase in osmolality in saltwater fishes (Carmichael et al., 1984; Robertson et al., 1988). In the absence of hematologic data, failure of live fish to orient properly in the water column during or after transport is an indication of transport-induced stress. Signs of transport stress may not appear until a few days after the transport (Tomasso et al., 1980).

Most work on transport stress has concentrated on prevention of the stress rather than treating the problem. The predominant strategy is to reduce transport stress by adding substances to the transport water to (1) reduce the osmotic gradient between plasma and environment and/or (2) induce light anesthesia.

Transportation-induced mortality in largemouth bass is reduced by fasting them for 72 hours prior to transport. Treatment with 10 mg/L copper sulfate for 1 hour/day for 10 days prior to transport, and anesthesia with 50 mg/L MS-222 prior to loading also reduces mortality (Carmichael et al., 1984). A density of 180 g fish/L in a solution of salts similar to those found in fish plasma during transport is also bene-

TABLE 21–4. Water Quality Characteristics of Transport Tank Water for Transport of Largemouth Bass

Characteristics	Value
Calcium	92 mg/L
Magnesium	40 mg/L
Potassium	179 mg/L
Bicarbonate	320 mg/L
Sulfate	114 mg/L
Chloride	3825 mg/L
Phosphate	116 mg/L
Oxytetracycline	10 mg/L
Temperature	16 or 20°C
Dissolved Oxygen	>7 mg/L

With permission from Carmichael, G.J., Tomasso, J.R., Simco, B.A., and Davis, K.B. (1984) Characterization and alleviation of stress associated with hauling largemouth bass. Trans. Am. Fish. Soc. 113:778–785.

ficial (Table 21–4). Bass transported at 16°C are less stressed than those transported in 20°C water.

Threadfin shad transport survival increases using 5 g/L sodium chloride and about 130 mg/L MS-222 (Collins and Hulsey, 1963). The reported MS-222 concentration is high when compared to other species (20 to 50 mg/L is normal for most other species). Care should be taken when using high levels of anesthetics.

Blueback herring are difficult to transport without excessive mortality (Guest and Prentice, 1982). However, transport in 12°C water containing 10 g/L marine salt, 0.05 mg/L etomidate, 0.5 mg/L Furanace, Clinoptiolite, and Corning No Foam has been successful. Transportation of herring by air has been accomplished in 12°C water containing 10 g/L marine salt, 0.5 mg/L Furanace, and either 25 mg/L MS-222 or 0.2 mg/L etomidate.

Striped bass fingerlings should be transported in water below 21°C containing 10 g/L sea salt and either 21 mg/L MS-222 or 0.25 mg/L quinaldine (Bonn et al., 1976). Acriflavin (1 mg/L) is also added routinely. Hauling densities should range from 30.4 to 60.8 g/L, with the lower density being used for smaller fish and longer transport periods.

Red drum that are feeding well and acclimated to holding tanks can be transported in various salinities at a density of 23 to 30 g/L with little or no mortality. Red drum fingerlings transported immediately after harvest from a pond are another matter. Mortality 10 days after a 5-hour transport of small (less than 0.5 g) fish ranged from 12 to 51% (Tomasso and Carmichael, 1988). Addition of MS-222 to the transport water may or may not reduce stress. Initially cortisol levels rise dramatically, but serum levels are decreased at the end of the transport (Robertson et al., 1988).

Readers seeking more information on hauling techniques used by North American fish hatcheries are referred to Carmichael and Tomasso (1988), which offers insight into how fish are actually transported by hatchery workers.

LITERATURE CITED

Angel, N.B., and Jones, W.R. (1974) Aquaculture of the American eel (*Anguilla rostrata*). Industrial Extension Service, Raleigh, North Carolina.

Bennett, G.W. (1962) Management of Artificial Lakes and Ponds. Reinhold, New York.

Bonn, E.W., Bailey, W.M., Bayless, J.D., Erickson, K.E., and Stevens, R.E. (eds.) (1976) Guidelines for Striped Bass Culture. American Fisheries Society, Bethesda, Maryland.

Boyd, C.E. (1979) Water Quality in Warmwater Fish Ponds. Auburn University, Auburn, Alabama.

Broderius, S., Drummond, R., Fiandt, J., and Russom, C. (1985) Toxicity of ammonia to early life stages of the smallmouth bass at four pH values. Environ. Toxicol. Chem. 4:87–96.

Campeau, S., Guderley, H., and Fitzgerald, G. (1984) Salinity tolerances and preferences of fry of two species of sympatric sticklebacks: Possible mechanisms of habitat segregation. Can. J. Zool. 62:1048–1051.

Carmichael, G.J., and Tomasso, J.R. (1988) A survey of fish transportation and techniques. Progressive Fish Culturist 50:155–159.

Carmichael, G.J., Tomasso, J.R., Simco, B.A., and Davis, K.B. (1984) Characterization and alleviation of stress associated with hauling largemouth bass. Trans. Am. Fish. Soc. 113:778–785.

Chamberlain, G.W., Miget, R.J., and Haby, M.G. (1987) Manual on Red Drum Aquaculture (Conference draft). Texas Agricultural Extension Service, College Station.

Collins, J.L., and Hulsey, A.H. (1963) Hauling mortality of threadfin shad reduced with MS-222 and salt. Progressive Fish Culturist 25:105–106.

Colt, J., and Tchobanoglous, G. (1978) Chronic exposure of channel catfish, *Ictalurus punctatus*, to ammonia: Effects on growth and survival. Aquaculture 15:353–372.

Coutant, C.C. (1985) Striped bass, temperature, and dissolved oxygen: A speculative hypothesis for environmental risk. Trans. Am. Fish. Soc. 114:31–61.

Coutant, C.C., and DeAngelis, D.L. (1983) Comparative temperature-dependent growth rates of largemouth and smallmouth bass fry. Trans. Am. Fish. Soc. 112:416–423.

Cox, D.K., and Coutant, C.C. (1981) Growth dynamics of juvenile striped bass as functions of temperature and ration. Trans. Am. Fish. Soc. 110:226–238.

Emerson, K., Russo, R.C., Lund, R.E., and Thurston, R.V. (1975) Aqueous ammonia equilibrium calculations: Effect of pH and temperature. J. Fish. Res. Bd. Can. 32:2379–2383.

European Inland Fisheries Advisory Commission. (1969) Water quality criteria for European freshwater fish—Extreme pH values and inland fisheries. Water Res. 3:593–611.

Fanta-Feofiloff, E., De Brito Eiras, D.R., Boscardium, A.T., and Lacerda-Krambeck, M. (1986) Effect of salinity on the behavior and oxygen consumption of *Mugil curema* (Pisces, Mugilidae). Physiol. Behav. 36:1029–1034.

Ferguson, R.G. (1958) The preferred temperature of fish and their midsummer distribution in temperate lakes and streams. J. Fish. Res. Bd. Can. 15:607.

Fields, R., Lowe, S.S., Kaminski, C., Whitt, G.S., and Phillip, D.P. (1987) Critical and chronic thermal maxima of northern and Florida largemouth bass and their reciprocal F_1 and F_2 hybrids. Trans. Am. Fish. Soc. 116:856–863.

Fromm, P.O. (1980) A review of some physiological and toxicological responses of freshwater fish to acid stress. Environ. Biol. Fish. 5:79–93.

Gerking, S.D., and Lee, R.M. (1980) Reproductive performance of the desert pupfish (*Cyprinodon n. nevadensis*) in relation to salinity. Environ. Biol. Fish. 5:375–378.

Grizzle, J.M., Mauldin, A.C., Young, D., and Henderson, E. (1985) Survival of juvenile striped bass (*Morone saxatilis*) and morone hybrid bass (*Morone chrysops* × *Morone saxatilis*) increased by addition of calcium to soft water. Aquaculture 46:167–171.

Guest, W.C., and Prentice, J.A. (1982) Transportation techniques for blueback herring. Progressive Fish Culturist 44:183–185.

Haines, T.A. (1981) Acid precipitation and its consequences for aquatic ecosystems: A review. Trans. Am. Fish. Soc. 110:669–707.

Hokanson, K.E.F. (1977) Temperature requirements of some percids and adaptations to the seasonal temperature cycle. J. Fish. Res. Bd. Can. 34:1524–1550.

Holt, G.J., and Arnold, C.R. (1983) Effects of ammonia and nitrite on growth and survival of red drum eggs and larvae. Trans. Am. Fish. Soc. 112:314–318.

Holt, J., Godbout, R., and Arnold, C.R. (1981) Effects of temperature and salinity on egg hatching and larval survival of red drum, *Sciaenops ocellata*. NOAA Fish. Bull. 79:569–573.

Hunn, J., Godbout, R., and Arnold, C.R. (1981) Effects of temperature and salinity on egg hatching and larval survival of red drum, *Sciaenops ocellata*. NOAA Fish. Bull. 79:569–573.

Kerby, J.H. (1986) Striped bass and striped bass hybrids. In Culture of

Nonsalmonid Freshwater Fishes (Stickney, R.R., ed.). CRC Press, Boca Raton, Florida, pp. 127–147.

Koenst, W.M., and Smith, L.L. (1976) Thermal requirements of the early life history stages of walleye and sauger. J. Fish. Res. Bd. Can. 33:1130.

Kramer, W.M., and Smith, L.L. (1960) First year growth of largemouth bass, *Micropterus salmoides*, and some related ecological factors. Trans. Am. Fish. Soc. 89:222.

Lachance, S., Magnan, P., and Fitzgerald, G.J. (1987) Temperature preferences of three sympatric stickle backs (Basterosteidae). Can. J. Zool. 65:1573–1576.

Lee, C.S., and Menu, B. (1981) Effects of salinity on egg development and hatching in grey mullet *Mugil caphalus*. J. Fish Biol. 19:179–188.

Lemke, A. (1977) Optimum temperature for growth of juvenile bluegills. Progressive Fish Culturist 39:55–57.

Lewis, W.M., and Morris, D.P. (1986) Toxicity of nitrite to fish: A review. Trans. Am. Fish. Soc. 115:183–195.

Mayes, M.A., Alexander, H.C., Hopkins, D.L., and Latvaitis, P.B. (1986) Acute and chronic toxicity of ammonia to freshwater fish: A site specific study. Environ. Toxicol. Chem. 5:437–442.

Meade, J.W. (1985) Allowable ammonia for fish culture. Progressive Fish Culturist 47:135–145.

Middaugh, D.P., Hemmer, M.J., and Lamadrid-Rose, Y. (1986) Laboratory spawning cues in *Menidid beryllina* and *M. penisulae* with notes on survival and growth of larvae at different salinities. Environ. Biol. Fish 15:107–117.

Mitchell, S.J., and Cech, J.J. (1983) Ammonia-caused damage in channel catfish *(Ictalurus punctatus)*: Confounding effects of residual chlorine. Can. J. Fish Aquatic Sci. 40:242–247.

Morgan, R.P., and Rasin, V.J. (1982) Influence of temperature and salinity on development of white perch eggs. Trans. Am. Fish. Soc. 111:396–398.

Morgan, R.P., Rasin, V.J., and Copp, R.L. (1981) Temperature and salinity effects on development of striped bass eggs and larvae. Trans. Am. Fish. Soc. 110:95–99.

Neill, W.H. (1987) Environmental requirements of red drum. In Manual on Red Drum Culture (Conference draft) (Chamberlain, G.W., Midget, R.J., and Haby, M.G., eds.). Texas Agricultural Extension Service, College Station, pp. IV1–IV8.

Nelson, J.T., Bowken, R.G., and Robinson, J.D. (1974) Rearing pellet-fed largemouth bass in a raceway. Progressive Fish Culturist 36:108–110.

Pic, P., and Maetz, J. (1981) Role of external calcium in sodium and chloride transport in the gills of seawater adapted *Mugil capito*. J. Comp. Physiol. 141:511–521.

Piper, R.G., McElwain, I.B., Orme, L.E., McCraren, J.P., Fowler, L.G., and Leonard, J.R. (1982) Fish Hatchery Management. U.S. Fish and Wildlife Service, Washington, D.C.

Roberts, D.E. (1987) Photoperiod/temperature control in commercial production of red drum *(Sciaenops ocellatus)* eggs. In Manual on Red Drum Aquaculture (Conference draft) (Chamberlain, G.W., Miget, R.J., and Haby, M.G., eds.). Texas Agricultural Extension Service, College Station, pp. II10–II26.

Robertson, L., Thomas, P., and Arnold, C.R. (1988) Plasma cortisol and secondary stress responses of cultured red drum *(Sciaenops ocellatus)* to several transportation procedures. Aquaculture 68:115–130.

Russo, R.C. (1985) Ammonia, nitrite and nitrate. In Fundamentals of Aquatic Toxicology (Rand, G.M., and Pertocelli, S.R., eds.). Hemisphere, New York, pp. 455–471.

Sadler, K. (1981/1982) The toxicity of ammonia to the European eel (*Anguilla anguilla* L.). Aquaculture 26:173–181.

Saroglia, M.G., Scarano, G., and Tibaldi, E. (1981) Acute toxicity of nitrite to sea bass (*Dicentrarchus labrax*) and European eel (*Anguilla anguilla*). J. World Mariculture Soc. 12:121–126.

Schwedler, T.E., Tucker, C.S., and Beleau, M.H. (1985) Noninfectious diseases. In Channel Catfish Culture (Tucker, C.S., ed.). Elsevier, New York, pp. 497–541.

Siefert, R.E. (1968) Reproductive behavior, incubation and mortality of eggs and postlarval food selection in the white crappie. Trans. Am. Fish. Soc. 97:252–259.

Simco, B.A., Williamson, J.H., Carmichael, G.J., and Tomasso, J.R. (1986) Centrarchids. In Culture of Freshwater Fishes (Stickney, R.R., ed.). CRC Press, Boca Raton, Florida, pp. 73–89.

Smith, T.I.J., Jenkins, W.E., and Haggerty, R.W. (1986) Growth and survival of juvenile striped bass (*Morone saxatilis*) × white bass (*M. chrysops*) hybrids reared at different salinities. Proc. Annu. Conf. Southeast Assoc. Fish Wildlife Agens. 40:143–151.

Spotte, S. (1979) Fish and Invertebrate Culture. 2nd ed. Wiley-Interscience, New York.

Stickney, R.R. (1986) Culture of Nonsalmonid Freshwater Fishes. CRC Press, Boca Raton, Florida.

Swingle, H.S. (1969) Methods of Analysis for Waters, Organic Matter and Pond Bottom Soils Used in Fisheries Research. Auburn University, Auburn, Alabama.

Tebo, L.B., and McCoy, E.G. (1964) Effect of sea-water concentration on the reproduction and survival of largemouth bass and bluegills. Progressive Fish Culturist 26:99–106.

Tomasso, J.R. (1986) Comparative toxicity of nitrite to freshwater fishes. Aquat. Toxicol. 8(2):129–137.

Tomasso, J.R., and Carmichael, G.J. (1986) Acute toxicity of ammonia, nitrite and nitrate to the Guadelupe bass, *Micropterus treculi*. Bull. Environ. Contam. Toxicol. 36:866–870.

Tomasso, J.R., and Carmichael, G.J. (1988) Handling and transport-induced stress in red drum fingerlings *(Sciaenops ocellatus)*. Contrib. Marine Sci. 30(Suppl.):133–137.

Tomasso, J.R., Simco, B.A., and Davis, K.B. (1979) Chloride inhibition of nitrite-induced methemoglobinemia in channel catfish *(Ictalurus punctatus)*. J. Fish. Res. Bd. Can. 36:1141–1144.

Tomasso, J.R., Davis, K.B., and Parker, N.C. (1980) Plasma corticosteroid and electrolyte dynamics of hybrid striped bass (white bass × striped bass) during netting and hauling stress. Proc. World Mariculture Soc. 11:303–310.

Tomasso, J.R., Davis, K.B., and Parker, N.C. (1981) Plasma corticosteroid dynamics in channel catfish, *Ictalurus punctatus* (Rafinesque), during and after oxygen depletion. J. Fish Biol. 18:519–526.

United States Fish and Wildlife Service (1978) Manual of Fish Culture. U.S. Printing Office, Washington, D.C.

Wedemeyer, G. (1970) The role of stress in disease resistance of fishes. In A Symposium on Diseases of Fishes and Shellfishes (Snieszko, S.F., ed.). American Fisheries Society, Bethesda, Maryland, pp. 30–35.

Westers, H. (1986) Northern pike and muskellunge. In Culture of Nonsalmonid Freshwater Fishes (Stickney, R.R., ed.). CRC Press, Boca Raton, Florida, pp. 91–101.

Wohlschlag, E.E., and Wakeman, J.M. (1978) Salinity stresses, metabolic responses and distribution of the coastal spotted seatrout, *Cynoscion nebulosus*. Contrib. Marine Sci. 21:171–185.

Chapter 22

NUTRITION AND NUTRITIONAL DISEASES OF TEMPERATE FRESHWATER FISHES

MARGIE LEE GALLAGHER

Good nutrition is vital to fish health. Underfed or nutrient-deficient fish exhibit nutritional diseases and are also more likely to contract diseases caused by other agents, such as bacteria or protozoa. Nutritional strategies for the support of healthy fish are simple: (1) supply all nutrients, (2) make sure each nutrient is available, and (3) feed at optimum rate and amount (Cho, 1983). There is a lack of information on the requirements of many temperate-water fishes such as the *Micropterus* basses perch, pike, muskellunge, and walleye (Milliken, 1982a). However, some temperate-water species have received considerable attention, specifically the eels and, to a lesser degree, the *Morone* basses, their hybrids, and the sturgeons.

MACRONUTRIENT REQUIREMENTS

Protein requirements for fish are a function of the quantitative requirements for each of the essential amino acids and the protein-to-energy ratio of the diet. Diets that are too high in energy will cause fish to stop feeding before enough protein is consumed to meet the needs of the animal unless the diet is excessively high in protein. Diets that are too low in energy will cause dietary protein to be used to meet energy needs. In both cases, poor growth and excessive feed cost are likely to occur.

The same 10 amino acids, arginine, histidine, isoleucine, lysine, leucine, methionine, phenylalanine, threonine, tryptophan, and valine, are required for temperate-water eels, red sea bream, and sea bass (Wilson, 1985). In addition, specific quantitative requirements of some of the essential amino acids have been determined for gilthead bream and sea bass. Japanese and European eels in temperate water have significantly increased requirements for leucine, methionine, threonine, tryptophan, and valine compared to either cold-water salmon or warm-water carp (Arai et al., 1972).

The symptoms of deficiencies vary from species to species. For example, although methionine deficiencies have been reported to cause bilateral cataracts in rainbow trout, this symptom has not been reported for temperate-water species studied. Likewise, although tryptophan deficiency causes scoliosis and lordosis in sockeye salmon and scoliosis, caudal fin erosion, cataracts, and short gill opercula in rainbow trout, none of these symptoms have been reported in temperate-water fish (Wilson, 1985).

Total protein requirements have been determined for only a few temperate-water species and appear to range from 35 to 45% of the total diet. The dietary protein level required for largemouth bass is near 40% (Anderson et al., 1981). The best growth is obtained in striped bass on a diet containing 55% protein (Milliken, 1982b, 1983). However, the energy levels in the particular diet used in those studies may have been too high (4.0 kcal/g). Other results for striped bass and their hybrids indicate that they require no more than 35% dietary protein when the diet contains 3.5 kcal/g (Gallagher, 1991). The optimum protein requirement of juvenile white sturgeon using four separate statistical manipulations of percentage body weight increase is 40% (Moore et al., 1988).

Because of the high cost of fishmeal there is a continued interest in the use of alternative protein sources for diets of fish. In some cases, poultry-meat meal has been used successfully in diets that retained sufficient amounts of fishmeal or fish oil to provide essential fatty acids (Tiews et al., 1976; Degani, 1986; Gallagher and Degani, 1988). Lupin seed meal has been used in diets for rainbow trout (De la Higuera et al., 1988). However, reviews of conventional and unconventional protein sources for fish diets point out the negative effects of such factors as antivitamins, enzyme inhibitors, and toxic substances found in cereals, legumes, oilseeds, and root tubers (Tacon and Jackson, 1985). Even with extensive autoclaving, legumes often retain nonthermolabile toxins that cause severe growth reduction and mortality (Olvera et al., 1988).

Other factors may also influence the protein requirements in fish. Generally, protein requirements decrease with age, and at least in some species, increasing temperature may increase the protein requirement (Milliken, 1982a). Meal size apparently has an effect on the heat increment in walleye (Beamish and MacMahon, 1988). As meal size increases so does the heat increment. In addition, carbohydrate contributes to the heat increment as well as the deamination of proteins. Inattention to these factors can lead to decreased growth and decreased feed efficiency.

Lipids and carbohydrates are sources of energy in the diet and must be balanced with protein to provide the optimum protein-to-energy ratio. Optimum ratios for species studied range from 73 mg protein/kcal of diet for channel catfish fingerlings to 100 mg protein/kcal of diet for striped bass. Whether or not lipid or carbohydrates are used in the diet depends upon the ability of the particular fish species to utilize the source. Generally, increasing carbohydrates in the diets of carnivorous species decreases the digestibility of all dietary ingredients, resulting in decreased growth (Shimeno et al., 1979). These differences may be due to changes in enzymes that digest carbohydrate. For example, amylase levels are lower in eels than in carp (Fischer, 1979). Increased dietary lipid increases the digestibility of feed in rainbow trout. Red drum fed diets with lipid levels ranging from 1.7 to 18.8% obtain best growth and feed conversions on diets with 7.4 and 11.2% lipid (Williams and Robinson, 1988). However, weight gains and feed conversion decrease when lipid levels reach 18.8% of the diet.

The source of lipid is also important. It must provide essential fatty acids. Evidence is mounting to support the essential nature of omega$_3$ (ω_3) fatty acids in diets for fish. Although the Japanese eel can use both 18:3ω_3 and 18:3ω_6 in its diet (Takeuchi et al., 1980), bioconversion of 18:3ω_3 to 20:5ω_3 or 22:6ω_3 is low (Kanazawa et al., 1979). A lack of essential ω_3 fatty acids in first-year sea bass (Mosconi-Bac, 1987) and European eels (Affandi and Biagianti, 1987) causes cellular abnormalities and accumulation of fat in liver cells. These abnormalities are apparently due to the presence of ω_9 fatty acids of terrestrial animal origin and the lack of ω_3 fatty acids from marine sources.

VITAMINS

The vitamin requirements of eels have received more attention than other temperate-water fishes. Thiamine, riboflavin, pyridoxine, pantothenic acids, folacin, and biotin all are required by the eel (Hashimoto, 1975) (Fig. 22–1). The symptoms of thiamine

deficiencies in eels include poor appetite, growth retardation, fin hemorrhage, ataxia, and flexion of the trunk (Hashimoto et al., 1970). Little is known of vitamin requirements in other temperate-water species (Halver, 1979, 1985).

MINERAL REQUIREMENTS

The mineral requirements for finfishes are complicated by the fact that some species of fish absorb minerals from the water as well as the diet (Koening, 1985; Milliken, 1982a; Lall, 1979; Halver, 1972). Therefore, in some fishes, water uptake may be sufficient, but in other fishes, dietary supplementation is necessary. In addition, studies of mineral requirements need to be conducted over long periods of time, since the overt effects of mineral deficiencies, especially trace mineral deficiencies, may take several months to develop.

CALCIUM AND PHOSPHORUS

The ratio of calcium to phosphorus is important whether minerals are obtained from the water or the diet. The optimum calcium-to-phosphorus ratio in many fish has been shown to be 1:2 (Lall, 1979). In eels, the optimum ratio also appears to be around 1:1 (Lall, 1979). Eels require higher total amounts of calcium than some other fishes. Symptoms of calcium or phosphorus deficiency include poor appetite with accompanying growth depression. In some species, decreased bone calcification and cranial and skeletal deformities have been noted (Lall, 1979).

The source of dietary calcium and phosphorus can be important. Phosphorus from plant sources may not be as available to fish as phosphorus from animal sources (Ketola, 1975a,b; Viola et al., 1986). However, these results may be due to a more favorable calcium-to-phosphorus ratio. In addition, phosphorus requirements are higher in faster-growing fish (Viola et al., 1986).

In some species, dietary sources of phosphorus may be more important than calcium. Chum salmon held in fresh water require 0.5 to 0.6% phosphorus supplements in the diet (Wantanabe et al., 1980). No calcium is required if the calcium in the water supply is sufficient. Fish fed diets without supplemental phosphorus have decreased bone development and decreased food conversions.

OTHER TRACE MINERALS

At least 11 other minerals have been shown to have demonstrable biological functions in fish (Lall, 1979). However, specific requirement studies are rare. Deficiencies of iron, copper, or cobalt can produce anemia in fish (Halver, 1972). Decreased growth, feed efficiency, hemoglobin, hematocrit, plasma iron, transferrin, and erythrocyte count occur in fish fed iron-poor diets (Gatlin and Wilson, 1986a).

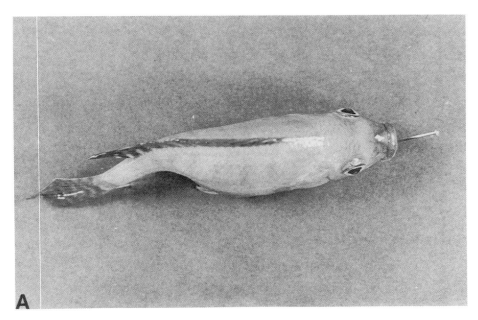

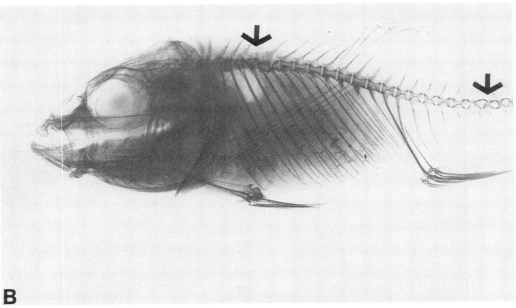

FIGURE 22–1. *A, B.* Nile tilapia fed a vitamin C–deficient diet lose color and develop cataracts and spinal deformities such as those evident in the thoracic and coccygeal vertebrae shown in the radiograph. (From Roberts, R. J. [1989] Fish Pathology. 2nd ed. Bailliere Tindall, London.)

Selenium deficiency in Atlantic salmon causes muscular dystrophy and exudative diathesis, and may be a factor in Hitra disease in salmonids (Ringdal and Julshamn, 1985). Decreases in superoxide dismutase and cytochrome oxidase are seen in channel catfish fed copper-deficient diets (Gatlin and Wilson, 1986b), but overt deficiency symptoms are not seen (Murai et al., 1981). Toxic effects are seen in catfish fed 16 and 32 mg copper/kg diet. Signs include decreased growth and decreased food conversion with an accompanying anemia.

Zinc is required in fish (Ogino and Yong, 1979; Koening, 1985). Deficiency symptoms include low growth rate, cataracts, and skin and fin erosions.

Eels fed purified diets require mineral mix supplementation at 2% of the diet (Arai et al., 1974). However, mineral mixes or bone meal should not be added indiscriminately to diet formulas. Higher levels of supplementation suppress growth. Excess calcium can decrease absorption of other minerals, such as zinc (Koening, 1985). Nephrocalcinosis has also been associated with increased mineral content in feed.

Many minerals may be toxic in fish. For example, structural changes occur in striped bass larvae exposed to aluminum (608 µg/L) for 20 hours (Rulifson et al., 1986). Although no clear morphologic changes are apparent using light microscopy, scanning electron micrographs clearly show reduction of epidermal microridges on the head and caudal fin.

Before temperate-water fishes can be cultured successfully, a much clearer knowledge of nutritional requirements must be available. Without such knowledge, nutritional deficiencies and the accompanying diseases and losses are inevitable.

LITERATURE CITED

Affandi, R., and Biagianti, S. (1987) A study of the liver of eels kept in captivity: Disturbances induced in hepatocytes by artificial diets. Aquaculture 67:226–228.

Anderson, R.J., Kienbrolz, E.W., and Flickinger, S.A. (1981) Protein requirements of smallmouth and largemouth bass. J. Nutr. 111:1085–1097.

Arai, S., Nose, T., and Hashimoto, Y. (1972) Amino acids essential for the growth of eels, *Anguilla anguilla* and *A. japonica*. Bull. Jpn. Soc. Sci. Fish. 38(7):753–759.

Arai, S., Nose, T., and Kawatsu, H. (1974) Effect of minerals supplemented to the fishmeal diet on growth of eel, *Anguilla japonica*. Bull. Freshwater Fish. Res. Lab. 24(2):95–100.

Beamish, F.W.H., and MacMahon, P.D. (1988) Apparent heat increment and feeding strategy in walleye, *Stizostedion viteum viteum*. Aquaculture 68:73–82.

Cho, C.Y. (1983) Nutrition and fish health. In: A Guide to Integrated Fish Health Management in the Great Lakes Basin (Meyer, F.P., Warren, J.W., and Carey, T.G., eds.). Great Lakes Fishery Comm., Ann Arbor, Michigan. Published by GLFC, Ann Arbor, Michigan, April 1983, pp. 63–73. Special PHBL GLEC No. 83–2.

Cowey, C.B., and Sargent, J.R. (1979) Nutrition. In: Fish Physiology. Vol. VIII, Bioenergetics and Growth (Hoar, W.S., Randall, D.J., and Brett, J.R., eds.). Academic Press, New York, pp. 1–69.

Degani, G. (1986) Dietary effect of lipid source, lipid level and temperature on growth of glass eels (*Anguilla anguilla* L.). Aquaculture 56:207–214.

De la Higuera, M., Garcia-Gallego, M., Sanz, A., Cardenete, G., Suarez, M.D., and Moyano, F.J. (1988) Evaluation of lupin seed meal as an alternative protein source in feeding of rainbow trout (*Salmo gairdneri*). Aquaculture 71:37–50.

Fisher, A. (1979) Selected problems of fish bioenergetics. In: Finfish Nutrition and Feed Technology. Vol. 1 (Halver, J.E., and Tiews, K., eds.). Heenemann Gmbh, Berlin, pp. 17–44.

Gallagher, M.L. (1991) Dietary formulations for striped bass and its hybrids: Interactions of dietary energy and protein. UNC Sea Grant Technical Report.

Gallagher, M.L., and Degani, G. (1988) Poultry meal and poultry oil as sources of protein and lipid in the diet of European eels (*Anguilla anguilla*). Aquaculture 73:177–187.

Gatlin, D.M., and Wilson, R.P. (1986a) Characterization of iron deficiency and the dietary iron requirement of fingerling channel catfish. Aquaculture 52(3):191–198.

Gatlin, D.M., and Wilson, R.P. (1986b) Dietary copper requirement of fingerling channel catfish. Aquaculture 54(4):277–285.

Halver, J.E. (1972) Fish nutrition. Academic Press, New York, p. 713.

Halver, J.E. (1979) Vitamin requirements of finfish. In: Finfish Nutrition and Fishfeed Technology. Vol. 1 (Halver, J.E., and Tiews, K., eds.). Heenemann Gmbh, Berlin, pp. 45–58.

Halver, J.E. (1985) Recent advances in vitamin nutrition and metabolism in fish. In: Nutrition and Feeding in Fish (Cowey, C.B., Mackie, A.M., and Bell, J.G., eds.). Academic Press, Orlando, Florida, pp. 415–429.

Hashimoto, Y., Arai, S., and Nose, T. (1970) Thiamine deficiency symptoms experimentally induced in the eel. Bull. Jpn. Soc. Sci. Fish. 36(8):791–797.

Hashimoto, Y. (1975) Nutritional requirements of warm water fish. Proc. 9th Int. Cong. Nutr. 3:158–175.

Kanazawa, A., Teshima, S.I., and Ono, K. (1979) Relationship between essential fatty acid requirement of aquatic animals and capacity for bioconversion of linolenic acid to highly unsaturated fatty acids. Comp. Biochem. Physiol. 63B:295–298.

Ketola, H.G. (1975a) Mineral supplementation of diets containing soybean meal as a source of protein for rainbow trout. Progressive Fish Culturist 37:73–75.

Ketola, H.G. (1975b) Requirements of Atlantic salmon for dietary phosphorus. Trans. Am. Fish. Soc. 104:548–551.

Koening, J. (1985) Besoins mineraux chez les poissons. Ichthyophysiol. Acta 9:93–104 (in French).

Lall, S.P. (1979) Minerals in finfish nutrition. In Finfish Nutrition and Fishfeed Technology. Vol. 1 (Halver, J.E., and Tiews, K., eds.). Heenemann Gmbh, Berlin, pp. 85–97.

Milliken, M.R. (1982a) Qualitative and quantitative nutrient requirements of fishes: A review. Fish. Bull. 80(4):655–686.

Milliken, M.R. (1982b) Effects of dietary protein concentration on growth, feed efficiency, and body composition of age-0 striped bass. Trans. Am. Fish. Soc. 111:373–378.

Milliken, M.R. (1983) Interactive effects of dietary protein and lipids on growth and protein utilization of age-0 striped bass. Trans. Am. Fish. Soc. 112:185–193.

Moore, B.J., Hung, S.S.O., and Medraus, J.F. (1988) Protein requirement of hatchery-produced juvenile white sturgeon (*Acipenser transmontanus*). Aquaculture 71:235–245.

Mosconi-Bac, N. (1987) Hepatic disturbances induced by an artificial feed in the sea bass (*Dicentrarchus labrox*) during the first year of life. Aquaculture 67:93–99.

Murai, T., Andrews, J.W., and Smith, R.G. (1981) Effects of dietary copper on channel catfish. Aquaculture 22(4):353–357.

Ogino, C., and Yong, G.Y. (1979) Requirement of rainbow trout for dietary zinc. In: Finfish Nutrition and Fishfeed Technology. Vol. 1 (Halver, J.E., and Tiews, K., eds.). Heenemann Gmbh, Berlin, pp. 105–111.

Olvera, N., Martinez, P., Galvan, C., and Chavez, S. (1988) The use of seed of the leguminous plant *Sesbania grandiflora* as a partial replacement for fish meal in diets for tilapia (*Oreochromis mossambicus*). Aquaculture 71:51–60.

Ringdal, O., and Julshamn, K. (1985) Selenium an important nutrient for salmonids. Canadian Translations in Fisheries and Aquaculture Sciences, No. 5195. Translated from Fisk. Gang. 9(8):317–318.

Rulifson, R.A., Cooper, J.E., and Colombo, G. (1986) Development of fed and starved striped bass (*Morone saxatilis*) larvae from the Roanoke River, North Carolina. North Carolina Department of Natural Resources and Community Development, Division of Marine Fisheries, Completion Report for East Carolina contract No. 5-21431, pp. 1–41.

Shimeno, S., Hosokawa, H., and Takeda, M. (1979) The importance of carbohydrate in the diet of carnivorous fish. In: Finfish Nutrition and Feed Technology. Vol. 1 (Halver, J.E., and Tiews, K., eds.). Heenemann Gmbh, Berlin, pp. 127–143.

Tacon, A.G.J., and Jackson, A.J. (1985) Utilization of conventional and unconventional protein sources in practical fish feeds. In: Nutrition and Feeding in Fish (Cowey, C.B., Mackie, A.M., and Bell, J.G., eds.). Academic Press, Orlando, Florida, pp. 119–145.

Takeuchi, T., Arai, S., Watanabe, T., and Shimma, Y. (1980) Requirements of eel *Anguilla japonica* for essential fatty acids. Bull. Jpn. Soc. Sci. Fish. 46:345–353.

Tiews, K., Gropp, J., and Koops, H. (1976) On the development of optimal rainbow trout pellet feeds. Arch. Fisch. Wiss. 27(1):1–29.

Viola, S., Zohar, G., and Arieli, Y. (1986) Phosphorus requirements and its availability from different sources for intensive pond culture species in Israel. Part 1, Tilapia, Bamidgeh 38(1):3–12.

Watanabe, T., Murakami, A., Taheuchi, L., Nose, T., and Ogino, C. (1980) Requirements of chum salmon held in freshwater for dietary phosphorus. Bull. Jpn. Soc. Sci. Fish. 46(3):361–367.

Williams, C.D., and Robinson, E.H. (1988) Response of red drum to various dietary levels of menhaden oil. Aquaculture 70:107–120.

Wilson, R.P. (1985) Amino acid and protein requirements of fish. In: Nutrition and Feeding in Fish (Cowey, C.B., Mackie, A.M., and Bell, J.G., eds.). Academic Press, Orlando, Florida, pp. 1–16.

Chapter 23

REPRODUCTION IN TEMPERATE FRESHWATER AND ESTUARINE FISHES

J. HOWARD KERBY

This chapter concentrates on a few species endemic to the United States that are representative of families frequently cultured for research, fisheries management, or aquaculture. In addition, this chapter covers species that must be artificially induced to ovulate and reproduce rather than fish with reproductive strategies that require little human assistance.

REPRODUCTION OF TEMPERATE BASSES

The genus *Morone* contains four species in the United States and is the principal genus in the family. The striped bass is an anadromous species that customarily migrates from estuarine areas up freshwater streams to spawn. Spawning typically occurs when temperatures are in the range of 15.6 to 21°C. The eggs are semibouyant and require sufficient flow and distance to keep them in suspension until the larvae hatch (Talbot, 1966). The white perch is also estuarine but does not normally inhabit higher salinities. The eggs are smaller than those of the striped bass and are demersal and adhesive. The white bass and the yellow bass are freshwater species that also lay demersal, adhesive eggs. The white perch and white and yellow basses all move upstream to spawn over a substrate in flowing streams or rivers.

Hybrids of female striped bass and male white bass were first produced in 1965 (Bishop, 1968). Several other crosses, such as the reciprocal of the above cross (female white bass X male striped bass), striped bass X white perch, striped bass X yellow bass, and various back crosses have also been made (Smith et al., 1967; Bayless, 1968, 1972; Bishop, 1968; Kerby, 1972, 1986; Ware, 1975; Harrell and Dean, 1987; Kerby and Harrell, 1990). Some of these hybrids have become important for stocking inland reservoirs for recreational and management purposes and are on the verge of becoming important aquaculture "fish." Comprehensive guidelines for spawning and culturing these fish are available (Bayless, 1972; Bonn et al., 1976; Harrell et al., 1990).

All material in this chapter is in the public domain, with the exception of any borrowed figures.

Production of Larvae

Currently, there are two principal methods for producing striped bass larvae for culture. In both, wild broodfish are collected, usually with electrofishing gear to minimize stress, and transported to the hatchery (Fig. 23–1). In the first method, the females are injected intramuscularly with 275 to 300 IU of human chorionic gonadotropin hormone (HCG) per kilogram of body weight. Injection of males with 110 to 165 IU/kg will increase semen volume by hydrating the testes, but may not actually increase spermatozoa production (Kerby, 1986). From 20 to 28 hours following injection, a small egg sample is taken with a 1.5-mm (outside diameter) plastic catheter (Smith and Jenkins, 1988) or a 3-mm (outside diameter) glass tube (Fig. 23–2) (Bayless, 1972). Approximate time to ovulation is determined by microscopic examination of the eggs (Fig. 23–3). Actual time of ovulation is verified by exerting manual pressure on the abdomen. Freely flowing eggs indicate that ovulation has occurred. Sometimes it is difficult to know if the female is fully ovulated. For fish over 12 kg, insert the little finger into the genital pore and feel whether all eggs have been released from the ovarian wall (J. E. Van Tassel, personal communication). It is

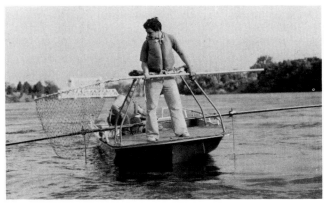

FIGURE 23–1. Electrofishing for striped bass broodstock.

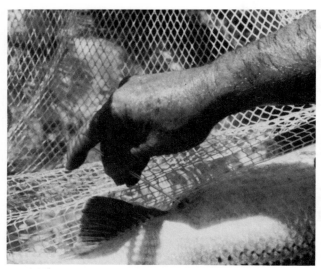

FIGURE 23–2. A 3-mm glass catheter is inserted into the ovary of a female striped bass to obtain an egg sample for use in predicting ovulation. (Courtesy of J.D. Bayless, South Carolina Wildlife and Marine Resources Department.)

extremely important to predict the time of ovulation accurately because, as ovulation occurs, the eggs separate from the ovarian tissue and from the parental oxygen supply. Anoxia results within about an hour and the eggs become overripe and cannot be fertilized (Stevens, 1966, 1967; Bayless, 1972).

Artificial Spawning

In a method sometimes called the jar method, the female fish is either sacrificed or anesthetized. The eggs are manually stripped into a spawning pan (Fig. 23–4). Semen from a male is then stripped into the pan, water is added, and the eggs, water, and semen are mixed. This is the dry method of fertilization. An alternate method adds the water and semen together. Some culturists prefer to strip the semen into water containing a low concentration of salt (3 to 5 ppt) before mixing it with the eggs.

After fertilization, the eggs are placed in hatching jars (Fig. 23–5) or into circular fiber glass tanks for incubation. A continuous flow of oxygenated water is introduced at a rate sufficient to keep the eggs in motion. Care must be taken to prevent air bubbles from floating eggs out of the water (Fig. 23–6). After 40 to 48 hours, depending on the water temperature, larvae hatch and swim over the lip of the jars into an aquarium or holding tank (Fig. 23–7). Since Chesapeake Bay striped bass eggs have much lower specific gravity than other stocks, hatchery jars cannot be used or the eggs float out. Eggs from these fish must be allowed to hatch in circular tanks equipped with appropriate screens. Larvae are normally held for 2 to 5 days before they are shipped or stocked (Kerby, 1986; Rees and Harrell, 1990).

Hybridization of female striped bass with males of other species is easily accomplished by using a male of the desired cross species to fertilize the eggs. However, production of hybrids with females of the other species requires additional procedures. Both males and females are normally injected with HCG at doses ranging from 1100 to 2200 IU/kg to induce ovulation and to increase semen flow (Kerby and Harrell, 1990). When eggs are taken, they should be fertilized dry with copious quantities of semen. Just enough water is added to activate the sperm and the mixture is stirred for 1 or 2 minutes. The fertilized eggs are then poured into a hatching jar with about 5 L of water containing 150 mg/L of tannic acid. The mixture is bubbled rather violently for a period of 6 or 7 minutes, using a weighted airstone placed in the bottom of the jar. Then, water is exchanged for the tannic acid water, and the eggs are incubated (Starling, 1983, 1985; Rottmann et al., 1988; Kerby and Harrell, 1990). Care should be taken not to leave the eggs in the tannic acid solution too long, as it tends to toughen the chorion, making it difficult for larvae to break through, resulting in lowered hatch rates.

Natural Spawning

The natural method of spawning allows broodfish to spawn naturally in tanks (Bishop, 1975; Smith and Whitehurst, 1990). Both males and females are injected with HCG at the rates described for artificial spawning. Females are normally catheterized before injection to determine when the eggs appear to be 7 to 12 hours before ovulation. Normally, two females and four males are placed in a 1.2- to 2.4-m diameter circular tank, about 1.2 m deep. Water is supplied through two or more 13-mm (ID) tubes under slight pressure at a rate of 30 to 38 L/minute. This creates a circular velocity of 10 to 15 cm/second at the perimeter of the tank. A 10-cm diameter center standpipe, encircled by a 45-cm diameter fine-mesh screen barrier, controls water depth and prevents the loss of eggs and larvae. A bubble curtain constructed from perforated airline tubing around the base of the screen keeps eggs and larvae from impinging on the screen.

The fish normally spawn in this system from 36 to 60 hours after injection, depending on water temperature. The fish should not be disturbed immediately before or during spawning. Some culturists isolate the tanks with partitions of black plastic. After the broodfish have spawned, they are removed and released. They are normally in excellent health. Eggs typically remain in the tank until they hatch. The larvae are then collected with scoops or a siphon attached to a large fine-mesh funnel placed so water in the tank flows through the funnel (Bishop, 1975; Smith and Whitehurst, 1990).

Both methods have advantages and disadvantages (Kerby et al., 1983). The jar method is more labor intensive and requires much more expertise in predicting time of ovulation. It is also more expensive than the tank culture method. At least three persons

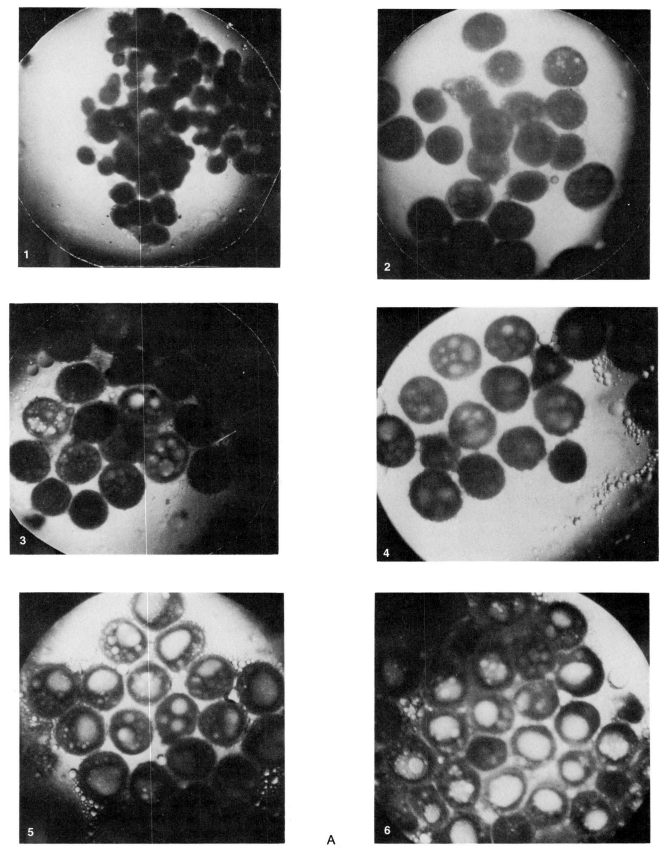

FIGURE 23–3. *A.* From maturity to 11 hr before ovulation. *B.* From 10 hr before ovulation. *C.* From 5 hr before ovulation to ripeness. *D.* Eggs that have ovulated and become ripe. (Courtesy of J.D. Bayless, South Carolina Wildlife and Marine Resources Department.)

Illustration continued on following page

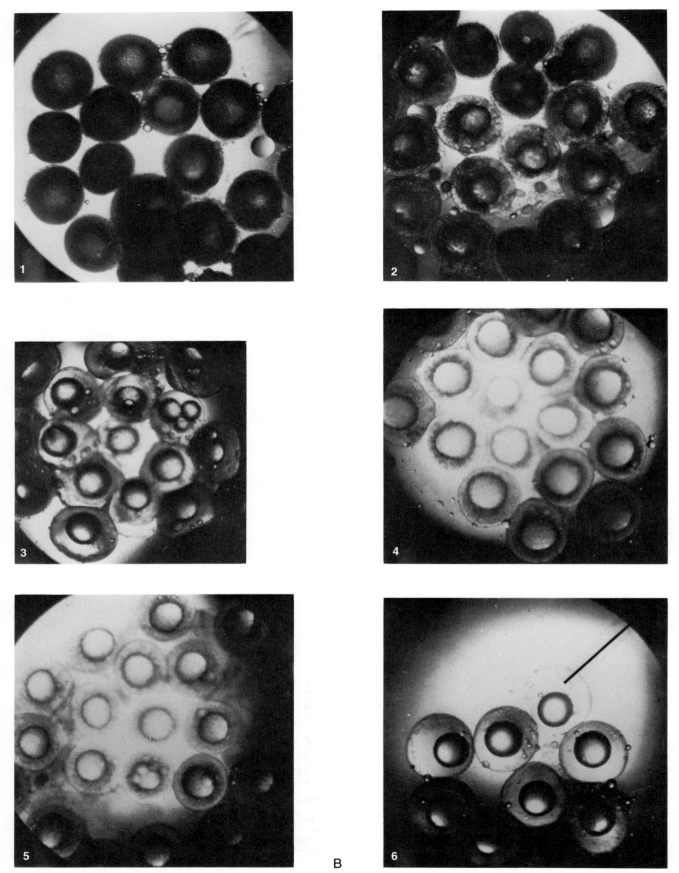

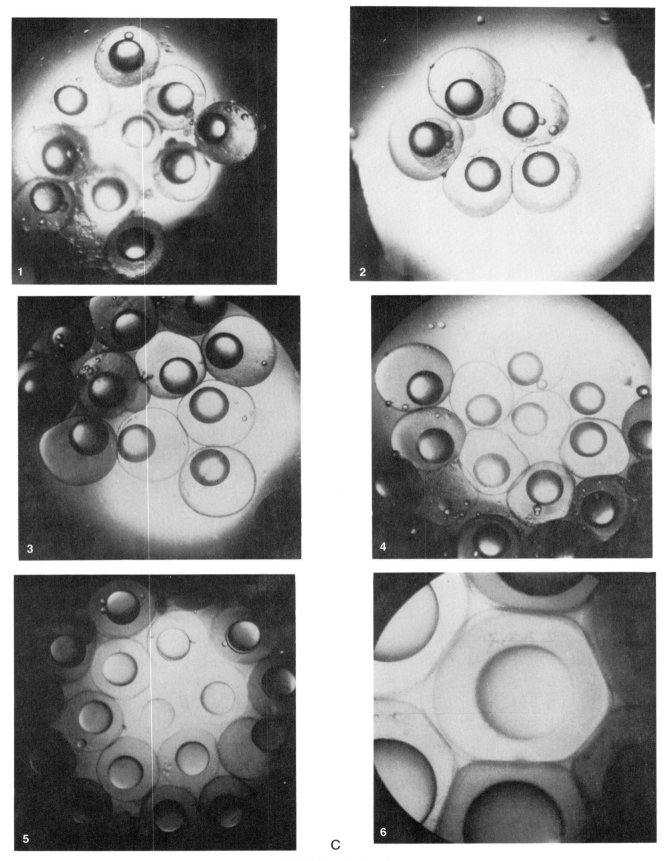

FIGURE 23–3 *Continued*

Illustration continued on following page

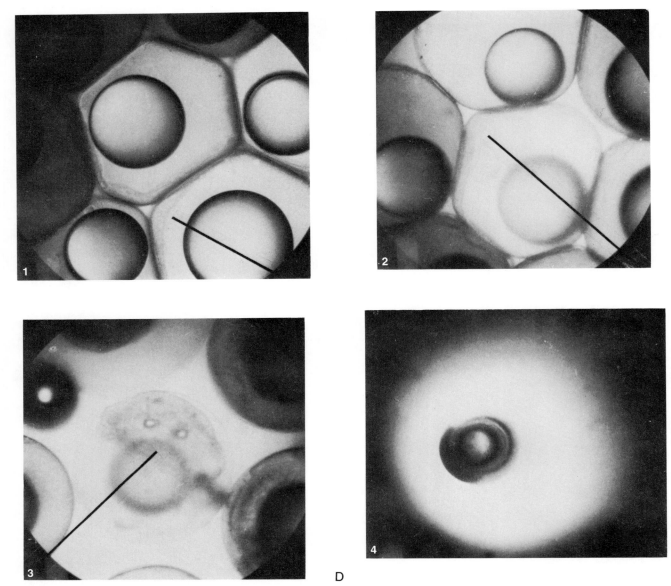

FIGURE 23–3 *Continued*

are required on a 24-hour basis for efficient operation. There is also much more stress on the broodfish because of frequent handling, anesthesia, and manual stripping. As a result, many broodfish are ultimately lost. In contrast, most broodfish can be released unharmed after tank spawning. On the other hand, because jar culture requires less space than tank culture, production per unit of space is much higher. It is also easier to predict the number of larvae produced, and the culturist has greater control of the developing eggs and larvae. Because dead eggs often have a lower specific gravity than live eggs, they either are flushed out of the jars or can easily be removed by siphoning. Their removal reduces fungal infections.

In the tank method, the removal of larvae from the tanks requires considerable time, but use of the screen-funnel-siphon arrangement reduces the amount of labor needed. A major disadvantage of natural spawning is that hybrids cannot be produced. Even after they have ovulated, female striped bass do not release their eggs in the presence of male white bass (Bishop, 1975). Thus, hybrid production requires prediction of ovulation and manual stripping procedures.

Culture of Larvae

Most larval culture takes place in freshwater or brackish water ponds that range from 0.04 to more than 2 hectares, but more intensive tank culture is also being successfully employed. Although procedures vary in different areas, recommendations by Braschler (1975) and Bonn et al. (1976) or Geiger and Turner (1990) are usually followed. A number of

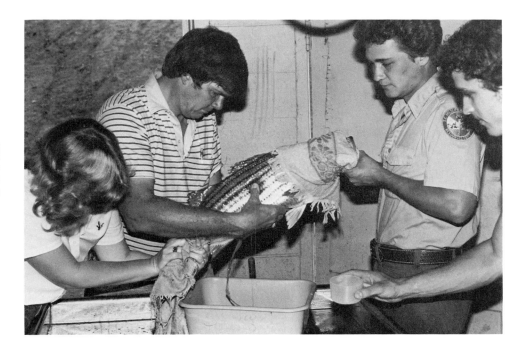

FIGURE 23–4. Manually stripping eggs from a female striped bass into a spawning pan. (Courtesy of J.D. Bayless, South Carolina Wildlife and Marine Resources Department.)

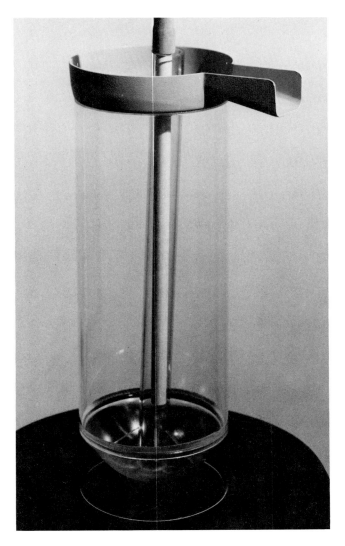

FIGURE 23–5. Modified MacDonald hatching jar showing tube-within-a-tube method of introducing water flow that prevents air bubbles from lifting eggs out of jars. (Courtesy of M. Stuckey.)

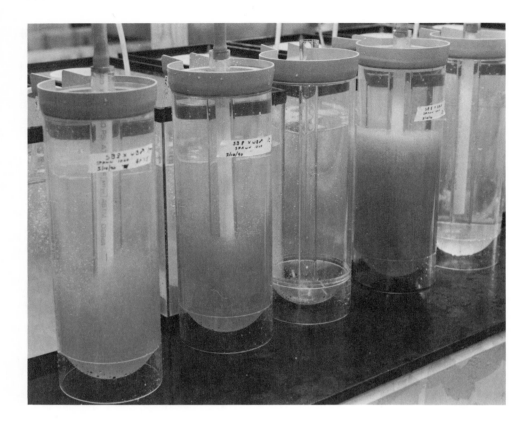

FIGURE 23–6. Striped bass eggs incubating in a modified MacDonald hatching jar. (Courtesy of M. Stuckey.)

food-habit and selectivity studies have clearly shown the importance of copepods and cladocerans to the young fish until they reach a length of 80 to 120 mm (Sandoz and Johnston, 1966; Harper et al., 1969; Meshaw, 1969; Harper and Jarman, 1972; Humphries and Cumming, 1972; Harrell et al., 1977).

Fertilization can help provide adequate food for the young fish by providing necessary nutrients. Organic fertilizers, such as alfalfa, Bermuda, milo, soybean, and cotton seed pellets or meals, which provide nutrients for both phyto- and zooplankton production, are generally believed to be preferable to inorganic types. The slower decay of organic materials appears to provide a more sustained pro-

duction of zooplankton. Inorganic fertilizers, especially when used alone, often produce dense phytoplankton blooms that tend to produce high pH and may cause oxygen depletion or a dominant blue-green algae production or both (Braschler, 1975; Bonn et al., 1976; Geiger, 1983). Application rates vary. Guidelines for fertilization regimens have been published (Geiger and Turner, 1990).

Larvae were previously stocked into ponds at 5 to 10 days of age, following the swim-up stage and an initial period of feeding on brine shrimp nauplii. More recently, the practice of holding larvae for any length of time has been questioned, and many agencies are stocking larvae at the age of 5 days or less

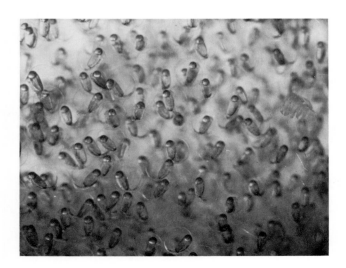

FIGURE 23–7. Striped bass embryos immediately before hatch. (Courtesy of T. Borg.)

without prior feeding of brine shrimp. Higher stocking rates can produce survival rates comparable to those from lower stocking rates, thus yielding more fingerlings per hectare (Harper and Jarman, 1972; Parker, 1979; Rees and Cook, 1985a). This relation holds true up to a point, but since any system has a maximum biomass-carrying capacity, larger numbers of fish may result in a correspondingly smaller average size (Rees and Cook, 1985a). The rule-of-thumb stocking rate is still 247,000 larvae/hectare (Bonn et al., 1976; Harrell et al., 1990). Fingerlings are normally harvested 30 to 50 days after stocking, when they are 25 to 50 mm long and weigh 0.3 to 1.5 g.

Intensive culture of striped bass to a fingerling stage in aquaria, troughs, tanks, or raceways is also practiced, but to a much lesser extent. This type of culture is still largely experimental (Nicholson, 1973; McIlwain, 1976; Lewis et al., 1981; Nicholson et al., 1990). Intensive culture has some distinct advantages but also has problems. It is very space efficient. Many more fish can be grown per unit space than in ponds. Closed and semiclosed systems permit precise control over physical and chemical water-quality characteristics. The fish are readily observable, which facilitates detection of disease and parasite infestations. Growth, survival, and condition can be more closely monitored, which results in more appropriate feeding rates. On the negative side, even closed recirculating systems require a constant and adequate supply of high-quality replacement water. Water quality must be monitored frequently so corrective measures can be taken immediately. Most closed systems are relatively complex, and the threat of mechanical or electrical failures requires extensive alarm and back-up systems. Cleaning tanks and filters can be a major problem and may be labor intensive. Because of high densities, disease and cannibalism can become problems. Finally, provision of sufficient quantities of an adequate diet for fry is difficult in intensive systems.

The early postlarval stage requires an abundance of food organisms small enough to be consumed. At this stage, early instars of cladocera and copepods are selected, and larger organisms are avoided (Sandoz and Johnston, 1966; Harper et al., 1969; Humphries and Cumming, 1972, 1973). In general, copepods constitute the most important food of striped bass less than 30 mm long (Regan et al., 1968; Meshaw, 1969; Harrell et al., 1977). Cladocerans become increasingly important as fish length increases. Early postlarvae do not accept prepared diets well (Bowman, 1979; Falls, 1983). Brine shrimp nauplii are widely used because they can easily be hatched from dry cysts in 24 to 48 hours and are readily accepted by striped bass fry as a first food. Some investigators have suggested that brine shrimp may not provide adequate nutrition (Regan et al., 1968; Braschler, 1975). High densities of brine shrimp (50 to 120 nauplii per milliliter) have been suggested as a means of increasing survival and reducing cannibalism (Lewis et al., 1981). Feeding should begin as soon as the digestive tract is developed and the

larvae are capable of feeding, usually at 4 to 5 days of age, depending on water temperature. Feeding at least every 3 hours or continuous feeding is recommended (Bonn et al., 1976). Brine shrimp nauplii can only be used as a diet for early postlarvae of striped bass and hybrids produced from female striped bass and males of other species. The other three species and hybrids produced with females of the other species are unable to utilize brine shrimp nauplii as a first food because of their small mouth size.

Water Quality

Water-quality requirements necessary for striped bass culture are not well understood, although the effects of specific factors have received considerable attention in the laboratory. Striped bass appear to have a wide tolerance for a number of factors, and in general, the fish become tolerant to a wider range of water-quality variables with age (Humphries and Cumming, 1973).

Temperature is one of the most important factors affecting the survival and growth of striped bass at all stages of development. The optimum spawning range for striped bass in the Roanoke River, North Carolina, is 16.7 to 19.4°C, but spawning occurs at temperatures as low as 12.8°C (Shannon, 1970). Sex products of both males and females are adversely affected by temperatures of 21 to 24°C (Barkuloo, 1967). Striped bass eggs and larvae survive temperatures ranging from 12.8 to 23.9°C. At temperatures above or below this range, mortality increases drastically (Albrecht, 1964; Doroshev, 1970; Shannon and Smith, 1968; Shannon, 1970; Otwell and Merriner, 1975; Morgan et al., 1981). Temperature tolerances of larvae can be increased by acclimation (Davies, 1973a). Water temperatures from 14.4 to 21.1°C are recommended until larvae are 9 days old, when they can be acclimated to higher pond temperatures (Bonn et al., 1976).

Dissolved oxygen is a major critical factor in striped bass culture. Mean survival of eggs at 18.4°C decreased when dissolved oxygen fell to 5 mg/L, and was 50% of control survival (22.2°C) at 4 mg/L (Turner and Farley, 1971). Incubation time can increase at lower oxygen concentrations, and subsequent survival of larvae is reduced in direct relation to the length of time the eggs are exposed to low oxygen concentrations. A number of abnormalities were also noted in larvae from eggs incubated at low oxygen levels (Harrell and Bayless, 1983). The minimum oxygen concentration necessary for normal morphologic development is 3 mg/L (Harrell and Bayless, 1983).

Although striped bass usually spawn in fresh water, some salinity is beneficial. Survival of striped bass eggs and larvae is enhanced by a salinity of 1.7 ppt and salinities of 8.3 to 8.6 ppt are not detrimental (Albrecht, 1964). Survival of eggs water-hardened in fresh water is higher after transfer to salinities up to 10 ppt than survival of eggs water-hardened directly in more saline water (Turner and Farley, 1971). Larvae subjected to 28 ppt salinity die, but significant numbers survive and grow in 21 ppt (Bayless, 1972). Growth and survival are better in salinities of 3.5 to 14.0 ppt than in fresh water (Bayless, 1972). Salinity can also affect other factors. For example, striped bass are more resistant to ammonia toxicity in 23°C brackish water (about 11 ppt salinity) than in either fresh water or undiluted seawater. At 15°C, this resistance is equal in fresh water and brackish water but is lower in seawater (Hazel et al., 1971).

Striped bass tolerances to pH have not been well defined. Striped bass larvae are extremely sensitive to pH changes and 100% mortality can occur after transfer of larvae to water with a pH difference of only 0.8 to 1.0 (Doroshev, 1970). In recirculating systems, pH values of 7.0 to 8.0 ensure optimum conditions for biofiltration, and pH values of 7.5 to 8.5 are considered optimum for striped bass culture (Bonn et al., 1976; Lewis et al., 1981). Values should not be outside the range of 7.0 to 9.5 (Bonn et al., 1976). Alkalinity should be maintained above 150 mg/L (as $CaCO_3$) to compensate for nitrous and nitric acids released by nitrifying bacteria (Lewis et al., 1981). Hard water appears to be beneficial to striped bass. Osmotic shock following stress may be a major cause of mortalities. Total hardness should exceed 150 mg/L, and 200 to 250 mg/L is considered very good (Bonn et al., 1976).

Ammonia, nitrites, and nitrates represent a more significant factor in intensive culture systems than in pond culture. Ammonia is the primary nitrogenous metabolite produced by fish. The un-ionized form (NH_3) is much more toxic than the ionized form (NH_4^+), and the balance between the forms depends on temperature and pH. As pH increases, the ratio of NH_3 to NH_4^+ is increased, whereas as the pH decreases, the ratio shifts in the other direction. As temperature increases, the ratio shifts in favor of NH_3 (Parker, 1984). Ammonia is probably second only to oxygen depletion as a cause of mortality in cultured striped bass (Lewis et al., 1981). Ammonia concentrations should not exceed 0.6 mg/L in intensive culture systems (Bonn et al., 1976; Lewis et al., 1981).

Nitrites and nitrates, the intermediate and end breakdown products of ammonia oxidation, are not normally a problem in pond culture unless the ponds are very intensively stocked or are very heavily fertilized. However, a diel shift in pH can alter the relative toxicity of ammonia and nitrates during each 24-hour period and may sometimes cause problems (Parker, 1984). Nitrite levels should be kept below 0.2 mg/L, and although striped bass are reported to tolerate nitrate concentrations in excess of 800 mg/L, larvae are stressed at levels as low as 200 mg/L (Bonn et al., 1976).

Most streams where striped bass spawn are turbid, but turbidity is probably not a requirement (Talbot, 1966). Direct sunlight adversely affects survival of 6.5-day-old larvae and fingerlings (Bonn et al., 1976; Rees and Cook, 1985b).

REPRODUCTION OF THE CENTRARCHIDAE

Members of the family Centrarchidae (the sunfishes) are probably the best-known fishes in the United States because of their ubiquitous distribution, and because they have long been favorites for recreational fishing. The family includes such well-known species as largemouth bass, smallmouth bass, bluegill, redear sunfish, green sunfish, and the black and white crappies. They are spring spawners, and the males construct shallow depressions in the bottom that are used as nests. Males do guard the eggs and young (Lagler, 1956). Eggs are demersal and adhesive. They have long been cultured in hatchery ponds for use in stocking lakes and ponds for recreational and management programs. More recently, refinement of spawning and rearing techniques has provided the means to intensively culture several species in the family, although emphasis has been placed on the largemouth bass (Simco et al., 1986). Several centrarchids, including the largemouth bass and black crappie, have been induced to spawn naturally in the laboratory (Carlson, 1973; Siefert and Herman, 1977). Basic culture techniques are similar for many members in the family, so this section will emphasize largemouth bass.

Production of Larvae

Largemouth bass broodstock can be collected from the wild using various nets or electrofishing. The fertility of largemouth bass is not significantly affected by capturing broodstock with an electroshocker (Jackson, 1979). Most broodstock are reared and held in captivity, although many hatchery managers like to collect wild fish or bring in fish from other hatcheries to introduce heterozygosity. As with any cultured species, it pays to maintain healthy broodfish and to turn over stock regularly.

Sexual maturity of largemouth bass is a function of size rather than age (Moorman, 1957), and eggs can normally be obtained from 1-year-old fish that weigh approximately 300 to 450 g (Piper et al., 1982). Broodfish can be expected to spawn satisfactorily for three or four seasons, so about one-third of the broodstock should be replaced each year. Enough food should be provided to yield a weight gain of 50% per year. Normally, forage fishes such as fathead minnows are supplied, but Oregon moist pellet (Hublou, 1968) has been used successfully with fish trained to artificial food (Snow, 1971). In addition to normal sexing techniques based on distended abdomens for females and emission of semen from ripe males when pressure is applied to the abdomen, female largemouth bass larger than 355 mm long have an elliptical or pear-shaped scaleless area surrounding and adjacent to the urogenital opening. The area in similar-sized males is nearly circular (Parker, 1971).

Largemouth bass spawn in the spring when

temperatures range from 15 to 24°C. They are intermittent spawners that may spawn several times if conditions are correct, but subsequent spawns normally contain about half the number of eggs of the preceding spawn (Simco et al., 1986). A sharp drop in water temperature followed by a rise provides stimulus for repeated spawning (Kramer and Smith, 1962). Largemouth bass can be induced to spawn later than normal in the laboratory by controlling photoperiod and temperature (Carlson and Hale, 1972). The natural spawning period can be extended by holding broodstock in water that averages 16°C and transferring them directly to ponds that average 23°C (Jackson, 1979).

Smallmouth bass usually spawn earlier than largemouth bass, when temperatures reach about 16.7°C, and hatching takes from 3 to 7 days at 18.3 to 23.3°C (Inslee, 1975; Piper et al., 1982). These fish are also multiple spawners and can be induced to spawn as many as eight times during a season. Bluegills usually begin spawning when water temperatures reach 21°C and will spawn several times. The crappies begin spawning at temperatures of about 18°C.

Although largemouth bass can be induced to ovulate with HCG (Stevens, 1970; Wilbur and Langford, 1975) and be strip-spawned like striped bass, most culturists spawn them naturally in hatchery ponds. Ponds should be prepared according to standard hatchery practices (Huet, 1972; Snow, 1975; Piper et al., 1982; Simco et al., 1986). Recommendations include placement of gravel or light-colored rocks in specific sites as an inducement to nesting and to facilitate locating larvae. Nylon mats can be used as spawning sites (Chastain and Snow, 1966). Ponds should be stocked with male-to-female ratios of 2:1 to 3:1 (Snow, 1975; Bishop, 1968). Stocking adults of the same year class together provides more uniformity in time of spawning and size of fry (Snow et al., 1964).

Hormones can be injected intramuscularly to provide more precise control of spawning. The threshold level of human choriogonadotropin for successful stimulation of ovulation is 4000 IU/kg (Stevens, 1970). Other hormones (such as luteinizing hormone, follicle-stimulating hormone, and thyroid-stimulating hormone) are also effective in inducing ovulation, but HCG is the hormone of choice based on effectiveness and cost. Females injected with HCG will usually ovulate within 48 hours (Wilford and Langford, 1975). If not stripped within 12 to 16 hours of ovulation, eggs become nonviable. Injection of males with similar levels of HCG often increases semen production. The rates of successful ovulation induction are higher early in the spawning season (Wilbur and Langford, 1975).

Eggs laid on nylon spawning mats can be transferred to a hatchery or laboratory where they can be separated from the mats by washing, cleaned, and incubated in a vertical incubator (Snow, 1973). During this period they can be prophylactically treated to control fungi. Sodium sulfite can be used to dissolve the gelatinous matrix that causes the adhe-

siveness of the eggs if desired (Simco et al., 1986). Eggs become less adhesive with time, but if eggs are too old when separated from the spawning mats, premature hatching occurs (Snow, 1973). Fry should be transferred to holding tanks within 48 hours after hatch. Swim-up occurs from 3 to 7 days following hatch, depending on temperature (Snow, 1973). Fry are ready for food at swim-up and probably should make the transition to outside energy sources within 24 hours (Toetz, 1966).

Smallmouth bass spawn naturally in nests built on gravel or rocky areas, so artificial nests can be provided in ponds with a silt bottom to control where the fish spawn (Inslee, 1975). Portable nests, constructed from wood and filled with rocks, can be designed to allow for easy collection of the fry after hatch (Inslee, 1975; Simco et al., 1986). This type of collection device should be used for greatest efficiency, as smallmouth bass larvae do not school well and scatter following swim-up. Another excellent method involves spawning broodstock in raceways, which provides the advantages of increased control of spawning, and the ability to obtain multiple spawns from the same broodfish. It also eliminates egg losses associated with males abandoning nests when the temperature drops. Artificial nests are collected daily, and eggs are hatched artificially by placing the nests in catfish hatching troughs under the paddles. Additional aeration can be supplied, water temperature can be controlled, and chemical treatments for disease can be applied as needed (Simco et al., 1986). Rearing is normally accomplished in fertilized ponds. MacDonald jars and Heath incubators have also been used successfully, but MacDonald jars are superior because dead or fungus-infected eggs are carried out of the jars with the water flow (Inslee, 1975). Similar methods can be used for bluegills if needed. They readily spawn in gravel-filled pans (Wrenn and Grannemann, 1980).

Culture of Larvae

There are three primary culture methods for larvae (Snow, 1975; Simco et al., 1986). In the spawning-rearing pond system, broodstock are lightly stocked at 25 to 100 adults/hectare, and the pond is fertilized to produce a zooplankton bloom. Adults and young stay in the pond until the young are harvested, usually at 25 to 50 mm. Bluegills, crappies, and other sunfishes are most often spawned and cultured in this manner. According to Simco et al. (1986), crappies are extremely susceptible to columnaris disease and shock, so harvesting and handling can be a problem.

The most commonly used method is the fry transfer method, which allows increased production through more efficient management. Broodstock are stocked in unfertilized ponds at a rate of about 100 to 250/hectare when water temperatures reach 17 to 20°C. The ponds are often treated with herbicides to prevent problems with filamentous algae and rooted aquatic weeds. Schools of fry are captured using traps or small mesh seines after they become free-swimming. Then they are transferred to rearing ponds that have been fertilized to provide an abundant zooplankton bloom. Recommended stocking rates vary from 100,000/hectare to 240,000/hectare, and fingerlings are normally harvested for distribution when they are 25 to 50 mm long.

Intensive culture of largemouth bass is possible, although first-feeding fry still require a natural diet. However, 10-mm or larger fry can be trained to accept common carp eggs (Brandenburg et al., 1979) and can be gradually weaned to a prepared diet. Although scoliosis and lordosis often develop in fish fed carp eggs, the condition is not permanent and disappears when the fish are later trained to a prepared diet. A variety of diets prepared for larvae, including some that contained up to 30% carp eggs, have met with little success (Brandt et al., 1987; Willis and Flickinger, 1981). Oregon moist pellet provides excellent survival, growth, and production of fingerling largemouth bass, and is also adequate for broodstock (Snow, 1968, 1970). Largemouth bass are primarily sight feeders, and olfactory stimuli play a minor role, if any (Brandt et al., 1987).

Water Quality

As with other fish species, water quality is of utmost importance for the successful reproduction and culture of centrarchids. Largemouth bass do best if pH is from 6.5 to 8.5, dissolved oxygen is greater than 6 mg/L, CO_2 is less than 10 mg/L, and total hardness is from 60 to 180 mg/L as $CaCO_3$ (Snow, 1975). Hatching and survival of smallmouth bass was reduced in dissolved oxygen concentrations less than 4.2 mg/L, and no fish survived after 2 weeks at 2.8 mg/L (Siefert et al., 1974). Yet, largemouth bass eggs can withstand dissolved oxygen levels as low as 2.8 mg/L (Dudley and Eipper, 1975). Black crappie can spawn naturally in laboratory tanks at constant dissolved oxygen concentrations as low as 2.5 mg/L (Carlson and Herman, 1978). Largemouth bass eggs spawned at 17 to 21°C can have more than 75% survival when exposed to 10 to 24°C, but survival drops above 24°C (Kelley, 1968). All of the commonly cultured centrarchids are freshwater species, but largemouth bass eggs can tolerate up to 3.9 ppt (Tebo and McCoy, 1964).

Little is known about the effects of un-ionized ammonia and nitrite concentrations on the centrarchids, apart from LC_{50} values (Simco et al., 1986). Calculations based on catfish data indicate that chronic levels as low as 0.01 and 0.0006 mg/L un-ionized ammonia may reduce growth of largemouth bass and bluegills, respectively. Similar computations estimate that 10.7 mg/L nitrite should inhibit growth in bluegill at pH 7.2, and 17.5 mg/L should inhibit largemouth bass growth at pH 8 (Simco et al., 1986).

REPRODUCTION OF THE PERCIDAE

The family Percidae contains a large number of species, but reproductive and culture research has been directed primarily at the walleye and the yellow perch. In addition, sauger X walleye hybrids have been produced and widely stocked for recreational fisheries. These species are commonly considered to be cool-water species (Trandahl, 1978), preferring temperatures ranging from 7.2 to 23°C (Piper et al., 1982; Nickum, 1986). Yellow perch and walleye are highly valued both recreationally and commercially, and represent two of the most exploited species in North American fisheries (Ney, 1978). Both reproduce in the spring, spawning over a broad temperature range from 3 to 16°C, but timing and location differ. Male walleye normally mature at 2 to 4 years and females at 3 to 6 years of age. Yellow perch mature somewhat earlier, with males typically maturing at 1 to 3 years and females maturing at age 3 (Ney, 1978; Clugston et al., 1978; Nickum, 1986). Both species require an extended period of winter chill at temperatures below 10°C for gonadal maturation (Hokanson, 1977).

Walleye produce demersal and adhesive eggs that are normally spawned over rocky or gravel areas (Huet, 1972; Piper et al., 1982). Yellow perch produce a unique gelatinous ribbonlike egg mass or tube that may be several meters long and 100 mm wide. They normally spawn over submerged vegetation and brush, which anchors the egg mass (Muncy, 1962; Mansueti, 1964; Heidinger and Kayes, 1986).

Production of Larvae

Techniques for producing eggs and larvae from wild-caught walleye are well established, dating from the nineteenth century (Nickum, 1986). Broodstock are often collected from trap nets set in areas where water temperatures are 7.2 to 10°C, but they may be collected with other types of gear, including gill nets and electroshockers. Broodstock are often stripped at the location of capture, or females that are not yet ripe may be held in pens or tanks until ovulation occurs (Huet, 1972; Colby et al., 1979). Some authors (Lessman, 1978; Hearn, 1980) report that held walleye often do not become ripe. Methods for taking yellow perch broodstock are similar to those for walleye, although naturally spawned egg ribbons may be collected from the environment and brought to a hatchery for incubation (Hinshaw, 1985). Yellow perch are normally considered to be lake and river spawners, but successful maturation and reproduction of fingerlings stocked in a 1.6-hectare irrigation pond in North Carolina has been observed. Both wet and dry fertilization methods are used. Fertilization in yellow perch can be improved by stripping into a 0.5% NaCl solution (Kayes, 1977). Fertilization percentages are drastically reduced, and most larvae are deformed if fertilization is delayed 5 minutes (Kayes, 1977).

Optimum temperatures, determined from laboratory experiments, for walleye fertilization, incubation, and culture through yolk-sac absorption are 6 to 12°C, 9 to 15°C, and 9 to 21°C, respectively (Smith and Koenst, 1975). When broodstock are collected from, and eggs are fertilized in, water temperatures above 12°C, hatch rates are reduced. Stripping and fertilizing eggs in water chilled to 7.2°C results in significantly increased hatch rates (Prentice and Dean, 1979). Optimum temperatures for yellow perch fertilization to hatching are considered to be 10 to 20°C, with a temperature rise of about 0.5°C/day resulting in maximum survival and hatch (Heidinger and Kayes, 1986). Manipulations of temperature and photoperiod to change the natural spawning cycle of yellow perch have met with little success. The onset of spawning apparently depends more on the intrinsic maturation state of the gonads than on photoperiod or temperature cues (Hokanson, 1977; Kayes and Calbert, 1979).

Hormones are not usually required for spawning walleye or yellow perch, but ovulation has been induced in walleye using a variety of hormones (Nelson et al., 1965; Lessman, 1978). Two intraperitoneal injections of carp pituitary at doses from 7.7 to 22 mg/kg at 72-hour intervals will induce ovulation in most walleye (Lessman, 1978). Chorionic gonadotropin, 152 IU/kg, is effective when administered in two injections, and HCG combined with low levels of luteinizing hormone and carp pituitary is effective in single doses (Lessman, 1978). Use of hormones too far in advance of natural spawning results in free-flowing but nonviable eggs (Nickum, 1986). The use of hormones to induce ovulation in yellow perch is not well documented (Heidinger and Kayes, 1986). However, the role of steroids in in vitro maturation of yellow perch oocytes has been studied (Goetz and Bergman, 1978; Goetz, 1979; Thoefan and Goetz, 1983).

Because walleye eggs are adhesive, various treatments have been used to prevent clumping. Three methods commonly used to eliminate adhesiveness include stirring with a large turkey feather, physical scouring with abrasive particles, and chemical treatment with tannic acid (Davis, 1953; Dumas and Brand, 1972; Waltemyer, 1976; Colesante and Youmans, 1983; Krise et al., 1986; Nickum, 1986). Exposure to a protease may be a superior method (Krise et al., 1986). In tests comparing eggs treated with 0.01% protease, tannic acid, bentonite, or constant stirring, both bentonite and stirred eggs reaggregate following treatment. No reclumping occurs in the protease- or tannic acid–treated eggs. Protease treatments give the best survival to hatch (83%), followed by tannic acid treatment (64%). Hatching duration is increased in tannic acid–treated eggs, and many larvae hatch with their egg shell lodged over their head and midsection. These larvae have difficulty freeing themselves. Similar phenomena have been observed when tannic acid is used on white bass eggs (Kerby and Harrell, 1990).

The adhesive layer on the eggs may provide a nutrient base for bacteria and fungi (Krise et al., 1986). Several species have a layer external to the chorion, which may be susceptible to enzymatic removal by protease. Stripping this layer might drastically reduce the prevalence of bacterial, fungal, or viral pathogens carried in this layer. For example, *Renibacterium salmoniarum* has been demonstrated to be vertically transmitted in a mucoproteinlike layer external to the chorion in eggs of chinook salmon (Krise et al., 1986).

After water-hardening, eggs are placed in hatching jars at densities of about 30,000/L, and water flow is adjusted to gently roll the eggs. A layer of gravel is sometimes added to the bottom of the jars to provide a diffuse upwelling of water (Colesante and Youmans, 1983; Nickum, 1986). Hatching is temperature dependent, ranging from about 1 week at 20°C to 3 weeks at 10°C. Walleye eggs do not require substantial care during incubation, although clumps of dead or fungal-infected eggs are normally removed. Prophylactic treatments with formalin have been used to control fungi during incubation (Nickum, 1986).

The yellow perch egg mass has a tendency to rise prior to hatch, so hatching jars do not work well. Vertical incubators have been used successfully because they do contain the egg mass, but they do not completely eliminate the floating problem (West and Leonard, 1978). Ranges in time to hatch are similar to those of walleye (Heidinger and Kayes, 1986).

Culture of Larvae

Most walleye culture is now done in freshwater ponds using fertilization methods similar to those used for other species. However, neither large numbers nor predictable production can be consistently obtained. Larvae are often stocked at swim-up, although some culturists wait an extra 1 to 3 days before stocking (Nickum, 1986). Because cannibalism is especially prevalent in walleye ponds, survival typically decreases with an increase in fish size. Harvesting when fingerlings reach 60 to 80 mm can increase survival and size uniformity (Nickum, 1986).

Yellow perch can also be reared in ponds, but little information is available on survival rates or production (Heidinger and Kayes, 1986). Perch from 8 to 50 mm are positively phototaxic, and a significant percentage of fingerlings can be harvested using lights and lift nets (Manci et al., 1983).

Intensive culture of walleye fry is presently limited. Although fry will feed on nonliving foods, survival is typically less than 1% for periods longer than a month (Nickum, 1978, 1986; Krise and Meade, 1986). Walleye eat, but slowly die after a few weeks, suffering what is termed the "dwindles" (Nickum, 1986). Survival rates are poor. Continuous feeding of size-graded zooplankton and brine shrimp nauplii as starter diets may help (Krise and Meade, 1986). A formulated diet based on the nutrient composition of unfertilized walleye eggs looks promising

(Nickum, 1986). Cannibalism is a significant problem but can be reduced by adjusting fish and food density and timing of first feeding. Color and light intensity within culture tanks can have a profound effect on the larvae. Walleye are so attracted to the sides of white tanks that all live or formulated foods are ignored (Corazza and Nickum, 1981). Uniform dispersal occurs in dark or neutral colored tanks. First feeding of yellow perch larvae occurs sooner, and feeding, growth, and survival are enhanced when prey have higher contrast, and light levels are higher (Hinshaw, 1985). After walleye reach 25 mm in length, they can be readily converted to prepared diets developed for cool-water species (Reinitz and Austin, 1980; Nickum, 1986; Westers, 1986).

Little is known about disease problems related to walleye fry culture. Myxobacteria and fungi have been reported, but not confirmed, at various hatcheries (Nickum, 1986). Walleye larvae appear unusually sensitive to many standard therapeutic agents, making maintenance of high water quality an even greater necessity. At least 68 parasites and diseases have been identified in walleye populations. The most important in fingerling culture are myxobacterial infections (especially columnaris), parasites such as *Ichthyophthirius multifiliis*, *Trichodina* sp., *Scyphidia* sp., bacterial gill disease, furunculosis, fin rot, and fungal infections. Minimizing handling when water temperatures exceed 20°C, strict sanitation, and maintenance of high water quality reduces disease problems (Nickum, 1986).

REPRODUCTION OF THE ESOCIDAE

The Northern pike is normally cultured to augment sport and commercial fisheries, whereas the muskellunge is produced to provide a trophy sport fishery (Westers, 1986). The tiger muskellunge, a sterile hybrid between the Northern pike and the muskellunge, is also frequently cultured and has become an important sport fish (Buss et al., 1978; Westers, 1986). The other native species (including the chain pickerel, the redfin pickerel, and the grass pickerel) are not normally cultured, although it has been demonstrated that all of the species can be artificially hybridized (Buss et al., 1978).

The pikes are also cool-water species, inhabiting temperatures from 0.5 to 26.7°C. The optimum temperature range is from 4.4 to 18.3°C with the muskellunge preferring slightly warmer temperatures (Casselman, 1978; Piper et al., 1982). Northern pike typically spawn just after ice melt, when water temperatures are from 4.4 to 11.1°C, whereas muskellunge usually spawn a little later, at temperatures of 9.4 to 15°C, with the optimum at 12.8°C (Scott and Crossman, 1973; Westers, 1986).

Eggs of both species are about 3 mm in diameter, but those of the pike are demersal and highly adhesive, whereas those of the muskellunge are semidemersal and nonadhesive. Both species spawn in shallow, heavily vegetated areas (Scott and Cross-

man, 1973; Hess and Heartwell, 1979). Low hatchability, cannibalism, and highly variable production are the main barriers to successful propagation of these species, but new culture techniques and the development of successful prepared diets have resulted in significant progress (Westers, 1986).

In the southern part of their range, Northern pike occasionally spawn at 1 year of age, but most do not spawn until they are at least 2 years old. Males usually mature a year earlier than females (Scott and Crossman, 1973). Male muskellunge mature at ages 3 to 4, at lengths greater than 610 mm. Females mature at 4 to 6 years and at lengths greater than 660 mm (Miles, 1978). Male broodstock held in ponds reach maturity at 3 years, and females mature at 4 or 5 years of age (Phillips and Graveen, 1973).

Production of Larvae

As with many of the piscivorous fishes, virtually all esocid broodstock are taken from the wild (Graff, 1978). Collecting methods include trap nets, pound nets, and electrofishing. Anesthetizing large broodfish improves fertilization owing to fewer broken eggs (Sorenson et al., 1966; Westers, 1986). The use of anesthetics results in less stress to both fish and the culturists handling them. MS-222, methyl pentynol, or a mixture of 1 part trichloro-trimethylpropanol:4 parts ethanol are three anesthetics that have been used.

Females can be spawned using a blood pressure cuff (Sorenson et al., 1966). Anesthetized fish are placed on an inclined rack and the cuff inflated to gently apply pressure and force egg expulsion.

Because male esocids produce low volumes of semen, various refinements have been developed to improve success. Surgical removal of the testes and forcing the semen through cheesecloth increases semen volume (Sorenson et al., 1966; Graff, 1978). Male muskellunge can also be catheterized to obtain urine-free semen without sacrificing the fish. Semen can be refrigerated and stored for up to 5 days before use.

Fertilization is improved by dry fertilization. Sperm are prematurely activated by urine contamination, resulting in lower fertilization rates (Sorenson et al., 1966). The duration of sperm viability increases in a saline diluent (de Montalembert et al., 1978). Saline solutions, including a 5.9-ppt solution of NaCl, prolongs sperm motility and fertilization in Northern pike (Rieniets and Millard, 1987).

Exogenous hormones have been used successfully for both male and female pike. Injecting male Northern pike with 100 mg/kg of progesterone results in a threefold semen volume increase with no effect on spermatocrit or fertilization rate (de Montalembert et al., 1978). Injecting males with 0.1 mg/kg of partially purified salmon gonadotropin results in semen increases up to 11 times that of controls (Billard and Marcel, 1980). Treatment with carp and pike pituitary also results in increased semen production. Carp pituitary has been used with some success to ovulate female esocids at doses ranging from 4.4 to 8.8 mg/kg (Sorenson, 1966; Phillips and Graveen, 1973). Salmon gonadotropin (0.1 mg/kg) results in complete or partial ovulation in female pike (de Montalembert et al., 1978; Billard and Marcel, 1980). Fertilization rates drop the second or third day following ovulation.

Esocid eggs are fragile and should be handled very carefully. Fertilized eggs can be handled 1 hour after fertilization but should not be jarred (Westers, 1986). The eggs are normally incubated in hatching jars, but should not be rolled during the first few days of incubation. Placement of gravel in the hatching jars similar to the method described for percids is recommended to prevent rolling while maintaining high-volume water flow (Westers, 1986).

Optimum incubation temperatures range from 9 to 13°C, but viable fry can be produced at temperatures from 5 to 21°C. Temperatures of 3 and 24°C are lethal for Northern pike embryos and sac fry. Dissolved oxygen should remain near saturation (Westers, 1986).

Daily prophylactic treatments of eggs with formalin (1666 mg/L for 17 minutes or 167 to 250 mg/L for 1 hour) are common during incubation (Sorenson et al., 1966; Pecor, 1978; Westers, 1986).

Approximately 120 degree days and 180 degree days are required to hatch Northern pike and muskellunge eggs, respectively. Yolk-sac absorption and initiation of feeding requires an additional 160 to 180 degree days (Johnson, 1958; Huet, 1972; Westers, 1986). It is advantageous to force-hatch eggs when hatching first begins by rapidly elevating the temperature 5 to 7°C. This reduces overall hatching time significantly (Sorenson et al., 1966; Westers, 1986).

After fry hatch, they are separated from egg shells and other debris and transferred to rearing units. A method for rearing fry in vertical incubators during yolk-sac absorption can eliminate the need to treat for fungi and results in significant savings in man-hours compared to rearing in troughs or tanks (Westers, 1986). Bacterial gill disease is one of the most serious problems in young fry (Graff, 1978). Immediately after feeding begins, the gills are invaded by fungi. Rapid water exchange prevents bacterial infections and avoids problems with gill fungi (Westers, 1986). Northern pike larvae have adhesive papillae on the anterior part of their head that are used to attach to substrates. Various substrates are provided in culture troughs, but the lack of such substrates in incubators does not appear to be detrimental (Westers, 1986).

Culture of Larvae

Esocids have typically been reared in freshwater ponds, although recent advances have resulted in substantially increased intensive culture. Ponds are fertilized with both organic and inorganic fertilizers to promote zooplankton blooms. Swim-up fry are stocked into ponds after the yolk sac is almost gone, at 13 to 21 days of age, depending on temperature (Hess and Heartwell, 1979; Westers, 1986). Muskellunge should be stocked at 16 to 17°C. Recommended stocking rates for fry are 80,000 to 125,000/hectare (Westers, 1986). Climatic factors, such as sudden temperature drops to less than 9°C, can have substantial effect on culture success (Graff, 1978; Westers, 1986). Because esocids are highly voracious and cannibalistic, zooplankton populations in the ponds should be carefully and frequently monitored (Westers, 1986).

Fingerlings are normally harvested when they reach 80 to 100 mm in length. Survival to this size is highly variable, ranging from 0 to more than 50%. Rates of 10 to 20% are generally considered satisfactory for fingerlings about 80 mm long. Culture beyond this size requires very high concentrations of forage fish, but if forage is sufficient, survival increases considerably. Common white sucker fry are usually provided daily at a ratio of 10 suckers to 1 esocid until the suckers can no longer be obtained. Common carp fry or fathead minnows are subsequently fed (Hess and Heartwell, 1979; Westers, 1986). Optimum temperatures for growth of Northern pike range from 19 to 25°C (Westers, 1986).

Substantial progress in intensive culture techniques and the development of artificial diets for esocids have allowed some state hatcheries to go exclusively to intensive culture (Sorenson et al., 1966; Hess and Heartwell, 1979; Westers, 1986). Pennsylvania has cultured esocid fry intensively in tanks for many years. Typically, the procedures involve culturing *Daphnia magna* in special ponds and grading them according to size of the fry. When muskellunge and Northern pike reach about 30 mm and 40 to 45 mm, respectively, appropriately sized fathead minnows are provided at a rate of 10 minnows to 1 fry. Use of graded food appears to reduce differential growth and cannibalism (Sorenson et al., 1966). Esocid fingerlings should be graded as necessary to reduce cannibalism. Prophylactic treatments with formalin at 333 mg/L for 20 minutes are normally provided three times weekly to control fungi and external parasites (Sorenson et al., 1966). Small esocid fingerlings raised intensively to 20 to 30 mm are sometimes stocked in ponds and provided with forage for culture up to 100 to 175 mm.

Successful conversion of Northern pike and tiger muskellunge from live foods to prepared trout starter diets (Graff and Sorenson, 1970) was a momentous discovery that has considerably altered the intensive culture of esocids in many hatcheries. Diets specially formulated to yield adequate nutrition and acceptance by fry and fingerlings have been developed for Northern pike and tiger muskellunge, but success has been limited for muskellunge (Orme, 1978; Pecor, 1978; Westers, 1986).

Fry are most vulnerable while they are being trained to accept prepared diets. Care should be taken not to stress them, and food should be offered at 3- to 5-minute intervals for at least 16 hours daily (Westers, 1986). Preferred feeding temperatures range from 18 to 22°C, with Northern pike preferring the lower range (Westers, 1986). Production and feed conversion of small (30 to 40 mm) tiger muskellunge fingerlings is best at 20 to 22°C, whereas 23°C is best for fingerlings between 120 and 130 mm. Increased dietary protein levels are required by this fish to achieve maximum growth at lower temperatures (Mead et al., 1983; Meade and Lemm, 1986).

In general, culture temperatures for esocids should be relatively constant, and should be maintained below those for optimum growth (23 to 24°C) to reduce problems with pathogens. A highly successful rearing program in Michigan operates at 18°C, but fish are treated daily with formalin (Westers, 1986).

Intensive culture of esocids appears to be more desirable than pond culture and will most likely become the prevalent means of culturing large numbers of fingerlings (Westers, 1986). However, the stress imposed by a highly artificial environment and the close proximity of individuals increases their susceptibility to pathogens. Careful attention must be given to providing proper quantities of food and to maintaining rigorous sanitation procedures (Westers, 1986). Bacteria, particularly *Pseudomonas fluorescens* and *Aeromonas hydrophila*, may cause significant losses (Schachte, 1979). These bacteria were implicated as the cause of total or near-total losses of muskellunge fry over several years in a New York hatchery. Treatment of incoming water supplies with ultraviolet irradiation during incubation and yolk absorption provide effective control of fry losses (Colesante et al., 1981).

Other important bacterial diseases include bacterial gill disease, furunculosis, and columnaris. Other pathogens, such as fungi and a variety of external parasites, can normally be controlled by formalin treatments (Westers, 1986).

LITERATURE CITED

Albrecht, A.B. (1964) Some observations on factors associated with survival of striped bass eggs and larvae. CA Fish Game 50:100–113.

Barkuloo, J.M. (1967) Florida striped bass. Florida Game and Fresh Water Fish Commission Fishery Bulletin 4, Tallahassee.

Bayless, J.D. (1968) Striped bass hatching and hybridization experiments. Proc. Ann. Conf. Southeast. Assoc. Game Fish Commiss. 21:233–244.

Bayless, J.D. (1972) Artificial Propagation and Hybridization of Striped Bass, *Morone saxatilis* (Walbaum). South Carolina Wildlife and Marine Resources Department, Columbia.

Billard, R., and Marcel, J. (1980) Stimulation of spermiation and induction of ovulation in pike (*Esox lucius*). Aquaculture 181–195.

Bishop, R.D. (1968) Evaluation of the striped bass (*Roccus saxatilis*) and white bass (*R. chrvsops*) hybrids after two years. Proc. Ann. Conf. Southeast. Assoc. Game Fish Commiss. 21:245–254.

Bishop, R.D. (1975) The use of circular tanks for spawning striped bass (*Morone saxatilis*). Proc. Ann. Conf. Southeast. Assoc. Game Fish Commiss. 28:35–44.

Bonn, E.W., Bailey, W.M., Bayless, J.D., Erickson, K.E., and Stevens, R.E. (1976) Guidelines for Striped Bass Culture. Striped Bass Committee, Southern Division, American Fisheries Society, Bethesda, Maryland.

Bowman, J.R. (1979) Survival and Growth of Striped Bass, *Morone saxatilis* (Walbaum), Fry Fed Artificial Diets in a Closed Recirculation System. Ph.D. Thesis, Auburn University, Auburn, Alabama.

Brandenburg, A.M., Ray, M.S., and Lewis, W.M. (1979) Use of carp eggs as a feed for fingerling largemouth bass. Progressive Fish Culturist 41:97–98.

Brandt, T.M., Jones, Jr., R.M., and Anderson, R.J. (1987) Evaluation of prepared feeds and attractants for largemouth bass fry. Progressive Fish Culturist 49:198–203.

Braschler, E.W. (1975) Development of pond culture techniques for striped bass *Morone saxatilis* (Walbaum). Proc. Ann. Conf. Southeast. Assoc. Game Fish Commiss. 28:44–48.

Buss, K., Meade III, J., and Graff, D.R. (1978) Reviewing the esocid hybrids. In: Selected Coolwater Fishes of North America (Kendall, R.L., ed.). Special Publication No. 11, American Fisheries Society, Washington, D.C., pp. 210–216.

Carlson, A.R. (1973) Induced spawning of largemouth bass, *Microoterus salmoides* Lacépède. Trans. Am. Fish. Soc. 102:442–444.

Carlson, A.R., and Hale, J.G. (1972) Successful spawning of largemouth bass, *Microoterus salmoides* (Lacépède), under laboratory conditions. Trans. Am. Fish. Soc. 101:539–542.

Carlson, A.R., and Herman, L.J. (1978) Effect of long-term reduction and diel fluctuation in dissolved oxygen on spawning of black crappie, *Pomoxis nigromaculatus*. Trans. Am. Fish. Soc. 107:742–746.

Casselman, J.M. (1978) Effects of environmental factors on growth, survival, activity, and exploitation of northern pike. In: Selected Coolwater Fishes of North America (Kendall, R.L., ed.). Special Publication No. 11. American Fisheries Society, Washington, D.C., pp. 114–128.

Chastain, G.A., and Snow, J.R. (1966) Nylon mats as spawning sites for largemouth bass, *Micropterus salmoides*, Lac. Proc. Ann. Conf. Southeast. Assoc. Game Fish Commiss. 19:405–408.

Clugston, J.P., Oliver, J.L., and Ruelle, R. (1978) Reproduction, growth, and standing crops of yellow perch in southern reservoirs. In: Selected Coolwater Fishes of North America (Kendall, R.L., ed.). Special Publication No. 11. American Fisheries Society, Washington, D.C., pp. 89–99.

Colby, P.J., McNicol, R.E., and Ryder, R.A. (1979) Synopsis of Biological Data on the Walleye *Stizostedion v. vitreum* (Mitchill 1818). FAO Fisheries Synopsis 119. Food and Agriculture Organization of the United Nations, Rome.

Colesante, R.T., Engstrom-Heg, R., Ehlinger, N., and Youmans, N. (1981) Cause and control of muskellunge fry mortality at Chautauqua hatchery 6, New York. Progressive Fish Culturist 43:17–21.

Colesante, R.T., and Youmans, N.B. (1983) Water-hardening walleye eggs with tannic acid in a production hatchery. Progressive Fish Culturist 45:126–127.

Corazza, L., and Nickum, J.G. (1981) Possible effects of phototactic behavior on initial feeding of walleye larvae. In: Proceedings of the Bio-Engineering Symposium for Fish Culture (Allen, L.J., and Kinney, E.C., eds.). Fish Culture Section, American Fisheries Society, and Northeast Society of Conservation Engineers, Bethesda, Maryland, pp. 48–52.

Davies, W.D. (1973a) Rates of temperature acclimation for hatchery reared striped bass fry and fingerlings. Progressive Fish Culturist 35:214–217.

Davis, H.S. (1953) Culture and Diseases of Game Fishes. University of California Press, Los Angeles.

de Montalembert, G., Bry, C., and Billard, R. (1978) Control of reproduction in northern pike. In: Selected Coolwater Fishes of North America (Kendall, R.L., ed.). Special Publication No. 11. American Fisheries Society, Washington, D.C., pp. 217–225.

Doroshev, S.I. (1970) Biological features of the eggs, larvae and young of the striped bass (*Roccus saxatilis* [Walbaum]) in connection with the problem of its acclimatization in the USSR. J. Ichthyol. 10:235–248.

Dudley, R.G., and Eipper, A.W. (1975) Survival of largemouth bass embryos at low dissolved oxygen concentrations. Trans. Am. Fish. Soc. 104:122–128.

Dumas, R.F., and Brand, J.S. (1972) Use of tannin solution in walleye and carp culture. Progressive Fish Culturist 34:7.

Falls, W.W. (1983) Food Habits and Feeding Selectivity of Larvae of the Striped Bass *Morone saxatilis* (Walbaum) (Osteichthyes; Percichthyidae) Under Intensive Culture Conditions. Ph.D. Dissertation, University of Southern Mississippi, Hattiesburg.

Geiger, J.G. (1983) A review of pond zooplankton production and fertilization for the culture of larval and fingerling striped bass. Aquaculture 35:353–369.

Geiger, J.G., and Turner, C.J. (1990) Pond fertilization and zooplankton management techniques for production of fingerling striped bass and hybrid striped bass. In: Culture and Propagation of Striped Bass and Hybrid Striped Bass and Its Hybrids (Harrell, R.M., Kerby, J.H., and Minton, R.V., eds.). Striped Bass Committee, Southern Division, American Fisheries Society, Bethesda, Maryland, pp. 79–98.

Goetz, F.W. (1979) The role of steroids in the control of oocyte final maturation and ovulation in yellow perch (*Perca flavescens*). Proc. Ind. Natl. Sci. Acad. 45:497–504.

Goetz, F.W., and Bergman, H.L. (1978) The effects of steroids on final maturation and ovulation of oocytes from brook trout (*Salvelinus fontinalis*) and yellow perch (*Perca flavescens*). Biol. Reprod. 18:293–298.

Graff, D.R. (1978) Intensive culture of esocids: the current state of the art. In: Selected Coolwater Fishes of North America (Kendall, R.L., ed.).

Special Publication No. 11. American Fisheries Society, Washington, D.C., pp. 195–201.

Graff, D.R., and Sorenson, L. (1970) The successful feeding of a dry diet to esocids. Progressive Fish Culturist 32:31–35.

Harper, J.L., and Jarman, R. (1972) Investigation of striped bass, *Morone saxatilis* (Walbaum), culture in Oklahoma. Proc. Ann. Conf. Southeast. Assoc. Game Fish Commiss. 25:501–512.

Harper, J.L., Jarman, R., and Yacovino, J.T. (1969) Food habits of young striped bass, *Roccus saxatilis* (Walbaum), in culture ponds. Proc. Ann. Conf. Southeast. Assoc. Game Fish Commiss. 22:373–380.

Harrell, R.M., and Bayless, J.D. (1983) Effects of suboptimal dissolved oxygen concentrations on developing striped bass embryos. Proc. Ann. Conf. Southeast. Assoc. Fish Wildlife Agen. 35:508–514.

Harrell, R.M., and Dean, J.M. (1987) Pterygiophore interdigitation patterns and morphometry of larval hybrids of *Morone* species. Trans. Am. Fish. Soc. 116:719–727.

Harrell, R.M., Kerby, J.H., and Minton, R.V. (eds.). (1990) Culture and Propagation of Striped Bass and Its Hybrids. Striped Bass Committee, Southern Division, American Fisheries Society, Bethesda, Maryland.

Harrell, R.M., Loyacano, Jr., H.A., and Bayless, J.D. (1977) Zooplankton availability and feeding selectivity of fingerling striped bass. GA J. Sci. 35:129–135.

Hazel, C.R., Thomsen, W., and Meith, S.J. (1971) Sensitivity of striped bass and stickleback to ammonia in relation to temperature and salinity. CA Fish Game 57:138–153.

Hearn, M.C. (1980) Ovulation of pond-reared walleyes in response to various injection levels of human chorionic gonadotropin. Progressive Fish Culturist 42:228–230.

Heidinger, R.C., and Kayes, T.B. (1986) Yellow perch. In: Culture of Nonsalmonid Freshwater Fishes (Stickney, R.R., ed.). CRC Press, Boca Raton, Florida, pp. 103–113.

Hess, L., and Heartwell, C. (1979) Literature review of large esocids (muskellunge, northern pike, hybrid tiger muskellunge). In: Proceedings of the 10th Warm Water Workshop (Dubé, J., ed.). Northeast Division, American Fisheries Society, Bethesda, Maryland, pp. 139–181.

Hinshaw, J.M. (1985) Effects of illumination and prey contrast on survival and growth of larval yellow perch *Perca flavescens*. Trans. Am. Fish. Soc. 114:540–545.

Hnath, J.G. (1975) A summary of the fish diseases and treatments administered in a cool water diet testing program. Progressive Fish Culturist 37:106–111.

Hokanson, K.E.F. (1977) Temperature requirements of some percids and adaptations to the seasonal temperature cycle. J. Fish. Res. Bd. Can. 34:1524–1550.

Hublou, W.F. (1963) Oregon pellets. Progressive Fish Culturist 25:175–180.

Huet, M. (1972) Textbook of fish culture: Breeding and cultivation of fish. Fishing News Books, Farnham, Surrey, England.

Humphries, E.T., and Cumming, K.B. (1972) Food habits and feeding selectivity of striped bass fingerlings in culture ponds. Proc. Ann. Conf. Southeast. Assoc. Game Fish Commiss. 25:522–536.

Humphries, E.T., and Cumming, K.B. (1973) An evaluation of striped bass fingerling culture. Trans. Am. Fish. Soc. 102:13–20.

Inslee, T.D. (1975) Increased production of smallmouth bass fry. In: Black Bass Biology and Management (Clepper, H., ed.). Sport Fishing Institute, Washington, D.C., pp. 357–361.

Jackson, U.T. (1979) Controlled spawning of largemouth bass. Progressive Fish Culturist 41:90–95.

Johnson, L.J. (1958) Pond Culture of Muskellunge in Wisconsin. Wisconsin Conservation Department Technical Bulletin 17.

Kayes, T.B. (1977) Reproductive biology and artificial propagation methods for adult perch. In: Advisory Report 421 (Soderberg, R.W., ed.). University of Wisconsin Sea Grant College Program, Madison, pp. 6–23.

Kayes, T.B., and Calbert, H.E. (1979) Effects of photoperiod and temperature on the spawning of yellow perch (*Perca flavescens*). J. World Mariculture Soc. 10:306–316.

Kelley, J.W. (1968) Effects of incubation temperature on survival of largemouth bass eggs. Progressive Fish Culturist 30:159–163.

Kerby, J.H. (1972) Feasibility of artificial propagation and introduction of hybrids of the *Morone* complex into estuarine environments, with a meristic and morphometric description of the hybrids. Ph.D. Dissertation, University of Virginia, Charlottesville.

Kerby, J.H. (1986) Striped bass and striped bass hybrids. In: Culture of Nonsalmonid Freshwater Fishes (Stickney, R.R., ed.). CRC Press, Boca Raton, Florida, pp. 127–147.

Kerby, J.H., and Harrell, R.M. (1990) Hybridization, genetic manipulation, and gene pool conservation of striped bass. In: Culture and Propagation of Striped Bass and Its Hybrids (Harrell, R.M., Kerby, J.H., and Minton, R.V., eds.). Striped Bass Committee, Southern Division, American Fisheries Society, Bethesda, Maryland, pp. 159–190.

Kerby, J.H., Woods, III, L.C., and Huish, M.T. (1983) Culture of the striped bass and its hybrids: A review of methods, advances and problems. In: Proceedings of the Warmwater Fish Culture Workshop (Stickney, R.R., and Meyers, S.P., eds.). World Mariculture Society Special Pub-

lication Number 3. Louisiana State University, Baton Rouge, Louisiana, pp. 23–54.

Kerby, J.H., Huish, M.T., Klar, G.T., and Parker, N.C. (1987) Comparative growth and survival of two striped bass hybrids, a backcross, and striped bass in earthen ponds. J. World Aquaculture Soc. 18:10A (abstract).

Kramer, R.H., and Smith, Jr., L.L. (1962) Formation of year classes in largemouth bass. Trans. Am. Fish. Soc. 91:29–41.

Krise, W.F., and Meade, J.W. (1986) Review of the intensive culture of walleye fry. Progressive Fish Culturist 48:81–89.

Krise, W.F., Bulkowski-Cummings, L., Shellman, A.D., Kraus, K.A., and Gould, R.W. (1986) Increased walleye egg hatch and larval survival after protease treatment of eggs. Progressive Fish Culturist 48:95–100.

Lagler, K.F. (1956) Freshwater Fishery Biology. William C. Brown, Dubuque, Iowa.

Lessman, C.A. (1978) Effects of gonadotropin mixtures and two steroids on inducing ovulation in the walleye. Progressive Fish Culturist 40:3–5.

Lewis, W.M., Heidinger, R.C., and Tetzlaff, B.L. (1981) Tank culture of striped bass production manual. Illinois Striped Bass Project IDC F-26-R. Fisheries Research Laboratory, Southern Illinois University, Carbondale.

Manci, W.E., Malison, J.A., Kayes, T.B., and Kuczyski, T.E. (1983) Harvesting photopositive juvenile fish from a pond using a lift net and light. Aquaculture 34:157–164.

Mansueti, A.J. (1964) Early development of the yellow perch *Perca flavescens*. Chesapeake Sci. 5:46–66.

McIlwain, T.D. (1976) Closed circulating system for striped bass production. Proc. World Mariculture Soc. 7:523–534.

Meade, J.W., and Lemm, C.A. (1986) Effects of temperature, diet composition, feeding rate, and cumulative loading level on production of tiger muskellunge. Am. Fish. Soc. Spec. Publ. 15:292–299.

Meade, J.W., Krise, W.F., and Ort, T. (1983) Effect of temperature on production of tiger muskellunge in intensive culture. Aquaculture 32:157–164.

Meshaw, Jr., J.C. (1969) A study of feeding selectivity of striped bass fry and fingerlings in relation to zooplankton availability. Master's Thesis, North Carolina State University, Raleigh, North Carolina.

Miles, R.L. (1978) A life history study of the muskellunge in West Virginia. In: Selected Coolwater Fishes of North America (Kendall, R.L., ed.). Special Publication No. 11. American Fisheries Society, Washington, D.C.

Moorman, R.B. (1957) Reproduction and growth of fishes in Marion Co., Iowa farm ponds. Ia. St. Coll. J. Sci. 32:71–88.

Morgan, II, R.P., Rasin, Jr., V.J., and Capp, R.L. (1981) Temperature and salinity effects on development of striped bass eggs and larvae. Trans. Am. Fish. Soc. 110:95–99.

Muncy, R.J. (1962) Life history of the yellow perch, *Perca flavescens*, in estuarine waters of Severn River, a tributary of Chesapeake Bay, Maryland. Chesapeake Sci. 3:143–159.

Nagel, T.O. (1976) Intensive culture of fingerling walleyes on formulated feeds. Progressive Fish Culturist 38:90–91.

Nelson, W.R., Hines, N.R., and Beckman, L.G. (1965) Artificial propagation of saugers and hybridization with walleyes. Progressive Fish Culturist 27:216–218.

Ney, J.J. (1978) A synoptic review of yellow perch and walleye biology. In: Selected Coolwater Fishes of North America. Special Publication No. 11 (Kendall, R.L., ed.). American Fisheries Society, Washington, D.C., pp. 1–12.

Nicholson, L.C. (1973) Culture of striped bass (*Morone saxatilis*) in raceways under controlled conditions. Proc. Ann. Conf. West. Assoc. St. Game Fish Commiss. 53:393–394.

Nicholson, L.C., Woods, L.C., III, and Woiwode, J.G. (1990) Intensive culture techniques for the striped bass and its hybrids. In: Culture and Propagation of Striped Bass and Its Hybrids (Harrell, R.M., Kerby, J.H., and Minton, R.V., eds.). Striped Bass Committee, Southern Division, American Fisheries Society, Bethesda, Maryland, pp. 141–157.

Nickum, J.G. (1978) Intensive culture of walleyes: the state of the art. In: Selected Coolwater Fishes of North America. Special Publication No. 11 (Kendall, R.L., ed.). American Fisheries Society, Washington, D.C., pp. 187–194.

Nickum, J.G. (1986) Walleye. In: Culture of Nonsalmonid Freshwater Fishes (Stickney, R.R., ed.). CRC Press, Boca Raton, Florida, pp. 115–126.

Orme, L.E. (1978) The status of coolwater fish diets. In: Selected Coolwater Fishes of North America (Kendall, R.L., ed.). Special Publication No. 11. American Fisheries Society, Washington, D.C., pp. 167–171.

Otwell, W.S., and Merriner, J.V. (1975) Survival and growth of juvenile striped bass, *Morone saxatilis* in a factorial experiment with temperature, salinity and age. Trans. Am. Fish. Soc. 104:560–566.

Parker, W.D. (1971) Preliminary studies on sexing adult largemouth by means of an external characteristic. Progressive Fish Culturist 33:55–56.

Parker, N.C. (1979) Striped bass culture in continuously aerated ponds. Proc. Ann. Conf. Southeast. Assoc. Fish Wildlife Agen. 33:353–360.

Parker, N.C. (1984) Culture requirements for striped bass. In: The Aquaculture of Striped Bass: A Proceedings (McCraren, J.P., ed.). Maryland Sea Grant Publication UM-SG-MAP-84-01. University of Maryland, College Park, pp. 29–44.

Pecor, C.H. (1978) Intensive culture of tiger muskellunge in Michigan during 1976 and 1977. In: Selected Coolwater Fishes of North America. Special Publication No. 11 (Kendall, R.L., ed.). American Fisheries Society, Washington, D.C., pp. 202–209.

Phillips, R.A., and Graveen, W.J. (1973) A domestic muskellunge broodstock. Progressive Fish Culturist 35:176–178.

Piper, R.G., McElwain, I.B., Orme, L.E., McCraren, J.P., Fowler, L.G., and Leonard, J.R. (1982) Fish Hatchery Management. U.S. Fish and Wildlife Service, Washington, D.C.

Prentice, J.A., and Dean, W.J. (1979) Effect of temperature on walleye egg hatch rate. Proc. Ann. Conf. Southeast. Assoc. Fish Wildlife Agen. 31:458–462.

Rees, R.A., and Cook, S.F. (1985a) Evaluation of optimum stocking rate of striped bass × white bass fry in hatchery rearing ponds. Proc. Ann. Conf. Southeast. Assoc. Fish Wildlife Agen. 37:257–266.

Rees, R.A., and Cook, S.F. (1985b) Effects of sunlight intensity on survival of striped bass × white bass fry. Proc. Ann. Conf. Southeast. Assoc. Fish Wildlife Agen. 36:83–94.

Rees, R.A., and Harrell, R.M. (1990) Artificial spawning and fry production of striped bass and hybrids. In: Culture and Propagation of Striped Bass and Its Hybrids (Harrell, R.M., Kerby, J.H., and Minton, R.V., eds.). Striped Bass Committee, Southern Division, American Fisheries Society, Bethesda, Maryland, pp. 43–72.

Regan, D.M., Wellborn, Jr., T.L., and Bowker, R.G. (1968) Striped Bass, *Roccus saxatilis* (Walbaum): Development of Essential Requirements for Production. U.S. Fish and Wildlife Service, Atlanta.

Reinitz, G., and Austin, R. (1980) Practical diets for intensive culture of walleyes. Progressive Fish Culturist 42:212–214.

Rieniets, J.P., and Millard, J.L. (1987) Use of saline solutions to improve fertilization of northern pike eggs. Progressive Fish Culturist 49:117–119.

Rottmann, R.W., Shireman, J.V., Starling, C.C., and Revels, W.H. (1988) Eliminating adhesiveness of white bass eggs for the hatchery production of hybrid striped bass. Progressive Fish Culturist 50:55–57.

Sandoz, O., and Johnston, K.H. (1966) Culture of striped bass *Roccus saxatilis* (Walbaum). Proc. Ann. Conf. Southeast. Assoc. Game Fish Commiss. 19:390–394.

Schachte, J.H. (1979) Iodophor disinfection of muskellunge eggs under intensive culture in hatcheries. Progressive Fish Culturist 41:189–190.

Scott, W.B., and Crossman, E.J. (1973) Freshwater Fishes of Canada. Fisheries Research Board of Canada Bulletin 184.

Shannon, E.H. (1970) Effect of temperature changes upon developing striped bass eggs and fry. Proc. Ann. Conf. Southeast. Assoc. Game Fish Commiss. 23:265–274.

Shannon, E.H., and Smith, W.B. (1968) Preliminary observations on the effect of temperature on striped bass eggs and sac fry. Proc. Ann. Conf. Southeast. Assoc. Game Fish Commiss. 21:257–260.

Siefert, R.E., and Herman, L.J. (1977) Spawning success of the black crappie *Pomoxis nigromaculatus* at reduced dissolved oxygen concentrations. Trans. Am. Fish. Soc. 106:376–378.

Siefert, R.E., Carlson, A.R., and Herman, L.J. (1974) Effects of reduced oxygen concentrations on the early life stages of mountain whitefish, smallmouth bass, and white bass. Progressive Fish Culturist 36:186–190.

Simco, B.W., Williamson, J.H., Carmichael, G.J., and Tomasso, J.R. (1986) Centrarchids. In: Culture of Nonsalmonid Freshwater Fishes (Stickney, R.R., ed.). CRC Press, Boca Raton, Florida, pp. 73–89.

Smith, J.M., and Whitehurst, K.D. (1990) Tank spawning methodology for the production of striped bass. In: Culture and Propagation of Striped Bass and Its Hybrids (Harrell, R.M., Kerby, J.H., and Minton, R.V., eds.). Striped Bass Committee, Southern Division, American Fisheries Society, Bethesda, Maryland, pp. 73–77.

Smith, L.L., and Koenst, W.M. (1975) Temperature Effects on Eggs and Fry of Percoid Fishes. U.S. Environmental Protection Agency Report EPA-660/3-75-017.

Smith, T.I.J., and Jenkins, W.E. (1988) Culture and controlled spawning of striped bass (*Morone saxatilis*) to produce striped bass and striped bass × white bass (*Morone chrysops*) hybrids. Proc. Ann. Conf. Southeast. Assoc. Fish Wildlife Agen. 40:152–162.

Smith, W.B., Bonner, W.R., and Tatum, B.L. (1967) Premature egg procurement from striped bass. Proc. Ann. Conf. Southeast. Assoc. Game Fish Commiss. 20:324–330.

Snow, J.R. (1968) The Oregon moist pellet as a diet for largemouth bass. Progressive Fish Culturist 30:235.

Snow, J.R. (1970) Culture of the largemouth bass. In: Report of the 1970 Workshop on Fish Feed Technology and Nutrition. Resource Publication 102, U.S. Bureau of Sport Fisheries and Wildlife, Washington, D.C., pp. 86–102.

Snow, J.R. (1971) Fecundity of largemouth bass, *Micropterus salmoides* (Lacépède), receiving artificial food. Proc. Ann. Conf. Southeast. Assoc. Game Fish Commiss. 24:550–559.

Snow, J.R. (1973) Controlled culture of largemouth bass fry. Proc. Ann. Conf. Southeast. Assoc. Game Fish Commiss. 26:392–398.

Snow, J.R. (1975) Hatchery propagation of the black bass. In: Black Bass Biology and Management (Clepper, H., ed.). Sport Fishing Institute, Washington, D.C., pp. 344–356.

Snow, J.R., Jones, R.O., and Rogers, W.A. (1964) Training Manual of Warm-Water Fish Culture. Bureau of Sport Fisheries and Wildlife, Washington, D.C.

Sorenson, L., Buss, K., and Bradford, A.D. (1966) The artificial propagation of esocid fishes in Pennsylvania. Progressive Fish Culturist 28:133–141.

Starling, C.C. (1983) Fish Hatcheries Review and Annual Progress Report for 1983–84. Florida Game and Fresh Water Fish Commission, Tallahassee.

Starling, C.C. (1985) Striped bass × white bass *Morone* spp. hybrids (sunshine bass) production at Florida state fish hatcheries. In: Fish Hatcheries Review and Annual Report for 1984–1985. Florida Game and Fresh Water Fish Commission, Tallahassee, pp. 65–112.

Stevens, R.E. (1966) Hormone-induced spawning of striped bass for reservoir stocking. Progressive Fish Culturist 28:19–28.

Stevens, R.E. (1967) A final report on the use of hormones to ovulate striped bass, *Roccus saxatilis* (Walbaum). Proc. Ann. Conf. Southeast. Assoc. Game Fish Commiss. 18:525–538.

Stevens, R.E. (1970) Hormonal relationships affecting maturation and ovulation in largemouth bass *Micropterus salmoides* (Lacépède). Ph.D. Dissertation. North Carolina State University, Raleigh, North Carolina.

Talbot, G.B. (1966) Estuarine environmental requirements and limiting factors for striped bass. In: A Symposium on Estuarine Fisheries. American Fisheries Society, Special Publication 3 (Smith, R.F., Swartz, A.H., and Massman, W.H., eds.). American Fisheries Society, Washington, D.C., pp. 37–49.

Tebo, Jr., L.B., and McCoy, E.G. (1964) Effect of sea-water concentration on the reproduction and survival of largemouth bass. Progressive Fish Culturist 26:99–106.

Theofan, G., and Goetz, F.W. (1983) The in vitro synthesis of final maturational steroids by ovaries of brook trout (*Salvelinus fontinalis*) and yellow perch (*Perca flavescens*). Gen. Comp. Endocrinol. 51:84–95.

Toetz, D.W. (1966) The changes from endogenous to exogenous sources of energy in bluegill sunfish larvae. Invest. Ind. Lakes Streams 7:115–146.

Trandahl, A. (1978) Preface. In: Selected Coolwater Fishes of North America (Kendall, R.L., ed.). American Fisheries Society, Washington, D.C., pp. ix–x.

Turner, J.L., and Farley, T.C. (1971) Effects of temperature, salinity, and dissolved oxygen on the survival of striped bass eggs and larvae. CA Fish Game 57:268–273.

Waltemyer, D.L. (1976) Tannin as an agent to eliminate adhesiveness of walleye eggs during artificial propagation. Trans. Am. Fish. Soc. 105:731–736.

Ware, F.J. (1975) Progress with *Morone* hybrids in fresh water. Proc. Ann. Conf. Southeast. Assoc. Game Fish Commiss. 28:48–54.

West, G., and Leonard, J. (1978) Culture of yellow perch with emphasis on development of eggs and fry. In: Selected Coolwater Fishes of North America (Kendall, R.L., ed.). Special Publication No. 11. American Fisheries Society, Washington, D.C., pp. 172–176.

Westers, H. (1986) Northern pike and muskellunge. In: Culture of Nonsalmonid Freshwater Fishes (Stickney, R.R., ed.). CRC Press, Boca Raton, Florida, pp. 91–101.

Wilbur, R.L., and Langford, F. (1975) Use of human chorionic gonadotropin (HCG) to promote gametic production in male and female largemouth bass. Proc. Ann. Conf. Southeast. Assoc. Game Fish Commiss. 28:242–250.

Willis, D.W., and Flickinger, S.A. (1981) Intensive culture of largemouth bass fry. Trans. Am. Fish. Soc. 110:650–655.

Wrenn, W.B., and Grannemann, K.L. (1980) Effects of temperature on bluegill reproduction and young-of-the-year standing stocks in experimental ecosystems. In: Microcosms in Ecological Research (Giesy, J.P., ed.). Technical Information Center, U.S. Department of Energy, Symposium Series 52 (CONF-781101), pp. 703–714.

Chapter 24

BACTERIAL DISEASES OF TEMPERATE FRESHWATER AND ESTUARINE FISHES

EDWARD J. NOGA

Temperate freshwater and estuarine fishes may inhabit a wide range of environments, including widely varying temperatures and salinity. As such, they are apt to encounter a diverse array of bacterial pathogens (Tables 24–1 and 24–2). This is especially true in estuaries, which represent an interface between marine and freshwater ecosystems. While a general-purpose medium such as trypticase soy agar, brain heart infusion agar, or blood agar is usually suitable for isolating most pathogens in low-salinity (less than 10 ppt) environments, the addition of 1 to 3% NaCl or 30 to 100% seawater is usually advisable to recover halophilic organisms. Not all differential media used for freshwater organisms are reliable in estuarine environments. For example, Rimmler-Shotts medium (Shotts and Rimmler, 1973), a useful selective medium for identifying *Aeromonas hydrophila* in freshwater, cannot differentiate between *A. hydrophila* and some vibrios in estuarine waters (Kaper et al., 1981).

EUBACTERIAL MENINGITIS

SYNONYM. *Catenabacterium* sp. infection.

Host and Geographic Distribution

Eubacterium tarantellus has been reported from several species of estuarine fishes from the northern Gulf of Mexico (Henley and Lewis, 1976) and southeast Florida (Udey et al., 1977) (see Tables 24–1 and 24–2).

Clinical Signs

Eubacterium tarantellus has caused epidemics of neurologic disease in fish of all ages, although most epidemics have primarily involved mature individuals. Experimental infections have a slow onset, with clinical signs developing 14 to 30 days after challenge. Affected fish are darkly pigmented and appear disoriented. Some swim while rotating along their long axis. Some fish may be either hypopneic and lie quiescent on the bottom or assume a vertical, head-up, floating position.

Diagnosis

Presumptive diagnosis is based on the observation of filamentous, gram-positive rods in brain

TABLE 24–1. Bacterial Diseases of Temperate Freshwater and Estuarine Fishes

Disease	Bacteria	Host(s)
Eubacterial meningitis	*Eubacterium tarantellus*	Striped mullet, snook, flounder, redfish
Columnaris disease	*Flexibacter columnaris*	All freshwater fishes
Pasteurellosis	*Pasteurella piscicida*	*Morone* spp., Atlantic menhaden, striped mullet
Edwardsiellosis	*Edwardsiella tarda*	Striped bass, striped mullet, eels, largemouth bass
Furunculosis	*Aeromonas salmonicida*	Eels, *Morone* spp., lamprey, smallmouth bass, Northern pike, yellow perch, brook stickleback, sablefish
Streptococcosis	*Streptococcus* spp.	Striped mullet, Atlantic menhaden, pinfish, Atlantic croaker, spot, sea trout
Epitheliocystis	Chlamydialike agent	Bluegill, gray mullet, striped bass, white perch

TABLE 24–2. Bacterial Diseases Reported in North American Temperate Freshwater and Estuarine Fishes*

Agent	Disease	Species	Ecological Location†	References
Anaerobes				
Eubacterium tarantellus	Eubacterial meningitis	Striped mullet	ES	Udey et al. (1977)
		Snook		"
		Gulf flounder		"
		Red drum		"
Aerobes—Gram-Positive Rods				
Mycobacterium marinum	Mycobacteriosis	Striped bass	FW	Hedrick et al. (1987)
Aerobes—Gram-Positive Cocci				
Streptococcus sp.	Streptococcosis	Gulf menhaden	ES	Plumb et al. (1974)
		Striped mullet		"
		Pinfish		"
		Atlantic croaker		"
		Spot		"
		Silver sea trout		"
		Bluefish		Baya et al. (1990a)
		Striped bass		"
		Weakfish		"
Aerobes–Aeromonads/Vibrios/ Pseudomonads				
Aeromonas hydrophila	Red-sore disease, Motile *Aeromonas* septicemia	Striped bass	FW, ES	Miller and Chapman (1976)
		White bass		"
		White perch		"
		Gizzard shad		"
		Redbreast sunfish		"
		Green sunfish		"
		Warmouth		"
		Bluegill		"
		Redear sunfish		"
		Largemouth bass		"
		Walleye		
Aeromonas sobria		Gizzard shad		Toranzo et al. (1989)
Aeromonas salmonicida	Ulcer disease Furunculosis	Sablefish	FW, ES	Hall (1963)
		Yellow bass		Herman (1968)
		American eel		"
		Smallmouth bass		Noga and Berkhoff (1990)
		Northern pike		LeTendre et al. (1972)
		Yellow perch		Economon (1960)
		Brook stickleback		McFadden (1970)
		Striped bass × white bass		Noga (unpublished data)
Vibrio anguillarum	Vibriosis	Striped bass	ES	Toranzo et al. (1983)
Pseudomonas sp.		Muskellunge	FW	Colesante et al. (1981)
Aerobes—Enterobacteriaceae				
Edwardsiella tarda	Edwardsiellosis	American eel	FW	Bullock and Herman (1985)
		Striped bass		"
		Striped mullet		"
		Largemouth bass		
Aerobes—Gram-Negative Pigmented Rods				
Flexibacter columnaris	Columnaris	Bluegill	FW	Davis (1922)
		Basses		"
		Yellow perch		"
		White bass		"
		Striped bass		Mitchell (1984)
		Gizzard shad		Isom (1960)
		Mummichog		Nigrelli and Hutner (1945)
Aerobes—Miscellaneous				
Pasteurella piscicida	Pasteurellosis	Striped bass	ES	Hawke et al. (1987)
		White perch		Snieszko et al. (1964)
		Menhadens		Lewis et al. (1970)
		Striped mullet		"
Moraxella sp.		Striped bass		Baya et al. (1990b)

*Many of these diseases may also occur in the marine environment (e.g., vibriosis, Streptococcus spp., M. marinum).
†ES = estuaries; FW = fresh water.

smears of fish showing typical clinical signs. Spinal cord and liver also appear to be major targets of infection. Definitive diagnosis is based on immunodiagnosis or culture characteristics. All isolates are antigenically similar and can be identified by direct fluorescent antibody.

Culture and Identification

Eubacterium tarantellus is an asporogenous anaerobe. Primary isolation requires the use of anaerobic media such as fluid thioglycolate medium with 1% NaCl and 100 μg/mL gentamicin incubated at 20°C. Culture on sheep or bovine blood agar with 100 μg/ml gentamicin produces colonies in 3 to 5 days that are β-hemolytic and arborescent. Other key features include production of lecithinase and deoxyribonuclease (DNAase), weak fermentation of glucose, fructose, and lactose, and the presence of acetate, lactate, and pyruvate in fermentation products, as determined by gas chromatography.

Transmission, Epidemiology, and Pathogenesis

The mode of transmission of *Eubacterium tarantellus* is uncertain. Direct fish-to-fish transmission has not been demonstrated, suggesting that ectoparasites may be important vectors. The organism has been found subclinically in several marine and estuarine fishes, which may act as reservoirs. The disease usually first appears sometime between December and April and then occurs sporadically until August. Outbreaks are most severe in May through June in the Gulf of Mexico and in December through February in southern Florida.

Treatment and Control

Intraperitoneal chloramphenicol injection is reported to be curative of eubacterial meningitis, although its efficacy in crossing the blood-brain barrier in fish is unknown. Oral administration of erythromycin, chloramphenicol, chlortetracycline, oxytetracycline, or novobiocin eliminates clinical signs of the disease from experimentally infected fish, but does not eliminate the infection from brain or liver (Lewis and Udey, 1978).

COLUMNARIS DISEASE

SYNONYMS. Peduncle disease, saddleback, fin rot, cotton wool disease.

Host and Geographic Distribution

Flexibacter columnaris (*Chondrococcus columnaris, Bacillus columnaris*) appears to have a worldwide distribution in fresh water and can probably infect most freshwater fishes (see Tables 24–1 and 24–2).

Clinical Signs

Flexibacter columnaris is most commonly associated with erosive or necrotic skin and gill lesions, which may become systemic. It typically presents as an acute infection, with lesions on the head, back (saddleback lesion), and/or fins, especially the caudal fin. Lesions typically begin as white plaques, which may have a red periphery. Lesions rapidly (often within 24 hours) progress to ulcers, which may be yellow or orange due to masses of pigmented bacteria. Ulcerations spread by radial expansion and may penetrate into muscle, eventually producing a bacteremia. Gill infections can cause severe necrosis and are very virulent. A less common peracute syndrome presents as a sudden death with systemic infection.

Diagnosis

Rapid presumptive identification of *Flexibacter columnaris* can be made by examining wet mounts of lesions, which have long, thin rods (0.50 to 1.0 × 4 to 10 μm) with a peculiar flexing or gliding motion. Organisms may aggregate into masses of writhing bacteria that appear like columns or haystacks on wet mounts (Fig. 24–1). Definitive diagnosis is based on biochemical tests or agglutination, although po-

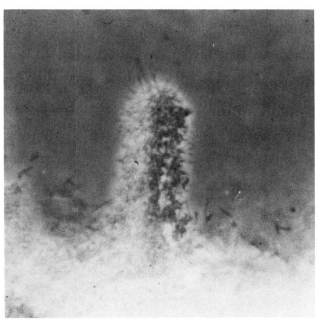

FIGURE 24–1. Wet mount of a lesion infected with *Columnaris* sp. showing the classic "haystack" appearance of aggregated bacteria. (From Noga, E.J. [1988] Determining the relationship between water quality and infectious disease in fishery populations. Water Resources Bull. 24:967–973.)

tential cross-reactivity with related organisms has not been fully determined. Some strains autoagglutinate. This is remedied by sonication or heating to 50°C for 5 minutes.

Culture and Identification

Culture of *F. columnaris* is best done at room temperature using media with a low nutrient and high moisture content (cytophaga agar [Anaker and Ordal, 1959]; a 1:10 dilution of nutrient broth in 1% agar is also satisfactory). Selective media containing antibiotics can also be used to enhance isolation (Bullock et al., 1986). These gram-negative bacteria form colonies that are usually orange- or yellow-pigmented, rhizoid, and spreading.

Transmission, Epidemiology, and Pathogenesis

Flexibacter columnaris is a very important fish pathogen in warm-water environments. It can rapidly infect a population and cause large mortalities (Becker and Fujihara, 1978; Fijan, 1968; Chen et al., 1982). *Flexibacter columnaris* is most pathogenic in high (greater than 18°C) water temperatures, especially when temperatures are suddenly increased. There is no apparent relationship between serotype and virulence. Virulence mechanisms are unclear, but the mineral content of the water may be very important. Other risk factors include low dissolved oxygen (Chen et al., 1982), hard, alkaline water (Fijan, 1968), organic pollution (Fijan, 1968), and high nitrite levels (Hanson and Grizzle, 1985). Exposure to high arsenic levels increases the susceptibility of striped bass to columnaris (MacFarlane et al., 1986). Lesions often begin at sites of previous injury (net damage, etc.).

Strain virulence and water temperature are usually considered to be the most important factors determining severity of columnaris disease, but the importance of mineral content to pathogenicity should not be ignored. In experimental trials, *Flexibacter columnaris* is nonpathogenic in distilled water and most pathogenic in a combination of salts having 14.9 ppm Na^+, 1.4 ppm K^+, 22.1 ppm Ca^{2+}, and 4.5 ppm Mg^{2+} as chloride salts, equivalent to a total hardness of 33.3 ppm as $CaCO_3$ (Chowdhury and Wakabayashi, 1988b). These data parallel the survival of the bacterium in various waters (Chowdhury and Wakabayashi, 1988a). Surprisingly, survival is poor in $CaCl_2$ levels greater than 55 ppm even though *Flexibacter columnaris* is considered most pathogenic in hard water (Fijan, 1968).

Treatment and Control

Early cases of columnaris may be successfully treated with waterborne treatments such as disinfectant dips (e.g., quaternary ammonium) or prolonged immersion in potassium permanganate or copper sulfate. However, advanced cases warrant systemic antibiotics. Most strains are susceptible to oxytetracycline, but not to ormetoprim-sulfadimethoxine (Anonymous, 1986). Vaccination may be feasible, since convalescent fish are resistant to reinfection. Medical therapy must always be accompanied by an improvement in environment.

OTHER YELLOW-PIGMENTED BACTERIA

Not all flexibacteria associated with fish disease are actually *Flexibacter columnaris*. Several different *Flexibacter* spp. may be involved (Pyle and Shotts, 1980, 1981; Starliper et al., 1988). In addition, a large number of other yellow-pigmented gram-negative bacterial rods have been isolated from fish epithelial lesions, including *Cytophaga, Flavobacterium, Sporocytophaga,* and "*Myxobacterium.*" Most notable among these are *Cytophaga psychrophila (Flexibacter aurianticus),* the cause of cold-water disease in salmonids, and *Flavobacterium branchiophila,* a cause of proliferative gill disease (Wakabayashi et al., 1989). There are also increasing reports of columnarislike infections in marine fishes (Wakabayashi et al., 1986). It is likely that new taxa will continue to emerge.

Isolation methods for these bacteria are similar to those for *Flexibacter columnaris* except that salt or seawater should be added to media when attempting isolations from high-salinity environments. Both *Flexibacter* and *Cytophaga* spp. exhibit gliding motility, whereas flavobacteria are nonmotile. Key differentiating features of the currently known pathogens have been summarized by Austin and Austin (1987). Susceptibility to antibiotic therapy is not well known for many of these yellow-pigmented bacteria; however, there is evidence that oxytetracycline, among other antibiotics, may be effective. It is likely that many of the yellow-pigmented bacteria infecting fish may occur naturally in healthy fish and in aquatic ecosystems, since many can be routinely isolated from such sources.

PASTEURELLOSIS

SYNONYMS. Tuberculosis, pseudotuberculosis.

Host and Geographic Distribution

Pasteurella piscicida has caused epidemics in white perch and striped bass in Chesapeake Bay (Snieszko et al., 1964; Paperna and Zwerner, 1976), striped bass in Long Island Sound (Robohm, 1983), striped bass from culture ponds in coastal Alabama (Hawke et al., 1987), and gulf menhaden in Galveston Bay, Texas (Lewis et al., 1970) (see Table 24–2). Its common presence in Japan suggests that it is widely distributed.

Clinical Signs

Pasteurella piscicida causes a bacteremic septicemia that takes one of two forms. In the acute form, few clinical signs are present, ranging from small hemorrhages around the gill covers or the bases of the fins in white perch (Snieszko et al., 1964) to abnormal skin pigmentation and enlarged spleens and kidneys in striped bass (Hawke et al., 1987). Histologically, there is acute necrosis of the spleen, liver, and pancreas with no inflammation.

In the chronic form, striped bass show 1- to 2-mm miliary lesions in the kidney and spleen that represent a chronic inflammatory response incited by bacteria. The appearance of this latter lesion has led to the names tuberculosis or pseudotuberculosis for this disease in cultured yellowtail.

Diagnosis

Presumptive diagnosis of *Pasteurella piscida* is based on observation of gram-negative, nonpigmented, nonmotile rods (0.5 to 0.75 $\times$ 1 to 2 μm), which stain bipolarly. Confirmatory diagnosis can be performed using slide agglutination or immunofluorescence.

Culture and Identification

The agent of pasteurellosis can be isolated from affected organs, especially kidney and spleen, using nutrient agar at room temperature. Shiny gray-yellow, entire, convex, 1- to 2-mm colonies develop after 48 to 72 hours. In culture, *Pasteurella piscida* most closely resembles nonpigmenting strains of *Aeromonas salmonicida*. Gelatinase is not produced and acid, but no gas, is produced with glucose media.

Transmission, Epidemiology, and Pathogenesis

The mode of transmission of *Pasteurella piscicida* is unknown, although fish-to-fish contact and an invertebrate vector have both been suggested. The reservoir of infection is uncertain, although striped bass are believed to be the major source of infection in the Chesapeake Bay. There is evidence that host susceptibility varies significantly, since spotted seatrout, red drum, gulf killifish, striped mullet, sheepshead minnow, pinfish, and sheepshead were not clinically affected during a striped bass epidemic (Hawke et al., 1987). Risk factors include high (greater than 10 ppt) salinity and high (greater than 25°C) temperatures.

Treatment and Control

Oxytetracycline was not very effective in controlling an outbreak of pasteurellosis in striped bass;

however, this was felt to be due to inadequate tissue levels attained in target organs, not resistance of the bacterial isolate (Hawke et al., 1987). Experimental infections in yellowtail have been controlled by ampicillin (Kusuda and Inoue, 1977) and sulfisozole/trimethoprim (Fujihara et al., 1984). Experimental vaccines also show promise (Fukuda and Kusuda, 1981).

EDWARDSIELLOSIS

SYNONYM. *Paracolobactrum anguillimortiferum* infection.

Host and Geographic Distribution

Edwardsiella tarda (called formerly *E. anguillimortifera*) is an economically important problem in channel catfish in the United States (Waltman et al., 1986). While not yet reported from American eels, it causes serious losses in Japanese eels (Waltman et al., 1986). The bacterium has been isolated from the gastrointestinal tract of numerous cold-blooded animals, from mussels to alligators. Reptiles and amphibians are especially common carriers (Waltman et al., 1986). It has caused disease in catfish, eels, goldfish, grass carp, Pacific salmon, and aquarium fish. Up to 100% of the crayfish, frogs, and turtles in ponds having infected catfish are infected with *E. tarda* (Wyatt, 1979).

Clinical Signs

Clinical signs of edwardsiellosis vary with the species affected. Lesions commonly have masses of bacteria, both surrounded by inflammatory cells and free within lesions. In channel catfish, lesions are initially seen as small 3- to 5-mm red cutaneous lesions on the flanks and caudal peduncle. They are caused by fistulas originating deep in the muscle that extend from malodorous fluctuant subdermal abscesses. There is also petechiation and malodorous liquefactive necrosis of the viscera with fibrinous peritonitis. Characteristically, fish may continue to eat even when severely affected.

Japanese eels exhibit one of two forms (Miyazaki and Egusa, 1976a,b). The nephric form (suppurative interstitial nephritis) is most common and is associated with necrotic renal foci that spread to the spleen, liver, gills, stomach, and heart. In the hepatic form (suppurative hepatitis), microabscesses form in the liver and spread to other organs. These lesions appear as light-colored nodules on the viscera. Abscesses may ulcerate through the body musculature.

In striped bass, unusual features include epithelial hyperplasia, which can give the fish a tattered appearance, and necrosis in the lateral line and on the body surface and gills (Herman and Bullock, 1986). Anemia and hypoxia also occur.

Diagnosis

Definitive diagnosis of pasteurellosis is based on standard biochemical tests and agglutination. Fluorescent antibody has also been used to identify the pathogen in tissues (Amandi et al., 1982).

Culture and Identification

Edwardsiella tarda can be isolated from affected tissues, especially the kidney, using trypticase soy agar. However, the frequent inability of *Edwardsiella tarda* to grow in selenite brilliant green or tetrathionate broth enrichments indicates that *Salmonella* isolation methods are inappropriate (Waltman et al., 1986). Isolates grow best at 37°C, but will appear after 2 to 4 days at 25°C as small, gray, circular, transparent colonies composed of motile gram-negative rods. Diagnostic biochemical features include lack of cytochrome oxidase activity and fermentation of glucose with production of acid and gas. Production of indol, a positive methyl red reaction and motility at 37°C, differentiates *E. tarda* from *E. ictaluri*, the only other member of *Edwardsiella* pathogenic to fish (Shotts and Teska, 1989). *Edwardsiella tarda* is a relatively homogeneous genus-species that has limited biochemical or enzymatic capabilities.

Transmission, Epidemiology, and Pathogenesis

Edwardsiella tarda is an important zoonotic problem and is a serious cause of enteric disease in humans. It can be isolated from the urine and feces of many mammals, including man (Clarridge et al., 1980) and marine mammals (Coles et al., 1978), although it is typically associated with freshwater environments. In humans, it has been implicated in meningitis, liver abscesses, wound infections, and most commonly gastroenteritis. The bacterium is often recovered from catfish fillets in processing plants and may spread to man via the oral route.

Transmission and the source of *E. tarda* infection during outbreaks in fish are uncertain, although it is known to remain dormant in fish tissues. Carrion-eating birds may also be an important source of infection (Winsor et al., 1981).

The organism is highly pathogenic under the proper conditions, including high temperatures (greater than 30°C) and organic pollution. It can cause high mortalities. Hemolysin and chondroitin sulfate activities may play roles in the pathogenesis of the disease.

Treatment and Control

As with many fish bacterial pathogens, *Edwardsiella tarda* is associated with polluted environments.

Thus, systemic antibiotic treatment (oxytetracycline) should be accompanied by an improvement in water quality. Some strains of *Edwardsiella tarda* are resistant to tetracyclines (Hilton and Wilson, 1980). Drug-resistant strains of *Edwardsiella tarda* carrying transferrable R-plasmids appear at high frequency in cultured Japanese eels (Aoki et al., 1987).

FURUNCULOSIS

SYNONYM. Ulcer disease.

Host and Geographic Distribution

While *Aeromonas salmonicida* has been classically associated with a bacterial septicemia of salmonids, it is also a very important pathogen of nonsalmonid fishes (see Tables 24–1 and 24–2).

Clinical Signs

The classic lesion of furunculosis in nonsalmonid fishes is the skin ulcer. This has led to the common term, ulcer disease. Skin lesions may vary grossly from white discolorations to shallow hemorrhagic ulcers to deep lesions that expose underlying muscle or bone. Lesions are often secondarily infected with other agents, including other bacteria and fungi.

Unlike typical furunculosis of salmonids, *Aeromonas salmonicida* infections in nonsalmonid fishes are often localized to the skin (Fig. 24–2) and may only become systemic in the late stages of the disease. Such was the case for ulcer disease outbreaks in wild smallmouth bass (LeTendre et al., 1972) and in American eels (Noga and Berkhoff, 1990).

Infections in eels begin as depigmented foci, which spread to form large patches of necrotic skin

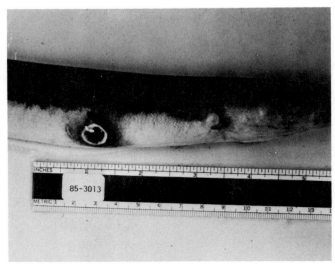

FIGURE 24–2. Ulcer disease in an American eel. Note skin ulcer on the flank.

up to 16 cm² in area. The depigmented patches detach at the dermoepidermal junction, forming large ulcers that rapidly expose underlying muscle. The infection commonly affects the head, producing cranial swelling and corneal edema. A mild to severe, primarily mononuclear infiltrate is seen, most prominently in large ulcers. Many lesions have extensive collagen deposition, which contributes to the tissue swelling. Both feral and impounded eels have been affected. A similar disease has also been described in European and Japanese eels.

Systemic lesions are common in some cases of nonsalmonid furunculosis (McFadden, 1970). Posttraumatic septicemia of yellow bass is similar to peracute or acute furunculosis, with organisms in the internal organs in the early stages (Bulkley, 1969). Major features include depression, high mortality, and secondary fungal infection of the skin.

Diagnosis

While *Aeromonas salmonicida* subspecies *salmonicida* ("typical" salmonicida) has been isolated from some outbreaks, many cases are associated with "atypical" strains that do not conform to the typical biochemical profile for this species. Definitive diagnosis requires immunologic confirmation such as by latex bead agglutination or fluorescent antibody (Austin and Austin, 1987).

Culture and Identification

Atypical strains of *Aeromonas salmonicida* are often fastidious, and thus it is best that an enriched medium such as brain-heart infusion agar or blood agar be used for primary isolation from ulcer disease lesions. Opportunists such as *Aeromonas hydrophila* can rapidly outcompete *Aeromonas salmonicida*, so primary cultures must be watched carefully daily. It is advisable to sample at least six fish, especially those with early lesions, where the primary pathogen is more likely to be isolated. Colonies are typically small, circular, gray, and up to 1.5 mm in diameter after 4 to 7 days at room temperature. Characteristically, colonies can be "pushed" along the agar surface with an inoculating loop (Shotts and Teska, 1989). Depending upon the strain, pigment may not be produced or may be inhibited owing to the presence of competing opportunists. Thus, pigmentation cannot be relied upon for presumptive identification.

Treatment and Control

Treatment has not been attempted in most cases of nonsalmonid furunculosis, although many *Aeromonas salmonicida* isolates are sensitive to oxytetracycline and potentiated sulfonamides. Interestingly, addition of estuarine water reduces morbidity in eels held in freshwater impoundments in North Carolina.

STREPTOCOCCOSIS

SYNONYMS. Popeye, yellowtail disease, streptococcicosis.

Host and Geographic Distribution

Streptococcosis has been associated with acute to chronic mortalities of several estuarine fishes in coastal Alabama and Florida (Plumb et al., 1974) (see Table 24–1).

Clinical Signs

Fishes dying of streptococcosis display a disoriented, whirling motion at the surface. There are hemorrhages on the operculum, around the mouth, at the base of the fins, and around the anus. The abdomen is often distended with serosanguineous fluid, and exophthalmia is observed. The liver is pale, and the spleen is deep red. Serosanguineous fluid is present in the intestine.

Diagnosis

Presumptive diagnosis of streptococcosis is based on clinical signs and the observation of grampositive cocci in internal organs. Definitive diagnosis requires the determination of cultural characteristics of the isolate and serology.

Culture and Identification

The agent of streptococcosis is easily cultured on blood agar or brain-heart infusion agar, producing dull gray, 1- to 2-mm colonies after 48 hours at 22 to 37°C. Lancefield groupings of isolates vary (see Chap. 78).

Transmission, Epidemiology, and Pathogenesis

Ingestion and water-borne transmission of streptococci may both be important. These organisms can survive in the environment, so stress may be important in precipitating clinical disease. Similar organisms are known human pathogens (Wilkinson et al., 1973), but the zoonotic importance of fish isolates is uncertain.

Treatment and Control

Studies with yellowtail in Japan, where streptococcosis is a very serious problem, showed that oral erythromycin was more effective than either oxytetracycline or ampicillin (Shiomitsu et al., 1980).

OTHER BACTERIAL AGENTS

Vibriosis has been reported in striped bass in the Chesapeake Bay (Toranzo et al., 1983) and is probably capable of infecting a wide range of other species in this ecologic group. What was tentatively considered a *Moraxella* sp. was identified as the cause of a bacterial septicemia in feral striped bass in the Chesapeake Bay (Baya et al., 1990b). *Aeromonas hydrophila* has been associated with widespread epidemic skin lesions, especially in the southeastern United States. Although red-sore lesions have been classically attributed to a primary *Aeromonas hydrophila* infection followed by a secondary infestation of the protozoan *Epistylis* (Esch and Hazen, 1980), there is evidence that many skin lesions attributed to red-sore may actually be due to one of several different types of parasitic infestation (Noga, 1986) (see Table 24–2).

EPITHELIOCYSTIS

SYNONYM. Mucophilosis.

Host and Geographic Distribution

Epitheliocystis is a chronic disease of varying pathogenicity that has been reported from several freshwater and marine fishes worldwide, including bluegill, gray mullet, striped bass, and white perch (Herman and Wolf, 1987).

Clinical Signs

In epitheliocystis, the gills and, rarely, the skin are the primary target organs. Lesions present as white miliary nodules up to 1 mm in diameter on the skin or gills.

Diagnosis

The lesions of epitheliocystis may grossly resemble those produced by *Ichthyophthirius multifiliis*, those associated with lymphocystis, or other nodular skin lesions, but they are easily distinguished with histopathology. Epitheliocystis infects skin and gill epithelial cells, resulting in the cells enlarging to 20 to 400 μm in diameter. The hypertrophic nucleus and cytoplasm are peripheral to a granular basophilic inclusion containing large numbers of coccoid or coccobacillary bodies (Fig. 24–3). Histologically, the

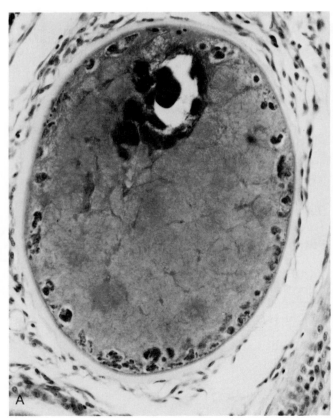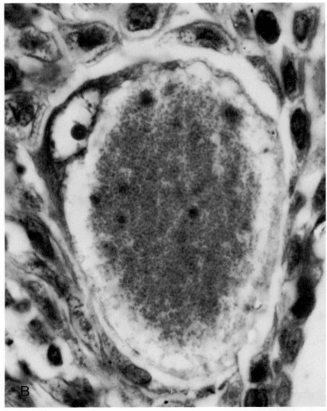

FIGURE 24–3. Histological sections comparing cells infected with epitheliocystis (*A*) and lymphocystis (*B*). (From Herman, R.L., and Wolf, K. [1987] Epitheliocystis infection in fishes. FDL #75, U.S.D.O.I., F.W.S., Div. of Fisheries and Wetlands Research, Washington, D.C.)

major differential is lymphocystis virus infection, which can be distinguished based upon its infection of dermal fibroblasts, the presence of irregular inclusions, and an undisplaced nucleus.

Culture and Identification

Epitheliocystis is tentatively considered to be caused by a chlamydialike organism, although it has never been cultured to confirm this hypothesis.

Transmission, Epidemiology, and Pathogenesis

When present in small numbers, the agent of epitheliocystis may be an incidental finding, but in high concentrations it has been associated with considerable mortality. Details of the organism's life cycle and pathogenesis are largely unknown.

Treatment and Control

There is no known treatment for epitheliocystis. Disinfection and quarantine are the only methods for control.

LITERATURE CITED

Amandi, A., Hiu, S.F., Rohovec, J.S., and Fryer, J.L. (1982) Isolation and characterization of *Edwardsiella tarda* from chinook salmon (*Oncorhynchus tsawyscha*). Appl. Environ. Microbiol. 43:1380–1384.

Anaker, R.L., and Ordal, E.L. (1959) Studies on the myxobacterium *Chondrococcus columnaris*. 1. Serological typing. J. Bacteriol. 78:25–32.

Anonymous. (1986) Treatment of columnaris disease. For Fish Farmers No. 86-1. Mississippi Cooperative Extension Service, Mississippi State University, pp. 1–2.

Aoki, T., Sakaguch, T., and Kitao, T. (1987) Multiple drug-resistant plasmids from *Edwardsiella tarda* in eel culture ponds. Nippon Suisan Gakkaishi 53:1821–1825.

Austin, B., and Austin, D. (1987) Bacterial fish pathogens: Disease in farmed and wild fish. Ellis Horwood, Chichester, England.

Baya, A.M., Lupiani, B., Hetrick, F.M., Roberson, B.S., Lukacovic, R., May, E., and Poukish, C. (1990a) Association of *Streptococcus* sp. with fish mortalities in Chesapeake Bay and its tributaries. J. Fish Dis. 13:251–253.

Baya, A., Toranzo, A.E., Nunez, S., Barja, J.L., and Hetrick, F.M. (1990b) Association of a *Moraxella* sp. and a reo-like virus with mortalities of striped bass, *Morone saxatilis*. In: Pathology in Marine Science (Perkins, F., and Cheng, T.C., eds.). Academic Press, New York, pp. 91–100.

Becker, C.D., and Fujihara, M.P. (1978) The Bacterial Pathogen *Flexibacter Columnaris* and Its Epizootiology Among Columbia River Fish. Monograph No. 2, American Fisheries Society.

Bulkley, R.V. (1969) A furunculosis epizootic in Clear Lake yellow bass. Bull. Wildlife Dis. Assoc. 3:322–327.

Bullock, G.L., Hsu, T., and Shotts, E.B. (1986) Columnaris disease of fishes. FDL # 72, U.S.D.O.I., F.W.S., Div. of Fisheries and Wetlands Research, Washington, D.C.

Chen, C-R.L., Chung, Y.Y., and Kuo, G-H. (1982) Studies on the pathogenicity of *Flexibacter columnaris*-1. Effect of dissolved oxygen and ammonia on the pathogenicity of *Flexibacter columnaris* to eel (*Anguilla japonica*). CAPD Fisheries series No. 8. Rep. Fish Dis. Res. 4:57–61.

Chowdhury, M.B.R., and Wakabayashi, H. (1988a) Effects of sodium, calcium and magnesium ions on the survival of *Flexibacter columnaris* in water. Fish Pathol. 23:231–235.

Chowdhury, M.B.R., and Wakabayashi, H. (1988b) Effects of sodium, calcium and magnesium ions on *Flexibacter columnaris* infection in fish. Fish Pathol. 23:237–241.

Clarridge, J.E., Musher, D.M., Fanstein, V., and Wallace, R.J. (1980)

Extraintestinal human infection caused by *Edwardsiella tarda*. J. Clin. Microbiol. 11:511–514.

Coles, B.M., Stroud, R.K., and Sheggeby, S. (1978) Isolation of *Edwardsiella tarda* from three Oregon sea mammals. J. Wildlife Dis. 14:339–341.

Colesante, R.T., Engstrom-Heg, R. Ehlinger, N., and Youmans, N. (1981) Cause and control of muskellunge fry mortality at Chautauqua Hatchery, New York. Progressive Fish Culturist 43:17–20.

Davis, H.S. (1922) A new bacterial disease of freshwater fishes. Bull. U.S. Bur. Fish. 1921–22. 38:261–280.

Economon, P. (1960) Furunculosis in northern pike. Trans. Am. Fish. Soc. 89:240–241.

Esch, G.W., and Hazen, T.C. (1980) The ecology of *Aeromonas hydrophila* in Albemarle Sound, North Carolina. University of North Carolina Water Resources Research Institute Final Report No. 80-153.

Fijan, N. (1968) The survival of *Chondrococcus columnaris* in waters of different quality. Bull. l'Office Inter. des Epizooties 69:1159–1166.

Fujihara, Y., Kano, T., and Fukui, H. (1984) Sulfisozole/trimethoprim as a chemotherapeutic agent for bacterial infections in yellowtail and eel. Fish Pathol. 19:35–44.

Fukuda, Y., and Kusuda, R. (1981) Efficacy of vaccination for pseudotuberculosis in cultured yellowtail by various routes of administration. Bull. Jpn. Soc. Sci. Fish. 47:147–150.

Hall, J.D. (1963) An ecological study of the chestnut lamprey, *Ichthyomyzon castaneus* Girard, in the Manistee River, Michigan. Ph.D. Thesis, University of Michigan, Ann Arbor.

Hanson, L.A., and Grizzle, J.M. (1985) Nitrite-induced predisposition of channel catfish to bacterial diseases. Progressive Fish Culturist 47:98–101.

Hawke, J.P., Plakas, S.M., Minton, R.V., McPherson, R.M., Snider, T.G., and Guarino, A.M. (1987) Fish pasteurellosis of cultured striped bass (*Morone saxatilis*) in coastal Alabama. Aquaculture 65:193–204.

Hedrick, R.P., McDowell, T., and Groff, J. (1987) Mycobacteriosis from cultured striped bass from California. J. Wildlife Dis. 23:391–395.

Henley, M.W., and Lewis, D.H. (1976) Anaerobic bacteria associated with mortality in grey mullet (*Mugil cephalus*) and red fish (*Sciaenops ocellata*) along the Texas Gulf Coast. J. Wildlife Dis. 12:448–453.

Herman, R.L. (1968) Fish furunculosis 1952–1966. Trans. Am. Fish. Soc. 97:221–230.

Herman, R.L., and Bullock, G.L. (1986) Pathology caused by *Edwardsiella tarda* in striped bass. Trans. Am. Fish. Soc. 115:232–235.

Herman, R.L., and Wolf, K. (1987) Epitheliocystis infection of fishes. FDL #75, U.S.D.O.I., F.W.S., Div. of Fisheries and Wetlands Research, Washington, D.C.

Hilton, L.R., and Wilson, J.L. (1980) Terramycin-resistant *Edwardsiella tarda* isolated from an epizootic among channel catfish. Progressive Fish Culturist 42:159.

Isom, B.G. (1960) Outbreaks of columnaris in Center Hill and Old Hickory Reservoirs, Tennessee. Progressive Fish Culturist 22:43–45.

Kaper, J.B., Lockman, H., and Colwell, R.R. (1981) *Aeromonas hydrophila*: Ecology and toxigenicity of isolates from an estuary. J. Appl. Bacteriol. 50:359–377.

Kusuda, R., and Inoue, K. (1977) Studies on the application of ampicillin for pseudotuberculosis in cultured yellowtails. III. Therapeutic effect of ampicillin on yellowtails artificially infected with *Pasteurella piscicida*. Fish Pathol. 12:7–10.

LeTendre, G.C., Schneider, C.P., and Ehlinger, N.F. (1972) Net damage and subsequent mortality from furunculosis in smallmouth bass. N.Y. Fish Game J. 19:73–82.

Lewis, D.H., and Udey, L.R. (1978) Meningitis in fish caused by an asporogenous anaerobic bacterium. Fish Disease Leaflet 56, U.S. Fish and Wildlife Service.

Lewis, D.H., Grumbles, L.C., McConnell, S., and Flowers, A.I. (1970) *Pasteurella*-like bacteria from an epizootic in menhaden and mullet in Galveston Bay. J. Wildlife Dis. 6:160–162.

MacFarlane, R.D., Bullock, G.L., and McLaughlin, J.J.A. (1986) Effects of five metals on susceptibility of striped bass to *Flexibacter columnaris*. Trans. Am. Fish. Soc. 115:227–231.

McFadden, T.W. (1970) Furunculosis in nonsalmonids. J. Fish. Res. Bd. Can. 27:2365–2370.

Miller, R.W., and Chapman, W.R. (1976) *Epistylis* and *Aeromonas hydrophila* infections in fishes from North Carolina reservoirs. Progressive Fish Culturist 38:165–168.

Mitchell, A.J. (1984) Parasites and diseases of striped bass. In: The Aquaculture of Striped Bass: A Proceedings (McCraren, J.P., ed.). University of Maryland Sea Grant Publication # UM-SG-MAP-84-01, pp. 177–204.

Miyazaki, T., and Egusa, S. (1976a) Histopathological studies of edwardsiellosis of the Japanese eel (*Anguilla japonica*)—I. Suppurative interstitial nephritis form. Fish Pathol. 11:33–44.

Miyazaki, T., and Egusa, S. (1976b) Histopathological studies of edwardsiellosis of the Japanese eel (*Anguilla japonica*)—I. Suppurative interstitial hepatitis form. Fish Pathol. 11:67–76.

Nigrelli, R.F., and Hutner, S.H. (1945) The presence of a myxobacterium, *Chondrococcus columnaris* (Davis) Ordal and Rucker (1944), on *Fundulus heteroclitus* (Linn.). Zoologica 30:101–104.

Noga, E.J. (1986) The importance of *Lernaea cruciata* (LeSeuer) in the initiation of skin lesions in largemouth bass *Micropterus salmoides* (Lacepede) in the Chowan River, North Carolina. J. Fish Dis. 9:295–302.

Noga, E.J. (1988) Determining the relationship between water quality and infectious disease in fishery populations. Water Resources Bull. 24:967–973.

Noga, E.J., and Berkhoff, H.A. (1990) Pathological and microbiological features of *Aeromonas salmonicida* infection in the American eel (*Anguilla rostrata*). Fish Pathol. 25:127–132.

Paperna, I., and Zerner, D. (1976) Parasites and diseases of striped bass, *Morone saxatilis* (Walbaum), from the lower Chesapeake Bay. J. Fish Biol. 9:267–287.

Plumb, J.A., Schachte, J.H., Gaines, J.L., Peltier, W., and Carroll, B. (1974) *Streptococcus* sp. from marine fishes along the Alabama and northwest Florida coast of the Gulf of Mexico. Trans. Am. Fish. Soc. 103:358–361.

Pyle, S.W., and Shotts, E.B. (1980) A new method of differentiating *Flexibacteria* from cold-water and warmwater fish. Can. J. Fish Aquatic Sci. 37:1040-1042.

Pyle, S.W., and Shotts, E.B. (1981) DNA homology studies of selected flexibacteria associated with fish disease. Can. J. Fish Aquatic Sci. 38:146–151.

Robohm, R.A. (1983) *Pasteurella piscida*. In: Antigens of Fish Pathogens (Anderson, D.P., Dorson, M., and Daborget, P., eds.). Collection Foundation Marcel Merieux, Lyon, pp. 161–175.

Shiomitsu, K., Kusuda, R., Osuga, H., and Munekiyo, M. (1980) Studies on chemotherapy of fish disease with erythromycin—II. Its clinical studies against streptococcal infection in cultured yellowtails. Fish Pathol. 15:17–23.

Shotts, E.B., and Rimler, R. (1973) Medium for the isolation of *Aeromonas hydrophila*. Appl. Microbiol. 26:550–553.

Shotts, E.B., and Teska, J.D. (1989) Bacterial pathogens of aquatic vertebrates. In: Methods for the Microbiological Examination of Fish and Shellfish (Austin, B., and Austin, D.A., eds.). John Wiley and Sons, New York, pp. 164–186.

Snieszko, S.F., Bullock, G.L., Hollis, E., and Boone, J.G. (1964) *Pasteurella* species from an epizootic of white perch (*Roccus americanus*) in Chesapeake Bay tidewater areas. J. Bacteriol. 88:1814–1815.

Starliper, C.E., Shotts, Jr., E.B., Hsu, T., and Schill, W.B. (1988) Genetic relatedness of some gram-negative yellow pigmented bacteria from fishes and aquatic environments. Microbios 56:181–198.

Toranzo, A.E., Barja, J.L., Potter, S.A., Colwell, R.R., Hetrick, F.M., and Crosa, J.H. (1983) Molecular factors associated with virulence of marine vibrios isolated from striped bass in Chesapeake Bay. Infect. Immun. 39:1220–1227.

Toranzo, A.E., Baya, A.M., Romalde, J.L., and Hetrick, F.M. (1989) Association of *Aeromonas sobria* with mortalities of adult gizzard shad, *Dorosoma cepedianum* LeSueur. J. Fish Dis. 12:439–448.

Udey, L.R., Young, E., and Sallman, B. (1977) Isolation and characterization of an anaerobic bacterium, *Eubacterium tarantellus* sp. nov., associated with striped mullet *Mugil cephalus* mortality in Biscayne Bay, Florida. J. Fish Res. Bd. Can. 34:402–409.

Wakabayashi, H., Hikida, M., and Masumura, K. (1986) *Flexibacter maritimus* sp. nov., a pathogen of marine fishes. Int. J. Syst. Bacteriol. 36:396–398.

Wakabayashi, H., Huh, G.J., and Kimura, N. (1989) *Flavobacterium branchophila* sp. nov., a causative agent of bacterial gill disease of freshwater fishes. Int. J. Syst. Bacteriol. 39:213–216.

Waltman, W.D., Shotts, E.B., and Hsu, T.C. (1986) Biochemical and enzymatic characterization of *Edwardsiella tarda* from the United States and Taiwan. Fish Pathol. 21:1–8.

Wilkinson, H.W., Thacker, L.G., and Facklam, R.R. (1973) Nonhemolytic group B streptococci of human, bovine and ichthyic origin. Infect. Immun. 7:496–498.

Winsor, D.K., Bloebaum, A.P., and Mathewson, J.M. (1981) Gram-negative aerobic, enteric pathogens among intestinal microflora of wild turkey vultures (*Cathartes aura*) in west central Texas. Appl. Environ. Microbiol. 42:1123–1124.

Wyatt, L.E., Nickelson, II, R., and Vanderzant, C. (1979) *Edwardsiella tarda* in freshwater catfish and their environment. Appl. Environ. Microbiol. 38:710–714.

Chapter 25

FUNGAL AND ALGAL DISEASES OF TEMPERATE FRESHWATER AND ESTUARINE FISHES

EDWARD J. NOGA

Temperate freshwater and estuarine fishes are susceptible to fungal and algal disease organisms that also affect fishes in other environments. Considerable study is needed in the taxonomy, pathogenesis, pathology, and clinical management of these diseases, as our understanding of their impact on the health of individual fishes and economically important populations remains incomplete. The fungal and algal diseases examined in this chapter are listed in Table 25–1. Additional relevant information can be found in Chapters 37, 68, and 79.

WATER MOLD INFECTION

SYNONYMS. Saprolegniosis, ulcerative mycosis, cotton mouth disease.

Host and Geographic Distribution

Oomycetes are increasingly being recognized as important pathogens of estuarine fishes. They are distributed worldwide; virtually every freshwater fish

TABLE 25–1. Fungal and Algal Diseases of Temperate Freshwater and Estuarine Fishes*

Disease	Agent	Host(s)
Water mold infection	Oomycetes	All freshwater species
Branchiomycosis	*Branchiomyces* spp.	Largemouth, smallmouth, and striped bass
Algal infections	*Cladophora* sp.	Largemouth bass
	Chlorella sp.	Bluegill

See also sections on saprolegniasis, branchiomycosis, and ichthyophoniasis in Chapter 37; ichthyophoniasis in Chapter 68; and ichthyophoniasis in Chapter 79.

is probably susceptible to at least one species of the class Oomycetes. The class is divided into four orders, three of which have been shown to have species capable of infecting living fishes (Saprolegniales, Leptomitales, and Peronosporales) (Table 25–2). Some of these agents also infect other aquatic vertebrates such as amphibians and are important pathogens of aquatic invertebrates.

Clinical Signs

The most common presentation of water mold infection is as a relatively superficial, cottony growth on the skin or gills. Such lesions usually begin as small, focal infections that can rapidly spread over the surface of the body. It is not unusual for large lesions to suddenly appear within 24 hours. Newly formed lesions are white owing to the presence of the mycelia of the fungus. With time, the lesions often become red, brown, or green as a result of trapping of algae or debris in the mycelial mat. If observed on a fish removed from the water, the mycelia appear as a slimy, matted mass (Fig. 25–1).

In contrast to typical saprolegniosis, ulcerative mycosis is a much more invasive disease, affecting primarily Atlantic menhaden. Lesions usually begin as a small, 5 mm in diameter focus of reddening on the skin, which rapidly enlarges to form a deep, necrotic ulcer up to 25 mm in diameter. Lesions contain white, friable material (Fig. 25–2) with numerous hyphae interspersed with necrotic muscle. Lesions often extend deep into the body and frequently affect internal organs. Eventually, the necrotic, infected tissue sloughs, leaving a crater-shaped cavity surrounded by dark red to white muscle.

Species of *Aphanomyces* are most commonly isolated from ulcerative mycosis lesions, but *Saprolegnia* species also have been cultured (Noga et al., 1988).

TABLE 25–2. Host Range of Parasitic Oomycetes in North American Temperate Freshwater Fishes*

Host	Agent	Reference
Anguillidae		
American eel	*Saprolegnia* sp.	Inman and Bland (1980)
Esocidae		
Northern pike	*Saprolegnia* sp.	Scott and O'Bier (1962)
	Saprolegnia delica	Scott and O'Bier (1962)
	Leptomitus lacteus	Scott and O'Bier (1962)
Centrarchidae		
Green sunfish	*Saprolegnia* sp.	Scott and O'Bier (1962)
Pumpkinseed	*Saprolegnia* sp.	Tiffney (1939b)
Bluegill	*Saprolegnia parasitica*	Scott and O'Bier (1962)
	Saprolegnia sp.	Scott and O'Bier (1962)
	Saprolegnia moneica	Scott and O'Bier (1962)
	Achlya americana	Scott and O'Bier (1962)
	Pythium ultimum	Scott and O'Bier (1962)
	Pythium sp.	Scott and O'Bier (1962)
Smallmouth bass	*Saprolegnia parasitica*	Bangham (1933)
Largemouth bass	*Saprolegnia* sp.	Scott and Bier (1962)
Cyprinodontidae		
Mummichog	*Saprolegnia* sp.	Tiffney (1939b)
Percichthyidae		
Striped bass	*Saprolegnia* sp.	Mitchell (1984)
Striped bass X white bass	*Saprolegnia* sp.	Noga (unpublished data)
Percidae		
Yellow perch	*Saprolegnia* sp.	Tiffney (1939b)

Clinton (1894) also listed the following fish as being susceptible to Saprolegnia sp.: small mouthed black bass, rock bass, dogfish, paddle-fish, moon-eye, long-nosed gar, short-nosed gar, black bass, white bass, yellow bass, calico bass, yellow perch, pike, pike perch, sheepshead, sand pike, bream, blue sunfish, and warmouth. Species names were not given.

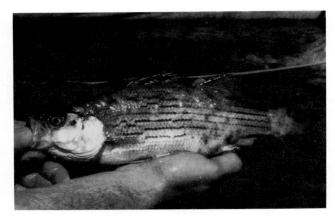

FIGURE 25–1. *Saprolegnia* sp. infection on a hybrid striped bass. When a fish is removed from the water, mycelia appear as a slimy mat.

While ulcerative mycosis has only been definitively identified from Atlantic menhaden and gizzard shad, many other estuarine fishes have been observed with similar skin lesions. These include southern flounder, ocellated flounder, topminnows, striped bass, white perch, bluefish, Atlantic croaker, weakfish, red drum, spot, silver perch, black drum, hogchoker, and pinfish (TeStrake and Lim, 1987; Grier and Quintero, 1987; Roberts et al., 1986).

Oomycetes are very important pathogens of fish eggs. Infections are believed to begin in unfertilized or nonviable eggs. However, once established, fungi rapidly spread to adjacent normal healthy eggs, eventually resulting in complete loss of the brood.

Diagnosis

Diagnosis of oomycete infection requires that affected fish be alive at the time of examination, because water molds are ubiquitous saprophytes in soil, fresh water and, to some extent, estuarine environments, and dead fish are fertile substrates for colonization. It is also important to realize that oomycetes are common secondary invaders of wounds that may be initiated by other pathogens.

Observation of a cottony, proliferative growth on the skin or gills should alert the clinician to a possible diagnosis of typical saprolegniosis. Some bacteria (e.g., *Cytophaga*) and colonial protozoa (e.g., *Heteropolaria*) can also produce similar gross lesions, so presumptive diagnosis of an oomycete infection is made by observing broad (7 to 40 μm), aseptate hyphae in wet mounts. Histologically, presumptive diagnosis of typical saprolegniosis is based upon the presence of relatively shallow lesions containing broad, aseptate hyphae. Hyphae are usually visible with hematoxylin and eosin stain. There is little inflammation, and the fungi usually do not extend past the superficial muscle layers.

A presumptive diagnosis of ulcerative mycosis is based upon the presence of deep skin ulcers

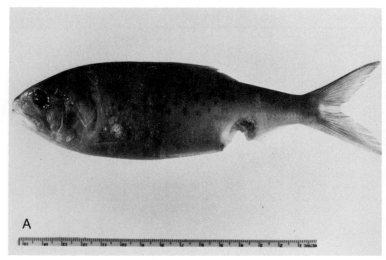
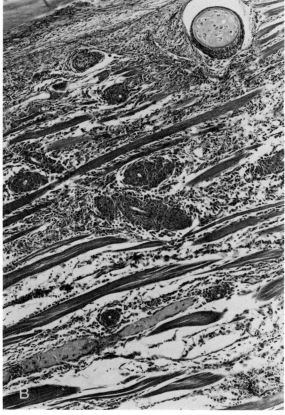

FIGURE 25–2. Ulcerative mycosis in Atlantic menhaden. *A.* A large, typical crater-shaped ulcer. *B.* Fungal hyphae surrounded by chronic inflammation (Gomori methenamine silver stain).

containing broad (at least 7 μm in diameter), colorless, aseptate hyphae associated with a chronic inflammatory response. Hyphae may be difficult to see with hematoxylin and eosin, but can be seen easily with silver stains (e.g., Gomori's methenamine silver). Other fungi can also cause chronic ulcers in fish, and this type of response is common in other deep mycoses (Richards et al., 1978). Other fungal infections can be differentiated from ulcerative mycosis on the basis of hyphal size and color and the presence of septae. *Ichthyophonus* hyphae have similar morphology, but other developmental stages (cysts, etc.) are usually also apparent. Oomycetes can be identified ultrastructurally by their tubular mitochondrial cristae, which differentiate them from all other broad, aseptate fungi, which have platelike cristae (Dykstra et al., 1986).

Historically, presumptive diagnosis has been used as the basis for most treatment decisions; however, oomycetes vary in drug susceptibility (see section on Treatment and Control below), and thus determining the type of oomycete(s) involved is an important consideration.

Culture and Identification

Definitive identification of an oomycete infection requires the observation of asexual sporangia. While these may be seen occasionally on infected fish, culture is usually required. Culture is best accomplished using a nutrient-poor medium such as corn meal agar or YpSs agar (Seymour and Fuller, 1987), which tends to reduce the growth of bacterial contaminants. Culturing oomycetes from ulcerative mycosis lesions is especially difficult because of the many bacteria also present. In heavily contaminated lesions, adding penicillin (about 500 U/ml) and/or streptomycin (about 0.2 μg/ml) may improve yields; however, some oomycetes (especially *Aphanomyces*) are significantly inhibited by antibiotics. *Saprolegnia* and *Achlya*, the two genera most commonly isolated from fishes, are usually not significantly inhibited.

Plates should be inoculated with a small (about 12 mm³) mass of infected tissue and incubated at room temperature. Once growth of the fungus is noticeable, usually within 48 hours, transfer the growing edge of the mycelium to a fresh culture plate by aseptically excising a small portion of the agar. This will reduce or eliminate bacterial contaminants introduced with the tissue sample. More than one pathogen may be present in lesions (Pickering and Willoughby, 1977).

Identification to genus or species requires the induction of asexual or sexual sporulation, respectively (Figs. 25–3 and 25–4). Unfortunately, many isolates fail to produce sexual stages in culture. Details of culture methodology and induction of reproductive stages are provided in Fuller and Jaworski (1987). Immunologic methods also hold promise as future diagnostic tools (Bullis et al., 1990).

Of all the oomycetes, *Saprolegnia parasitica* and *S. diclina* are probably the two species most commonly isolated from fishes. They are closely related

and are often referred to as the *S. diclina–S. parasitica* complex (Neish and Hughes, 1980). Most studies of this complex have involved salmonids (see Chap. 37).

Transmission, Epidemiology, and Pathogenesis

The water molds require water for growth and sporulation and do not produce aerial spores. The motile zoospore produced by the vegetative hyphae of water molds allows dissemination to distant sites and is probably the primary means for infecting fish.

Although typical saprolegniosis lesions grow rapidly over the surface of the skin, they usually do not penetrate deeply into muscle. However, the damage to the skin or gills from superficial lesions is sufficient to kill fish. The severity of the disease is generally related to the surface area of skin or gills affected. The larger the area affected, the greater the osmotic stress and electrolyte imbalance (Richards and Pickering, 1979).

Skin wounds due to mechanical trauma or other pathogens increase the risk of infection (Tiffney, 1939a; Scott and O'Bier, 1962). Careful handling during transport or other procedures should be exercised. The importance of other risk factors is poorly understood. Many oomycetes display a seasonal periodicity; for example, many *Saprolegnia* species are most active in the cooler months of the year (Hughes, 1962). Most saprolegniaceous oomycetes are inhibited by even moderate salt concentrations, which is probably why they do not affect marine fishes. As in other animals, there is increasing evidence that fungal infections in fish are more likely to develop if a host is stressed, which may result in immunosuppression. Thus, a diagnosis of saprolegniosis should always include a thorough search for underlying predisposing factors. There is evidence that water molds may require the presence of at least one other pathogen, possibly one or more bacterial agents, in order to cause ulcerative mycosis. There may also be primarily parasitic strains of *Saprolegnia*. For example, *Saprolegnia parasitica* appears to be highly pathogenic, whereas *Pythium* and *Leptomitus* are only weakly pathogenic (Scott and O'Bier, 1962).

Of the oomycetes, only *Pythium insidiosum* has been shown to be of zoonotic importance. It causes a granulomatous infection of the extremities in horses, cattle, and dogs and has been reported occasionally as a skin infection in humans (De Cock et al., 1987). The inability of oomycetes to survive at 37°C limits their potential pathogenicity to mammals.

Treatment and Control

Water molds are among the most difficult diseases to treat because legally approved therapeutic agents are of limited effectiveness. Potassium permanganate pond treatment has been occasionally successful. Salt dips are useful because, as mentioned

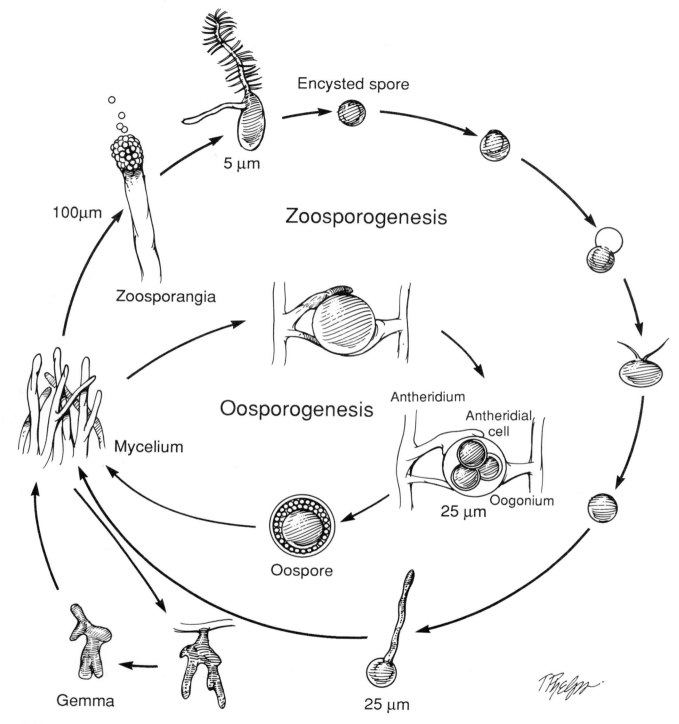

Encysted spore

Zoosporogenesis

5 μm

100μm

Zoosporangia

Oosporogenesis

Antheridium

Antheridial cell

Mycelium

Oogonium

25 μm

Oospore

Gemma

25 μm

FIGURE 25–3. The life cycle of *Saprolegnia*. (After Neisch, G. A., and Hughes, G. C. [1980] Fungal Diseases of Fish. T. F. H. Publications, Neptune City, New Jersey.)

previously, most saprolegniaceous molds are usually inhibited by even low (less than 10 ppt) concentrations of salt. Salt also helps to counteract osmotic stress in affected fish with skin damage and subsequent salt loss. However, usually neither treatment will totally arrest fungal growth. The only agent presently approved for use in food fishes is formalin (Schnick et al., 1986). However, formalin is not very

effective in most cases. Malachite green is an effective agent for treating fungal infections in fish, but it is not approved for food fishes because of its teratogenic and mutagenic properties.

In recent years, a wide range of agents have been tested in an unsuccessful search for candidates to replace malachite green (Bailey, 1984; Alderman and Polglase, 1984; Scott and Warren, 1964; Olah

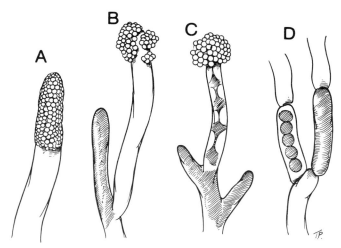

FIGURE 25–4. Zoosporangia of some Oomycetes pathogenic to fishes. *A. Saprolegnia. B. Achyla. C. Aphanomyces. D. Leptolegnia.* (*A* and *B*, After Webster, J. [1970] Introduction to Fungi. Cambridge University Press, London; *C*, After Cutter, V.M., Jr. [1941] Observations on certain species of *Aphanomyces.* Mycologia 33:220–240, copyright 1941, The New York Botanical Garden; *D*, After Coker, W.C. [1923] The Saprolegniaceae, with notes on other water molds. University of North Carolina Press, Chapel Hill.)

and Farkas, 1978), including numerous agricultural fungicides, medical antimycotic agents, and various disinfectants and miscellaneous compounds. There does appear to be some species differences among oomycetes in their tolerance to antifungal agents. For example, *Saprolegnia* species are usually resistant, whereas *Aphanomyces* species are much less so. Whether these are clinically relevant differences is unknown.

Branchiomycosis

Branchiomyces sanguinis has been reported from largemouth, smallmouth, and striped bass in Arkansas (Meyer and Robinson, 1973). Clinicopathologic features are similar to that described for cyprinids (see Chap. 49). Other fish genera in Europe and elsewhere, having related taxa in the United States, are also affected. They include northern pike, three-spined stickleback, Eurasian perch, topminnows, and eels.

Algal Infections

Cladophora sp. have been reported infecting the maxillary bone of a largemouth bass in Lake Texoma, Oklahoma (Vinyard, 1953). There has been a report of *Chlorella* sp. within the orbit of a bluegill in West Virginia (Hoffmann et al., 1965).

LITERATURE CITED

Alderman, D.J., and Polglase, J. (1984) A comparative investigation of the effects of fungicides on *Saprolegnia parasitica* and *Aphanomyces astaci.* Trans. Br. Mycol. Soc. 83:313–318.

Bailey, T.A. (1984) Effects of 25 compounds on 4 species of aquatic fungi (Saprolegniales) pathogenic to fish. Aquaculture 38:97–104.

Bangham, R.V. (1933) Parasites of spotted bass, *Micropterus pseudaplites* Hubbs, and summary of parasites of smallmouth and largemouth black bass from Ohio streams. Trans. Am. Fish. Soc. 63:220–225.

Bullis, R.A., Noga, E.J., and Levy, M.G. (1990) Immunological relationship of the fish-pathogenic oomycete, *Saprolegnia parasitica*, to other oomycetes and unrelated fungi. J. Aquatic Anim. Health 2:223–227.

Clinton, G.P. (1894) Observations and experiments on *Saprolegnia* infesting fish. Bull. U.S. Fish Comm. 13:163–172.

Coker, W.C. (1923) The Saprolegniaceae, with notes on other water molds. University of North Carolina Press, Chapel Hill.

Cutter, V.M., Jr. (1941) Observations on certain species of *Aphanomyces.* Mycologia 33:220–240.

De Cock, A.W.A.M., Mendoza, L., Padhye, A.A., Ajello, L., and Kaufman, L. (1987) *Pythium insidiosum* sp. nov., the etiological agent of pythiosis. J. Clin. Microbiol. 25:344–349.

Dykstra, M.J., Noga, E.J., Levine, J.F., Hawkins, J.H., and Moye, D.F. (1986) Characterization of the *Aphanomyces* sp. involved with ulcerative mycosis. Mycologia 78:664–672.

Fuller, M.S., and Jaworski, A. (1987) Zoosporic Fungi in Teaching and Research. Southeastern Publishing, Athens, Georgia.

Grier, H., and Quintero, I. (1987) A microscopic study of ulcerated fish in Florida. Fl. Bur. Marine Fish. Rep. WM-164.

Hoffmann, G.L., Prescott, G.W., and Thompson, C.R. (1965) *Chlorella* parasitic in bluegills. Progressive Fish Culturist 27:175.

Hughes, G.C. (1962) Seasonal periodicity of the Saprolegniaceae in the southeastern United States. Trans. Br. Mycol. Soc. 45:519–531.

Inman, A.O., and Bland, C.E. (1980) Bacterial and fungal pathogens of cultured American eels. Progressive Fish Culturist 43:53–54.

Meyer, F.P., and Robinson, J.A. (1973) Branchiomycosis: A new fungal disease of North American fishes. Progressive Fish Culturist 35:74–77.

Mitchell, A.J. (1984) Parasites and diseases of striped bass. In: The Aquaculture of Striped Bass: A Proceedings (McCraren, J.P., ed.). University of Maryland Sea Grant Publication # UM-SG-MAP-84-01.

Neisch, G.A., and Hughes, G.C. (1980) Fungal Diseases of Fish. T.F.H. Publications, Neptune City, New Jersey.

Noga, E.J., Levine, J.F., Dykstra, M.J., and Hawkins, J.H. (1988) Pathology of ulcerative mycosis in Atlantic menhaden *Brevoortia tyrannus.* Dis. Aquatic Org. 4:189–197.

Olah, L., and Farkas, J. (1978) Effect of temperature, pH, antibiotics, formalin, and malachite green on the growth and survival of *Saprolegnia* and *Achlya* parasitic on fish. Aquaculture 13:273–288.

Pickering, A.D., and Willoughby, L.G. (1977) Epidermal lesions and fungal infection on the perch, *Perca fluviatilis* L., in Windermere. J. Fish Biol. 11:349–354.

Richards, R.H., and Pickering, A.D. (1979) Changes in serum parameters of *Saprolegnia*-infected brown trout, *Salmo trutta* L. J. Fish Dis. 2:197–206.

Richards, R.H., Holliman, A., and Helgason, S. (1978) *Exophiala salmonis* infection in Atlantic salmon *Salmo salar* L. J. Fish Dis. 1:357–368.

Roberts, R.J., MacIntosh, D.J., Tonguthai, K., Boonyaratpalin, S., Tayapuch, N., Phillips, M.J., and Millar, S.D. (1986) Field and laboratory investigations into ulcerative fish diseases in the Asia-Pacific region. FAO, Tech. Rept. FAO Proj. TCP/RAS/4508, Bangkok.

Schnick, R.A., Meyer, F.P., and Walsh, D.F. (1986) Status of fishery chemicals in 1985. Progressive Fish Culturist 48:1–17.

Scott, W.W., and O'Bier, A.H., Jr. (1962) Aquatic fungi associated with diseased fish and fish eggs. Progressive Fish Culturist 24:3–15.

Scott, W.W., and Warren, C.O. (1964) Studies of the host range and chemical control of fungi associated with diseased tropical fish. Va. Agric. Exp. Sta., Blacksburg, Tech. Bull. 171.

Seymour, R., and Fuller, M.S. (1987) Collection and isolation of water molds (Saprolegniaceae) from water and soil. In Zoosporic Fungi in Teaching and Research. (Fuller, M.S., and Jaworski, A., eds.). Southeastern Publishing, Athens, Georgia, pp. 125–127.

TeStrake, D., and Lim, D.V. (1987) Bacterial and fungal studies of ulcerative fish in the Saint Johns River. Report of Contract WM 138 to Florida Department of Environmental Regulation.

Tiffney, W.N. (1939a) The host range of *Saprolegnia parasitica.* Mycologia 31:310–321.

Tiffney, W.N. (1939b) The identification of certain species of the Saprolegniaceae parasitic to fish. J. Elisha Mitch. Scient. Soc. 55:134–151.

Vinyard, W.C. (1953) Epizoophytic algae from molluscs, turtles, and fish in Oklahoma. Proc. Ok. Acad. Sci. 34:63–65.

Webster, J. (1970) Introduction to Fungi. Cambridge University Press, London.

Chapter 26

FRESHWATER TEMPERATE FISH VIRUSES

PHILIP E. McALLISTER

Freshwater temperate fish viruses can have quite specific host ranges or affect diverse species. Their health and economic impact varies; some infections result in epizootic mortality, others chronic low-level losses, and still others cause little mortality, but fish are disfigured and cannot be marketed. In several instances, a virus has been isolated that apparently causes no clinical disease or pathology. The viruses in Table 26–1 have been detected in freshwater temperate fishes.

WHITE STURGEON ADENOVIRUS DISEASE

SYNONYM. Sturgeon-wasting disease.

Host and Geographic Distribution

Wild, sexually mature white sturgeon were captured from the Sacramento River, California, for use as broodstock. After several years of successfully rearing progeny, severe levels of mortality occurred in young-of-the-year fish at several culture stations. Some mortalities were attributed to bacterial infections, but a new viral disease was also detected (Hedrick et al., 1985).

Clinical Signs and Pathology

Diseased juvenile white sturgeon (about 0.5 g) are lethargic, inappetent, and emaciated. Internally, the liver is pale and alimentary tract devoid of food, but no other gross signs of clinical disease are evident. Epithelial cells lining the intestine and spiral valve show progressive enlargement of nuclei, and eventually rupture into the lumen of the intestine. In one instance, similar changes were seen in hepatocytes.

TABLE 26–1. Viral Diseases in Freshwater Temperate Fishes*

Disease	Virus	Host
Sturgeon wasting disease	White sturgeon adenovirus	White sturgeon
Epidermal hyperplasia	Esocid herpesvirus 1	Northern pike
Epidermal hyperplasia	*Herpesvirus vitreum*	Walleye
Squamous cell carcinoma	Rainbow smelt herpesvirus	Rainbow smelt
Unnamed mortality	Japanese eel iridovirus	Japanese eel
Lymphocystis	Lymphocystis virus	At least 125 species
Epizootic hematopoietic necrosis	Epizootic hematopoietic necrosis virus	Redfin perch, rainbow trout
Unnamed epizootic mortality	Rainbow smelt picornalike virus	Rainbow smelt
Hepatic necrosis	13p₂ reovirus	Bluegill, golden shiner, rainbow trout, American oyster
Epidermal hyperplasia	Esox epidermal hyperplasia retrovirus	Muskellunge, northern pike
Lymphosarcoma	Esox lymphosarcoma retrovirus	Muskellunge, northern pike
Sarcoma	Esox sarcoma retrovirus	Northern pike
Dermal sarcoma	Walleye dermal sarcoma retrovirus	Walleye
Epidermal hyperplasia	Walleye discrete epidermal hyperplasia retrovirus	Walleye
Epidermal papilloma	White sucker epidermal papilloma retrovirus	White sucker
Unnamed mortality	Perch rhabdovirus	Northern pike perch
Pike fry rhabdovirus disease	Pike fry rhabdovirus	Bream, brown trout, grass carp, gudgeon, northern pike, tench, white bream
Unnamed mortality	Cichlid rhabdovirus	Rio Grande perch, convict cichlid, Zilli cichlid
Unknown	Bluegill virus	Bluegill

See also sections on Infectious Pancreatic Necrosis in Chapter 38; Carp Pox, Golden Shiner Virus Disease, and Spring Viremia of Carp in Chapter 50; Channel Catfish Virus Disease and Catfish Reovirus Disease in Chapter 59; and Eel Rhabdovirus Disease and Stomatopapilloma of Eel in Chapter 88.

Diagnosis and Virus Detection

Diagnosis is based on clinical signs. The virus has been seen in electron micrographs but has not been isolated in cell culture in spite of repeated attempts (Hedrick et al., 1985). Electron micrographs of affected intestine and spiral valve show intranuclear arrays of electron-dense icosahedral virus particles about 74 nm in diameter. The particles are found almost exclusively in the nucleus and exhibited many morphologic characteristics of an adenovirus (Hedrick et al., 1985).

Transmission, Epidemiology, and Pathogenesis

Disease results in chronic mortality with losses up to 50% over 4 months. Juvenile white sturgeon experimentally inoculated with membrane-filtered visceral homogenate from infected fish developed nuclear hypertrophy identical to, but not as severe as, naturally infected fish.

Treatment and Control

Nothing is known about treatment or control of the infection. Culturists should avoid introductions of fish, fish products, and so forth, from stations known to have experienced unusual levels of mortality.

ESOCID HERPESVIRUS 1 EPIDERMAL HYPERPLASIA

SYNONYMS. Blue spot disease, esocid herpesvirus 1 infection, pike herpesvirus infection.

Host, Geographic Distribution, and Clinical Signs

Blue spot disease appears as hyperplastic epidermal lesions seen in northern pike taken from lakes in Manitoba and Saskatchewan, Canada (Yamamoto et al., 1984). The lesions are flat, bluish white, granular or "gritty," 3 to 10 mm in diameter, and about 0.25 mm thick. They occur primarily on the dorsal skin and fins. No lesions are seen on internal organs or gills. The "blue spot" is composed of grossly hypertrophied epidermal cells about 0.15 mm in diameter, interspersed with normal epidermal cells. Larger infected cells subsequently lyse near the periphery of the lesions.

Diagnosis

Blue spot disease can be presumptively diagnosed by correlating clinical signs and histologic examination. The lesion superficially resembles lymphocystis disease, but lacks a hyaline layer and no connective tissue involvement. Hematoxylin and eosin staining shows an enlarged, dark nucleus, and an enlarged cytoplasm filled with dark staining, granular inclusions. Deoxyribonucleic acid (DNA) accumulation in the cytoplasm can be demonstrated with Feulgen or bisbenzimide staining.

Virus Detection

Attempts to isolate virus from the blue spot proliferation have been unsuccessful using WC-1, We-2, and WO cells (Yamamoto et al., 1984). Electron micrographs of affected cells show accumulations of herpesviruslike capsids 100 to 110 nm in diameter in the nucleus and capsids budding from the nuclear membrane. The hypertrophied cytoplasm is filled with granular inclusions containing virus particles (Yamamoto et al., 1984).

Epidemiology and Pathogenesis

Blue spot lesions are observed in feral fish captured in early May when the fish return to streams to spawn. During a 5-year survey, the highest annual prevalence was 7.4%. The disease is considered widespread, seasonal, and variable from year to year. Apparently, no unusual mortality is associated with the disease, and no attempts to transmit the disease have been reported.

Treatment and Control

The disease has been observed only in feral fish. No method of treatment or control is known.

WALLEYE DIFFUSE EPIDERMAL HYPERPLASIA

SYNONYMS. Percid herpesvirus 1 infection, walleye herpesvirus infection.

Geographic Distribution, Clinical Signs, and Pathology

Diffuse epidermal hyperplasia occurs in walleye populations throughout North America. It appears as a flat, laterally spreading, indistinct cell proliferation several centimeters in diameter that resembles translucent, thickened slime. The normal epidermal structure is disorganized and underlying tissue mildly edematous. Cell nuclei are slightly enlarged, contain granular inclusions, and occasionally form syncytia (Yamamoto et al., 1985a). There is no involvement of internal organs, and mortality is rare.

Electron micrographs of hyperplastic tissue show intracellular and extracellular accumulations of herpesvirus particles (Kelly et al., 1983).

Diagnosis

Walleye diffuse epidermal hyperplasia can be distinguished from walleye dermal sarcoma and walleye discrete epidermal hyperplasia by clinical appearance. A herpesvirus has been isolated from diffuse epidermal hyperplasia, but the etiologic significance of the virus has not been proven. Serologic tests for virus identification have not been reported.

Virus Isolation

Herpesvirus vitreum can be isolated from homogenates of hyperplastic tissue inoculated onto walleye cell cultures WO, WC-1, and We-2. The virus replicates at 4 and 15°C, but not at 20°C. Syncytia form about 2 weeks after infection and then lyse (Kelly et al., 1983).

Epidemiology and Pathogenesis

Lesions are most prevalent at spawning in the spring and disappear during the summer (Yamamoto et al., 1985a). The disease repeatedly has been observed in the same populations, indicating the virus persists. Winter temperature stress and physiologic changes associated with spawning may activate latent infection (Yamamoto et al., 1985a). Diffuse epidermal hyperplasia can occur in fish concurrently showing lymphocystis, dermal sarcoma, and discrete epidermal hyperplasia.

Treatment and Control

Walleye diffuse epidermal hyperplasia occurs in feral fish, and no method of treatment or control has been reported.

RAINBOW SMELT SQUAMOUS CELL CARCINOMA

SYNONYM. Rainbow smelt herpesvirus infection.

Host and Geographic Distribution

A noninvasive squamous cell carcinoma occurs in landlocked rainbow smelt in several lakes in New Hampshire and may occur in other areas of the northeastern United States. Electron micrographs of tumor tissue show herpesviruslike particles (R. L. Herman, National Fish Health Research Laboratory, personal communication).

Clinical Signs

Multiple gray, jellylike masses of variable size and shape occur on the body and fins of rainbow smelt. The tumors are discrete and detach easily, and are sometimes hyperemic or hemorrhagic. Apparently, the tumor is not overtly injurious to the fish because no unusual mortality has been reported. The physical appearance of this carcinoma differs from another squamous cell carcinoma in rainbow smelt that is more solid, has an irregular surface, and is invasive (Herman, 1988).

Pathology

The noninvasive tumor is a squamous cell carcinoma consisting of pleomorphic epithelial cells with intercellular bridges. No mitotic figures are seen, and the tumor does not invade the dermis. Varying degrees of lymphocytic infiltration and necrosis occur.

Diagnosis and Virus Detection

The diagnosis is based on clinical signs and confirmed by histology. Electron micrographs of tumor tissue from the noninvasive tumor show herpesviruslike particles developing in the nucleus and complete virions in the cytoplasm and intercellular spaces. The virus has not been isolated in cell culture.

Epidemiology and Pathogenesis

The tumor is seen prior to and during the spring spawning runs but has not been reported in summer. Prevalence varies annually from less than 10 to more than 30%. The tumor occurs with similar frequency in both male and female fish.

The etiologic significance of the virus seen in tumor tissue is unknown, and experimental transmission of the tumor has not been reported. Physiologic stresses associated with overwintering or spawning might activate latent viral infection or promote uncontrolled cell proliferation.

Treatment and Control

The noninvasive squamous cell carcinoma occurs in feral fish, making treatment or control impractical.

JAPANESE EEL IRIDOVIRUS INFECTION

SYNONYM. EV-102 infection.

Geographic Distribution

During a routine disease survey of eel pond-culture facilities in Shizuoka Prefecture, Japan, an iridovirus was isolated from Japanese eels (Sorimachi and Egusa, 1982; Sorimachi, 1984). The virus is found only in Japan.

Clinical Signs and Transmission

When eels are exposed to cell culture–grown virus by immersion or by intramuscular or intraperitoneal injection, lethal infection occurs in all age classes of Japanese eel, but no mortality occurs in European eel (Sorimachi, 1984). By 3 to 5 days after virus exposure, affected eels become light in color and show congested fins and increased surface mucus. During 2 weeks of monitoring, 40 to 75% of the eels held at 14.5 to 18.5°C died, 15% of those at 22.8°C died, and no eels died at 24.1°C.

Virus Detection

This iridovirus was one of several viruses isolated from Japanese eels during a disease survey in which kidney homogenates were inoculated onto RTG-2 and EPC cells and incubated at 20°C for 10 to 15 days. The iridovirus was isolated in both cell lines. The isolate is an unenveloped, icosahedral DNA virus 180 to 205 nm in diameter (Sorimachi and Egusa, 1982; Sorimachi, 1984).

Treatment and Control

Based on results of experimental challenges, mortality from viral infection might be prevented if Japanese eels were reared at water temperatures greater than 24°C (Sorimachi, 1984). However, maintaining ponds at 24°C might not be practical.

Virus Stability

The Japanese eel iridovirus is inactivated by exposure to ether, chloroform, and acid (pH 3.0) and by heating at 60°C for 30 min.

LYMPHOCYSTIS

Synonym. Lymphocystis virus infection.

Host and Geographic Distribution

Lymphocystis is recognized worldwide, occurring in at least 125 species of teleosts belonging to 34 families and 9 orders (Anders and Darai, 1985; Duijn, 1967; Lawler et al., 1977; Nigrelli and Ruggieri, 1965; Wolf, 1988). The disease occurs in warm-, cool-, and cold-water fish species from freshwater, estuarine, and marine environments.

Clinical Signs

Fish with lymphocystis develop macroscopic nodules (0.3 to 2.0 mm or more in diameter) that occur primarily on the body surface but can also develop on the internal organs (Dukes and Lawler, 1975; Dunbar and Wolf, 1966; Russell, 1974). The nodules appear cream to pink or gray depending on the condition of the overlying epithelium and the degree of vascularity of the lesion. They take a week to a year or more to develop depending on the host species and environmental conditions. The lesions eventually heal, leaving little evidence of scar tissue. Lymphocystis is a chronic but seldom fatal disease.

Pathology

Lymphocystis virus infection causes a unique cellular hypertrophy (Dunbar and Wolf, 1966; Lopez et al., 1969; Midlige and Malsberger, 1968; Nigrelli and Ruggieri, 1965). Infected cells do not divide, but both the cytoplasm and nucleus become greatly enlarged as the infection develops. Degenerative changes in the nucleus include chromatin condensation and fragmentation and enlargement. Nucleoli are distorted or indistinct. Within the expanding cytoplasm, Feulgen-positive inclusion bodies develop as weblike filaments or more dense vacuolated bodies depending on the host species (Wolf, 1962). Associated with the inclusions are icosahedral viral particles 150 to 250 nm in diameter. As the infected cell develops, a thick hyaline capsule forms at the periphery (Howse and Christmas, 1970; Pritchard and Malsberger, 1968). Proliferating fibroblasts isolate the infected cell, and plasma cells, lymphocytes, macrophages, and polymorphonuclear leukocytes accumulate at its periphery.

Diagnosis

Lymphocystis can be diagnosed by histologic examination. Lymphocystis virus can be isolated in cell culture, and antisera have been prepared in rabbits. However, no attempts to evaluate antigenic relationships among the various lymphocystis isolates have been reported. Also, virus-specific precipitating antibody has been detected in the sera of infected fish (Roberts, 1976; Russell, 1974).

Virus Isolation

Lymphocystis virus replicates in a variety of cell lines having fibroblastlike morphology, including the freshwater fish cell lines (BF-2, BF-W, and LBF-1) and marine fish cell lines (CrF, CyA-1, CyA-2, CyN-1, GF, SP-1, blue striped grunt kidney, and lane snapper fin). The virus does not replicate in BB, FHM, RTG-2, or bluegill ovary cells (Beasley et al., 1967; Durham and Anderson, 1981; Lopez et al., 1969; Middlebrooks et al., 1979, 1980, 1981; Midlige and Malsberger, 1968; Walker and Hill, 1980; Wharton et al., 1977; Wolf, 1962; Wolf et al., 1966).

Transmission

In nature, lymphocystis virus appears to be transmitted by exposure of surface wounds to water-borne virus or by ingestion of virus or virus-infected cells (Lawler et al., 1974; Stephens et al., 1970). Lymphocystis can be transmitted experimentally by cohabitation, exposure to water containing the virus, feeding lesion tissue and lesion homogenate, and by applying lesion homogenate to gills or scarified skin. The disease can also be experimentally transmitted by subcutaneous or intraperitoneal lesion implantation and subdermal or intramuscular injection of lesion homogenate or medium from virus-infected cell cultures (Dunbar and Wolf, 1966; Rasin, 1927; Wolf et al., 1966, 1979).

Lymphocystis can be experimentally transmitted with relative ease within a genus, but with difficulty between families. This limited degree of host specificity may indicate various types of lymphocystis viruses exist.

Epidemiology and Pathogenesis

The disease occurs with equal frequency in both sexes and can occur in fish of any age, although the prevalence appears higher in young fish.

Treatment and Control

Lymphocystis is a chronic, nonfatal disease. The lesions are unsightly and affect marketability. In culture situations, lesion-bearing fish should be removed. The antineoplastic drug, 6-mercaptopurine, inhibits virus-specific synthesis and the appearance of virus-induced cytopathic effects in cell culture and has been used to experimentally control lymphocystis in fish (Beasley et al., 1967; Lopez et al., 1970).

Lymphocystis virus is remarkably stable under a variety of storage conditions. Significant levels of infectivity were recovered after 15 years from infected tissue dried over P_2O_5 at 4°C (Wolf et al., 1979). Lymphocystis virus is inactivated when exposed to ether or chloroform, heat (56 to 60°C), or pH 3.0. The virus is progressively inactivated by sonication, but it is stable to multiple cycles of freezing and thawing.

EPIZOOTIC HEMATOPOIETIC NECROSIS

SYNONYMS. EHN, epizootic hematopoietic necrosis virus (EHNV) infection, Nillahcootie redfin perch virus infection, perch iridovirus infection.

Geographic Distribution

In November and December 1984, large numbers of juvenile redfin perch died in Lake Nillahcootie, Victoria, Australia, of a disease designated epizootic hematopoietic necrosis. An iridovirus was isolated from the affected fish and is now known to be widespread in Victoria. This virus is the first virus isolated from fish in Australia (Langdon et al., 1986), and it is found only there.

Clinical Signs

Juvenile and adult redfin perch with epizootic hematopoietic necrosis appear listless and ataxic, swim slowly on or spiraling to the surface, and respire weakly. Sometimes the fish are seen "head-standing" (Langdon and Humphrey, 1987). The brain and nostril areas of the head become reddened and the caudal trunk pallid. Petechial hemorrhages occur at the base of the fins, and the vent is reddened. Cutaneous ulcers with fungal invasion sometimes develop. Epizootic mortality is common.

Affected rainbow trout become dark in color, ataxic, and inappetent and sometimes react with erratic, hyperactive, spiral swimming. Abdominal distension, anal protrusion, and sharply defined 3- to 8-mm skin ulcers are seen. Morbidity approaches 100%, but mortality is low (Langdon et al., 1988).

Juvenile Atlantic salmon experimentally infected by intraperitoneal injection of cell culture grown virus are initially quiescent, dark, inappetent, and apparently blind, but later they become hyperactive and show an increased coughing reflex. The infection is not lethal, and fish recover normal color and behavior (Langdon et al., 1986).

Pathology

Gross examination of affected redfin perch shows focal mottling of the liver, an enlarged, bright red, gelatinous spleen, and diffuse hyperemia of the kidneys and swimbladder. Histologic examination shows necrotic changes in the liver, kidney, spleen, and sometimes the pancreas. The most severe lesions occur in the hematopoietic tissue of the kidney and in the liver; lesions in the spleen and pancreas are variable (Langdon and Humphrey, 1987).

Gross examination of affected rainbow trout shows edema and protrusion of the kidney and edema and pallor of the spleen. Multiple necrotic foci occur in the gastrointestinal epithelium; focal to diffuse necrosis is evident in the liver, hematopoietic tissue of the kidney, and the spleen. Vacuolating encephalopathy is present in the optic lobes, cerebral hemispheres, and thalamus (Langdon et al., 1988).

Histologic examination of convalescent Atlantic salmon shows severe vacuolating encephalopathy of the optic lobe, focal vacuolation in the cerebellar fiber tracts and optic nerve, and focal hepatocyte necrosis (Langdon et al., 1986).

Diagnosis

Presumptive diagnosis is based on clinical signs and isolation of virus in cell culture. Electron micrographs of infected cell cultures show iridoviruslike particles 150 to 170 nm in diameter in cytoplasmic arrays. Antisera produced to date are of low titer and cannot be used for serologic identification of the virus (Langdon and Humphrey, 1987).

Virus Isolation

Virus can be isolated from brain, liver, kidney, spleen, and whole viscera (Langdon and Humphrey, 1987; Langdon et al., 1986, 1988). The virus has been isolated only occasionally from eggs from suspect virus-carrying adults. The virus replicates in BB, BF-2, FHM, and RTG-2 cells. FHM cells give the highest virus yield. When infected cell cultures are incubated at 15 to 22°C, cytopathic effects consisting of focal cell rounding and lysis generally appear in 24 to 48 hours, but up to 10 days incubation may be needed for primary isolation (Langdon and Humphrey, 1987; Langdon et al., 1986, 1988). Basophilic, cytoplasmic inclusions can be seen in infected cells by light microscopy, and cytoplasmic arrays of iridoviruslike particles are seen in electron micrographs.

Transmission

In limited transmission trials, adult redfin perch injected with cell culture–grown virus developed clinical signs and histopathologic changes indistinguishable from natural infection (Langdon and Humphrey, 1987). The virus can be transmitted to, but is not highly pathogenic for, young rainbow trout (Langdon et al., 1988). Juvenile Atlantic salmon experimentally infected by intraperitoneal injection show transient clinical signs, but no mortality.

Epidemiology and Pathogenesis

Outbreaks of epizootic hematopoietic necrosis in juvenile and adult redfin perch occur between November and January (early summer in Australia) and continue for 2 to 3 weeks. Adult fish are suspect carriers, but the virus is isolated only infrequently from juveniles and adults after epizootics (Langdon and Humphrey, 1987). Introductions of subclinically infected or carrier fish into previously pristine watersheds has probably augmented the natural spread of the virus via water, fish migration, and possibly by predators (Langdon and Humphrey, 1987; Langdon et al., 1988).

Treatment and Control

Avoidance of suspect fish and fish products, quarantine, and viral examination of new fish stocks, disinfection of culture facilities, and eradication of subclinically infected or diseased fish are prudent steps toward disease control. No treatment or control methods are practical for feral fish. Further spread of the disease might be limited by restricting distribution of fish stocks (Langdon et al., 1988).

RAINBOW SMELT PICORNALIKE VIRUS INFECTION

SYNONYMS. None.

Host and Geographic Distribution

In 1986, epizootic mortality occurred in landlocked rainbow smelt in New Brunswick, Canada, and a picornalike virus was recovered from affected fish (Moore et al., 1988). The etiologic significance of the virus to the mortality in the rainbow smelt is unknown. The disease is known to occur only in landlocked rainbow smelt in Canada.

Clinical Signs and Pathology

Other than mortality, no clinical signs of infection or disease are discernible in affected rainbow smelt. When young brook trout are exposed to cell culture–grown virus, no clinical signs of disease or infection and no mortality occur. No histologic examinations have been reported.

Diagnosis

At present, diagnosis requires isolation of the virus in cell culture. No serologic tests have been developed. Although virus has been isolated in cell culture from affected fish, the etiologic significance of the virus has not been proved. Electron micrographs of infected cell cultures show cytoplasmic accumulations of unenveloped icosahedra 20 to 30 nm in diameter. The virus has tentatively been classified as picornaviruslike.

Virus Isolation

The rainbow smelt picornalike virus can be isolated from homogenates of pooled kidney, spleen, and pyloric ceca. The virus replicates in AK, BF-2, CHSE-214, GF, and SH cell lines and after several blind passages also replicates in FHM, GFT, and RTG-2. No virus replication occurs in A549 or VERO cells. At 15°C, cytopathology consists of focal syncytia that vacuolate, aggregate, and then detach and become evident in 12 days for primary isolation and in 38 to 48 hours for subsequent passages.

Transmission, Epidemiology, Pathogenesis, and Treatment and Control

No experimental infections of rainbow smelt with this virus have been reported. Young brook trout experimentally infected by intraperitoneal injection of cell culture–grown virus show no clinical signs and no mortality. The etiologic relationship between the virus isolate and the mortality is unproven. Treatment and control of disease or infection in feral fishes is impractical.

13p$_2$ REOVIRUS INFECTION

SYNONYMS. Oyster reovirus 13p$_2$ infection, bluegill hepatic necrosis reovirus infection.

Host and Geographic Distribution

A virus designated 13p$_2$ was isolated from apparently healthy juvenile American oysters collected at mollusk hatcheries on Long Island Sound, New York (Meyers, 1979). The primary host of the virus remains unknown. The oyster may have merely accumulated sufficient virus by filter feeding to make virus isolation possible (Meyers, 1980, 1983). The virus is considered of possible piscine origin because of the more virulent pattern of disease and mortality that occurs in experimentally infected fish.

Clinical Signs

No clinical signs of infection or disease are seen in the oysters, but rainbow trout develop a transient subclinical infection, which is evidenced by increasing virus titer and production of virus-specific antibody (Meyers, 1980). The virus also replicates in golden shiners with no clinical signs. In contrast, experimentally infected fingerling bluegills become lethargic and inappetent, show loss of equilibrium, and remain prostrate on the bottom of the aquarium prior to death.

Pathology

Experimentally infected juvenile American oysters develop no pathology, whereas fingerling and adult rainbow trout develop multifocal reticuloendothelial granulomatous hepatitis and occasionally fibrosing pancreatitis (Meyers, 1983). Experimentally infected fingerling bluegills develop diffuse multifocal hepatitis characterized by formation of large syncytial cells, coagulative necrosis of hepatocytes, and diffuse infiltration of phagocytic macrophages. Primary lesions occur around major hepatic blood vessels, but hepatic regeneration occurs while necrosis is in progress. Virus titer in the liver increases, and electron micrographs of liver tissue show intracytoplasmic arrays of reoviruslike particles (Meyers, 1980).

Diagnosis and Virus Isolation

Presumptive diagnosis is based on correlating clinical signs and pathology, but definitive diagnosis requires isolation and serologic identification of the virus. The 13p$_2$ virus was originally isolated from homogenates of whole juvenile oysters inoculated onto BF-2 cells and incubated at 15°C. Large syncytia developed 6 days after infection and progressively involved the entire monolayer. In subsequent passages, cytopathic effects appeared 2 to 12 days after infection depending on the cell line. The virus replicates in AS, BB, BF-2, CHH-1, CHSE-214, GE-4, and WF-2 cell lines, to a limited extent in ASH cells, and not at all in RTG-2, FHM, or RTS cells (piscine), CKC cells (avian), or FBS, LK, MDCK, PK, RK, or VERO cells (mammalian) (Meyers, 1979; Winton et al., 1987). The virus replicates at 15 and 23°C, but not at 9 or 30°C. The 13p$_2$ virus is not neutralized by antiserum to infectious pancreatic necrosis virus, Tellina virus, feline reovirus type 3, canine reovirus type 1, or chicken FDO reovirus.

Transmission, Epidemiology, and Pathogenesis

No instance of naturally occurring disease has been linked to infection with 13p$_2$ virus, and the role of the virus in nature is unknown. In fingerling and adult rainbow trout challenged by intraperitoneal and subcutaneous injection of virus, self-limiting, subclinical infection develops. Virus titers increase in the liver, kidneys, spleen, and pancreas, and the fish produce precipitating and virus-neutralizing antibody (Meyers, 1980, 1983).

In bluegills exposed by intraperitoneal inoculation, mortality begins 13 days after exposure, and 44% of fish die by day 50. No mortality was reported in bluegills exposed to virus by immersion, but hepatic lesions and increased virus titers were observed. The immersion challenge experiments might not have been of sufficient duration to allow mortality to develop (Meyers, 1980). No methods of treatment or control have been described.

ESOX EPIDERMAL HYPERPLASIA

SYNONYMS. Esox epidermal hyperplasia retrovirus infection, pike epidermal proliferation retrovirus infection.

Host and Geographic Distribution

An epidermal hyperplasia has been observed in northern pike and muskellunge in Canada and in northern pike inhabiting the Baltic coast of Sweden (Ljungberg, 1976; Sonstegard, 1976; Yamamoto et al., 1984; Winqvist et al., 1968). The effect of the proliferation on the host is unknown. Electron micrographs show retroviruslike particles associated with the affected tissue, but virus has not been isolated in cell culture.

Clinical Signs

The epidermal lesions are transparent to whitish-gray plaques 5 to 10 mm in diameter and 1 to 3 mm thick and occur on the head, trunk, or fins (Sonstegard, 1976; Winqvist et al., 1968). The proliferations can occur on fish that also have lymphosarcoma or sarcoma.

Pathology

Lesions are confined to the epidermis and are composed of homogeneous masses of polygonal cells apparently derived from the middle epidermis (Winqvist et al., 1968). The mucus-forming cells and the stratified structure of the normal epidermis are absent.

Diagnosis and Virus Detection

Presumptive diagnosis is based on clinical signs. The type C retrovirus is detected by electron microscopy. Electron microscopic examination of the epithelial lesions reveals type C retroviruslike particles 120 to 150 nm in diameter (Sonstegard, 1976; Winqvist et al., 1968). Particles are seen in intercellular spaces, in the cell cytoplasm, and budding from cytoplasmic membranes.

Transmission, Epidemiology, Pathogenesis, and Treatment and Control

No experimental transmission of the disease has been reported; thus the etiologic significance of the virus is unproven. The effect of the proliferation on the host is unknown. The lesion is found with equal frequency in mature fish of both sexes, and its prevalence in captured escoids can approach 6%. No methods of treatment and control have been described.

ESOX LYMPHOSARCOMA

SYNONYMS. Esocid lymphosarcoma, esocid leukosarcoma, esocid lymphoma, esox lymphosarcoma retrovirus infection.

Host and Geographic Distribution

Lymphosarcoma in esocids was described in the late 1890s and early 1900s. Population surveys show that the prevalence of the disease can approach 21%, the highest for a malignant tumor in a free-living vertebrate (Mulcahy, 1963; Sonstegard, 1975, 1976). Lymphosarcoma occurs in northern pike and muskellunge. The disease in northern pike has been documented in Canada, Ireland, Finland, Sweden, and the United States, but northern pike throughout the world may be affected (Ljungberg, 1976; Mulcahy, 1976; Mulcahy and O'Rourke, 1964; Sonstegard, 1976; Thompson, 1982; Wellings, 1969). Lymphosarcoma in muskellunge has been reported only in Canada (Sonstegard, 1976).

Clinical Signs

Esocids affected by lymphosarcoma show single or multiple nodular external lesions on the head, trunk, or fins. As tumor volume increases, the surface scales slough, and the epidermis is breached, exposing a cream to pinkish-red soft proliferation. The lesion can heal, producing a sharply delineated gray area on the epidermis, but generally metastasizes (Mulcahy, 1963, 1976; Sonstegard, 1975, 1976; Wellings, 1969). Lymphosarcoma usually results in death. The disease seems to be more fulminating in muskellunge than in northern pike, and spontaneous regression occurs with greater frequency in northern pike (Sonstegard, 1976).

Pathology

The tumor initially develops in the connective tissue between the muscle and epidermis and then metastasizes sequentially to the muscle, kidneys, spleen, and liver, and possibly other internal organs. Epidermal infiltration and external lesion expression precede muscle involvement. Neoplastic cells infiltrate the underlying musculature via intracellular spaces along reticular fibers and capillaries. Eventually individual muscle fibers are surrounded by neoplastic cells (Mulcahy, 1963; Mulcahy et al., 1970;

Sonstegard, 1975). Thereafter, the kidneys and spleen undergo neoplastic replacement. Later, hepatic stroma is similarly affected. Involvement of the connective tissue of the thymus, swim bladder, intestine, pancreas, rectum, and stomach has been reported (Mulcahy, 1963, 1969, 1976; Wellings, 1969). The affected organs become enlarged and can develop solid sarcomatous masses. Death often occurs before the internal organs become extensively involved.

Pathologic changes also occur in the blood. Erythrocyte counts and serum protein levels decrease, but leukocyte concentrations remain stable until terminal stages (Mulcahy, 1975). Little fibroblastic or inflammatory response is seen during the course of the disease. Immunodeficiency may be a factor in tumor development (Mulcahy, 1963, 1969, 1976; Sonstegard, 1975; Wellings, 1969).

Esocid lymphosarcoma is a stem cell lymphoreticular neoplasm in which tissues are infiltrated by masses of isomorphic undifferentiated hemocytoblasts (Mulcahy, 1963; Mulcahy et al., 1970; Sonstegard, 1975, 1976; Wellings, 1969). The neoplastic cells have a round to oval nucleus with a single identation. The chromatin can be uniformly dispersed or aggregated at the periphery of the nuclear membrane. No intranuclear inclusions are evident, but multinucleated cells are occasionally seen. The cytoplasm contains many mitochondria and free ribosomes and a few fat droplets and vacuoles. Cylindroid lamellaparticle complexes and nucleoid bodies also occur in the cytoplasm (Dawe et al., 1976; Sonstegard, 1976). Similar structures are seen in cells from several types of lymphomas and leukemias (Dawe et al., 1976). Nucleoid bodies are less frequently seen and appear to be spheroids 2 to 8 μm in diameter with a densely staining chromatinlike periphery and an unstained or diffusely stained center.

Diagnosis and Virus Detection

Esox lymphosarcoma is diagnosed based on clinical signs and histologic examination. Virus has not been detected in cell culture. Cell-free extracts of tumor homogenates contain ribonucleic acid (RNA)–dependent DNA polymerase (reverse transcriptase) activity, an indicator of retrovirus infection (Papas et al., 1976, 1977). The thermal profile of the enzyme indicates that reverse transcriptase activity is high below 25°C and reduced above 25°C, which correlates with field observations that marked reduction in tumor prevalence and development occur in middle and late summer when water temperatures range to 30°C.

The etiologic significance of the viruslike particles has not been proved. Attempts to identify virus particles in tumor tissue are generally unsuccessful, as are attempts to induce virogenesis in cultured neoplastic cells (Mulcahy, 1976; Mulcahy et al., 1970; Sonstegard, 1976). Electron-dense particles 60 to 80 nm in diameter can be seen, albeit infrequently, in tumor tissue and cultured tumor cells and are suggestive of retroviruses (Thompson, 1982). Transformation assays using primary and established fish cell cultures inoculated with cell-free tumor extract or suspensions of viable neoplastic cells have produced negative results (Sonstegard, 1976).

Transmission

Empirical evidence suggests that in nature, esox lymphosarcoma is transmitted horizontally, possibly by contact at spawning. At other times, northern pike and muskellunge are solitary (Sonstegard, 1976).

Lymphosarcoma can be experimentally transmitted by intraperitoneal injection of membrane-filtered (0.22 μm average pore diameter [apd]) tumor homogenates, by intramuscular and intraperitoneal implantation of neoplastic tissue, and by cohabitation (Brown et al., 1976; Mulcahy and O'Leary, 1970; Schlumberger, 1957; Sonstegard, 1976). In experimentally infected adults and fingerlings, clinical signs develop after prolonged incubation (1 to 7 months for transplants and 1 to 18 months for filtrate injection). Variations in host response affect natural and experimental transmission (Brown et al., 1976; Mulcahy, 1976; Sonstegard, 1976).

Epidemiology and Pathogenesis

Seasonal variations in the disease are evident in geographic areas where annual temperature fluctuations are pronounced. In North America, tumor prevalence and development are low in winter and in middle and late summer and are high in spring, early summer, and fall, suggesting tumorigenesis is adversely affected by high and low water temperatures (Papas et al., 1976; Sonstegard, 1976). In Ireland, no seasonal periodicity is observed (Mulcahy, 1976). Water quality does not appear to be etiologically significant. Tumors occur with high frequency in both polluted and unpolluted water (Brown et al., 1973; Mulcahy, 1976; Sonstegard, 1976).

Lymphosarcoma occurs in 1- to 11-year-old fish and at the same relative frequency in males and females. The relationship between frequency and age is not clearly understood. Some suggest the prevalence increases with age and peaks in 4-year-old fish (Mulcahy, 1963, 1976). Others report that the disease occurs only in fish older than 4 years (Sonstegard, 1976). Experimental transmission suggests that maturity is not requisite for tumor development.

Treatment and Control

No methods for treatment or control of esox lymphosarcoma have been described. The disease is widespread in nature. Fish with a history of infection or exposure to the virus should not be stocked into pristine watersheds.

ESOX SARCOMA

SYNONYM. Esox sarcoma retrovirus infection.

Host and Geographic Distribution

A sarcoma restricted to the skin and underlying musculature occurs in northern pike along the Baltic coast of Sweden (Ljungberg, 1976; Ljungberg and Lange, 1968; Sonstegard, 1976; Winqvist et al., 1973). The tumor was first reported in 1953 and has been observed with increasing frequency in polluted brackish water (Ljungberg, 1976). Esox sarcoma occurs along the Baltic coast of Sweden. The disease has not been reported in North America.

Clinical Signs

Tumors develop in the skin as single or multiple yellow-gray to yellow-red lesions that become 4 to 5 cm in diameter and 1 cm thick. Petechial hemorrhaging sometimes occurs in the soft tumor tissue (Ljungberg and Lange, 1968). The lesions can involve up to 25% of the total skin surface, and are not covered by scales or skin.

Pathology

The undifferentiated sarcoma develops in the cutaneous layers of the skin and connective tissue and is not separated from the underlying tissue by fibroblastic encapsulation (Ljungberg and Lange, 1968). Infiltration of the muscle is not seen. The tumor appears to be well vascularized and contains little or no connective tissue or reticulin fibers between the tumor cells.

The round to slightly elongated neoplastic cells are poorly differentiated. The nucleus appears round to slightly indented and contains finely dispersed chromatin and distinct nucleoli. In contrast to lymphosarcoma cells, the skin sarcoma cells contain many lipid droplets and lack the cylindroid lamella-particle complex and nucleoid bodies (Winqvist et al., 1973). Chromosome analysis of cultured neoplastic cells indicates abnormal chromosome types and numbers (Ljungberg, 1976).

Diagnosis and Virus Detection

Presumptive diagnosis is based on appearance of clinical signs and histopathologic examination. Virus has not been isolated in cell culture, but type C retroviruslike particles are occasionally seen in the cytoplasm of sarcoma cells. Extracellular and budding particles are not observed. The intracytoplasmic particles are 100 nm in diameter and contain a centrally placed, electron-dense nucleoid 50 nm in diameter

(Winqvist et al., 1973). The etiologic significance of these viruslike particles is unknown.

Transmission

The sarcoma can be experimentally transmitted by intraperitoneal, intracutaneous, and subcutaneous injections of tumor cells and by cohabitation, but attempts to transmit the tumor by intraperitoneal injection of cell-free tumor homogenates have not been successful (Ljungberg, 1976).

Epidemiology, Pathogenesis, and Treatment and Control

The tumors seem to occur at the same relative frequency in both sexes. Prevalence to 10% is reported (Ljungberg, 1976). Seasonal fluctuations in prevalence and severity of tumor development are not pronounced, but high tumor frequency occurs in polluted brackish water, suggesting that environmental interactions affect tumorigenesis. Esox sarcoma occurs in feral fish. No methods of treatment or control are practiced.

WALLEYE DERMAL SARCOMA

SYNONYMS. Walleye dermal sarcoma retrovirus infection, walleye dermal sarcoma virus infection.

Host and Geographic Distribution

A dermal sarcoma is often seen in walleyes in the United States and Canada (Walker, 1958, 1961, 1969; Yamamoto et al., 1976). The tumor can occur in walleyes concurrent with lymphocystis and diffuse and discrete epidermal hyperplasia (Yamamoto et al., 1985a, b). Viral etiology is presumed because retroviruslike particles are associated with tumor tissue.

Clinical Signs

Affected walleyes show single or multiple dermal nodules covered by a thin layer of epidermis. The nodules are smooth and firm, develop to about 10 mm in diameter, and occur predominantly on the trunk. The nodules appear pink to white depending on the level of fibroreticulation and vascularity.

Pathology

The sarcoma is confined to the skin, and there is no evidence of invasiveness or metastasis. The lesions appear similar in gross morphology to lymphocystis, but the hyperplasic sarcoma cells can be readily distinguished from the hypertrophied lymphocystis cells.

The neoplastic cells vary in morphology and are extensively conjoined by interdigitating cytoplasmic processes. The cytoplasm is highly vesiculated, and the chromatin often marginated (Walker, 1961, 1969; Yamamoto et al., 1976, 1985a). Tumor composition varies from a highly proliferative, irregularly arranged sarcoma to a densely whorled, well-organized fibroma.

Diagnosis and Virus Detection

Diagnosis requires histopathologic examination. Dermal sarcoma can be confused with lymphocystis and discrete epidermal hyperplasia. Virus has not been isolated in cell culture, but electron micrographs of tumor tissue show accumulations of viruslike particles (Walker, 1961, 1969). The type C retroviruslike particles are approximately 135 nm in diameter and contain a centrally placed, electron-dense nucleoid approximately 75 nm in diameter (Yamamoto et al., 1976, 1985a). Virus particles were seen in intercellular spaces and cytoplasmic vesicles and budding from cytoplasmic membranes. The retrovirus particles from walleye dermal sarcoma seem to be ultrastructurally different from those from walleye discrete epidermal hyperplasia (Yamamoto et al., 1985b).

Transmission, Epidemiology, Pathogenesis, and Treatment and Control

Walleye dermal sarcoma can be experimentally transmitted by injection of cell-free filtrates of sonicated tumor cells, supporting the etiologic significance of the tumor-associated retrovirus (Martineau et al., 1990). The incidence of dermal sarcoma can approach 10%, and the lesions are observed in females more frequently than in males and in younger fish more frequently than in older fish. No methods of treatment or control have been described.

WALLEYE DISCRETE EPIDERMAL HYPERPLASIA

SYNONYMS. Walleye discrete epidermal hyperplasia retrovirus infection, walleye epidermal hyperplasia retrovirus infection.

Host and Geographic Distribution

Walleyes in the provinces of Saskatchewan and Manitoba (Canada) and in Lake Oneida, New York (United States) can develop a discrete epidermal

hyperplasia of putative viral etiology (Yamamoto et al., 1985a, b; Walker, 1969). In addition to the discrete epidermal hyperplasia, three other skin lesions of proven or putative viral etiology are seen in walleyes—lymphocystis, dermal sarcoma, and diffuse epidermal hyperplasia. Discrete epidermal hyperplasia can develop in fish concurrent with the other three diseases (Yamamoto et al., 1985a, b).

Clinical Signs

The discrete epidermal hyperplasia is a firm, smooth lesion that is a translucent, clear to gray, sharply delineated plaque, 0.25 to 1.5 mm thick and several centimeters in diameter. The single or multiple proliferations can occur on any body surface, but involvement of the fins seems most common.

Pathology

Discrete epidermal hyperplasia shows no evidence of invasiveness, metastasis, or necrosis of the dermal or subcutaneous layers, including the musculature. The hyperplastic cells are uniformly homogeneous undifferentiated cuboidal cells with long cytoplasmic extensions that leave large spaces between cells. Mucous cells are present at the periphery of the lesion but are infrequent in the body of the hyperplasia.

Diagnosis and Virus Detection

Diagnosis is based on clinical signs coupled with histopathologic examination. Virus has not been isolated in cell culture, but electron micrographs show type C retroviruslike particles 80 to 120 nm in diameter throughout the hyperplastic epidermis (Walker, 1969; Yamamoto et al., 1985a, b). Virions are seen budding from cell surface membranes, but not in the interior of the cells. No viruslike particles are observed in the dermis or in normal epidermis.

Transmission, Epidemiology, and Treatment and Control

Experimental transmission of discrete epidermal hyperplasia in walleyes has not been reported. In sampled populations the disease varies in prevalence to 20% (Yamamoto et al., 1985a, b; Walker, 1969). No methods of treatment or control have been described.

WHITE SUCKER EPIDERMAL PAPILLOMA

SYNONYMS. White sucker epidermal papilloma retrovirus infection, sucker papilloma retrovirus infection.

Host and Geographic Distribution

White sucker epidermal papilloma is widely distribued in Canada and the United States (Sonstegard, 1977a, b). Tumor prevalence is highest in heavily polluted areas.

Clinical Signs

Single or multiple papillomatous growths can occur at any site on the body surface. In heavily polluted waters, the growths appeared most frequently on the lips. The white to pink tumor is firm with a nodular, undulating texture.

Pathology

The papilloma is confined to the epidermis and shows no invasiveness or metastasis (Sonstegard, 1977b). No histopathologic description of the tumor or tumor development has been reported.

Diagnosis and Virus Detection

Diagnosis is based on clinical signs. Virus has not been isolated in cell culture, but in electron micrographs of papilloma tissue, type C retrovirus-like particles approximately 100 nm in diameter are seen in cytoplasmic aggregates and budding from cytoplasmic membranes. RNA-dependent DNA polymerase (reverse transcriptase) activity can be detected in tumor preparations fractionated on sucrose gradients. Attempts to demonstrate cell transformation in vitro using BB, BF-2, FHM, and RTG-2 cell lines have been unsuccessful (Sonstegard, 1977b). No attempts to culture papilloma cells have been reported.

Transmission

Attempts to experimentally transmit the tumor by cohabitation, percutaneous transplantation of tumor tissue, percutaneous injection of cell-free tumor homogenates, and exposure of abraded surfaces to tumor tissue have not been successful (Sonstegard, 1977b).

Epidemiology, Pathogenesis, and Treatment and Control

The proliferations occur in sexually mature 4-year-old fish and increase in size and prevalence with age, suggesting that the benign tumor might be borne throughout life. Results from epidemiologic investigations in the Great Lakes region suggest that environmental factors, such as water- and sediment-borne carcinogens, might affect tumor development by triggering the expression of horizontally or vertically transmitted virus (Sonstegard, 1977a, b). In heavily polluted areas of Lake Ontario, tumor prevalence approaches 51% in certain collections, whereas in other areas, the prevalence is 0.7% or less. No methods for treatment or control have been described.

PERCH RHABDOVIRUS DISEASE

SYNONYM. Perch rhabdovirus infection.

Host and Geographic Distribution

Only a single outbreak has been reported. Affected perch were taken from a pond near Sologne, France (Dorson et al., 1984). Experimental challenges show that northern pike fry are susceptible to infection (Dorson et al., 1987).

Clinical Signs and Pathology

In perch, clinical signs of infection are loss of equilibrium, disorganized swimming, and death (Dorson et al., 1984). Histopathologic changes have not been described. Experimentally infected northern pike become exophthalmic and develop hemorrhages in the intermuscular spaces at the bases of the fins and in the body cavity (Dorson et al., 1987).

Diagnosis and Virus Isolation

Diagnosis requires isolation and serologic identification of the virus. The perch rhabdovirus can be isolated from pooled anterior kidney and spleen and from brain using RTG-2 cells incubated at 14°C. The virus replicates poorly, if at all, in EPC cells. By infectivity neutralization assays, the virus is distinct from infectious hematopoietic necrosis and viral hemorrhagic septicemia viruses.

Transmission, Epidemiology, Pathogenesis, and Treatment and Control

Mortality occurs in young perch inoculated intracranially, and virus is recovered from the brain (Dorson et al., 1984). Fish challenged by immersion or intraperitoneal injection do not die, and virus is not recovered. Northern pike fry experimentally infected by immersion exposure begin to die after 8 days, and 40% of challenged fish die in 15 days. Virus can be recovered from homogenates of whole fry (Dorson et al., 1987). No mortality occurs in experimentally challenged rainbow trout fry (Dorson et al., 1984). No methods of treatment or control have been described.

PIKE FRY RHABDOVIRUS DISEASE

SYNONYMS. Hydrocephalus, head disease of pike, red disease of pike, pike fry rhabdovirus (PFR) infection, grass carp rhabdovirus infection.

Host and Geographic Distribution

The northern pike is the principal host species for pike fry rhabdovirus, but the virus has been isolated from brown trout, grass carp, gudgeon, tench, and white bream (Adair and McLoughlin, 1986; Ahne, 1975; Ahne and Thomsen, 1986; Ahne et al., 1982; Bekesi et al., 1984; Bootsma et al., 1975). Pike fry rhabdovirus also replicates in insects (*Drosophila melanogaster*) (Bussereau et al., 1975). The pike fry rhabdovirus disease occurs throughout eastern and western Europe but does not occur in North America (Bekesi et al., 1984; Bootsma, 1976).

Clinical Signs

Diseased pike show a large hemorrhagic swelling on the trunk or on the side of the skull, or show a prominent unilobate or bilobate swelling from the middle of the skull (Fig. 26–1). Affected fish are exophthalmic, the gills are pale, and the abdomen is distended with ascites. Behavior varies from lethargic to hyperactive.

Grass carp and white bream show hemorrhages on the ventral body surface and at the scale bases and ascites. Tench show hemorrhages in the skin and at scale bases, and in the gudgeon PFR infection is inapparent (Ahne, 1975; Ahne et al., 1982).

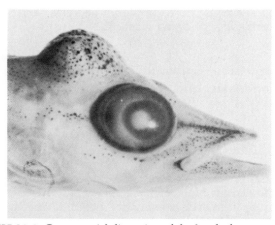

FIGURE 26–1. Gross cranial distention of the head of a young pike infected with pike fry rhabdovirus. (Courtesy of R. Bootsma. From Roberts, R. J. [1989] Fish Pathology. 2nd ed. Bailliere Tindall, London.)

Pathology

In diseased pike fry, petechial hemorrhages are evident in the brain, spinal cord, spleen, and kidneys. There is extensive degeneration and necrosis in the kidney tissue, but pathologic changes in other tissues are inconsistent (Bootsma, 1971, 1976). Cells in the proximal tubules of the kidneys undergo lytic and coagulative necrosis, characterized by nuclear pyknosis or margination of the chromatin. Necrotic detritus collects in the lumina and the distal tubules. Glomeruli are less affected, but the nuclei of the vascular cells appear swollen. Petechial hemorrhages occur in the kidney hemopoietic tissue. Hepatic cells can exhibit necrobiotic changes similar to those observed in the tubule and vascular cells of the kidneys. Hemorrhages occur in muscle connective tissue and can extend into the muscle fibers. Muscle cell degeneration can accompany severe hemorrhaging. The swelling of the head results from the overproduction of cerebral fluid. No inclusion bodies are evident in any organ or tissue. Electron microscopy indicates significant concentrations of viral particles in renal hematopoietic tissue, but not in muscle, spinal cord, or skin (Bootsma and Van Vorstenbosch, 1973).

In young grass carp and white bream, the spleen is swollen and the liver pale, and the swim bladder shows petechial hemorrhages. In tench and gudgeon, infection is inapparent (Ahne, 1975; Ahne et al., 1982). No description of histopathology has been reported for adult pike, grass carp, gudgeon, tench, or white bream.

Diagnosis

In northern pike, presumptive diagnosis is based on clinical signs. In other species, clinical signs are not sufficient for presumptive diagnosis. Diagnosis is confirmed by isolation and serologic identification of the virus.

Virus Isolation and Identification

The pike fry rhabdovirus is isolated from homogenates of pooled internal organs or whole northern pike fry. It is isolated from homogenates of pooled liver, kidneys, and spleen of grass carp, gudgeon, tench, and white bream (Ahne, 1975, 1985; Ahne et al., 1982; de Kinkelin et al., 1973). Virus cannot be isolated from liver, kidneys, spleen, intestine, gonads, ovarian fluid, or fertilized or unfertilized eggs from adults (Bootsma et al., 1975).

Pike fry rhabdovirus replicates in piscine (BB, CaPi, EPC, FHM, RF, and RTG-2) and mammalian (BHK-21) cell lines (Hill et al., 1975; de Kinkelin et al., 1973; Roy et al., 1975). The temperature range for virus replication in cell culture is 10 to 31°C, and the optimum temperature range is 16 to 23°C. The virus is most commonly identified using infectivity neutralization assay, but other serologic tests, such as fluorescent antibody staining, are applicable (Ahne, 1981). Grass carp rhabdovirus is antigenically indistinguishable from pike fry rhabdovirus (Ahne, 1975; Hill et al., 1975).

Transmission

Horizontal transmission to young-of-the-year pike can be demonstrated under natural and experimental conditions (Bootsma et al., 1975; de Kinkelin et al., 1973). Pike fry and grass carp are experimentally infected by feeding virus-carrying forage, by immersion, and by intraperitoneal injection. Preliminary infectivity trials with rainbow trout and tench are inconclusive. Yearling pike are infected by feeding virus-carrying forage fish, but do not develop disease (Ahne, 1985). The virus is not recovered from spawning fish or their sex products, but the potential for egg-associated transmission has been shown using experimentally contaminated eggs (Bootsma et al., 1975). Pike fry rhabdovirus replicates in the fly *Drosophila melanogaster,* indicating the potential for insect transmission (Bussereau et al., 1975). Further investigations are needed to elucidate the mechanisms of transmission and to ascertain the carrier status of adult fish.

Epidemiology and Pathogenesis

Several observations, but few experimental data, are available concerning interactions between the host, the virus, and the environment. The disease occurs in fry and fingerling pike up to 6 cm in length, and susceptibility decreases with age. Neutralizing antibody can be stimulated in adult pike by injection of virus (Clerx et al., 1978), but no other data on host immune or interferon response have been reported.

Pike develop the disease naturally at temperatures from 10 to 20°C and experimentally to 24°C (Bootsma, 1976; de Kinkelin et al., 1973). Physiologic stress from overcrowding, low oxygen, or handling may predispose fish to infection (Bootsma, 1971, 1976).

Treatment and Control

No treatment methods are effective. To control pike fry rhabdovirus disease, contact between the virus and the host must be prevented by ensuring that the facility, water supply, and fish are virus free. Because the carrier status of adult pike is uncertain, decontamination of eggs with iodophor should be performed (Bootsma et al., 1975). Management and environmental factors that promote physiologic stress should be avoided. Immunized pike show an increase in virus-neutralizing activity in their serum (Clerx et al., 1978), but the significance to the epidemiology or control of the disease has not been determined.

RIO GRANDE PERCH RHABDOVIRUS INFECTION

SYNONYMS. Rio Grande cichlid rhabdovirus infection, cichlid rhabdovirus infection.

Host and Geographic Distribution

Convict and Zilli cichlids and Rio Grande perch are susceptible to lethal viral infection. The virus was isolated at Bethlehem, Pennsylvania, from fish shipped by an undesignated U.S. commercial supplier (Malsberger and Lautenslager, 1980).

Clinical Signs, Pathology, Diagnosis, and Virus Isolation

Clinical signs of the disease are lethargy and death. No histopathologic changes have been reported. Diagnosis requires isolation and serologic identification of the virus. Initially, the virus was recovered from homogenates of whole fish. Subsequently, the virus was recovered only from skin and muscle. The virus replicates in FHM, RTG-2, LBF-2, and BHK-21 cells (Malsberger and Lautenslager, 1980). The temperature range for virus replication is 13 to 31.5°C, and the optimum temperature for virus replication in FHM cells is 29°C. Infectivity neutralization assays indicate that the virus is distinct from infectious hematopoietic necrosis, viral hemorrhagic septicemia, and pike fry rhabdovirus disease viruses.

Transmission, Epidemiology, Pathogenesis, and Treatment and Control

Mortality exceeding 80% occurs in convict and Zilli cichlids and Rio Grande perch experimentally challenged by intraperitoneal injection of cell culture–grown virus. Virus could be recovered from mortalities of all three species of fishes. No methods of treatment or control have been described. The disease has been reported on only this one occasion.

BLUEGILL VIRUS INFECTION

Geographic Distribution, Clinical Signs, and Pathology

Only two instances of virus isolation are known, the original isolation at Leetown, West Virginia (Hoffman et al., 1969), and a second at Frankfort, Kentucky (Wolf, 1988). No clinical signs or pathology are evident in either natural or experimental infections (Beckwith and Malsberger, 1979; Hoffman et al., 1969; Wolf, 1976).

Electron micrographs of infected BF-2 cells show spheroidal viral particles about 90 nm in diameter in extracellular arrays, in cytoplasmic vacuoles, and budding from cell membranes (Beckwith and Malsberger, 1979; Berthiaume et al., 1982). Presumptive diagnosis is based on isolation of virus in cell culture that causes elongate, fusiform cytopathic effects.

Virus Isolation and Identification

The bluegill virus was originally isolated from membrane-filtered (0.45 μm apd) homogenates of scrapings from the caudal fin of an adult bluegill (Hoffman et al., 1969) inoculated onto BF-2 cells and incubated at 23°C. Enlarged, rounded cells developed about 2 days after inoculation. Later, inoculation of infected medium onto fresh BF-2 cells after prolonged culture resulted in cytoplasmic and nuclear pyknosis with progressive vacuolation that produced extremely elongated fusiform cells (100 to 160 μm) (Hoffman et al., 1969; Wolf and Quimby, 1973). In the second isolation at Frankfort, Kentucky, the virus was recovered from homogenates of pooled kidneys and spleen. The same unique cytopathology was seen.

The virus replicates only in fibroblastic cells of piscine origin (Beckwith and Malsberger, 1979; Nicholson and Byrne, 1973; Wolf and Quimby, 1973). Other piscine cell lines are refractory, as are cells of mammalian (BHK-21, HeLa, WI-38, and WISH), amphibian (A6), or reptilian (IgH-2) origin (Beckwith and Malsberger, 1979). The temperature range of virus replication has not been determined, but infected cell cultures are usually incubated at 20 to 25°C. No cross-neutralization infectivity trials have been reported.

Transmission, Epidemiology, and Pathogenesis

Bluegills injected intramuscularly, intraperitoneally, or subdermally with infected cell culture supernatants or exposed per os or by swabbing virus on gill lamellae show no evidence of disease. Bluegills immunosuppressed by corticosteroids, or stressed by elevated temperature or by experimentally induced bacterial infections, are also refractory (Beckwith and Malsberger, 1979; Hoffman et al., 1969; Wolf, 1976). No methods of treatment or control are known.

Bluegill virus is completely inactivated by exposure to ether, ultraviolet irradiation, and acid (pH 3.0) but appears to be stable at pH 7.2 and is only partly inactivated at pH 5.0 and 9.5 (Beckwith and Malsberger, 1979). When suspended in cell culture medium supplemented with 10% serum, no loss of infectivity occurs during 90 days storage at −70°C, and after 1 year infectivity can still be recovered.

LITERATURE CITED

Adair, B.M., and McLoughlin, M. (1986) Isolation of pike fry rhabdovirus from brown trout (*Salmo trutta*). Bull. Eur. Assoc. Fish Pathol. 6:85–86.

Ahne, W. (1975) A rhabdovirus isolated from grass carp (*Ctenopharyngodon idella* Val.). Arch. Virol. 48:181–185.

Ahne, W. (1981) Serological techniques currently used in fish virology. Dev. Biol. Stand. 49:3–27.

Ahne, W. (1985) Viral infection cycles in pike (*Esox lucius* L.). J. Appl. Ichthyol. 1:90–91.

Ahne, W., and Thomsen, I. (1986) Isolation of pike fry rhabdovirus from *Pseudorasbora parva* (Temminck & Schlegel). J. Fish Dis. 9:555–556.

Ahne, W., Mahnel, H., and Steinhagen, P. (1982) Isolation of pike fry rhabdovirus from tench, *Tinca tinca* L., and white bream, *Blicca bjoerkna* (L.). J. Fish Dis. 5:535–537.

Anders, K., and Darai, G. (1985) Genome analysis of fish lymphocystis disease virus. In: Fish and Shellfish Pathology (Ellis, A.E., ed.). Academic Press, London, pp. 301–306.

Beasley, A.R., Sigel, M.M., and Lopez, D.M. (ca. 1967). Virological and related problems in marine animals. Final Report Contract NONR 4008 (05), not published.

Beckwith, D.G., and Malsberger, R.G. (1979) Characterization and morphology of the bluegill virus. J. Gen. Virol. 43:489–501.

Bekesi, L., Majoros, G., and Szabo, E. (1984) Mass appearance of a rhabdovirus in pike fry (*Esox lucius* L.) in Hungary. Magy. Allatory. Lapja 39:231–234.

Berthiaume, L., Robin, J., and Alain, R. (1982) Electron microscopic study of bluegill virus. Can. J. Microbiol. 28:398–402.

Bootsma, R. (1971) Hydrocephalus and red-disease in pike fry *Esox lucius* L. J. Fish Biol. 3:417–419.

Bootsma, R. (1976) Studies on two infectious diseases of cultured freshwater fish, rhabdovirus disease of pike fry, *Esox lucius* L., columnaris disease of carp, *Cyprinus carpio* L. Ph.D. Dissertation, State University of Utrecht, The Netherlands.

Bootsma, R., and Van Vorstenbosch, C.J.A.H.V. (1973) Detection of a bullet-shaped virus in kidney sections of pike fry (*Esox Lucius* L.) with red-disease. Neth. J. Vet. Sci. 98:86–90.

Bootsma, R., de Kinkelin, P., and Le Berre, M. (1975) Transmission experiments with pike fry (*Esox lucius* L.) rhabdovirus. J. Fish. Biol. 7:269–276.

Brown, E.R., Hazdra, J.J., Keith, L., Greenspan, I., Kwapinski, J.B.G., and Beamer, P. (1973) Frequency of fish tumors found in a polluted watershed as compared to nonpolluted Canadian waters. Cancer Res. 33:189–198.

Brown, E.R., Sinclair, T.F., Keith, L., Hazdra, J.J., Callaghan, O.H., and Inch, W.R. (1976) Lymphoma in *Esox lucius* (northern pike): Viral and environmental interactions. Proc. Am. Assoc. Cancer Res. Abstr. 17:2.

Bussereau, F., de Kinkelin, P., and Le Berre, M. (1975) Infectivity of fish rhabdoviruses for *Drosophila melanogaster*. Ann. Microbiol. 126:389–395.

Clerx, J.P.M., Horzinek, M.C., and Osterhaus, A.D.M.E. (1978) Neutralization and enhancement of infectivity of non-salmonid fish rhabdoviruses by rabbit and pike immune sera. J. Gen. Virol. 40:297–308.

Dawe, C.J., Banfield, W.G., Sonstegard, R., Lee, C.W., and Michelitch, H.J. (1976) Cylindroid lamella-particle complexes and nucleoid intracytoplasmic bodies in lymphoma cells of northern pike (*Esox lucius*). Prog. Exp. Tumor Res. 20:166–180.

de Kinkelin, P., Galimard, B., and Bootsma, R. (1973) Isolation and identification of the causative agent of "red disease" of pike (*Esox lucius* L. 1766). Nature 241:465–467.

Dorson, M., de Kinkelin, P., Torchy, C., and Monge, D. (1987) Sensibilite du brochet (*Esox lucius*) a differents virus de salmonides (NPI, SHV, NHI) et au rhabdovirus de la perche. Bull. Fr. Peche Piscis 307:91–101.

Dorson, M., Torchy, C., Chilmonczyk, S., de Kinkelin, P., and Michel, C. (1984) A rhabdovirus pathogenic for perch, *Perca fluviatilis* L.: Isolation and preliminary study. J. Fish Dis. 7:241–245.

Duijn, C. van. (1967) Diseases of Fishes. Iliffe Books, London.

Dukes, T.W., and Lawler, A.R. (1975) The ocular lesions of naturally occurring lymphocystis in fish. Can. J. Comp. Med. 39:406–410.

Dunbar, C.E., and Wolf, K. (1966) The cytological course of experimental lymphocystis in the bluegill. J. Infect. Dis. 116:466–472.

Durham, P.J.K., and Anderson, C.D. (1981) Lymphocystis disease in imported tropical fish. N.Z. Vet. J. 29:88–91.

Hedrick, R.P., Speas, J., Kent, M.L., and McDowell, T. (1985) Adenovirus-like particles associated with a disease of cultured white sturgeon, *Acipenser transmontanus*. Can. J. Fish. Aquatic Sci. 42:1321–1325.

Herman, R.L. (1988) Squamous cell carcinoma in rainbow smelt *Osmerus mordax*. Dis. Aquatic Org. 5:71–73.

Hill, B.J., Underwood, B.O., Smale, C.J., and Brown, F. (1975) Physicochemical and serological characterization of five rhabdoviruses infecting fish. J. Gen. Virol. 27:369–378.

Hoffman, G.L., Dunbar, C.E., Wolf, K., and Zwillenberg, L.O. (1969) Epitheliocystis, a new infectious disease of the bluegill (*Lepomis macrochirus*). J. Microbiol. Serol. 35:146–158.

Howse, H.D., and Christmas, J.Y. (1970) Lymphocystis tumors: histochemical identification of hyaline substances. Trans. Am. Microscop. Soc. 89:276–282.

Kelly, R.K., Nielsen, O., Mitchell, S.C., and Yamamoto, T. (1983) Characterization of *Herpesvirus vitreum* isolated from hyperplastic epidermal tissue of walleye, *Stizostedion vitreum vitreum* (Mitchill). J. Fish Dis. 6:249–260.

Langdon, J.S., and Humphrey, J.D. (1987) Epizootic haematopoietic necrosis, a new viral disease in redfin perch, *Perca fluviatilis* L., in Australia. J. Fish Dis. 10:289–297.

Langdon, J.S., Humphrey, J.D., and Williams, L.M. (1986) First virus isolation from Australian fish: An iridovirus-like pathogen from redfin perch, *Perca fluviatilis* L. J. Fish Dis. 9:263–268.

Langdon, J.S., Humphrey, J.D., and Williams, L.M. (1988) Outbreaks of an EHNV-like iridovirus in cultured rainbow trout, *Salmo gairdneri* Richardson, in Australia. J. Fish Dis. 11:93–96.

Lawler, A.R., Howse, H.D., and Cook, D.W. (1974) Lymphocystis infections in the silver perch, *Bairdiella chrysura*. J. Miss. Acad. Sci. 19:183.

Lawler, A.R., Ogle, J.T., and Donnes, C. (1977) *Dascyllus* spp.: New hosts for lymphocystis and a list of recent hosts. J. Wildlife Dis. 13:307–312.

Ljungberg, O. (1976) Epizootiological and experimental studies of skin tumours in northern pike (*Esox lucius* L.) in the Baltic Sea. Prog. Exp. Tumor Res. 20:156–165.

Ljungberg, O., and Lange, J. (1968) Skin tumours of northern pike (Esox lucius L.) I.—Sarcoma in a Baltic pike population. Bull. Off. Int. Epizoot. 69:1007–1022.

Lopez, D.M., Sigel, M.M., Beasley, A.R., and Dietrich, L.S. (1969) Biochemical and morphologic studies of lymphocystis disease. Natl. Cancer Inst. Monograph. 31:223–236.

Lopez, D.M., Sigel, M.M., Beasley, A.R., and Dietrich, L.S. (1970) DNA synthesis in lymphocystis-infected cells: Effect of 6-mercaptopurine. Bacteriol. Proc. 1970:190–191.

Malsberger, R.G., and Lautenslager, G. (1980) Fish Viruses: Rhabdovirus isolated from a species of the family cichlidae. Fish Health News 9(2):i–ii.

Marineau, D., Bowser, P.R., Wooster, G.A., and Armstrong, L.D. (1990) Experimental transmission of a dermal sarcoma in fingerling walleyes (*Stizostedion vitreum vitreum*). Vet. Pathol. 27:230–234.

Meyers, T.R. (1979) A reo-like virus isolated from juvenile American oysters (*Crassostrea virginica*). J. Gen. Virol. 43:203–212.

Meyers, T.R. (1980) Experimental pathogenicity of reovirus 13p₂ for juvenile American oysters (*Crassostrea virginica* (Gmelin) and bluegill fingerlings *Lepomis macrochirus* (Rafinesque). J. Fish Dis. 3:187–201.

Meyers, T.R. (1983) Serological and histopathological responses of rainbow trout, *Salmo gairdneri* Richardson, to experimental infection with the 13p₂ reovirus. J. Fish Dis. 6:277–292.

Middlebrooks, B.L., Ellender, R.D., and Wharton, J.H. (1979) Fish cell culture: A new cell line from *Cynoscion nebulosus*. In Vitro 15:109–111.

Middlebrooks, B.L., Po, C.M., and Ellender, R.D. (1980) Properties of an established cell line from the Atlantic croaker (*Micropogon undulatus*). Proc. Soc. Exp. Biol. Med. 165:123–128.

Middlebrooks, B.L., Stout, D.L., Ellender, R.D., and Safford, S. (1981) Fish cell lines: Two new cell lines derived from explants of trunk musculature of *Cynoscion arenarius*. In Vitro J. Tissue Cult. Assoc. 17:427–430.

Midlige, F.H., Jr., and Malsberger, R.G. (1968) In vitro morphology and maturation of lymphocystis virus. J. Virol. 2:830–835.

Moore, A.R., Li, M.F., and McMenemy, M. (1988) Isolation of a picorna-like virus from smelt, *Osmerus mordax* (Mitchill). J. Fish Dis. 11:179–184.

Mulcahy, M.F. (1963) Lymphosarcoma in the pike, *Esox lucius* L. (Pisces; Esocidae) in Ireland. Proc. R. Irish Acad., Sect. B. 63:103–129.

Mulcahy, M.F. (1969) The thymus glands and lymphosarcoma in the pike *Esox lucius* L. (Pisces; Esocidae) in Ireland. Comp. Leukemia Res. 36:600–609.

Mulcahy, M.F. (1975) Fish blood changes associated with disease: A hematological study of pike lymphoma and salmon ulcerative dermal necrosis. In: The Pathology of Fishes. (Ribelin, W.E., and Migaki, G., eds.). The University of Wisconsin Press, Madison, pp. 925–944.

Mulcahy, M.F. (1976) Epizootiological studies of lymphomas in northern pike in Ireland. Prog. Exp. Tumor Res. 20:129–140.

Mulcahy, M.F., and O'Leary, A. (1970) Cell-free transmission of lymphosarcoma in northern pike *Esox lucius* L. (Pisces; Esocidae). Experientia 26:891.

Mulcahy, M.F., and O'Rourke, F.J. (1964) Lymphosarcoma in the pike *Esox lucius* L., in Ireland. Life Sci. 3:719–720.

Mulcahy, M.F., Winqvist, G., and Dawe, C.J. (1970) The neoplastic cell type in lymphoreticular neoplasms of the northern pike, *Esox lucius* L. Cancer Res. 30:2712–2717.

Nicholson, B.L., and Byrne, C. (1973) An established cell line from the Atlantic salmon (*Salmo salar*). J. Fish Res. Bd. Can. 30:913–916.

Nigrelli, R.F., and Ruggieri, G.D. (1965) Studies on virus diseases of fishes. Spontaneous and experimentally induced cellular hypertrophy (Lymphocystis disease) in fishes of the New York Aquarium, with a report of new cases and an annotated bibliography (1874–1965). Zoologica 50:83–96.

Papas, T.S., Dahlberg, J.E., and Sonstegard, R.A. (1976) Type C virus in lymphosarcoma in northern pike (*Esox lucius*). Nature 261:506–508.

Papas, T.S., Pry, T.W., Schafer, M.P., and Sonstegard, R.A. (1977) Presence of DNA polymerase in lymphosarcoma in northern pike (*Esox lucius*). Cancer Res. 37:3214–3217.

Pritchard, N.H., and Malsberger, R.G. (1968) A cytochemical study of lymphocystis tumors in vivo. J. Exp. Zool. 169:371–380.

Rasin, K. (1927) Prispevek k pathogenesi *Lymphocystis johnstonei* Woodcock. I. Biologicke spisy vysoke skoly zverolekarske Brno, CSR 6:11–38.

Roberts, R.J. (1976) Experimental pathogenesis of lymphocystis in the plaice (*Pleuronectes patessa*). In: Wildlife Diseases. (Page, L.A., ed.). Plenum Press, New York, pp. 431–441.

Robin, J., and Lariviere-Durand, C. (1983) Bluegill virus is a ribovirus of positive-strand polarity. Arch. Virol. 77:119–125.

Roy, P., Clark, H.F., Madore, H.P., and Bishop, D.H.L. (1975) RNA polymerase associated with virions of pike fry rhabdovirus. J. Virol. 15:338–347.

Russell, P.H. (1974) Lymphocystis in wild plaice *Pleuronectes platessa* (L.), and flounder *Platichthys flesus* (L.) in British coastal waters: A histopathological and serological study. J. Fish Biol. 6:771–778.

Schlumberger, H.G. (1957) Tumors characteristic for certain animal species. Cancer Res. 17:823–832.

Sonstegard, R. (1975) Lymphosarcoma in muskellunge (*Esox masquinongy*). In: The Pathology of Fishes (Ribelin, W.E., and Migaki, G., eds.). The University of Wisconsin Press, Madison, pp. 907–924.

Sonstegard, R.A. (1976) Studies of the etiology and epizootiology of lymphosarcoma in *Esox* (*Esox lucius* L. and *Esox masquinongy*). Prog. Exp. Tumor Res. 20:141–155.

Sonstegard, R.A. (1977a) The potential utility of fishes as indicator organisms for environmental carcinogens. In: Wastewater Renovation and Reuse (D'Itri, F.M., ed.). Marcel Dekker, New York, pp. 561–577.

Sonstegard, R.A. (1977b) Environmental carcinogenesis studies in fishes of the Great Lakes of North America. Ann. N.Y. Acad. Sci. 298:261–269.

Sorimachi, M. (1984) Pathogenicity of ICD virus isolated from Japanese eel. Bull. Nat. Res. Inst. Aquaculture 6:71–75.

Sorimachi, M., and Egusa, S. (1982) Characteristics and distribution of viruses isolated from pond-cultured eels. Bull. Nat. Res. Inst. Aquaculture 3:97–105.

Stephens, J.S., Johnson, R.K., Key, G.S., and McCosker, J.E. (1970) The comparative ecology of three sympatric species of California blennies of the genus *Hypsoblennius* gill (Teleostomi, Blenniidae). Ecol. Monograph 40:213–233.

Templemann, W. (1965) Lymphocystis disease in American plaice of the eastern Grand Bank. J. Fish. Res. Bd. Can. 22:1345–1356.

Thompson, J.S. (1982) An epizootic of lymphoma in northern pike, *Esox lucius* L., from the Aland Islands of Finland. J. Fish Dis. 5:1–11.

Walker, D.P., and Hill, B.J. (1980) Studies on the culture, assay of infectivity and some in vitro properties of lymphocystis virus. J. Gen. Virol. 51:385–395.

Walker, R. (1958) Lymphocystis warts and skin tumors of walleyed pike. Rensselaer Rev. Grad. Stud. 14:1–5.

Walker, R. (1961) Fine structure of a virus tumor of fish. Am. Zool. 1:395–396.

Walker, R. (1969) Virus associated with epidermal hyperplasia in fish. Natl. Cancer Inst. Monograph 31:195–207.

Wellings, S.R. (1969) Environmental aspects of neoplasia in fishes. In: Fish in Research (Neuhaus, O.W., and Halver, J.E., eds.). Academic Press, New York, pp. 3–22.

Wharton, J.H., Ellender, R.D., Middlebrooks, B.L., Stocks, P.K., Lawler, A.R., and Howse, H.O. (1977) Fish cell culture: Characteristics of a cell line from the silver perch *Bairdiella chrysura*. In Vitro 13:389–397.

Winqvist, G., Ljungberg, O., and Hellstroem, B. (1968) Skin tumours of northern pike (*Esox lucius* L.) II. Viral particles in epidermal proliferations. Bull. Off. Int. Epizoot. 69:1023–1031.

Winqvist, G., Ljungberg, O., and Ivarsson, B. (1973) Electron microscopy of sarcoma of the northern pike (*Esox lucius* L.). Bibl. Haematol. 39:26–30.

Winton, J.R., Lannan, C.N., Fryer, J.L., Hedrick, R.P., Meyers, T.R., Plumb, J.A., and Yamamoto, T. (1987) Morphological and biochemical properties of four members of a novel group of reoviruses isolated from aquatic animals. J. Gen. Virol. 68:353–364.

Wolf, K. (1962) Experimental propagation of lymphocystis disease of fishes. Virology 18:249–256.

Wolf, K. (1976) Fish viral diseases in North America, 1971–1975, and recent research of the Eastern Fish Disease Laboratory, U.S.A. Fish Pathol. 10:135–154.

Wolf, K. (1988) The Viruses and Viral Diseases of Fish. Cornell University Press, Ithaca, New York.

Wolf, K., and Carlson, C.P. (1965) Multiplication of lymphocystis virus in the bluegill (*Lepomis macrochirus*). Ann. N.Y. Acad. Sci. 126:414–419.

Wolf, K., and Quimby, M.C. (1973) Fish viruses: Buffers and methods for plaquing eight agents under normal atmosphere. Appl. Microbiol. 25:659–664.

Wolf, K., Gravell, M., and Malsberger, R.G. (1966) Lymphocystis virus: Isolation and propagation in centrarchid fish cell lines. Science 151:1004–1005.

Wolf, K.E., Quimby, M.C., Carlson, C.P., and Owens, W.J. (1979) Lymphocystis virus: Infectivity of lesion preparations stored after lyophilization or simple desiccation. J. Fish Dis. 2:259–260.

Yamamoto, T., Kelly, R.K., and Nielsen, O. (1984) Epidermal hyperplasias of northern pike (*Esox lucius*) associated with herpesvirus and C-type particles. Arch. Virol. 79:255–272.

Yamamoto, T., Kelly, R.K., and Nielsen, O. (1985a) Morphological differentiation of virus-associated skin tumors of walleye (*Stizostedion vitreum vitreum*). Fish Pathol. 20:361–372.

Yamamoto, T., Kelly, R.K., and Nielsen, O. (1985b) Epidermal hyperplasia of walleye, *Stizostedion vitreum vitreum* (Mitchill), associated with retrovirus-like type-C particles: prevalence, histologic and electron microscopic observations. J. Fish. Dis. 8:425–436.

Yamamoto, T., Macdonald, R.D., Gillespie, D.C., and Kelly, R.K. (1976) Viruses associated with lymphocystis disease and dermal sarcoma of walleye (*Stizostedion vitreum vitreum*). J. Fish. Res. Bd. Can. 33:2408–2419.

Chapter 27

PARASITES OF TEMPERATE FRESHWATER GAME FISHES, INCLUDING ESTUARINE BAIT FISHES

SARAH L. POYNTON   GLENN L. HOFFMAN

Parasites of game and bait fishes from temperate freshwater and brackish environments are a diverse assembly, owing in part to the broad range of ecologic conditions with widely differing salinities and temperatures in which the hosts are found. In this chapter, attention is focused on problematic parasites affecting economically important families of fishes. The families and their importance are as follows: eels in international trade; killifishes as baitfish; perch and pike in commerce and recreation; smelt and herring as forage fishes; sturgeon in commerce; and sunfishes in recreation.

The chapter discusses six parasites of particular importance and provides a table (Table 27–1) listing problematic parasites in wild or intensively cultured North American fish. Additional information on the parasites can be found in works dedicated to teleost parasitology (Bykhovskaya-Pavlovskaya et al., 1962; Hoffman, 1960, 1967, 1973; Lee et al., 1985; Lom, 1986, McClelland et al., 1983; Shulman, 1966; Yamaguti, 1959, 1963, 1971). Many fishes in this ecologic group are euryhaline. When in salt water, they are often susceptible to marine parasites. For example, *Amyloodinium ocellatum* causes severe epidemics in striped bass and their hybrids (Lawler, 1980). These parasites are covered in Chapters 81 and 89.

HETEROPOLARIA SPP.

SYNONYMS. *Epistylis* sp., red-sore disease, part of the A-E complex (*Aeromonas hydrophila–Epistylis* sp.).

Members of the genus *Heteropolaria* are attached sessile, colonial ciliates belonging to the subclass Peritrichia, family Epistylididae (Lee et al., 1985), which infect the body, fins, and gills of fishes (Fig. 27–1). Usually these organisms are ectocommensals, but they have been associated with fish in poor condition (Lom, 1973b). *Heteropolaria colisarum* is often associated with *Aeromonas hydrophila* in red-sore disease, but it is not clear which organism is the primary invader (Foissner et al., 1985). Infections are unsightly and may reach epidemic proportions, killing numerous game fish (Esch et al., 1976).

Life Cycle, Transmission, and Epidemiology

Heteropolaria has a direct life cycle, requiring only the fish host. Asexual reproduction is by binary fission. The resulting young forms, called telotrochs,

TABLE 27–1. Problematic Parasites in Temperate Freshwater Game Fishes, Including Bait Fishes in North America

Parasite	Hosts	Location on/in Host	Method of Infection	Prevalence
Apicomplexa				
Eimeria	Freshwater eels Killifishes Sticklebacks	Liver Intestine	Unknown, First intermediate host = grass shrimp for killifishes	Unknown
Microspora				
Glugea	Herrings Smelts Sticklebacks	Body cavity	Direct	Common
Ciliata				
Heteropolaria	Sunfishes Temperate basses	Skin	Direct	Common in southern United States
Ichthyophthirius	Freshwater eels Sunfishes	Gills Skin	Direct	Common
Trichodina	Freshwater eels Perch Pike Sunfishes	Fins Gills Skin	Direct	Common
Trichophrya	Sunfishes	Gills	Direct	Can be common in local regions
Myxozoa				
Henneguya	Pikes	Eye	Life cycle poorly known, some may need intermediate hosts	Uncommon
Myxidium	Freshwater eels	Gills Skin	Life cycle poorly known, some may need intermediate hosts	Common
Myxobolus	Killifishes Pikes Sunfishes	Mouth Many organs	Life cycle poorly known, some may need intermediate hosts	Common
Coelenterata				
Polypodium	Sturgeons	Ova	Direct	Common
Monogenea				
Gyrodactylus	Cavefish Freshwater eels Sunfishes	Gills Skin	Direct	Common
Digenea				
Ascocotyle	Killifishes	Gills Heart Liver Many other organs	Definitive host = mammals	Most common in southern United States
Clinostomum	Killifishes Sunfishes	Gills Skin	Definitive host = heron First intermediate = snail Second intermediate = fish	Common
Diplostomum	Freshwater eels Sticklebacks Sunfishes	Eye	Definitive host = gull First intermediate = snail Second intermediate = fish	Common
Neascus	Numerous hosts	Eye Fins Skin	Definitive host = bird First intermediate = mollusc Second intermediate = fish	Common
Posthodiplostomum	Temperate basses	Viscera	Definitive host = heron First intermediate = snail Second intermediate = fish	Common
Cestoda				
Diphyllobothrium	Smelts Pikes	Liver Muscle	Definitive host = bird mammal First intermediate = copepod Second intermediate = fish	Common in smelts Uncommon in pikes

Table continued on following page

**TABLE 27–1. Problematic Parasites in Temperate Freshwater Game Fishes,
Including Bait Fishes in North America** *Continued*

Parasite	Hosts	Location on/in Host	Method of Infection	Prevalence
Ligula	Sticklebacks	Body cavity	Definitive host = bird First intermediate = copepod Second intermediate = fish	Common
Proteocephalus	Cavefish	Intestine	Definitive host = fish First intermediate = unknown Second intermediate = unknown	Unknown
Schistocephalus	Sticklebacks	Body cavity	Definitive host = birds First intermediate = copepod Second intermediate = fish	Common
Triaenophorus	Perches Pikes Trout-perches	Intestine Muscle Viscera	Definitive host = fish First intermediate = copepod Second intermediate = fish	Common
Nematoda *Anguilicola*	Freshwater eels	Swim bladder	Definitive host = eels First intermediate = copepods	Unknown
Anisakis	Herrings	Muscle	Definitive host = cetacean First intermediate = crustacean Second intermediate = fish or squid Transport host = fish	Common
Contracaecum	Herrings Sunfishes	Viscera	Definitive host = birds or mammals First intermediate = copepod Second intermediate = fish	Common
Eustrongylides	Killifishes	Viscera	Definitive host = birds First intermediate = tubificid worms Second intermediate = fish	Common
Goezia	Sunfishes Temperate basses	Stomach wall	Definitive host = fish First intermediate = unknown Second intermediate = fish	Unknown
Philometra	Temperate basses	Muscle	Definitive host = fish First intermediate = copepods Second intermediate = fish	Common
Pseudoterranova	Herrings	Muscle	Definitive host = seal First intermediate = invert. Second intermediate = fish	More common in marine fishes
Spinitectus	Sunfishes	Intestine	Definitive host = fish First intermediate = mayfly larvae	Common
Hirudinea *Myzobdella*	Sunfishes	Skin, oral cavity	Direct	Common
Copepoda *Ergasilus*	Temperate basses	Gills	Direct	Common
Lernaea	Sunfishes	Skin	Direct, occasionally infests amphibians	Common
Branchiura *Argulus*	Gars	Skin	Direct	Common

The most important parasites for each host family are given. This list is therefore not a comprehensive parasite-host inventory. The location on or in the hosts, method of infection, and prevalence are summarized for all fish hosts.

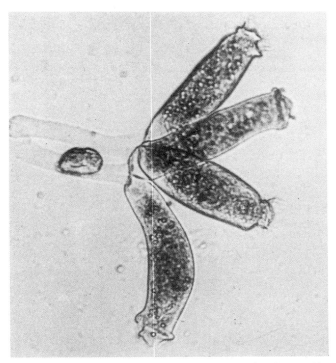

FIGURE 27–1. A small colony of *Heteropolaria* sp. showing zooids. (Courtesy of R. Wooten. In Roberts, R. J. [1989] Fish Pathology. 2nd ed. Bailliere Tindall, London.)

are free swimming. The mature stage, the trophont, is sessile (Hoffman, 1967; Lee et al., 1985).

Sessile peritrichs such as *Heteropolaria* spp. may become very numerous in waters containing high levels of organic matter. As soon as stress conditions prevail against the hosts' resistance, populations of these protozoa flourish (Lom, 1973b). In largemouth bass, there is a positive correlation between total length of the fish and the prevalence of infection (Esch et al., 1976). *Heteropolaria* spp. infestations may be most common in winter months in some areas (Lom, 1966), but outbreaks of red-sore disease are more common during warmer months (Esch et al, 1976).

Hosts and Geographic Distribution

Heteropolaria is ubiquitous in fresh water, both in the water column and in sediments (Esch et al., 1976), and has been reported from a variety of fishes in North America. Of particular note are problematic infestations on sunfishes and temperate basses in the southeastern United States (Esch et al., 1976; Hazen et al., 1978). The genus has also been reported from darters (Hoffman, 1967).

Clinical Appearance

Heavy infections of *Heteropolaria* are characterized by white-gray cottonlike patches on the body surface. Dermal ulcers may develop. Infected fish may roll on their sides or "flash." Red-sore disease, or A-E complex, is characterized by scale erosion, pitting lesions on the body surface, and hemorrhagic septicemia.

Microscopic Appearance and Diagnosis

Heteropolaria can be seen in wet mounts of scrapings from the body surface or gills. The colony is made up of numerous bodies, or zooids, each borne on part of a branched, noncontractile stalk (see Fig. 27–1). The zooid may be shaped like an inverted bell or may be cylindroid and elongated, depending on the species. In *H. colisarum*, the extended cylindrical zooids are 150 to 300 μm long and 40 to 60 μm wide (Foissner et al., 1985). In *H. lwoffi*, the conical zooids are approximately 50 to 80 μm long and 20 to 30 μm wide (Cone and Odense, 1987). There is a spiral of oral cilia at the anterior end of each zooid and a stalk at the posterior, or aboral, end. Stalks of adjacent zooids are usually joined together.

Pathologic Effects and Pathogenesis

Heteropolaria uses the fish only as a substrate for attachment, and feeds on bacteria and organic debris from the surrounding water (Hazen et al., 1978; Wootten, 1989). The base of the *Heteropolaria* colony is attached to epithelial cells. The exact mode of attachment varies between different species of peritrich. Attachment of *H. lwoffi* is superficial, and there is no evidence of serious damage to the host cells (Cone and Odense, 1987; Lom, 1973b). Yet in *H. colisarum*, the terminal platelet of the stalk is embedded in the epidermis, which may allow secondary invasion by bacteria (Foissner et al., 1985). Conversely, it is believed that *Heteropolaria* sp. may be a secondary invader of bacterial lesions, being present as a benign ectocommensal in red-sore disease (Hazen et al., 1978).

There have been suggestions that the presence of numerous peritrichs may cause irritation or suffocation (Hoffman, 1978; Lom, 1973b), and the efforts of the fish to remove them may result in bruising or open wounds on the skin, through which bacteria and fungi can enter. The main problem with *H. colisarum* infection in North American freshwater fishes is not mortality of fish, but rejection by anglers because of the diseased appearance of the fish (Foissner et al., 1985).

Treatment and Control

A salt bath is recommended and effective for treatment and control of *Heteropolaria* if repeated three times at weekly intervals (Foissner et al, 1985). Formalin will retard the spread of this protozoan. A copious flow of water low in organic content may be sufficient to reduce the numbers of the organisms (Hoffman, 1978). There are no public health concerns with these parasites.

TRICHODINIDS

SYNONYMS. *Trichodinella* and *Tripartiella* are other genera of mobile peritrichs that may be referred to as trichodinids or the *Trichodina* complex. *Trichodina* is a mobile ciliate belonging to the subclass Peritrichia, family Trichodinidae (Fig. 27–2) (Lee et al., 1985). Although often found incidentally on the gills, fins, and skin, *Trichodina* spp. can become harmful parasites (Hoffman, 1967). The closely related genera *Trichodinella* and *Tripartiella* are also found on the gills (Lom and Haldar, 1977). Less frequently, *Trichodina* and the closely related genus *Vauchomia* may be found in the urinary tract (Lom and Haldar, 1976). Additional information is provided in Chapter 70.

Life Cycle, Transmission, and Epidemiology

Trichodina has a direct life cycle, requiring only the fish host. Reproduction is normally asexual, by binary fission, but conjugation may also occur (Van As and Basson, 1987). The ciliates can move about on the surface of the fish and through the water. Hyperinfestation is indicative of poor water quality and/or excess stocking, as may occur under intensive culture conditions (Wootten, 1989). Striped bass are prone to severe infections with these parasites. Larvae and fry are especially vulnerable, and many mortalities may occur (Van As and Basson, 1987). Trichodinids often occur in conjunction with other ectoparasites.

Hosts and Geographic Distribution

Trichodinids infect wild, cultured, and laboratory fishes in many parts of the world and occur in fresh, brackish, and salt water. In North America, they are frequently reported from perch, pike, sunfishes, and striped bass (Hoffman, 1967, 1978). Opportunistic species, with a broad host range, tend to be larger skin parasites; specialized species are smaller and usually only parasitize the gills of specific hosts (Van As and Basson, 1987).

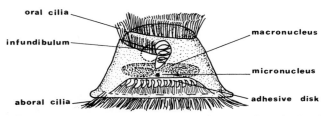

FIGURE 27–2. Schematic representation, side view, of a trichodinid.

Clinical Appearance

Trichodinid infections may cause a variety of dermal lesions, including epithelial erosion, loosened scales, and excess mucus production, giving fish a grayish sheen. Fins may become frayed (Hoffman, 1978; Wootten, 1989). Hyperplastic gill epithelium and respiratory difficulties can occur (Hoffman, 1987). Heavily infected fish "flash," become anorectic, listless, and finally die (Hoffman, 1978; Roberts and Shepherd, 1979).

Microscopic Appearance and Diagnostic Basis

Trichodina can be identified in wet mounts of scrapings by its characteristic motion and shape. In side view, the organisms range from barrel to saucer shaped, with a spiral of oral cilia at the anterior end, and a band of cilia at the posterior (aboral) pole surrounding the denticular ring. The ring, the most distinct feature of *Trichodina*, comprises radially arranged articulated denticles (each with a blade, central part, and thorn), and associated fibrils. This structure is sometimes called the saw-toothed structure. *Trichodinella* and *Tripartiella* are much smaller than *Trichodina*.

Pathologic Effects and Pathogenesis

Although trichodinids neither invade nor permanently attach to epithelial cells, they do cause irritation. During attachment, the movement of the proteinaceous elements of the denticular ring allows the organism to form a cuplike sucker pressed to the host surface. Injury to the host may be caused by the sharp edge of the border membrane of the disc, and by the pulling of epithelial cells into the vaulted disc (Lom, 1973a). Subsequent to the epithelial damage, there may be secondary invasion by waterborne fungi and bacteria (Van As and Basson, 1987).

The injury and disintegration of host cells resulting from hyperinfestation provides cell debris and bacteria to feed the protozoans, thus they behave as parasites. In low-density infections, this food is not available, and trichodinids are believed to feed on material in the water, behaving more like symphobionts, and using the host solely for attachment (Lom, 1973a).

Treatment and Control

Trichodinids can often be controlled by improvements in husbandry. Decreasing organic loads in the water is usually sufficient. Chemical treatments are normally not required, but the parasites can be controlled with copper sulfate or formalin (Wootten, 1989). There are no public health concerns with this parasite.

BLACK SPOT DISEASE

SYNONYMS. *Neascus, Apophallus.*

Many species of fishes can have pinhead-sized black spots in their skin, branchial arches, eyes, fins, mouth, and muscle caused by the metacercariae of digenean trematodes. These parasites belong to the family Diplostomatidae, superfamily Strigeoidea (strigeoids). The metacercariae are often referred to by the generic name *Neascus*, and an individual metacercaria as a neascus (Hoffman, 1960), for example, *Neascus* of *Crassiphiala bulboglossa, Neascus* of *Uvulifer ambloplitis* (both cause black spot). The metacercaria of *Posthodiplostomum minimum* (white grub) is a neascus *(Neascus vancleavei)* (Hoffman, 1967; Schell, 1985). Metacercariae of certain species of *Apophallus*, a member of the family Heterophyidae, are also found in pigmented spots (Hoffman, 1967).

Life Cycle, Transmission, and Epidemiology

The digenean flukes have an indirect life cycle requiring three hosts. The definitive host, usually a bird, harbors adult flukes in its digestive tract. Eggs, in which miracidia develop, are shed in the bird's feces. When miracidia pentrate or are eaten by the first intermediate host, a mollusc, they develop and multiply to become cercariae. The cercariae are shed from the mollusc, and become free swimming. After locating the second intermediate host, a fish, the cercariae penetrate the skin, and transform into metacercariae. The life cycle is completed when the fish is eaten by a bird.

Hosts and Geographic Distribution

Black spot is a common infection in freshwater fishes. Hosts of *Neascus* include killifishes, perches, pikes, sunfishes, and others (Hoffman, 1960, 1967). Hosts of *Apophallus* include perches (Hoffman, 1967).

Clinical Appearance

Black spots, 1 to several millimeters in diameter, are present in the skin, fins, and eyes of infected fishes. The spots are most easily seen in fish with white or silver skin.

Microscopic Appearance and Diagnosis

The metacercaria, which is frequently contained in a cyst of parasite origin, usually lies just beneath the epidermis. The metacercaria resembles an adult fluke, with one oral and one ventral sucker, and a bifurcate gut. Larval members of the Diplostomatidae are characterized by a large, oval forebody, and a smaller hindbody (Hoffman, 1967). Larvae of *Apophallus* are not divided into fore and hind body but are small, flattened, and elongated (Hoffman, 1967). Melanin pigment is deposited around the parasite by the host, giving rise to the black spots.

Pathologic Effects and Pathogenesis

When a cercaria penetrates a fish, it causes mechanical damage and hemorrhage (Hoffman, 1967). The presence of metacercariae in the skin of a fish does not usually cause serious harm, although young fish may be killed by heavy infections (Wootten, 1989). Stimulation of melanocytes is prompted by the presence of the metacercaria, with the size and intensity of the pigmentation being dependent on the length of time after invasion. Some metacercariae are not surrounded by black pigment until 2 to 3 weeks after infection (Ferguson, 1989; Hoffman 1967; Sindermann et al., 1978). The presence of a parasitic capsule tends to limit the amount of host response to the metacercaria (Ferguson, 1989).

Treatment and Control

The best treatment for black spot infections is control of the first intermediate hosts; i.e., the mollusc populations. Copper sulfate is officially cleared for use as an algicide and has been used as a molluscicide in fish culture facilites. Public health concerns for these parasites are unclear. *Apophallus* species may be able to develop in man (Hoffman, 1967).

ERGASILUS SPP.

SYNONYMS. Fish lice, fish crabs, members of this genus may be referred to as ergasilids.

The members of the genus *Ergasilus* are small copepod crustaceans that have recently evolved to the parasitic way of life. Their morphologic adaptions to this way of life include antennae modified for attachment, and a large trunk providing space for reproductive products (Kabata, 1988). These parasites, members of the suborder Poecilostomatoida, family Ergasilidae, most frequently attach to the gills but also are found on the body surface.

Life Cycle, Transmission, and Epidemiology

Copulation occurs while the copepods are free swimming, and subsequently the male dies. The female then seeks out and settles on a fish host, attaching by clasperlike claws (Hoffman, 1967; Kabata, 1988). Eggs are laid in egg sacs, where embryonic development takes place, and the free-swimming nauplii hatch from the egg. The larvae pass through four copepodid stages, accompanied by moulting. Reproduction occurs in the summer, leading to outbreaks of disease as parasite numbers increase (Wootten, 1989).

Hosts and Geographic Distribution

The genus is widespread in fresh water, brackish water, and ocean habitats in many parts of the world (Kabata, 1979). In temperate fresh water and brackish habitats in North America, the hosts of *Ergasilus* include freshwater eels, gars, herrings, killifishes, paddlefishes, perches, pirate perch, smelts, sticklebacks, sunfishes, temperate basses, and troutperches (Hoffman, 1967).

Clinical Appearance

Ergasilus species are found on the gills, and less frequently the body surface. Severely affected gills may be anemic. The parasites are usually visible to the naked eye as dark bodies.

Microscopic Appearance and Diagnosis

Ergasilus shows only a slight degree of adaption to parasitism, maintaining many of the features of a free-living copepod. The mature female is characterized by a cephalothorax that is slightly flattened dorsoventrally. It is longer than wide. The four thoracic leg-bearing segments are well delimited from one another, and gradually diminish in size posteriorly. The thoracic segments are followed by a genital segment with two long egg sacs, and finally three abdominal segments. The first antennae have five or six segments, and the second antennae are modified for attachment as long stout clasping organs ending in a single claw (Kabata, 1979). *Ergasilus* can be up to 1.5 mm long (Kabata, 1988).

Pathologic Effects and Pathogenesis

Ergasilus damages its host during attachment and feeding. The copepod attaches firmly to the gill filaments with its modified second antennae. The organism can change position, causing additional damage to the host. The feeding activity of *Ergasilus* causes severe gill damage (Wootten, 1989). Lysis of tissue and hyperplasia at the point of attachment is caused by the extrabuccal digestion characteristic of ergasilid copepods (Ferguson, 1989). The lesions caused by the copepod can become foci for secondary infections by bacteria (Wootten, 1989).

Treatment and Control

Treatment and control of copepod parasites is discussed in Chapters 70, 81, and 100.

LERNAEA SPP.

SYNONYMS. Anchor worm, anchor parasite; in part *Lernaeocera*.

Members of the genus *Lernaea* are highly specialized parasitic copepods, with a high degree of structural departure from ancestral free-living crustaceans (Kabata, 1988). Adult females are permanently fixed to a fish and can be very damaging. *Lernaea* is a member of the suborder Cyclopoida, family Lernaeidae (Kabata, 1988). Additional information is provided in Chapter 70.

Life Cycle, Transmission, and Epidemiology

Usually only the postmetamorphosis adult female is parasitic. Young stages comprise nauplii (I–III) and copepodids (I–IV). Morphologic development of one stage to the next is marked mainly by the addition of segments and the appearance of additional swimming appendages (Kabata, 1979). Larval stages are free swimming (Kabata, 1988). At the stage of copepodid V, male and female parasites can be distinguished. This stage is succeeded by the adult male and premetamorphosis female stages. After copulation, the male of many species dies, and the female enters into a close and intimate relationship with the fish host, then undergoes metamorphosis (Kabata, 1979). Outbreaks of disease usually occur in the summer months in temperate regions (Wootten, 1989).

Hosts and Geographic Distribution

Lernaea is a very successful freshwater genus, capable of fully exploiting mesoparasitism and adapting to a large variety of habitats offered by different hosts and by different sites on these hosts. Its hosts include drums, gars, perch, sunfishes, and temperate basses (Hoffman, 1967). An important species is *L. cyprinacea*, a non–host-specific species of worldwide distribution, that also infects amphibians (Hoffman, 1967; Kabata, 1979).

Clinical Appearance

The posterior, wormlike, part of the body of *Lernaea* species protrudes above the site of attachment. The holdfast organ, or anchor, attaches under the body surface, fins, gills, or mouth. Its location may be indicated by the presence of an ulcer, and/or a nodule. The copepod can reach approximately 20 mm in length.

Microscopic Appearance and Diagnosis

The body of the postmetamorphosis female that has lost segmentation has three parts: the cephalothorax, neck, and posterior part. The small cephalo-thorax is followed by a symmetric holdfast organ consisting of two simple or subdivided branches on each side. The diversity of holdfast forms is partly due to the nature of the tissues in which the holdfast is embedded (Kabata, 1979). The neck is subcylindrical, and gradually expands posteriorly into the trunk, terminating in a swelling or swellings, and a subconical abdomen. The paired egg sacs are multiseriate, and contain spherical eggs. The vestigial swimming appendages are minute (Kabata, 1979, 1988).

Pathologic Effects and Pathogenesis

Lernaea species penetrate into the tissues of the host fish and then develop the large holdfast, or attachment, organ. Penetration is often into the body musculature but can extend into the body cavity and liver of small fish (Wootten, 1989). The embedded copepod causes extensive tissue damage, including ulceration, formation of a fibrous hillock, and severe acute inflammation (Ferguson, 1989; Wootten, 1989). Infected fish may lose weight, and there can be mass mortalities in fish stocks (Kabata, 1988).

These parasites are considered mesoparasites, being partly internal (the anterior end is buried in the host) and partly external (the posterior end of the body protrudes above the site of penetration) (Kabata, 1988). Mesoparasites exert a profound negative influence on their hosts, regardless of their abundance (Kabata, 1988). Young fish may be killed by only a few parasites (Wootten, 1989).

Treatment and Control

The standard treatments of *Lernaea* infections have been baths in organophosphatase pesticides. Although not approved for fish use, Dimilin (a chemical cleared for use in insect control) has been found to be very effective experimentally (Hoffman, 1985). Dimilin is effective at warm summer temperatures, in contrast to organophosphates. There are no public health concerns with these parasites.

ARGULUS SPP.

SYNONYMS. Fish lice, fish crabs.

Argulus belongs to a small group of parasitic crustaceans called Branchiura. These ectoparasites, common on the skin, fins, and gills of fish, are particularly important in freshwater aquaculture, where they can be significant pathogens (Kabata, 1988).

Life Cycle, Transmission, and Epidemiology

The life cycle is direct, with only the fish host being required. Although unequivocally parasitic,

Argulus can spend prolonged periods swimming free, and mating takes place while the male and female are swimming (Post, 1987). Clusters of eggs are deposited on submerged objects, and after hatching, juveniles must locate a suitable host within 2 to 3 days (Wootten, 1989). *Argulus* can transfer from fish to fish (Kabata, 1988). Additional information is provided in Chapter 70.

Hosts and Geographic Distribution

Argulus has been reported from a wide range of freshwater fishes throughout North America. Host families include bowfins, drums, gars, herrings, killifishes, perches, pikes, sticklebacks, sturgeons, sunfishes, and temperate basses (Hoffman, 1967). Host specificity is low.

Clinical Appearance

Argulus can be seen moving rapidly around on the surface of the fish but will often swim away as soon as the fish is netted out for examination. The skin of the fish may be erythemic, hemorrhagic, and edematous; and excess mucus may be secreted. Necrotic and ulcerated lesions may be present at the site of old wounds. The fish will show behavioral changes consistent with ectoparasitic infection, including scraping along the bottom of the tank or pond, "flashing," jumping at the inflow, and reduced appetite. Mortality may result (Roberts and Shepherd, 1979).

Microscopic Appearance and Diagnosis

The most distinctive feature of a branchiuran is an oval, flat dorsal shield, which covers all appendages except one or two posterior pairs of legs. The animal is dorsoventrally flattened, with two pairs of antennae, first and second maxillae, and four pairs of legs. The abdomen is bilobed. The genus *Argulus* is characterized by first maxillae that are modified to form cuplike suckers with reinforced walls, and a preoral stylet and mouth situated in the midventral line (Kabata, 1988). The body of an adult ranges from 5 to 20 mm long. Recently attached juveniles are small (1 to 3 mm).

Pathologic Effects and Pathogenesis

Parasitic crustaceans damage their host during attachment and feeding. *Argulus* attaches to the fish by its appendages, modified as suckers and curved hooks. The second maxillae bear spines and armed plates, and there are accessory spines between the second maxillae and the first pair of legs (Kabata, 1988). The feeding apparatus is inserted into the epidermis and underlying host tissues, releasing blood, which the parasite ingests (Wootten, 1989). The stylet causes local mechanical injury, and releases digestive enzymes, causing systemic as well as local effects (Ferguson, 1989). Wounds inflicted by *Argulus* can become necrotic and ulcerated, and may provide a site for secondary attacks by microorganisms. Heavy infections can cause mass mortalities, especially of young fish (Wootten, 1989).

Treatment and Control

Treatment and control of *Argulus* infections are generally through the use of pesticide baths or dips. Additional information is provided in Chapter 70. There are no public health concerns with this parasite.

LITERATURE CITED

Bykhovskaya-Pavlovskaya, I.E., Gusev, A.V., Dubinina, M.N., Izyamova, N.A., Smirnova, T.S., Sokolovskaya, I.L., Shtein, G.A., Shulman, S.S., and Epshtein, V.M. (1962) Key to parasites of freshwater fish of the USSR (in Russian). English translation in 1964, Israel Program for Scientific Translations, Jerusalem.

Cone, D.K., and Odense, P.H. (1987) Occurrence of *Heteropolaria lwoffi* (Faure-Fremiet, 1943) and *Apiosoma piscicola* (Blanchard, 1885) (Ciliata) on *Salvelinus fontinalis* (Richardson in Nova Scotia, Canada). Can. J. Zool. 65:2426–2429.

Esch, G.W., Hazen, T.C., Dimock, R.V., Jr., and Gibbons, J.W. (1976) Thermal effluent and the epizootiology of the ciliate *Epistylis* and the bacterium *Aeromonas* in association with centrarchid fish. Trans. Am. Microscop. Soc. 95:687–693.

Ferguson, H. W. (1989) Systemic Pathology of Fish. Iowa State University Press, Ames.

Foissner, W., Hoffman, G.L., and Mitchell, A.J. (1985) *Heteropolaria colisarum* (Foissner and Schubert, 1977) (Protozoa: Epistylididae) of North American freshwater fishes. J. Fish Dis. 8:145–160.

Hazen, T.C., Raker, M.L., Esch, G.W., and Fliermans, C.B. (1978) Ultrastructure of red-sore lesions on largemouth bass *(Micropterus salmoides)*: Association of the ciliate *Epistylis* sp. and the bacterium *Aeromonas hydrophila*. J. Protozool. 25:351–355.

Hoffman, G.L. (1960) Synopsis of Strigeoidea (Trematoda) of fishes and their life cycles. U.S. Fish Wildlife Serv. Fish. Bull. 175, (60): i–iv, 439–469.

Hoffman, G.L. (1967) Parasites of North American Freshwater Fishes. University of California Press, Berkeley and Los Angeles.

Hoffman, G.L. (1973) Parasites of Laboratory Fishes. In: Parasites of Laboratory Animals. (Flynn, R.J., ed.). Iowa State University Press, Ames, pp. 645–768.

Hoffman, G.L. (1978) Ciliates of freshwater fishes. In: Parasitic Protozoa, Vol. II. (Kreier, J.P., ed.). Academic Press, New York, pp 583–632.

Hoffman, G.L. (1985) Anchor parasite *(Lernaea cyprinacea)* control. Fish Health Section, American Fisheries Society, Newsletter 13(4):4.

Kabata, Z. (1979) Parasitic Copepoda of the British Isles. The Ray Society, London.

Kabata, Z. (1988) Copepoda and Branchiura. In: Guide to the Parasites of Fishes of Canada. Part II. Crustacea. (Margolis, L., and Kabata, Z., eds.). Canadian Special Publication of Fisheries and Aquatic Sciences No. 101, pp. 3–127.

Lawler, A.R. (1980) Studies on *Amyloodinium ocellatum* (Dinoflagellata) in Mississippi Sound: Natural and experimental hosts. Gulf Res. Rep. 6:403–413.

Lee, J.J., Hutner, S.H., and Bovee, E.C. (1985) An Illustrated Guide to the Protozoa. Society of Protozoologists, Lawrence, Kansas.

Lom, J. (1966) Sessiline peritrichs from the surface of some freshwater fishes. Folia Parasitol. (Praha) 13:36–56.

Lom, J. (1973a) The adhesive disc of *Trichodinella epizootica*—Ultrastructure and injury to the host tissue. Folia Parasitol. (Praha) 20:193–202.

Lom, J. (1973b) The mode of attachment and relations to the host in *Apiosoma piscicola* Blanchard and *Epistylis lwoffi* Faure-Fremiet, ectocommensals of freshwater fish. Folia Parasitol. (Praha) 20:105–112.

Lom, J. (1986) Protozoan infections in fish. In: Pathology in Marine Aquaculture. (Vivares, C.P., Banami, J.R., and Jaspers, E., eds.) European Aquaculture Society, Special Publication No. 9, Bredene, Belgium, pp. 95–104.

Lom, J., and Haldar, D.P. (1976) Observations on trichodinids endocommensal in fishes. Trans. Am. Microscop. Soc. 95:527–541.

Lom, J., and Haldar, D.P. (1977) Ciliates of the genera *Trichodinella*, *Tripartiella* and *Paratrichodina* (Peritricha, Mobilina) invading fish gills. Folia Parasitol. (Praha) 24:193–210.

McClelland, G., Misra, R.K., and Marcogliese, D.J. (1983) Variations in abundance of larval anisakines, sealworm *(Phocanema decipiens)* and related species in cod and flatfish from the southern gulf of St. Lawrence (4T) and the Breton Shelf (4Vn). Canadian Technical Report of Fisheries and Aquatic Sciences No. 1201.

Noga, E.J., Bullis, R.A., and Miller, G.C. (1990) Epidemic oral ulceration in largemouth bass *(Micropterus salmoides)* associated with the leech *Myzobdella lngubris*. J. Wildlife Dis. 26:132–134.

Post, G. (1987) Textbook of Fish Health. T.F.H. Publications, Neptune City, New Jersey.

Roberts, R.J., and Shepherd, C.J. (1979) Handbook of trout and salmon diseases. Fishing News Books, Farnham, England.

Robins, C.R., Bailey, R.M., Bond, C.E., Brooker, J.R., Laschner, E.A., Lea, R.N., and Scott, W.B. (1980) A list of common and scientific names of fishes from the United States and Canada. 4th ed. American Fisheries Society, Special Publication No. 12, Bethesda, Maryland.

Schell, S.C. (1985) Handbook of Nematodes of North America North of Mexico. University Press of Idaho, Moscow, Idaho.

Shulman, S.S. (1966) Myxosporidian fauna of USSR. Akad. Nauk SSSR. Moscow-Leningrad. English translation TT–52043, Amerind Publishing Company, New Delhi, India, and Fish Farming Experimental Station, United States Department of the Interior, Stuttgart, Arkansas.

Sindermann, C.J., Ziskowski, J.J., and Anderson, V.T. (1978) A Guide to the Recognition of Some Disease Conditions and Abnormalities in Marine Fish. U.S. National Marine Fisheries Service, Technical Series Report No. 14.

Van As, J.G., and Basson, L. (1987) Host specificity of trichodinid ectoparasites of freshwater fish. Parasitol. Today 3:88–90.

Wootten, R. (1989) The parasitology of teleosts. In: Fish Pathology. 2nd ed. (Roberts, R.J., ed.). Balliere Tindall, London, pp. 242–288.

Yamaguti, S. (1959) Systema Helminthum. Vol. 2. The Cestodes of Vertebrates. Interscience Publishers, New York.

Yamaguti, S. (1963) Systema Helminthum: Monogenea and Aspidocotylea. Vol. 4. Interscience Publishers, New York.

Yamaguti, S. (1971) Synopsis of Digenetic Trematodes of Vertebrates. Vols. I and II. Keigaku Publishing, Tokyo.

Chapter 28

NEOPLASIA OF FRESHWATER TEMPERATE FISHES

MICHAEL K. STOSKOPF

Tumors or neoplastic diseases of freshwater temperate fishes, including the game fishes, have been reasonably well represented in the literature, particularly those of the yellow perch and the northern pike. Game fishes have been of interest because of the possibility that they may serve as environmental monitors and that a high prevalence of neoplasia in these fishes may signal problems of water contamination. Although environmental, genetic, and nutritional factors are known to be involved in predisposing fish to tumors (Mix, 1985), the relative roles of each of these factors are yet to be established. Examples of neoplasias reported in these species are listed in Table 28–1.

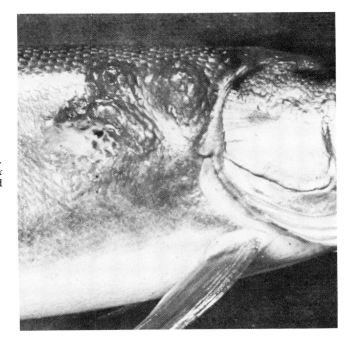

FIGURE 28–1. Early skin lesions of lymphosarcoma in muskellunge. (From Sonstegard, R. [1975] Lymphosarcoma in muskellunge *(Esox masquinongy)*. In: The Pathology of Fishes [Ribelin, W. E., and Migaki, G., eds.]. University of Wisconsin Press, Madison.)

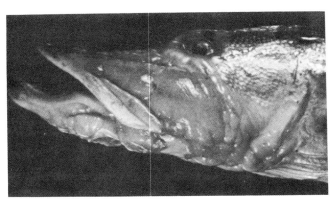

FIGURE 28–2. Lymphosarcoma of the face in a muskellunge. (From Sonstegard, R. [1975] Lymphosarcoma in muskellunge *(Esox masquinongy)*. In: The Pathology of Fishes [Ribelin, W. E., and Migaki, G., eds.]. University of Wisconsin Press, Madison.)

TABLE 28–1. Neoplasia Reported in Various Species of Freshwater Temperate Fish

Neoplasia	Fish	Reference
Nervous System		
Schwannoma	Redfish perch	Finkelstein and Danchenko-Ryzchkova, 1965
Ganglioneuroma	Yellow perch	Budd et al., 1975
Cardiovascular System		
Lymphosarcoma	Northern pike	Mulcahy, 1963
		Sonstegard, 1975
Gastrointestinal System		
Cholangioma	Rivulus	Park and Kim, 1984
Urinary System		
Adenocarcinoma, renal	American eel	Schmey, 1911
		Plehn, 1924
Fibrosarcoma, renal	Northern pike	Plehn, 1906
Lymphosarcoma, renal	Northern pike	Nigrelli, 1947
Nephroblastoma	Striped bass	Helmboldt and Wyand, 1971
Carcinoma, urinary bladder	Yellow perch	Budd et al., 1975
Endocrine System		
Thyroid carcinoma	Yellow perch	Budd et al., 1975
Reproductive System		
Adenocarcinoma, ovarian	Northern pike	Haddow and Blake, 1933
Unidentified, testicular	Yellow perch	Budd and Schroder, 1969
Leiomyoma, testicular	Yellow perch	Budd et al., 1975
Ovarian, unidentified	Yellow perch	Budd et al., 1975
Musculoskeletal System and Connective Tissues		
Fibrosarcoma	American eel	Wolff, 1912
		Plehn, 1924
	Northern pike	Ohlmacher, 1898
	Walleye pike	Walker, 1958
Lipoma	Northern pike	Bergman, 1921
Lipoma	Large mouth bass	Mawdesley-Thomas, 1972
Osteoma	Northern pike	Bland-Sutton, 1885
Osteosarcoma	Northern pike	Walgren, 1876
Rhabdomyoma	Redfish perch	Finkelstein and Danchenko-Ryzchkova, 1965
Integumentary System		
Papilloma	American eel	Schäperclaus, 1953
		Christiansen and Jensen, 1947
Squamous cell carcinoma	Yellow perch	Budd et al., 1975
Respiratory System		
None reported		

LITERATURE CITED

Bergman, A.M. (1921) Einige geschwulste bei fischen: Rhabdomyom, lipome und melanom. Z. Krebsforsch. 18:292–302.
Bland-Sutton, J. (1885) Tumours in animals. J. Anat. Physiol. (Lond.) 19:415–475.
Budd, J., and Schroder, J.D. (1969) Testicular tumors of yellow perch, Perca flavescens (Mitchill). Bull. Wildlife Dis. Assoc. 5:315–318.
Budd, J., Schroder, J.D., and Dukes, K.D. (1975) Tumors of the yellow perch. In: The Pathology of Fishes (Ribelin, W.E., and Migaki, G., eds.). University of Wisconsin Press, Madison, pp. 895–906.
Christiansen, M., and Jensen, A.J.C. (1947) On a recent and frequently occurring tumor disease in eel. Rep. Dan. Biol. Stn. No. 50:31–44.
Finkelstein, E.A., and Danchenko-Ryzchkova, L.K. (1965) [Neurinoma in the perch Perca fluviatilis.] Arkh. Patol. 27:81–84. (In Russian, cited in Mawdesley-Thomas, 1975.)
Haddow, A., and Blake, I. (1933) Neoplasms in fish: A report of six cases with a summary of the literature. J. Pathol. Bacteriol. 36:41–47.
Helmboldt, C.F., and Wyand, D.S. (1971) Nephroblastoma in a striped bass. J. Wildlife Dis. 7:162–165.
Mawdesley-Thomas, L.E. (1972) Some tumours of fish. In: Diseases of Fish (Mawdesley-Thomas, L.E. ed.), Symp. Zool. Soc. Lond. 30:191–284.
Mawdesley-Thomas, L.E. (1975) Neoplasia in fish. In: The Pathology of Fishes. (Ribelin, W.E., and Migaki, G., eds.). University of Wisconsin Press, Madison, pp. 805–870.
Mix, M.C. (1985) Cancerous Diseases in Aquatic Animals and Their Association with Environmental Pollutants: A Critical Review of the Literature. American Petroleum Institute.
Mulcahy, M.F. (1963) Lymphosarcoma in the pike, Esox lucius L. (Pices; Esocidae) in Ireland. Proc. R. Ir. Acad. (B) 63:103–129.
Nigrelli, R.F. (1947) Spontaneous neoplasms in fishes. III. Lymphosarcoma in Astyanax and Esox. Zoologica 33:133–137.
Ohlmacher, H. (1898) Several examples illustrating the comparative pathology of tumors. Bull. Ohio Hosp. Epilep. 1:223–226.
Park, E.H. and Kim, D.S. (1984) Hepatocarcinogenicity of diethylnitrosamine to the self-fertilizing hermaphroditic fish Rivulus marmoratus. J. Natl. Cancer Inst. 73:871–876.
Plehn, M. (1906) Uber geschwulste bei kaltblutern. Z. Krebsforsch. 4:525–564.
Plehn, M. (1924) Praktikum der Fischkrankheiten: E. Schweizerbart, Stuttgart, pp. 301–479.
Schäperclaus, W. (1953) Die blumenkohlkrankheit der aale und anderer fische der ostsee. Z. Fisch. (Neth.) 2:105–124.
Schmey, M. (1911) Uber neubildungen bei fischen. Frankf. Z. Pathol. 6:230–253.
Sonstegard, R. (1975) Lymphosarcoma in muskellunge (Esox masquinongy). In: The Pathology of Fishes (Ribelin, W.E., and Migaki, G., eds.). University of Wisconsin Press, Madison, pp. 907–924.
Wahlgren, E. (1876) Osteoid sarcoma in the anal fin of a pike (cited by Schmey, M., 1911).
Walker, R. (1958) Lymphocystic warts and skin tumors of walleyed pike. Rennsselaer Rev. Grad. Stud. 14:1–5.
Wolff, B. (1912) Uber ein bastom bei einem Aal (Anguilla vulgaris) nebst bemerkungen zur vergleichenden pathologie der geschwulste. Virchows Arch. Pathol. Anat. Physiol. 210:365–385.

Chapter 29

TOXICOLOGY AND PHARMACOLOGY OF TEMPERATE FRESHWATER FISHES

JOHN A. PLUMB

Water is the receiving point of many natural and synthesized substances that are either intentionally or accidentally put there by man. Heavy metals, pesticides, therapeutic agents, industrial and municipal waste products, and naturally occurring toxins occur in open and confined waters used in fish husbandry. Some chemicals have very little effect on the resident aquatic communities, whereas others have immediate, severe effects resulting in overt signs of toxicity and high mortality. Although the death of large numbers of fish is obvious to the casual observer, other changes may be less apparent. Substances that do not kill immediately, or within a short period of time, may still have adverse effects on the health of exposed fish. Less noticeable effects on fish include increased disease susceptibility, decreased handling tolerance, or reduced fecundity. This chapter examines the toxicity of some of the most commonly reported chemicals to fish that inhabit temperate fresh water. The topic can be pursued in more depth by examining any of several reviews or textbooks (Alabaster, 1969; Driesbach, 1983; Hurlbert, 1975; Murphy, 1980; Mayer and Ellersieck, 1986; U.S. Environmental Protection Agency, 1986; Heath, 1987; Law, 1981; Rand and Petrocelli, 1985).

GENERAL TOXICOLOGIC PROBLEMS

One of the most difficult problems in aquatic toxicology is to differentiate problems in fish caused by toxins from the effects of low dissolved oxygen or infectious diseases. Each type of fish kill has a signature that provides some clue to the cause. For example, fish kills caused by chemicals are usually characterized by very rapid onset (a matter of hours) and high morbidity and mortality affecting many species that continues throughout the day. Fish kills due to oxygen depletion are also characterized by rapid onset, high morbidity, and mortality and affect many species, but such fish kills are most acute in the early morning. Conditions improve during the day as photosynthesis becomes greater than oxygen demand. Infectious disease–caused fish kills usually but not always begin more slowly, and the mortality rate gradually increases over a period of days. Obviously these guidelines are not clear-cut, and when fish kills occur, investigators should not be content to examine only one cause, particularly in natural fish populations. Water samples should be tested for toxins, dissolved oxygen should be checked, and fish should be examined for pathogens.

Factors of primary importance that affect the toxicity of chemicals are the temperature, pH, hardness and alkalinity of the water, the formulation of the toxic chemical, and the species, size, and life stage of the fish (Mayer and Ellersieck, 1986). Temperature contributes to respiration rate, absorption, excretion, and detoxification of chemicals. A positive or negative temperature effect will depend on the type of chemical and species of fish. A change in pH may either increase or decrease toxicity. Predicting the effects of pH on the acute toxicity of chemicals to fish is difficult and thus far has been poorly analyzed (Mayer and Ellersieck, 1986). Generally, embryos near hatching are the least sensitive stage and larvae the most sensitive stage to chemical toxicities (Mayer and Ellersieck, 1986). Once larvae develop into juveniles, the toxicity of many chemicals decreases as the fishes' weight increases.

Methods and terminology have been standardized so that the toxicity of chemicals can be compared (American Public Health Association, 1981). The most common term used to compare toxicity of chemicals is *lethal concentration–50* (LC$_{50}$) in which 50% of the exposed animals die in a specified time, usually 48 or 96 hours. Other terms are *medial tolerance limit* (T$_{Lm}$, *effective concentration–50* (EC$_{50}$), or *maximum allowable toxicant concentration* (MATC). When these values are given for a specific chemical, environmental conditions such as water temperature, pH, oxygen concentration, water hardness, alkalinity, organic content of the water, and fish species and life stage should be specified. Each of these variables can affect the toxicity of many chemicals.

Most sources of toxins in inland water and estuaries are associated with people. Common events that result in toxicants entering water are industrial or municipal activities, runoff from forestry or agricultural lands, accidental chemical spills, intentional application of compounds to water for pest control, and application of therapeutics to aquaculture facilities. Fish toxicants may also occur in water because of naturally occurring events, such as heavy rains. The introduction of toxicants into water can occur instantaneously, such as contamination as a result of accidental spills of pesticides or chemicals, accidental contamination from aerial spraying, accidental release of industrial pollutants, or an overdose of therapeutics. This sort of exposure usually results in an acute, rapidly developing mortality among exposed fish. Acute toxicity usually is a response of fish to relatively large doses of chemicals.

A gradual contamination may occur, in which small amounts of substances are released in the environment and concentrations accumulate in the water, bottom mud, and fish flesh. Often the compounds involved in this type of toxicity (mercury, lead, DDT, polychlorinated biphenyls [PCBs], and others) are not easily degraded. Effects of such toxicants are often chronic and are not as spectacular as those seen with sudden contamination, but they are usually longer lasting and have an insidious impact on the fish population. Chemicals in stream or pond sediments may cause toxicity problems to fish. Toxicants in sediment may degrade before they have an opportunity to kill fish, but in some circumstances where they degrade slowly or not at all, the food chain becomes contaminated and toxicants accumulate in fish (Norris et al., 1983).

Bioaccumulation, the uptake of chemicals from the environment by organisms, is a significant problem in the aquatic system. This occurs through the food chain or absorption through the gills or skin. The degree of bioaccumulation depends heavily on the lipid solubility of the chemical in question (Norris et al., 1983). Compounds that have high bioaccumulation capability include mercury, DDT, PCBs, and organophosphate pesticides. Concentrations of chemicals bioaccumulated in fish have been reported to be as high as 100,000 times those found in the water (Nebecker et al., 1971). Although bioaccumulation may not produce any overt clinical signs in fish, accumulated toxins may pose a significant hazard to humans eating contaminated fish.

OXYGEN-DEPLETING MATERIALS

Oxygen-depleting materials usually come from domestic sewage, paper mill effluents, runoff from animal feed lots, animal product processing plants, or, in aquaculture ponds, excess feed. Oxygen depletions in water also occur when algicidal chemicals, such as formalin, are added to water, resulting in reduced photosynthesis (Allison, 1962). Affected fish gasp at the surface, move into shallow water, or swim lethargically. Oxygen-depletion problems are characterized by rapid onset and high fish morbidity and mortality. These problems often begin just before daylight when oxygen concentrations are lowest. In order to diagnose oxygen depletions, it is helpful to determine the dissolved oxygen concentration along with other water-quality variables, such as temperature, pH, carbon dioxide concentration, and ammonia concentration. Marginally low oxygen may not be lethal unless there is a compounding problem, such as high ammonia or CO_2 (Walters and Plumb, 1980). Oxygen depletions in fish ponds are often accompanied by a change in color of the water from some shade of green to brown because of phytoplankton die-off.

TOXIC METALS

Some of the most common metal toxicities in fish are associated with copper, iron, manganese, mercury, lead, or zinc (Table 29–1). Sources of these metals vary, but the most serious problems with fish occur as a result of mining operations and industrial release of metals. Also, metal toxicity has sometimes occurred as a result of ground water flowing through subsurface seams of the metals (Grizzle, 1981).

Water-quality factors, such as hardness, alkalinity, pH, and temperature, affect the solubility and toxicity of many metals. For example, copper is more toxic and more soluble in water with low alkalinity (15 mg/L) and pH (pH 6) than in waters with high alkalinity (100 mg/L) and pH (pH 9) (McKim and Benoit, 1971; Phelps, 1975). Metals may cause toxemias that result in death, bioaccumulation in the flesh, loss of reproductive capability, skeletal deformities, or increased susceptibility to infectious agents (Benoit, 1975; Crandall and Goodnight, 1962;

TABLE 29–1. Toxicity (48- to 96-Hour LC$_{50}$) of Selected Metals to Freshwater Fish

Metal	Toxicity[1] (mg/L)
Copper (McKim and Benoit, 1971; Hodson et al., 1979; U.S. EPA, 1980a)	10–10,000
Iron (Duodoroff and Katz, 1953)	0.1–10.0
Lead (U.S. EPA, 1973; Pickering and Henderson, 1966; U.S. EPA, 1980c)	1000–500,000
Manganese (Duodoroff and Katz, 1953)	2.2–4.1
Mercury (U.S. EPA, 1980d)	3–20,000
Zinc (U.S. EPA, 1973; Pickering and Henderson, 1966; Woltering, 1984; U.S. EPA, 1980b)	50–50,000

[1]*The LC$_{50}$ will depend on pH, water hardness, alkalinity, temperature, and species of fish.*
From Post, G. (1987) Textbook of Fish Health, Revised and Expanded. T.F.H. Publications, Neptune, New Jersey.

McFarlane and Franzin, 1978; Pickering and Henderson, 1966). Mercury, in particular, accumulates in the flesh of fish and can be passed on to humans who eat the contaminated fish (Rucker, 1968; Amend, 1970).

Microscopic pathologic changes can occur in liver, kidney, gill, bone, and other tissues where the metals accumulate. Higher than normal concentrations of metals can be detected in fish tissues with laboratory assays. Subtle clinical signs indicative of metal toxicity are reduced reproduction and altered blood parameters (Gardner, 1975; Gardner and LaRoche, 1973; Gardner and Yevich, 1970).

TOXIC GASES

Toxic gases in water can come from animal waste, industrial or domestic pollution, water-treatment plants, or natural sources. Decomposition of organic material in water, bacterial metabolism, fish metabolism, and deep wells are sources of naturally occurring toxic gases in water. The most common gases in water that can develop concentrations toxic to fish are ammonia, hydrogen sulfide, chlorine, and carbon dioxide, and even supersaturation of oxygen or nitrogen can be toxic to fish. Un-ionized ammonia is the most toxic form of ammonia, and it increases in concentration as the pH rises (Boyd, 1979). Nitrification of ammonia creates problems if nitrites are not rapidly metabolized into nitrates, leading to nitrite toxicity. High nitrite levels in water result in methemoglobinemia, or "brown blood" (Huey et al., 1980). The addition of sodium chloride at a rate of 3 parts NaCl to 1 part nitrite is sometimes used to reduce the methemoglobin in fish to safe levels, but does not reduce the nitrite concentration in the water (Schwedler and Tucker, 1983).

Hydrogen sulfide gas is usually associated with sewage pollution, chemical contamination, or is a result of anaerobic decomposition in bottom sediments. This gas is highly soluble in water and very toxic to fish. Hydrogen sulfide interferes with fish eggs hatching and survival of juveniles near pond bottoms (Post, 1987).

Chlorine and its derivatives are usually associated with release of treated waters from sewage-treatment plants, industries, or the use of chlorinated municipal water for fish culture. Fish are highly sensitive to small concentrations of chlorine, so municipal water supplies should be neutralized with sodium thiosulfate or the water should be exposed to the atmosphere for several days to allow the chlorine to dissipate. The U.S. Environmental Protection Agency (EPA) (1973) recommends that effluents into natural waters have no more than 0.03 mg/L of residual chlorine when released. Fish affected by chlorine try to avoid the area, lose equilibrium, and die following rapid swimming. Unidentified chemicals formed in chlorinated waste water may also cause tumors in fish exposed to them over long periods (Grizzle et al., 1984, 1981).

Oxygen is an essential element necessary for fish life, but it is possible to have a supersaturation of oxygen that will kill fish. Supersaturated oxygen causes "gas-bubble disease," which is similar to the "bends" of deep sea divers caused by nitrogen supersaturation in the blood. Supersaturation of nitrogen causes a similar problem in fish. Gas-bubble disease attributed to supersaturation by nitrogen has been reported in fish in a 150 km^2 reservoir (Crunkilton et al., 1980). The supersaturation of gas in water results in minuscule bubbles of the gas in the blood blocking the flow of blood in the gills, and macroscopic air bubbles in the skin and eyes (Bouck, 1980). The supersaturation of gases can often be corrected by agitation of the water column.

ORGANIC TOXICANTS

A large array of substances, including oil, phenolics, and PCBs, are produced by industries and released into water where they may be toxic to fish (Post, 1987). Oil spills often cause extensive damage to aquatic life, especially in the marine environment. Oil may cover the external surfaces of the fish and cause suffocation (U.S. EPA, 1973), or it may be absorbed by the fish and cause toxicosis (Tagatz, 1961).

The organic carbon absorbables are an ill-defined group of chemicals that are readily absorbed onto activated carbon. These include chloroform and alcohol-extractable compounds. The effects of these chemicals on fish are not clearly defined.

Phenolic compounds, derived from coal, petroleum, and other industrial procedures, may cause a direct mortality or a sublethal effect in fishes.

The PCBs, used in a variety of lubricants, hydraulic fluids, and electrical transformers, have become well known in recent years as aquatic contaminants. They are very stable and, once in the environment, do not readily degrade, thus persisting for years. They bioaccumulate up to 100,000-fold in animal tissue (Nebecker et al., 1971) and have been found in body tissues of fish from around the world (Peakall and Lincer, 1970). Mortality of PCB-exposed fish is not usually seen, but bioaccumulation in the tissues leads to discrete physiologic damage. The greatest danger of PCBs to freshwater temperate fishes is their adverse affect on reproduction (Nebecker et al., 1971).

AGRICULTURAL TOXINS

Since the early part of the twentieth century, pesticides have been used in great quantities to aid mankind. Pesticides include insecticides, herbicides, rodenticides, miticides, and fungicides, of which there are many formulations (U.S. EPA, 1973). Their benefit to the world is immeasurable in terms of increased crop production, decreased insect pests, and improved human and domestic animal health.

However, many pesticides have harmful side effects to nontarget organisms. Agricultural practices are a major source of pesticide contamination in the aquatic environment. Pesticides generally have low solubility in water and adsorb onto particulate matter. They have an affinity for animal tissues, especially fat, and bioaccumulate in fish. Many of these compounds are very stable and are not subject to rapid biodegradation. Once they are in the environment, they stay for a long time.

INSECTICIDES

Common insecticides include the chlorinated hydrocarbons, organophosphates, carbamates, and pyrethroids. Chlorinated hydrocarbons are synthetic organic compounds that are fat soluble, but have low solubility in water. Fat solubility allows the chlorinated hydrocarbons to be absorbed into animal flesh, where bioaccumulation occurs. They persist for long periods, because of their resistance to oxidation (Post, 1987). The best known chlorinated hydrocarbon insecticide is DDT. It does gain access to the aquatic environment, and fish become contaminated (Menzie, 1978).

Fish may accumulate small quantities of chlorinated hydrocarbons during the summer when the chemicals are in use. Fish store the compounds in their fat without any obvious serious effect. However, following sublethal exposure during the summer, fish may develop toxicosis in the winter when they are not feeding and are using their fat for energy (Plumb and Richburg, 1977). As their fat is metabolized, bioaccumulated pesticide is mobilized, and a toxicosis occurs.

Toxaphene is one compound that acts this way in freshwater temperate fishes. Toxaphene toxicosis causes fish to be more susceptible to infectious disease and interferes with collagen formation, causing spinal deformities (Mayer et al., 1978; Stickel and Hickey, 1977). Other effects of chlorinated hydrocarbons include poor growth, reduced survivability, and lowered egg production (Allison et al., 1964). Different species of fishes vary in their sensitivity to chlorinated hydrocarbons; however, most of these compounds are toxic at low concentrations. The

TABLE 29–3. Toxicity of Commonly Used Chlorinated Hydrocarbon Insecticides to Fish

Common Name of Insecticide	96-Hour LC$_{50}$ (μg/L) to Fish
Chlordane	44–56
DDT	7–19
Endrin	0.6–1.0
Lindane	27–67
Toxaphene	11–14

From U.S. Environmental Protection Agency (1973) Water quality criteria (1972). Series EPA-PR-236-199. Washington, D.C.

sensitivities of four species of salmonids to DDT and endrin are compared in Table 29–2 (Post, 1987). The comparative toxicities of several chlorinated hydrocarbons to fish are listed in Table 29–3. For acute toxicities, water analysis may be preferable, because the potential for bioaccumulation in tissues makes it difficult to determine whether an insecticide is a recent contaminant. In more chronic cases, the bioaccumulation in fish tissues may be useful in detecting exposures to extremely low levels of pesticides.

Organophosphate insecticides are oily and relatively insoluble in water. They can be absorbed through the skin, gills, and digestive tract of fishes. Most organophosphate insecticides are not stable and lose their toxicity shortly after application in water. Toxicity of organophosphates is derived from their ability to inhibit acetylcholinesterases, enzymes essential in the degradation of acetylcholine (Driesback, 1983). Organophosphates interfere with the function of somatic motor neurons and parasympathetic and sympathetic nerves of the autonomic nervous system (Murphy, 1980). Typical clinical signs of organophosphate poisoning include muscle contraction (tetany), dark pigmentation, reduced stamina, and deformities of the spine. Some organophosphate insecticides, malathion for example, cause hematologic, immunologic, and histologic alterations (Areechon, 1987). Toxicity of organophosphates does not occur at as low a concentration as the chlorinated hydrocarbons, and toxic levels are usually measured in milligrams per liter. Table 29–4 lists some common organophos-

TABLE 29–2. Comparative Toxicity of Endrin and DDT to Four Species of Salmonids

Fish Species	96-H Medial Tolerance Limit (μg/L) DDT	96-H Medial Tolerance Limit (μg/L) Endrin
Cutthroat trout	1.37	0.19
Rainbow trout	1.72	0.40
Brook trout	11.90	0.59
Coho salmon	18.65	0.77

Data derived from Post, G., and Schroeder, T. R. (1971) The toxicity of four insecticides to four salmonid species. Bull. Environ. Contam. Toxicol. 6:144–149; and Post. G. (1987) Textbook of Fish Health, Revised and Expanded. T.F.H. Publications, Neptune, New Jersey.

Table 29–4. Toxicity of Selected Organophosphate Insecticides to Several Species of Fish

Insecticide	96-Hour LC$_{50}$ (mg/L) Channel Catfish	Fathead Minnow	Rainbow Trout	Largemouth Bass
Trichlorfon*	—	7.8	—	—
Guthion	—	0.093	0.014	0.005
Methylparathion	—	8.9	2.750	5.22
Malathion	9.65	9.0	0.170	0.285
Parathion	—	1.6	—	0.19

*Used in fish ponds for parasitic copepod control.

Data derived from U.S. Environmental Protection Agency (1973) Water quality criteria (1972). Series EPA-PR-236-199. Washington, D.C.; and Areechon, N. (1987) Acute and Subchronic Toxicity of Malathion in Channel Catfish. Ph. D. Dissertation. Auburn University, Alabama.

phate insecticides and their toxicity to several species of fish. The effects of organophosphate insecticides on fish food organisms must also be considered because many of these compounds are highly toxic to copepods, other zooplankters, and insect larvae (Moore, 1970; Gaufin et al., 1965). Reviews of the impact of organophosphate insecticides on aquatic ecosystems are available for more in-depth study (Mulla and Mian, 1981).

Carbamate insecticides are cholinesterase inhibitors. They function similarly to the organophosphates but are not as potent toxins to fish. The toxicities of two common carbamates to several fish species are listed in Table 29–5. Diagnosis of carbamate poisoning in fish requires detection of the insecticides in fish tissue or in the water, but the assays must be done soon after exposure. Carbamates have intermediate persistence compared to the highly persistent chlorinated hydrocarbons and the rapidly degraded organophosphates (Mauck et al., 1977).

HERBICIDES

There are many herbicides used in agriculture that may contaminate the aquatic environment. Some are specifically designed for use in water (Schnick et al., 1986). Herbicides vary in their persistency in the environment following application, but some remain in sediments or bottom muds for months (Frank and Comes, 1967). The common herbicide 2,4-D is easily absorbed by fish, but it is rapidly excreted (Carpenter and Eaton, 1983). Diagnosis of herbicide poisoning in fish is difficult but can be accomplished with tissue or water analysis (Menzie, 1978).

FISH ERADICANTS

There are a number of compounds of synthetic or natural origin that are used as fish eradicants or piscicides. The most widely known are rotenone, antimycin, and 3-trifluoromethyl-4-nitrophenol (Schnick et al., 1986).

TABLE 29–5. Toxicity of Two Common Carbamate Insecticides to Several Species of Fish

	96-Hour LC$_{50}$ (mg/L)	
Fish Species	Sevin	Zectran
Rainbow trout	1.47–4.34	10.2
Largemouth bass	6.4	14.7
Bluegill	6.7–11.0	11.4–16.7
Yellow perch	0.75	2.48
Channel catfish	15.8	11.45

Data derived from U.S. Environmental Protection Agency (1973) Water quality criteria (1972). Series EPA-PR-236-199. Washington, D.C.; Post, G., and Schroeder, T. R. (1971) The toxicity of four insecticides to four salmonid species. Bull. Environ. Contam. Toxicol. 6:144–149; and Post, G. (1987) Textbook of Fish Health, Revised and Expanded. T.F.H. Publications, Neptune, New Jersey.

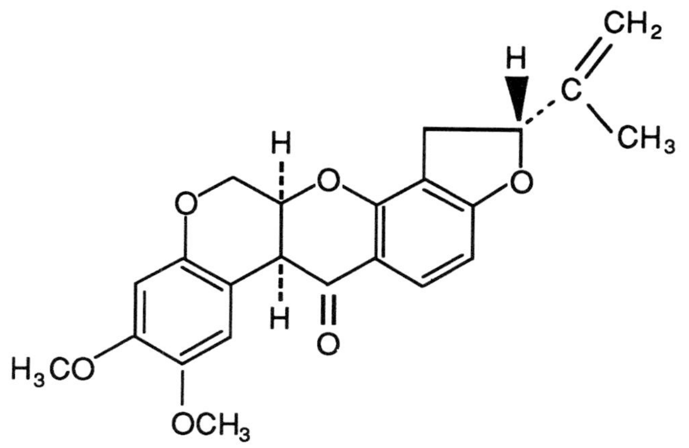

FIGURE 29–1. Structure of rotenone.

Rotenone is a naturally occurring product derived from cube and derris root plants (Fig. 29–1). It is the most widely used piscicide and is also used as an insecticide. Rotenone products have been used as a dip to rid farm animals of insects, and rotenone from treated cattle has killed fish in a stream 14 miles below the point of contamination (Post, 1987). A concentration of 0.02 mg/L is toxic to some species of fishes, but for fish eradication, 0.05 to 0.5 mg/L of active ingredient is normally used, depending on the target species. For example, the 96-hour LC$_{50}$ for fathead minnow is 0.006 mg/L, and the 96-hour LC$_{50}$ for channel catfish is 0.47 mg/L (Clemens and Sneed, 1959; Cohen et al., 1960). Rotenone kills fish by blocking electron transport by the cytochrome system in the gill. Affected fish gasp at the surface, and lose equilibrium (Lindahl and Oberg, 1961).

Rotenone degrades fairly rapidly. High temperature, high alkalinity, and light exposure speed up rotenone degradation. Turbidity slows rotenone degradation. Concentrations of 2 mg/L degrade in 3 days at 20°C, but at 11.5°C up to 16 days is required for total degradation (Meadows, 1973). When required, rotenone can be detoxified with potassium permanganate (KMnO$_4$) (Lawrence, 1956). A ratio of 2 parts of KMnO$_4$ is required to detoxify 1 part of rotenone in 30 minutes (Hepworth and Mithcum, 1967). Chlorine (Jackson, 1957) and activated charcoal (Bonn and Holbert, 1961) will also detoxify rotenone.

Antimycin is an antifungal agent isolated from *Streptomyces* sp. (Danshee et al., 1949) (Fig. 29–2). It has piscicidal activity for a variety of cold-water and warm-water fish species (Walker et al., 1964). The recommended concentration of antimycin for fish eradication is 5 to 50 mg/L. Some species are completely eradicated with concentrations of less than 1 mg/L (shad), whereas other species (black bullheads for example) survive concentrations of 100 mg/L. Owing to its reduced toxicity to catfishes, antimycin is used to remove unwanted scaled fishes from catfish culture ponds. The pH and temperature of the water affects the toxicity of antimycin. It is less

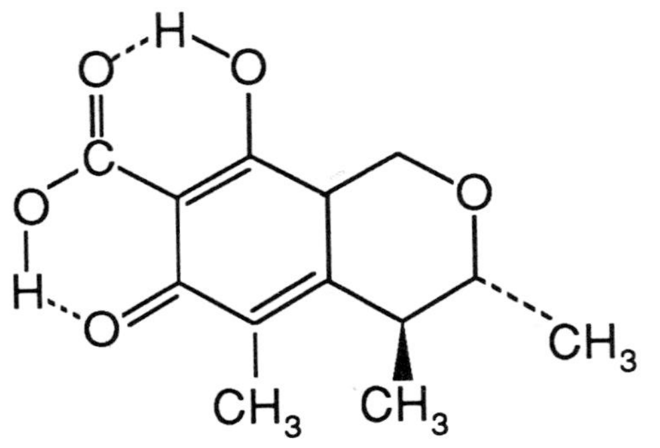

FIGURE 29–2. Structure of antimycin.

toxic at higher pH (8.5 to 9.5) and lower water temperatures (10 to 12°C) (Gilderhus, 1972).

PARASITICIDES

Reviews of the literature related to the use of malachite green in fisheries report its broad use and efficacy against external protozoan and fungal infections (Nelson, 1974). Malachite green has carcinogenic properties and causes chromosome defects (Lieden, 1961; Nelson, 1974) and leukopenia (Glagoleva and Malikova, 1968, from Nelson, 1974) in treated trout. It is not approved by the U.S. Food and Drug Administration (FDA) for use on fishes, and its registration for such purposes is highly unlikely. It is still widely used in some parts of the world. Concentrations of malachite green ranging from 0.1 to 0.5 mg/L in a variety of application methods, from a dip of a few seconds to an indefinite exposure, have been used as protozoan treatments. The 24-hour LC_{50}s of malachite green (Table 29–6) range from 0.11 mg/L for rainbow trout to 0.62 mg/L for common carp. The toxicity of malachite green is not affected by pH (pH 6 to 9), total hardness (15 to 100 mg/L $CaCO_3$), or iron concentration (0 to 1 mg/L), but malachite green is slightly more toxic at temperatures above 21°C (Phelps, 1975). Malachite green causes injury to the gills (Waluga, 1971, from Nelson, 1974). Clinical signs include lethargy, pale gills, and mottled skin coloration (Wood, 1968). Fish are at risk of toxicity if exposed to concentrations greater than 0.11 mg/L (Willford, 1967) and concentrations of 15 mg/L for more than 30 minutes are highly toxic (Martin, 1968).

Potassium permanganate is used in the aquatic environment as an oxidizing agent and chemical detoxifier, for which it is approved by the EPA. It is also used as a parasiticide and for external bacterial infections. Although not approved by the FDA for disease treatment, $KMnO_4$ is used at levels of 2 to 10 mg/L, depending on the organic matter content of the water and duration of the treatment (Tucker and Boyd, 1977). Being an oxidizing agent, the higher the organic load in the water, the higher the concentration of $KMnO_4$ that must be used to obtain control for either protozoan parasites or bacterial infection.

The organic oxidizing demand must be exceeded by 2 mg/L to control *Flexibacter columnaris* (Jee and Plumb, 1981). A spectrophotometric technique for measuring potassium permanganate organic demand in water is available (Engstrom-Heg, 1971). A visual method for determining potassium permanganate demand has been developed and gives comparable results to the spectrophotometric method (Boyd, 1979). Owing to the narrow safety factor of $KMnO_4$, the organic potassium permanganate demand should be determined before it is used.

Potassium permanganate is slightly more toxic at pH 5 to 8 than at pH 9, and slightly more toxic at 16 to 21°C than at 27 to 32°C. Total hardness of 25 to 100 mg/L does not affect $KMnO_4$ toxicity (Phelps, 1975). Although the toxic action of potassium permanganate is not fully understood, it is generally thought that a manganese by-product of $KMnO_4$ injures the gill tissues of fish. Repeated exposure to $KMnO_4$ will result in cumulative gill injury.

Trichlorfon, sold under the trade names Masoten, Dylox, or Neguvon, is used to control parasitic copepods and monogenetic trematodes on fish. Developed as an insecticide, this organophosphate functions to inhibit acetylcholinesterase. Trichlorfon has a 96-hour LC_{50} of 50 mg/L for fathead minnows (McKee and Wolf, 1963). The toxicity of trichlorfon is significantly higher at pH 8 or above than at pH 7 or below (Phelps, 1975). Similarly, toxicity increases with increased temperature (16 to 32°C). Fish exposed to toxic levels of trichlorfon develop typical signs of organophosphate poisoning and show tetany and loss of equilibrium.

FUNGICIDES

There are no effective FDA-approved fungicides for fish and fish eggs. Chemicals that are fungicidal are often also toxic to fish at or near their effective concentrations. Historically, malachite green has been used to treat fungi (water mold) on fish eggs and fish. Owing to reasons previously discussed, malachite green is no longer used extensively for fish in the United States, but it is used in other regions of the world. The concentration used to treat eggs is usually 5 mg/L for 15 minutes to 1 hour (Burrows, 1949; Hoffman and Meyer, 1974). Exposure of rainbow trout eggs to 1, 3, and 5 mg/L of malachite green results in three times the incidence of deformities in

TABLE 29–6. Twenty-four Hour LC_{50} of Malachite Green for Selected Species of Fishes

Species of Fish	mg/L	Reference
Rainbow trout	0.11	Alabaster, 1969
Brown trout	0.45	Willford, 1967
Common carp	0.62	Anonymous, 1972
Channel catfish	0.21	Willford, 1967
Striped bass	0.25	Hughes, 1973
Bluegill	0.13	Anonymous, 1972
Smallmouth bass	0.15	Anonymous, 1972

21-day-old fry as in the untreated controls (Meyer and Jorgenson, 1983). Channel catfish treated with 0.1 mg/L for 4 consecutive days still have the chemical in their muscle 36 days after exposure (Poe and Wilson, 1983), and if the fish are treated with 0.3 mg/L for 24 hours, some fish still have malachite green tissue concentrations for 60 days. Formalin is also used to treat fungi on fish eggs and fish.

LITERATURE CITED

Alabaster, J.S. (1969) Survival of fish in 164 herbicides, insecticides, fungicides, wetting agents and miscellaneous substances. Int. Pest Cont. 11(2):29–35.

Allison, D.T., Kallman, B.J., Cope, O.B., and Van Valen, C. (1964) Some chronic effects of DDT on cutthroat. Res. Rep 64. U.S. Fish and Wildlife Service, Washington, D.C.

Allison, R. (1962) The effects of formalin and other parasiticides upon oxygen concentration in ponds. Proc. S.E. Assoc. Game Fish Comm. 16:446–449.

Amend, D.F. (1970) Retention of mercury by salmon. Progressive Fish Culturist 32:192–194.

American Public Health Association (1981) American Water Works Association, and Water Pollution Control Federation (1980) Standard Methods for Examination of Water and Waste Water. 15th ed. American Public Health Association, Washington, D.C.

Anonymous (1972) Quarterly Progress Report (July–September) Fish Control Laboratory. U.S. Department of the Interior, La Crosse, Wisconsin.

Areechon, N. (1987) Acute and Subchronic Toxicity of Malathion in Channel Catfish. Ph.D. Dissertation. Auburn University, Alabama.

Benoit, D.A. (1975) Chronic effects of copper on survival, growth, and reproduction of the bluegill (Lepomis macrochirus). Trans. Am. Fish. Soc. 104:353–358.

Bonn, E.W., and Holbert, L.R. (1961) Some effects of rotenone products on municipal water supplies. Trans. Am. Fish. Soc. 90:287–297.

Bouck, G.R. (1980) Etiology of gas bubble disease. Trans. Am. Fish. Soc. 109:703–707.

Boyd, C.E. (1979) Water Quality in Warmwater Fish Ponds. Alabama Agricultural Experiment Station. Auburn University, Alabama.

Burrows, R.E. (1949) Prophylactic treatment for control of fungus (Saprolegnia parasitica) on salmon eggs. Progressive Fish Culturist 11:97–103.

Carpenter, L.A., and Eaton, D.L. (1983) The disposition of 2, 4-dichlorophenoxyacetic acid in rainbow trout. Arch. Environ. Contam. Toxicol. 12:169–173.

Clemens, H.R., and Sneed, K.E. (1959) Lethal doses of several commercial chemicals to fingerling channel catfish. Special Scientific Report on Fish No. 316. U.S. Fish and Wildlife Service, Washington, D.C.

Cohen, J.M., Kamphake, L.J., Lamke, A.E., Henderson, C., and Woodward, R.L. (1960) Effects of fish poisons on water supplies. Part 1. Removal of toxic materials. J.A. Water Works Assoc. 52:1551–1566.

Crandall, C.A., and Goodnight, C.J. (1962) Effects of sublethal concentrations of several toxicants on the common goby, Lehistes reticulatus. Trans. Am. Microsoc. Soc. 82:59–73.

Crunkilton, R.L., Czarnezki, J.M., and Trial, L. (1980) Severe gas bubble disease in a warmwater fishery in the midwestern United States. Trans. Am. Fish. Soc. 109:725–733.

Danshee, B.R., Leben, C., Keitt, G.W., and Strong, F.M. (1949) Isolation and properties of antimycin A. J. Am. Chem. Soc. 71:2436–2437.

Dreisbach, R.H. (1983) Handbook of Poisoning: Prevention, Diagnosis and Treatment. 11th ed. Lange, Los Altos, California.

Duodoroff, P., and Katz, M. (1953) Critical review of literature on the toxicity of industrial wastes and their components to fish. II. The metals, as salts. Sewage Ind. Wastes 25:802–839.

Engstrom-Heg, R. (1971) Direct measurement of potassium permanganate demand and residual potassium permanganate. N.Y. Fish and Game J. 18:117–122.

Frank, P.A., and Comes, R.D. (1967) Herbicidal residues in pond water and hydrosoil. Weeds 15:210–213.

Gardner, G.R. (1975) Chemically induced lesions in estuarine or marine teleosts. In: The Pathology of Fishes (Ribelin, W.E., and Migaki, G., eds.). University Wisconsin Press, Madison, pp. 657–693.

Gardner, G.R., and LaRoche, G. (1973) Copper induced lesions in estuarine teleosts. J. Fish. Res. Bd. Can. 30:363–368.

Gardner, G.R., and Yevich, P.P. (1970) Histological and hematological responses of an estuarine teleost to cadmium. J. Fish. Res. Bd. Can. 27:2185–2196.

Gaufin, A.R., Jensen, L.D., Nebekor, A.V., Nelson, T., and Ted, R.W. (1965) The toxicity of ten organic insecticides to various aquatic invertebrates. Water and Sewage Works 112:276.

Gilderhus, P.A. (1972) Exposure times necessary for antimycin and rotenone to eliminate certain freshwater fish. J. Fish. Res. Bd. Can. 29:199–202.

Glagoleva, T.P., and Malikova, E.M. (1968) Effect of malachite green on the composition of blood in Baltic salmon fingerlings (in Russian). Ryhnoe Khoziastvo. 45:15–18.

Grizzle, J.M. (1981) Effects of hypolimnetic discharge on fish health below a reservoir. Trans. Am. Fish. Soc. 110:29–43.

Grizzle, J.M., Melius, P., and Strength, D.R. (1984) Papillomas on fish exposed to chlorinated wastewater effluent. J. Natl. Conc. Inst. 73:1133–1142.

Grizzle, J.M., Schwedler, T.E., and Scott, A.L. (1981) Papillomas of black bullheads, Ictalurus melas (Rafinesque), living in a chlorinated sewage pond. J. Fish Dis. 4:345–351.

Heath, A.G. (1987) Water pollution and fish physiology. CRC Press, Boca Raton, Florida.

Hepworth, W.G., and Mitchum, D.L. (1967) Study of fish toxicants. Wyoming Job Compl. Report, Project No. FS-3-R-13, Work Plan 9. Job No. 2F.

Hodson, P.V., Borgmann, U., and Shear, H. (1979) Toxicity of copper to aquatic biota. In: Copper in the Environment. Part II. Health Effects. (Nriagu, J.O., ed.). Wiley Interscience, New York, pp. 307–372.

Hoffman, G.L., and Meyer, F.P. (1974) Parasites of Freshwater Fishes: A Review of Their Control and Treatment. T.F.H. Publications, Neptune City, New Jersey.

Huey, D.W., Simco, B.A., and Criswell, D.W. (1980) Nitrite-induced methemoglobin formation in channel catfish. Trans. Am. Fish. Soc. 109:558–562.

Hughes, J.S. (1973) Acute toxicity of thirty chemicals to striped bass (Morone saxatilis). Western Association of State Game and Fish Commission, Salt Lake City, Utah.

Hurlbert, S.H. (1975) Secondary effects of pesticides on aquatic systems. Residue Rev. 57:81–148.

Jackson, C.F. (1957) Detoxification of rotenone-treated water. N.H. Fish Game Dept. Tech. Circ. 14:1–28.

Jee, L.K., and Plumb, J.A. (1981) Effects of organic load on potassium permanganate as a treatment for Flexibacter columnaris. Trans. Am. Fish. Soc. 90:264–268.

Law, E.A. (1981) Aquatic Pollution. John Wiley & Sons, New York.

Lawrence, J.M. (1956) Preliminary results on the use of potassium permanganate to counteract the effects of rotenone on fish. Progressive Fish Culturist. 18:15–21.

Lieden, U. (1961) On the effect of the carcinogen and mutagen malachite green (P-dimethylamino-fuchson-dimethylaminooxalate {sulfate}) on mitosis in fish and fish eggs (in German). Die Naturwissenschaften 48:437–438.

Lindahl, P.E., and Oberg, K.E. (1961) The effect of rotenone on respiration and its points of attack. Exp. Cell Reg. 23:228–237.

Martin, R.L. (1968) A comparison of effects of concentrations of malachite green and acriflavine on fungi associated with diseased fish. Progressive Fish Culturist 30:153–158.

Mauck, W.L., Olson, L.E., and Hogan, J.W. (1977) Effects of water quality on deactivation of mexacarbate (Zectran) to fish. Arch. Environ. Contam. Toxicol. 6:385–393.

Mayer, F.L., Jr., and Ellersieck, M.R. (1986) Manual of Acute Toxicity: Interpretation and Data Base for 410 Chemicals and 66 Species of Freshwater Animals. U.S. Department of the Interior, Fish and Wildlife Service Resource Publication No. 160.

Mayer, F.L., Mehrle, P.M., and Crutcher, P.L. (1978) Interactions of toxaphene and vitamin C in channel catfish. Trans. Am. Fish. Soc. 107:326–333.

McFarlane, G.A., and Franzin, W.G. (1978) Evaluated heavy metals: A stress on a population of white suckers (Catastomus commersoni), in Hamell Lake, Saskatchewan. J. Fish. Res. Bd. Can. 35:963–970.

McKee, J.E., and Wolf, H.W. (1963) Water quality criteria. Resource Agency of California, State Water Quality Control Board Publication No. 3-A.

McKim, J.M., and Benoit, D.A. (1971) Effects of long-term exposures to copper on survival, growth and reproduction of brook trout (Salvelinus fontinalis). J. Fish. Res. Bd. Can. 28:655–662.

Meadows, B.S. (1973) Toxicity of rotenone to some species of coarse fish and invertebrates. J. Fish Biol. 5:155–163.

Menzie, C.M. (1978) Metabolism of pesticides, update II. Special Scientific Report No. 212. U.S. Fish and Wildlife Service, Washington, D.C.

Meyer, F.P., and Jorgenson, T.A. (1983) Teratological and other effects of malachite green on development of rainbow trout and rabbits. Trans. Am. Fish. Soc. 112:818–824.

Moore, R.B. (1970) Effect of pesticides on growth and survival of Euglena gracilus. Z. Bull. Environ. Contam. Toxicol. 5:226.

Mulla, M.S., and Mian, L.A. (1981) Biological and environmental impacts of the insecticides malathion and parathion on nontarget biota in aquatic ecosystems. Residue Rev. 78:101–135.

Murphy, S.D. (1980). Pesticides. In: Casaraett and Doulls Toxicology: The Basic Science of Poisons. 2nd ed. (Doull, J., Klaassen, C.D., and Amdur, M.O., eds.). Macmillan, New York, pp. 357–408.

Nebecker, A.V., Publis, F.A., and Defoe, D.L. (1971) Toxicity of Polychlorinated Biphenyls (PCB) to Fish and Other Aquatic Life. Environmental

Protection Agency, National Water Quality Laboratory, Duluth, Minnesota.

Nelson, N.C. (1974) A Review of the Literature on the Use of Malachite Green in Fisheries. National Technical Information Service, U.S. Department of Commerce. PB-235450.

Norris, L.A., Lorz, H.W., and Gregory, S.V. (1983) Influence of Forest and Rangeland Management on Anadromous Fish Habitat in Western North America. U.S. Dept. of Agriculture, U.S. Forest Service. General Technical Report PNW-149.

Peakall, D.B., and Lincer, J.L. (1970) Polychlorinated biphenyls—another long-life widespread chemical in the environment. Bioscience 20:958–964.

Phelps, R. (1975) Toxicity and Efficacy of Five Chemotherapeutics Used in Aquaculture When Applied to Waters of Different Quality. Ph.D. Dissertation, Auburn University, Alabama.

Pickering, Q.H., and Henderson, C. (1966) The acute toxicity of some heavy metals to different species of warmwater fishes. Int. J. Air Water Pollut. 10:453–563.

Plumb, J.A., and Richburg, R.W. (1977) Pesticide levels in sera of moribund channel catfish from a continuous winter mortality. Trans. Am. Fish. Soc. 106:185–188.

Poe, W.F., and Wilson, R.P. (1983) Absorption of malachite green by channel catfish. Progressive Fish Culturist 45:228–229.

Post, G. (1987) Textbook of Fish Health, Revised and Expanded. T.F.H. Publications, Neptune, New Jersey.

Post, G., and Schroeder, T.R. (1971) The toxicity of four insecticides to four salmonid species. Bull. Environ. Contam. Toxicol. 6:144–145.

Rand, G.M., and Petrocelli, S.R. (1985) Fundamentals of Aquatic Toxicology. Hemisphere, Washington, D.C.

Rucker, R.R. (1968) Effects of mercurial compounds on fish and humans. Bull. Off. Intern. Epizool. 69(9–10):1431–1437.

Schnick, R.A., Meyer, F.P., and Gray, D.L. (1986) A Guide to Approved Chemicals in Fish Production and Fishery Resource Management. MP 241. University of Arkansas Cooperative Extension Service and U.S. Fish and Wildlife Service.

Schwedler, T.E., and Tucker, C.S. (1983) Empirical relationship between percent methemoglobin in channel catfish and dissolved nitrite and chloride in ponds. Trans. Am. Fish. Soc. 112:117–119.

Stickel, L.F., and Hickey, J.J. (1977) Toxicological Aspects of Toxaphene in Fish: A Summary. Trans. N. Amer. Wildl. Nat. Res. Conf., Wildlife Management Institute, Washington, D.C. 42:365–373.

Tagatz, M.E. (1961) Reduced oxygen tolerance and toxicity of petroleum products to juvenile American shad. Chesapeake Sci. 2:65–71.

Tucker, C.S., and Boyd, C.E. (1977) Relationship between potassium permanganate treatment and water quality. Trans. Am. Fish. Soc. 106:481–488.

U.S. Environmental Protection Agency (1973) Water quality criteria (1972). Series EPA-PR-236-199.

U.S. Environmental Protection Agency (1980a) Ambient water quality criteria for copper. EPA 440/5-80-036. Washington, D.C.

U.S. Environmental Protection Agency (1980b) Ambient water quality criteria for zinc. EPA 440/5-80-079. Washington, D.C.

U.S. Environmental Protection Agency (1980c) Ambient water quality criteria for lead. EPA 440/5-80-057. Washington, D.C.

U.S. Environmental Protection Agency (1980d) Ambient water quality criteria for mercury. EPA 440/5-80-058. Washington, D.C.

U.S. Environmental Protection Agency (1986) Quality criteria for water, 1986. EPA 440/5-86-001.

Walker, C.R., Lennon, R.E., and Berger, B.L. (1964) Preliminary observations on the toxicity of antimycin A to fish and other aquatic animals. Investigations in Fish Control. U.S. Fish & Wildlife Service Circular 185.

Walters, G.R., and Plumb, J.A. (1980) Environmental stress and bacterial infection in channel catfish, *Ictalurus punctatus* Rafinesque. J. Fish Biol. 17:177–185.

Waluga, D. (1971) Changes in the gills of rainbow trout (*Salmo giardneri*, Richardson) under the influence of malachite green (in Polish). Rocznik. Nauk. Roiniczyck. Tom. 93-H-4:172–31.

Willford, W.A. (1967) Toxicity of 22 therapeutic compounds to six fishes. U.S. Bureau of Sport Fish & Wildlife. Investigations in Fish Control. No. 18.

Woltering, D.M. (1984) The growth response in fish: chronic and early life stage toxicity tests: A critical review. Aquatic Toxicol. 5:1021.

Wood, J.W. (1968) Drugs and chemicals introduced directly into the water: Malachite green. In: Diseases of Pacific Salmon; The Prevention and Treatment. State of Washington, Department of Fisheries, p. B-4.6.

SECTION II

SALMONIDS

GEORGE W. KLONTZ, *Section Editor*

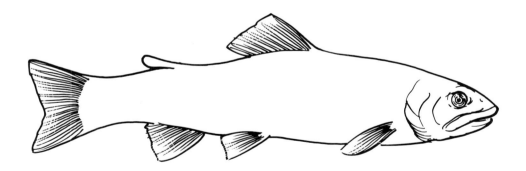

Chapter 30

TAXONOMY AND NATURAL HISTORY OF SALMONIDS

LYNWOOD S. SMITH

TAXONOMY AND EVOLUTION OF THE SALMONIDS

Among the bony fishes (Actinopterigii), the salmonids are somewhere in the middle of the evolutionary progression of increasing complexity. If one divides the bony fishes into three groups, an ancient group including the sturgeons and gars, a middle group including the herrings and true cods, and a specialized group with all of the spiny-rayed fishes (bass, perch, tunas, etc.), the salmonids fall in the middle group. One of the indications of their status is the position of the paired fins. In salmonids the pectoral fins are below the midline of the body, and the pelvic fins relatively far posterior, more or less under the dorsal fin (Fig. 30–1). In comparison, the spiny-rayed fishes have their pectoral fins on or near the midline. The pelvic fins of salmonids are ventral and sometimes even anterior to the pectorals. All salmonids have an adipose fin, although this fin also occurs in other groups.

The salmonids can be divided into several major groups (Table 30–1). Emphasis for further discussion has been placed on salmon and trout because of their commercial importance.

NATURAL HISTORY

Salmonids are now widely distributed throughout the world, but they originally inhabited only the colder waters of the northern hemisphere. Their temperature tolerance ranges from near freezing to 30°C. Transplanted salmonids are now found in the colder climates of the southern hemisphere, including New Zealand, southern Chile and Argentina, and even the higher altitudes of the northern Andes mountains.

All salmonids spawn in fresh water, producing eggs with large amounts of yolk. They fertilize them externally and produce large fry after a relatively long incubation. Much of the success of salmonids in aquaculture stems from the ease of handling the large eggs and of feeding the fry with artificial food. Most salmonids spawn several times, except Pacific salmon which spawn only once.

Many salmonid life histories include some kind of anadromous migration. There is general agreement that this is a feeding migration because the sea has greater food resources than the cold northern lakes and rivers. Catadromy prevails in the tropics where food resources are greater in fresh water (Gross et al., 1988; McDowall, 1987). The degree of migration varies widely. In Japan, only the male masou salmon migrates to sea for only about 3 months. Cutthroat trout may travel between fresh and salt water several times a year. At the other extreme, chum and pink salmon migrate to sea as soon as yolk absorption is complete and stay there until ready to spawn. One consensus has been that the evolutionary trend has been from full-time residence in fresh water to more and more of the life history in seawater. Another point of view suggests that chum and pink salmon are the least anadromous, with greater development of smolti-

TABLE 30–1. Optimal Rearing Temperatures

| Common Name | Max. Optimal Temp. (°C) | |
	Hatching	Rearing
Coho salmon	10	18
Sockeye salmon	10	18
Rainbow, steelhead trout	9	19
Atlantic salmon	5	19
Brook trout	9	18

From Wedemeyer, G. A., and Wood, J. W. (1974) Stress as a predisposing factor in fish diseases. Fish Disease Leaflet No. 38. U.S. Department of the Interior, Fish and Wildlife Service, Washington, D.C.

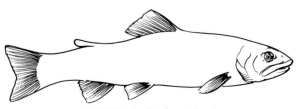

FIGURE 30–1. Cutthroat trout.

fication in coho, sockeye, and chinook salmon (Fig. 30–2).

The length of the migration also varies widely. The masou salmon and brown trout travel along the coastline near their river for tens or a few hundred miles. Stocks of coho and chinook salmon from Oregon and Washington usually occupy ocean areas within a few hundred miles of the mouths of their natal streams. In contrast, more northern stocks of Atlantic and Pacific salmon range over much of the northern portion of their respective oceans with fairly specific routes extending for 3000 miles or more across open sea. This results in mixing of stocks from both shores of each ocean, making regulation of the respective international fisheries complex.

Even in those salmonid species designated as anadromous, migration into seawater is not mandatory. Sockeye salmon have a landlocked strain called kokanee. Pink, coho, and chinook salmon have adapted to rearing in the Great Lakes and spawning in adjacent streams.

The complexities of migration require navigation and homing. In Bristol Bay sockeye salmon, tagging studies have shown that fish often swim downstream in the ocean currents and that they can home to a single point from several directions, performing bicoordinate navigation (Royce et al., 1968). Suggested mechanisms include sensing the electromagnetic characteristics of the ocean current, sun-compass orientation, and following odor trails (the latter proposed for Atlantic salmon only). Homing probably emphasizes olfactory identification of unique characteristics of water systems, but probably also includes other senses. Suggested odorants include leachates of organic materials unique to each watershed and bile salts in the feces of fish currently or recently residing in the water. An artificial odorant, morpholine, also produces homing behavior. Moving the odorant, even to a water system different from that where the stock was reared, results in homing (Hasler, 1971). While homing is crucial, it seems equally important to salmonid zoogeography that a few individuals stray from their home water so the species can colonize new streams.

Having returned from the sea to fresh water, neither Pacific nor Atlantic salmon feed, presumably as a way of reserving the freshwater food resources for juveniles. Differing lengths of migrations lead to stock specificities for the quantity of energy stored prior to the spawning migration. In a short stream, adult chum salmon may migrate upstream to barely above the high tide line to spawn and die in about 2 weeks. Therefore, they require only minimal energy reserves. Chum salmon in the Yukon River have maximal energy reserves, since they may migrate as much as 2700 km upstream, after which they spawn and die in about 2 weeks.

During starvation, the digestive tract and associated organs atrophy. The routine metabolic rate increases owing to the increased workload of swimming upstream. Most stress-related responses steadily increase during the upstream migration and peak on the spawning grounds. Pacific salmon typically die from reduced disease resistance produced by the extended stress, not from any inherent mechanism. Sockeye salmon have been kept alive for nearly a year after spawning by keeping them in a disease-free system, where they spontaneously started feeding again and regained their silvery, prespawning coloration. Their digestive histology also returned to normal (McBride et al., 1963).

While the death of the adults soon after spawning may seem to be a waste of biologic resource, the decay of their carcasses contributes significantly to the primary productivity of the ecosystem in which the eggs will hatch. The carcasses of an average escapement to Lake Illiamna in southwestern Alaska contributed about 30% of the total phosphorus budget of this 15,000-km^2 lake. In western British Columbia (Canada), preliminary results of a recent project to fertilize several large lakes suggested that the low levels of adult returns also limited the production of juveniles. The lack of enrichment from decaying adult salmon was thought to be limiting primary productivity and therefore also limiting the biomass of juvenile salmon. Once the adult escapement increases to historic levels, the expectation is that artificial fertilization becomes unnecessary.

Contemporary ecological problems in perpetuating natural salmon stocks are varied. Loss of spawning areas occurs when logging debris blocks access to streams. Increased runoff in both logged-off and urban areas causes siltation of gravel beds, preventing the upwelling of water through the gravel needed to provide oxygen to incubating eggs. Increased runoff in the spring also leads to increased water temperatures and decreased water flows in summer, thus negatively impacting those species that rear in fresh water through one or more summers. Rearing of fish in hatcheries typically reduces wild stocks owing to the increased survival rate of hatchery stocks in the early stages of the life cycle. At the same time, hatchery salmonids are seriously impacted by diseases such as infectious hemopoietic necrosis virus and bacterial kidney disease, both of which lack effective treatments. Thus, solving the loss of habitat for wild stocks simply by moving them into hatcheries is no solution for their long-term survival.

LITERATURE CITED

Gross, M.R., Coleman, R.M., and McDowall, R.M. (1988) Aquatic productivity and the evolution of diadromous fish migration. Science 239:1291–1293.

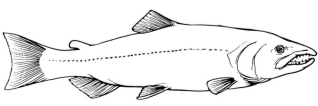

FIGURE 30–2. Chinook salmon.

Hasler, A.D. (1971) Orientation and fish migration. In: Fish Physiology. Vol. VI (Hoar, W.S., and Randall, D.J., eds.). Academic Press, New York, pp. 429–510.

McBride, J.R., Fagerlund, U.H.M., Smith, M., and Tomlinson, N. (1963) Resumption of feeding by and survival of adult sockeye salmon (*Oncorhynchus nerka*) following advanced gonad development. J. Fish. Res. Bd. Can. 20:95–100.

McDowall, R.M. (1987) Evolution and importance of diadromy. The occur-

rence and distribution of diadromy among fishes. Am. Fish. Soc. Symp. 1:1–13.

Royce, W.F., Smith, L.S., and Hartt, A.C. (1968) Models of oceanic migrations of Pacific salmon and comments on guidance mechanisms. Fish. Bull. 66:441–462.

Wedemeyer, G.A., and Wood, J.W. (1974) Stress as a predisposing factor in fish diseases. Fish Disease Leaflet No. 38. U.S. Department of the Interior, Fish and Wildlife Service, Washington, D.C.

Chapter 31

ANATOMY AND SPECIAL PHYSIOLOGY OF SALMONIDS

LYNWOOD S. SMITH

ANATOMY

Salmonids have many characteristics in common with higher vertebrates and few specialized features. The trout is used as the prototype fusiform fish in the chapter on fish anatomy in the general medicine section of this book (Chap. 1). All salmonids have fusiform, muscular bodies for their strong swimming lifestyle. Compared to catfishes, carp, or true cod, they have a relatively high aspect ratio (span/chord) caudal fin, denoting relatively high efficiency in swimming, but not nearly to the degree seen in tunas and mackerels. Salmonids have dark, lipolytic muscle laterally that is highly vascularized for aerobic, sustainable (marathon) swimming and light, glycolytic muscle medially for anaerobic, nonsustainable (burst, sprint) swimming (Smith and Bell, 1975).

The salmonid vertebral column appears similar to other vertebrates, but the compression load from the contraction of swimming muscles is born by dorsoventral ligaments acting like a bowstring between the hemal and neural spines and the centra, rather than directly by the centra and intervertebral discs. The skeleton has no hemopoietic tissue, which is typically found in the kidney and spleen as well as various other tissues, depending on species (Fange, 1986).

The internal organs of salmonids are typical of higher vertebrates with a few notable exceptions. The pancreas is diffuse as small nodules and is visible only histologically. The bile duct, therefore, does not have a branch from the pancreas, since the pancreatic secretions enter the intestine in separate ducts.

Sometimes the pancreatic globules reside in the liver, and secretions enter the gallbladder.

The urogenital system has evolved in a different manner from the higher vertebrates, with a single median kidney and urinary duct, which have a minimal relationship with the kidney evolution of the land vertebrates. Sperm in salmonids remains in an expanded testes and sperm duct, but the ova may become free in the coelomic cavity. The expanded oviduct, which some say contains the eggs, is so thin-walled at maturation that its presence is disputed.

The digestive tract is short and typical of vertebrates except for the numerous pyloric ceca. In salmonids, the numbers of the pyloric ceca have been used as a taxonomic character, and their abundance has excited speculation about their possessing unique functions. However, all tests have shown them to be functionally similar to the upper intestine with emphasis on lipid absorption (Buddington, 1987).

Salmonids have several hormone glands, arranged differently or not found at all in higher vertebrates. The adrenal and corticosteroid secretions come from the chromaffin tissue and the interrenal gland of the cranial kidney. Both of these tissues are identifiable only histologically. Calcium metabolism is regulated by two hormones, calcitonin and hypocalcin, secreted from the ultimobranchial gland and corpuscles of Stannius, respectively. The former is a faintly gray-white streak on the transverse membrane, and the latter consists of a pair of yellow dots on the posterior ventral surface of the kidney. The exact role of both hormones in regulating calcium metabolism in salmonids is unclear. The thyroid gland is diffuse in the muscles of the isthmus, whereas the thymus is visible on the medial surface of the gill covers in immature fish. Whether there are T and B lymphocytes comparable to those of higher vertebrates is still uncertain.

The circulatory system of salmonids is typical of other generalized fishes but is perhaps better known than that in most fishes. The serial arrangement of vessels, with three capillary beds in series, has some exceptions in the gills that may or may not be unique to salmonids. The general plan of blood flow through the gills is that arterial blood enters the trailing edge of the gill filaments and moves through the secondary gill lamellae against the direction of the water flow, providing maximal gas exchange by a countercurrent mechanism. At the same time, there is a need to minimize surface area and the osmoregulatory workload owing to passive diffusion of water and salts. Thus, fish physiologically appear to adjust their gill surface area to the minimum needed to meet their oxygen demand. However, detailed examinations of the vascular anatomy of several fishes using scanning electron microscopy show the arteriolar vasoconstrictive points to be downstream from the gill lamellae. Blood flows through all of the lamellae all of the time (Laurent and Dunel, 1976). All gills have arterioarterial and arteriovenous components that balance the respiratory and circulatory demands with the passive osmoregulatory workload at the gills (Jones and Randall, 1978; Laurent, 1984). In contrast to higher vertebrates, a coronary artery leaves the ventral portion of the second gill arch and returns posteriorly along the ventral surface of the ventral aorta to supply the ventricular muscle with oxygenated blood. The major function of the coronary artery may be something other than the anatomically obvious role of supplying blood to the ventricular muscle (Daxboeck, 1982).

PHYSIOLOGY

Eggs and Alevins

Salmonid eggs have relatively long, temperature-dependent incubation times. For coho salmon at 11°C, hatching may occur 38 days after fertilization, 48 days at 9°C, or 115 days or more at still colder temperatures. The concept of degree-days (number of degrees above some minimum temperature multiplied by the number of days at that temperature) seems to work over moderate ranges of temperature and latitude, but is not universal. Temperatures less than 5°C or greater than 15°C cause increased egg mortality.

Hatching involves escaping through the egg membranes with the help of a hatching enzyme. Typical hatching size is 20 to 30 mm. Salmonids stay in the gravel (photonegative orientation) after hatching for anywhere from 2 weeks to several months, a stage of larval development widely called alevin,

during which they grow to 30 to 40 mm. As alevins, they absorb most of the balance of their yolk material, close the midventral opening of the intestine (button-up), and may start to feed. After button-up, fish are then called fry. The fry emerge from the gravel with increased swimming activity and photopositive orientation and begin regular feeding. The increased swimming activity that occurs may result from the development of appropriate muscle cells. Similarly, gut development goes through a sequence of digestive enzymes, starting with proteolytic enzymes initially, and adding the rest of the normal complement over several weeks. Once into the fry stage, most salmonids have maximal swimming performance (velocity at which they fatigue), which is proportional to their size regardless of whether they are a species that migrates as fry (chum, pinks) or not (rainbow trout, coho and chinook salmon). This is in contrast to smolts, which show decreased swimming performance just before and during migration.

Juveniles and Smolts

Temperature is probably the most pervasive factor in the physiology of all fishes, but the effects of temperature change are best known in sockeye salmon (Brett, 1971; Brett and Groves, 1979) (Fig. 31–1). Fish normally operate in the lower middle of their temperature envelope (Brett and Groves, 1979).

Growth efficiency (growth as a percentage of body [dry] weight per day) changes with temperature and ration. As both temperature and ration decrease, the temperature of maximum growth efficiency also decreases. Sockeye juveniles in fresh water have nearly the same growth efficiency on 3% of body weight ration at 5°C as they have on 6% ration at 15°C (Brett, 1970). This is considered an adaptation to cold northern lakes with minimal productivity (Brett, 1971).

Extreme temperature changes cause puzzling effects. In contrast to the increased growth efficiency, rapid temperature changes close to either the upper or lower lethal temperatures can cause pH regulation problems, particularly for plasma bicarbonate. Low temperatures can also produce dormancy with discontinuous breathing and activity, but with no metabolic shutdown (Crawshaw, 1979).

Smolt is defined as the migratory stage of salmonids that are preadapted for entry into seawater. As one defines smolt in increasing detail, the characteristics of various species and stocks have more and more exceptions to the general rules. The most conspicuous indicator of smoltification is increasingly silver coloration, eventually with the parr marks being completely covered by deposition of guanine in the dermis and under the scales. However, some salmon stocks migrate to seawater without any color change. For many species and stocks within species, there is a minimum age and weight below which fish do not migrate downstream or adapt to seawater.

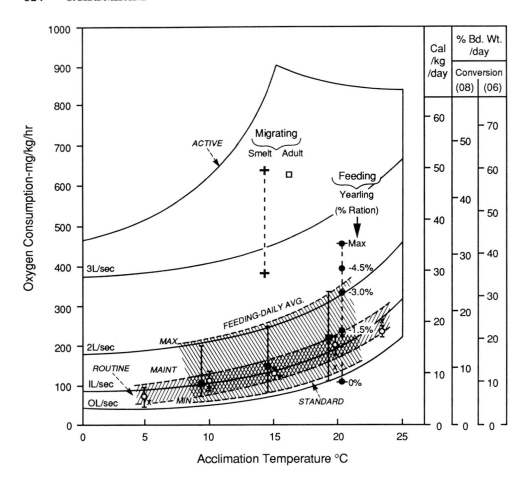

FIGURE 31–1. A performance polygon in which the boundaries are the upper and lower lethal temperatures, the minimal (standard or basal, depending on the data) metabolism, and the maximum sustainable (for 1 hour) swimming velocity. At temperatures below the maximum swimming velocity, the performance is temperature limited. Above the temperature of maximum sustainable swimming velocity, performance is limited by oxygen availability. (Adapted from Brett, J.R. [1964] The respiratory metabolism and swimming performance of young sockeye salmon. J. Fish Res. Bd. Can. [Department of Fisheries and Oceans] 21:1183–1226. Reproduced with the permission of the Minister of Supply and Services Canada, 1992.)

When migration begins, wild fish may change their orientation from the stream bottom or sides, to the surface, often preferring higher velocity water. Orientation often changes from holding position in the stream to moving downstream, either swimming head first or drifting tail first. In hatcheries, fish crowd together at the downstream end of their raceway and jump at the screens, a behavior described as migratory restlessness. Maximal sustainable swimming velocity also decreases by about a third in both wild and hatchery fish during smoltification. Downstream migration may be mostly passive drifting with the current, as in Atlantic salmon, or more active, as in Pacific salmon.

Since most hatcheries are too far from seawater to test the marine survival of their fish directly, various indicators have been developed to estimate the degree of readiness to enter seawater. The most obvious test is simulated entry into seawater. When fully smolted, the serum sodium level of salmon from many stocks will not increase to more than 175 mmol/L after 24 hours in seawater (Clarke and Blackburn, 1977). Different stocks under different circumstances may have different serum sodium limits.

There have been numerous attempts to control smolting. Short day lengths can delay smolting but cannot prevent it. Long photoperiod can accelerate smolting, but not by more than a few months. In some cases, added salt in the diet improves survival

at seawater entry (Zaugg et al., 1983). Body lipids, especially triglycerides, decrease greatly during smolting. This is more accentuated in coho than in chinook salmon, but the functional significance is unclear (Woo et al., 1978). Methods for feeding or injecting of hormones have given mixed results and have not been used in production.

Plasma thyroxin concentrations increase during smoltification, presumably producing migratory restlessness. In addition to a general increase in thyroxin, there can be a further sudden increase in thyroxin in phase with the moon (Grau et al., 1981). With the advent of a radioimmune assay for thyroxin, it has become a routine measure of smoltification (Folmar and Dickhoff, 1980).

Similarly, sodium-potassium ATPase activity increases in gill tissue during smolting, presumably in anticipation of the active transport of ions needed in seawater (Zaugg and McLain, 1972). This test is now often done at the same time as measurement of the plasma thyroxin level to provide a dual assessment of the degree of smoltification (Fig. 31–2). Using these apparently simple tests is complicated by the fish's distance upriver. In large systems such as the Columbia River, upriver fish may start downstream at lower thyroxin and ATPase levels than fish nearer the sea. However, fish released later with higher ATPase levels may come downstream faster than those released earlier from the same site (Fig. 31–3).

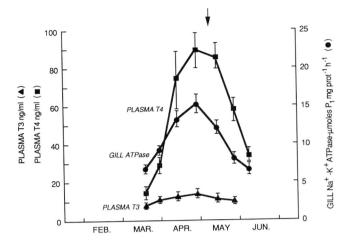

FIGURE 31–2. Relationships between mean gill sodium-potassium ATPase activities and plasma T_4 and T_3 concentrations of coho salmon in fresh water. The arrow indicates release from the hatchery. (Adapted from Folmar, L.C., and Dickhoff, W.W. [1981] The parr-smolt transformation (smoltification) and seawater adaptation in salmonids: A review of selected literature. Aquaculture 21:1–37.)

At the estuary, a smolt's problems are not over. Though forced entry into seawater, such as when cultured fish are put into seawater net pens, causes little or no immediate mortality, there may be an advantage to gradual entry. Chum salmon fry in Japan move slowly down the river estuary, and reach full-strength seawater only after 1 to 2 weeks. Wild coho smolts migrating through the Chehalis River (Washington) estuary remain in back eddies of the estuary for nearly a week before suddenly departing out to sea. Whether gradual entry into seawater is either normal or beneficial is unclear.

That entry into seawater can be stressful is indicated by outbreaks of disease soon after seawater entry. Diseases such as infectious hematopoietic necrosis or bacterial kidney disease may be carried in latent form from fresh water or may be picked up from the marine environment during a period of reduced resistance to disease. Part of the physiologic dysfunction involves increased absorption of seawater by the large intestine (Collie and Bern, 1982).

In instances of forced entry into seawater, some fish may survive for as long as 2 to 6 months, but they fail to grow as well as those fully adapted to seawater. Because of their small size, such fish are called runts, stunts, or reverts (Fig. 31–4). They are most readily recognized by their gold-black color and the reappearance of dark parr marks on the side of their body. If returned to fresh water until the following spring, these fish typically smolt again as abnormally large smolts and successfully enter seawater. However, increased feed and maintenance costs make most fish growers unwilling to do this.

Stress Response and Disease Effects

Stress responses in fishes have been best studied in salmonids. They follow generally the same pattern as in mammals. Briefly, a stress response in a fish can be described as increased levels of catechola-

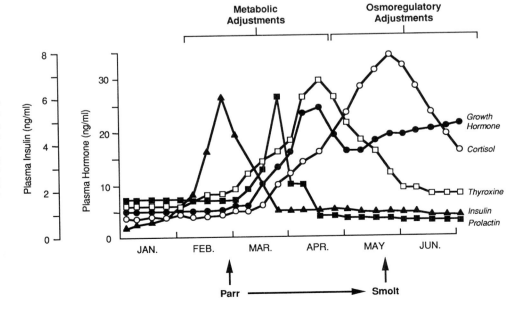

FIGURE 31–3. Composite scheme showing endocrine changes during smolting of yearling coho salmon. Initially insulin promotes deposition of lipid and carbohydrate stores, but then stores are mobilized to provide energy for smoltification and increased capacity for seawater osmoregulation.

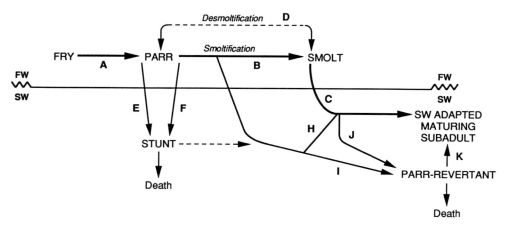

FIGURE 31–4. A diagram showing possible sources of "stunts" and "parr-revertants" during the smolting and postsmolting stages in coho salmon. *A, B, C.* The normal sequence in anadromous salmon. *D.* Smolts that do not enter seawater revert to fresh water parr condition. *E, F.* Premature transfer to seawater during the parr stage results in stunting. *G, I.* Transfer to seawater before the completion of smolting. *H, J.* The failure of smolts to make adequate growth may result in the death of undersized fish.

mines and later cortisol in response to circumstances that disturb homeostasis. The stages of a stress response include an alarm stage (initial increase), resistance (sustained output if stressor continues), and exhaustion of the capabilities of the fish to produce stress hormones. Cortisol levels increase as the fish progresses upstream, with peak cortisol concentrations coinciding with the fish's arrival on the spawning grounds. We now know that catecholamines are also involved, and fish exhibit similar responses to many different stressors (Wedemeyer et al., 1984).

Perhaps the most important effect of chronic stress is decreased resistance to disease. One mechanism involves cortisol stimulation of messenger ribonucleic acid (RNA), which is coded for synthesis of proteolytic enzymes. The enzymes destroy β-globulins in the plasma, the fish's antibodies. After stress, fish tend to more easily contract infectious diseases to which they are exposed.

Maturation, Spawning, and Death

In Pacific salmon, the spawning migration from the sea to the natal stream involves a combination of a change in osmoregulation, increased activity, starvation, sexual maturation, and stress responses. The cumulative stress debilitates the fish sufficiently that they come down with whatever disease is readily available and die soon after spawning. There is no mechanism that requires that these fish die. They can recover spontaneously and begin feeding again if kept free of disease. Such fishes have survived in fresh water for up to 11 months after spawning (McBride et al., 1963).

Atlantic salmon and steelhead (migratory rainbow trout) seem to stress themselves less severely than Pacific salmon. They return to seawater and may spawn for 2 or 3 successive years. The causes of death following spawning are complex. Continued activity of a proteolytic enzyme that frees the eggs from the ovary after spawning may cause lethal damage (Dickhoff, 1989). A gonadotropin-releasing

hormone analog also causes mortality when administered to fish.

Prior to spawning, ova develop individually in follicles under the control of a single leutenizing hormone–like substance. A possible second hormone may also be involved. Spawning is not commonly induced in salmonids, although it has been done successfully in pink salmon. As ova develop, the fluid around them resembles plasma but becomes more dilute as the ova mature (Satia et al., 1974). Ova remain in a compact mass until the day before spawning, when they suddenly loosen, perhaps through the activity of a proteolytic enzyme. Expulsion of ova occurs through contractions of the body wall. In rainbow trout, if a few eggs remain in the body cavity or if fish retain their eggs because of lack of suitable spawning gravel, fish attempt to resorb their eggs, often unsuccessfully. This leads to inflammation and probable infection, a condition often described as being egg-bound.

LITERATURE CITED

Brett, J.R. (1964) The respiratory metabolism and swimming performance of young sockeye salmon. J. Fish. Res. Bd. Can. 21:1183–1226.

Brett, J.R. (1970) Fish—The energy cost of living. In: Marine Aquaculture (McNeil, W.J., ed.). Oregon State University Press, Corvallis, pp. 37–52.

Brett, J.R. (1971) Energetic responses of salmon to temperature. A study of some thermal relations in the physiology and freshwater ecology of sockeye salmon (*Oncorhynchus nerka*). Am. Zool. 11:99–113.

Brett, J.R., and Groves, T.D.D. (1979) Physiological energetics. In: Fish Physiology. Vol. VIII (Hoar, W.S., Randall, D.J., and Brett, J.R., eds.). Academic Press, New York, pp. 280–352.

Buddington, R.K., and Diamond, J.M. (1987) Pyloric ceca of fish: A "new" absorptive organ. Am. J. Physiol. 252(1)P1:G65-G76.

Clarke, W.C., and Blackburn, J. (1977) A seawater challenge test to measure smolting in juvenile salmon. Department of the Environment, Fisheries and Marine Service Research Division Dir., Technical Report 705, Ottawa.

Collie, N.L., and Bern, H.A. (1982) Changes in intestinal fluid transport associated with smoltification and seawater adaptation in coho salmon, *Oncorhynchus kisutch* (Walbaum). J. Fish Biol. 21(3):337–348.

Crawshaw, L.I. (1979) Responses to rapid temperature change in vertebrate ectotherms. Am. Zool. 19:225–237.

Daxboeck, C. (1982) Effect of coronary artery ablation on exercise performance in *Salmo gairdneri*. Can. J. Zool. 60(3):375–381.

Dickhoff, W.W. (1989) Salmonids and annual fishes: Death after sex. In: Development, Maturation, and Senescence of the Neuroendocrine System (Schreibman, M.P., and Scanes, C., eds.). Academic Press, New York.

Fange, R. (1986) Physiology of haemopoiesis. In: Fish Physiology: Recent Advances (Nilsson, S., and Holmgren, S., eds.). Croom Helm, London, pp. 1–23.

Folmar, L.C., and Dickhoff, W.W. (1980) The parr-smolt transformation (smoltification) and seawater adaptation in salmonids: A review of selected literature. Aquaculture 21:1–37.

Folmar, L.C., and Dickhoff, W.W. (1981) Evaluation of some physiological parameters as predictive indices of smoltification. Aquaculture 23:309–324.

Grau, E.G., Dickhoff, W.W., Nishioika, R.S., Bern, H., and Folmar, L. (1981) Lunar phasing of the thyroxin surge preparatory to seaward migration of salmonid fish. Science 211:607–609.

Jones, D.R., and Randall, D.J. (1978) The respiratory and circulatory systems during exercise. In: Fish Physiology. Vol. VII (Hoar, W.S., and Randall, D.J., eds.). Academic Press, New York, pp. 425–501.

Laurent, P. (1984) Gill internal morphology. In: Fish Physiology: Gills, Anatomy, Gas Transfer, and Acid-Base Regulation. Vol. 11A (Hoar, W.S., and Randall, D.J., eds.). Academic Press, New York, pp. 73–183.

Laurent, P., and Dunel, S. (1976) Functional organizaton of the teleost gill. I. Blood pathways. Acta Zool. (Stockh.) 57:189–209.

McBride, J.R., Fagerlund, U.H.M., Smith, M., and Tomlinson, N. (1963) Resumption of feeding by and survival of adult sockeye salmon (Oncorhynchus nerka) following advanced gonad development. J. Fish. Res. Bd. Can. 20:95–100.

Rombout, J.H.W.M., Lamers, C.H.J., Helfrich, M.H., Dekker, A., and Taverne-Thiele, J.J. (1985) Uptake and transport of intact macromolecules in the intestinal epithelium of carp (Cyprinus carpio) and the possible immunological implications. Cell Tissue Res. 239(3):519–530.

Satia, B.P., Donaldson, L.R., Smith, L.S., and Nightingale, J.N. (1974) Composition of ovarian fluids and eggs of the University of Washington strain of rainbow trout (Salmo gairdneri). J. Fish. Res. Bd. Can. 31:1796–1799.

Smith, L.S., and Bell, G.R. (1975) A practical guide to the anatomy and physiology of Pacific salmon. Department of the Environment, Fisheries and Marine Service, Miscellaneous Special Publication 27, Ottawa.

Wedemeyer, G.A., McLean, D.J., and Goodyear, C.P. (1984) Assessing the tolerance of fish and fish populations to environmental stress: The problems and methods of monitoring. In: Contaminant Effects in Fisheries (Cairns, V.W., Hodson, P.V., and Nriagu, J.O., eds.). John Wiley and Sons, New York.

Woo, N.Y.S., Bern, H.A., and Nishioka, R.S. (1978) Changes in body composition associated with smoltification and premature transfer to seawater in coho salmon (Oncorhynchus kisutch Walbaum) and king salmon (O. tschawytscha Walbaum). J. Fish Biol. 13(4):421–428.

Zaugg, W.S., and McLain, L.R. (1972) Changes in gill adenosine-triphosphatase activity associated with parr-smolt transformation in steelhead trout, coho, and spring chinook salmon. J. Fish. Res. Bd. Can. 29:161–171.

Zaugg, W.W., Roley, D.D., Prentice, E.F., Rores, K.X., and Waknitz, F.W. (1983) Increased seawater survival and contribution to the fishery of chinook salmon (Oncorhynchus tshawytscha) by supplemental dietary salt. Aquaculture 32(1–2):183–188.

Chapter 32

CLINICAL PATHOLOGY OF SALMONID FISHES

PAUL R. BOWSER

A knowledge of the hematology of salmonids can provide information supportive of a wide variety of uses. There is a considerable body of literature on this topic, particularly with regard to the rainbow trout. This chapter summarizes the recent literature describing baseline hematology as well as that associated with various normal physiologic states, environmental stressors, and infectious and noninfectious diseases. The information is summarized, for presentation, in the form of seven tables. Table 32–1 presents reference hematology values for the rainbow trout. Table 32–2 contains serum biochemistry and electrolyte values for the rainbow trout and the Atlantic salmon. Table 32–3 shows the effects of various types of handling on hematologic and serum chemistry values of salmonids. The impact of nutritional and water-quality parameters are given in Table 32–4 and Table 32–5, respectively. The effects of infectious diseases on salmonid hemograms are summarized in Table 32–6. Table 32–7 contains the effects of a few toxicants on salmonid hematologic and serum chemistry values.

TABLE 32–1. Reference Hematologic Values for Rainbow Trout

Parameter	Value	References
Erythrocyte count (cells/ml)	1.2–1.7×10^6	Miller et al., 1983; Lane, 1979b
Hematocrit (%)	32–45	Miller et al., 1983; Lane, 1979b
Hemoglobin (g/dl)	7–9	Miller et al., 1983; Lane, 1979b
Reticulocyte count (cells/ml)	1.8–2×10^3	Moccia et al., 1984
Leukocyte count (cells/ml)	10–15×10^3	Hoffman and Lommel, 1984
Thrombocyte count (cells/ml)	2.5–3×10^3	Hoffman and Lommel, 1984

TABLE 32–2. Reference Serum Chemistry Values for Rainbow Trout and Atlantic Salmon

Parameter	Rainbow Trout	References	Atlantic Salmon	References
Na (mEq/L)	123–164	1	140–165	5
Cl (mEq/L)	120–147	2,4		
K (mEq/L)	3.2–3.5	7		
Ca (mEq/L)	11.1–12.8	1,2	7–25	5
Fe (mg/dl)	110	6		
Cu (mg/dl)	99	6		
Zn (g/dl)	1.6	6		
Mg (mEq/L)	1.1–4.8	1,3		
HCO₃ (mEq/L)	11.9	4		
Total protein (g/dl)	2.8–6.0	1,2	4–7.5	5
Albumin (g/dl)	1.7–1.9	2,3		
Triglyceride (mg/L)			600	5
Cholesterol (mg/dl)	150–575	1,2	200–600	5
Glucose (mg/dl)	63–144	2,3		
Alanine aminotransferase (μ/L)	7–12	1,2		
Aspartate aminotransferase (μ/L)	158–368	1,2		
Alkaline phosphatase (μ/L)	50–200	1,3	600–900	5
Lactate dehydrogenase (μ/L)	250–1000	1,2,3		
Hydroxybuterate dehydrogenase (μ/L)	150–350	1,2		
Total bilirubin (mg/dl)	0–2	1		
Lactate (mg/dl)	4–17	1		
Serum urea nitrogen (mg/dl)	3.5–4.1	2		
Creatinine (mg/dl)	0.2–0.5	2		
Cholinesterase (μ/L)	180–190	2		
pH	7.6	4		
pCO₂ (mmHg)	8.5	4		
pO₂ (mmHg)	98	8		
Osmolarity (mOsm/kg)	296–340	7,8		

References: 1, Hille, 1982; 2, Warner et al., 1978; 3, Miller et al., 1983; 4, Meade and Peronne, 1980; 5, Johnson et al., 1987; 6, Zeitoun, 1978; 7, Witters, 1986; 8, Kikuchi et al., 1985b.

TABLE 32–3. Effects of Handling on Salmonid Clinical Pathology

Treatment/Species (References)	Parameter	Values	Effect Related to Controls
Rainbow Trout			
Immediately postsurgery (Bry and Zohar, 1980)	Hematocrit (%)	35	Increase
	Glucose (mg/dl)	400	Increase
	Total leukocytes	—	Decrease
30 minutes postsurgery (Bry and Zohar, 1980)	Hematocrit (%)	21–26	Decrease
	Glucose (mg/dl)	350–1600	Increase
	Total leukocytes	–	Decrease
Splenectomy and 12% blood loss (Lane, 1979a)	RBC Count (mm³)		40% Decrease
	Hematocrit (%)		35% Decrease
Exercise (Kikuchi et al., 1985a)	Hematocrit (%)	17–18	Slight Increase
	Osmolality (mOsm/kg)	303–318	Increase
96 hours of crowding and temperature stress (McLeay and Gordon, 1977)	Hematocrit (%)	26–27	Increase
	Total leukocytes	—	Decrease
Coho Salmon			
96 hours of crowding and temperature stress (McLeay and Gordon, 1977)	Hematocrit (%)	27	Increase
	Total leukocytes	—	Decrease

TABLE 32–4. Effects of Nutrition on Rainbow Trout Clinical Pathology

Treatment/Species (References)	Parameter	Values	Effect Related to Controls
Vitamin C deficiency (Akand et al., 1987)	Hematocrit (%)	24–35	Decrease
	Hemoglobin (g/dl)	4.3–8.9	Decrease
	Ca (mg/dl)	13–18	No change
	P (mg/dl)	7–24	No change
	Albumin (g/dl)	0.7–1.7	No change
	Alanine aminotransferase (Karmen U)	51–201	No change
	Lactate dehydrogenase (Wroblewski U)	10,200–19,080	Increase
Carob seed protein source (Alexis et al., 1986)	Hematocrit (%)	35–45	Decrease
	Hemoglobin (g/dl)	6.3–9.9	Decrease
	Total protein (g/dl)	3.5–4.3	No change
	Total lipid (g/dl)	1.4–1.9	No change
	Cholesterol (mg/dl)	245–405	No change
	Glucose (mg/dl)	105–155	No change
Yeast protein source (Sanchez-Muniz et al., 1979)	Erythrocyte count (cells/ml)	0.76 mil.	No change
	Hematocrit (%)	37–40	No change
	Hemoglobin (g/dl)	6.5–7.6	No change
	Erythrocyte morphology		Poikilocytosis, anisocytosis
	Total protein (g/dl)	5.8–7.6	No change
	Albumin/globulin ratio	0.77	Decrease
Oxidized fish oils and low vitamin E diet (Moccia et al., 1984)	Erythrocyte count (cells/ml)	0.9–1.4 mil.	Decrease
	Hematocrit (%)	16–23	Decrease
	Hemoglobin (g/dl)	5.1–6.5	Decrease
Postprandial (Bry, 1982)	Cortisol (ng/ml)	15–50	Increase
Disturbance (Bry, 1982)	Cortisol (ng/ml)	2–100	Increase

TABLE 32–5. Effects of Water Quality on Salmonid Clinical Pathology

Water Condition/Species (References)	Parameter	Effect Related to Controls
Rainbow Trout		
Decreased pH (Giles et al., 1984; Milligan and Wood, 1982)	Erythrocyte count	Increase
	Hematocrit	Increase
	Hemoglobin	Increase
	Reticulocytes	Increase
	Na	Decrease
	Cl	Decrease
	Ca	Decrease
	Mg	Decrease
	Total protein	Increase
	Osmolarity	Decrease
Elevated nitrite (Margiocco et al., 1983)	Hemoglobin	Decrease
	Methemoglobin	Increase
	Cl	No change
Soft water (McDonald and Rogano, 1986)	Na	Decrease
	Cl	Decrease
	Ca	No change
Atlantic Salmon		
Elevated CO_2 (Borjeson, 1977)	Erythrocyte count	Increase
	Hematocrit	Increase
	Cl	Decrease
	CO_2	Increase
	pH	No change
Elevated nitrite (Bowser et al., 1989)	Hemoglobin	Decrease
	Methemoglobin	Increase
	Na	No change
	Cl	No change
	K	Decrease
	Total protein	Decrease
	Albumin	Decrease
	Globulin	No change
	Glucose	No change
	Alanine aminotransferase	Slight increase
	Alkaline phosphatase	Decrease

TABLE 32–6. Effects of Infectious Disease on Salmonid Clinical Pathology

Agent or Disease/Species (References)	Parameter	Effect Related to Controls
Aeromonas and *Streptococcus* Rainbow trout (Barham, 1980)	Erythrocyte count	Decrease
	Hematocrit	Decrease
	Hemoglobin	Decrease
	Na	Decrease
	Cl	Decrease
	K	Decrease
	Total protein	Decrease
	Glucose	Decrease
	pH	No change
	CO_2	No change
	pO_2	No change
Reinbacterium salmoninarum Rainbow trout (Bruno and Munro, 1986) Atlantic salmon (Iwama et al., 1986) Coho salmon (Suzumoto et al., 1977)	Erythrocyte count	Decrease
	Hematocrit	Decrease
	Hemoglobin	Decrease
	Erythrocyte sedimentation rate	Increase
	Leukocyte count	Decrease then increase
	Heterophils	Increase
	Monocytes	Increase
	Thrombocytes	Increase
	Na	Decrease
	K	Increase
	Fe	Decrease
	Total protein	Decrease
	Cholesterol	Decrease
	Glucose	Decrease
	Serum urea nitrogen	Increase
	Conjugated bilirubin	Increase
	Cortisol	Decrease
Noninfectious anemia Atlantic salmon (Groman and Miller, 1986)	Erythrocyte count	Decrease
	Hematocrit	Decrease
	Hemoglobin	Decrease
	Glucose-6-phosphate dehydrogenase	Increase
	Alanine aminotransferase	No change
	Aspartate aminotransferase	No change
	Alkaline phosphatase	No change
	Lactate dehydrogenase	Increase
	Total bilirubin	Increase
	Conjugated bilirubin	Increase
Proliferative kidney disease Rainbow trout (Hoffman and Lommel, 1984)	Erythrocyte count	Decrease
	Hematocrit	Decrease
	Hemoglobin	Decrease
	Reticulocytes	Increase
	Leukocyte count	No change
	Thrombocytes	No change
	Total protein	Decrease
	Serum urea nitrogen	No change
Cryptobia Rainbow trout (Lowe-Jinde, 1986)	Erythrocyte count	Decrease
	Leukocyte count	No change
	Heterophils	Increase
	Granuloblasts	Increase
Nephrocalcinosis Rainbow trout (Yurkowski et al., 1985)	Hematocrit	Decrease
	Hemoglobin	Decrease
	Total lipid	Decrease
	Aspartate aminotransferase	Increase
	Creatinine	Increase
Salmincola salmonus and *Saprolegniasis* Atlantic salmon (Johnson et al., 1987)	Leukocyte count	Increase

TABLE 32–7. Effects of Toxicants on Salmonid Clinical Pathology

Toxicant/Species (References)	Parameter	Effect Related to Controls
Aromatic hydrocarbons Rainbow trout (Zbanyszek and Smith, 1984)	Erythrocyte count Hematocrit Hemoglobin Prothrombin time Cl Glucose	Increase Increase Increase Increase Decrease Decrease
Benzo-(a)-pyrene Rainbow trout (Walczak et al., 1987)	Hematocrit Leukocyte count	No change Increase
bis-Tri-N-butyltin Rainbow trout (Chliamovitch and Kuhn, 1977)	Erythrocyte count Hematocrit Hemoglobin	No change Decrease Decrease
Cadmium Rainbow trout (Lowe-Jinde and Niimi, 1986)	Erythrocyte count	Decrease
Chlorine Rainbow trout (Zeitoun, 1978)	Hematocrit Hemoglobin Methemoglobin Na Ca P Mg Fe Cu Zn Total protein	Increase Increase Increase Decrease Increase Increase Increase Increase Increase Increase Increase
Dehydroabietic acid Rainbow trout (Soivio et al., 1983)	Na Cl Total protein Glucose	Decrease Decrease Decrease Increase
Ozone Rainbow trout (Wedemeyer et al., 1979)	Erythrocyte count Hematocrit Hemoglobin Heterophils Bands Lymphocytes Thrombocytes Na Cl Glucose	No change Increase No change No change No change Decrease No change Increase Increase No change
Thiocyanate Rainbow trout, Brook trout (Heming et al., 1985)	Cl	Decrease

LITERATURE CITED

Akand, A.M., Sato, M., Yoshinaka, R., and Ikeda, S. (1987) Haematological changes due to dietary ascorbic acid deficiency at various levels of calcium and phosphorus in rainbow trout. Curr. Sci. 56:298–301.

Alexis, M.N., Theochari, V., and Papaparaskeva-Papoutsoglou, E. (1986) Effects of diet composition and protein level on growth, body composition, hematological characteristics and cost of production of rainbow trout Salmo gairdneri. Aquaculture 58:75–85.

Barham, W.T., Smit, G.L., and Schoonbee, H.J. (1980) The hematological assessment of bacterial infection in rainbow trout Salmo gairdneri. J. Fish Biol. 17:275–281.

Barnhart, R.A. (1969) Effects of certain variables on hematological characteristics of rainbow trout. Trans. Am. Fish. Soc. 98:411–418.

Benfey, T.J., and Sutterlin, A.M. (1983) Production of triploid landlocked Atlantic salmon Salmo salar and the implications of their hematology of oxygen utilization. In Salmonid Reproduction: An International Symposium (Iwamoto, R.N., and Sower, S., eds.), Washington Sea Grant Program, Seattle, Washington, p. 64.

Benfey, T.J., and Sutterlin, A.M. (1984) The hematology of triploid landlocked Atlantic salmon Salmo salar salar. J. Fish Biol. 24:333–338.

Borjeson, H. (1977) Effects of hypercapnia on the buffer capacity and hematological values in Salmo salar. J. Fish Biol. 11:133–142.

Bowser, P.R., Wooster, G.A., Aluisio, A.L., and Blue, J.T. (1989) Plasma chemistries of nitrite-stressed Atlantic salmon (Salmo salar). J. World Aquaculture Soc. 20:173–180.

Bruno, D.W. (1986) Changes in serum parameters of rainbow trout, Salmo gairdneri Richardson, and Atlantic salmon Salmo salar L., infected with Renibacterium salmoninarum. J. Fish Dis. 9:205–211.

Bruno, D.W., and Munro, A.L.S. (1986) Hematological assessment of rainbow trout Salmo gairdneri and Atlantic salmon Salmo salar infected with Renibacterium salmoninarum. J. Fish Dis. 9:195–204.

Bry, C. (1982) Daily variation in plasma cortisol levels of individual female rainbow trout Salmo gairdneri: Evidence for a post-feeding peak in well-adapted fish. Gen. Comp. Endocrinol. 48:462–468.

Bry, C., and Zohar, Y. (1980) Dorsal aorta catheterization in rainbow trout Salmo gairdneri 2. Glucocorticoid levels, hematological data, and resumption of feeding for 5 days after surgery. Reprod. Nutr. Dev. 20:1825–1834.

Chliamovitch, Y.-P., and Kuhn, C. (1977) Behavioral, hematological and histological studies on acute toxicity of bis-tri-N-butyl tin oxide on Salmo gairdneri and Tilapia rendalli. J. Fish Biol. 10:575–585.

Florkin, M., and Stortz, E.H. (Eds.) (1973) Enzyme Nomenclature. Recommendations (1972) of the Commission on Biochemical Nomenclature. 3rd ed. Elsevier, Amsterdam.

Giles, M.A., Majewski, H.S., and Hobden, B. (1984) Osmoregulatory and hematological responses of rainbow trout Salmo gairdneri to extended environmental acidification. Can. J. Fish. Aquatic Sci. 41:1686–1694.

Groman, D.B., and Miller, K. (1986) Hemolytic anaemia of wild Atlantic salmon: Haematology and chemical pathology. Aquaculture 67:210–212.

Heming, T.A., Thurston, R.V., Meyn, E.L., and Zajdel, R.K. (1985) Acute toxicity of thiocyanate to trout. Trans. Am. Fish. Soc. 114:895–905.

Hille, S. (1982) A literature review of the blood chemistry of rainbow trout *Salmo gairdneri*. J. Fish Biol. 20:535–569.

Hoffman, R., and Lommel, R. (1984) Hematological studies in proliferative kidney disease of rainbow trout *Salmo gairdneri*. J. Fish Dis. 7:323–326.

Iwama, G.K., Greer, G.L., and Randall, D.J. (1986) Changes in selected hematological parameters in juvenile chinook salmon subjected to a bacterial challenge and a toxicant. J. Fish Biol. 28:563–572.

Johnson, C.E., Gray, R.W., McLennan, A., and Paterson, A. (1987) Effects of photoperiod, temperature and diet on the reconditioning response, blood chemistry and gonad maturation of Atlantic salmon kelts *Salmo salar* held in freshwater. Can. J. Fish. Aquatic Sci. 44:702–711.

Kikuchi, Y., Hughes, G.M., and Duthie, G.G. (1985a) Effects of moderate and severe exercise in rainbow trout on some properties of arterial blood, including red blood cell deformity. Jpn. J. Ichthyol. 31:422–426.

Kikuchi, Y., Hughes, G.M., Tomiyasu, K., Kakiuchi, Y., and Araiso, T. (1985b) Effects of temperature and transfer from seawater to freshwater on blood microrheology in Pacific salmon. Jpn. J. Physiol. 35:683–688.

Lane, H.C. (1979a) Some hematological responses of normal and splenectomized rainbow trout *Salmo gairdneri* to a 12 percent blood loss. J. Fish Biol. 14:159–164.

Lane, H.C. (1979b) Progressive changes in hematology and tissue water of sexually mature trout *Salmo gairdneri* during the autumn and winter. J. Fish Biol. 15:425–436.

Lone, K.P., Ince, B.W., and Matty, A.J. (1982) Changes in the blood chemistry of rainbow trout *Salmo gairdneri* in relation to dietary protein level and an anabolic steroid hormone ethyl estrenol. J. Fish Biol. 20:597–606.

Lowe-Jinde, L. (1986) Hematological changes in *Cryptobia* infection in rainbow trout *Salmo gairdneri*. Can. J. Zool. 64:1352–1355.

Lowe-Jinde, L., and Niimi, A.J. (1983) Influence of sampling on the interpretation of hematological measurements of rainbow trout *Salmo gairdneri*. Can. J. Zool. 61:396–402.

Lowe-Jinde, L., and Niimi, A.J. (1986) Hematological characteristics of rainbow trout *Salmo gairdneri* in response to cadmium exposure. Bull. Environ. Contam. Toxicol. 37:375–381.

Margiocco, C., Arillo, A., Mensi, P., and Schenone, G. (1983) Nitrite bioaccumulation in *Salmo gairdneri* Rich. and hematological consequences. Aquatic Toxicol. 3:261–270.

McDonald, D.G., and Rogano, M.S. (1986) Ion regulation by rainbow trout, *Salmo gairdneri*, in ion-poor water. Physiol. Zool. 59:318–331.

McLeay, D.J., and Gordon, M.R. (1977) Leucocrit: A simple hematological technique for measuring acute stress in salmonid fish including stressful concentrations of pulpmill effluent. J. Fish. Res. Bd. Can. 34:2164–2175.

Meade, T.L., and Perrone, S.J. (1980) Selective hematological parameters in steelhead trout *Salmo gairdneri*. J. Fish Biol. 17:9–12.

Miller, W.R., III, Hendricks, A.C., and Cairns, J., Jr. (1983) Normal ranges for diagnostically important hematological and blood chemistry characteristics of rainbow trout *Salmo gairdneri*. Can. J. Fish. Aquatic Sci. 40:420–425.

Milligan, C.L., and Wood, C.M. (1982) Disturbances in hematology fluid distribution and circulatory function associated with low environmental pH in the rainbow trout *Salmo gairdneri*. J. Exp. Biol. 99:397–415.

Moccia, R.D., Hung, S.S.O., Slinger, S.J., and Ferguson, H.W. (1984) Effect of oxidized fish oil, vitamin E and ethoxyquin on the histopathology and hematology of rainbow trout *Salmo gairdneri*. J. Fish Dis. 7:269–282.

Pickering, A.D. (1986) Changes in blood cell composition of the brown trout, *Salmo trutta* L., during the spawning season. J. Fish Biol. 29:335–347.

Pickering, A.D., and Pottinger, T.G. (1985) Cortisol can increase the susceptibility of brown trout, *Salmo trutta* L., to disease without reducing the white blood cell count. J. Fish Biol. 27:611–619.

Pickering, A.D., Griffiths, R., and Pottinger, T.G. (1987) A comparison of the effects of overhead cover on the growth, survival and hematology of juvenile Atlantic salmon *Salmo salar* Richardson. Aquaculture 66:109–124.

Sanchez-Muniz, F.J., De La Higuera, M., Mataix, F.J., and Varela, G. (1979) The yeast *Hansenula anomala* as a protein source for rainbow trout *Salmo gairdneri*—hematological aspects. Comp. Biochem. Physiol. Part A Comp. Physiol. 63:153–157.

Soivio, A., Lindgren, S., and Oikari, A. (1983) Seasonal changes in certain metabolic and hematologic responses of *Salmo gairdneri* acutely exposed to dehydro abietic acid. Comp. Biochem. Physiol. Part C Comp. Pharmacol. Toxicol. 75:281–284.

Steele, J.A., and Courtois, L.A. (1979) Hematological stress response of rainbow trout *Salmo gairdneri* to a simulated geo-thermal stream condensate spill. Ca. Fish Game 65:166–167.

Suzumoto, B.K., Schreck, C.B., and McIntyre, J.D. (1977) Relative resistances of 3 transferrin genotypes of coho salmon *Oncorhynchus kisutch* and their hematological responses to bacterial kidney disease. J. Fish. Res. Bd. Can. 34:1–8.

Walczak, B.Z., Blunt, B.R., and Hodson, P.V. (1987) Phagocytic function of monocytes and hematological changes in rainbow trout injected intraperitoneally with benzo-a-pyrene B-A-P and benzo-a-anthracene B-A-A. J. Fish Biol. 31(Suppl. A):251–253.

Warner, M.C., Diehl, S.A., and Tomb, A.M. (1978) Effects of dilution and temperature of analysis on blood serum values in rainbow trout *Salmo gairdneri*. J. Fish Biol. 13:315–319.

Wedemeyer, G.A., Nelson, N.C., and Yasutake, W.T. (1979) Physiological and biochemical aspects of ozone toxicity to rainbow trout (*Salmo gairdneri*). J. Fish. Res. Bd. Can. 36:605–614.

Witters, H.E. (1986) Acute acid exposure of rainbow trout *Salmo gairdneri* Richardson effects of aluminum and calcium on ion balance and hematology. Aquatic Toxicol. 8:197–210.

Witters, H., Vangenechten, J., Van Puymbroeck, S., and Vanderborght, O. (1987) Ionoregulatory and haematological responses of rainbow trout, *Salmo gairdneri*, to chronic acid and aluminum stress. Ann. Soc. Royale Zool. Belg. 117(Suppl. 1):411–420.

Yurkowski, M., Gillespie, D.C., Metner, D.A., and Lockhart, W.L. (1985) Nephrocalcinosis and blood chemistry in mature rainbow trout *Salmo gairdneri*. Canadian Technical Report of Fisheries and Aquatic Sciences No. 1348.

Zbanyszek, R., and Smith, L.S. (1984) The effect of water-soluble aromatic hydrocarbons on some hematological parameters of rainbow trout *Salmo gairdneri* during acute exposure. J. Fish Biol. 24:545–552.

Zeitoun, I.H. (1978) The recovery and hematological rehabilitation of chlorine-stressed adult rainbow trout *Salmo gairdneri*. Environ. Biol. Fishes 3:355–359.

Chapter 33

ENVIRONMENTAL REQUIREMENTS AND ENVIRONMENTAL DISEASES OF SALMONIDS

GEORGE W. KLONTZ

Salmonids live in a very complex, dynamic environment. A common misconception is that water is the total environment for fish. This is not the case. Other components of a fish's environment are listed in Table 33–1. Each has several subordinate factors that can function directly or indirectly to cause disease.

Salmonids are irrevocably oriented to their environment. Any quantitative change of an environmental condition is reflected in quantitative changes in the fish as it responds to maintain physiologic homeostasis. Also, a quantitative change in the environment usually sets into motion a sequential series of environmental changes, the environmental domino effect. For example, an increase of water temperature from 9 to 15°C generates the following changes in the environment of a 100-g rainbow trout:

Fish-associated changes:

- 67.5% increase in metabolic rate (oxygen demand)
- 97.8% increase in daily length gain potential
- 66.7% increase in daily weight gain potential
- 98.6% increase in ammonia generation
- 33.1% decrease in oxygen carrying capacity

Water-associated changes:

- 12.8% decrease in oxygen concentration
- 58.8% increase in environmental un-ionized ammonia
- 67.5% decrease in dissolved oxygen

Another example would be increasing the amount of daily feed to a population of fish. In this case, health-compromising changes could occur (Fig. 33–1). The first change would be increased metabolic activity that would result in (1) increased growth rate, (2) increased ammonia production, (3) increased carbon dioxide production, and (4) increased settleable and suspended solids production. The increased growth rate was the intended purpose of this change.

The increased ammonia, carbon dioxide, and solids production could have very serious negative impact on the fish. Thus, in certain cases, the desired effect can be masked by undesired effects.

As can be seen from these two examples, environmental diseases of fish can be quite complex. The investigator must be able to evaluate many causal factors, both qualitatively and quantitatively, and be able to establish cause and effect relationships among them. Most environmental factors have limits within which fish can function and outside of which the health of the fish is compromised.

DIRECT CAUSAL FACTORS IN ENVIRONMENTAL DISEASES OF SALMONIDS

Acidity

Acidity, or the degree to which water can neutralize hydroxyl ions, is often expressed as equivalents of calcium carbonate. An excess of 4.0 mg/L mineral acids is lethal for most salmonids. Acidity is closely related to pH and alkalinity, which are discussed under indirect causal factors.

TABLE 33–1. Direct and Indirect Causal Factors of Environmental Diseases of Salmonids

Direct Causal Factors	Indirect Causal Factors
Acidity	pH
Ammonia	Alkalinity
Nitrite	Hardness
Dissolved oxygen	Temperature
Organic contaminants	Velocity
Inorganic contaminants	Handling
Fecal solids	Population density
Suspended sediments	
Trauma	
Carbon dioxide	

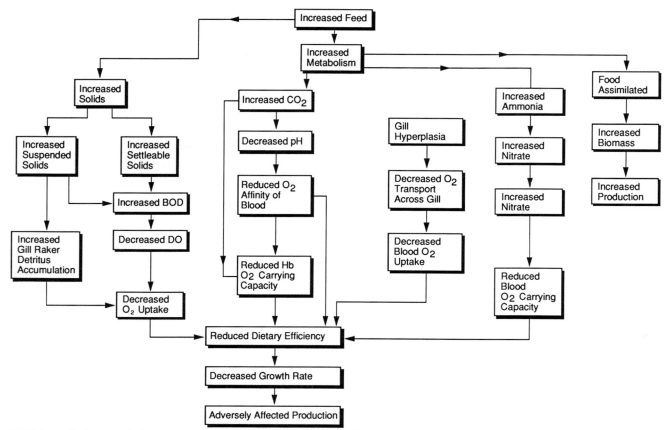

FIGURE 33–1. Pathways of changes initiated in an aquaculture system following an increase in feeding rate. (Adapted from Downey, P.C. [1978] Systems analysis of fish hatcheries. Proceedings 29th N.W. Fish Cult. Conf., Vancouver, WA. pp. 102–105.)

Ammonia

Ammonia is generated in the system as the end product of protein metabolism. The fish excretes ammonia across the gill membranes in exchange for Na^+. In the aquatic environment, ammonia occurs in two forms. Dissociated, or ionized ammonia (NH_4^+), is relatively nontoxic for fish. Undissociated, or unionized ammonia (NH_3), is very toxic for most finfishes. Salmonids exposed to continuous levels exceeding 0.03 mg/L NH_3 have reduced growth rates and can develop environmental gill disease (Stewart, 1983; Klontz et al., 1985). The ratio of NH_4^+ to NH_3 is both temperature and pH dependent (Trussel, 1972). The primary effect of long-term exposure to continuous levels of ammonia (as NH_3) exceeding 0.03 mg/L is to the gill tissues (D'Aoust and Ferguson, 1984). The lesions initially are lamellar epithelial hypertrophy, followed by epithelial-capillary separation and, ultimately, interlamellar hyperplastic occlusion (Stewart, 1983). In addition, blood ammonia levels become quite excessive because the uptake of Na^+, which is exchanged for NH_4^+, is impeded by the lamellar hyperplasia.

Nitrate

The accepted tolerance level of nitrite for salmonids is 0.55 mg/L. Levels exceeding this create methemoglobinemia in which the iron in the heme molecule is reduced and cannot transport oxygen (Bowser, 1983).

TABLE 33–2. Percentage of Dissolved Oxygen Saturation in Water When the pO_2 Is 90 mmHg

Temperature (°C)	Elevation (ft above sea level)				
	0	*1000*	*2000*	*3000*	*4000*
0	0.5687	0.5909	0.6140	0.6830	0.6619
5	0.5701	0.5924	0.6159	0.6397	0.6636
10	0.5718	0.5945	0.6178	0.6418	0.6663
15	0.5748	0.5975	0.6212	0.6462	0.6709
20	0.5782	0.6014	0.6250	0.6506	0.7019

TABLE 33–3. Life-Support Indices (kg fish/cm of length/L/minute) for Trout and Salmon as Related to Water Temperature and Elevation

Temperature (°C)	Elevation (m)					
	0	*300*	*600*	*950*	*1250*	*1500*
0.55	0.198	0.190	0.183	0.176	0.169	0.162
5.00	0.134	0.129	0.124	0.119	0.114	0.110
10.00	0.086	0.083	0.080	0.077	0.074	0.071
15.00	0.054	0.052	0.050	0.048	0.046	0.045
20.00	0.034	0.033	0.032	0.030	0.029	0.028

Modified from Piper, R. G. (1972) Managing hatcheries by the numbers. Am. Fishes and U.S. Trout News 17(3):10–15.

Oxygen

Dissolved oxygen is a primary life-support requirement for fish. A partial pressure difference of 12 to 15 mmHg between the water pO_2 and the lamellar pO_2 is required for transport across the gills (Randall and Daxboek, 1984). Since complete vascular oxygenation occurs at a pO_2 of 70 to 80 mmHg, the environmental pO_2 should not be less than 90 mmHg (Downey and Klontz, 1981; David, 1975). This is approximately 60% of saturation (Table 33–2). This is a departure from the traditionally accepted dissolved oxygen limit of 5 mg/L, which, under certain circumstances of temperature, is less than 90 mmHg pO_2.

The dissolved oxygen available for fish establishes the carrying capacity of a pond (Piper et al., 1982; Klontz, 1990). This is expressed as a relationship between the oxygen content (mg/L) of the inflowing water corrected for temperature, elevation, and the standard metabolic rate (mg O_2/hour) of the fish, corrected for temperature and fish weight (Klontz et al., 1983) (Table 33–3).

Organic and Inorganic Contaminants

Organic contaminants in water used in aquaculture systems come from municipal, industrial, and agricultural sources. The list of potential hazards is lengthy (Mayer and Ellersieck, 1986). The effects in most cases are dose dependent. Inorganic contaminants affecting salmonids in aquaculture systems are often of natural origin. Heavy metal contaminants include lead, zinc, copper, chromium, cadmium, and iron. Each metal has a unique dose-dependent response. The "no-effect" limits for salmonids are less than 0.1 mg/L for each of these metals.

Nitrogen Supersaturation

Nitrogen-supersaturated water is a common problem (Bell, 1986). Water from deep wells or plunge pools is frequently at 110 to 120% of nitrogen saturation. This necessitates the use of gas-stabilization chambers to reduce the supersaturation (Bell, 1986). Water supersaturated with nitrogen is unable to carry adequate oxygen for fish.

Fecal Solids

Fecal solids are excreted by fish into the aquatic environment, and if permitted to accumulate, cause a reduction in fish growth rate through one or more of the following changes: increased biologic oxygen demand (BOD); accumulation of solids and other detritus on the buccal aspect of the gill rakers; lamellar thickening resulting from the physical irritation due to solids passing over the lamellar tissues; and toxic by-products of fecal solid decomposition.

Suspended Sediments

Suspended sediments in the environment come from a variety of sources, the most common being surface run-off following a rainstorm. Depending on their nature, suspended sediments can cause gill problems. Most sediments are quite innocuous at levels less than 80 mg/L. Certain pollens and newly formed sediments such as volcanic ash have very irregular, sharp edges, and can cause lamellar inflammation, which results in reduced water flow through the interlamellar spaces.

Trauma

Trauma is a management-associated factor where fish being handled are physically injured during the process. In some cases, the injury is life threatening. Salmonids are susceptible to handling trauma.

Carbon Dioxide

Carbon dioxide is a product of aerobic and anaerobic decomposition of organic materials and a respiratory by-product of fish. Fresh water at equilibrium contains about 2 mg/L CO_2. Levels above 12 mg/L have a negative impact on fish growth. Such levels are common to waters from deep wells, which has a deficiency of dissolved oxygen, and an acid pH. Other than in closed, recycled water systems, CO_2 generated by fish should pose few deleterious effects. However, plasma carbon dioxide levels can influence the oxygen disassociation from hemoglobin, which can adversely affect productivity.

INDIRECT CAUSAL FACTORS OF ENVIRONMENTAL DISEASES

pH

The role of pH in environmental diseases is primarily indirect, but very low values (less than pH 6.0) and very high values (greater than pH 8.0) can have direct deleterious effects on salmonids. The most common indirect effect is the influence on the ratio of ionized ammonia (NH_4^+) to un-ionized ammonia (NH_3). At pH values below 7.0, the amount of NH_3 is very low. At pH values above 7.0, NH_3 levels become quite high.

Alkalinity

Alkalinity is the degree to which water can neutralize hydrogen ions and is expressed as equivalents of calcium carbonate. The alkalinity of water consists of carbonates, bicarbonates, hydroxides, and to a lesser extent silicates, borates, phosphates, and organics. Water suitable for supporting salmonids has carbonate/bicarbonate alkalinities of over 100 mg/L.

Hardness

Hardness of water is expressed as milligrams per liter total (calcium and magnesium) hardness. In freshwater situations, fish in hard water (over 200 mg/L) will spend less metabolic energy on osmoregulation than those in soft water (less than 30 mg/L), reserving more metabolic energy for growth (Wedemeyer et al., 1976).

Temperature

Water temperature is perhaps the single most important indirect factor in environmental disease (Roberts, 1975). The fish itself is directly influenced by water temperature. Each species has a preferred temperature. The standard environmental temperature (SET) is the optimum temperature for the species growth (Table 33–4). In salmonids at temperatures above or below the SET, there is a growth reduction of about 8% per degree Celsius (Table 33–5). Above the SET, the rate of performance decline increases as the thermal death point is reached. However, there is still some doubt about the thermal death point of rainbow trout. In certain parts of the world, rainbow trout are being raised in 26°C water without too many problems. The primary purpose of knowing the temperature-related growth rate of a species is that it can be used as a diagnostic aid. One of the

TABLE 33–4. Standard Environmental Temperatures (SET) and Upper Tolerance Limits of Water Temperature for Selected Salmonids

Species	SET (°C)	Tolerance Limit (°C)
Atlantic salmon	17	19
Brook trout	15	18
Rainbow trout	15	19
Pacific salmon	12	18

Modified from Wedemeyer, G. A., and Wood, G. W. (1974) Stress as a predisposing factor in fish diseases. U.S. Department and Wildlife Service, Fisheries Leaflet No. 38, Washington, D.C.

main early clinical signs of a low-grade toxicity is a reduction of growth rate with a concomitant decrease in feed conversion. Temperature also influences other direct causal agents. For example, the association-dissociation of ammonia-nitrogen is influenced by temperature. Also, the susceptibilities to potentially toxic compounds are influenced by temperature.

Water Velocity

Water velocity is a function of the water inflow rate and the style of pond. For most species of salmonids, it should not exceed 2.5 cm/second. High water velocity can cause mechanical trauma. Another cause of mechanical trauma is handling. Handling increases susceptibility of fish to other causal factors. For example, scale loss during rough handling can alter the osmoregulatory balance of fish. If scale loss is sufficient, the freshwater fish becomes severely edematous.

Population Density

Population density is the most common chronic stressor in an aquaculture system. All salmonids have rather well-defined spatial requirements. These are measured as density-carrying capacities and are expressed as kilograms of fish/per centimeter of mean body length per cubic meter of space (Piper, 1972) (Table 33–6). If the density-carrying capacity is exceeded, stress responses occur. Long-term exposure to high densities often results in the environmental gill disease syndrome, reduced growth rates, and increased susceptibility to latent infectious processes.

SPECIFIC ENVIRONMENTAL DISEASES

Epidemiologic aspects of environmental disease syndromes are quite similar. By and large, the onset, severity, and course of the episode are dose dependent. The lower the exposure, the slower the onset; the lower the morbidity and mortality, the longer the clinical course. Often, the earliest signs seen are

TALE 33–5. Temperature-Related Growth Rate Potential for Trout

	mm/Day Length Increase			
T (°C)	Shasta Rainbow Trout	Kamloops Rainbow Trout	Brook Trout	Brown Trout
25	0.193	0.222	0.088	0.140
20	0.646	0.746	0.480	0.470
15	1.100	1.270	0.872	0.800
10	0.646	0.746	0.637	0.470
5	0.193	0.222	0.245	0.140
2	0.000	0.000	0.010	0.000

From Klontz, G. W., and Klontz, D. I. (1989) AQUASYST: A Computer Program for Commercial Salmonid Production. S. H. Nelson and Sons, Murray, Utah.

reduced growth rates and depression. Identification of causal factors in these cases is quite difficult.

Stress is a complex physiologic response to an environmental condition (Wedemeyer, 1981; Wedemeyer et al., 1984). Causal factors in the acute stress response include day-to-day husbandry activities such as population inventorying and pond cleaning, as well as transportation and the administration of chemotherapeutants. Common causal factors in the chronic stress response are population density and water quality.

The main clinical feature of the acute stress response is hyperactivity. Physiologically, there are many alterations. Chief among them are the rapid depletion of intrarenal ascorbic acid, an increase in circulating cortisol, cessation of renal and intestinal activity, hemoconcentration, leukocytosis, and an increase in blood ammonia (Wedemeyer and Yasutake, 1977; Wedemeyer et al., 1983; McLeay and Gordon, 1977). This response, the alarm reaction, (Selye, 1950) is eliminated with the removal of the stressor from the system.

If stressors persist in the system, adaptation ensues. In this stage of the stress response, the fish "adjusts" its physiologic activities to cope with the situation. Most physiologic parameters remain within baseline values; however, the longer the fish must accommodate to stressors, the more pronounced are the deleterious effects. Growth rates begin to decline, and a generalized melanosis becomes apparent. Concomitant with this, the tissue between the fin rays loses integrity owing to ischemia. In this stage of the stress response, an acute stressor may cause fish to die suddenly by bringing them to the stage of exhaustion where they are no longer capable of mounting further adjustment.

TABLE 33–6. Recommended Population Densities for Salmonids in Aquaculture Systems

Species	kg/cm/m³	lb/in./ft³
Rainbow trout	3.0	0.5
Steelhead trout	1.5	0.25
Chinook salmon	1.8	0.3
Coho salmon	2.4	0.4
Atlantic salmon	1.8	0.3

From Klontz, G. W., and Klontz, D. I. (1989) AQUASYST: A Computer Program for Commercial Salmonid Production. S. H. Nelson and Sons, Murray, Utah.

Environmental Gill Disease

Many feel that environmental gill disase is one of the major production-limiting factors in farmed fishes (Klontz, 1990; Snieszko, 1974). Subclinical episodes are often difficult to detect because of their insidious onset. Clinical episodes, especially those complicated by secondary, opportunistic pathogens, are frequently dramatic in terms of the mortality, which has a rapid onset and often an exponential daily increase.

The environmental gill disease syndrome is perhaps more a debilitating process than it is lethal, since secondary invaders are often the ultimate cause of death. The inflammatory process ensuing from the initial exposure begins with lamellar epithelial hypertrophy. If the irritant exposure is short lived, the hypertrophic condition subsides within a few days and the condition usually goes unnoticed.

If the irritant exposure continues, the squamous epithelium of the lamellae becomes separated from the underlying capillaries, and the resultant space is filled with a serous exudate. At this point, especially if there is generalized involvement, the fish exhibit clinical respiratory distress, particularly during or immediately following physical handling. This condition can be diagnosed in wet mounts of gill tissues, following a 1-hour exposure to certain chemotherapeutants administered in the water such as formalin.

One of the major cost factors in this disease is inappropriately applied chemotherapeutic regimens. Fish with clinical signs of rapid, shallow respiratory movements, grossly enlarged gill tissues, and incomplete opercular closure are commonly "treated" with one of the many medicaments added to the pond water. Unfortunately, these treatments can exacerbate the problem and are a waste of money.

As the disease continues, the lamellar hypertrophy is replaced with epithelial hyperplasia of the primary lamellar epithelium and then the secondary lamellar epithelium. The hyperplastic response can be terminal, involving only the distal portions of the lamellae, or it can involve the entire lamella. This condition, over a period of 1 to 2 weeks, gradually worsens to become interlamellar hyperplastic occlusion, in which the interlamellar spaces are completely obliterated. At this point, gill tissues frequently protrude from the opercular cavity, and there is incomplete closure of the opercula. Grossly, the excised gill is quite characteristic, with filamental separation due to the increased mucus production and the entrapped aquatic particulates.

There are several approaches to preventing and controlling environmental gill disease episodes. The first is avoidance of the conditions that are conducive to the occurrence of subclinical and clinical disease. This is best accomplished by avoiding exposure of the fish to high settleable and suspended solids, ammonia-nitrogen, dissolved oxygen, and population density (Klontz et al., 1985). To accomplish this, measuring the environmental parameters and their effects on growth and gill tissues should begin with sac fry and continue throughout the production cycle. This is time consuming and often frustrating, but always rewarding in the long term.

If a clinical episode of gill disease occurs, then an accurate diagnosis must be made prior to initiating any therapeutic regimen. The sequence of changes occurring in the gill tissues is the best indicator of the nature of the causal factors involved. Lesions such as hypertrophy, epithelial-capillary separation, and occlusive hyperplasia all suggest basic physiologic upsets, which may be reflected by alterations in other systems. The presence of bacteria and gill parasites often is a reflection of an underlying environmental problem, the most common of which is "poor housekeeping." At this juncture, it might be apropos to present an oft-quoted saying by Frederick Fish, a fish pathologist of the 1930s, to wit: "In fish culture, cleanliness is not next to godliness—it supersedes it" (Fish, 1938).

Once the problem is defined, i.e., the major causal factors identified, the next step is to "rebalance" the system. This is best accomplished by, first, withholding feed for 3 to 4 days, if the fish are of sufficient size to permit this. This will (1) reduce the oxygen demand of the fish, (2) reduce the ammonia-nitrogen generation by the fish, and (3) reduce the fecal and uneaten solids in the system. Second, administer sufficient salt (as granulated NaCl) to the system to obtain a 1 to 2% solution. This will (1) reduce the blood ammonia-nitrogen levels, (2) stimulate mucus secretion, and (3) have an astringent effect on the gill tissues. Third, reduce the population density to approximately one-half the oxygen-related carrying capacity of the system. This should be accomplished without unduly stressing the fish.

Nephrolithiasis

This is a chronic inflammatory condition in which calcium and other minerals precipitate as hydroxyapatite within the distal renal and collecting tubules (Bendele and Klontz, 1975; Landolt, 1975). This condition is commonly seen in water high in carbon dioxide and phosphates. Some speculate the presence of a dietary-mediating factor (Landolt, 1975). It is more debilitating than lethal. Most cases are diagnosed coincidentally to examining a fish for other causal factors. In severe cases, the only sign

usually seen is bilateral exophthalmia. There is no known treatment.

Strawberry Disease

This is a nondebilitating disease of rainbow trout (Erickson, 1969; Olson et al., 1985) characterized by circumscribed reddened areas in the skin. These occur primarily below the lateral line, posterior to the dorsal fin. The morbidity is usually 10 to 15%. The condition is most frequently seen during the processing of the fish for market. Affected fish are discarded as unsuited for the marketplace, causing an economic concern.

For years, the causal factor was thought to be infectious because treating affected fish with an antibacterial drug reduced the lesions within a few days. Another theory was that the disease is an atopy or an allergic response to an unidentified allergin, presumably a substance released by a saprophytic bacterium. This theory had its basis in the observation that affected fish were often in an environment conducive to high populations of saprophytic bacteria with a high load of organics from uneaten feed and fecal material. The gastrointestinal tract of affected fish contain many saprophytes, which are reduced by feeding antibacterial drugs. This theory has yet to be proved, although subcutaneous injection of antihistamine into the reddened areas reduces the lesions considerably.

Fin-Nipping

Fin-nipping is a condition precipitated by overcrowding. It is commonly a problem in concrete raceways and is uncommon in earthen ponds. Rainbow trout are especially territorial and defend their territory by acts of aggression, primarily nipping the dorsal fin or pectoral fins of an intruder. Following the initial trauma, the affected fin becomes discolored and a "target" for further traumatization. The end result is "soreback" or "hamburger pectoral." Fin nipping is common in hatchery-raised trout and farmed trout destined for the marketplace. Such fish also are usually in the adaptive phase of the chronic stress response and are quite melanotic. The suggested treatment is to reduce the population by grading out the larger, more aggressive fish. Other methods have included increasing the water velocity to distract the fish. This works sometimes but not always.

Soreback

Soreback is a sequel to dorsal fin-nipping, especially in rainbow trout raised in concrete raceways. In this condition, the initially traumatized dorsal fin is a target for further aggression to the point that the skin and underlying musculature are eaten away.

Some cases are so severe that the dorsal vertebral spines are exposed. Such cases are occasionally secondarily infected with *Saprolegnia*, an opportunistic pathogenic aquatic fungus. The condition is probably quite painful but nonlethal. The morbidity can be 5 to 10% in highly crowded ponds. The recommended therapy is to move affected fish from the population to a pond by themselves and to reduce the general population by size grading. The lesions on affected fish will heal within a matter of weeks, depending upon the water temperature. If the environmental conditions permit, there should be no secondary problems.

Electrocution

In salmonid rearing facilities, the problem of electrocution should be termed an extraenvironmental disease. It is caused by electrical shock, usually from a lightening strike or faulty electrical devices. In either case, mortality is virtually 100%. The most common postmortem lesion is intramuscular hemorrhage. Of all the environmental and extraenvironmental diseases of salmonids, this problem presents the greatest health hazard to the aquaculturist. It is a general policy in modern hatchery construction to either eliminate all electrically operated equipment from the facility or to convert the necessary equipment to direct current to reduce the hazard to both fish and humans.

Handling Trauma

Handling trauma is the result of mishandling the fish. The morbidity and mortality are very low and are often written off as part of doing business. While cleaning a pond, fish get stepped on. While size-grading fish, they get caught by the gills in the grader. When crowding fish for population inventory, they get impinged between the crowding screen and the pond wall or bottom. Nonetheless, any of these acts, in addition to being lethal to a few fish, are quite stressful to the remainder and can result in many of the aforementioned syndromes.

Sestonosis

Sestonosis is the accumulation of organic material, including feed, fecal materials, and aquatic fungi along the buccal aspect of the gill rakers. The problem is quite common in sac-fry that spend their time on the bottom of the rearing units. There is usually very high morbidity (greater than 50%) and a high mortality (greater than 90%). The problem is untreatable by current technology. The best therapy is prophylaxis by constantly siphoning debris from rearing units.

Sunburn

Sunburn, or "back-peel," is common during midsummer in the northern latitudes (Fig. 33–2). The complete etiologic picture has not been demonstrated (Roberts, 1978). Some workers think there is a contributory nutritional imbalance, and others think there is a genotypic contribution. Sunburn is usually seen in populations of small (2- to 3-inch fish) within days of their being moved from the inside rearing units to small outside units containing very clear water. The morbidity can be greater than 50%, but the mortality is quite low in cases not complicated by bacterial infections. In secondarily infected cases, the mortality can be very high. The suggested treatment is to provide shade for the rearing units and to keep the fish on a high plane of nutrition fortified with extra vitamins, especially the B-complex and C vitamins. Recovery is usually uneventful and quite rapid. Prevention is easily accomplished by not stocking unshaded, outside rearing units.

Botulism

Botulism is a problem associated with deep earthen ponds from which the sediments have not

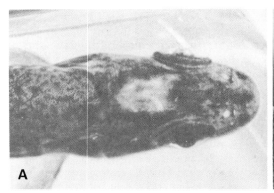 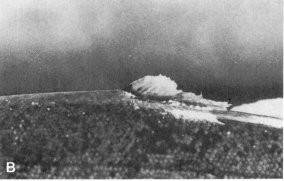

FIGURE 33–2. *A.* Sunburn lesions in American lake trout. (Courtesy of L.N. Allison.) *B.* Sunburn lesion on the dorsal fin and dorsum of a caged rainbow trout held at high altitude. (From Roberts, R.J. [1989] Fish Pathology, 2nd ed. Bailliere Tindall, London.)

been removed or stirred for a number of years. The benthos becomes anaerobic and covered with a thin layer of aquatic fungi, which provides an excellent medium for the production of anaerobic bacteria. If one of these is *Clostridium botulinum* (type E or type C), intoxications of the resident fish occur when the sediments are disturbed or the fish ingest sediments. This condition is seen most commonly in midsummer, although it could presumably occur at anytime during the year if the water temperatures are above 12 to 15°C.

The clinical signs of fish botulism are initially disorientation and erratic swimming, followed by complete ataxia, flaccid paralysis, and death. The postmortem lesions are not distinctive. The investigator must assemble the associated factors of earthen ponds, accumulated sediments, a history of disturbing the sediments, and analysis of the sediments and fish tissues for toxin.

There is no known treatment for botulism in fish. It is best prevented by removing accumulated sediments annually or by keeping the benthos well aerated. The latter does have the undesired effect of suspending the benthic materials and perhaps causing gill problems.

Brown Blood Disease

The common name for clinical methemoglobinemia in fishes is brown blood disease. The major causal factor is nitrite, the oxidation product of ammonia-nitrogen in the environment. Continuous levels greater than 0.55 mg/L are sufficient to start the process of oxidizing the ferrous iron (Fe^{2+}), thereby inhibiting the oxygen transport capabilities of hemoglobin.

The primary clinical sign is, as the common name implies, brown blood. The gill tissues are quite brown, rather than their normal rich, red color. Sampled blood is also brown. Methemoglobin levels exceeding 25% are considered clinically important and levels exceeding 50% are lethal. The suggested treatment is 1 to 2% sodium chloride followed by high dietary levels of ascorbic acid (Wedemeyer and Yasutake, 1977; Bowser, 1983).

Hypoxia

When the partial pressure of dissolved oxygen falls below 90 mmHg, the pressure differential between the water and the lamellar blood is insufficient to fully oxygenate the blood (David, 1975; Downey and Klontz, 1981).

The usual causal factors are (1) exceeding the oxygen-carrying capacity of the rearing unit; (2) nighttime or cloudy weather oxygen demands by phytoplankton/zooplankton populations in the rearing unit; (3) the biologic oxygen demand of the rearing unit. The morbidity is usually 100% and the mortality slightly elevated above baseline; however,

an increased mortality ensues as the condition persists.

The primary clinical sign is a reduction of growth rate followed by labored respiration as the condition worsens.

Anoxia

When the dissolved oxygen in the aquatic environment decreases to the point where there is insufficient dissolved oxygen to support life, anoxia results. This is often due to cessation of inflowing water to the rearing unit or the loss of water in the rearing unit. Anoxia also occurs when the lamellar epithelium is altered, so as not to permit oxygen uptake. This happens with sestonosis or complete interlamellar occlusion from the epithelial hyperplasia associated with environmental gill disease. Fish that have died of anoxia exhibit a typical posture. The mouth is agape, the opercula are extended, and the body is in rigor immediately at the time of death.

The suggested method of prevention is constantly to monitor the dissolved oxygen levels in the rearing units and be watchful of clinical signs of hypoxia. Also, cleanliness of the rearing units and proper attention to chronic stressors will prevent gill lamellar changes.

Herbicide, Pesticide, and Other Organic Toxicities

Herbicide, pesticide, and other organic compound toxicities are very difficult to define. In many cases, the investigator makes a tentative diagnosis of a chemical toxicity when all the other possibilities have been excluded. By this time, the offending chemical, if water borne, has long since left the system, making definitive diagnosis quite difficult (Wells and Moyse, 1981).

The effects range from mild paralytic signs at low-level exposures to death in high-level exposures. One of the main effects in low-grade toxicities is immunosuppression, which leaves the fish vulnerable to infectious agents (Zeeman and Brindley, 1981). Neoplasia is another effect of long-term, low-grade exposure to certain organic toxicants.

Diagnosis is based mainly on a history of toxicant release(s), paralytic signs in the fish, and histopathologic and chemical analyses of the tissues (see Chap. 41).

Heavy Metal Toxicities

Heavy metal toxicities in aquaculture systems are rare; however, there is always the potential for them to occur. This is especially true as traditional sources of water are replaced with water-replenishment systems. In these systems, copper or zinc plumbing fixtures can provide sufficient levels to be

TABLE 33–7. Levels of Dissolved Heavy Metals Toxic to Salmonids

Metal	Safe Limit (mg/L)	Comments
Copper	0.014	More toxic in soft water
		Zinc exacerbates toxicity
Zinc	0.01	Synergistic with copper
	0.15	In hard water
Cadmium	0.03	
Chromium	0.1	
Lead	0.01	In soft water
	4.0	In hard water
Silver	0.03	

From Post, G. (1987) Textbook of Fish Health (rev. ed.). T.F.H. Publications, Neptune, New Jersey.

toxic. Other metals that affect salmonids in culture are cadmium, chromium, lead, selenium, and silver (Bell, 1986; Post, 1987) (Table 33–7).

Death from chronic, low-level heavy metal intoxication usually occurs as a result of hepatic or renal failure. The diagnosis is based on analysis of tissues for levels of the suspected metal. It is then necessary to identify the source and remove it from the system.

Gas Bubble Disease

Gas bubble disease can be caused by gas supersaturation of the water in the rearing unit (Bouck, 1980; Marking, 1987). The factors giving rise to this condition are varied. Water passing tiny leaks in pipes creates a vacuum, drawing in atmospheric air. Water flowing into a plunge-pool entrains air and the pressure of the depth creates supersaturation. Water being pumped in a closed system from a deep well (greater than 300 ft) is usually supersaturated with nitrogen and deficient in oxygen (Colt et al., 1986). Whatever the cause, excess solubilized nitrogen in the water passes the lamellar epithelium and endothelium, only to come out of solution in the blood vascular system, creating gas emboli that can lead to death (Bouck, 1980). Nitrogen saturation levels of 101 to 105% affect sac fry. Levels greater than 110% affect juvenile fish (more than 100/kg), and levels greater than 125% affect adult fish (Wood, 1976).

Characteristic clinical signs in peracute cases are few. In acute cases, there is depression and bilateral exophthalmia. In chronic cases, the effects are not well documented and are of some concern to aquaculturists. Sac-fry dead of gas bubble disease usually float upside down owing to the gas in the yolk sac. Diagnosis is largely based on observing gas emboli in the vessels of the fins and periorbital tissues. In addition, water total gas pressures are markedly increased.

Prevention is accomplished easily by installing gas-stabilization chambers through which the inflowing water passes into the rearing unit. Other methods of gas reduction and oxygenation, such as cascading the inflow water over a series of boards or screens, have been successful (Bell, 1986).

Cyanide Toxicity

Cyanide toxicity occurs during the midsummer months when the water temperatures are at maximum. The warm water enhances the growth of cyanogenic blue-green algae, which release cyanide when they die. This is very rare in conditions of intensive management but can be an annual problem in fish being raised in net pens in large reservoirs. The signs of cyanide toxicity are indistinct. The diagnosis is based largely on recording a massive fish kill in a eutrophic condition, supporting the production of blue-green algae. Prevention is best focused on preventing environmental eutrophication through minimizing the organic load and by applying one of the commercial "shade" chemicals that restrict the sunlight needed by the algae.

Oxygen Supersaturation

This causes a massive distension of the swimbladder of salmonids in waters coming from highly vegetated streams on bright, sunny days. In this situation, vegetation produces copious quantities of oxygen that is not dissipated. The high oxygen loading of the water apparently results in the overfilling of the fishes' swimbladder.

The morbidity of this condition is often low. Affected fish swim in distress on their side, at the surface of the water. At sundown and on cloudy days, the condition disappears. Mortality is low. The suggested means of prevention is to provide a means of gas reduction in the water and/or reduce the vegetation in the source stream.

Therapeutant Toxicities

Unfortunately, therapeutant toxicities are quite common. The majority are an overdose of a chemical intended to treat a clinical condition. The most common chemicals involved are formalin and malachite green (Herwig, 1979). It has been said that therapeutants have killed more fish than the diseases they were intended to treat. There is probably much truth in this statement. One of the more common maladies attributed to the exuberant use of malachite green on embryonating eggs is "white spot" disease. The syndrome appears at the sac-fry stage in which the yolk material contains particles of cream-colored, coagulated yolk. As the clinical course progresses, the fins become rigidly extended and covered with a whitish film. Death ensues within days. There is no known treatment.

To prevent these situations, it is important to establish a rigid policy that no fish be treated with waterborne chemicals, until a bioassay for dose and efficacy have been completed. The dosages recommended in many texts and extension leaflets should only be considered as guides. The toxic levels of all chemotherapeutants administered in water are affected by exposure time, pH, temperature, hardness, fish species, and fish age.

LITERATURE CITED

Bell, M.C. (1986) Fisheries Handbook of Engineering Requirements and Biological Criteria. U.S. Army Corps of Engineers.

Bendele R.A., Jr., and Klontz, G.W. (1975) Histopathology of teleost kidney diseases. In: Pathology of Fishes (Ribelin, W.E., and Migaki, G., eds.). University of Wisconsin Press, Madison, pp. 365–383.

Bouck, G.R. (1980) Etiology of gas bubble disease. Trans. Am. Fish. Soc. 109:703–707.

Bowser, P.R. (1983) Brown blood disease in channel catfish. Information Sheet 1314. Mississippi Agriculture Forestry Experimental Station, Mississippi State University.

Bullock, G.L. (1972) Studies on selected Myxobacteria pathogenic for fishes and on bacterial gill disease in hatchery-raised salmonids. Bureau of Sport Fish and Wildlife, Technical. Paper No. 60.

Colt, J., Bouck, G.R., and Fidler, L. (1986) Review of current literature and research on gas supersaturation and gas bubble trauma. Special Publication No. 1, B.P.A. and Bioengineering Section, American Fisheries Society.

D'Aoust P.-Y., and Ferguson, H.W. (1984) The pathology of chronic ammonia toxicity in rainbow trout, Salmo gairdneri Richardson. J. Fish Dis. 7:199–205.

David, J.C. (1975) Minimal dissolved oxygen requirements of aquatic life with emphasis on Canadian species: A review. J. Fish. Res. Bd. Can. 32(12):2295–2332.

Downey, P.C., and Klontz, G.W. (1981) Aquaculture techniques: Oxygen (pO$_2$) requirements for rainbow trout. Technical Compl. Report, Idaho Water Resources Research Institute, University of Idaho, Moscow.

Eller, L.L. (1975) Gill lesions in freshwater teleosts. In: Pathology of Fishes (Ribelin, W.E., and Migaki, G., eds.). University of Wisconsin Press, Madison, pp. 305–331.

Ellis, M.M., Westfall, B.A., and Ellis, M.D. (1948) Determination of water quality. Research Report No. 9, Fish and Wildlife Service, U.S. Government Printing Office, Washington, D.C.

Erickson, J.D. (1969) An investigation on strawberry disease in trout. Am. Fish. U.S. Trout News, p. 26.

Fish, F. (1938) Treat, think and be wary—For tomorrow they may die. Progressive Fish Culturist. Memorandum I–131: No. 139.

Herwig, N. (1979) Handbook of Drugs and Chemicals Used in the Treatment of Fish Diseases. Charles C Thomas, Springfield, Illinois.

Jagoe, C.H., and Haynes, T.A. (1983) Alterations in gill epithelial morphology of yearling sunapee trout exposed to acute acid stress. Trans. Am. Fish. Soc. 112:689–695.

Klontz, G.W. (1990) Intensive Aquaculture Technology (A Syllabus). College of Forestry, Wildlife and Range Experimental Station, University of Idaho, Moscow.

Klontz, G.W., and Klontz, D.I. (1989) AQUASYST: A Computer Program for Commercial Salmonid Production. S.H. Nelson and Sons, Murray, Utah.

Klontz, G.W., Herr, C., and McArthur, T.J. (1983) Aquaculture techniques: Preliminary studies on carrying capacities and census-taking in serial reuse ponds. Technical Compl. Report, Idaho Water Resources Research Institute, University of Idaho, Moscow.

Klontz, G.W., Stewart, B.C., and Eib, D.W. (1985) On the etiology and pathophysiology of environmental gill disease in juvenile salmonids. In: Fish and Shellfish Pathology (Ellis, A.E., ed.). Academic Press, New York, pp. 199–211.

Landolt, M. (1975) Visceral granuloma and nephrocalcinosis of trout. In: Pathology of Fishes (Ribelin, W.E., and Migaki, G., eds.). University of Wisconsin Press, Madison, pp. 793–805.

Marking, L.L. (1987) Gas supersaturations in fisheries: Causes, concerns, and cures. Fish and Wildlife Leaflet 9, U.S. Department of the Interior Fish and Wildlife Service, Washington, D.C.

Mawdesley-Thomas, L.E. (ed.) (1972) Some tumors of fish. In: Diseases of Fish. Academic Press, New York, pp. 191–285.

Mayer, F.L., and Ellersieck, M.R. (1986) Manual of acute toxicity: Interpretation and data base for 410 chemicals and 66 species of freshwater animals. Resource Publication 160. U.S. Department of the Interior Fish and Wildlife Service, Washington, D.C.

McLeay, D.J., and Gordon, M.R. (1977) Leucocrit: A simple hematological technique for measuring acute stress in salmonid fish, including stressful concentrations of pulpmill effluent. J. Fish. Res. Bd. Can. 34(11):2164–2175.

Olson, D.P., Beleau, M.H., Busch, R.A., Roberts, S., and Kreiger, R.I. (1985) Strawberry disease in rainbow trout, Salmo gairdneri Richardson. J. Fish Dis. 8:103–111.

Paulson, L.J. (1980) Models of ammonia excretion for brook trout, Salvelinus fontinalis, and rainbow trout, Salmo gairdneri. Can. J. Fish. Aquatic Sci. 37:1421–1425.

Piper, R.G. (1972) Managing hatcheries by the numbers. Am. Fishes U.S. Trout News 17(3):10–15.

Piper, R.G., McElwain, I.B., Orme, L.E., McCraren, J.P., Fowler, L.G. and Leonard, J.R. (1982) Fish hatchery management. U.S. Department of the Interior Fish and Wildlife Service, Washington, D.C.

Post, G. (1987) Textbook of Fish Health (rev. ed.). T.F.H. Publications, Neptune, New Jersey, pp. 250–285.

Randall, D., and Daxboek, C. (1984) Oxygen and carbon dioxide transfer across fish gills. In: Fish Physiology. Vol. X. Part A. (Hoar, W.S., and Randall, D.J., eds.). Academic Press, New York, pp. 263–315.

Roberts, R.J. (1975) The effects of temperature on diseases and their histopathological manifestations in fish. In: Pathology of Fishes (Ribelin, W.E., and Migaki, G., eds.). University of Wisconsin Press, Madison, pp. 463–477.

Roberts, R.J. (1978) Miscellaneous Non-infectious Diseases. In: Fish Pathology (Roberts, R.J., ed.). Bailliere Tindall, London, pp. 227–235.

Selye, H. (1950) Stress and the general adaptation syndrome. Br. Med. J. 1:1383–1392.

Smith, C.E., and Piper, R.G. (1975) Lesions associated with chronic exposure to ammonia. In: Pathology of Fishes (Ribelin, W.E., and Migaki, G., eds.). University of Wisconsin Press, Madison, pp. 497–515.

Snieszko, S. (1974) The effects of environmental stress on outbreaks of infectious diseases of fishes. J. Fish Biol. 6(2):197–208.

Stewart, B.C. (1983) Environmental gill disease in salmonids: The role of environmental unionized ammonia. M.S. Thesis, Fishery Resources, University of Idaho, Moscow.

Trussel, R.P. (1972) The percent un-ionized ammonia in aqueous ammonia solutions at different pH levels and temperatures. J. Fish. Res. Bd. Can. 29(10):1505–1507.

Wedemeyer, G.A. (1981) The physiological response of fishes to the stress of intensive aquaculture in recirculation systems. Proceedings of the World Symposium on Aquaculture in Heated Effluents and Recirculation Systems, Vol. II, pp. 4–18.

Wedemeyer, G.A., and Wood, J.W. (1974) Stress as a predisposing factor in fish diseases. U.S. Department of the Interior Fish and Wildlife Service, Fisheries Leaflet No. 38, Washington, D.C.

Wedemeyer, G.A., and Yasutake, W.T. (1977) Clinical methods for the assessment of the effects of environmental stress on fish health. Technical Papers of the U.S.F.W.S., No. 89. U.S. Department of Interior, Washington, D.C.

Wedemeyer, G.A., Meyer, F.P., and Smith, L. (1976) Book 5: Environmental Stress and Fish Diseases. In: Diseases of Fishes (Snieszko, S.F., and Axelrod, H.R., eds.). T.F.H., Neptune, New Jersey.

Wedemeyer, G.A., Gould R.W., and Yasutake, W.T. (1983) Some potentials and limits of the leucocrit test as a fish health assessment method. J. Fish Biol. 23:711–716.

Wedemeyer, G.A., McLeay, D.J., and Goodyear, C.P. (1984) Assessing the tolerance of fish and fish populations to environmental stressors: The problems and methods of monitoring. In: Contaminant Effects of Fisheries (Cairns, V.W., Hodson, P.V., and Nriagu, J.O., eds.). Wiley and Sons, New York, pp. 164–195.

Wells, P.G., and Moyse, C. (1981) A selected bibliography on Salmo gairdneri Richardson (rainbow, steelhead, Kamloops trout), with particular reference to studies with aquatic toxicants (Second Edition). Economic and Technical Review Report (EPS–3–AR–81–1) Environmental Protection Service, Environment Canada.

Wood, J.W. (1976) Diseases of Pacific Salmon. (2nd ed.). Washington Department of Fisheries. Seattle, Washington.

Wood, E.M., and Yasutake, W.T. (1957) Histopathology of fish: V. Gill disease. Progressive Fish Culturist 19:7–13.

Zeeman, M.G., and Brindley, W.A. (1981) Effects of toxic agents upon fish immune systems: A review. In: Immunologic Considerations in Toxicology. Vol. II. (Sharma, R.P., ed.). CRC Press, Boca Raton, Florida, pp. 1–60.

Chapter 34

NUTRITION AND NUTRITIONAL DISEASES OF SALMONIDS

GEORGE W. POST

Malnutrition is often implicated in the disease processes of salmonid fishes, either as direct malnutrition or through reduced resistance to opportunistic pathogenic organisms. This holds true among confined or free-ranging fishes. However, free-ranging fishes usually have a wide choice of foods from which to select a well-balanced diet, and if the food supply is not overutilized, malnutrition rarely occurs. The discussion here will be concerned primarily with the feeding of intensively reared, confined fishes where the ration being fed must contain all essential nutrients necessary to maintain health, satisfactory growth, and successful reproduction. Disease conditions relating directly to malnutrition and food toxins will be discussed.

GENERAL ASPECTS OF SALMONID NUTRITION

Propagation of salmonids has been practiced since the late nineteenth century. Salmonid culture can be classified into two categories: (1) fish confined to an ecosystem that supplies part of the required nutrients, leaving the remainder to be supplied by supplemental feeding; and (2) fish confined under intensive rearing conditions in which all required nutrients must be supplied by rations offered. Completely balanced rations for intensively reared fishes are much more difficult to formulate and prepare. Not only must the formulation contain all nutritional requirements for the fish, but also they must be available (digestible and absorbable). Care is necessary in processing the ingredients into food particles, and palatability is a major concern.

Salmonids are poikilothermic, and their body temperature remains near that of their environment. Changes in environmental temperatures cause alterations of metabolic rates and subsequent increases or decreases in the required intake of nutrients (Fig. 34–1). Size and age also affect metabolic rate. Young fish of any species have a higher metabolic rate than older fish (Fig. 34–2). Fish activity also alters metabolic rate. A salmonid reared in rapidly flowing water must work constantly to maintain its position in the water. Such fish require more energy in their diet to maintain adequate growth than less active fish.

Basic research on salmonid nutrition began in the middle 1940s. Earlier, feeding confined salmonids involved the use of meat and body organ products obtained from slaughter houses or rendering plants. These were ground and mixed with sodium chloride, carboxymethylcellulose, grain meals, or other compounds to reduce losses of water soluble nutrients. These diets did not prevent diet-related sporadic and extensive mortality.

A purified diet from gelatin, casein, fat, dextrin, and crystalline vitamins and minerals developed in 1951 (Wolf, 1951), and more highly refined test diets for trout and salmon prepared entirely from crystalline and highly purified ingredients devised in 1957 (Halver and Coates, 1957; Halver, 1957) have been used with minor modifications to establish many of the nutrient requirements of salmonids and other fish species. Much of the research on nutrient requirements of salmonids has been done on rainbow trout and chinook salmon. Data obtained on these two species can often be used directly, or with minor

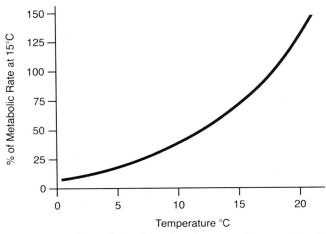

FIGURE 34–1. The relationship of environmental temperature to the metabolic rate of rainbow trout.

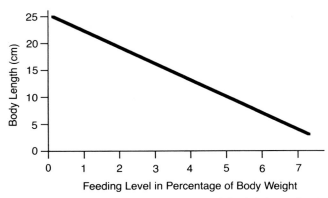

FIGURE 34–2. The approximate quantity of food fed per day in percentage of body weight for rainbow trout of various body sizes at an environmental temperature of 15°C.

TABLE 34–1. Recommended Percentage of Total Protein (as Fed Basis) for Chinook Salmon and Rainbow Trout

Fish Size	Chinook Salmon (% Total Protein)	Rainbow Trout (% Total Protein)
Young	47–56	38–40
Subadult	43–47	36–38
Adult	40–42	34–36

Protein must contain the necessary amino acid profile and availability; reduced protein quality must be compensated by additional protein or supplemented amino acids.

Data derived from Post, G. (1987) Textbook of Fish Health, Revised and Expanded. T.F.H. Publications, Neptune, New Jersey; Poston, H. A. (1986) Response of lake trout and rainbow trout to dietary cellulose. U.S. Fish and Wildlife Service Technical Report No. 5:1–6, Washington, D.C.; Kim et al. (1984) Requirements for sulfur-containing amino acids by rainbow trout. Fed. Proc. 43:856 (Abs. 3338); Rumsey et al. (1983) Methionine and cystine requirements of rainbow trout. Progressive Fish Culturist 45:139–143; Walton et al. (1982) Methionine metabolism in rainbow trout fed diets of differing methionine and cystine content. J. Nutr. 112:1525–1535; and Ogino et al. (1980) Requirements of carp and rainbow trout for essential amino acids. Bull. Jpn. Soc. Sci. Fish. 44:1015–1018.

alterations, for other salmonid species, but not always, possibly because of minor differences in species nutritional requirements.

NUTRITIONAL REQUIREMENTS FOR SALMONIDS

Salmonids are carnivores and their nutritional requirements reflect this. The major nutrients in salmonid diets include high protein levels and relatively low-digestible carbohydrate. The requirements for lipids are also relatively high. Salmonids require all of the essential vitamins and certain vitaminlike substances required by other vertebrates. Unlike terrestrial mammals, however, salmonids and other fishes are capable of absorbing certain minerals from their environmental water. Thus, the nutritional requirements of salmonids have similarities and dissimilarities to other vertebrates.

Protein and Amino Acids

The quantitative protein requirement for salmonids is dependent on the amino acid profile of the protein being fed. General requirements for good-quality gross protein in salmonids is quite high, depending to some extent on age. Young fish require higher dietary protein than older fish of the same species. The salmons generally have a greater dietary requirement for gross protein than the trout of the same age. Young chinook salmon require up to 56% of a good-quality protein in the ration. Older chinook may require as low as 40% gross protein in the diet. Small rainbow trout require up to 40% quality protein, and large rainbow may require as low as 34% gross protein in the diet (Phillips and Brockway, 1956). The protein fraction must have the necessary amino acid profile and amino acid availability. Reduced protein quality must be compensated for by adding additional protein or supplementing necessary amino acids (Table 34–1).

The essential amino acid requirements for salmonids have been established through the use of amino acid test diets (Halver and Coates, 1957; Halver, 1957). Research has demonstrated an essential need for 10 amino acids in these animals (Table 34–2). Two nonessential amino acids will reduce the quantitative requirements for two essential amino acids. Cystine can replace up to one-third of the methionine requirement, and tyrosine can replace up to one-fifth of the required phenylalanine (National Academy of Sciences, 1978). All other amino acids can be synthesized by the fish if required amounts of essential amino acids are available from the ration.

Fats and Fatty Acids

The major source of energy for salmonids is dietary fats. Dietary fats are also essential for synthe-

TABLE 34–2. Recommended Essential Amino Acid Content (as Fed Basis) for Salmonids

Amino Acid	% of Diet
Arginine	2.4
Histidine	0.7
Isoleucine	0.9
Leucine	1.6
Lysine	2.0
Methionine*	1.5
Phenylalanine†	2.1
Threonine‡	0.9
Tryptophan	0.2
Valine	1.3

*Up to one-third of methionine may be supplied by cystine, L-methionine may yield better growth than the DL analog.

†Up to one-fifth of phenylalanine may be supplied by tyrosine.

‡Chum salmon fry require 1.1 to 1.2% threonine (Akiyama et al., 1985).

TABLE 34–3. Percentage of Essential Fatty Acids in Fat Sources Used as Ingredients in Salmonid Ration Formulas

Source	Average % 18:3ω3	18:3ω6
Herring oil	21.6	1.4
Menhaden oil	29.3	3.0
Cod liver oil	25.9	2.3
Salmon oil	27.1	2.6
Soybean oil	7.1	50.3
Corn oil	1.1	55.8
Lard	0.8	9.9
Beef tallow	0.4	2.5

Data derived from Post, G. (1987) Textbook of Fish Health, Revised and Expanded. T.F.H. Publications, Neptune, New Jersey; and National Academy of Sciences (1973) Nutrient Requirements of Trout, Salmon, and Catfish. National Research Council, Washington, D.C.

sis of phospholipids and steroids and for specific structural elements in cell walls. Trout and salmon have one essential fatty acid, an 18-carbon fatty acid with an 18:3ω3 configuration. Rainbow trout require no less than 1% of the diet as this ω3 fatty acid. A similar fatty acid, 18:3ω6, can substitute for the ω3 fatty acid up to 0.1% of the diet (Lee and Sinnhuber, 1972). Other trout species may be similar to rainbow trout in this sparing action.

The essential fatty acid requirement for coho salmon has been established as 1 to 2.5% of the diet being 18:3ω3 fatty acid (Cowey et al., 1985). Other salmon species may have similar essential fatty acid requirements. Quantitative fatty acids in a salmonid ration can be estimated from the known fatty acid profile of each fat-bearing ingredient in the ration formula (Table 34–3).

Carbohydrates

The use of carbohydrates for energy appears to be limited in trout and salmon. Enzymatic metabolism of carbohydrate is similar to higher animals (Phillips and Brockway, 1956). However, quantities of carbohydrates that can be assimilated by salmonids is apparently limited by the ability of the fish to

TABLE 34–4. Digestibility of Certain Carbohydrates by Trout

Carbohydrate	Percentage Digestibility
Glucose	99
Glycogen	99
Maltose	92
Dextrin	80
Sucrose	73
Lactose	60
Starch (cooked)	57
Starch (raw)	38
Cellulose	Less than 10

From Post, G. (1987) Textbook of Fish Health, Revised and Expanded. T.F.H. Publications, Neptune, New Jersey.

metabolize them. Insulin activity in trout, for example, is similar to that of a diabetic mammal. Large-molecule carbohydrate (raw starch and cellulose) is poorly digested by most salmonids. Thus, rations containing relatively large amounts of raw starch or cellulose may produce reduced utilization and reduced growth in these fishes (Bromley and Adkins, 1984).

Carbohydrate can be used in ration formulation to reduce protein required for energy (Edwards et al., 1977). There is no specific requirement established for carbohydrates in the diet of salmonids. However, the maximum digestible carbohydrate for trout has been suggested as 20% of the ration (Post, 1987). Quantitative digestibility of the carbohydrate fraction of the ration formulation can be estimated from the known digestibility of various carbohydrates by trout (Table 34–4). Digestibility of carbohydrate cannot be equated to the total nitrogen-free extract of a ration, it must be estimated from each carbohydrate-bearing ingredient in the ration formula.

Minerals

Fish require the same mineral elements to maintain metabolism and health as mammals (Phillips and Podoliak, 1957). Mineral elements are used for the same biologic purposes, such as metalloenzymes, oxygen-bearing substances, neurotransmitters, and skeletal stability. A major difference between dietary mineral requirements in fish and terrestrial animals is that some of the required minerals are absorbed from the water by diffusion across the gill membrane. Part or all requirements for some minerals, if present in the environmental water, can be supplied by this route rather than from the alimentary tract. Calcium, bicarbonate, chloride, iodine, potassium, sodium, sulfate, and other minerals are more efficiently absorbed from the aqueous environment than from the gut. Other ions such as aluminum, cobalt, copper, iron, magnesium, molybdenum, phosphorus, and zinc may be less diffusible from water and all or part of the requirement for each should be supplied in the diet (Post, 1987; National Academy of Sciences, 1981).

Data on the complement of dissolved ions in a water supply may be used to elevate or reduce quantities of highly diffusible elements in the ration formula. However, most formulations of salmonid rations have a full-complement mineral supplement to assure there will be no mineral deficiencies. Quantitative requirements for known essential minerals in salmonid nutrition are difficult to state accurately. Information on fishes other than salmonids is often used to indicate a probable full complement of essential mineral elements in practical natural ingredient rations (Table 34–5).

Vitamins

There are 11 water-soluble and four fat-soluble vitamins and vitaminlike substances essential in sal-

TABLE 34–5. Known Quantitative Mineral Requirements of Certain Fish Species

Mineral	Fish Species	Requirement	Reference
Copper	Rainbow trout	3.0 mg/kg ration	Cowey et al., 1985
Iodine	Chinook salmon	0.6–1.1 mg/kg ration	Woodall and LaRoche, 1964
Iron	Fishes	80–100 mg/kg ration	Cowey et al., 1985
Magnesiun	Channel catfish	0.6–0.7% of ration	Gatlin et al., 1982
Maganese	Channel catfish	2.4 mg/kg ration	Gatlin and Wilson, 1984
Selenium	Rainbow trout	0.15–0.38 mg/kg ration	Hilton et al., 1980
Zinc	Rainbow trout	15–30 mg/kg ration	Ogino and Yand, 1978

monid nutrition (Table 34–6). There is some doubt about the absolute salmonid dietary requirements for two water-soluble vitaminlike substances, choline, and inositol (myoinositol), since salmonids can synthesize their requirements for these compounds. However, practical diet formulas for salmonids usually assure an adequate content of choline and inositol or their precursors.

Water-Soluble Vitamins

Ascorbic acid (vitamin C) is required by all salmonids. Unlike most higher animals, they have no means of ascorbic acid synthesis. Ascorbic acid is essential for maintaining the integrity of supporting tissues, especially the biosynthesis of cartilage and collagen (Fig. 34–3). It is also necessary for the maintenance of capillary integrity. Ascorbic acid is a physiologic antioxidant and hydrogen acceptor through nicotinamide diphosphate, but does not serve as a coenzyme. It enhances iron absorption from the intestine and is involved in erythrocyte maturation.

Vitamin B_{12} (cyanocobalamin) may be universally required by vertebrates, including fishes. Bacteria synthesize the compound and it is usually passed in the food chain through plants to animals. Cyanocobalamin has a major role in hematopoiesis, acting with folic acid in the development of erythroid cells. It is required for erythrocyte formation in higher vertebrates and possibly in fishes. Vitamin B_{12} is also essential for reduction of formyl groups to methyl groups and the formation of choline. It is important in sulfhydryl metabolism.

Biotin is active in the function of several important enzymes. It is essential for specific carboxylation and decarboxylation reactions in glycolysis and acts in the same capacity in the elongation of fatty acids and in conversion of unsaturated fatty acids to more stable cis forms (Fig. 34–4). It also is active in reactions leading to synthesis of nicotinamide and the biosynthesis of citrulline from ornithine.

Folic acid, like vitamin B_{12}, is essential for normal erythropoiesis, being essential in nucleic acid synthesis. Folic acid becomes part of the coenzyme tetrahydrofolic acid (formalhydrofolic acid, or FH–4), which acts with tranformylases and tranformaminases in the metabolism of serine, methionine, and other amino acids to yield one-carbon units. Supplementation with folic acid improves growth and hatchability of salmonid eggs.

Niacin (nicotinic acid) is a component of two coenzymes, nicotinamide adenine dinucleotide and its phosphate, which are important in managing oxidation-reduction states in salmonid tissues (Fig. 34–5). Nicotinamide adenine dinucleotide phosphate and its reduced form, NADPH, is important in the metabolism of glucose. Nicotinamide adenine dinucleotide is active in oxidative deamination of amino acids, and is essential in lipid metabolism. Because of its biofunctions involving carbohydrate, lipids, and amino acids at the cellular level, niacin is essential in all cells of salmonids. Some niacin can be synthesized by salmonids through the metabolism of tryptophan, but not enough to meet all requirements. Additional dietary niacin is essential in salmonid nutrition.

Pantothenic acid is an integral part of coenzyme A (CoA), and is essential for any reaction involving CoA in the tricarboxylic acid cycle of carbohydrate metabolism, the oxidation and synthesis of fatty acids, or in amino acid metabolism. It is especially important in benzyl transfer to hippuric acid. Pantothenic acid is essential for the development of the central nervous system of salmonids.

Pyridoxine or one of its active coenzymes, pyridoxal phosphate and pyridoxamine phosphate, is essential for amino acid, carbohydrate, and lipid

TABLE 34–6. Vitamin Requirements of Salmonids

Vitamin*	mg/kg Fish Body Weight/Day	mg/kg Ration
Water-Soluble		
Ascorbic acid	3–5	100
B_{12}	0.0005–0.0007	0.02
Biotin	0.03–0.07	1
Choline	50–60	3000
Folic acid	0.15–0.20	5
Inositol	18–20	400
Niacin	3–7	150
Pantothenic acid	1.0–1.5	40
Pyridoxine	0.2–0.4	10
Riboflavin	0.5–1.0	20
Thiamin (B_{12})	0.15–0.20	10
Fat-Soluble		
A	75 IU	2500 IU
E	1.0 IU	30 IU
K	0.1 IU	5–10 IU
D	72 IU	2400 IU

*Based on requirements of young fish.

Data derived from Post G. (1987) Textbook of Fish Health, Revised and Expanded. T.F.H. Publications, Neptune, New Jersey. National Academy of Sciences (1981) Nutrient Requirements of Cold Water Fishes. National Research Council, Washington, D.C.

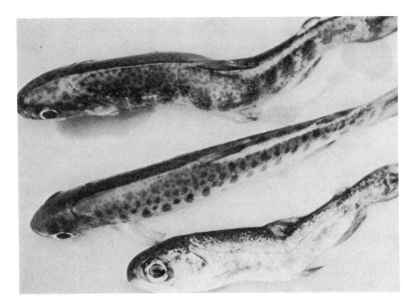

FIGURE 34–3. Coho salmon showing lordosis due to a diet deficient in vitamin C. (From Halver, J.E., Ashley, L.M., and Smith, R.R. [1969] Ascorbic acid requirements of coho salmon and rainbow trout. Trans. Am. Fish. Soc. 98:762–771.)

metabolism. Pyridoxal phosphate is the coenzyme for several transaminases and other reactions involving amino acids. It is active in the conversion of phenylalanine and tyrosine to dehydroxyphenylalanine and of tryptophan to serotonin. In this capacity pyridoxine is directly related to nervous disorders of salmonids and other fishes. It is essential for the utilization of not only these two amino acids but also glutamic acid, lysine, methionine, cystine, glycine, and alanine. Pyridoxal phosphate is also involved in lipid metabolism, especially of the essential unsaturated fatty acids.

Riboflavin is an essential coenzyme with many oxidases and reductases in the tricarboxcylic acid cycle, fatty acid metabolism, and metabolism of several amino acids. It is essential, working in conjunction with coenzymes of niacin, in the transfer of labile hydrogen in the cytochrome system. It is involved with pyridoxine in the conversion of tryptophan to nicotinic acid. Riboflavin is important in the respiration of poorly vascularized tissues, the cornea for example, and is a component of porphyropsin, a retinal pigment necessary for adaptation to light. Porphyropsin is found in the retina of most freshwater fishes and is a conjugated flavonoid protein. This flavonoid protein is responsible for reflecting light from the retinal tapetum.

Thiamine or its active coenzyme, thiamine pyrophosphate, participates in carbohydrate metabolism. Thiamine pyrophosphate acts in conjunction with pyruvate dehydrogenase in the decarboxylation of pyruvic acid. Thiamine is essential for normal nervous tissue function. It participates in decarboxylation reactions leading to the formation of carbon dioxide, and is essential for good appetite, normal digestion, growth, and fertility.

Choline acts as a methyl donor for metabolic reactions requiring single-carbon units, the formation

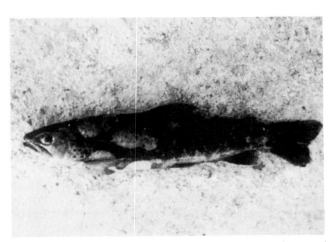

FIGURE 34–4. Biotin deficiency in a brown trout. Note the round edges of the lesions.

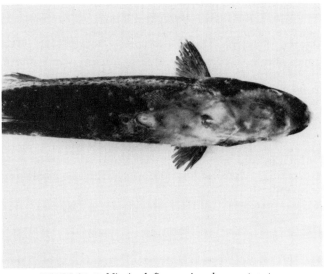

FIGURE 34–5. Niacin deficency in a brown trout.

of acetylcoenzyme A, for example. It is a major component of the neurotransmitter acetylcholine, and is essential for lipid transport.

Inositol is a structural component of certain tissues in which it acts as a lipotropic agent in the prevention of cholesterol accumulation. It serves as a carbohydrate reserve in muscle (myoinositol).

Lipoic acid is often mentioned as a water-soluble vitaminlike active biocatalyst. It participates in the decarboxylation of pyruvic acid, but it is not directly associated with thiamine pyrophosphate. It is both lipid and water soluble. Lipoic acid is widely distributed in lower vertebrates, and it can be synthesized by fishes and is, therefore, not a dietary essential.

Fat-Soluble Vitamins

The fat-soluble vitamins are covered in more detail in the chapter on nutrition in koi, carp, and goldfish (Chap. 46). Vitamin A is essential to maintain the integrity of epithelial cells, particularly the gill epithelium. Excessive dietary vitamin A can be toxic, and may result in slow growth, anemia, and caudal fin necrosis (Poston, 1977). Conversion of carotenes to vitamin A is limited in cold-water fishes, thus salmonids may have an absolute requirement for vitamin A.

Vitamin D is stored in large quantities in the liver of fishes. The calciferols are biologically active in the absorption of dietary calcium and, to a lesser degree, phosphorus. Although it has been known for many years that this vitamin is required by terrestrial animals, it did not receive recognition as essential in the diet of salmonids until the late 1970s, probably because most environmental waters contain dissolved calcium and phosphorus ions. Since both ions can be absorbed via the gills, there is often no requirement for absorption from the alimentary tract. Active forms of vitamin D are known to enhance transport and utilization of calcium and phosphorus in the fish body. It activates alkaline phosphatase, and is directly involved in phosphorus metabolism.

Vitamin E has been called the "antisterility" vitamin, which is probably a misnomer. The biologic activity of vitamin E is through eight naturally occurring compounds, with α-tocopherol being the most active. Deficiencies lead to a form of myomeric dystrophy. Tocopherol, cystine, and selenium act in unison to prevent the problem. Vitamin E acts as a biologic antioxidant and protects fish against oxidative agents.

Vitamin K is essential for the synthesis of prothrombin. This is extremely important for an aquatic animal in which small external wounds could be fatal from blood loss unless blood clotting is especially efficient.

Fiber

Fiber describes a number of nondigestible complex polysaccharides and carbohydrates (celluloses, pentosans, lignins, and others) in the diet. The small amounts of some of these compounds digested by higher animals is accomplished by bacterial flora in the gut. Salmonids have no stable bacterial flora in the alimentary tract and there is little or no digestion of fibrous compounds (National Academy of Sciences, 1981).

Eight percent or greater fiber in the diet of rainbow trout results in an apparent inability to absorb required nutrients. Excess dietary fiber prevents the fish from consuming enough energy to maintain satisfactory growth (Poston, 1986a). The rations of trout and salmon are formulated to reduce fiber as much as possible. Vegetable ingredients in salmonid rations add fiber to the diet. It is recommended that diets contain no more than 4% fiber (Post, 1987).

Dietary Energy

Fish require a caloric intake that will support their metabolism. Salmonid body temperature is maintained near the environmental temperature and the metabolic rate is altered by changes in the environmental temperature.

There is little need for dietary intake when salmonids are at low temperatures. The metabolic rate increases parabolically with environmental temperature (see Fig. 34–1), so salmonids require an ever-increasing caloric intake as the environmental temperature increases (Winberg, 1956). The size of salmonids also affects their caloric intake. Larger fish require fewer calories than small fish of the same species (see Fig. 34–2). Table 34–7 provides a guide to daily food intake in percentage of body weight (Duel et al., 1952). Salmonid caloric intake requirements have not been specifically determined because of the rapid changes in the metabolic rate with fish size and environmental temperature. However, practical experience indicates that between 3000 and 3500 kcal of metabolizable energy per kilogram of ration, and approximately 100 mg of well-balanced protein per kilocalorie of metabolizable energy is appropriate (National Academy of Sciences, 1981; 1973).

Fish have no single basal metabolic rate with which to establish a basic energy intake. There have been attempts to label a specific environmental temperature in which the fish appear to be most comfortable. This is called the standard environmental temperature for a species and the metabolic rate of a resting fish at that temperature is called the standard or routine metabolic rate. Changes in feed requirements with temperature and fish size have been determined for several salmonid species and incorporated into feed charts. The modified New York Feeding Chart (see Table 34–7) continues to be used as a guide to formulate rations to be fed to varioussized salmonids at various water temperatures (Deuel et al., 1952; Post, 1987; National Academy of Sciences, 1981).

Other methods of estimating food quantities fed

TABLE 34–7. Feeding Chart Guide (Ration to Feed per Day in Percentage of Body Weight)

Water Temperature (°C)	Number of Fish/kg (length in cm)										
	5600 or less (<2.5)	5600–670 (2.5–5.0)	670–190 (5.0–7.5)	190–83 (7.5–10)	83–43 (10–13)	43–26 (13–15)	26–16 (15–18)	16–11 (18–20)	11–8 (20–23)	8–6 (23–25)	6 or less (>25)
6	3.6	3.0	2.5	1.9	1.4	1.2	1.0	0.9	0.8	0.7	0.6
7	4.0	3.3	2.7	2.1	1.6	1.3	1.1	1.0	0.9	0.8	0.7
8	4.3	3.6	3.0	2.3	1.7	1.4	1.2	1.0	0.9	0.8	0.7
9	4.5	3.8	3.1	2.4	1.8	1.5	1.3	1.1	1.0	0.9	0.8
10	5.2	4.3	3.4	2.7	2.0	1.7	1.4	1.2	1.1	1.0	0.9
11	5.4	4.5	3.6	2.8	2.1	1.8	1.5	1.3	1.2	1.0	0.9
12	5.8	4.9	3.9	3.0	2.3	1.9	1.6	1.4	1.3	1.1	1.0
13	6.1	5.1	4.2	3.2	2.4	2.0	1.7	1.5	1.3	1.2	1.0
14	6.7	5.5	4.5	3.5	2.6	2.1	1.8	1.6	1.4	1.2	1.1
15	7.3	6.0	5.0	3.7	2.8	2.3	1.9	1.7	1.5	1.3	1.2
16	7.8	6.5	5.3	4.1	3.1	2.5	2.0	1.8	1.6	1.4	1.3
17	8.4	7.0	5.7	4.5	3.4	2.7	2.1	1.9	1.7	1.5	1.4
18	9.0	7.5	6.1	4.9	3.6	2.9	2.2	2.0	1.8	1.6	1.5
19	9.2	7.7	6.2	5.0	3.7	3.0	2.3	2.1	1.9	1.7	1.6
20	9.3	7.9	6.3	5.1	3.8	3.1	2.4	2.2	2.0	1.8	1.7

Adapted from Deuel C.R., et al., (1952) The New York State Feeding Chart. New York Conservation Commission Fisheries Research Bulletin No. 3.

to fishes to maximize production include adjusting the amount of feed to the amount of biologically available oxygen in the water. Food quantities are fed to use as much of the available oxygen as possible without depleting the aqueous dissolved oxygen below a critical level. This requires experience with a particular water supply and acceptable loading of fish biomass per unit water (Buterbaugh and Willoughby, 1967). Food quantity estimation can also be based on food conversion to fish body weight gain, or net energy conversion. An acceptable feeding level should provide about 70% of the calories for body maintenance and 30% for growth. Energy requirements can also be used to establish feeding levels, based on the body surface area of the fish and water temperature. For example, an actively growing rainbow trout requires 60 cal/dm² of body surface area per hour at 15°C.

$$\text{Body Surface Area} = \frac{(\text{Body Weight})^{2/3}}{10}$$

Special ration formulations and feeding levels can also include adjustments for fish activity and the corresponding metabolic rate change. However, most ration formulations do not account for activity-induced metabolic rate alterations, leaving food quantity adjustments to practical experience of the husbandryman.

RATIONS FOR INTENSIVELY REARED SALMONIDS

Salmonid diet preparations are of three major types: wet (moist), semidry (semimoist), and dry. Wet rations have approximately 70% moisture and they are prepared from fresh meat or fish products.

Semidry rations are prepared from a ground meat or fish fraction and a dry meal fraction; the moisture content is approximately 35%. Dry rations contain approximately 10% moisture and are prepared from dry animal and vegetable products with crystalline vitamin and minerals added (Post, 1987).

Wet Rations

Wet rations are used for rearing salmonids in many parts of the world where fresh meat and/or fish products are inexpensive. The meat is ground to a consistency commensurate with the size of fish. Crystalline vitamins may be added to the mix to make up for losses during processing or storage. Also, a binding agent may be added to reduce loss of nutrients while the food is in the water prior to being ingested by the fish. This type of ration is the least desirable because it is difficult to prepare, requires continuous refrigerated storage, and is inconsistent from day to day. All fish products should be pasteurized to eliminate potential pathogens before being fed to fishes.

Semidry Rations

Semidry salmonid rations are formulated from a meat and/or fish fraction and a dry meal fraction. The meat fraction is ground and mixed with approximately equal parts of dry, ground animal, or vegetable products. Crystalline vitamins and minerals are added to supply requirements for essential nutrients. The mixture is stored either chilled or frozen. Chilled semidry rations are usually fed from the hand by forming boluses to be thrown into the water. Semidry rations to be frozen are usually pressed into the desired pellet or particle size first. The ration is fed while frozen, either by hand or mechanical feeder. An example of frozen, moist pellets is the Oregon moist pellet, one of the first formulations of this ration type used. Semidry rations can be formulated to exacting specifications, but they require refrigerated storage. Nonfrozen semidry rations containing up to 35% moisture are prepared using humectants and mold inhibitors, and stored at room temperatures. Propylene glycol is usually the humectant of choice because it also has mold-inhibiting properties. Sorbates or propionates may also be added to assist in mold inhibition (Hughes, 1988). These rations are usually more expensive than other semidry rations and are used primarily as fry or fingerling diets (Ketola and Rumsey, 1985; Lemm, 1983).

Dry Rations

Dry rations are widely used for the feeding of salmonids in those parts of the world where major milling technology is available. Dry animal and vegetable meals and other natural products such as animal fats, fish oils, fish solubles, raw sugar, specific crystalline amino acids, crystalline vitamins, minerals, antioxidants, and other specific compounds are mixed and processed into pellets or particles commensurate with the size of fish being fed. Two forms of dry particulate rations are prepared: (1) solid, sinking pellets/particles, or (2) floating pellets mixed with air and extruded. Dry rations are usually prepared with slight excesses of fragile nutrients so they can be stored at room temperature for up to 90 days and remain complete and balanced. Dry rations are fed by hand or from mechanical automatic feeders adjusted to release desired quantities of ration at specified times. These rations are also fed from demand feeders.

FORMULATION PROCEDURES

The first step in formulating a ration is to establish the type of ration and the size (age) of fish to be fed (Post, 1975). Specifications are made for total protein (amino acid profile), maximum fat, maximum digestible carbohydrate, metabolizable energy content, maximum ash, maximum fiber, and the presence of required quantities of all essential vitamins and minerals to support health.

An arithmetic approach to formulation can be used by constructing a chart listing each selected ingredient, the percentage of each ingredient in the final formulation, and an expression of each nutrient contributed to the final ration by each ingredient (Post, 1975). This procedure is difficult and time consuming but can be used when sophisticated computers are not available.

Computers and computer programs are used in the milling industry to prepare a wide variety of least-cost domestic animal ration formulations and

can be used for fish rations. Many linear computer programs have simplified the difficult procedure of matching nutritional requirements of the fish to nutrient availability in ingredients. Constraints must be given to direct the computer away from using large quantities of certain ingredients because of palatability. It may also be necessary to set minimum levels of nutritionally desirable and expensive ingredients the computer would pass over because of cost.

The final formulation will be no better than the information given in the feedstuffs tables. Technologies for manufacturing some feedstuffs change and yield moderately disadvantageous qualities to the ingredient. The addition of salt to high seas–caught fish to reduce autolysis between the time of catch and processing into fishmeal is an example. The additional salt reflects as increased ash when large quantities of the fishmeal are incorporated into fish rations. Another example is the difference in the protein digestibility coefficient for rainbow trout between flame-dried blood with a digestibility coefficient near zero, and ring- or spray-dried blood with a digestive coefficient of approximately 65%.

The method used to establish a ration formulation does not matter as long as the information reflects a nutritionally acceptable and millable mixture of ingredients. Proximate analyses, vitamin and amino acid assays, mineral analyses, and calorimetry should be a part of the evaluation of the first milling of an untried ration formulation. Combinations of these analyses with nutritional evaluation when fed to fish may suggest minor changes in the formula. Computer- or hand calculator–derived ration formulations are only an estimate of nutritional performance when fed to fish.

Feedstuffs for Salmonid Rations

The choice of ingredients in a ration will vary depending on the type of diet being prepared, semidry, moist pellet, or dry pellet. Also, availability and cost of each ingredient must be considered; locally available products are usually less expensive. Digestibility coefficients and metabolizable energy values of each ingredient should be compared. A poor-quality, less expensive product, even though locally available, may yield less growth potential for fish than a more efficiently digested and absorbed product costing more per unit weight.

Protein and Amino Acids

To start, dietary protein and amino acid profiles are balanced to the requirements of the fish. Salmonid rations usually include good-quality fishmeal and feed grain meals such as soybean meal, cottonseed meal, corn gluten meal, rapeseed meal, peanut meal, or other high-protein seedmeals. Various other high-quality animal by-products (shrimp meal, poultry by-product meal, hydrolyzed feather meal, meat meals, blood flour, dried or condensed fish solubles, fish silage) rich in one or more of the indispensable amino acids are added to balance the amino acid requirements. Crystalline DL-methionine is the only economically available amino acid added to formulations when methionine is limiting.

Fat

Dietary fat is the next important consideration in salmonid ration formulation. Fish oils are rich in the required fatty acids (see Table 34–3). Thus, a quantity of good-quality fish oil to supply the minimum daily requirement of essential fatty acids is a basic ingredient of most formulations. Other dietary fat requirements can then be made up from economically available animal or vegetable fats. Beef tallow, lard, rendered poultry fat, and other animal fats are usually acceptable. Corn oil, soybean oil, and safflower oil are most desirable of the vegetable oils for salmonid rations. Cottonseed oil and other oilseed oils have also been used, but they are less acceptable nutrients.

Carbohydrate

Feedstuffs supplying the carbohydrate fraction of the ration include a wide variety of feed grains (wheat, corn, milo, sorghum, rice, brewer's grains, sesame seed), yeast, whey products, molasses, dried distiller's solubles, and many other low-fiber products. These products may also enhance the milling qualities of the ration.

Vitamins

Certain feedstuffs can be used in salmonid ration formulations to supply all or part of the vitamin requirements. Dried brewer's yeast, torula yeast, wheat germ meal, dried whey, and other products are good sources of B vitamins. Rice polishings, dried distiller's solubles, and similar products are sources of water-soluble vitamins and vitamins E and K. Quantitative vitamin requirements not present in the major ingredients of the ration formula must be supplied by crystalline vitamins, usually in the form of a vitamin premix. Calcium pantothenate and ascorbic acid tend to be depleted rapidly in a premix. They may be withheld and be added at feeding or can be microencapsulated to protect them in the premix.

Minerals

Mineral elements inherent in basic ingredients, or known to be present and available in the water supply, can be used to make up all or a large part of the quantitative mineral requirements. Dried yeasts are rich in zinc, phosphorus, manganese, and copper. Whey products can supply much of the required calcium and phosphorus. Feed-grade molasses is a relatively good source of iron. Most seed grains can supply much if not all of the requirements for selenium, magnesium, manganese, iron, and zinc. Steamed bone meal or meat and bone meal in which a high percentage of the meal is bone is of little value as a mineral source for salmonids. Undigested bone particles end up on the bottom of holding ponds along with undigestible particles of flame-dried blood meal. These products should be replaced with ingredients of greater nutritional value. Fishmeals manufactured from filleted fish carcasses, often referred to as white fishmeal, should be avoided because of the high bone content.

Mineral requirements not present in the ingredients in the ration are supplied by a mineral mix containing specific quantities of those elements known to be below requirements. Care must be taken to use absorbable mineral compounds and those of acceptable palatability. Organomineral compounds (gluconates, lactates) of the required element are more expensive than inorganic compounds but do not alter palatability when used in relatively large quantities. More absorbable compounds such as magnesium chloride rather than the less soluble magnesium sulfate should be used. Some mineral supplements are such a small part of the mineral mix that they cause no alteration in palatability, for example, iodates or iodides, whereas others are used in relatively large amounts and palatability can be a concern. Also mineral mix supplementation should be kept to a minimum to minimize the ash content of the ration. Addition of large quantities of salt or calcium carbonate do not enhance nutrition, but may increase ration cost per unit of weight gain in the fish being fed.

Fiber

As mentioned earlier, dietary fiber is of no nutrient value to salmonids. Selecting reduced fiber ingredients such as dehulled soybean or cottonseed meal will reduce the undigestible, bulk material. Oat hulls, alfalfa meal, and beet pulp meal offer few nutrients for salmonids and add to the dietary fiber fraction of the ration.

Products To Avoid

Products containing adventitious toxins should be avoided in ration formulation. Soybean meal should be autoclaved properly to remove the trypsin inhibitor. Cottonseed meal should have been treated to remove gossipol. Canola (rapeseed) meals should be treated to reduce or eliminate gluconate and eurcic acid, which can cause thyroid malformation and malfunction (Hardy and Sullivan, 1983; Rapeseed Association of Canada, 1978). Fish oils and other highly unsaturated oils should be protected with antioxidants to reduce autoxidation and formation of peroxidation products. Any product with mold growth, especially those molds known to produce mycotoxins, should be avoided.

Special Ingredients

A wide variety of special ingredients are routinely or occasionally added to salmonid rations. Algin or lignin sulfonate enhance the milling, handling, and storage qualities of the finished ration. Mold inhibitors decrease mold growth on the finished ration during storage, especially in a warm, moist environment. Antioxidants reduce autoxidation of unsaturated fats and other easily oxidizable nutrients. Natural and synthetic carotenoids and xanthophyll pigments are sometimes added to the ration formula to produce desired skin or flesh pigmentation (Storebakken et al., 1987), or, in the case of broodfish ration, to produce a more marketable bright orange-red salmonid egg. This is discussed in more detail in the chapter on nutrition of koi, carp, and goldfish (Chap. 46).

Milling

Salmonids do not masticate food; therefore, special care must be taken to facilitate feedstuff digestion and absorption. Large particle–size feedstuffs must be pulverized before addition to the mixer. The size of the fish to be fed determines the size of the finished ration particle (Table 34–8). Each particle or pellet should contain a quantitative representation of each ingredient used to make up the formulation, so pulverization and mixing are extremely important.

The type of ration desired determines the milling equipment required. Moist pellet rations and dry floating rations are processed through extrusion machines. Ingredients for moist particle rations are mixed, passed through an extrusion plate with correct size openings, quick frozen, bagged, and stored frozen. Dry floating particles are manufactured by entraining air and moisture in the mixer. The ration is then passed through an extrusion plate, dried, bagged, and stored at room temperature. The ingredients for dry, sinking rations are mixed, treated with steam, processed through a standard pellet mill,

TABLE 34–9. Food Particle Size and Sieve Size Correlation

Particle Size Designation	U.S. and Canadian Standard Sieve Number		Sieve Opening (mm)
#1 Fry (starter)	Over	No. 40	0.42
	Through	No. 28	0.64
#2 Fry Ration	Over	No. 28	
	Through	No. 16	1.19
#3 Crumbles	Over	No. 16	
	Through	No. 12	1.68
#4 Crumbles	Over	No. 12	
	Through	No. 10	2.04
#5 Crumbles	Over	No. 10	
	Through	No. 7	2.82
#6 Crumbles	Over	No. 7	
	Through	No. 5	3.80

cooled, dried, bagged, and stored at room temperature.

The pellet size used is related to the size of the fish being fed. Rations for salmonids averaging 120 or fewer fish per kilogram (fish longer than 14 cm) are produced by specific size pelleting dies, and cut into short, intermediate, or long lengths. Smaller salmonids with more than 120 fish per kilogram (shorter than 14 cm) are fed particulate diets processed from dried pellets. The pellets are crumbled in a roller mill and then passed through a specific screen size to produce desired size "crumbles" (Table 34–9).

Dry rations of all types (floating particulate or sinking pellet) should be hard enough to resist abrasion while stored as stacked bags, in bulk feed bins, or during shipping. Crumbles or pellets not resisting abrasion lose small particles (fines) that will be lost in the feeding process. A milled ration formula that through normal handling, storage, and shipping yields fines of greater than 1% of its weight is considered unsatisfactory.

A pellet or particle that is too soft not only loses nutrients by abrasion and production of fines but also may soak apart in the water before it can be taken in by the fish. However, the pellet or particle should not be so hard that it will not soak apart within a reasonable time in the fish stomach. A properly milled and satisfactory ration formulation for salmonids should hold together 4 to 5 minutes in water, yet fall apart within at least 12 to 15 minutes. Slight formulation changes may be necessary to yield a pellet or particle of satisfactory consistency (Post, 1975). The best devised formulation will yield poor results if it is not milled properly.

Commercial Milling

Not all laboratories or fish producers have equipment to mill rations. These facilities must rely on commercially produced, closed-formula rations, or locate a commercial feed miller to prepare rations. A closed-formula ration is devised to be generally satisfactory under most water quality conditions. These

TABLE 34–8. Food Particle Size Correlation with Fish Size

Particle Size Designation	Acceptable Fish Sizes (No. of Fish/kg)
#1 Fry Stater	4400–2200
#2 Fry Ration	2200–1100
#3 Crumbles	1100–770
#4 Crumbles	770–220
#5 Crumbles	220–190
#6 Crumbles	190–120
3/32" Pellets	120–85
1/8" Pellets	85–50
5/32" Pellets	50–20
3/16" Pellets	20–4
7/32" Pellets	4–2
3/8" Pellets	Fewer than 2

All pellets can be cut to short, intermediate, and long lengths.

formulations are guarded by the miller, so fish producers must rely on the miller to maintain ration quality, and have no input on sources or quality of ingredients used. Usually commercial millers will not continue to sell smaller-particle rations without orders for pelleted rations. There is less profit on small-particle (fry starter through #6 Crumbles) rations because of additional handling and the special equipment necessary to prepare them.

Feeding Practices

Methods of feeding are an extremely important part of the success or failure of a well-formulated salmonid ration. Misfeeding of a well-balanced, carefully milled ration may reflect erroneously on the biologic performance of the ration. There are many methods of feeding salmonids including feeding by hand, using time-set automatic feeding devices, mechanical feeding devices, or demand feeding devices. There are advantages and disadvantages to each method.

Feeding from the hand is labor intensive and time consuming but has the advantage of personal observation for overfeeding or underfeeding and acceptance or rejection of the ration. Also, the ration is offered to the fish where they are in the pond.

Automatic feeding devices feed the fish at predetermined times. Disadvantages of these devices include their high initial cost. They can also become clogged, so no ration is released at the prescribed time. Power failures may interfere with feeding intervals.

Mechanical feeding devices are usually attached to a vehicle, driven by the husbandryman, or a robot vehicle guided by electronic relays. Those operated by the husbandryman have the advantage of personal observation, but are labor intensive.

Demand feeding devices are suspended above the water. A long wire "trigger" extends from the bottom of the device into the water. Fish learn to bump the trigger and release a small quantity of ration. The fish do this until satiated. Demand feeders are much less labor intensive than other feeding devices. They do require that the containment vessel be stocked as it empties. Disadvantages of these devices are only fish large enough to activate the trigger can be fed, and some belligerent fish tend to keep timid fish away from the feeding area below the device.

The procedure by which the ration is offered to the fish is a matter of choice; distribution so each fish receives a fair share of the offering is essential. Nutritionally related diseases may result if excessive or inadequate quantities of diet are received by some or all fish.

Monitoring Clinical Parameters Related to Nutritional Status

Normal, healthy and nutritionally balanced salmonids being fed a satisfactory ration using acceptable feeding practices, and residing in an acceptable environment, should be resistant to infectious and other types of disease. These fish should continue satisfactory and economic growth. The population should demonstrate a minimum mortality level. External appearance should meet acceptable standards, and blood parameters should be within normal ranges.

Biologic and/or clinical standard values are essential to the judgment of health in these animals. Collecting data on representative samples of a population can be used to evaluate nutritional health. Table 34–10 lists biologic and clinical values frequently used to assess nutrition-related health status. Careful scrutiny should be given to diet and diet-related factors if a population of fish fail to meet these values.

TABLE 34–10. Parameters used to Evaluate Nutritional Status of Salmonids

Parameter	Range of Acceptable Values
Conversion ratio	< 2.0 kg ration/kg gain
Protein: gain ratio	475–650 g dietary protein/kg gain
Energy: gain ratio	3600–5500 kcal dietary energy/kg gain
Percent gain	5–300%/month (depending on age and environmental temperature)
Percent mortality	< 0.1% per month
Blood hematocrit	≥ 42%
Blood hemoglobin	≥ 10 g/dl
Erythrocyte count	≥ 1 million/cu^3
Blood glucose	70–120 mg/dl
Serum protein	≥ 3.5 g/dl

NUTRITIONAL DISEASES

Protein Deficiency

Gross protein deficiency in salmonids is usually a deficiency of one or more essential amino acids. The first sign is usually reduced growth. Long-term deficiency results in malfunction of hepatic, hematopoietic, endocrine, and other organ systems relying on enzymes, hormones, or intermediates synthesized from the essential amino acid which is deficient.

Specific diagnosis of gross protein and/or essential amino acid deficiency is difficult because of the broad impact on many body functions. Early changes are subtle and nonspecific. Food conversion becomes less efficient and the conversion ratio will exceed 2 kg of ration per kilogram gain. The mortality rate will increase slowly in the early stages of deficiency and become more pronounced if the deficiency is not corrected. Grams of protein and kilocalories per kilogram of body weight gain will increase.

Clinical findings include moderate to severe anemia, with a decreased hematocrit, erythrocyte count, and blood hemoglobin content. Serum total protein will be reduced (see Table 34–10).

Gross protein or essential amino acid deficiency resembles other noninfectious diseases as well as diseases caused by certain infectious agents. Exami-

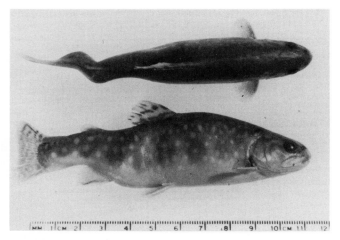

FIGURE 34–6. Scoliosis and lordosis due to tryptophan deficiency.

nation of the ration formulation is essential to diagnosis. The use of poor-quality protein in a ration without increasing the percent of protein-bearing feedstuffs is a common finding. Response to treatment can be a valuable diagnostic observation in early cases. Growth will be restored if the essential amino acids are replaced in the diet prior to onset of severe damage to vital body functions (see Fig. 34–1) (Halver et al., 1957; Shanks et al., 1962; Post, 1987). Specific essential amino acid deficiencies may also have specific clinical signs other than reduced growth.

Tryptophan deficiency causes transient scoliosis in rainbow trout (Kloppel and Post, 1975; Poston and Rumsey, 1983), and scoliosis and lordosis in sockeye salmon (Halver and Shanks, 1960) and brook trout (Fig. 34–6). Replacement of required amounts of tryptophan to the diet of scoliotic or lordotic fish results in complete reversal of the syndrome and return to normal growth. Probably all salmonids will be affected similarly in cases of tryptophan deficiency.

Another specific syndrome associated with an essential amino acid deficiency is the tendency toward cataracts in trout fed diets with reduced tryptophan or methionine. The condition is increased when the diet has limited zinc (Poston and Rumsey, 1983; Poston, 1986b). Eye lens abnormalities may be the result of reduced growth of epithelial tissues. Caudal fin and opercular growth may also be affected.

Diseases Related to Dietary Lipids

There are four general pathologic syndromes involving dietary lipids in salmonids: obesity, fatty infiltration of organs, deficiency of essential fatty acids, and toxicity from autoxidation of unsaturated fats.

Obesity

Obesity is common in fish fed high-fat rations. Many commercial trout and salmon rations contain up to 18% ether extract (crude fat). These rations may yield satisfactory body weight gain, some or much of which will be weight gain of adipose tissue. Normal, well-nourished salmonids should have a trim external appearance and moderate fat storage in adipose tissues surrounding ceca, intestine, spleen, and stomach. Obese salmonids will have distended abdomens with masses of adipose fat, which in many cases may limit visibility of the abdominal organs. Adipose tissue may extend into the upper abdominal cavity, surrounding the liver and possibly the heart.

Fatness or trimness of salmonids can be judged mathematically using the formula below, where C represents a condition index, W is the weight of the fish in grams, and L is the length of the fish in centimeters.

$$C = \frac{(W \times 10)^2}{L^3}$$

This condition index should be near unity for a fish of desirable general robustness (Lagler, 1956).

Fatty Infiltration of the Liver

Fatty infiltration of the liver may accompany obesity and may be the result of feeding high-fat diets. The liver appears yellow to ochre and sometimes mottled. The cut surface of the liver from a fish with fatty infiltration appears greasy and a film of oil will appear when the cut liver surface is touched to the surface of water. Intracellular fat droplets will be observed microscopically in thin frozen sections stained with Sudan-IV, Oil Red O, or Sudan Black B (Preese, 1972). Intracellular fat droplets will usually appear round or oval. The clinician must distinguish between intracellular fat droplets and those lying extracellularly between liver cells. The severity of fatty infiltration must be judged by the relative quantities of intracellular fat droplets. A few are acceptable, but the condition is pathologic when large amounts are observed in the cytoplasm of most liver cells in a hepatic lobule. Liver fatty infiltration may also result from biotin and/or choline deficiency, toxemias, or other causes, all of which must be ruled out in the diagnosis.

Elimination of fatty liver syndrome in a population of fish can often be accomplished by reducing dietary fat intake or alteration of the saturation level of dietary fat. Highly saturated fats, especially tallows, fed to small salmonids in cold water (10°C or less) may exacerbate fatty infiltration of the liver. Rations containing greater than 15 to 18% ether extract (crude fat) may also be predispose to the condition. Adding more choline chloride to the ration fed to the fish may assist in eliminating excess intracellular fat by increasing hepatic fat metabolism.

Essential Fatty Acid Deficiency

The pathologic syndrome associated with deficiency of essential fatty acid(s) in rainbow trout includes reduced growth, depigmentation, fin erosion, and fainting, and possibly similar conditions in other salmonids. Rainbow trout receiving a ration with less than 1.0% 18:3ω3 (or 0.9% 18:3ω3 plus at least 0.1% 18:3ω6) may become pale. The greater the deficiency, the greater the depigmentation, to the point where not only is the red-pink pigmentation lost, but the gray to blue to black as well. The fish appear pale silver-white, with no "rainbow," parr marks, or other normal body pigmentation. Also, the severity of growth reduction and fin erosion is related to the degree and duration of the deficiency (Phillips and Podoliak, 1957; Post, 1987; Castell et al., 1972).

The fainting, or shock, syndrome in rainbow trout fed rations deficient in essential fatty acids begins by rapid or frantic swimming when excited or netted. This is followed by immobility and/or loss of consciousness. Fish demonstrating either condition float on the water surface or sink to the tank bottom and remain in an immobile state for a few minutes.

They either recover by swimming up or die. These fish do not survive routine handling (Castell et al., 1972). A similar condition may occur in other salmonids but has not been reported. The condition can be alleviated on addition of fish oils or other items high 18:3ω3 fatty acid to the ration.

Lipid Autoxidation Toxicity

Salmonid rations generally contain relatively high levels of polyunsaturated fats and oils. This is because fish receiving the ration are classified as cold-water fishes and their environmental temperature is generally less than 15°C. Saturated fats become hard and difficult to digest, especially for small (young) salmonids. Unsaturated fats are subject to autoxidation (peroxidation or rancidification). Peroxides, aldehydes, and other similar compounds are formed. These compounds are extremely toxic to trout and possibly all salmonids. Toxic effects from feeding rations containing small quantities of these compounds include necrosis of renal hematopoietic tissue, resulting in an extreme megaloblastic anemia. Hepatic ceroid accumulation, nephrosis (see Plate 28A–D in Post, 1987) and nutritional muscular dystrophy are also seen. Affected fishes become emaciated, dark, lose scales, develop fin necrosis, and have pale gills. Mortality levels increase and all fish will die if rations containing greater than 10 mg of the toxic compounds per kilogram of dietary fat continue to be fed. The condition is usually much more pronounced in small fish (12 cm or less).

Affected fish have light, straw-colored ascitic fluid, enlarged spleens, pale yellow livers, moderately swollen kidneys, which ooze pale pink blood when cut, and a general appearance of extreme anemia in all organs. The stomach and intestine may be free of food and filled with bile-stained fluid.

The syndrome associated with the feeding of relative high levels of rancidification products resembles vitamin E deficiency, and well it should, because dietary vitamin E is destroyed in the autoxidation process. Diagnosis of this toxic condition is based on external and internal appearances. Hematologic findings include hematocrits as low as 7%, hemoglobin content as low as 2.5 g/dl, and erythrocyte counts as low as 0.15 million/mm^3. Analysis of the ration for autoxidation products is confirmational. Quantities of thiobarbituric acid greater than 10 mg/kg of fat are considered pathognomonic. Thiobarbituric acid levels of 2 to 5 mg/kg of fat should not be fed to small trout or small salmon. Larger fish (greater than 20 cm) may be capable of withstanding the toxic effects of small amounts in the ration. However, larger fish fed a ration known to contain 2 to 5 mg of thiobarbituric acid per kg of dietary fat should be watched closely for signs of anemia and the ration should be withdrawn if anemia is noted.

Prevention of thiobarbituric acid toxicity to susceptible fish can be accomplished by protecting the ration with antioxidants (ethoxyquin, santoquin, butylated hydroxyanisole, or butylated hydroxytoluene). The antioxidant should be added to susceptible ration formulations to the maximum allowable level of 0.02% of the ration. Vitamin E acts as an antioxidant within the mixed ration and will be destroyed if other sources of antioxidant are depleted on storage.

Formulating rations with ingredients containing catalyzing agents should be avoided. Hemoglobin is known to catalyze autoxidation in dry rations. Therefore, ingredients containing hemoglobin such as blood or blood products, dried meat scrap meal, and dried liver meal should be held to a minimum or eliminated. The hemoglobin present in whole fishmeals may possibly catalyze autoxidation in the ration. Cold storage, even frozen storage, will not prevent hemoglobin catalyzation in dry ration mixtures. Rations known to contain relatively large amounts of hemoglobin-bearing ingredients, combined with polyunsaturated fats, should be fed soon after preparation, usually within 2 weeks.

Diseases Related to Dietary Carbohydrates

Carbohydrate Overload

Excess digestible carbohydrate in the ration of salmonids causes hyperglycemia, hepatohyperglyconeogenisis, and hepatomegaly. Blood glucose is normally 70 to 120 mg/dl of blood (see Table 34–10). Blood glucose levels may exceed 300 mg/dl of blood when relatively high levels of digestible carbohydrates are fed. Hyperglycemia is usually accompanied by excessive quantities of glycogen stored in hepatic cells. The significance of this condition is not known in salmonids. Liver glycogen is normally 0.5 to 5.0% of the liver mass, but may increase to as high as 17% of the liver mass when the fish are fed rations high in digestible carbohydrate. Trout with hyperglycemia of approximately 300 mg glucose per deciliter of blood, accompanied by glycogen storage approaching 15% of the liver mass, will usually be lethargic, become dark, seek the sides of the holding facility or swim near the surface of the water, and may refuse to take food. These fish may spontaneously resume feeding after several days of refusing food when blood glucose and liver glycogen reduces. There may or may not be increased mortality (National Academy of Sciences, 1978).

Diagnosis of the condition is by blood glucose and liver glycogen analyses. There will be an increase in liver size as liver glycogen storage increases. Normal rainbow trout have a liver mass to body weight ratio of between 0.8 and 1.5%. A ratio of greater than 3% has been observed in rainbow trout with hyperglycemia (Post, 1987).

Liver histopathology can be used to estimate the severity of the condition. Hepatocyte vacuolation is common in salmonids, but glycogen will stain magenta with periodic acid–Schiff reagent and can be digested and removed from histologic sections by treatment with diastase (see Plates 7M and 28E in Post, 1987).

Vitamin Deficiencies

Basic ration ingredients may not always contain the expected level of each vitamin because the source of an ingredient, methods of processing it, or methods of storing either the ingredients or the finished ration may change. Fish receiving a deficient ration will gradually become deficient as they deplete stored vitamins. Thus, vitamin deficiency syndromes are usually chronic conditions that develop slowly. These conditions are summarized in Table 34–11.

Dietary Mineral Deficiencies and Toxicities

There are few known syndromes in salmonids related to specific dietary mineral deficiencies or toxicities. Research on dietary mineral deficiency is difficult because certain minerals in the water may reduce or eliminate the need for them in the diet.

Iodine Deficiency

Probably the first known disease in fish involving a mineral deficiency was endemic goiter from reduced iodine in both food and water. The condition was reported in brook trout in 1910. It was mistaken for thyroid carcinoma, but further studies and addition of about 2% iodized salt to the diet prevented the condition and proved it to be goiter (Marine and Lenhart, 1910; Gaylord and Marsh, 1912).

Definitive diagnosis of iodine deficiency can be

TABLE 34–11. Vitamin Deficiency Syndromes in Salmonids

Vitamin Deficiency	Signs
Water-Soluble	
Ascorbic acid	Scoliosis; lordosis; impaired collagen formation; altered support cartilage in eye, fin, and gill; capillary fragility especially of gill; hemorrhagic exophthalmos; intramuscular hemorrhage; anemia; ascites; anorexia; reduced growth; reduced liver ascorbic acid; reduced serum thyroid hormone (T_3); reduced cholinesterase; elevated plasma cholesterol and triglycerides.
Vitamin B_{12}	Hematologic disorders; anemia; microcytic easily fragmented erythrocytes; reduced hemoglobin.
Biotin	Skin lesions (blue slime); muscle atrophy; degeneration of gill lamellae; reduced growth and food conversion; liver fatty infiltration; altered fatty acid synthesis; glycogen storage in kidney tubules; degeneration of pancreatic acinar cells; reduced liver acetyl CoA carboxylase and pyruvate carboxylase.
Choline	Reduced growth; reduced food conversion; liver fatty degeneration.
Folic acid	Macrocytic anemia; pale colored gills; anorexia; reduced growth; reduced food conversion.
Inositol	Anorexia reduced growth and food conversion; slow gastric emptying time with distended stomach; reduced cholinesterase and transaminase activity; increased neutral lipids and triglycerides in liver.
Niacin	Anemia; anorexia; reduced growth and food conversion; skin lesions with hemorrhage; lesions in lower intestine.
Pantothenic acid	Clubbed exudate–covered gills; proximal lamellar hyperplasia; anorexia; reduced growth; anemia; atrophy of pancreatic acinar cells; vacuoles and hyaline droplets in kidney tubules.
Pyridoxine	Nervous disorders (epileptiform convulsions); anorexia, anemia; erratic, spiral swimming; rapid breathing and gasping; blue-violet iridescent skin color; flexing of opercles; rapid rigor mortis.
Riboflavin	Corneal vascularization with lens to corneal adhesion; reduced vision; dark skin; cataract; anorexia; reduced growth.
Thiamin	Convulsions followed by body flexure and possible death; instability and loss of equilibrium; anorexia, reduced growth; low transketolase activity in erythrocytes and kidneys.
Fat-Soluble	
Vitamin A	Retinal degeneration; exophthalmos with eye lens displacement; depigmentation; edema with ascites, reduced growth.
Vitamin D	Tetany of white skeletal muscle; impaired calcium homeostasis.
Vitamin E	Muscular dystrophy; microcytic anemia; reduced activity and growth; ascites; depigmentation.
Vitamin K	Prolonged blood clotting time; reduced hematocrit; anemia.

Data derived from Poston-Roche Information Service (1986); Sato et al. (1983) Effect of water temperature on the skeletal deformity in ascorbic acid deficient rainbow trout. Bull. Jpn. Soc. Sci. Fish. 49:443–446; Poston, H. A., and Page, J. W. (1982) Gross and histological signs of dietary deficiencies of biotin and pantothenic acid in lake trout Salvelinus namaycush. Cornell Vet. 72:242–261; and National Academy of Sciences (1981) Nutrient Requirements of Cold Water Fishes. National Research Council, Washington, D.C.

made by the external appearance and histologic examination of thyroid tissue. Analysis for stored iodine in thyroid tissue may also be used (Woodall and LaRoche, 1964). Advanced goiter will be observable as a swelling in the thyroid gland region from the base of the tongue to near the atrium of the heart. The extent of the hyperplasia will depend on the severity of iodine deficiency and the length of time the condition has been evolving.

Zinc Deficiency

Deficiency of zinc has been associated with cataracts in salmonids. Addition of calcium, phosphorus, sodium, or potassium to cataractogenic diets will increase the severity of the condition (Poston et al., 1978; Ketola, 1979).

Iron Deficiency

Feeding iron-deficient rations (less than 1 mg iron/kg ration) will probably produce a microcytic, hypochromic anemia in salmonids as it occurs in other fishes (Sakamoto and Yone, 1978). Diagnosis of suspected iron deficiency is by hematologic examination and analysis of the ration for quantitative iron. The ration should contain 80 to 100 mg iron/ kg. Iron is poorly absorbed from environmental water and should be supplied in the ration.

Other Mineral Deficiencies

Deletion or deficiency of dietary manganese in rainbow trout causes reduced growth, cataracts, and dwarfism (Yamamoto et al., 1983). Deletion of magnesium also causes cataracts (Satoh et al., 1983). Deficiencies of other dietary macromineral elements or ions (calcium, potassium, sodium, chloride, and sulfate) have not been studied in salmonids, nor have the trace minerals aluminum, copper, cobalt, or molybdenum. The fish disease diagnostician should be aware that these elements or ions are essential to fish health and must either be present in the diet or available from environmental water.

Mineral Toxicities

Some macro- or trace minerals may produce adverse effects if present in food for the fish. Dietary mercury may contribute to the body burden of mercury. The problem is not so much reaching toxic levels, but the United States Food and Drug Administration (FDA) tolerance for food fish tissues is for a maximum of 0.5 mg mercury/kg of fish tissue. Salmonids are not acceptable as food for humans if mercury exceeds this level.

Rainbow trout have been fed rations as high as 13 mg selenium per kilogram of diet without toxic effects. This dietary level produces elevated blood levels of the selenium-bearing enzyme glutathione peroxidase (Hilton et al., 1980). Rainbow trout have been fed diets containing as high as 170 mg of zinc per kilogram of ration without toxic effects (Ogino and Yand, 1978; Wekell et al., 1983). Maximum dietary copper levels tolerated by rainbow trout have been found to be 665 mg copper per kilogram of diet. No specific signs of dietary toxicosis are noted at this level, although there may be initial growth depression followed by compensatory growth (Lanno et al., 1985).

LITERATURE CITED

Akiyama, T., Arai, S., and Murai, T. (1985) Threonine, histidine and lysine requirements of chum salmon. Bull. Jpn. Soc. Sci. Fish. 51:635–639.

Bromley, G., and Adkins, T.C. (1984) The influence of cellulose filler on feeding, growth and utilization of energy in rainbow trout, Salmo gairdneri, Richardson. J. Fish Biol. 24:235–244.

Buterbaugh, G.L., and Willoughby, H. (1967) A feeding guide for brook, brown and rainbow trout. Progressive Fish Culturist 29:210–215.

Castell, J.D., Sinnhuber, R.O., Wales, J.H., and Lee, D.J. (1972) Essential fatty acids in the diet of rainbow trout (Salmo gairdneri): Growth, feed conversion and some gross deficiency symptoms. J. Nutr. 102:77–85.

Cowey, C.B., Mackie, A.M., and Bell, J.G. (1985) Nutrition and feeding of fish. Academic Press, Orlando, Florida.

Deuel, C.R., Haskell, D.C., Brockway, D.R., and Kingsbury, O.R. (1952) The New York State Feeding Chart. N.Y. Cons. Comm. Fish. Research Bulletin No. 3.

Edwards, D.J., Austeng, E., Risa, S., and Gjedrem, T. (1977) Carbohydrate in rainbow trout diets. I. Growth of fish of different families fed diets containing different proportions of carbohydrate. Aquaculture. 11:31–38.

Gatlin, D.M., III, and Wilson, R.P. (1984) Studies on manganese requirements of fingerling channel catfish. Aquaculture 41:85–92.

Gatlin, D.M. III, Robinson, E.H., Poe, W.E., and Wilson, R.P. (1982) Magnesium requirements of fingerling channel catfish and signs of magnesium deficiency. J. Nutr. 112:1182–1187.

Gaylord, H.R., and Marsh, M.C. (1912) Carcinoma of the thyroid in salmonid fishes. U.S. Bull. Bur. Fish. 32:364–524.

Halver, J.E. (1957) Nutrition of salmonid fishes. IV. An amino acid test diet for chinook salmon. J. Nutr. 62:245–254.

Halver, J.E. (ed.) (1972) Fish Nutrition. Academic Press, New York.

Halver, J.E., and Coates, J.A. (1957) A vitamin test diet for long term feeding studies. Progressive Fish Culturist 19:112–118.

Halver, J.E. and Shanks, W.E. (1960) Nutrition of salmonid fishes. VIII. Indispensible amino acids for sockeye salmon. J. Nutr. 72:340–346.

Halver, J.E., Ashley, L.M., and Smith, R.R. (1969) Ascorbic acid requirements of coho salmon and rainbow trout. Trans. Am. Fish. Soc. 98:762–771.

Hardy, R. (1987) Fish silage and liquified fish products. Aquaculture 13:48–50.

Hardy, R.W., and Sullivan, C.V. (1983) Canola meal in rainbow trout (Salmo gairdneri) production diets. Can. J. Fish. Aquatic Sci. 40:281–286.

Hilton, J.W., Hodson, P.V., and Slinger, S.J. (1980) The requirements and toxicity of selenium in rainbow trout (Salmo gairdneri). J. Nutr. 110:2527–2535.

Hilton, J.W., Atkinson, J.L., and Slinger, S.J. (1983) Effects of increased dietary fiber on the growth of rainbow trout (Salmo gairdneri). Can. J. Fish. Aquatic Sci. 40:81–85.

Hoar, W.S. (1966) General and Comparative Physiology. Prentice-Hall, Englewood Cliffs, New Jersey.

Hoar, W.S., and Randall, D.R. (1969) Fish Physiology. Vol I. Excretion, Ionic Regulation and Metabolism. Academic Press, New York.

Hughes, S.G. (1988) Effect of dietary propylene glycol on growth, survival, histology and carcass composition of Atlantic salmon. Progressive Fish Culturist 50:12–15.

Ketola, H.G. (1979) Influence of dietary zinc on cataracts in rainbow trout (Salmo gairdneri). J. Nutr. 109:965–969.

Ketola, H.G., and Rumsey, G.L. (1985) Starter diets compared. Salmonid 9:9,19.

Kim, K.I., Kayes, T.B., and Amundsen, C.H. (1984) Requirements for sulfur-containing amino acids by rainbow trout. Fed. Proc. 43:856 (Abs. 3338).

Kloppel, T.M., and Post, G. (1975) Histological alteration in tryptophan-deficient rainbow trout. J. Nutr. 105:861–866.

Lagler, K.F. (1956) Freshwater fishery biology. Wm. C. Brown, Dubuque, Iowa.

Lanno, R.P., Slinger, S.J., and Hilton, J.W. (1985) Maximum tolerable and toxicity levels of dietary copper in rainbow trout (Salmo gairdneri, Richardson). Aquaculture 49:257–268.

Lee, D.L., and Sinnhuber, R.O. (1972) Lipid requirements. In: Fish Nutrition (Halver, J. E., ed). Academic Press, New York, pp. 145–180.

Lemm, C.A. (1983) Growth and survival of Atlantic salmon fed semimoist or dry starter diets. Progressive Fish Culturist 45:72–75.

Marine, D., and Lenhart, C.H. (1910) Observations and experiments on the so called thyroid carcinoma of the brook trout (Salvelinus fontinalis) and its relation to ordinary goitre. J. Exp. Med. 12:311.

National Academy of Sciences (1973) Nutrient Requirements of Trout, Salmon and Catfish. National Research Council, Washington, D.C.

National Academy of Sciences (1978) Nutrient Requirements of Laboratory Animals. 3rd rev. ed. National Research Council, Washington, D.C., pp. 85–89.

National Academy of Sciences (1981) Nutrient Requirements of Cold Water Fishes. National Research Council, Washington, D.C.

National Research Council (1969) United States and Canadian Tables of Feed Composition. National Academy of Sciences, Washington, D.C.

Ogino, C. (1980) Requirements of carp and rainbow trout for essential amino acids. Bull. Jpn. Soc. Sci. Fish. 46:171–174.

Ogino, C., and Yand, G.Y. (1978) Requirements of rainbow trout for dietary zinc. Bull. Jpn. Soc. Sci. Fish. 44:1015–1018.

Phillips, A.M., Jr., and Brockway, D.R. (1956) The nutrition of trout II. Proteins and carbohydrates. Progressive Fish Culturist 18:159–161.

Phillips, A.M., Jr., and Podoliak, H.A. (1957) The nutrition of trout III. Fats and minerals. Progressive Fish Culturist 19:68–75.

Post, G. (1966) Response of rainbow trout (Salmo gairdneri) to antigens from Aeromonas hydrophila. J. Fish. Res. Bd. Can. 23:1481–1494.

Post, G. (1975) Ration formulation for intensively reared fishes. Proceedings of the 9th International Congress on Nutrition In: Foods for the Expanding World. Vol. 3. Kargar, Basel, pp. 199–207.

Post, G. (1987) Textbook of Fish Health, Revised and Expanded. T.F.H. Publ. Neptune, New Jersey.

Poston, H.A. (1977) The role of nutrition on preventing ocular lesions in salmonid fishes. Proceedings of the 1977 Cornell Nutrition Conference for Feed Manufacturers, Syracuse, New York, pp. 83–86.

Poston, H.A. (1986a) Response of lake trout and rainbow trout to dietary cellulose. U.S. Fish and Wildlife Service Technical Report. No. 5:1–6, Washington, D.C.

Poston, H.A., (1986b) Response of rainbow trout to source and level of supplemental dietary methionine. Comp. Biochem. Physiol. 85A:739–744.

Poston, H.A., and Page, J.W. (1982) Gross and histological signs of dietary deficiencies of biotin and pantothenic acid in lake trout, Salvelinus namaycush. Cornell Vet. 72:242–261.

Poston, H.A., and Rumsey, G.L. (1983) Factors affecting dietary requirements and deficiency signs of L-tryptophan in rainbow trout. J. Nutr. 113:2568–2577.

Poston, H.A., Riis, R.C., Rumsey, G.L., and Ketola, H.G. (1977). The effect of supplemental dietary amino acids, minerals and vitamins on Atlantic salmon fed cataractogenic diets. Cornell Vet. 67:472–509.

Poston, H.A., Riis, R.C., Rumsey, G.L., and Ketola, H.G. (1978) Nutritionally induced cataracts in salmonids fed purified and practical diets. Marine Fish Rev. 40:45–46.

Preese, A. (1972) A Manual for Histological Technicians. Little, Brown, Boston, Massachusetts.

Rackis, J.J., McGhee, J.E., Honig, D.H., and Booth, A.N. (1975) Processing soybeans into food: Selective aspects of nutrition and flavor. J. Am. Oil Chem. Soc. 52:249A–253A.

Rapeseed Association of Canada (1978) Canadian rapeseed meal. Poultry and animal feeding. Publication No. 51

Rohovec, J.S., Garrison, R.L., and Fryer, J.L. (1975) Immunization of fish for control of vibriosis. Proceedings of the 3rd U.S.–Japanese Aquaculture Special Publication Reg. Jpn. Fish. Res. Lab. Nigato, pp. 105–112.

Rumsey, G.L., Page, J.W., and Scott, M.L. (1983) Methionine and cystine requirements of rainbow trout. Progressive Fish Culturist 45:139–143.

Sakamoto, S., and Yone, Y. (1978) Iron deficiency symptoms in carp. Bull. Jpn. Soc. Sci. Fish. 44:1157–1160.

Sato, M., Kondo, T., Yoshinaka, R. and Ikeda, S. (1983) Effect of water temperature on the skeletal deformity in ascorbic acid deficient rainbow trout. Bull. Jpn. Soc. Sci. Fish. 49:443–446.

Satoh, S., Yamamoto, H., Tekeuchi, T., and Watanabe, T. (1983) Effects on growth and mineral composition of rainbow trout of deletion of trace elements magnesium from fish meal diet. Bull. Jpn. Soc. Sci. Fish. 49:425–429.

Satoh, S., Takeuchi, T., and Watanabe, T. (1987) Availability to rainbow trout of zinc in white fish meal and of various zinc compounds. Nip. Suis. Gak. 53:595–599.

Shanks, W.E., Gahimer, G.D., and Halver, J.E. (1962) The indispensable amino acids for rainbow trout. Progressive Fish Culturist 22:68–73.

Snieszko, S.F. (1970) Immunization of fishes: A review. J. Wildlife 6:24–30.

Storebakken, T., Foss, P., Schiedt, K., Austreng, E., Liaaen-Jensen, S., and Manz, U. (1987) Carotenoids in diets for salmonids. IV. Pigmentation of Atlantic salmon with astaxanthin, astaxanthindipalmitate and canthaxanthin. Aquaculture 65:279–292.

Walton, M.J., Cowey, C.B., and Adron, J.W. (1982) Methionine metabolism in rainbow trout fed diets of differing methionine and cystine content. J. Nutr. 112:1525–1535.

Wekell, J.C., Shearer, K.D., and Houle, C.R. (1983) High zinc supplementation of rainbow trout. Progressive Fish Culturist 45:144–147.

Winberg, G.G. (1956) Rate of metabolism and food requirements of fishes. Fisheries Research Board of Canada Trans. Series No. 194. Queens Printer, Ottawa.

Wolf, L.E. (1951) Diet experiments with trout: I. A synthetic formula for diet studies. Progressive Fish Culturist 13:17–24.

Woodall, A.N., and LaRoche, G. (1964) Nutrition of salmonid fishes. XI. Iodine requirements for chinook salmon. J. Nutr. 82:475–482.

Yamamoto, H., Satoh, S., Takeuchi, T., and Watanabe, T. (1983) Effects on rainbow trout of deletion of manganese or trace elements from fish meal diet. Bull. Jpn. Soc. Sci. Fish. 49:287–293.

Chapter 35

SALMONID REPRODUCTION

GEORGE POST

Capture of wild-ranging salmonids by net or trap as they migrate to spawn has been a way of obtaining reproductive products for hatchery propagation. There is little or no means of controlling egg or milt productivity from these captured wild-ranging fishes. The spawn is taken, eggs fertilized, water hardened and disinfected, and both placed into a fish hatchery. Spent broodfish are released following spawning in the case of some salmon, trout, char, and grayling. The only control the hatcheryman has is control of disease problems associated with fertilized and incubating eggs.

The first scientific approach to the rearing of salmonid broodfish strictly for spawn production does not appear to have been practiced prior to the early part of the nineteenth century. Surprisingly, there have been few scientific approaches to the husbandry of salmonid broodfish since that time. Most advances have been made by trial and error, with satisfactory procedures passed to colleagues and friends. Salmonid hatchery manuals and handbooks usually contain a section on broodfish management with descriptions of procedures used for their genetic selection, maintenance, spawning, and egg handling. Most of these are derived from practical experience (Laird and Needham, 1988; Brown, 1980; Huet, 1973; Hickling, 1962; Greenberg, 1962; Davis, 1953).

The rearing of salmonid broodfish in fish cultural facilities is undertaken by many state and federal agencies and by commercial fish farmers. Some facilities are used primarily for the production of "eyed" eggs, others combine this crop with the rearing of fish for sale or release for sport fishing, or to enhance wild populations. Broodfish rearing offers different health management problems than does rearing of fish for market or release. The main objective in the rearing of salmonid broodfish is the production of milt with high numbers of normal sperm from the male and high fecundity from females producing acceptable eggs.

Prevention of health problems in salmonid broodfish begins with attention to the immature fish that will be held for spawn production. The selected fish should be given the best care and environmental quality possible from early in life and throughout their reproductive life.

BROODFISH FACILITIES AND DISEASE

Satisfactory rearing facilities and the best possible quality of water are essential throughout the reproductive life of broodfish to achieve the highest egg numbers, egg hatchability, and alevin survival. Unfortunately, broodfish are often placed at the bottom of all rearing facilities at fish hatcheries, especially when production of eyed eggs is a secondary product from the fish cultural operation. They are then exposed to water that may have been passed through several stages of fish rearing prior to reaching broodfish ponds. This practice can be responsible for numerous gill, fin, and skin diseases among the broodfish. Reduced dissolved oxygen and high levels of dissolved excretory products from the fish above can cause mild to severe health problems. Transmissable diseases in populations of fish above the broodfish result in either disease in broodfish or the carrying of communicable organisms to the egg, causing disease in alevins or more advanced stages of young fish.

ASSESSMENT OF ACCEPTABLE SALMONID REPRODUCTION

There are many variables in the production of acceptable eggs and milt. These include heredity, age, and environmental quality factors such as temperature, water volume to fish biomass ratio, and water-quality parameters. Egg and milt production is also affected by time of spawning, disease problems, and nutritional status. Estimates of the ex-

TABLE 35–1. An Example of Female Age versus Average Eggs per Female and Average Egg Size from Cultured Rainbow Trout*

Spawning Age	Eggs per Female	Egg Size (g/1000)	Egg Size (no./oz)
First spawn (2-year-old)	3763	86	342
Second spawn (3-year-old)	5126	88	333
Third spawn (4-year-old)	6028	99	396
Fourth spawn (5-year-old)	6866	96	306

Four years of data from all females at a commercial trout egg production operation in the United States.

pected egg numbers per female, acceptable egg size, and average hatchability of eggs for several salmonid species are given in Tables 35–1 and 35–2 to aid assessment of productivity from broodfish, and evaluation of possible reproductive problems.

BROODFISH NUTRITION

A high-quality, balanced ration must be used throughout the productive life of broodfish to prevent reduced fecundity, poor egg or milt quality, and weak alevins (Scott, 1962). Broodfish ration formulations have usually been established by experiments where ingredients are varied until satisfactory egg numbers, egg quality, egg hatchability, and alevin survivability are reached. Most salmonid broodfish rations contain a higher (35 to 50%) gross protein level, a more balanced essential amino acid profile, a higher fat (10 to 18%) level, a more carefully selected fatty acid make-up, and generally higher available energy per unit ration than rations used for general fish production of the same species. The vitamin premix used for rearing a certain fish species is usually doubled for broodfish. There is no proven scientific reason for the increased vitamin levels in broodfish rations. They are provided on the basis of a suspected need to supply intrinsic quantities of these essential nutrients to the egg for acceptable sac-fry survival, growth, and metabolism until fry are capable of taking food containing extrinsic vitamins. Several studies have been completed on salmonid broodfish dietary mineral intake effects on egg quality, with conflicting results. Most broodfish rations are compounded with the general salmonid mineral requirements (Post, 1987).

Broodfish feeding management is extremely important, particularly for females. Large quantities of nutrients and nutrient products of female metabolism are deposited in the developing egg mass. Most female salmonids lay 15 to 25% of their body mass as eggs. This large loss of body reserves occurs at each spawning, which is an annual event in all salmonids except the Pacific salmons, which spawn only once in a lifetime.

Proper nutrition can be measured by successful egg production from each female. Age, heredity of the female, and certain environmental factors must

TABLE 35–2. Guidelines for Expected Fecundity of Selected Salmonids

Species		No. of Females	Eggs/Oz		No. of Eggs/Female	
			Average	*Range*	*Average*	*Range*
Rainbow trout	W*	1194	256	238–304	1484	1484–2229
	D*	12,083	258	237–311	1641	1381–2297
	W*	7519	267	240–369	1756	1519–1974
Brown trout	D	—	284	253–334	1554	580–2585
	W	4437	427	393–516	1569	1404–1886
Brook trout	D	—	582	367–831	536	203–1056
	W	1394	497	423–536	898	836–904
Cutthroat trout	D	4265	358	216–572	3639	2649–4816
Lake trout	D	958	281	353–218	3812	2294–4974
	W	652	398	342–479	512	445–621
Golden trout	D	—	364	334–423	641	566–720
Kokanee salmon	W	306	245	228–297	1195	1000–1510
Grayling	W	410	744	700–788	7315	6168–8400

*Wild or Domestic
Data courtesy W. Huggins (Wyoming Game and Fish Department).

be considered in the evaluation. Also used to evaluate female broodfish nutrition programs are the variables of egg size and egg quality, including egg viability, egg hatchability, or alevin viability (Orr et al., 1982). Nutritional condition of the male salmonid is also important, even though production of milt does not require the same vast quantities of body nutrients as does egg production. Normal milt should be thick and creamy, with a high viable sperm count. Poor nutrition can be responsible for watery, opalescent milt with small numbers of sperm per unit volume. Such milt will be limited in egg-fertilization capabilities (Small, 1978; Smith et al., 1979). A normal male rainbow trout should have approximately 58 billion spermatozoa per gram of testis during the peak of the spawning period (Billard et al., 1971). These numbers are extremely variable. There may be between 0.2 and 1.0 trillion spermatozoa available from a 1-kg male rainbow trout during a spawning season (Billard, 1985).

The color of salmonid eggs is affected by nutrition. Wild fish choose a variety of natural food items, some of which are high in carotenoid pigments. These pigments are passed to the lipids within the eggs. Some fish husbandrymen mistakenly believe highly colored eggs produce higher-quality sac-fry. This idea is so firmly entrenched in salmonid hatchery operators that they are willing to pay a premium for highly colored eyed eggs. Carotenoid pigments, usually xanthins (canthaxanthin, astaxanthin, and others), are added to rations fed to broodfish between spawnings. There is no indication that addition of these pigments affects hatchability of the egg or viability of sac-fry as long as adequate vitamin A or carotene precursors of vitamin A have been passed from female to egg (Quantz, 1980). Experiments have demonstrated reduced survival of highly pigmented eggs and sac-fry of Atlantic salmon when exposed to certain wavelengths of light during incubation. Survival is not affected if these eggs are incubated in darkness (Torrissen, 1985).

DIETARY TOXICOLOGY AND EGG QUALITY

Broodfish rations should be prepared from quality ingredients. Toxic substances in broodfish rations may not cause noticeable effects in the broodfish, but egg survivability may be altered. Feeding a ration containing lipid peroxidation products greater than 10 mg of malonaldehyde (thiobarbituric acids, or TBAs) per killigram of dietary fat may cause reduced percent eye-up, hatch, and/or alevin survival. Transfer of certain foodborne pesticides (chlorinated hydrocarbon insecticides), polychlorobiphenyls, petrochemicals, cresols, and heavy metals, including lead, mercury, cadmium, and copper to broodfish may cause poor-quality spawn. Addition of certain antibiotic compounds to the diet of broodfish may affect eggs and subsequent alevins and cause abnormalities. Chlortetracycline, for example, may cause skeletal deformities in alevins derived from spawn of broodfish fed this compound (Seaman et al., 1959).

EGG PRODUCTION

The size and numbers of eggs produced per female of specific age and size may be an indication of a satisfactory ration. Older, heavier females will, on average, produce more and larger eggs than their younger, smaller counterparts (see Table 35–1). Also, alevins and fingerlings produced from larger eggs grow more rapidly (Table 35–3), (Pitman, 1979; Gall, 1974). Other parameters used to estimate a satisfactory ration include percent eyed eggs per female and viable eggs per killigram of fish body weight.

The diagnostician must realize there are nondietary variables other than hereditary background of the fish that alter fecundity in salmonids. Environmental temperature has a direct effect on average egg size and total numbers of eggs per female. In

TABLE 35–3. An Example of Female Age as It Relates to
Egg Numbers, Egg Size, and Alevin Growth
in Rainbow Trout

	2-Year-Old	3-Year-Old
Total eggs per female	3230	4537
Average egg size (No./fl oz)	484	315
Eyed eggs produced (%)	81.0	85.8
Average alevin body weight (g)		
25 days	0.41	0.51
50 days	1.20	1.34
75 days	2.46	2.97

*From Gall, G. A. E. (1974) Influence of size of egg and age of female
on hatchability and growth in rainbow trout. Ca Fish Game 11(1):26–
35.*

Table 35–4, the positive effect of a constant warmer
(12.1°C) water temperature compared to water temperatures gradually reduced from 14.2 to 2.0°C over
5 months prespawn is apparent. Females held at the
higher prespawn temperatures yield an average of
nearly 100 more and 10% larger eggs, even though
all fish were fed the same ration. The economics of
increased egg production for salmonid hatcheries
with large numbers of spawning females is evident.
Water temperature, water quality, and other environmental factors must be considered when assessing
general fecundity patterns in spawning salmonids.

BROODFISH DISEASE RELATED TO REPRODUCTION

Netting, sorting, stripping, and handling broodfish prior to and during spawning procedures can
cause injury to the integument. Pathogenic *Cytophaga*, fungi, and certain ecoparasites invade injured
skin where the mucous layer has been scuffed away.
The use of 1-minute dips in 5% sodium chloride
solution following netting and handling may reduce
invasion of these organisms. A bath treatment using
formalin or a combination of 1% NaCl and formalin
solution may reduce fungal or protozoan infection.
Malachite green is no longer recommended for fungal
control on fishes in the United States.

Salmonid broodfish are susceptible to bacterial
kidney disease, enteric redmouth disease, furuncu-

TABLE 35–4. Fecundity of a Divided First Spawn Group
of Rainbow Trout in Which the Two Resultant
Subgroups Were Held at Different Environmental
Temperatures and Fed the Same Diet

	12.1°C	14.2 to 2.0°C*
Number of females	2489	3161
Peak spawn time	10 December	11 December
Average female body weight (kg)	1.86	1.82
Average egg volume per fish (ml)	315	285
Average egg size (No./fl oz)	363	407

*July to December water temperatures.
From J. C. Povey, personal communication.

losis, motile aeromonad disease, and other bacterial
diseases. Control measures for these diseases are
covered in the chapters on bacterial diseases; however, precaution is needed to use only those therapeutic compounds accepted by the U.S. Food and
Drug Administration in broodfish to reduce the possibility of transfer of drug to eggs and alevins.

PROBLEMS AT EGG TAKING AND WATER HARDENING

Eggs of female rainbow trout have been found
to lose viability if they are not taken within 4 to 6
days of ovulation. Hatchability reduces rapidly, especially if eggs are not taken for 18 or more days
after ovulation. Eggs of other salmonids may be
similarly affected (Hoar et al., 1988). Spawn takers
should not attempt to remove all eggs from the fish.
Attempting to do so may be more traumatic than
resorption of hold-over eggs.

An acceptable fertilization process must be followed or egg hatchability will be reduced. Experiments have demonstrated that fish sperm is activated
by ovarian fluid surrounding the eggs and by calcium
ions in hatchery water. Sperm activity lasts from a
few seconds to as much as 15 seconds. Sperm activity
is more prolonged in ovarian fluid than when hatchery water is added to the milt-egg mixture (Rucker
et al., 1962). The use of buffered saline diluted with
hatchery water also prolongs sperm motility (Petit et
al., 1973). The use of highly mineralized water for
sperm activation in milt-egg mixtures causes frantic
but short-lived motility and reduced fertilization.

Substances dissolved in water may be taken into
eggs during the water-hardening process, the process
in which water infiltrates through pores in the egg
shell to equalize osmotic pressure and expand the
egg. Aflatoxin from *Aspergillus flavus* crosses the
eggshell barrier during water hardening of rainbow
trout eggs and subsequently causes liver tumors as
fish develop from the eggs (Hendricks et al., 1980).
Heavy metals, such as the chlorides of mercury and
lead, enter the egg at this time and cause embryo
malformations or death. Certain therapeutic compounds are thought to pass the eggshell. Erythromycin phosphate and the free iodine radical from
povodine-iodine are examples (Evelyn et al., 1984).

EFFECTS OF STRESSES DURING INCUBATION

Control of environmental conditions and certain
pathogenic organisms is essential during incubation
of salmonid eggs. Cold water increases incubation
time and the time of vulnerability to pathogens. For
example, brown trout eggs require approximately
100 days to hatch at 4.3°C and only 40 days at 10°C.
Rainbow trout hatch in 80 days at the colder temperature and 30 days at the warmer, and lake trout
hatch in 100 days and 50 days, respectively (Green-

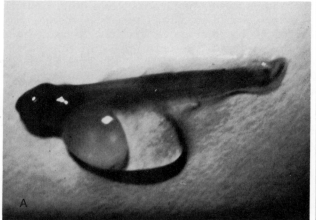 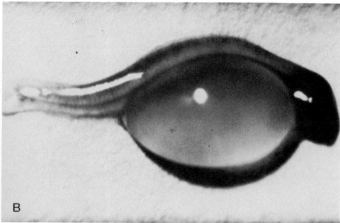

FIGURE 35–1. *A,* Blue sac disease in a rainbow trout fry. Note the cloudiness and separation of yolk material. *B,* Normal rainbow trout sac fry. Note uniform color of yolk material.

berg, 1962; Davis, 1953). The primary pathogens affecting eggs during incubation include *Saprolegnia* spp., *Achlya* spp., and other water molds. These organisms do not attack living eggs, but invade and grow on dead eggs. Heavy growth of these filamentous organisms reduces water circulation around living eggs, often to the point where other eggs die. Thus, all eggs in a redd or tray may be destroyed by advancing fungal mycelia.

Control of fungal growth can be accomplished by the periodic elimination of dead eggs or the regular use of fungicidal chemicals during the entire incubation process (Benoit and Matlin, 1966; Alderman, 1985). Incubating salmonid eggs in jars or cans in which water enters at the bottom and keeps eggs in gentle motion is less conducive to fungal growth on dead eggs, but does not eliminate the problem completely, especially in cold water with long-term incubations.

Circulation of adequate amounts of well-oxygenated water is essential to successful incubation. Accumulation of metabolic wastes from the eggs and reduced dissolved oxygen around the eggs is the cause of blue-sac disease (hydrocoele embryonalis) in alevins (Fig. 35–1A, B) (Greenberg, 1962).

Developing salmonid eggs become sensitive to physical shock shortly after the blastoderm forms. This sensitivity continues until the germ ring closes or nearly closes over the yolk (Fig. 35–2). However, gentle movement and moderate physical stress can be tolerated. For example, there was no significant reduced survival of rainbow trout embryos subjected to physical shocks up to 50 times gravity at various stages of development between newly fertilized eggs and the eyed stage (Post et al., 1974).

Incubating salmonid eggs are sensitive to direct sunlight and to certain wavelengths of light produced from artificial lighting. This is especially true of the blue-violet emissions of cool-white fluorescent tubes (Leitriz, 1976; Perlmutter, 1962). If eggs are incubating in open trays or small glass jars, they should be

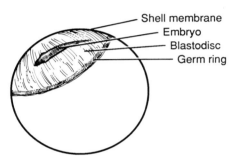

20 % Incubation Time

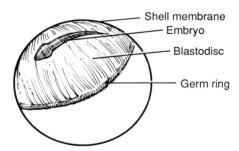

30 % Incubation Time

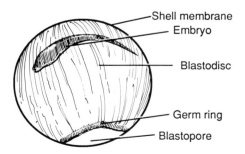

45 % Incubation Time

FIGURE 35–2. Sensitivity of incubating salmonid eggs to physical shock is related to closure of the blastodermal membrane over the yolk. Physical shock sensitivity reduces as the germ ring closes or nearly closes over the yolk.

kept as far away from lighting fixtures as possible and the exposure to light minimized.

Rapid temperature changes of incubating eggs reduces survivability. Eyed eggs are usually transported under wet ice. The egg temperature in styrofoam shipping containers is often near the freezing temperature of water. Eggs should be warmed at the rate of approximately 0.5°C/ minute to reduce temperature shock.

Disinfection of very late incubation stages of salmonid eggs with povidone-iodine at the recommended rate of 100 mg iodine/L for 15 minutes (Post, 1987) may cause early pip. When this premature hatch occurs, the alevin cannot force itself from the shell, and the young fish dies. The use of these compounds for egg disinfection in the last 3 days of incubation is not recommended.

SPECIAL EGG DISEASES

White Spot Disease

Late stages of incubating salmonid eggs and sac-fry are subject to white spot disease. The primary sign is coagulation of the yolk or small white spots or flecks in the normally orange-colored yolk. The problem has been investigated thoroughly, but no specific cause is known. Attempts have been made to duplicate the condition by subjecting incubating eggs to temperature extremes, deficiency of dissolved oxygen, treatment with malachite green or other fungicidal compounds, paint on hatchery equipment, spawn-taking and egg-washing methods, rough handling, and bacterial, fungal, and protozoan infections. Physical trauma is the most promising suspect but does not consistently induce the disease (Davis, 1953).

Constricted Yolk Disease

Constricted yolk disease has occurred sporadically in some Pacific salmon hatcheries in the United

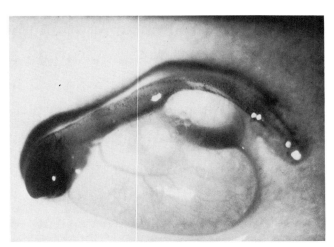

FIGURE 35–3. Constricted yolk disease; note constriction in the posterior portion of the yolk. Compare this to Figure 35–1B.

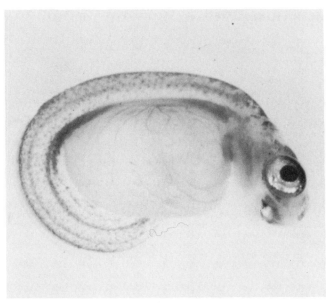

FIGURE 35–4. Anomalies may be the result of contact with toxic substances during formation of the egg in ovary or during spawning or incubation.

States. The yolk sac becomes constricted at the posterior end (Fig. 35–3). Sac-fry with this condition usually die. The cause of the condition is unknown.

Soft Shell Disease

Soft shell disease has been reported at some salmonid hatcheries in the western United States. Eggs water-harden properly but become soft and flaccid during incubation. The condition is caused by minute openings in the shell membrane that allow fluids to pass from the egg. Some yolk material may escape if the condition arises prior to closing of the blastopore (see Fig. 35–2). The cause is thought to be an amebic infection on the outside of eggs. Control is by careful disinfection of all hatchery facilities and equipment (Davis, 1953).

Anomalies and Teratologic Diseases

Anomalies and teratologic problems have been reported in relatively high numbers (<1% to >30%) in some spawns (Fig. 35–4). Their etiology is often difficult to determine. Heavy metal toxicity or toxicity of other organic or inorganic compounds, extreme environmental factors during incubation, heredity, and many others causes must be considered. The diagnostician may have difficulty determining the cause or which preventive measures must be taken to eliminate the problem among subsequent spawns. Prespawn factors, spawning operations, water-hardening practices, incubation procedures, and sac-fry handling must be examined as well as heredity, history of the spawning population, and environmental factors.

LITERATURE CITED

Alderman, D.J. (1985) Malachite green: a review. J. Fish Dis. 8:289–298.

Benoit, R.F., and Matlin, N.A. (1966) Control of *Saprolegnia* on eggs of rainbow trout *(Salmo gairdneri)* with ozone. Trans. Am. Fish. Soc. 95:430–432.

Billard, R. (1985) Artificial insemination of salmonids. In: Salmonid Reproduction: An International Symposium. (Iwamoto, R.N., and Sower, S., eds.). University of Washington Sea Grant Program, Seattle, pp. 117–125.

Billard, R., Breton, B., and Jalabert, B. (1971) La production spermatogenetique chez la truite. Ann. Biol. Anim. Biochem. Biophys. 11:190–212.

Brown, E.E. (1980) Fish Farming Handbook. AVI Publishing Co. Westport, Connecticut, pp. 91–105.

Brown, E.E., and Gratzek, J.R. (eds) (1980) Fish Farming Handbook. Van Nostrand Reinhold, New York, p. 392.

Davis, H.S. (1953) Culture and Diseases of Game Fishes. University of California, Berkeley and Los Angeles. p. 332.

Evelyn, T.P.T., Ketcheson, J.E., and Prosperi-Porta, L. (1984) Further evidence of *Renibacterium salmoninarium* in salmonid eggs and the failure of providone-iodine to reduce the intra-ovum infection rate in water-hardened eggs. J. Fish Dis. 7:173–182.

Gall, G.A.E. (1974) Influence of size of egg and age of female on hatchability and growth in rainbow trout. Ca. Fish Game 11(1):26–35.

Gall, G.A.E. (1985) Quantitative genetic aspects of reproduction in salmonids. In: Salmonid Reproduction, An International Symposium, (Iwamoto, R.N., and Sower, S., eds.). University of Washington Sea Grant Program, Seattle, pp. 44–51.

Greenberg, D.B. (1962) Trout Farming. Chilton, Philadelphia.

Hendricks, J.D., Wales, J.H., Sinnhuber, E.O., Loveland, P.M., and Scanlan, R. A. (1980) Rainbow trout *(Salmo gairdneri)* embryos: a sensitive animal model for experimental carcinogenesis. Fed. Proc. 39:3222–3229.

Hickling, C.F. (1962) Fish Culture. Faber & Faber, London.

Hoar, W.S., Randall, D.J., and Donaldson, E.M. (1988) Fish Physiology. Vol. XIA. Academic Press, New York, pp. 17–23.

Huet, M. (1973) Textbook of Fish Culture—Breeding and Cultivation of Fish. Fishing News (Books), West Byfleet, Surrey, England, pp. 67–85.

Laird, L., and Needham, T. (1988) Salmon and Trout Farming. John Wiley & Sons, Somerset, New Jersey.

Leitritz, C. (1976) Trout and salmon culture. California Fish & Game Fish Bulletin No. 164.

Orr, W., Call, J., Brooks, J., Holt, E., and Mainwaring, J. (1982) Effect of feeding ratios on spawning performance of two-year-old rainbow trout brood stock. U.S. Fish & Wildlife Service Fish Development Center, Bozeman, Montana, Information Leaflet No. 24.

Perlmutter, A. (1962) Lethal effect of fluorescent light on the eggs of brook trout. Progressive Fish Culturist 25:26–30.

Petit, J., Jalabert, B., Chevasous, B., and Billard, R. (1973) L'insemination artificielle de la truite: I. Effects du taux de dilution, du pH et de pression osmotique de dilueur sur la fecundation. Ann. Hyrobiol. 4:201–210.

Pitman, R.W. (1979) Effects of female age and egg size on growth and mortality in rainbow trout. Progressive Fish Culturist 41:203–204.

Post, G. (1987) Textbook of Fish Health. T.F.H. Publications Inc, Neptune, New Jersey.

Post, G., Powers, D.V., and Kloppel, T.M. (1974) Survival of rainbow trout eggs after receiving physical shocks of known magnitude. Trans. Am. Fish. Soc. 103:711–716.

Quantz, G. (1980) The influence of carotenoid-enriched dry feed on egg fertilization of rainbow trout. Arch. Fischereiwissenschaft. 31:29–40 (Tran. in German).

Rucker, R.R., Conrad, J.F., and Dickerson, C.W. (1962) Ovarian fluid, its role in fertilization. Progressive Fish Culturist 25:77–78.

Scott, D.P. (1962) Effects of food quantity on fecundity of rainbow trout, *Salmo gairdneri*. J. Fish. Res. Bd. Can. 19:715–730.

Seaman, E.A., Norton, V.J., and DeVaney, T.E. (1959) Registration and clearance of chemicals for fish culture and fishery management. Transactions of the 99th Annual Meeting of the American Fish Society.

Small, T. (1978) Trout eggs—look for size and service. Fish Farmer 1(3):14–15.

Smith, C.E., Osborne, M.E., Piper, R.G., and Dwyer, P. (1979) Effects of diet composition on performance of rainbow trout brood stock during a three-year period. Progressive Fish Culturist 41:185–188.

Torrissen, O. (1985) Pigmentation of salmonids: effects of carotenoids in eggs and startfeeding diets on survival and growth rate. Abstracts—Nutrition. In: Salmonid Reproduction: An International Symposium, (Iwamoto, R.N., and Sowers, S., eds.). University of Washington Sea Grant Program, Seattle.

Chapter 36

SELECTED BACTERIAL DISEASES OF SALMONIDS

EMMETT B. SHOTTS, JR.   THOMAS G. NEMETZ

Salmonids have been a mainstay in aquaculture, particularly in the early days of this emerging industry. This group of fish has been extensively farmed and represents a large portion of the fish eaten in the United States. Salmonids, like other fishes, are susceptible to a variety of bacterial infections. Some of these are quite host specific, whereas others are not. In this chapter, we will restrict our comments to diseases unique primarily to salmonids. These diseases include examples of infections that cause epizootic mortalities, others that are chronic and have low losses, and still others that disfigure individual fishes, making them unmarketable. For the purposes of this chapter, we will concentrate on the diseases listed in Table 36–1.

FURUNCULOSIS

SYNONYMS. Ulcer disease, Dee disease, *Aeromonas salmonicida* infection, ulcerative furunculosis, ulcerative disease of goldfish, carp erythrodermatitis.

Snieszko et al. (1950) described *Haemophilus piscium* as the etiologic agent of an ulcerative condition

TABLE 36–1. Selected Bacterial Diseases of Salmonids

Disease	Organism	Host
Furunculosis	*Aeromonas salmonicida* (*Haemophilus piscium*)	Salmonids and all freshwater and marine fishes
Enteric Redmouth	*Yersinia ruckeri*	Salmonids, goldfish, dace, largemouth bass, cisco
Bacterial Gill Disease	*Flavobacterium* spp.	Salmonids, other freshwater fishes
Bacterial Kidney Disease	*Renibacterium salmoninarum*	Salmonids, possibly herring
Lactobacillosis (Pseudokidney Disease)	*Lactobacillus piscicola*	Salmonids

in trout. Several years later, it was demonstrated that the organism did not belong to the genus *Haemophilus* and differed significantly from the type species, *Haemophilus influenzae* (Kilian, 1976). Similar questions about the organism's taxonomic position were raised by several other investigators (Austin and Austin, 1987). In 1980, using multiple criteria, including bacteriophage typing and serologic relationships, it was conclusively demonstrated that *Haemophilus piscium* associated with ulcer disease of trout is in fact atypical *Aeromonas salmonicida* (Paterson et al., 1980; Shotts et al., 1980). It appears that *Haemophilus piscium* is a synonym for *Aeromonas salmonicida*.

Host and Geographic Distribution

While *Aeromonas salmonicida* is usually associated with salmonid species, all species of freshwater and marine fishes are considered susceptible. A number of "noncharacteristic" species are discussed in detail by several authors (McCarthy, 1975a; McCarthy and Roberts, 1980; Austin and Austin, 1987). One of the most recent significant epizootics in nonsalmonids occurred in goldfish in the United States (Elliott and Shotts, 1980; Shotts et al., 1980).

Aeromonas salmonicida is known to be present and cause disease problems in various species of fishes in North America, South America, Europe, Asia, Australia, and Africa.

Clinical Signs

Typical furunculosis is caused by *Aeromonas salmonicida* var. *salmonicida*, and may be observed clinically in several forms or stages of severity. The peracute form, that in which very few, if any, outward signs are seen, is noted most frequently in fingerlings, and the etiology cannot be readily established without necropsy and/or culture. In the more commonly seen acute form of the disease, there is very little, if any, size discrimination noted in the disease. In most situations, there are some subtle indications of the pending die-off 2 or 3 days before the beginning of mortality. This is usually seen as a darkening of the skin pigmentation and refusal to eat (Austin and Austin, 1987). When affected fish are necropsied, the primary gross pathology includes hemorrhagic viscera, mushy kidneys, pale liver, and enlarged spleen. Most of these signs are compatible with septicemic disease.

A more protracted, subacute form that allows the organism a longer incubation in the host, results in a gradual onset of mortality, with the appearance of classic furunculelike skin lesions that often rupture, producing open lesions. Internally, the gross pathologic findings are similar to those noted in the acute form. In some populations, one might encounter a chronic form that will have signs similar to the subacute form, but may be distinguished by evidence of healed or healing lesions. In the chronic form of the disease, the morbidity is usually very significant, but the mortality low. Recovered fish, however, are often not marketable because of scarring. Fish may be affected by strains of low virulence, but show no outward evidence of disease, although cultures are positive. Such populations are considered to be suffering from a latent form. A method often used to confirm latent infection is fluorescent antibody testing, which is used in lieu of culture (Bullock et al., 1983a).

Diagnosis

Determination of the etiology of suspected outbreaks of furunculosis should be based on necropsy and culture of at least five moribund fish from each pond showing disease signs. Freshly dead fish may be used if moribund specimens are not available. The use of multiple samples from multiple sites enhances the validity of the diagnosis.

Pathology

In its most common form (i.e., subacute or chronic), furunculosis is characterized by darkened pigmentation, a slight exophthalmia, lethargy, bloodshot fins, and often bloody discharges from the vent and/or nares. External lesions may be noted on affected fish that resemble boils in some respects (McCarthy, 1975b). In the acute form, lack of appetite, subtle hemorrhages at the base of finage, and darkening of skin color are often noted. Internal pathology is usually more pronounced in the subacute and chronic forms and may include, but not be restricted to, kidney necrosis, enlargement of the spleen, liver hemorrhage, and hemorrhaging in the muscles. The internal pathology noted in the acute form more closely resembles a classic septicemia (McCarthy and Roberts, 1980; Snieszko, 1958).

In nonsalmonids, *Aeromonas salmonicida* has been

associated with a chronic skin condition that has been referred to by a number of names, including carp erythrodermatitis, ulcerative furunculosis, and goldfish ulcer disease (Bootsma et al., 1977; Elliott and Shotts, 1980).

Culture and Identification

Clinical diagnosis can be made visually or by necropsy, but the final diagnosis requires culture, isolation, and identification of the causative organism. Culture from the caudal kidney on appropriate media such as trypticase soy agar, brain heart infusion agar, or 5% bovine blood agar, and incubate at 20 to 25°C for 24 to 48 hours. When skin involvement is suspected, we have found that blood agar plates inoculated from early lesions have yield growth at 20 to 25°C after 72 to 96 hours.

It should be pointed out that although by deoxyribonucleic acid (DNA) homology, organisms from ulcerative disease and furunculosis are identical, they are grossly different phenotypically. *Aeromonas salmonicida* is a short (1 to 2 × 0.8 μm), nonmotile, gram-negative rod. The organism is oxidase positive, and the classic type produces a brown water-soluble pigment that is readily noted. The atypical usually does not produce this pigment unless maintained on artificial media for long periods. Although extensive comparative identification criteria are available, the most time-efficient means of confirmatory identification is by serologic means using either direct fluorescent antibody techniques or agglutination procedures.

Transmission, Epidemiology, and Pathogenesis

It is commonly accepted that lateral transmission of *Aeromonas salmonicida* occurs via contaminated water, infected fish, and fish intestinal tracts; however, the actual portal of entry into the fish host remains a mystery. Several studies have demonstrated rapid uptake of the organism into susceptible hosts. The final answers regarding the transmission mechanism remain unsolved after 90 years of investigations.

Basic unsolved epidemiologic questions relate to the ability of the organism to exist as a free-living entity in the natural environment, what the host entry mechanisms are, and the natural predisposing environmental factors which might start an epidemic (Austin and Austin, 1987).

It is well established that the pathogenesis of *Aeromonas salmonicida* is an extremely complex process, which includes components of the outer cell membrane and a multitude of extracellular products resulting from the growth of the organism in the host. These include, but are not restricted to, several proteases, hemolysins, lipopolysaccharides, leukoci-

dins, and other growth products. The primary knowledge available indicates that probably the key factors are proteases, hemolysins, leukocytotoxic factors, and outer membrane adhesions.

Treatment and Control

Control of the disease is directed primarily at management practices, which include both the development of resistant stock as well as adequate control of sanitary practices and quality of the environment.

If disease occurs, the use of chemotherapy should be considered. The effectiveness of treatment depends on the route of administration and drug selection.

Selection of the drug is best based on drug sensitivities established for the isolate encountered in an outbreak. The occurrence of drug-resistant plasmids associated with *Aeromonas salmonicida* have been known for over 30 years. With that in mind, it is important to judiciously select drugs for disease control. Along with the use of chemotherapy, vaccines are another important aspect of control. Unfortunately, the development of a suitable vaccine for use against *Aeromonas salmonicida* represents one of the great challenges remaining for researchers.

ENTERIC REDMOUTH

SYNONYMS. ERM, Hagerman redmouth disease, redmouth, salmonid blood spot, *Yersinia ruckeri* infection.

Host and Geographic Distribution

Most clinical disease has been reported from salmonids. Isolations and disease have been reported in Atlantic salmon, brown trout, brook trout, coho salmon, chinook salmon, sockeye salmon, cutthroat trout, rainbow trout, and steelhead. Isolations have also been reported from goldfish, emerald dace, large mouth bass, and cisco. Geographically, the organism has been reported associated with disease in North America and Europe.

Clinical Signs

The predominant signs of enteric redmouth disease, which set it apart, are the reddening in the mouth and darkening of the skin pigmentation with cutaneous petechiae. Enteric redmouth, like other bacterial septicemias, occurs in varying severity (peracute, acute, subacute, or chronic). At necropsy, the most characteristic observations include hemorrhages of the large intestine, diffuse petechial hemorrhages of the musculature, hypertrophy of the spleen, and a yellowish discharge in the vent area.

Diagnosis

While gross observation of affected fish is helpful, diagnosis of enteric redmouth disease ultimately rests with the recovery of the etiologic agent, *Yersinia ruckeri*. This task is complicated by the other members of the Enterobacteriaceae, notably *Serratia liquefaciens* and *Hafnia alvei*. These organisms not only have similar phenotypic characteristics but also are serologically similar to the point of cross-reactivity.

In North America, the use of a selective medium based upon Tween 80 (+) and sucrose utilization (−) is helpful (Waltman and Shotts, 1984). However, the medium has not proved of great use in Europe, and particularly in Great Britain, where most strains are Tween negative (Austin and Austin, 1987). Other advances in diagnosis include the use of bacteriophage typing (Stevenson and Airdrie, 1989).

Concomitant to diagnosis by isolation of the etiologic agent is the recognition of certain salient clinical signs. As would be assumed from the name, there is a reddening of the mouth and throat. This may be accompanied by a darkening of the skin pigment and erosion of the jaw. Other helpful signs include the presence of hemorrhages at the base of the fins and often exophthalmia (Busch, 1973; Bullock and Anderson, 1984).

Pathology

Internal signs suggest a classic bacteremia accented with profuse petechial hemorrhages throughout the internal organs, musculature, and fat. The intestines are flaccid and in most cases contain a yellowish fluid. In cases where disease has persisted for several days, the kidney and spleen may be enlarged (Fuhrmann et al., 1983).

Culture and Identification

The culture of the organism from the caudal kidney is usually accomplished without problem on an array of enteric medias. A selective medium (SW) (Waltman and Shotts, 1984) is available; however, its use is limited to areas where isolates are Tween 80 positive. Growth is achieved after incubation at 35°C for 24 hours.

Once colonies are selected for identification, care must be taken to rule out phenotypically similar organisms such as *Hafnia alvei* and *Serratia liquefaciens*. There are at least five serologic groups, all of which are capable of producing experimental disease. Despite literature to the contrary, sorbitol fermentation cannot be used to differentiate among serovars (O'Leary, 1977). When using API20E, this organism often keys as *Hafnia alvei*, and working with conventional biochemicals, several secondary reactions are necessary to avoid confusion with *Serratia liquefaciens*.

Transmission, Epidemiology, and Pathogenesis

As early as 1975, the presence of carrier fish was established (Busch and Lingg, 1975). It was also observed that stressed fish are more susceptible, and that the organism is commonly present in the environment (Rucker, 1966). This organism can be recovered from a variety of sources in the environment, including sewage (Dudley et al., 1980), muskrats (Stevenson and Daly, 1982), and goldfish (McArdee and Dooley-Martin, 1985). Unstressed carrier fish do not shed organisms into the environment (Hunter et al., 1980). However, when temperatures are between 15 and 18°C and stress occurs in inapparent carrier populations, mortalities begin within 5 to 20 days after the stress. These mortalities continue for a month or more (Rucker, 1966).

Factors associated with virulence are not well understood. Pathogenic mechanisms may be associated with plasmids, but conclusive evidence of mechanisms have not been proven (De Grandis and Stevenson, 1985).

Treatment and Control

A number of antimicrobics have been used successfully against enteric redmouth disease, including tetracycline, sulfa drugs, tiamulin, and oxalinic acid (Rucker, 1966; Bosse and Post, 1983; Bullock et al., 1983b; Rodgers and Austin, 1982). Most therapy should be continued for approximately 14 days for maximum effectiveness. At times, the presence of R-plasmids alters the usefulness of antimicrobics (De Grandis and Stevenson, 1985).

Vaccines have proven valuable in the control of enteric redmouth disease. The effectiveness varies somewhat depending upon the route of administration. The least effective route is oral, and the best administration route is either injection or spray (Austin and Austin, 1987).

BACTERIAL GILL DISEASE

The genus *Flavobacterium* has been reported as a cause of bacterial gill disease in salmonids. A great deal of confusion surrounds the exact taxonomic status and the species responsible for the disease (Austin and Austin, 1987; Wakabayashi et al., 1980; Kimura et al., 1978). Bacterial gill disease caused by *Flavobacterium* sp. has also been reported in the Netherlands and Hungary (Farkas, 1985).

Currently, it is our opinion that the identification and classification methodology available for these organisms is not defined to an extent that it provides a valid means of determination of the magnitude of the disease problem caused by this group. There has been, and still is, extensive confusion of classification at the generic level. Further research will be necessary to both determine the etiology and define the pathogenesis. An organism referred to as *Flavobacterium branchiophila* has been described as a cause of bacterial gill disease in this country and Japan; however, its association with clinical disease has not been demonstrated with regularity (Wakabayashi et al., 1980). Disease caused by this group of organisms is discussed in more detail in Chapter 67.

BACTERIAL KIDNEY DISEASE

SYNONYMS. BKD, Dee disease, *Renibacterium salmoninarum* infection, *Corynebacterium salmonarum* infection.

Host and Geographic Distribution

Renibacterium salmoninarum is the etiologic agent of bacterial kidney disease in salmonid fishes. It is a gram-positive, nonmotile, non–acid-fast aerobic rod (0.3 to 1.5 × 0.1 to 1.0 μm), which is frequently seen in pairs. Bacterial kidney disease was first reported as a clinical entity in Scotland in 1930. The first report of disease in the United States was in 1935. The organism has been isolated from fish in North America, Chile, Japan, and Europe (Austin and Austin, 1987). Originally classified as a *Corynebacterium*, the organism was designated as a unique genus in 1980 (Sanders and Fryer, 1980).

Clinical Signs

Clinical presentation of bacterial kidney disease has been recently reviewed (Bruno, 1986; Austin and Austin, 1987). The organism produces disease only in salmonid fishes, although a carrier state has been suggested to occur in herring (Traxler and Bell, 1988). Infection may result in a chronic progressive systemic infection, with potentially high rates of mortality among affected fish.

External signs are variable. Some fish may appear to be clinically normal. Others appear listless and off feed, and their body color may darken. Exophthalmia, abdominal distension, and petechial hemorrhages of the bases of fins have been observed. Vesicle formation, with consequent ulceration and abscesses, may develop in the musculature.

Gross internal lesions may include the accumulation of ascitic fluid. The spleen and/or liver may be enlarged. Pseudomembrane formation may occur around the swimbladder and other internal organs. The kidney often appears to be pale, swollen, and granular, with white or gray nodular patches visible on the surface.

Diagnosis

Culture and serology are used to diagnose bacterial kidney disease. The causative organism has an absolute requirement for cysteine, and a number of selective media have been developed (Evelyn, 1977; Austin et al., 1983; Daly and Stevenson, 1985). The organism grows slowly in culture, and visualization of colonies may require 3 to 6 weeks. Slow growth on media has been attributed to the fastidious nature of the organism and to potential toxicants present within infected host tissues, since tissue samples are homogenized prior to inoculation (Daly and Stevenson, 1988). It has been suggested that enzymatic digestion and prefiltration of homogenized samples prior to inoculation may lower tissue toxicity and increase the sensitivity of culture techniques in detecting the organism (Lee, 1989).

Slow growth of *Renibacterium salmoninarum* in culture has been an obstacle to rapid and accurate diagnosis. As a result, a variety of serologic diagnostic tests have been developed (Elliott et al., 1989). Techniques include immunodiffusion (Chen et al., 1974), fluorescent antibody (Bullock and Stuckey, 1975; Bullock et al., 1980; Elliott and Barila, 1987; Lee and Gordon, 1987; Smith et al., 1987), counterimmunoelectrophoresis, and coagglutination techniques (Cipriano et al., 1985). However, problems with these techniques include potentially low sensitivity, variable specificity, and requirements for specialized equipment and/or labor-intensive procedures (Bruno, 1987; Pascho et al., 1987; Armstrong et al., 1989; Sakai et al., 1989a).

Rapid and accurate diagnosis of bacterial kidney disease has recently been facilitated by use of enzyme-linked immunosorbent assay (ELISA) and monoclonal antibody (Mab) techniques. ELISA tests capable of detecting minute amounts of bacterial kidney disease-specific soluble antigens have been evaluated (Sakai et al., 1987a,b; Pascho and Mulcahy, 1987; Turaga et al., 1987a). Two Mabs have been generated which specifically react with a 57-kD soluble antigen protein found in sera of infected fish (Wiens and Kaattari, 1989). Significantly, this protein may be an important factor in the pathogenesis of bacterial kidney disease.

Pathology

Histologically, the disease is characterized by diffuse granulomatous reactions that often occur within reticuloendothelial tissues (Bruno, 1986). The organism is initially observed in phagocytes of the spleen and kidney. As the disease progresses, bacterial aggregates and/or aggregates of macrophages containing *Renibacterium salmoninarum* may be seen in the spleen, pancreas, and liver. The heart may be infiltrated with macrophages, and extensive myocarditis may ensue. The kidney is typically affected, with the appearance of bacteria within tissue macrophages early in the infection. Later, the organism spreads both intra- and extracellularly into the interstitium. Granulomas may develop and result in focal areas of necrosis in the kidney and other tissues. In advanced infections, normal kidney tissue may be obliterated. The disease often produces high morbidity and mortality among infected fish. Death is ascribed to liver or kidney failure, myocarditis and heart failure, and possible direct damage to tissues by elaborated substances (Bruno, 1986).

Culture and Identification

Selective media containing cysteine is required for successful culture. Incubation is done at 15°C, and the organism requires 3 to 6 weeks before colony growth is visible. KDM2 (Evelyn, 1977) is the medium most often employed. One problem with KDM2 is lot-to-lot variation in the peptone component (Evelyn and Prosperi-Porta, 1989). A second difficulty is that inoculation of media with low numbers of bacteria may inhibit growth. This inhibition is believed to be due to elaboration of small amounts of unidentified growth factors by bacteria and/or an inability to effect biochemical changes in the medium conducive to growth (Evelyn et al., 1989). Inoculation of the center of a culture plate with large numbers of *Renibacterium salmoninarum* (nurse culture technique), or use of "spent" KDM2 culture broth in the preparation of new culture media, has been shown to stimulate more rapid colony growth (Evelyn et al., 1989, 1990).

Transmission and Epidemiology

Bacterial kidney disease may be transmitted horizontally by contact with contaminated water, via skin abrasions, or by ingestion of contaminated food (Frerichs and Roberts, 1989). The organism can be recovered from feces and other organically rich tank sediment (Austin and Rayment, 1985). Fish with subclinical infections may serve as carriers or reservoir hosts (Austin and Austin, 1987; Traxler and Bell, 1988). *Renibacterium salmoninarum* is also transmitted vertically. Bacteria have been demonstrated within ova exposed to contaminated coelomic (ovarian) fluid (Evelyn et al., 1984). An increased incidence of intraovum infection, and subsequent infection of juvenile salmonids (smolts), have been correlated with high bacterial counts in coelomic fluid; however, infections in smolts are also seen when low numbers of bacteria are present in these fluids (Lee and Evelyn, 1989).

Bacterial kidney disease has only been found in salmonid species of North America, Chile, Europe, and Japan. Data are contradictory as to the effects of seasonality and water temperature on disease incidence (Austin and Austin, 1987). Rates of mortality are highest during transfer from fresh to salt water and during spawning (Fryer and Sanders, 1981). Stressor stimuli during these activities may compromise immune function and precipitate disease outbreaks (Frerichs, 1989).

Pathogenesis

Infection with *Renibacterium salmoninarum* results in a chronic, systemic disease. Upon entry into the host, the bacteria are phagocytosed by tissue macrophages, where they apparently survive and proliferate (Bruno, 1986). Survival within cells of the immune system is obviously a part of the pathogenesis.

Development of the disease may be stress mediated. The organism may exist in a quiescent state and may even be a normal resident of kidney tissues (Austin and Austin, 1987). Bacterial growth may be impeded in unstressed fish by toxins found in liver and kidney tissues (Lee, 1989). Stressor stimulus may lower immune defense mechanisms and allow bacterial proliferation and overt clinical disease.

Pathogenic mechanisms at the molecular level are incompletely understood. There are reports that *Renibacterium salmoninarum* produces several soluble protein antigens (including an "F" antigen), which can be recovered from culture supernatants (Getchell et al., 1985). Also, soluble protein(s) suppress antibody responses in vitro (Turaga et al., 1987b). Different bacterial strains are hydrophobic and agglutinate rabbit erythrocytes (hydrophobicity renders bacteria "sticky" and facilitates attachment to host cells) (Daly and Stevenson, 1987). Heating bacterial suspensions results in loss of hemagglutination activity, and it has been established that the hemagglutinin and the F antigen are identical 57-kD proteins (Daly and Stevenson, 1990). A positive correlation between hydrophobicity, agglutination, and virulence of bacterial strains has also been noted, strengthening the concept that the protein plays an important role in disease pathogenesis (Bruno, 1988). Monoclonal antibodies generated against *Renibacterium salmoninarum* recognize a 57-kD protein (Wiens and Kaattari, 1989), and they may be of use in elucidating pathogenic mechanisms at the molecular level.

Treatment and Control

Literature concerning treatment and control of bacterial kidney disease has been recently reviewed (Elliott et al., 1989). The ability to colonize host phagocytes and vertical transmission of the bacteria have hindered the development of effective therapeutic regimens. However, some treatment protocols show promise in limiting disease outbreaks.

Antibiotics have been evaluated as chemoprophylactic and therapeutic agents, and as a means of preventing vertical transmission. Erythromycin appears to be particularly effective, but it is not presently approved for use by the Food and Drug Administration. Oral administration (100 mg/kg body weight, 10 to 21 days) has been advocated to prevent disease outbreaks or to treat early infections (Austin, 1985; Moffitt and Schreck, 1988; Moffitt and Bjornn, 1989). The drug has also been administered by injection (11 mg/kg, once every 20 to 30 days) to treat adult salmonids (Peterson, 1982). Problems with erythromycin treatment may include palatability at high oral dosages (Schreck and Moffitt, 1987) and the potential for development of resistant bacterial strains (Bell et al., 1988).

Injection of prespawning female salmonids with erythromycin may be a practical and efficacious means of preventing vertical transmission. Povidone-iodine egg baths did not eliminate intraovum infections (Evelyn et al., 1984; Evelyn et al., 1986b). In contrast, single injections of erythromycin (11 to 20 mg/kg, 14 to 60 days prior to spawning) result in deposition of therapeutic levels of the drug in ova and in reducing the incidence of infection in hatched eggs (Bullock and Leek, 1986; Evelyn et al., 1986a; Brown et al., 1990).

Diet modification and vaccination have been evaluated in the control of bacterial kidney disease. Low levels of zinc, manganese, and ascorbate increased survival times of sockeye salmon (Oncorhynchus nerka) experimentally challenged with Renibacterium salmoninarum (Bell et al., 1984). Increasing dietary ascorbate levels results in decreased survivability, possibly due to enhancement of iron absorption from the gut with subsequent saturation of transferrin and facilitation of bacterial growth. Increased dietary levels of fluoride have been correlated with decreased mortality in rainbow trout (Bowser et al., 1988).

Vaccination using whole cell or antigen preparations has been attempted, but no protective effects have been observed (Evelyn et al., 1988; Sakai et al., 1989b). Molecular biology techniques may prove useful in the future development of subunit vaccines. However, development of a safe and effective vaccine may be hindered by the immunosuppressive activity of proteins produced by the bacterium (Turaga et al., 1987b).

LACTOBACILLOSIS

SYNONYMS. Pseudokidney disease, Lactobacillus piscicola infection, Carnobacterium piscicola infection.

Host and Geographic Distribution

Lactobacillus piscicola has been associated with postspawning mortalities for a number of years in vague die-off situations and has been referred to as pseudokidney disease (Ross and Toth, 1974). It was not until 1984 that definitive classification of the isolate was done and the name Lactobacillus piscicola proposed as the etiologic agent (Hiu et al., 1984). The disease has been described only in salmonids, and predominantly in the United States; however, reports of a disease with similar signs has been reported in England (Austin and Austin, 1987).

Clinical Signs

Affected fish are usually in the 1- to 2-year class and have been stressed. A number of outward signs may be noted, including septicemia and ascites. In some cases, no outward signs are seen. Internally, there may be damage to the organs, especially the kidney, spleen, and liver. Often petechial hemorrhages are noted on the air bladder and in the musculature (Herman et al., 1985).

Diagnosis

In light of the often vague clinical signs, diagnosis rests with the isolation of the organism using either trypticase soy agar or brain heart infusion agar incubated at 20 to 25°C for 48 hours. The resulting organisms, which are small, nonmotile, gram-positive rods, then must be characterized (Hiu et al., 1984).

Pathology

The pathology associated with lactobacillosis is rather unremarkable and vague. There is nothing currently available regarding the pathogenesis. The only common findings are dead and dying fish with swollen kidneys and ascites. The inability to produce disease by injection of cell-free extracts suggests that exotoxins are probably not involved (Austin and Austin, 1987).

Culture and Identification

The presence of a small nonmotile, non–spore-forming organism that is non–acid fast and catalase negative is highly suggestive of the organism (Hiu et al., 1984). This identification may be further verified by acid production with no gas from glucose, sucrose, maltose, and mannitol. The taxonomic position of this organism has been challenged (Collins et al., 1987). It has been proposed that the original isolates were not lactobacilli, but belonged to the genus Carnobacterium, and that the name should be changed to Carnobacterium piscicola. A detailed study recently completed of clinical isolates demonstrates a heterogeneity of isolates and presents evidence that both Lactobacillus sp. and Carnobacterium are capable of causing disease in salmonids (Starliper et al., 1991). Another cultural characteristic helpful in identification is the isolate's ability to grow on medias containing 7% NaCl.

Transmission, Epidemiology, and Pathogenesis

Currently, the mechanisms of transmission of Lactobacillus piscicola are not known. It is currently thought that the organism may be a part of the normal flora and become an opportunistic pathogen when the host is stressed. The epidemiology is fragmentary. Since the first description in 1967, disease outbreaks have been reported throughout North America and in England (Ross and Toth, 1974).

Treatment and Control

Currently, there is no information available in the literature with animal data to provide a basis for speculation. In most disease situations, it has been suggested that stress be reduced and chemotherapy of some type instituted based upon sensitivity to approved compounds for food fishes.

LITERATURE CITED

Armstrong, R., Martin, S., Evelyn, T., Hicks, B., Dorward, W., and Ferguson, H. (1989) A field evaluation of an indirect fluorescent antibody-based broodstock screening test used to control the vertical transmission of *Renibacterium salmoninarum* in Chinook salmon *(Onchorhynchus tshawytscha)*. Can. J. Vet. Res. 53:385–389.

Austin, B. (1985) Evaluation of antimicrobial compounds for the control of bacterial kidney disease in rainbow trout, *Salmo gairdneri* Richardson. J. Fish Dis. 8:209–220.

Austin, B., and Austin, D. (1987) Bacterial Fish Pathogens, Diseases in Farmed and Wild Fish. John Wiley & Sons, New York.

Austin, B., and Rayment, J. (1985) Epizootiology of *Renibacterium salmoninarum*, the causal agent of bacterial kidney disease in salmonid fish. J. Fish. Dis. 8:505–509.

Austin, B., Embley, T., and Goodfellow, M. (1983) Selective isolation of *Renibacterium salmoninarum*. FEMS Micro. Lett. 17:111–114.

Bell, G., Higgs, D., and Traxler, G. (1984) The effect of dietary ascorbate, zinc, and manganese on the development of experimentally induced bacterial kidney disease in sockeye salmon *(Oncorhynchus nerka)*. Aquaculture 36:293–311.

Bell, G., Traxler, G., and Dworschak, C. (1988) Development in vitro and pathogenicity of an erythromycin-resistant strain of *Renibacterium salmoninarum*, the causative agent of bacterial kidney disease in salmonids. Dis. Aquatic Organ. 4:19–25.

Bootsma, R., Fijan, N., and Blommaert, J. (1977) Isolation and identification of the causative agent of carp erythrodermatitis. Veterinarski Archiv. 47:291–302.

Bosse, M.P., and Post, G. (1983) Tribrissen and tiamulin for control of enteric redmouth disease. J. Fish Dis. 6:27–32.

Bowser, P., Landy, R., and Wooster, G. (1988) Efficacy of elevated dietary fluoride for the control of *Renibacterium salmoninarum* infection in rainbow trout, *Salmo gairdneri*. J. World Aquaculture Soc. 19:1–7.

Brown, L., Albright, L., and Evelyn, T. (1990) Control of vertical transmission of *Renibacterium salmoninarum* by injection of antibiotics into maturing female coho salmon, *Oncorhynchus kisutch*. Dis. Aquatic. Organ. 9:127–131.

Bruno, D. (1986) Histopathology of bacterial kidney disease in laboratory infected rainbow trout, *Salmo gairdneri* Richardson, and Atlantic salmon, *Salmo salar* L., with reference to naturally infected fish. J. Fish Dis. 9:523–537.

Bruno, D. (1987) Serum agglutinating titres against *Renibacterium salmoninarum* the causative agent of bacterial kidney disease in rainbow trout, *Salmo gairdneri* Richardson, and Atlantic salmon, *Salmo salar* L. J. Fish Biol. 30:327–334.

Bruno, D. (1988) The relationship between auto-agglutination, cell surface hydrophobicity and virulence of the fish pathogen *Renibacterium salmoninarum*. FEMS Microbiol. Lett. 51:135–140.

Bullock, G.L., and Anderson, D.P. (1984) Immunization against *Yersinia ruckeri*, cause of enteric redmouth disease. In: Symposium on Fish Vaccination; Theoretical Background and Practical Results on Immunization Against Infectious Diseases (De Kinklen, P., ed.). Office International des Epizooties, Paris, pp. 151–166.

Bullock, G.L., and Leek, S. (1986) Use of erythromycin in reducing vertical transmission of bacterial kidney disease. Vet. Hum. Toxicol. 28 (Suppl. 1):18–20.

Bullock, G.L., and Stuckey, H. (1975) Fluorescent antibody identification and detection of the *Corynebacterium* causing kidney disease of salmonids. J. Fish. Res. Bd. Can. 32:2224–2227.

Bullock, G.L., Griffin, B., and Stuckey, H. (1980) Detection of *Corynebacterium salmoninus* by direct fluorescent antibody test. Can. J. Fish. Aquatic. Sci. 37:719–721.

Bullock, G.L., Cipriano, R.C., and Snieszko, S.F. (1983a) Furunculosis and other diseases caused by *Aeromonas salmonicida*. U.S. Fish and Wildlife Service, Fish Disease Leaflet 66.

Bullock, G.L., Maestrone, G., Starliper, C., and Schill, B. (1983b) Potentiated sulfa therapy of enteric redmouth disease. Can. J. Fish. Aquatic Sci. 40:101–102.

Busch, R.A. (1973) The Serological Surveillance of Salmonid Populations for Presumptive Evidence of Specific Disease. Ph.D. Dissertation, University of Idaho, Moscow, Idaho.

Busch, R.A., and Lingg, A. (1975) Establishment of an asymptomatic carrier state infection of enteric redmouth disease in rainbow trout. J. Fish. Res. Bd. Can. 32:2429–2432.

Chen, P., Bullock, G., Stuckey, H., and Bullock, A. (1974) Serological diagnosis of corynebacterial kidney disease of salmonids. J. Fish. Res. Bd. Can. 21:1939–1940.

Cipriano, R., Starliper, C., and Schachte, J. (1985) Comparative sensitivities of diagnostic procedures used to detect bacterial kidney disease in salmonid fishes. J. Wildlife Dis. 21:144–148.

Collins, M.D., Farrow, J.A.E., Phillips, B.A., Ferusu, S., and Jones, D. (1987) Classification of *Lactobacillus divergens*, *Lactobacillus piscicola*, and come catalase-negative asporagenous, rod shaped bacteria from poultry in a new genus, *Carnobacterium*. Int. J. Syst. Bacteriol. 37:310–316.

Daly, J., and Stevenson, R. (1985) Charcoal agar, a new growth medium for the fish disease bacterium *Renibacterium salmoninarum*. Appl. Environ. Microbiol. 50:868–871.

Daly, J., and Stevenson, R. (1987) Hydrophobic and hemagglutinating properties of *Renibacterium salmoninarum*. J. Gen. Microbiol. 133:3575–3580.

Daly, J., and Stevenson, R. (1988) Inhibitory effects of salmonid tissue on the growth of *Renibacterium salmoninarum*. Dis. Aquatic Organ. 4:169–171.

Daly, J., and Stevenson, R. (1990) Characterization of the *Renibacterium salmoninarum* hemagglutinin. J. Gen. Microbiol. 136:949–953.

De Grandis, S.A., and Stevenson, R.W.W. (1985) Antimicrobial susceptibility patterns and R plasmid–mediated resistance of the fish pathogen *Y. ruckeri*. Antimicrob. Agents Chemother. 27:938–942.

Dudley, D.J., Guentzel, M.N., Ibarra, M.J., Moore, B.E., and Sagik, B.P. (1980) Enumeration of potentially pathogenic bacteria from sewage sludges. Appl. Environ. Microbiol. 39:118–126.

Elliott, D., and Barila, T. (1987) Membrane filtration-fluorescent antibody staining procedure for detecting and quantifying *Renibacterium salmoninarum* in coelomic fluid of chinook salmon *(Onchorhynchus tshawytscha)*. Can. J. Fish. Aquatic. Sci. 44:206–210.

Elliott, D., and Shotts, E.B. (1980) Aetiology of an ulcerative disease in goldfish, *Carassius auratis* (L.): Microbiological examination of diseased fish from seven locations. J. Fish Dis. 3:133–143.

Elliott, D., Pascho, R., and Bullock, G. (1989) Developments in the control of bacterial kidney disease of salmonid fishes. Dis. Aquatic Organ. 6:201–215.

Evelyn, T. (1977) An improved growth medium for the kidney disease bacterium and some notes on using the medium. Bull. Off. Int. Epizoot. 87:511–513.

Evelyn, T., and Prosperi-Porta, L. (1989) Inconsistent performance of KDM2, a culture medium for the kidney disease bacterium *Renibacterium salmoninarum*, due to variation in the composition of its peptone ingredient. Dis. Aquatic Organ. 7:227–229.

Evelyn, T., Ketcheson, J., and Prosperi-Porta, L. (1984) Further evidence for the presence of *Renibacterium salmoninarum* in salmonid eggs and for the failure of povidone-iodine to reduce the intraovum infection rate in water-hardened eggs. J. Fish Dis. 7:173–182.

Evelyn, T., Ketcheson, J., and Prosperi-Porta, L. (1986a) Use of erythromycin as a means of preventing vertical transmission of *Renibacterium salmoninarum*. Dis. Aquatic Organ. 2:11.

Evelyn, T., Prosperi-Porta, L., and Ketcheson, J. (1986b) Persistence of the kidney-disease bacterium, *Renibacterium salmoninarum*, in coho salmon, *Oncorhynchus kisutch* (Walbaum), eggs treated during and after water-hardening with povidone-iodine. J. Fish Dis. 9:461–464.

Evelyn, T., Ketcheson, J., and Prosperi-Porta, L. (1988) Trials with antibacterial kidney disease vaccines in two species of Pacific salmon. In: Conference Handbook, International Fish Health Conference, Vancouver, B.C., Canada, 1988. Fish Health Section, American Fisheries Society, Washington, D.C.

Evelyn, T., Bell, G., Prosperi-Porta, L., and Ketcheson, J. (1989) A simple technique for accelerating the growth of the kidney disease bacterium *Renibacterium salmoninarum* on a commonly used culture medium (KDM2). Dis. Aquatic Organ. 7:231–234.

Evelyn, T., Prosperi-Porta, L., and Ketcheson, J. (1990) The new techniques for obtaining consistent results when growing *Renibacterium salmoninarum* on KDM2 culture medium. Dis. Aquatic. Organ. 9:209–212.

Farkas, J. (1985) Filamentous *Flavobacterium* sp isolated from fish with gill diseases in cold water. Aquaculture 44:1–10.

Frerichs, G. (1989) Bacterial diseases of marine fish. Vet. Rec. 125:315–318.

Frerichs, G., and Roberts, R. (1989) Fish Pathology (Roberts, R., ed.). Bailliere Tindall, London.

Fryer, J., and Sanders, J. (1981) Bacterial kidney disease of salmonid fish. Annu. Rev. Microbiol. 35:273–298.

Fuhrmann, H., Bohm, K.H., and Schlotfeldt, H.J. (1983) An outbreak of enteric redmouth disease in West Germany. J. Fish Dis. 6:309–311.

Getchell, R., Rohovec, J., and Fryer, J. (1985) Comparison of *Renibacterium salmoninarum* isolates by antigenic analysis. Fish Pathol. 20:149–159.

Herman, R.L., McAllister, K., Bullock, G.L., and Shotts, E.B. (1985) Post-spawning mortality of rainbow trout *(Salmo gairdneri)* associated with *Lactobacillus*. J. Wildlife Dis. 21:358–360.

Hiu, S.F., Holt, R.A., Sriranganathan, N., Seidler, R.J., and Fryer, J.L.

(1984) *Lactobacillus piscicola*, a new species from salmonid fish. Int. J. Syst. Bacteriol. 34:393–400.

Hunter, V.A., Knittel, M.D., and Fryer, J.L. (1980) Stress-induced transmission of *Yersinia ruckeri* infection from carriers to recipient steelhead trout. J. Fish Dis. 3:467–472.

Kilian, M. (1976) A taxonomic study of the genus *Haemophilus* with the proposal of a new species. J. Gen. Microbiol. 93:9–62.

Kimura, T., Wakabayashi, H., and Kudo, S. (1978) Studies on bacterial gill disease in salmonids I. Selection of bacterium transmitting gill disease. Fish Pathol. 12:233–242.

Lee, E. (1989) Technique to enumerate *Renibacterium salmoninarum* in fish kidney tissues. J. Aquatic Anim. Health 1:25–28.

Lee, E., and Evelyn, T. (1989) Effect of *Renibacterium salmoninarum* levels in the ovarian fluid of spawning chinook salmon on the prevalence of the pathogen in their eggs and progeny. Dis. Aquatic Organ. 7:179–184.

Lee, E., and Gordon, M. (1987) Immunofluorescence screening of *Renibacterium salmoninarum* in the tissues and eggs of farmed chinook salmon spawners. Aquaculture 65:7–14.

McArdee, J.F., and Dooley-Martin, C. (1985) Isolation of *Y. ruckeri*, type 1 (Hagerman strain) from goldfish. Bull. Eur. Assoc. Fish Pathol. 5:10–11.

McCarthy, D.H. (1975a) Fish furunculosis. J. Inst. Fish Mgt. 6:13–18.

McCarthy, D.H. (1975b) Fish furunculosis caused by *Aeromonas salmonicida* var. *Achromogenes*. J. Wildlife Dis. 11:489–493.

McCarthy, D.H., and Roberts, R.J. (1980) Furunculosis of fish—The present state of our knowledge. In: Advances in Aquatic Microbiology. Vol. 2 (Droop, M.R., and Jounasch, H.W., eds.). Academic Press, London, pp. 293–341.

Moffitt, C., and Bjornn, T. (1989) Protection of chinook salmon smolts with oral doses of erythromycin against acute challenges of *Renibacterium salmoninarum*. J. Aquatic Anim. Health 1:227–232.

Moffitt, C., and Schreck, J. (1988) Accumulation and depletion of orally administered erythromycin thiocyanate in tissues of chinook salmon. Trans. Am. Fish Soc. 117:394–400.

O'Leary, P.J. (1977) Enteric Redmouth of Salmonids: A Biochemical and Serological Comparison of Selected Isolates. M.S. Thesis, Oregon State University, Corvallis.

Pascho, R., and Mulcahy, D. (1987) Enzyme-linked immunosorbent assay for a soluble antigen of *Renibacterium salmoninarum*, the causative agent of bacterial kidney disease. Can. J. Fish. Aquatic Sci. 44:183–191.

Pascho, R., Elliott, D., Mallett, R., and Mulcahy, D. (1987) Comparison of five techniques for the detection of *Renibacterium salmoninarum* in adult coho salmon. Trans. Am. Fish. Soc. 11:882–890.

Paterson, W.D., Doney, D., and Desautels, D. (1980) Relationships between selected strains of typical and atypical *Aeromonas salmonicida*, *Aeromonas hydrophila*, and *Haemophila piscium*. Can. J. Microbiol. 26:588–598.

Peterson, J. (1982) Analysis of bacterial kidney disease (BKD) and BKD control measures with erythromycin phosphate among cutthroat trout (*Salmo clarki bouveri*). Salmonid 5:12–15.

Rodgers, C.J., and Austin, B. (1982) Oxolinic acid for control of enteric redmouth disease in rainbow trout. Vet. Rec. 112:83.

Ross, A.J., and Toth, R.J. (1974) *Lactobacillus*—New fish pathogen. Progressive Fish Culturist 36:191.

Rucker, R.R. (1966) Redmouth disease of rainbow trout. Bull. Off. Int. Epizoot. 65:825–830.

Sakai, M., Atsuta, S., and Kobayashi, M. (1989a) Comparison of methods used to detect *Renibacterium salmoninarum*, the causative agent of bacterial kidney disease. J. Aquatic Anim. Health 1:21–24.

Sakai, M., Atsuta, S., and Kobayashi, M. (1989b) The immune response of rainbow trout, *Salmo gairdneri* Richardson, vaccinated by *Renibacterium salmoninarum*. In: Program of the First International Marine Biotechnology Conference (IMBC '89), Baltimore, Maryland, p. 71.

Sakai, M., Amaaki, N., Atsuta, S., and Kobayashi, M. (1987a) Comparative sensitivity of dot blot methods used to detect *Renibacterium salmoninarum*. J. Fish Dis. 10:415–418.

Sakai, M., Koyama, G., Atsuta, S., and Kobayashi, M. (1987b) Detection of *Renibacterium salmoninarum* by a modified peroxidase-antiperoxidase (PAP) procedure. Fish Pathol. 22:1–5.

Sanders, J., and Fryer, J. (1980) *Renibacterium salmoninarum* gen. nov., sp. nov., the causative agent of bacterial kidney disease in salmonid fishes. Int. J. Syst. Bacteriol. 30:496–502.

Schreck, J., and Moffitt, C. (1987) Palatability of feed containing different concentrations of erythromycin thiocyanate to chinook salmon. Progressive Fish Culturist 49:241–247.

Shotts, E.B., Talkington, F.D., Elliott, D.G., and McCarthy, D.H. (1980) Aetiology of an ulcerative disease in goldfish *Carassius auratis* (L.): Characterization of the causative agent. J. Fish Dis. 3:181–186.

Smith, A., Goldring, O., and Dear, G. (1987) The production and methods of use of polyclonal antisera to the pathogenic organisms *Aeromonas salmonicida*, *Yersinia ruckeri*, and *Renibacterium salmoninarum*. J. Fish Biol. 31(Suppl. A):225–226.

Snieszko, S.F. (1958) Fish furunculosis. U.S. Fish and Wildlife Service Fishery Leaflet 467, Washington, D.C.

Snieszko, S.F., Griffin, P.J., and Friddle, S.B. (1950) A new bacterium (*Hemophilus piscium* v. sp.) from ulcer disease of trout. J. Bacteriol. 59:699–710.

Starliper, C.E., Shotts, E.B., and Brown, J. (1991) Isolation of *Carnobacterium* and *Lactobacillus* spp. from juvenile and post-spawning mortalities in rainbow trout (*Oncorhynchus mykiss*). Submitted.

Stevenson, R.M.W., and Airdrie, D.E. (1989) Isolation of *Yersinia ruckeri* bacteriophages. Appl. Environ. Microbiol. 47:1201–1205.

Stevenson, R.M.W., and Daly, J.G. (1982) Biochemical and serologic characteristics of Ontario isolates of *Y. ruckeri*. Can. J. Fish. Aquatic Sci. 39:870–876.

Traxler, G., and Bell, G. (1988) Pathogens associated with impounded Pacific herring *Clupea harengus pallasi*, with emphasis on viral erythrocytic necrosis (VEN) and atypical *Aeromonas salmonicida*. Dis. Aquatic Organ. 5:93–100.

Turaga, P., Wiens, G., and Kaattari, S. (1987a) Analysis of *Renibacterium salmoninarum* antigen production in situ. Fish Pathol. 22:209–214.

Turaga, P., Wiens, G., and Kaattari, S. (1987b) Bacterial kidney disease: The potential role of soluble protein antigen(s). J. Fish Biol. 31(Suppl. A):191–194.

Wakabayashi, H., Egusa, S., and Fryer, J.L. (1980) Characteristics of filamentous bacteria isolated from a gill disease of salmonids. Can. J. Fish. Aquatic Sci. 37:1499–1504.

Waltman, W.D., and Shotts, E.B. (1984) A medium for the isolation and differentiation of *Yersinia ruckeri*. Can. J. Fish. Aquatic Sci. 41:804–806.

Wiens, G., and Kaattari, S. (1989) Monoclonal antibody analysis of common surface protein(s) of *Renibacterium salmoninarum*. Fish Pathol. 24:1–7.

Chapter 37

FUNGAL AND ALGAL DISEASES OF SALMONIDS

A. JIM CHACKO

A number of species of fungi, including organisms that produce motile spores and true fungi without motile spores, are associated with disease processes in salmonid fishes. The fungal infections in Table 37–1 have been diagnosed in salmonid fishes.

SAPROLEGNIASIS

SYNONYM. Integumentary mycosis.

Host and Geographic Distribution

Saprolegniasis affects all adult salmonids and their eggs. The disease is worldwide in distribution and affects a wide range of species other than salmonids.

Etiology

Saprolegniasis in salmonids is caused by a number of genera of parasitic fungi belonging to the orders Saprolegniales, Peronosporales, and Leptomitales. These are common water molds, present mostly in fresh and brackish water. They are ubiquitous in nature and are also present in moist soil. The hyphal walls contain chiefly glucagon, but cellulose may also be present (Alexopoulos and Mims, 1979). The mycelium is composed of branched nonseptate hyphae of varying diameter.

Clinical Signs

In salmonids, saprolegniasis produces characteristic lesions. During the initial stages, lesions are usually circular, although later in the course of the disease, they merge to produce large irregular patches. Grayish-white, focal, cotton-like masses on the skin are characteristic. The fungal hyphae can also be seen on the gills, and *Saprolegnia ferax* has been reported in the lumen of the gut of brook trout (Agersborg, 1933). In advanced cases of saprolegniasis, skin destruction can cause considerable musculature to be exposed (Fig. 37–1).

TABLE 37–1. Fungal Infections in Salmonid Fishes

Disease	Fungus	Host
Saprolegniasis	*Achyla flagellata*	Brook trout
	A. racemosa var. *stelligera*	Trout eggs
	A. radiosa	Brook trout
	Aphanomyces laevis	Rainbow trout eggs
	Saprolegnia australis	Rainbow trout
	S. diclina	Brook trout, rainbow trout, brown trout
	S. ferax	Brook trout and eggs
	S. monoica	Brown trout eggs, rainbow trout, brook trout, Atlantic salmon
	S. shikotsuensis	Coho salmon
Branchiomycosis	*Branchiomyces* spp.	Brown trout, Arctic char, rainbow trout
Candidiasis	*Candida sake*	Biwa Salmon
Cerebral mycetoma	*Exophiala salmonis*	Cutthroat trout, Atlantic salmon
Ichthyophoniasis	*Ichthyophonus hoferi*	Coho salmon, sockeye salmon, Chinook salmon, rainbow trout, Brown trout, brook trout
	Leptomitus lacteus	Rainbow trout eggs
Phaeohyphomycosis	*Ochroconis humicola*	Coho salmon, rainbow trout
	O. tshawytschae	Chinook salmon
Paecilomycosis	*Paecilomyces farinosus*	Atlantic salmon
Phomamycosis	*Phoma herbarum*	Coho salmon, Chinook salmon, rainbow trout

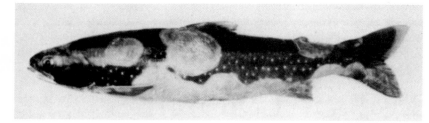

FIGURE 37–1. Windermere char severely infected with *Saprolegnia diclina* Type 1. (From Pickering, A.D., and Willoughby, L.G. [1982] *Saprolegnia* infections of salmonid fish. In: Microbial Diseases of Fish. [Roberts, R.J., ed.]. Academic Press, New York, p. 284.)

Pathology

Histologically the hyphae can be seen penetrating to the dermis and even to the area between the muscle fibers. The hyphae are weakly PAS-positive (periodic acid–Schiff stain) (Wolke, 1975).

Diagnosis

The various fungi responsible for this disease will grow on a variety of fungal culture media. Diagnosis is made by culture and identification of the organism.

Epidemiology and Pathogenesis

The common genera of fungi causing saprolegniasis in salmonids are *Saprolegnia*, *Achyla*, *Aphanomyces,* and *Leptolegnia*. Saprolegnia reproduces by way of asexual reproduction. During this process, the free terminals of the hyphae develop into long, dilated zoosporangia. These special structures contain biflagellated zoospores (sporangiospores). Many genera produce zoospores sexually that will give rise to new hyphae. The released zoospores landing on an egg or an injured part of the host will germinate to produce hyphae (Fig. 37–2).

Morbidity among salmonids varies, depending on the primary cause. It may affect all fish in a hatchery or only a very few. All salmonids and salmonid eggs are susceptible. The majority of saprolegniasis in salmonids is considered secondary to stress (Richards and Pickering, 1978). Temperature plays a major role in the infection process (Roberts, 1978). Death due to saprolegniasis in salmonids may occur in less than 36 hours (Roberts, 1978).

Even though most of the earlier literature dealing with saprolegniasis in fish refers to the saprophytic nature of the fungus, recent work suggests that under intensive rearing conditions, Saprolegnia may act as a primary pathogen (Willoughby and Pickering, 1977). The pathogenicity of *S. diclina* may be attributed to the presence of bifurcate hooks on the secondary zoospore cysts that may help them attach to the fish surface (Pickering et al., 1979). Experimental results indicate that spores of the pathogenic form, *Saprolegnia parasitica*, attach to salmonid fish more rapidly than spores of the saprophyte *S. diclina* (Wood, Willoughby and Beakes 1988). Salmonid mu-

cus may contain a morphagen capable of inhibiting spore germination (Wood et al., 1988).

Treatment and Control

A wide variety of chemicals and drugs have been used to control saprolegniasis in fish. Biologic control has been suggested using macrobenthic crustaceans (Oseid, 1977). Zinc-free malachite green was the chemical of choice for fish culturists until its carcinogenic nature resulted in denial of approved

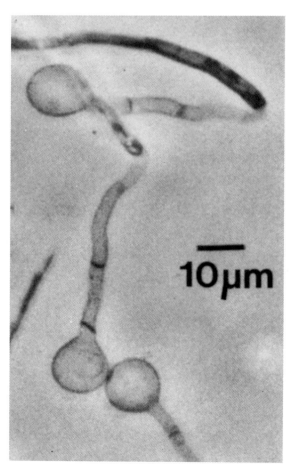

FIGURE 37–2. Secondary zoospore cysts of *Saprolegnia diclina* Type 1 showing attached zoospore cyst and initial germ tube with several cross walls (wet mount). (From Pickering, A.D., and Willoughby, L.G. [1982] *Saprolegnia* infections of salmonid fish. In: Microbial Diseases of Fish. [Roberts, R.J., ed.]. Academic Press, New York, p. 281.)

use in many countries. Formalin as a dip treatment is now generally used against saprolegniasis. This treatment may face a similar regulatory fate.

Dead salmonid eggs serve as a rich nutrient medium for *Saprolegnia* in hatcheries. Removal of dead eggs will prevent the spreading of *Saprolegnia* among eggs. Formalin has been effective in controlling the disease in hatcheries.

ICHTHYOPHONUS DISEASE

SYNONYMS. Taumelkrankheit, reeling disease.

Host and Geographic Distribution

Ichthyophonus disease has a worldwide distribution and appears able to infect all salmonids. Rainbow trout seem to be particularly susceptible. Major outbreaks have been reported in Idaho. Organisms described as *Ichthyophonus hoferi* have been reported to infect a wide variety of freshwater and marine fish.

Etiology

The agent of *Ichthyophonus* disease is *Ichthyophonus hoferi,* an obligate fungal parasite present in both fresh and marine waters. It is frequently described as very pleomorphic. In infected salmonids 10 to 300 μm in diameter, spherical, thick and double- or triple-walled multinucleate spores, cysts, and resting stages are found. The taxonomy of the genus is not well established.

Clinical Signs

Originally *Ichthyophonus* disease was called "Taumelkrankheit," or "reeling disease," because of the spiral or corkscrew-fashion swimming pattern exhibited by the infected fish. Fish with light infections may not show any external signs. In fish with extreme infection, a characteristic sandpaper effect is seen, resulting from a subcutaneous granulomatous response. Salmonids often exhibit scoliosis and lordosis, which inhibits their swimming performance.

Pathology

Internally the kidney, liver, spleen, heart, and muscles may be infected. These organs will have granulomatous gray-white lesions. The walls of the resting stages of the fungus are strongly PAS-positive.

Diagnosis

Ichthyophonus can be cultured on Sabouraud's dextrose agar medium with 1% beef serum (Sinder-

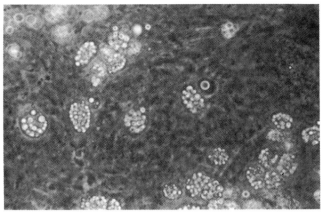

FIGURE 37–3. Endospores of *Ichthyophonus* from the intestine of a rainbow trout (wet mount). (From McVicar, A.H. [1982] *Ichthyophonus* infections of fish. In: Microbial Diseases of Fish. [Roberts, R.J., ed.]. Academic Press, New York, p. 256.)

mann and Scattergood, 1954). Optimum growth is at 10°C within 7 to 10 days. After attaining a diameter of 5 to 15 mm in 30 to 60 days the growth ceases. The hyphae are nonseptate.

Epidemiology and Pathogenesis

Salmonids are infected by the ingestion of fungal elements sometimes referred to as cysts (Dorier and Degrange, 1961). These cysts then transform into ameboblasts in the stomach, which release ameboid forms into the salmonid intestine. Many of the ameboid forms are inactivated into spherical bodies, which can be identified in the feces. Some of the ameboid forms gain access into the host fish's bloodstream by penetrating the intestinal wall and migrate into the visceral organs and musculature. At these sites they become the typical multinucleate cysts. Some cysts produce plasmodia, and others produce endospores (Fig. 37–3), which then infect the host tissue. Water temperature influences the maturation of the cysts into infective forms.

Rainbow trout appear to be the most susceptible salmonid species. There are reports of transmission of the disease to rainbow trout through dietary contamination (Dorier and Degrange, 1961) with 100% infection and low mortality.

Treatment and Control

No known therapeutic agents are available for *Ichthyophonus* disease. Prevention can be achieved by sterilization of raw fish fed to the hatchery fish, if that is the source of infection.

CEREBRAL MYCETOMA

SYNONYMS. Exophialiosis, phaeohyphomycosis.

Hosts and Geographic Distribution

Susceptible salmonid species include cutthroat trout, lake trout, and Atlantic salmon. Naturally occurring or experimentally induced disease due to a related organism, *Exophiala pisciphilia*, has been reported in channel catfish, white catfish, bluegill, mummichog, Atlantic cod, scup, sargassum trigger-fish, clownfish, and the lined sea horse.

Etiology

This is an internal mycotic disease of salmonids caused by *Exophiala salmonis*. The life cycle of the organism and predisposing conditions for the disease are not known. The disease has never been repro-duced by inoculating *Exophiala salmonis* into unin-fected salmonids. The taxonomy of the genus *Exo-phiala* is not yet well described. Another organism, *Exophiala pisciphilia*, has been described as an agent of naturally occurring disease in a variety of fresh-water and marine species of fish.

Clinical Signs

Affected salmonids exhibit signs similar to those produced by whirling disease, including ataxia, whirling swimming patterns, exophthalmus, and cra-nial cutaneous ulcers. Clinical signs are not pathog-nomonic.

Pathology

Histopathologic examination of lesions in in-fected fish reveal a chronic granulomatous response with many giant multinucleated cells. Lesions are often confined to the brain.

Diagnosis

The fungal mycelia cultured from lesions of this disease are mouse-gray with a dark gray reverse. They grow at 25°C, reaching 5 to 8 mm in diameter on Sabouraud's, Czapek's, or cornmeal agars (Neish and Hughes, 1980) (Fig. 37–4). There is no growth at 37°C. Attempts to reproduce the disease have failed.

Epidemiology and Pathogenesis

The life cycle of the organism isolated from fish affected with this disease is not fully known. Since the original description of the disease in fish did not refer to any fungal masses comprising granules, it has been suggested that the term *mycetoma* is inap-propriate (Ajello, 1975; Wolke, 1975). Cerebral my-cetoma has caused fall and winter epizootics in young cutthroat and lake trout from Calgary, Canada (Car-

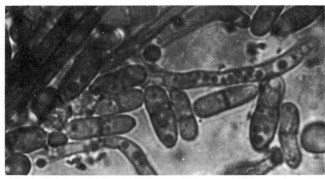

FIGURE 37–4. Wet mount of *Exophiala salmonis* showing two-celled conidia. (From Alderman, D.J. [1982] Fungal diseases of aquatic animals. In: Microbial Diseases of Fish. [Roberts, R.J., ed.]. Aca-demic Press, New York, p. 228.)

michael, 1966). The incidence of infection in these outbreaks may have been as high as 40%.

Treatment and Control

There is no reported treatment or control meas-ure for cerebral mycetoma.

PHAEOHYPHOMYCOSIS

SYNONYMS. Ochromomycosis, blister disease.

Hosts and Geographic Distribution

This disease has been reported in rainbow trout and coho salmon and is thought to affect frogs. The causative organisms were originally isolated from soil. The geographic range is unknown.

Etiology

There are two fungal pathogens reported as causative agents for phaeohyphomycosis among sal-monid fishes. One, *Ochroconis humicola* (syn. *Scoleco-basidium humicola*), is a dematiaceous hyphomycetous fungus (pigmented cell wall; mycelial) reported to cause mortalities in coho salmon (Ross and Yasutake, 1973) and rainbow trout (Ajello et al., 1977). Another agent, *Ochroconis tshawytschae* (syn. *Scolebasidium tshawytschae*), has been reported from the kidneys of Chinook salmon in a single outbreak in California (Doty and Slater, 1946).

Clinical Signs

External symptoms of phaeohyphomycosis in-clude blister-like areas on the sides of fish, exo-phthalmus, and pale edematous gills (Fig. 37–5). Ulceration of the skin can also be seen in *Ochroconis humicola* infections.

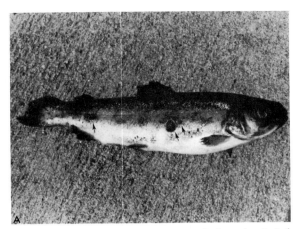

FIGURE 37–5. Rainbow trout with cutaneous lesions due to infection with *Ochroconis humicola*. (From Ajello, L., McGinnis, M.R., and Camper, J.: An outbreak of phaeohyphomycosis in rainbow trout caused by *Scolecobasidium humicola*. Mycopathologia 62:15–22, 1977.)

Pathology

Grossly, the disease is characterized by enlarged kidneys, a pale, hemorrhagic liver, and a pale spleen with hemorrhages. Mycelial aggregates can be observed in dark areas of visceral organs. Histologic changes include granulomas with heavy lymphocyte and mononuclear infiltration in various organs. The lesions can be very extensive in the kidneys.

Diagnosis

Ochroconis humicola grows on potato dextrose agar, V–8 juice agar, and cereal agar at 25°C. On these media, the fungal colonies are flat and dark olive brown. The fungus has septate, pigmented hyphae bearing conidiophores that produce olive-brown conidia (Fig. 37–6). There is no growth at 37°C.

Epidemiology and Pathogenesis

Ochroconis tshawytscha infection was present in fewer than 1% of yearling salmon in the reported outbreak in which it appeared the fungus reached the posterior kidney through the mesonephric ducts via the cloaca (Doty and Slater, 1946). Epizootics of *Ochroconis humicola* among rainbow trout occur in the fall and winter and have been associated with contaminated seepage from a septic tank. Experiments to infect rainbow trout by exposing them to suspensions of *Ochroconis humicola* have failed, but intraperitoneal injections of preparations of the fungus grown on culture medium successfully transmit the disease (Ajello et al., 1977).

Treatment and Control

No therapeutic controls have been reported for *Ochroconis* infections. Since epizootics in rainbow trout are attributed to contaminated water sources, it is recommended that water sources be kept clean and free of excessive organics.

PHOMAMYCOSIS

SYNONYMS. Coelomycosis, swim bladder disease, air bladder disease, swollen vent disease.

Hosts and Geographic Distribution

This disease has been reported in Chinook salmon, coho salmon, and rainbow trout. All reports are from the Pacific northwestern United States.

Etiology

Phoma herbarum was first suggested as a fish pathogen after isolation and culture from affected salmon and trout (Ross et al., 1975). It is a ubiquitous fungus that will grow on a wide variety of substrates, including paint, rubber, cement, and butter.

Clinical Signs

Externally, affected fish develop a "pinched" area in front of the vent. They may have swollen hemorrhagic vents. Fish may swim on their sides or in a vertical upside-down position. In acute cases, affected fish rest on their sides and resume swimming activity when disturbed.

Pathology

Affected young fry may have a flooded swim bladder. Older fish may have watery fluid in their

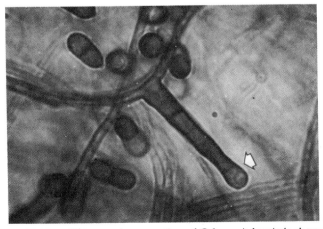

FIGURE 37–6. Wet mount preparation of *Ochroconis humicola* showing conidiophore *(arrow)* and two-celled conidia. (From Alderman, D.J. [1982] Fungal diseases of aquatic animals. In: Microbial Diseases of Fish. [Roberts, R.J., ed.]. Academic Press, New York, p. 227.)

stomachs. A tuft of mycelia may be visible free in the lumen of the swim bladder. Histologic lesions include the presence of mycelia in the swim bladder, often penetrating the wall in areas of extensive inflammatory reaction. The fungus invades other organs, including the kidneys, stomach, and gonads, in advanced cases.

Diagnosis

Phoma herbarum develops superficially formed, globular pycnidia, (mycelial structures resembling fruiting bodies) that are either simple or compound (Fig. 37–7). It will grow on oatmeal agar, potato dextrose agar, malt, or Sabouraud's dextrose agar. Growth is influenced by the composition and acidity of the nutrient substrate. On cornmeal agar there will be a pink or orange-red pigment formation.

Epidemiology and Pathogenesis

It is assumed that the fungal spores are taken in by young fish during the initial stages of the filling up of the swim bladder. The spores find their way to the swim bladder via the pneumatic duct and grow inside the swim bladder. In spring Chinook salmon, the reported mortality is less than 3%. The fungus appears to invade only fish less than 100 days old.

Treatment and Control

Some fish recover spontaneously, and losses in older fish are rare. No therapeutic or control measures are reported.

PAECILOMYCOSIS

SYNONYMS. Swim bladder disease.

Hosts, Geographic Distribution, and Etiology

Paecilomyces farinosus is reported as the cause of the low-level mortalities among farmed Atlantic salmon in Scotland (Bruno, 1989). A member of the same genus, *P. marquandii* has been reported to cause renal mycosis in a nonsalmonid fish (Lightner et al., 1988).

Clinical Signs

Moribund infected fish exhibit reddened vents and swollen abdomens (Bruno, 1989).

Diagnosis

Growth at 25°C is reported on Sabouraud's maltose agar. After 10 days the colonies are white and produce conidiophores and conidia.

Epidemiology and Pathogenesis

Details of the life cycle of these fungi in fish are not available. It has been suggested that the fungus gains entry into fish by way of the infected insect larvae the fish ingest (Bruno, 1989). *Paecilomyces farinosus* is pathogenic to a variety of insect larvae. Reported mortalities are low in farmed Atlantic salmon. Branching septate hyphae penetrate the wall

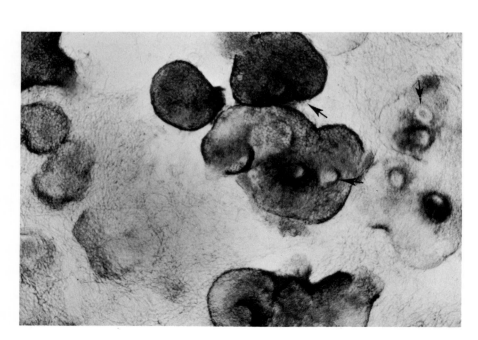

FIGURE 37–7. Mature pycnidia of *Phoma* sp. with visible ostioles *(arrows)* (350×). (From Rippon, J.W. [1988] Appendix. In: Medical Mycology. 3rd ed. Saunders, Philadelphia, p. 766.)

of the swim bladder. The fungus has not been detected in other organs.

Therapy and Control

No therapy or control measures are reported.

LITERATURE CITED

Agersborg, H.P.K. (1933) Salient problems in the artificial rearing of salmonid fishes, with special reference to intestinal fungisitosis and the cause of white-spot disease. Trans. Am. Fish. Soc. 63:240–250.

Ajello, L. (1975) Phaeohyphomycosis: definition and etiology. Proceedings of the Third International Conference on the Mycoses, Sao Paolo, Brazil, 1974. Pan. Am. Health Organ. Sci. Publ. 304:126–130.

Ajello, L., McGinnis, M.R., and Camper, J. (1977) An outbreak of phaeohyphomycosis in rainbow trout caused by *Scolecobasidium humicola*. Mycopathologia 62:15–22.

Alexopoulos, C.J., and Mims, C.W. (1979) Introductory Mycology. John Wiley & Sons, New York.

Amlacher, E. (1965) Pathologische und histochemische Befunde bei Ichthyosporidiumbefall der Regenbogenforelle *(Salmo gairdneri)* und am "Aquarienfisch Ichthyophonus." Z. Fisch. 13:85–112.

Barthelmus, D., Matheis, T., and Meyer, J. (1968) Kiemenfaule bei Regenbogenforellen. Deut. Fisch Zeit., Radebeul. 15:296–300.

Bruno, D.W. (1989) Observations on a swim bladder fungal infection of farmed Atlantic salmon, *Salmo salar* L. Bull. Eur. Assoc. Fish Pathol. 9:7–8.

Bruno, D.W., and Stamps, D.J. (1987) Saprolegniasis of Atlantic salmon, *Salmo salar* L., fry. J. Fish Dis. 10:513–517.

Carmichael, J.W. (1966) Cerebral mycetoma of trout due to a *Phialophora*-like fungus. Sabouraudia 5:120–123.

Dorier, A., and Degrange, C. (1961) L'evolution de *L'Ichthyosporidium (Ichthyophonus) hoferi* (Plehn et Mulsow) Chez les salmonides d'elevage (truite arc-en-ciel et saumon de fontaine). Trav. Lab. Hydrobiol. Pisci. Univ. Grenbole 1960/1961:7–44.

Doty, M.S., and Slater, D.W. (1946) A new species of *Heterosporium* pathogenic on young chinook salmon. Am. Midl. Nat. 36:663–665.

Grimaldi, E., Peduzzi, R., Cavicchioli, G., Giussani, G., and Spreafico, E. (1973) Diffusa infezione branchiale da funghi attribuiti al genere *Branchiomyces* Plehn (Phycomycetes Saprolegniales) a carico dell'ittiofauna di laghi situati a nord e a sud delle Alpi. I. Epidemiologia dell'infezione da *Branchiomyces* in ambiente lacustre. Mem. Ist. ital. Idrobiol. 30:61–80.

Gustafson, P.V., and Rucker, R. R. (1956) Studies on an *Ichthyosporidium* infection in fish: transmission and host specificity. Spec. Scient. Rep. U. S. Fish Wildl. Serv. 166:1–8.

Hatai, K., and Egusa, S. (1975) *Candida sake* from gastro-tympanites of amago, *Oncorhynchus rhodurus*. Bull. Jpn. Soc. Scient. Fish. 41:993.

Hatai, K., Egusa, S., and Awakura, T. (1977) *Saprolegnia shikotsuensis* sp. nov. isolated from kokanee salmon associated with fish saprolegniasis. Fish Pathol. 12:105–110.

Hatai, K., Egusa, S., and Nomura, T. (1977) *Saprolegnia australis* Ellis isolated from body surface lesions of rainbow trout fingerlings. Fish Pathol. 11:201–206.

Humphrey, J.E. (1893) The Saprolegniaceae of the United States, with notes on other species. Trans. Am. Phil. Soc. 17:63–148.

Laveran, A., and Petit, A. (1910) Sur un'epizootie des truites. C. r. hebd. Se'anc. Acad. Sci., Paris 151:421–423.

Lightner, D., Redman, R.M., Mohney, L., Sinski, J., and Priest, D. (1988) A renal mycosis of an adult hybrid red tilapia *Oreochromis mossambique* X *O. hornorum*, caused by the imperfect fungus, *Paecilomyces marquandii*. J. Fish Dis. 11:437–444.

Maurizio, A. (1899) Beitrage zur Biologie der Saprolegnieen. Mitt. dt. Fisch Ver. 7:1–66.

McGinnis, M.R. (1977) *Exophiala spinifera*, a new combination for *Phialophora spinifera*. Mycotaxon 5:337–340.

Neish, G.A., and Hughes, G.C. (1980) Diseases of Fishes: Book 6: Fungal Diseases of Fishes. T.F.H. Publications, Neptune, New Jersey.

Neresheimer, E., and Clodi, C. (1914) *Ichthyophonus hoferi* Plehn u. Mulsow, der Erreger der Taumelkrankheit der Salmoniden. Arch. Protintenk. 34:217–248.

Oseid, D. M. (1977) Control of fungus growth on fish eggs by *Asellus militaris* and *Gammarus pseudolimnaeus*. Trans. Am. Fish. Soc. 106:192–195.

Pickering, A.D., Willoughby, L.G., and McGrory, C.B. (1979) Fine structure of secondary zoospore cyst cases of *Saprolegnia* isolates from infected fish. Trans. Br. Mycol. Soc. 72:427–436.

Plehn, M., and Mulsow, K. (1911) Der Erreger der "Taumelkrankheit" der Salmoniden. Zentbl. Bakt. ParasitKde., Abt. 1, 58:63–68.

Richards, R.H., and Pickering, A.D. (1978) Frequency and distribution pattern of *Saprolegnia* infection in wild and hatchery-reared brown trout *Salmo trutta* L. and char *Salvelinus alpinus* (L.). J. Fish Dis. 1:69–82.

Richards, R.H., Holliman, A., and Helgason, S. (1978) Naturally occurring *Exophiala salmonis* infection in Atlantic salmon *(Salmo salar* L.). J. Fish Dis. 1:357–369.

Roberts, R.J. (1978) Fish Pathology. Bailliere Tindall, London.

Ross, A.J., and Yasutake, W.T. (1973) *Scolecobasidium humicola*, a fungal pathogen of fish. J. Fish. Res. Bd. Can. 30:994–995.

Ross, A.J., Yasutake, W.T., and Leek, S. (1975) *Phoma herbarum*, a fungal saprophyte as a fish pathogen. J. Fish. Res. Bd. Can. 32:1648–1652.

Schnetzler, J.B. (1887) Infection d'une larve de grenouille par *Saprolegnia ferax*. Archs Sci. Phys. Nat., Ser. 3, 18:492.

Scott, W.W., and O'Bier, A.H.J. (1962) Aquatic fungi associated with diseased fish and fish eggs. Progressive Fish Culturist 24:3–15.

Sindermann, C.J., and Scattergood, L.W. (1954) Diseases of fishes of the western North Atlantic II. *Ichthyosporidium* disease of the sea herring *(Clupea herengus)*. Res. Bull. Dept. Sea Shore Fish. Me. 19:1–40.

Tiffney, W.N. (1939) The identity of certain species of Saprolegniaceae parasitic to fish. J. Elisha Mitchell Scient. Soc. 55:134–151.

Tiffney, W.N., and Wolf, F.T. (1937) *Achlya flagellata* as a fish parasite. J. Elisha Mitchell Scient. Soc. 53:298–300.

Tomanek, J. (1962) Plisnova' na'kaza pstruhu duhovy'ch. Cslke'. Ryb. 3:36.

Willoughby, L.G., and Pickering, A.D. (1977) Viable Saprolegniaceae spores on the epidermis of salmonid fish *Salmo trutta* and *Salvelinus alpinus*. Trans. Br. Mycol. Soc. 68:91–95.

Witala, B., and Zielonke, M. (1974) Zgorzel skrzeli (branchiomycosis) u pstraga tcczowego *(Salmo gairdneri* Rich.). Medycyna Weter. 30:603–605.

Wolke, R.E. (1975) Pathology of bacterial and fungal diseases affecting fish. In: The Pathology of Fishes (Ribelin, W.E., and Migaki, G. eds.). University of Wisconsin Press, Madison, Wisconsin, pp. 33–116.

Wood, S.E., Willoughby, L.G., and Beakes, G.W. (1988) Experimental studies on uptake and interaction of spores of the *Saprolegnia diclina-parasitica* complex with external mucus of brown trout *(Salmo trutta)*. Trans. Br. Mycol. Soc. 90:63–73.

Chapter 38

SALMONID FISH VIRUSES

PHILIP E. McALLISTER

Salmonid fishes are susceptible to a variety of viral infections. Some infections cause epizootic mortality, whereas others have no readily apparent effect on the overall health of the fish. Some of the viruses are associated with and shown to be the cause of neoplastic conditions. Because of the economic and recreational importance of salmonid fishes, the salmonid fish viruses have received sustained, intense research emphasis. The following viruses in Table 38–1 are detected in salmonid fishes.

STRAWBERRY DERMATITIS

SYNONYMS. Strawberry disease, rainbow trout adenovirus disease.

Host and Geographic Distribution

Strawberry dermatitis occurs in rainbow trout and has been recognized for almost 30 years as endemic to certain hatcheries in the northwest United States. The disease has occurred in France (Fleury et al., 1985; Olson et al., 1985). The etiology is unknown, but speculations vary from infectious agents (strawberry disease virus, rainbow trout virus) to local allergic reactions (Olson et al., 1985).

Clinical Signs and Pathology

Strawberry dermatitis is a nonfatal, inflammatory skin condition. The only clinical signs associated with the disease are bright red skin lesions that develop over the central and caudal body. Initially, lesions appear as single or multiple, small, circular to oval raised areas on the skin. Fully developed lesions are bright red, nonhemorrhagic ulcerations several millimeters to several centimeters in diameter. When the ulcers heal, normal skin pigmentation returns. Morbidity of 80% has been reported.

Histologically, the disease is a progressive inflammatory response. Infiltration of lymphocytes and monocytes into the dermis, hypodermis, and underlying fascial planes separates muscle blocks and forms an almost continuous layer separating dermis from epidermis. Focal necrosis and sloughing of the epidermis and scales and focal necrosis and lysis of muscle fibers occur. Dilation and congestion of blood vessels give lesions their bright red appearance.

Diagnosis and Virus Detection

Strawberry dermatitis can be presumptively diagnosed by correlating clinical signs and histologic examination. An adenoviruslike agent can be isolated from strawberry disease lesions (Fleury et al., 1985). When lesion tissue is dispersed and inoculated onto the chorioallantoic membrane of 9-day embryonated chicken eggs, pocks 1 mm in diameter become evident after 7 days incubation at 37°C. Electron microscopy of pocks and lesion tissue shows morphologically identical, unenveloped icosahedral virus particles 65 nm in diameter. The particles have six capsomeres on each peripheral edge, but no vertex fibers are seen. The piscine origin of the putative virus is questioned because only adenoviruses of avian origin are known to replicate in embryonated chicken eggs, and because no virus isolated from salmonid fishes is known to replicate at 37°C.

Transmission and Epidemiology

The disease has been transmitted only by cohabitation. Affected fish usually recover after about 2 months, and the disease does not recur. No experimental challenges have been made using the adenoviruslike agent recovered from strawberry lesions (Fleury et al., 1985).

Treatment and Control

No methods of treatment or control have been adequately described. Oral treatment with oxytetracycline reportedly shortens recovery time (Olson et al., 1985).

SALMONID HERPESVIRUS

SYNONYMS. *Herpesvirus salmonis*, (HSV, HPV), *H. salmonis*, steelhead herpesvirus (SHV), salmonid herpesvirus group I.

Host and Geographic Distribution

Herpesvirus salmonis was first isolated in 1971 from spawning rainbow trout and confirmed in 1975

TABLE 38–1. Viral Diseases of Salmonid Fishes*

Disease	Virus	Host
Strawberry dermatitis	Rainbow trout adenovirus	Rainbow trout
Salmonid herpesvirus mortality	*Herpesvirus salmonis* and Steelhead herpesvirus	Chinook salmon Rainbow trout Steelhead trout
Japanese salmonid herpesvirus epizootic mortality	Nerka virus	Kokanee salmon Masou salmon
Epithelial papilloma	*Oncorhynchus masou* virus and Yamame tumor virus	Chum salmon Rainbow trout Lake trout
Epidermal hyperplasia	Lake trout herpesvirus	Lake trout Lake trout × Brook trout
Infectious pancreatic necrosis	Infectious pancreatic necrosis virus	Many species of fishes Crustaceans Molluscs
Landlocked salmon disease	Landlocked salmon virus	Masou salmon
Focal necrotizing hepatitis	Chum salmon reovirus	Chinook salmon Chum salmon Kokanee salmon
Atlantic salmon leiomyosarcoma	Atlantic salmon fibrosarcoma retrovirus	Atlantic salmon
Epidermal papilloma	Atlantic salmon papilloma retrovirus	Atlantic salmon
Infectious hematopoietic necrosis	Infectious hematopoietic necrosis virus	Various species of salmonids
Salmonid hepatitis	Rhabdovirus of salmonid hepatitis	Rainbow trout
Viral hemorrhagic septicemia	Viral hemorrhagic septicemia virus	Various species of fish
Unknown	Chinook salmon paramyxovirus	Chinook salmon
Erythrocytic inclusion body syndrome	Erythrocytic inclusion body syndrome virus	Chinook salmon Coho salmon
Coho anemia	Intraerythrocytic virus of Coho salmon	Coho salmon
Hemorrhagic trout disease	Intraerythrocytic virus of rainbow trout	Rainbow trout
Unknown	Picornalike virus of Atlantic salmon	Atlantic salmon
Unknown	Picornalike virus of salmonids from California	Brook trout Brown trout Cutthroat trout Rainbow trout
Ulcerative dermal necrosis	Ulcerative dermal necrosis–associated virus	Atlantic salmon Brown trout

See also sections on Epizootic Hematopoietic Necrosis Virus, 13p₂ Reovirus, and Pike Fry Rhabdovirus in Chapter 26; and Erythrocytic Necrosis Virus, Eel Virus—American, Eel Virus—European X, and Rhabdovirus olivaceus in Chapter 88.

(Wolf, 1976). The virus has not been reisolated since. Rainbow trout less than 6 months old develop clinical disease and die when experimentally challenged. Young Atlantic salmon, brook trout, brown trout, yearling rainbow trout, and kokanee are refractory to infection (Wolf, 1976, 1983; Wolf and Smith, 1981). *Herpesvirus salmonis* was isolated at only one location, the Winthrop National Fish Hatchery in the state of Washington. A 2-year survey of stations that had received Winthrop eggs and fry showed no further dissemination of the virus.

Recently, however, a closely related herpesvirus was isolated from spawning steelhead trout returning to the Warm Spring Hatchery in Northern California. Fingerling rainbow trout and chinook salmon are susceptible to experimental infection with the steelhead trout herpesvirus, but brown trout and coho salmon are not (Eaton et al., 1989; Hedrick et al., 1987a). The steelhead herpesvirus has been isolated from seven hatcheries and two lakes in California (Eaton et al., 1989).

Clinical Signs

In fry and fingerling rainbow trout experimentally challenged with *Herpesvirus salmonis*, clinical signs of disease appear 2 to 3 weeks after infection, and mortality ranges from 50 to 100% (Wolf, 1976, 1983; Wolf et al., 1975). Affected fish are initially hyperactive, but become increasingly lethargic and die. External signs include darkened color, exophthalmia, abdominal distension, and pale gills. White mucoid casts trail from the vent, and hemorrhages are evident in the eyes and at the base of the fins. Internally, the peritoneal cavity is filled with ascitic fluid, and the digestive tract contains little food. Hematocrits are often 30% of normal. Adult rainbow trout carrying *Herpesvirus salmonis* show no clinical signs other than excessive postspawning mortality ranging from 30 to 50%. No clinical signs are reported for fingerling fish exposed to or adult steelhead carrying the steelhead herpesvirus.

Pathology

In rainbow trout experimentally infected with *Herpesvirus salmonis*, the internal organs appear edematous, yet flaccid. The liver, heart, and spleen are mottled with areas of hyperemia, and the kidneys sometimes appear pale (Wolf, 1983; Wolf and Smith, 1981). The cranial kidney shows edema and hyperplasia of hematopoietic tissue. In the caudal kidney, pronounced edema and necrosis is seen in hematopoietic tissue and renal tubules, whereas glomeruli are only slightly edematous. There is hepatic edema, necrosis, and hemorrhage or congestion. The small intestine and pyloric ceca appear normal, but the large intestine shows extensive necrosis, sloughing of the mucosa, and leukocyte infiltration into the submucosa. The heart is edematous and necrotic and infiltrated with lymphocytes, polymorphonuclear leukocytes, and macrophages. Edema and congestion of the spleen and brain are evident and hemorrhage and necrosis are occasionally observed in skeletal muscle. Large syncytia form in the pancreas. Gills show edema, hypertrophy, and hemorrhage and structural separation of epithelium from connective tissue.

Steelhead herpesvirus causes liver inflammation and focal hepatic syncytia in young rainbow trout—pathologic changes appear 6 to 31 weeks after experimental infection. The fused hepatocytes contain enlarged nuclei with Feulgen-positive, eosinophilic Cowdry Type A inclusions (Eaton et al., 1989).

Diagnosis, Virus Isolation, and Identification

Viral infection is diagnosed by isolation of virus in cell culture and its subsequent identification by reactivity with virus-specific immune serum.

Both *Herpesvirus salmonis* and the steelhead herpesvirus can be isolated from ovarian fluid and from internal organ homogenates. The steelhead herpesvirus can also be recovered from semen (Eaton et al., 1989).

Herpesvirus salmonis replicates in CHSE-214, KF-1, RTG-2, and RTF-1 cells, but not in BB, BF-2, and FHM cells. The steelhead herpesvirus replicates in CHSE-214 and RTG-2 cells. For greatest sensitivity of detection, cell culture inoculum should be adsorbed for 2 hours. The optimum temperature for replication

of either virus is 10°C. Virus replication is inconsistent at 15°C and does not occur at temperatures above 15°C. Cells infected with *H. salmonis* coalesce to form syncytia in 7 to 14 days after inoculation (Wolf et al., 1978).

Cytopathic effects (syncytia) from steelhead herpesvirus are apparent in 3 to 4 weeks. Viral deoxyribonucleic acid (DNA) can be detected in liver, kidney, and pancreatic tissue using hybridization, DNA-probe techniques (Eaton et al., 1989).

Infectivity neutralization assays show that *Herpesvirus salmonis* and the steelhead herpesvirus are very closely related. These North American isolates comprise a serogroup distinct from the Japanese salmonid herpesvirus isolates, but all share some common antigens associated with neutralization (Eaton et al., 1989; Hedrick et al., 1987a).

Transmission and Epidemiology

The mode of transmission of *Herpesvirus salmonis* and steelhead herpesvirus is unknown. Both viruses are carried as latent infections ostensibly activated at spawning. Survivors of infection can become long-term virus carriers.

Only fish less than 6 months old have been infected experimentally. *Herpesvirus salmonis* can be experimentally transmitted by intramuscular and intraperitoneal injection, but not by cohabitation (Wolf, 1976, 1983). The steelhead herpesvirus can be experimentally transmitted by immersion challenge and by injection (Eaton et al., 1989; Hedrick et al., 1987a).

Temperature profoundly affects the course of infection. Disease and mortality occur only if infected fish are held at about 10°C. Under optimal conditions several weeks may elapse before the first mortalities occur.

Treatment and Control

Control of *Herpesvirus salmonis* was achieved by destruction of the affected captive broodstock and by the disinfection of the Winthrop National Fish Hatchery. For the steelhead herpesvirus, no methods of treatment or control are known. The virus was isolated from apparently healthy feral fish.

The antiviral drugs 9-(2-hydroxyethoxymethyl) guanine (acycloguanosine) and 5-iodo-2'-deoxyuridine suppress the replication of *Herpesvirus salmonis* in cell culture, but have not been tested in fish (Kimura et al., 1983a).

JAPANESE SALMONID HERPESVIRUS

SYNONYMS. *Nerka* virus, *Oncorhynchus masou* virus (OMV), yamame tumor virus (YTV), NeVTA, Japanese salmonid herpesviruses, salmonid herpesvirus group II.

Host and Geographic Distribution

Three herpesviruses can be isolated from salmonid fishes in Japan, the nerka virus in Towada Lake, Akita and Aomori Prefecture from kokanee or himemasu (Sano, 1976), *Oncorhynchus masou* virus from masou salmon or yamame (Kimura et al., 1981a), and yamame tumor virus from yamame (Sano et al., 1983; Hedrick et al., 1987a). Chum salmon, kokanee, and rainbow trout can be experimentally infected with OMV, as can chum salmon with YTV.

Clinical Signs and Pathology

Kokanee fry infected with Nerka virus become dark, lethargic, and inappetent. The kidneys show syncytia and cytoplasmic inclusions in interstitial cells, necrotic tubules, and serous fluid accumulation in Bowman's space. Pancreatic acinar cells become vacuolated, epithelial cells in the gills show swelling and sloughing, and degenerative changes occur in skeletal muscle (Sano, 1976). Losses during epizootic mortality can exceed 80% in young-of-the-year fish.

Oncorhynchus masou virus was originally isolated from apparently healthy yamame, but experimentally infected fry and fingerling fish become exophthalmic, inappetent, hyperactive, and ultimately die. Petechial hemorrhages are evident particularly under the jaw. Internally, the liver is mottled white to completely blanched and shows severe multifocal necrosis and syncytium formation. Necrosis also occurs in the spleen, and edema in cardiac muscle. Herpesvirus particles are seen in electron micrographs of liver tissue. Perioral and renal epithelial papillomas develop in some survivors of experimental infection (Kimura et al., 1981a,b; Yoshimizu et al., 1988b).

Yamame tumor virus has been isolated from a spontaneous tumor consisting of undifferentiated spindle and cylindrical basal cells in an alveolar array seen in the perioral region of otherwise healthy-appearing fish. Mortality occurs in experimentally infected fish. Moribund fish show exophthalmia, abdominal distension, and hyperemia particularly at the vent. Some survivors of infection develop perioral tumors that are histologically similar to the spontaneous neoplasm (Sano et al., 1983).

Diagnosis, Virus Isolation, and Identification

Diagnosis of NeVTA infection requires isolation of the virus in cell culture and its identification by reactivity with specific immune serum. For OMV and YTV, histologic examination of perioral tumors can be used to formulate a presumptive diagnosis in the species of concern, but confirmed diagnosis requires isolation of virus in cell culture coupled with serologic identification using specific immune serum. These viruses replicate only in salmonid cell cultures (RTG-

2 and CHSE-214 are used most frequently) (Kamei et al., 1987; Kimura et al., 1981a,b; Sano, 1976; Sano et al., 1983). All three viruses can be isolated from homogenates of internal organs. Infected cells form syncytia at temperatures from 5 to 18°C. Virus replication is optimum at 15°C.

Infectivity neutralization assays indicate that the three viruses have strong serologic similarity. The salmonid herpesviruses from Japan and the United States are serologically distinct, but share some common antigens (Hedrick et al., 1987a).

Transmission and Epidemiology

Both horizontal and vertical transmission may play roles in the annual epizootics in young-of-the-year kokanee, in the low survivability of progeny from carrier broodstock, and in the persistence of basal cell epitheliomas in various yamame populations. The OMV can be experimentally transmitted to fry and fingerling chum salmon, kokanee, and rainbow trout by immersion and by cohabitation (Kimura et al., 1981a,b). Three-month-old fish are more susceptible to infection than 5-month-old fish, and 7-month-old fish become infected but do not die. Survivors of experimental infection produce OMV-neutralizing antibody (Kimura et al., 1981b). Five-month-old yamame and chum salmon can be experimentally infected by intraperitoneal injection of YTV (Sano et al., 1983). Epithelial perioral tumors develop 4 to 13 months after exposure to OMV or YTV.

Treatment and Control

Fish health survey programs are routinely used to identify fish populations that harbor pathogens, and restrict distribution of infected fish.

Replication of OMV in RTG–2 cells is inhibited most effectively by 9-(2-hydroxyethoxymethyl) guanine (acycloguanosine) and to a lesser extent by 5-iodo–2'-deoxyuridine (IUdR) and phosphonoacetate (Kimura et al., 1983a,b). Experimentally challenged fish that are immersed daily in acycloguanosine show 30% greater survival than untreated controls, and similar results are seen in fish given daily oral treatments of IUdR. Both acycloguanoside and IUdR suppress the development of virus-induced tumors.

LAKE TROUT EPIDERMAL HYPERPLASIA

SYNONYMS. Lake trout herpesvirus, salmonid herpesvirus 3, epizootic epitheliotropic disease (EED).

Host and Geographic Distribution

Sporadic incidents of epizootic mortalities involving lake trout occur at hatcheries in the Lake

Superior and Lake Michigan basins of the United States (Bradley et al., 1989; McAllister and Herman, 1989). The epizootics date to the mid-1980s.

Lake trout and lake trout hybrids are the target species of this herpesvirus (salmonid herpesvirus 3, epizootic epitheliotropic disease virus [EEDV]). Backcross lake trout hybrids (75% lake trout, 25% brook trout) and splake lake trout hybrids (50% lake trout, 50% brook trout) can be experimentally infected. Brook trout, brown trout, rainbow trout, Atlantic salmon, and chinook salmon are refractory.

Clinical Signs and Pathology

Affected fish are lethargic and swim near the surface showing sporadic flashing and diving, spiral swimming. The fins have a frayed appearance. Hemorrhages develop in the lower quadrant of the eyes and occasionally at the mouth and base of the fins, and gray-white blotches of mucuslike material accumulate on the skin and fins. In survivors, secondary fungal infection occurs on the eyes and fins and in patches on other body surfaces. Hematocrit values are elevated (ave. 45.6) in acutely infected lake trout. Blood chemistry profiles show reduced ion levels consistent with osmotic imbalance. In fingerling to yearling fish the level of mortality can approach 100%.

Histopathologic examination shows consistent epidermal hyperplasia with lymphocytic infiltrates, hydrophic cells, and necrosis on the snout, inside the mouth, and on the oral flap. In some severely affected fish the hyperplasia occurs over most of the body. Eosinophilic intranuclear inclusion bodies are sometimes seen in epidermal cells. Gill pathology is inconsistent.

The kidneys contain macrophages filled with cell debris, and the proximal tubules and glomerular capillaries are dilated. Tubular degeneration is sometimes seen. Liver sinusoids may contain debris-laden macrophages late in the infection. Hepatocytes show depleted glycogen reserves.

Diagnosis and Virus Detection

Presumptive diagnosis is based on correlating the species of concern, clinical signs, and pathologic changes. Diagnosis is confirmed by detection of herpesvirus particles in electron micrographs of thin sections of epidermal tissue or herpesvirus capsids in fractionated, purified skin homogenates. Virus has not been isolated in cell culture.

Attempts made to isolate virus from samples of skin, whole heads, gills, kidneys, and spleen using CHSE-214, EPC, FHM, RTG-2, RTH-149, RTM, and McCoy cells incubated at 9, 15, and 18°C were unsuccessful, as were attempts to isolate virus using primary and established cells from lake trout. No evidence of cytopathogenic virus is seen either on primary inoculation or blind passage.

Transmission, Epizootiology, and Pathogenesis

The disease is experimentally transmitted by immersion in or injection of filtered (0.22 or 0.45 μm apd) skin scrapings or skin homogenates, and by cohabitation with or exposure to water from virus-infected fingerling, yearling, or adult fish. The virus can also be transmitted mechanically via contaminated culture equipment. Death occurs 7 to 14 days after exposure.

Natural epizootics occur predominately in the spring of the year at a water temperature of about 9°C, although outbreaks can occur at temperatures from 6 to 15°C. In yearling fish, the onset of mortality often occurs 7 to 14 days after some culture or environmental stress event, e.g., fin clipping, tagging, excessive handling, large-scale bird predation, or nitrogen supersaturation. Epizootics continue for several months, and the level of mortality can approach 100%. Death is seemingly the result of osmoregulatory dysfunction resulting in the loss of essential ions. Survivors of infection almost always develop secondary fungal infections. Isolations of various bacteria are incidental to the viral infection, as are instances of epitheliocystis infection. The clinical and histopathologic profile of epitheliocystis is very different from the lake trout epidermal hyperplasia.

Treatment and Control

Infection with the lake trout herpesvirus cannot be effectively treated and those fish that survive become long-term carriers of the virus. The only effective way to control the infection is to remove all fish stocks and completely disinfect the facility. Water supplies can be effectively disinfected using ozone or ultraviolet irradiation.

INFECTIOUS PANCREATIC NECROSIS

SYNONYMS. Infectious pancreatic necrosis (IPN), IPNV, Aquatic birnavirus.

Host and Geographic Distribution

The earliest isolations of the infectious pancreatic necrosis virus (IPNV) (aquatic birnavirus) were from brook trout (Wolf et al., 1960), but since then IPN and IPN-like viruses have been recovered from at least 65 species of fishes and shellfish (Table 38–2).

The IPN and IPN-like viruses are distributed essentially worldwide. Isolations have been reported in North America (Canada and the United States), in South America (Chile), in most of eastern and western Europe, and in Asia (Japan, Korea, Taiwan, and Thailand).

TABLE 38–2. Fish and Shellfish Species from Which IPN and IPN-Like Viruses Have Been Recovered*

Fishes		Shellfish
Salmonids	Nonsalmonids	
Arctic char	Barbel	Hard clam
Japanese char	Sea bass	Limpet
Grayling	Striped bass	Blue mussel
Atlantic salmon	Bream	American oyster
Chinook salmon	Silver bream	Flat oyster
Chum salmon	Common carp	Pacific oyster
Coho salmon	Crucian carp	Common
Danube salmon	Discus fish	periwinkle
(Huchen)	European eel	Shore crab
Pink salmon	Japanese eel	Kuruma shrimp
Kokanee	Southern flounder	Tellina tenuis
(Himemasu)	Goldfish	Asian clam
Amago trout	Gudgeon	
Brook trout	Blueback herring	
Brown trout	Hogchoker	
Cutthroat trout	Lamprey	
Lake trout	Loach	
Rainbow trout	Atlantic menhaden	
	Minnow	
	Nase	
	Perch	
	Northern pike	
	Chain pickerel	
	Roach	
	Rudd	
	Sand goby	
	Atlantic shad	
	Atlantic silverside	
	Dover sole	
	Spot	
	White sucker	
	Tilapia	
	Turbot	
	Walleye	
	Yellowtail	
	Zebra danio	
	Dab	
	Gizzard shad	

Isolations of IPN virus from salmonid fish have been reported by Bellet (1969), Dorson (1983), Hill (1982), Ljungberg and Jorgensen (1973), MacKelvie and Artsob (1969), McAllister (1983), McAllister and Reyes (1984), McMichael et al. (1973), Munro and Duncan (1977), Olesen et al. (1988), Parisot et al. (1963), Sano (1973), Swanson and Gillespie (1979), Wolf and Pettijohn (1970), and Yulin and Zhengqiu (1987). Recovery of IPN and IPN-like viruses from nonsalmonid fishes and the susceptibility of nonsalmonid fishes to IPN and IPN-like viruses have been reported by Adair and Ferguson (1981), Ahne (1977, 1978), Bonami et al. (1983), Castric and Chastel (1980), Daud and Agius (1987), Diamant et al. (1988), Dorson (1983), Dorson et al. (1987), Hah et al. (1984), Hedrick et al. (1983a,b, 1985a, 1986a), Hill (1982), Mangunwiryo and Agius (1987), McAllister (1983), McAllister et al. (1984), Munro et al. (1976), Olesen et al. (1988), Sano (1976), Sano et al. (1981), Schutz et al. (1984), Sorimachi and Hara (1985), Sonstegard et al. (1972), and Stephens et al. (1980). IPN and IPN-like viruses recovered from shellfish have been reported by Bovo et al. (1984), Hill (1976a,b, 1982), and Underwood et al. (1977).

Clinical Signs and Pathology

In salmonids, acute infection occurs in 1- to 4-month-old fish and can result in cumulative mortality approaching 100%. Fish 6 months old or older undergo subclinical or inapparent infection, but experience no significant loss. Disease outbreaks in older fish involve virus carriers and are usually stress activated.

The affected fry and fingerlings appear darkly pigmented; show exophthalmia, abdominal distention, and mucoid fecal pseudocasts; and swim erratically, rotating about their long axis or whirling violently. Hematocrit values are depressed.

Internally, the liver and spleen appear pale, and the stomach and intestine are devoid of food but filled with mucoid fluid. Petechial hemorrhages are evident throughout the pyloric and pancreatic tissues. Pancreatic acinar cells, and occasionally islet tissue, undergo massive necrosis characterized by pyknosis, karyorrhexis, and intracytoplasmic inclusions (Kudo et al., 1973; McKnight and Roberts, 1976; Wood et al., 1955; Yasutake, 1970). The pylorus, pyloric ceca, and anterior intestine show extensive necrosis. The sloughing intestinal epithelium combines with excess mucus to form a whitish catarrhal exudate (McKnight and Roberts, 1976). Degenerative changes also occur in renal hematopoietic and excretory tissue and in the liver (Besse and de Kinkelin, 1965; Kudo et al., 1973; Sano, 1971a,b; Wolf and Quimby, 1971). Pancreatic and hepatic tissues are infiltrated by macrophages and polymorphonuclear leukocytes (Kudo et al., 1973; Swanson and Gillespie, 1979). Electron microscopy reveals viral particles in pancreatic, hepatic, renal, and splenic tissue (Kudo et al., 1973; Lightner and Post, 1969; Mulcahy and Fryer, 1976; Yamamoto, 1975c).

In nonsalmonid fishes, IPN and IPN-like viruses are generally isolated from fish showing no clinical signs; however, notable exceptions are the viruses isolated from branchionephritis in eels, from "spinning disease" in menhaden, and from viral ascites in yellowtail. In some other cases, IPN and IPN-like viruses have been isolated in association with disease but have not been proved to be the cause of the disease.

The clinical signs of branchionephritis or viral kidney disease in European and Japanese eels are body rigidity, abdominal retraction, and congestion or diffuse petechial hemorrhaging on the gills and ventral body surface and at the anal fin (Sano, 1976; Sano et al., 1981). Internally, the intestine is devoid of food, the body cavity contains ascites, and the kidney is somewhat hypertrophied. Histopathologic changes include hyperplasia, fusion, and clubbing in the gills, glomerular nephritis, hyaline droplet degeneration in renal tubule epithelial cells, and varying levels of necrosis in the liver, spleen, lymphoid tissue, and renal elements. The disease can be experimentally transmitted in eels but not in rainbow trout.

Menhaden with "spinning disease" become dark and swim in an erratic, uncoordinated manner (Stephens et al., 1980). Hemorrhages develop at the base of the fins, in the eyes, and along the body. Internally, the spleen and vessels of the brain are congested and hemorrhages are sometimes seen in the lumen of the gut. Histopathologic lesions include focal necrosis, pyknosis, and sloughing of the mucosae of the duodenum and pyloric ceca, inflammation of adipose tissue, focal necrosis of the exocrine pancreas and glandular stomach, and slight meningitis with edema and focal demyelinating lesions in the brain. The disease can be experimentally transmitted to menhaden and brook trout.

A disease called viral ascites occurs in yellowtail (Egusa and Sorimachi, 1986; Fujimaki et al., 1986; Isshiki et al., 1989; Miyazaki, 1985; Sorimachi and Hara, 1985). The disease causes high levels of mortality in hatchery- and pen-cultured fry and fingerling yellowtail in several prefectures in Japan. Affected fish show abdominal distension, pale gills, and quiescent behavior. The body cavity is filled with clear to blood-tinted ascites. Hemorrhages are evident in the liver, pyloric ceca, and stomach, and the kidneys and spleen are pale. Histologic examination shows focal and diffuse necrosis in hepatic parenchymal cells, pancreatic acinar cells, kidney tubule cells, and splenic pulp and arteries, degeneration of the intestinal epithelium, and edema of the spleen and submucosa of the stomach. The disease can be experimentally transmitted to yellowtail.

Evidence that the IPN and IPN-like viruses from marine molluscs and crustaceans cause disease is limited (Hill, 1976a,b, 1982; Underwood et al., 1977). Experimental infection of oyster (Ostrea edulis) and the bivalve mollusc (Tellina tenuis) induces pathologic changes in the digestive gland, which include edema, hemocyte infiltration, and connective tissue necrosis. Experimental infection of various crustaceans with an IPN-like virus from shore crab show that the virus can be recovered for several weeks after initial challenge.

Diagnosis, Virus Isolation, and Identification

Clinical signs combined with the age, species, and source of the fish and the geographic location and health history of the culture station are often used to formulate a presumptive diagnosis of IPN virus infection. Confirmed diagnosis requires isolation of the virus in cell culture and its identification based on serologic reactivity in neutralization, fluorescent antibody, immunoperoxidase, complement fixation, immunoelectrophoresis, coagglutination, or enzyme-linked immunosorbent assay (ELISA) tests (Ahne, 1981; Dea and Elazhary, 1983; Dixon and Hill, 1983; Faisal and Ahne, 1980; Finlay and Hill, 1975; Hattori et al., 1984; Hsu et al., 1989b; Kimura et al., 1984; Leintz and Springer, 1973; McAllister and Schill, 1986; Nicholson and Caswell, 1982; Piper et al., 1973; Rodak et al., 1988; Swanson, 1981; Swanson and Gillespie, 1981).

Infectivity neutralization is the standard to which other virus identification methods are compared. The results of IPN and IPN-like virus neutralization assays require careful consideration (McMichael et al., 1975). Some IPN virus isolates are sensitive to a single freeze-thaw cycle and require more acidic storage conditions to maintain infectivity (Wolf and Quimby, 1971).

A variety of salmonid and nonsalmonid cell lines and experimental conditions are used to isolate IPN and IPN-like viruses (Agius et al., 1982, 1983; Department of Fisheries and Oceans, 1984; Hedrick et al., 1986a,b; Hill, 1976a; Mangunwiryo and Agius, 1988; McAllister et al., 1987; Okamoto et al., 1985; Swanson and Gillespie, 1982; Wolf and Mann, 1980; Wolf and Quimby, 1973; Yu et al., 1982). Prolonged incubation and blind passage may be needed and the sensitivity of virus detection assays can be adversely affected by inhibitory factors in tissue extracts and by viral autointerference (Dixon, 1987; Nicholson and Dexter, 1975; Stephens et al., 1980; Yamamoto, 1974).

Internal organs and sex products are the clinical samples of choice (Billi and Wolf, 1969; Frantsi and Savan, 1971a; Mangunwiryo and Agius, 1988; Swanson and Gillespie, 1979; Wolf et al., 1963, 1968; Yamamoto 1975a,b). The caudal kidney yields virus more consistently than other tissues (Reno et al., 1978; Swanson and Gillespie, 1979; Yamamoto, 1974, 1975a,b; Yamamoto and Kilistoff, 1979). When nondestructive sampling is practiced, sex products (especially the particulate component recovered from the fluid associated with spawned eggs) are the preferred samples (McAllister et al., 1987). Blood, feces, and peritoneal washings can be assayed but are less reliable (Swanson and Gillespie, 1982; Yu et al., 1982). Virus can also be recovered from brain tissue (Stephens et al., 1980), and can be concentrated from water (Grinnell and Leong, 1979).

Specimens should be assayed as soon as possible, preferably within 24 hours of sampling. Infectivity is better if whole tissue is held on ice or at 4°C rather than frozen at −20 or −70°C. Conversely, infectivity in tissue homogenates is better preserved by freezing at −20 or −70°C. If bovine serum albumin is added to 2% final concentration, ovarian fluids can be held on ice or at 4, −20, or −70°C with minimal loss of infectivity. The probability of recovering virus is increased if fish are physiologically stressed (Frantsi and Savan, 1971a). No increased frequency of virus isolation occurs in fish stressed by injection of immunosuppressants (Bucke, 1977; Bucke et al., 1979).

A variety of salmonid and nonsalmonid cell lines support the replication of IPN and IPN-like viruses (Wolf and Mann, 1980). The cell lines most commonly used for virus isolation are BF-2, CHSE-214, PG, and RTG-2. EPC and FHM should not be used. Cell lines may vary in their comparative sensitivity for virus detection. Virus isolation may require specific host cells; for example, the IPN virus from menhaden can only be isolated using menhaden cells, but replicates in other cell lines after primary isolation (Stephens et al., 1980).

Isolates of IPN virus from salmonids replicate well at 10 to 26°C, poorly at 4°C, and not at all at 30°C. Isolates from nonsalmonid fishes show a similar temperature range profile, but some have the distinctive capability of replicating at 30°C (Hedrick et al., 1986a; Sorimachi and Hara, 1985).

The serologic relations among the IPN and IPN-like viruses are complex and multiple cross-reacting serotypes occur among isolates from salmonid and nonsalmonid fishes and freshwater and marine shellfish and crustaceans (Dorson, 1983; Okamoto et al., 1983). The nomenclature associated with IPN virus serotyping is in a state of flux. The basic salmonid serotypes are the North American VR-299 and the European Ab and Sp, also identified as serotypes 1, 2, and 3, respectively (Macdonald and Gower, 1981). The IPN-like viruses that replicate at 30°C may represent a fourth serotype (Hedrick et al., 1986a). Other groupings of virus isolates described as "He" and sero groups 1, 2, and 3 have been reported (Dorson, 1983; Hill, 1976b). Within each of the serotypes are a variety of cross-reacting isolates. Polyvalent antisera for diagnostic use may be a composite of antisera to as many as seven different virus isolates.

Transmission

Horizontal transmission occurs as a consequence of infected fish shedding virus with feces, urine, and sex products. Under epizootic conditions, hatchery water can contain 10^4 to 10^8 or more infectious units of virus per liter (Billi and Wolf, 1969; Desautels and MacKelvie, 1975; Wolf, 1966).

Homeotherms and poikilotherms can act as "mechanical" vectors. IPN virus has been recovered from the feces of chicken, great horned owl (*Bubo virginianus*), black-headed gull (*Laurus ridibundus*), heron (*Ardea cinerea*), and mink (*Mustella* sp.) (Eskildsen and Jorgensen, 1973; Peters and Neukirch, 1986; Sonstegard and McDermott, 1972), and from inoculated freshwater crayfish (*Astacus astacus*) (Halder and Ahne, 1988). Infectivity persists in two species of protozoans (*Mianiensis ovidus* and *Tetrahymena* sp.) that are fed virus-infected RTG-2 cells (Moewus-Knobb, 1965; Moewus, 1962).

Egg-associated, putative vertical transmission was proposed not long after the virus was first isolated (Wolf et al., 1963, 1968). The IPN virus can be transmitted with iodophor-treated brook trout eggs (Bullock et al., 1976), can be isolated from eyed rainbow trout eggs (Fijan and Giorgetti, 1978), and can be transmitted to the zebra fish egg (Seeley et al., 1977). Unfortunately, none of these studies differentiates between virus in the egg and virus that might be sequestered on the egg. The virus may possibly be carried inside the egg with the sperm (Dorson and Torchy, 1985). The virus appears to have an affinity for the eggshell, and can be recovered from the shells of eyed eggs for more than 3 weeks after infection, and can also be recovered from egg shells after hatching (Ahne and Negele, 1985a). If eggs are exposed to virus before fertilization, the virus appears to be washed off within 1 hour. Broodstock can possibly be inadvertently infected with IPN virus by injection of virus-contaminated pituitary extracts used to induce spawning (Ahne and Negele, 1985b).

Experimentally, IPN virus can be transmitted by injection, immersion, and feeding. The observed virulence in laboratory challenges is affected by the species and age of the fish, the method of exposure, the virus serotype, the cell culture passage history of the virus, and the culture history of the fish (Dorson et al., 1975; Dorson and Torchy, 1981; Hill, 1982; Hill and Dixon, 1977; Jorgensen and Kehlet, 1971; McAllister and Owens, 1986; Silim et al., 1982).

Epidemiology

The virus probably gains access by contact with the gills, ingestion with food, or passage through the sensory pores of the lateral line system. Some survivors of infection become virus carriers and are the reservoir of infection for contemporary and subsequent generations. The carrier prevalence can exceed 90% of the survivors of an epizootic. There are no indications of sex-related differences in carrier prevalence. The carrier state can continue for many years in both hatchery and natural environments, but some surveys suggest that the carrier prevalence decreases with time (Reno et al., 1978; Rosenlund, 1977; Yamamoto, 1975a; Yamamoto and Kilistoff, 1979). The carrier state may be affected by the host immune response because lower levels of virus occur in fish with circulating virus-neutralizing antibody (Billi and Wolf, 1969; Wolf and Quimby, 1969; Yamamoto, 1975b).

The prevalence of the carrier state can vary with different salmonid species. Rainbow trout appear to have a lower carrier prevalence and a carrier state of shorter duration than do brook trout (Yamamoto, 1974, 1975a; Yamamoto and Kilistoff, 1979). The lower frequency of virus isolation from the progeny of wild carrier fish and from virus-free fish introduced into carrier populations suggests that carrier-mediated transmission in nature may not be as significant as in the hatchery (Yamamoto, 1975a,b; Yamamoto and Kilistoff, 1979). Epizootics occur regularly in hatcheries that use eggs from virus-carrier broodstock or use surface waters inhabited by carrier fish. Nonsalmonid fishes can be reservoirs of infection (Munro and Duncan, 1977; Silim et al., 1982). Virus shed from carrier striped bass can infect brook trout and induce virus-neutralizing antibody (McAllister and McAllister, 1988). Feral striped bass may be exposed to IPN virus by consuming virus-carrier Atlantic menhaden (Wechsler et al., 1987).

Environmental conditions and stress factors affect IPN viral infection. Temperature influences both the host response to infection and the replication of the virus (Frantsi and Savan, 1971b; Sano, 1973; Dorson and Torchy, 1981). In general, high, rapidly developing mortality occurs at about 10 to 14°C, whereas high-level but delayed, protracted mortality occurs at about 6°C. At temperatures above 14°C, the level of mortality can be significant but is reduced. Recrudescence of infection can occur in apparently healthy IPN virus–carrier fish stressed by transport, crowding, increased temperature, or low oxygen concentration (Frantsi and Savan, 1971a; Roberts and McKnight, 1976), and nutritionally stressed fish are more susceptible to infection (McAllister and Owens, 1986). One study suggests that a soluble immuno-suppressive factor may be released when fish are crowded (Perlmutter et al., 1973).

Resistance to viral infection may correlate with developing immunocompetence (Klontz et al., 1965). High antibody levels in carrier fish correlate with reduced virus titers in organs and feces (Yamamoto, 1975b). Neutralizing antibody produced in response to natural infection or experimental inoculation is associated with an IgM-like immunoglobulin (Dorson, 1974; Jorgensen, 1973b). The carrier state may represent a balance between the persistent replication of defective and infectious virus and the production of virus-specific antibody (Hedrick and Fryer, 1982).

Treatment and Control

Infectious pancreatic necrosis is most effectively controlled by preventing contact between the host and the virus. There is no effective treatment for this viral infection. IPN virus is not inactivated by exposure to ether, chloroform, or glycerol, but is rapidly inactivated when exposed to chlorine, iodophor, ozone, or ultraviolet irradiation (Amend, 1976; Amend and Pietsch, 1972; Desautels and MacKelvie, 1975; Eskildsen and Jorgensen, 1974; Jorgensen, 1973a; MacKelvie and Desautels, 1975; Wedemeyer et al., 1978, 1979). With increasing water hardness, progressively higher concentrations and longer contact times are needed to inactivate the virus with chlorine and ozone (Wedemeyer et al., 1978, 1979). The virucidal activity of chlorine and iodophor are reduced by organic matter and at pH levels above pH 8 (Amend and Pietsch, 1972; Elliott and Amend, 1978). Exposure to ultraviolet irradiation (λ = 254 nm) causes rapid, exponential loss of infectivity at an intensity of 2000 μW/cm^2, but a slower curvilinear decrease in infectivity at 440 μW/cm^2 (MacKelvie and Desautels, 1975). The virus is progressively inactivated by exposure to β-propiolactone, formalin, drying, heating at 60°C, or pH 2 or 9 (Desautels and MacKelvie, 1975; Dixon and Hill, 1983; MacKelvie and Desautels, 1975; Vestergaard Jorgensen, 1973). If IPN virus is exposed to a 1:4000 dilution of formalin, the virus inactivation curve is multiphasic, and residual infectivity is detected after 14-day exposure at 4°C (MacKelvie and Desautels, 1975). When exposed to 1:200 dilution of formalin, the virus is completely inactivated in 4 days at 20°C, whereas residual infectivity can be detected after 7 days at 4°C (Dixon and Hill, 1983). Virus exposed to a 1:200 dilution of β-propiolactone loses all infectivity in 6 days at 4°C, but residual infectivity can be detected after 7 days at 20°C (Dixon and Hill, 1983). Treatment with formalin causes only slight reduction in the antigenicity of the virus, whereas over 50% of the antigenicity is lost by treatment with B-propiolactone (MacKelvie and Desautels, 1975).

A contaminated culture facility and hatchery implements can be disinfected by treatment with chlorine (200 mg/L for 1 hour). Chlorine treatment should be monitored because organic matter and pH affect the available chlorine concentration (Desautels and MacKelvie, 1975; Elliott and Amend, 1978). The water supply should be protected and controlled to the maximum extent possible by using enclosed spring and well water supplies. Ozone and ultraviolet irradiation can be used to decontaminate large volumes of water (MacKelvie and Desautels, 1975; Wedemeyer et al., 1978). Infectivity tends to persist longer in water that has been treated by filtration or autoclaving, suggesting that the stability of the virus can be affected by the resident microbial flora (Toranzo and Hetrick, 1982; Toranzo et al., 1983). Fish introduced into the facility should be assayed and determined to be specific pathogen–free, and eggs should originate from virus-free broodstock because IPN virus appears to be transmitted with eggs in spite of iodophor treatment (Bullock et al., 1976; Dorson and Torchy, 1985).

There is no evidence of maternally transferred immunity, but susceptible fry can be protected by passive transfer of antibody or interferon. Resistance to IPN viral infection appears to be heritable and can be enhanced by selective breeding.

Effective vaccines are only in the developmental stages. Inactivated IPN virus vaccines elicit a protective response when administered by injection and immersion, but not by hyperosmotic infiltration or feeding (Bootland et al., 1990; Dixon and Hill, 1983; Dorson, 1977; Hill and Dixon, 1977; Sano et al., 1981). Efforts to develop an attenuated IPN virus vaccine have not been successful. Live virus vaccines whether attenuated or naturally avirulent present diagnostic and regulatory problems that have thus far been insurmountable. More promising are the efforts to develop subunit vaccines using cloned components from virulent strains of IPN virus and from avirulent strains that cross-react with virulent strains.

The incidence of acute IPN and consequent mortality can be reduced if factors that promote physiologic stress are controlled. Reducing population density, following optimal feeding protocols, maintaining proper hatchery hygiene, and utilizing prophylactic treatments for bacterial diseases and parasites have been effective in moderating outbreaks of IPN.

No truly effective chemotherapeutics are available for treatment of IPN. The antiviral synthetic nucleoside virazole (1-D-ribofluranosyl-1, 2,4-triazole-3-carboxamide) inhibits IPN virus replication in cell culture and somewhat reduces the mortality in virus-infected rainbow trout fry (Migus and Dobos, 1980; Savan and Dobos, 1980). However, because virazole is a reversible inhibitor, effectiveness decreases with time, and repeated treatment is necessary. Cost analysis shows that antiviral chemotherapy is too costly. Interferon induction with tilorone elicits no protection. Polyvinylpyrrolidone-iodine, ϵ-aminocaproic acid, and tranexamic acid chemotherapy appear to reduce IPN virus mortality (Economon, 1963, 1973; Inoue, 1973), but in experimental challenge trials, the chemicals are generally ineffective.

LANDLOCKED SALMON VIRUS

SYNONYM. Aquareovirus.

Host and Geographic Distribution

The only reported isolation of landlocked salmon virus is from landlocked masu salmon from the upper basin of the Ta-Chia river in the Republic of China (Taiwan) (Hsu et al., 1989a).

Clinical Signs and Pathology

Other than epizootic mortality of fry and egg stages, no clinical signs are described. Virus was isolated from a fish showing necrosis of the pelvic fin and internal organs (Hsu et al., 1989a).

Diagnosis, Virus Isolation, and Identification

Diagnosis requires isolation of the virus in cell culture. At present, the virus is identified by comparative analysis of protein and ribonucleic acid (RNA) electrophoretic profiles (Hsu et al., 1989a).

The virus is isolated from homogenates of liver and gills. Cytopathic effects, consisting of plaquelike syncytia, appear about 14 days after inoculation in BB, BF-2, CCO, CHSE-214, AS, MHR, or PL cells. The virus grows to a limited extent in EPC, FHM, GK, PH, RTG-2, and TO-2 cells. The virus replicates at temperatures from 10 to 30°C, optimum 20 to 22°C (Hsu et al., 1989a).

Transmission, Epidemiology, and Pathogenesis

Little is known about the transmission, epidemiology, and pathogenesis of this virus. Epizootic losses of fry and egg stages suggest mechanisms involving horizontal and possibly vertical transmission may be involved.

Treatment and Control

No methods of treatment or control are known. Fish populations with a known history of landlocked salmon virus infection should be avoided.

FOCAL NECROTIZING HEPATITIS

SYNONYMS. Chum salmon virus hepatitis, chum salmon reovirus hepatitis, aquareovirus hepatitis.

Host and Geographic Distribution

A reovirus, designated the chum salmon virus (CSV), was recovered from adult chum and masou salmon returning to spawn at hatcheries in Hokkaido (Japan) (Winton et al., 1980, 1981). The virus can be experimentally transmitted to chum, chinook, and kokanee salmon and rainbow trout. The virus has been isolated only from fish and fish products originating in Japan.

Clinical Signs, Pathology, and Diagnosis

The chum salmon virus can be isolated from from apparently healthy adult chum and masou salmon at spawning and from apparently healthy chum, chinook, and kokanee salmon and rainbow trout following experimental challenge (Winton et al., 1980, 1981). No clinical signs of disease are observed in either naturally or experimentally infected fish, and little to no mortality occurs. In laboratory infected fish, small foci of hepatic necrosis are the histopathologic changes seen.

No presumptive diagnosis is possible based on clinical signs or pathologic changes. A presumptive diagnosis can be made based on the unusual plaque-like syncytial cytopathic effect in cell culture. Confirmed diagnosis requires serologic identification of the virus.

Virus Isolation and Identification

Kidney, spleen, or liver are the tissues of choice for isolation of virus in cell culture. The virus replicates in a variety of salmonid and nonsalmonid cell lines and at temperatures from 10 to 20°C; optimally at 15 to 20°C. Cytopathic effects become apparent in CHSE-214 cells after 6 days incubation at 18°C. The cytoplasm of adjacent infected cells fuse, but the nuclei remain intact and accumulate at the periphery of the expanding syncytium. Only one serotype of the virus is known. Cross-neutralization assays show that although chum salmon virus, golden shiner virus, and catfish reovirus share some common antigens, they are serologically distinct.

Transmission, Treatment, and Control

The virus can be experimentally transmitted by waterborne exposure and by intraperitoneal injection of cell culture–grown virus. No reservoirs of infection other than adult chum and masou salmon are known. The mechanisms of natural transmission are unknown.

No methods of treatment are known. Avoidance is the only known method for control of the dissemination of the virus.

Viral infectivity is unaffected by exposure to chloroform or acid conditions (pH 3.0), is stable for 24 hours at 18 to 37°C, but is rapidly inactivated by heating at 56°C (Winton et al., 1980, 1981).

ATLANTIC SALMON LEIOMYOSARCOMA

SYNONYMS. Atlantic salmon fibrosarcoma, Atlantic salmon leiomyosarcoma, Atlantic salmon fibrosarcoma-associated virus, Atlantic salmon fibrosarcoma retrovirus.

Host and Geographic Distribution

Atlantic salmon held in sea cages in Scotland are affected by a fibrosarcoma of the swim bladder (McKnight, 1978).

Clinical Signs and Pathology

The tumor is detected in dead and moribund 1- and 2-year-old Atlantic salmon (McKnight, 1978). Affected fish show no external lesions, but appear lethargic. Internally, multiple nodular tumors 5 to 30 mm in diameter are evident on the swimbladder and protrude into the abdominal cavity. There is no evidence of invasion or metastasis. The tumor develops at the interface of the areolar tissue and the inner smooth muscle of the swimbladder wall and is composed of well-differentiated, interdigitating spindle cells with tampering blunt to pointed nuclei. Little collagen is detected by histochemical staining. The neoplasm is classified as a leiomyosarcoma.

Diagnosis and Virus Detection

Presumptive diagnosis is based on histologic examination of the swimbladder tumor. Diagnosis is confirmed by detection of electron-dense, spheroidal retroviruslike particles in thin-section preparations of the neoplastic tissue (Duncan, 1978). The etiologic significance of the retroviruslike particles is not known because virus has not yet been isolated in cell culture. It has been designated Atlantic salmon fibrosarcoma–associated virus or Atlantic salmon fibrosarcoma reovirus. The type C–like virions are 120 nm in diameter and contain a centrally placed ringlike nucleoid, 90 nm in diameter. The particles appear to be assembled as they bud from the cell surface, and extracellular aggregates of particles are associated with semiordered fibrils, each 20 nm in thickness.

Transmission, Epidemiology, Treatment, and Control

The tumor has not been experimentally transmitted. In nature, the swimbladder tumor is observed in sea-caged Atlantic salmon at a prevalence of about 5% (McKnight, 1978). No methods of treatment or control are known.

ATLANTIC SALMON PAPILLOMA

SYNONYMS. Atlantic salmon papilloma-associated virus, Atlantic salmon papilloma retrovirus.

Host and Geographic Distribution

A benign epidermal papilloma occurs in Atlantic salmon in Great Britain, Norway, Sweden, and the United States (Carlisle and Roberts, 1977; Ljungberg, 1963; Wiren, 1971; Wolf, 1966).

Clinical Signs

The papillomas appear as single or multiple proliferations that have a smooth to nodular texture and are translucent to white. They may occur at any site on the body surface and are 2 to 5 mm thick and up to 4 cm in diameter. The tumor eventually sloughs, and the epidermal tissues heal with no evidence of invasion or metastasis. Mortality occurs principally as the result of secondary bacterial or fungal infection (Bylund et al., 1980).

Pathology

The papillomatous epidermis is 5 to 15 times thicker than normal and appears to be composed of cells derived from the middle epidermis. The hyperplastic cells are spindle shaped and weakly interdigitated, have poorly formed desmosomes, and contain a rounded nucleus with prominent nucleoli and aggregated, marginated chromatin. Numerous atypical mitotic figures are evident, as are occasional degenerating cells containing intracytoplasmic inclusions. Mucous cells and a distinct basal layer and basement membrane are lacking, but fibrovascular stalks of apparent dermal origin penetrate the papillomatous mass.

Mild inflammatory activity is associated with the papilloma. Tissues adjacent to the tumor become hyperemic, and the lesion is infiltrated by lymphocytes, macrophages, and neutrophils. The lesion may slough in a graft rejection–type reaction, ostensibly as the result of cell-mediated immunity (Carlisle, 1976, 1977).

Diagnosis and Virus Detection

Presumptive diagnosis is based on the detection and histologic examination of the tumor. Diagnosis is confirmed by electron microscopic examination of tumor tissue, which reveals, albeit infrequently, intracytoplasmic and extracellular retroviruslike particles, 125 to 150 nm in diameter, containing a centrally placed, electron-dense nucleoid, 70 to 95 nm in diameter (Carlisle, 1976, 1977; Wiren, 1971). Attempts to isolate the virus from homogenates of papillomas, kidneys, and spleens, and from primary cultures of papilloma cells have been unsuccessful (Carlisle, 1976, 1977; Wiren, 1971).

Transmission, Epidemiology, Treatment, and Control

Attempts to experimentally transmit the tumor have been unsuccessful (Carlisle, 1976, 1977; Wiren, 1971). In nature, the prevalence may approach 55% in 1- to 2-year-old freshwater hatchery fish, 10% in 2- to 3-year-old fish captured in salt water, and 1.5% in spawning adults. The papilloma has also been observed in 1- to 2-year-old feral Atlantic salmon. The epizootic occurrence of the lesions suggests infectious etiology, but genetic and hormonal factors may possibly affect the occurrence of the papilloma (Carlisle, 1977). In younger, freshwater fish, the epidermal papilloma appears in late summer and regresses in autumn. In the older, saltwater fish, the tumor persists for up to a year. No methods of treatment or control are known.

INFECTIOUS HEMATOPOIETIC NECROSIS

SYNONYMS. IHN, infectious hematopoietic necrosis virus, IHNV, Oregon sockeye salmon virus, OSV, Sacramento River Chinook disease virus, SRCDV.

Host and Geographic Distribution

Salmonid hatcheries in the Pacific Northwest of the United States have historically experienced devastating epizootics of viral etiology. Three viruses were isolated in association with different epizootics—the Oregon sockeye salmon virus (OSV) (Wingfield et al., 1969), the Sacramento River chinook disease virus (Ross et al., 1960) (SRCDV), and infectious hematopoietic necrosis virus (IHNV) (Amend et al., 1969). The three virus isolates caused diseases that were similar in clinical and histopathologic manifestations, and the viruses were very similar in biochemical, biophysical, morphologic, and antigenic characteristics (Amend et al., 1973; McCain et al., 1971; Yasutake, 1970). The single designation, infectious hematopoietic necrosis virus, accommodates all three isolates.

The IHN virus can be isolated from naturally infected anadromous and freshwater rainbow trout and sockeye salmon, from Atlantic, chinook, chum, and yamame salmon, and from amago, sea-run cutthroat, and kamloops trout (Amend et al., 1973; Follett et al., 1987; Grischkowsky and Amend, 1976; Mulcahy and Wood, 1986; Sano, 1976; Sano et al., 1977; Traxler and Rankin, 1989). Northern pike can be experimentally infected (Dorson et al., 1987). Coho

salmon, brook, brown, and cutthroat trout, and yellow perch are considered refractory to disease, although the virus has been isolated from asymptomatic coho salmon and brook and cutthroat trout (Amend et al., 1973; McMichael et al., 1973; Nicholson, 1983; Wolf, 1976).

The disease is endemic to the Pacific Coast of North America, from northern California through Alaska, and is well established in Japan. Outbreaks have recently occurred in Italy, France, and Germany (Ahne, 1988; Arkush et al., 1989). The virus has been disseminated to other areas of the United States and the world with contaminated fish and fish eggs from the Pacific Northwest of North America.

Clinical Signs

Epizootics of infectious hematopoietic necrosis can result in very high mortality in 3-week to 6-month-old fish (Mulcahy et al., 1983b; Williams and Amend, 1976). Mortality can occur in fish 7 to 14 months old, but the clinical signs seen in younger fish are generally absent (Yasutake, 1978).

Clinical signs evident in young fish include darkening and exophthalmia (Amend et al., 1973; Parisot et al., 1965; Yasutake, 1970). The abdomen is distended with ascites, gills appear pale, and white fecal casts trail from the vent. Affected fish are lethargic, but sporadically hyperactive. Hemorrhages are evident at the bases of the pectoral and pelvic fins and at the vent, but only occasionally in the skin, musculature, and mouth. A prominent subdermal hemorrhage can occur between the head and dorsal fin. The fish appear anemic. Scoliosis and lordosis occur in 1 to 5% of survivors.

Pathology

In fish younger than 6 months of age, extensive pathologic changes occur in the kidneys, spleen, liver, and pancreas and in the granular cells of the alimentary tract (Amend et al., 1969, 1973; Yasutake, 1970, 1978; Yasutake et al., 1965). Renal hematopoietic tissue is the primary focus of infection and becomes severely necrotic. Kidney tubules and glomeruli show little involvement. Similarly, the hematopoietic tissue of the spleen becomes severely necrotic. Pleomorphic intracytoplasmic and intranuclear inclusions are evident in the acinar and islet cells of the pancreas, and focal necrotic changes can occur in the liver. Necrosis of the granular cells in the lamina propria, stratum compactum, and stratum granulosum of the alimentary tract is a distinguishing pathologic characteristic of the disease found in fish 3 to 4 months old, but not in younger fish (Yasutake, 1978). Tissues contain large numbers of lymphocytes and polymorphonuclear leukocytes, and hyperemia contributes to petechiation and hemorrhage. Erythrocytes accumulate in the musculature, but there is no necrotic involvement of striated muscle.

In fish 7 to 14 months old, histopathologic changes are not severe (Yasutake, 1978). The anterior kidneys and spleen show subtle, focal areas of cellular degeneration and necrosis. Cells in kidney tubule epithelium contain intracytoplasmic droplets, and kidney imprints show necrobiotic bodies. Moderate sloughing of the epithelial lining of the small intestine occurs posterior to the ceca.

Diagnosis

Clinical signs cannot be used to distinguish infectious hematopoietic necrosis from the other salmonid viral diseases. Nevertheless, clinical signs combined with the age, species, and source of the fish and the geographic location and health history of the culture station are often used to formulate a presumptive diagnosis. Confirmed diagnosis requires isolation of the virus in cell culture and its identification by reactivity with specific antibody.

Virus Isolation and Identification

Virus is generally isolated only from acutely diseased young-of-the-year fish and from asymptomatic, virus-carrier adult fish at spawning (Burke and Grischkowsky, 1984; Mulcahy et al., 1984a). Although virus is rarely isolated from eggs or from alevins in the absence of acute disease (Mulcahy and Pascho, 1985; Mulcahy et al., 1983b), virus can be recovered from dead eggs and from dead, partly developed embryos. Virus is not recovered as a latent infection from the marine phase of freshwater fishes.

The comparative frequency of virus isolation at spawning from individual organs and sex products suggests that prevalence of infection and virus titer are usually higher in females than in males (Mulcahy and Pascho, 1986; Mulcahy et al., 1982, 1983a,c, 1984a, 1987). In prespawning fish, the prevalence of viral infection is very low, but virus can be isolated most frequently from the gills, with low frequency from the spleen and pyloric ceca, and rarely from other organs. Prevalence of infection can increase from undetectable to 100% within 2 weeks. In spawning fish, virus can be present in all organs and fluids. The highest prevalence of virus occurs in gills, ovarian fluid, lower gut, spleen, and pyloric ceca. Fewer isolations are made from the brain and blood (Yamamoto et al., 1989). Virus can also be detected in mucus collected from the external surface of infected fish (LaPatra, 1989). Because of the high prevalence of virus and ease of handling and processing, ovarian fluid from spawning or preferably spent fish is the sample of choice for diagnostic assays. When sampling male fish, kidney and spleen tissues are superior to sex products, but sex products should also be included (Mulcahy et al., 1987). Some evidence suggests that monitoring for IHN virus–neutralizing antibody can be used for general population surveillance (Hattenberger-Baudouy et al., 1989). Molecular

filtration systems can be used to recover IHN virus from water (Watanabe et al., 1988).

Sample composition and storage temperature and duration affect the level of infectivity in clinical specimens. Generally, infectivity is best preserved if tissues and fluids are stored at 4°C and processed as soon as possible (Burke and Mulcahy, 1983; Gosting and Gould, 1981).

A variety of piscine cell lines support the replication of infectious hematopoietic necrosis virus. The CHSE-214, EPC, FHM, RTG-2, and STE-137 are the more commonly used, but the virus will replicate in other freshwater and marine fish cell lines (Frerichs, 1989; McAllister, 1979; Nicholson, 1983; Watanabe et al., 1981). The virus replicates in mammalian (BHK-21 and WI-38) and reptilian (GL-1 and TH-1) cells, but virus yields are lower than in piscine cells (Clark and Soriano, 1974). The IHN virus replicates in cell culture at temperatures from 0.5 to 20°C, the optimum range is 10 to 15°C. The characteristics of the virus replication cycle can vary considerably (Mulcahy et al., 1984b). Detailed procedures for assay of IHN virus in cell culture have been published (Burke and Mulcahy, 1980; Okamoto et al., 1985). The sensitivity of virus detection can be enhanced by pretreating cells with polyethylene glycol (Batts and Winton, 1989; Brunson et al., 1988).

Although differences in the electrophoretic profiles of viral structural proteins suggest the existence of IHN virus strains, infectivity neutralization tests indicate only one IHN virus serotype. The virus can be identified by neutralization and fluorescent antibody reactions (Arkush et al., 1989; Hill et al., 1975; LaPatra et al., 1989; McAllister et al., 1974; McCain et al., 1971; Winton et al., 1988) and by plate, contact diffusion blotting, and immunoblot enzyme-linked immunosorbent assays (Dixon and Hill, 1984; Hsu and Leong, 1985; McAllister and Schill, 1986; Schultz et al., 1989). Formalin-inactivated virus remains serologically reactive for months and can be used for positive control reagents for plate and immunoblot ELISAs. Virus-neutralizing monoclonal antibodies can be used to differentiate antigenic variants of IHN virus (Winton et al., 1988). Other monoclonal antibodies have virus-binding activity (Ristow and Arnzen, 1989; Schultz et al., 1989). Virus-infected cells can be identified in tissue sections and smears of body fluids by immunofluorescent and immunohistochemical staining (Yamamoto et al., 1989), and the fluorescent antibody test can be used for rapid detection of IHN virus in blood smears, in organ imprints, and of IHN virus–infected cells in ovarian fluid (LaPatra et al., 1989).

Transmission

In nature, horizontal transmission of infectious hematopoietic necrosis occurs when infected fish shed virus with feces, urine, and sex products contaminating eggs, fry, and older fish. The virus can remain infectious for months in water (Toranzo and

Hetrick, 1982; Wedemeyer et al., 1978) and binds to stream and river sediments and to slime on egg incubator walls. Effective contact with the host is established through the gills and the gastrointestinal tract, and survivors of infection become virus carriers. In spawning fish, waterborne virus probably does not affect the infection rate (Mulcahy et al., 1983c).

Because virus can be present in ovarian fluid, eggs are at least superficially contaminated with virus. Virus can be detected in eggs at 3 hours, but not at 24 hours, after fertilization (Mulcahy and Pascho, 1985). Virus also binds very efficiently to sperm (Mulcahy and Pascho, 1984). In experimentally infected eggs, viral infectivity decreases and cannot be detected 1 month after infection, and similarly in vitro the virus is inactivated by homogenized egg yolk (Yoshimizu et al., 1989). Some contend that vertical transmission probably occurs, but involves a very small proportion of the eggs (Mulcahy and Pascho, 1985; Mulcahy et al., 1983c), whereas others hold that vertical transmission is doubtful because the virus cannot survive in the developing egg before the embryo reaches the eyed stage (Yoshimizu et al., 1989).

Virus can be recovered from dead eggs and from dead, partly developed embryos, indicating that eggs were infected before or during fertilization and that the virus replicated in embryonic tissue. Eggs killed by virus may be a reservoir of infection for alevins (Mulcahy and Pascho, 1985). Replication of infectious hematopoietic necrosis virus in developing embryos can be demonstrated experimentally (Yoshimizu et al., 1988a, 1989).

Hatchery implements can be mechanical vectors, and ectoparasites, such as leeches, may support replicaton of the virus and may be involved in transmitting or maintaining IHNV in a watershed (Mulcahy et al., 1990; Yamamoto et al., 1989). Although attempts to demonstrate IHN virus replication in the fly *Drosophila melanogaster* were unsuccessful (Bussereau et al., 1975), insects are considered potential vectors or reservoirs of infection (Scott et al., 1980). Experimentally, infection can be induced by cohabitation, immersion exposure, injection, and feeding.

Epidemiology

Clinical signs of infectious hematopoeitic necrosis become evident as early as 21 to 35 days after hatching (Amend, 1975; Mulcahy et al., 1983a), and the highest incidence of mortality occurs in fish 3 weeks to 6 months old. Although mortality has occurred in 12- to 16-month-old fish, epizootics in these and older fish are infrequent (Amend et al., 1973; Burke and Grischkowsky, 1984).

The optimum temperature for epizootic mortality is 12 to 15°C, as judged by high mortality and low mean time to death (Hetrick et al., 1979a). High levels of mortality occur at lower temperature, but the epizootic is protracted. In nature, disease outbreaks do not occur above 15°C (Amend (1970). As with other fish rhabdoviral infections, the effect of water temperature may be related to interferon production (de Kinkelin and Le Berre, 1974a). Virus-neutralizing antibody is produced in survivors of both natural epizootics and experimental infections (Amend and Smith, 1974; Fryer et al., 1976; Hattenberger-Baudouy et al., 1989), but there is little evidence of virus-neutralizing antibody in spawning adult fish (Mulcahy et al., 1984a).

The hatchery environment introduces stress factors—crowding, handling, nutrition, and chemical exposure—that increase the potential for virus expression and epizootic disease outbreaks. Relatively high concentrations of virus are found in water when fish are held at high density (Mulcahy et al., 1983c). When stressed by exposure to sublethal levels of copper in water, fish are significantly more susceptible to virus infection (Hetrick et al., 1979b).

Survivors of epizootics become latent virus carriers, and latent infection is ostensibly activated by stress associated with the rigors and physiologic changes of spawning. Virus replication seemingly increases because immune and general resistance mechanisms are weakened in spawning fish (Mulcahy et al., 1984a).

Pathogenesis

Viral infection is established through the gills and the gastrointestinal tract. The infection does not progress to the viscera until a threshold titer of about 105 PFU/g is reached in the gills (Mulcahy et al., 1983c).

Based on the hematologic and blood chemical characteristics of infected fish, the probable cause of death is severe electrolyte and fluid imbalance due to renal failure (Amend and Smith, 1974, 1975). Increasing histopathologic change correlates with increasing virus concentration (Yasutake and Amend, 1972). Electron microscopic examination reveals virus in the anterior kidneys, spleen, pancreas, and pyloric ceca (Amend and Chambers, 1970).

Treatment and Control

The most effective and economical means for controlling infectious hematopoietic necrosis is by preventing contact between the virus and the host. Broodstock culling and disinfection of eggs with iodophor are partly effective, but epizootics can occur despite such management strategy. Stocks of eggs should originate from virus-free broodstock, and stocks of young-of-the-year-fish should be assayed and determined to be free from IHN virus. Ideally, the water supply should be controlled and virus free; however, if this is not feasible, the water supply can be effectively disinfected using ozone or ultraviolet irradiation (Wedemeyer et al., 1978, 1979).

The virus is inactivated by exposure to ether, cholorform, formalin, glycerol, diethylpyrocarbonate, ozone, sodium hypochlorite, organic iodophors, gamma and ultraviolet irradiation, extremes of pH (below pH 4 or above pH 10), and heating (60°C for 15 minutes).

Early studies suggest that rearing fish at elevated water temperature (17°C or higher) reduces IHN mortality, but does not necessarily prevent development of the carrier state (Amend, 1970, 1976). In practice, probably only the Coleman (California), isolate of IHN virus can be effectively and practically controlled by raising the water temperature (Hetrick et al., 1979a; Mulcahy et al., 1984b).

Resistance to the disease can be heritable and enhanced by selective breeding (Amend and Nelson, 1977; McIntyre and Amend, 1978). Triploid hybridization (triploid rainbow trout female × coho salmon male) improves viability of the hybrid cross and increases relative resistance to virus challenge (Parsons et al., 1986).

Several antiviral drugs inhibit infectious hematopoietic necrosis virus in cell culture (Amend, 1976; Hasobe and Saneyoshi, 1985). Treatment of fishes with 6-thioinosine or 1-B-D-ribofuranosyl-5-hydroxyuracil promotes higher survival (Hasobe and Saneyoshi, 1985). As with other fish viruses, chemical and drug treatments have not proven to be economically feasible.

Immunization trials with the avirulent virus and inactivated and subunit vaccines show that fish are protected against lethal challenge when immunized by immersion or intraperitoneal injection (Engelking and Leong, 1989; Fryer et al., 1976; Nishimura et al., 1985; Leong, 1984). Research with subunit vaccines continues (Engelking and Leong, 1989; Koener and Leong, 1990), while research with live, attenuated virus vaccines has progressed little. Formalin-inactivated virus retains its immunogenicity and serologic reactivity.

RHABDOVIRUS OF SALMONID HEPATITIS

SYNONYM. Rhabdoviral hepatitis of salmonids (RHS).

Host and Geographic Distribution

A rhabdovirus was isolated from moribund fingerling and yearling rainbow trout and spawning rainbow trout in the Ukraine region of the Soviet Union (Osadchaya, 1981).

Clinical Signs and Pathology

Fish affected with rhabdoviral salmonid hepatitis are dark in color and hyperactive. The liver is grayish-yellow, the spleen is dark red and enlarged, and the kidneys are mottled and friable (Osadchaya, 1981).

Diagnosis, Virus Isolation, and Identification

Diagnosis requires isolation and identification of the virus. Clinical specimens are assayed using FHM and EPC cells. Infectivity-neutralization assays show that the virus is antigenically distinct from infectious hematopoietic necrosis, viral hemorrhagic septicemia, and infectious pancreatic necrosis viruses, but no assays have been performed using antisera to the other fish rhabdoviruses.

Transmission, Epidemiology, Treatment, and Control

Mechanisms for the natural transmission of this virus are not known, but spawning trout produce offspring that develop hepatitis. The disease occurs at 18 to 22°C. No methods of treatment or control are known.

VIRAL HEMORRHAGIC SEPTICEMIA

SYNONYMS. Infektiose nierenschwellung und leberdegeneration (INuL), Egtved virus, VHS, VHSV.

Host and Geographic Distribution

Viral hemorrhagic septicemia (VHS) is enzootic in most countries of continental eastern and western Europe, and in the United States the virus can be isolated in the Puget Sound area of Washington and in the Gulf of Alaska. No outbreaks or isolations of the viral hemorrhagic septicemia virus have been reported elsewhere.

In Europe, epizootics occur primarily in rainbow trout, brown trout, and to a lesser extent in northern pike (Ghittino, 1968; Jorgensen, 1980; de Kinkelin and Le Berre, 1977; Meier and Vestergard Jorgensen, 1980). Natural infections also occur in grayling and whitefish (Ahne and Thomsen, 1985a; Meier et al., 1986; Wizigmann et al., 1980) and are suspected in pollan and lake trout (Ghittino, 1973; Reichenbach-Klinke, 1959). The virus has also been isolated from Atlantic cod with ulcus syndrome (see Chap. 88) (Vestergard Jorgensen and Olesen, 1987). In the United States, natural infections occur in chinook and coho salmon, steelhead trout, and Pacific cod.

Fish shown by experimental challenge to be susceptible to viral hemorrhagic septicemia virus infection are Atlantic salmon, brook trout, golden trout, rainbow trout × coho salmon hybrids, giebel, sea bass, and turbot (Ahne et al., 1976; Castric and de Kinkelin, 1984; Ghittino, 1965; de Kinkelin and Castric, 1982; Ord et al., 1976; Pfitzner, 1966; Rasmussen, 1965; Wolf, 1988). Fish shown by experimental challenges to be refractory are common carp, chub, Eurasian perch, roach, and tench (de Kinkelin et al., 1974b; Ord, 1975; Tack, 1959; Zwillenberg et al., 1968).

Clinical Signs

Some fish show clinical signs, whereas others appear normal, and clinical signs reflect the severity of infection rather than progressive stages of the disease (Bellet, 1965; Ghittino, 1973; Meier, 1980; Yasutake, 1970). Acute signs are typically associated with a rapid onset of heavy mortality. Fish are lethargic, dark, exophthalmic, and anemic. Hemorrhages are evident in the eyes, skin, and gills and at the bases of the fins. In chronically infected fish, cumulative mortality is moderate, but protracted. Fish are also lethargic, dark, exophthalmic, and severely anemic, but not grossly hemorrhagic. The abdomen is markedly distended due to edema of the liver, kidneys, and spleen. In a latent infection, mortality is low, and the fish are nearly normal in appearance but may be hyperactive. Inapparent virus carriers show no clinical signs. In fish with viral hemorrhagic septicemia, total blood protein is reduced, but the immunoglobulin fraction is increased (Flondro et al., 1984; Georgiev and Kamenov, 1980; Hoffmann et al., 1979). The changes in the quantitative ratio of proteins are reflected in blood electrophoretic profiles. Low hematocrit and hemoglobin values are indicators of the severe anemia that occurs early in infection. Late in infection, immature erythrocytes increase in number. Acutely infected fish are leukopenic.

Pathology

Histopathologic changes are generally confined to the liver, kidneys, spleen, and muscle (Amlacher et al., 1980; Elger and Hentschel, 1983; Hofmann, 1971; Yasutake, 1970).

In acutely infected fish, liver sinusoids are engorged with blood, and hepatocytes show extensive focal changes, including cytoplasmic vacuoles, pyknosis, karyolysis, lymphocytic invasion, and occasionally intracytoplasmic and intranuclear inclusions. Similar changes occur in the spleen and in the hematopoietic and renal elements of the kidneys. Lymphoid tissue necrosis leads to leukopenia. In skeletal muscle, erythrocytes may accumulate in muscle bundles and fibers, but little muscle tissue damage occurs.

In chronically infected fish, liver sinusoids remain enlarged but contain coagulated plasma. Kidney and splenic hematopoietic tissues and mononuclear lymphoid cells are hyperplastic. Severe glomerular changes in the kidney resemble membranous glomerulonephritis in mammals. No remarkable histopathologic changes occur in inapparent virus carriers.

Diagnosis

Clinical signs combined with the age, species, and source of the fish and the geographic location and health history of the culture station are often used to formulate a presumptive diagnosis of viral hemorrhagic septicemia. Confirmed diagnosis requires isolation of the virus in cell culture and its identification by reactivity with specific antibody.

Virus Isolation and Identification

The viral septicemia virus can be recovered from internal organ homogenates, sex products, and urine. Virus concentrations are higher in the anterior kidney and spleen than in liver, heart, and muscle (Hoffman et al., 1970; Jorgensen, 1970, 1982a; de Kinkelin, 1983; Menezes, 1977; Neukirch and Glass, 1984). Brain samples should also be included when assaying for inapparent virus carriers (Castric and de Kinkelin, 1980; Kruse and Neukirch, 1989; Neukirch, 1984). Little virus can be recovered from feces.

Although infected fish can develop an immune response, the detection of anti-VHS virus antibody is not a reliable indicator of the presence or absence of current infection (Dorson and Torchy, 1979; Jorgensen, 1982b; Neukirch and Glass, 1984). Nevertheless, the detection of virus-specific neutalizing antibody can be a useful tool for surveillance (Enzmann and Konrad, 1990; Olesen and Vestergard Jorgensen, 1986).

The virus replicates in a variety of piscine cell lines, including BF-2, CaPi, CHSE-214, EPC, FHM, PG, RTG-2, RTM, STE-137, and primary cultures of sea bass, tench, carp ovary, and goldfish (de Kinkelin, 1983; McAllister, 1979). In addition, the virus replicates in some mammalian (BHK-21 and WI-38) and reptilian (GL-1 and TH-1) cell lines (Clark and Soriano, 1974). The optimal temperature for virus replication in cell culture is 14 to 15°C. Virus yield is reduced at 6°C and only slight replication occurs above 20°C (de Kinkelin and Scherrer, 1970). Replication of VHS virus in cell culture is greatly influenced by hydrogen ion concentration, a pH of 7.4 to 7.8 should be maintained in diagnostic assays (Campbell and Wolf, 1969; Wolf and Quimby, 1973). The detection of VHS virus in cell culture can be enhanced by pretreating cells with a 7% solution of polyethylene glycol or including DEAE-Dextran or polyethylene glycol in the inoculum (Batts and Winton, 1989; Campbell and Wolf, 1969). Detection of virus in tissue sections by fluorescent antibody staining is less sensitive than virus isolation in cell culture (Jorgensen and Meyling, 1972; Pfeil and Wiedemann, 1977).

The three currently recognized serotypes of viral hemorrhagic septicemia virus (F1, F2, and 23.75) are distinguished by infectivity neutralization (Le Berre et al., 1977). Viral antigen can be detected in inoculated cell cultures by indirect fluorescent antibody and immunoperoxidase staining (Faisal and Ahne,

1980; Meier and Jorgensen, 1975), and immunoblot and plate ELISA systems are used for detection and identification of virus in cell culture fluids. Binding and neutralizing monoclonal antibodies are available for identification of VHS virus (Lorenzen et al., 1988; de Kinkelin, unpublished data; McAllister, unpublished data).

Cross-reactivity occurs among the VHS virus serotypes in indirect fluorescent antibody assays and in some instances in infectivity neutralization assays (Jorgensen, 1980; Meier and Jorgensen, 1980). Similarly, all three VHS virus serotypes can be identified by immunoblot ELISA using antiserum only to the F1 serotype (McAllister and Owens, 1987).

Transmission and Epidemiology

The viral hemorrhagic septicemia virus is readily transmissible to fish of nearly all ages, and survivors of infection can become life-long virus carriers that shed virus with urine and sex products. Virus shed with sex products appears to be solely a surface contaminant of the egg and is readily dissipated. Although virus can be isolated from eggs for 3 to 4 hours after spawning, true vertical transmission has not been demonstrated. Experimentally, fish can be infected by cohabitation, immersion, intraperitoneal and intramuscular injection, brushing virus on the gills, and feeding (Ahne, 1985; Castric and de Kinkelin, 1984; de Kinkelin and Castric, 1982; Jorgensen, 1973b, 1980, 1982b; Neukirch, 1984).

The heron, *Ardea cinerea*, is ostensibly a mechanical vector of the virus (Olesen and Jorgensen, 1982; Peters and Neukirch, 1986), but the virus is inactivated in the gastrointestional tract of some birds (Eskildsen and Jorgensen, 1973). Viral hemorrhagic septicemia virus has not been recovered from potential parasitic vectors, so their role in the transmission of VHS virus is unknown. A study in the fruit fly, *Drosophila melanogaster*, failed to show replication in insects (Bussereau et al., 1975).

In the hatchery environment, mechanical transfer of virus on the surface of animate or inanimate objects presents a substantial hazard. Virus can persist in water for several days (de Kinkelin and Scherrer, 1970), and can be isolated from feral fish in waters receiving hatchery effluent (Jorgensen, 1980, 1982a; Enzmann and Konrad, 1985). Virus can be transmitted to predator fish via infected prey (Ahne, 1985).

The virus ostensibly gains access to the fish through the secondary gill lamellae with primary virus replication occurring in the gills and in vascular endothelial cells, principally of the kidney and spleen (Chilmonczyk, 1980; Chilmonzyk and Monge, 1980; Kruse and Neukrich, 1990; Neukrich, 1984). Epizootic losses occur at temperatures of 3 to 12°C, and mortality is greatest at 3 to 5°C. Mortality and the proportion of virus carriers decrease at higher temperatures (de Kinkelin, 1983; Neukirch, 1984). Deaths rarely occur at temperatures above 15°C.

In captive fish, culture and environmental stress seemingly enhance susceptibility and recurrence of infection (de Kinkelin, 1983; Ghittino, 1965, 1973; Tesarcik et al., 1968). In feral fish, inapparent infection is more common than disease (Enzmann and Konrad, 1985; Jorgensen, 1982b).

Treatment and Control

Preventing contact between the virus and the host is the most effective method for controlling viral hemorrhagic septicemia. A systematic program of hatchery disinfection, combined with restocking with specific pathogen–free fish and eggs, is used with considerable success (Enzmann, 1983; Jorgensen, 1974a; Kehlet, 1973). Eggs used for restocking are decontaminated by iodophor treatment (Conroy and Santacana, 1980; Eskildsen and Jorgensen, 1974; Fuhrmann and Savvidis, 1984). Ideally, the water supply should be controlled and virus free, but if not, ultraviolet irradiation can be used to inactivate the virus in the water supply (Maisse et al., 1980). Conditions that promote physiologic stress should be identified and alleviated. Selective breeding to increase host resistance is not successful (Margaritov, 1969; Ord et al., 1976).

Vaccination is a potential method for controlling this disease, and several avirulent vaccines are under development (Ellis, 1988; Jorgensen, 1976; de Kinkelin and Le Berre, 1977; Gerard, 1977). The attenuated vaccines prepared to date induce a protective response, but they also retain residual pathogenicity. Although the protective effects of attenuated vaccines can be demonstrated in the laboratory, their efficacy under production conditions is yet to be proven (Enzmann, 1983), and their value for controlling disease in healthy fish populations is under question (Ellis, 1988; Enzmann, 1983). Some work is underway to analyze the gene sequence and clone various genomic segments as a strategy for developing subunit vaccines (Bernard and de Kinkelin, 1989).

Viral hemorrhagic septicemia is inactivated by exposure to ether, chloroform, glycerol, formalin, sodium hypochlorite, iodophors, ultraviolet irradiation, heating (56 to 60°C), and drying. It is inactivated at pH 3.5, but is stable at pH 5.0 to 10.4 (de Kinkelin, 1983; McAllister, 1979; Pilcher and Fryer, 1980; Roberts, 1978; Vestergaard Jorgensen, 1973).

CHINOOK SALMON PARAMYXOVIRUS

Host, Geographic Distribution, and Clinical Signs

The only isolations of chinook salmon paramyxovirus (CSP) are from adult chinook salmon in Oregon (Winton et al., 1985). The virus is recovered from apparently healthy fish at spawning. No gross clinical or histopathologic signs of disease are evident in virus-infected fish. The virus has been isolated in consecutive years from separate river systems in Oregon.

Diagnosis and Virus Detection

Presumptive diagnosis is based on isolation of the virus in cell culture. Finding paramyxovirus particles by electron microscopic examination of infected cells strengthens the presumptive diagnosis. Definitive diagnosis is not possible because virus-specific antibody is not yet available.

From adult fish, the virus is isolated from homogenates of kidney and spleen, but not from ovarian fluids. The virus has not been recovered from progeny of infected adults. Samples are inoculated onto CHSE-214 cells and incubated at 18°C. After 14 to 28 days, cytopathic effects are seen and consist of rounded clusters of refractile cells that eventually detach. The virus replicates with cytopathic effects in CHH-1, CHSE-214, KO-6, and CSE-119 cells. The virus replicates at temperatures from 6 to 21°C (18°C optimum), but cytopathic effects are seen only at 15 to 21°C.

Transmission, Epidemiology, Treatment, and Control

Virus is not detected in chinook salmon experimentally challenged by intraperitoneal injection or waterborne exposure. Infection may result in a transient viremia.

No methods of treatment or control are known. Prudent management practice dictates that virus-contaminated fish and fish products should be avoided. The virus is inactivated by exposure to chloroform, pH 2, and heating (56°C for 6 hours or 37°C for 24 hours), but is stable from pH 3 to 11, and to a freeze-thaw cycle at −20 or −70°C. Virus replication in cell culture is inhibited by 5-iodo-2'-deoxyuridine.

ERYTHROCYTIC INCLUSION BODY SYNDROME

SYNONYMS. Erythrocytic inclusion disease (EIBS), salmonid anemia virus.

Host and Geographical Distribution

Erythrocytic inclusion body syndrome occurs in chinook and coho salmon in the Pacific Northwest of the United States (Arakawa et al., 1989; Holt and Piacentini, 1989; Holt and Rohovec, 1984; Leek, 1985, 1987), and a similar condition occurs in Atlantic salmon in Norway (Lunder et al., 1990). In addition, rainbow trout and cutthroat trout can be experimentally infected (Piacentini et al., 1989).

Clinical Signs and Pathology

Affected fish are anemic and lethargic and may show dark or variable pigmentation, or affected fish can have normal appearance and behavior. Internally, the organs and tissues are pale, and the spleen is enlarged. Hematocrit readings vary with the stage of infection and can range from 1 to 50% with lowest hematocrit values (1 to 4%) occurring late in infection when erythrocyte lysis is greatest. Histologic examination shows inclusions in erythrocytes and necrotic, inclusion-bearing hemoblasts as well as congestion of the kidneys, congestion, enlargement, and hemosiderosis of the spleen, and focal necrosis of kidney interstitial cells.

Diagnosis and Virus Detection

For presumptive diagnosis, blood films are examined microscopically for cytoplasmic inclusions in erythrocytes. To confirm the diagnosis, erythrocyte preparations are examined by electron microscopy to find cytoplasmic accumulations of 80 nm in diameter icosahedral virions. The virus has not been isolated in cell culture.

Intracytoplasmic erythrocytic inclusions are detected in blood films and kidney imprints using pinacyanol chloride or Leishman-Giemsa blood stains (Leek, 1987) (Figs. 38–1 and 38–2). Pinacyanol chloride stain gives the more consistent results (Leek, 1987). The cytoplasmic inclusions stain pale purple, lavender, or pink. When stained with acridine orange, inclusions fluoresce red, whereas viral erythrocytic necrosis inclusions fluoresce green (Holt and Piacentini, 1989). Each erythrocyte contains one round to ovoid inclusion, which measures 0.8 to 3.0 μm in diameter. Inclusions are found most frequently in fish with hematocrits of 20 to 40% and few inclusions are seen in fish with hematocrits of 1 to 4% (Leek, 1987).

Fish should be examined when water temperatures are cooler. If spawning fish are sampled, specimens should come predominantly from male fish and should be collected near the end of the spawning season (Holt and Piacentini, 1989).

Electron micrographs of thin-sectioned erythrocytes show single virions and membrane-bound aggregates of virus in the cytoplasm of affected erythrocytes. The virus particles measure 75 to 100 nm in diameter and are morphologically distinct from virions seen in erythrocytes from fish with viral erythrocytic necrosis that measure 140 to 500 nm in diameter (see Chap. 88), intraerythrocytic virus of coho salmon that measure about 106 nm in diameter, and intraerythrocytic virus of rainbow trout that measure 80 to 90 nm in diameter (Lunder et al., 1990). The EIBS virus (salmonid anemia virus) is tentatively placed in the togavirus group (Arakawa et al., 1989).

Attempts to isolate the EIBS virus using BB, CHSE-214, CHH-1, CSE-119, EPC, FHM, RTG-2, RTH-149, and SSE-5 cells are without success (Leek, 1987; Piacentini et al., 1989).

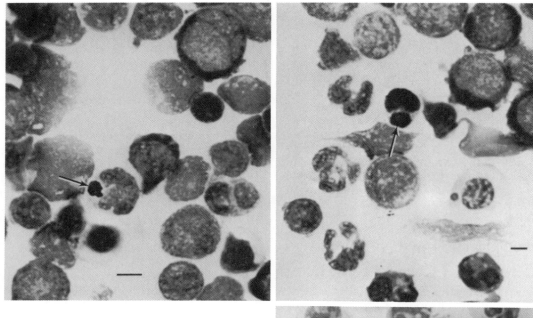

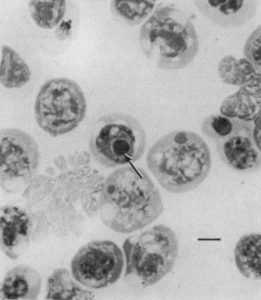

FIGURE 38–1. Erythrocytic necrosis virus (arrow) in a macrophage *(A)*, lymphocyte or thrombocyte *(B),* and an erythroid cell *(C)* from the pronephros of a chum salmon juvenile. (Leishman-Giemsa stain, bars represent 5 μ). (From MacMillan, J.R. et al. [1989] Cytopathology and coagulopathy associated with viral erythrocytic necrosis in chum salmon. J. Aquatic Anim. Health 1(4):260.)

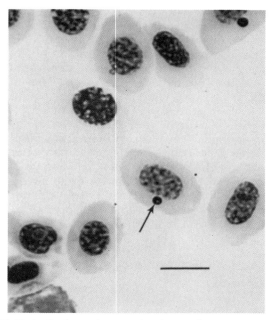

FIGURE 38–2. Erythrocytic necrosis virus inclusion (arrow) in a mature circulating erythrocyte of a chum salmon. (Leishman-Giemsa stain, bars represent 5 μ) (From MacMillan, J.R. [1989] Cytopathology and coagulopathy associated with viral erythrocytic necrosis in chum salmon. J. Aquatic Anim. Health 1(4):257.)

Transmission, Epidemiology, and Pathogenesis

Erythrocytic inclusion body syndrome can be transmitted horizontally by waterborne exposure, and by intraperitoneal injection of blood or kidney tissue (Arakawa et al., 1989; Pelton, 1987; Piacentini et al., 1989), and by oral intubation of homogenates of infected tissue (Leek, 1985). Under natural conditions, adult fish can be infected, but whether the virus can be transmitted vertically is unknown.

Losses are low, but the survivability of virus-infected fish is compromised by anemia, and the fish are thus predisposed to secondary bacterial, fungal, or parasitic infections (Arakawa et al., 1989). Because of these secondary infections, overall losses vary. Chronic to epizootic losses occur predominately in juvenile to yearling chinook and coho salmon.

Disease outbreaks occur most frequently during cool water–temperature months. Natural epizootics can persist for 5 months or more (Piacentini et al., 1989). At 2°C, inclusions become evident about 25 days after infection and persist in low numbers as a chronic infection. At 6 to 12°C, inclusions appear in 11 to 17 days postinfection, accumulate in great numbers, and persist for 19 to 32 days. At 15 to 18°C, inclusions can be detected about 7 days after initial exposure, are few in number, and persist for 5 to 13 days. Fish that recover are resistant to reinfection (Piacentini et al., 1989). This serum is protective.

Treatment and Control

No methods of treatment or control are known. Evidence from laboratory challenge studies shows that the time to recovery from infection is shortened if fish are held at temperatures of at least 15°C (Piacentini et al., 1989). Susceptible fish can be protected by intraperitoneal injection of serum from fish that have recovered from experimental infection (Piacentini et al., 1989). Management strategies to minimize losses include handling anemic fish as little as possible to prevent further stress and rearing fish in pathogen-free water supplies to minimize exposure to bacterial and fungal agents.

COHO ANEMIA

SYNONYM. Intraerythrocytic viral disease of coho salmon.

Host, Geographic Distribution, and Clinical Signs

An intraerythrocytic virus was detected in saltwater-reared coho salmon in northern California and in coho salmon from Washington state (Hedrick et al., 1987b). Severe anemia is the only clinical sign associated with the infection.

Diagnosis and Virus Detection

Principal pathologic changes occur in the kidney and spleen and consist of diffuse degeneration of the hematopoietic tissues and accumulation of hemosiderin in macrophages (Hedrick et al., 1987b). Macrophages containing degenerating erythrocytes are seen in the sinuses of the liver, kidney, and spleen. Circulating erythrocytes contain numerous cytoplasmic inclusion bodies. Nephrocalcinosis is sometimes seen, but its relationship to the infection is unknown.

Tentative diagnosis of an erythrocytic infection is based on detecting cytoplasmic inclusions in erythrocytes. Blood films are stained using Lieshman-Giemsa, which gives the inclusions a pink to red color. The inclusions are numerous, 1 to 2 μm in size, and often rod shaped.

The four recognized viral erythrocytic infections, i.e., erythrocytic inclusion body syndrome, intraerythrocytic viral infection of coho salmon, intraerythrocytic viral infection of rainbow trout, and viral erythrocytic necrosis (see Chap. 88), cannot be definitively distinguished based on inclusion body characteristics, although there are differences in the number and size of the inclusions. At present, the infections are differentiated by the morphologic characteristics of virus particles seen in affected erythrocytes by transmission electron microscopy (Hedrick et al., 1987b; Lunder et al., 1990). The intraerythrocytic virus of coho salmon is roughly spherical, about 106 nm in diameter, and appears to have surface projections. Virions accumulate in membrane-bound vacuoles in the cytoplasm and are sometimes seen near the nuclear membrane. The erythrocytic inclusion body syndrome virion is 75 to 100 nm in diameter; the intraerythrocytic virus of rainbow trout is 80 to 90 nm in diameter; and the viral erythrocytic necrosis virion is 140 to 500 nm in diameter.

Attempts to isolate the intraerythrocytic virus of coho salmon from affected kidney and spleen using various established fish cell lines have been unsuccessful (Hedrick et al., 1987b).

Transmission, Epidemiology, Treatment, and Control

The mechanism of transmission and the factors affecting the prevalence, distribution, and effects of the infection on individuals and on populations are unknown. Some evidence suggests that the virus may be transmitted with sex products (Hedrick et al., 1987b). No methods of treatment or control are known. Screening broodstock for cytoplasmic inclusions in circulating erythrocytes would be a prudent first step in an attempt to avoid contact with the virus.

HEMORRHAGIC TROUT DISEASE

SYNONYM. Intraerythrocytic viral disease of rainbow trout.

Host and Geographic Distribution

A fatal hemorrhagic disorder can occur in the Donaldson strain of rainbow trout, particularly in adult females. Only one instance of the infection has been reported (Landolt et al., 1977).

Clinical Signs and Pathology

The clinical signs are exsanguinating hemorrhage, hypoxia, and sudden death. Internally, the fish show either expansive hematomas in the liver or extravasated blood in the body cavity. Histopathologic examination shows diffuse necrotic hepatitis, eosinophilic intracytoplasmic inclusions in hepatocytes and in renal tubule epithelium, disseminated intravascular coagulation, and skeletal muscle dysfunction and deterioration. Peripheral blood contains unusually high levels of immature erythrocytes, and mature erythrocytes frequently contain small, basophilic, pleomorphic cytoplasmic inclusions.

Diagnosis and Virus Detection

Diagnosis is based on correlating clinical signs and the results of electron microscopic examination of erythrocytes. Attempts to isolate the virus in FHM and RTG-2 cells have been unsuccessful.

Electron micrographs of erythrocytes show cytoplasmic inclusions consisting of numerous vesicles about 900 nm in diameter that contain viruslike particles. The particles are spherical, 80 to 90 nm in diameter, with an electron-dense outer layer and a more electron-lucent reticulated core. The erythrocyte inclusions also contain membrane-bound electron-dense structures 1000 nm in diameter. Electron microscopic examination of hepatocytes and in renal tubule epithelial cells show their intracytoplasmic inclusions to be composed of membrane-bound accumulations of amorphous material. The virions are morphologically distinct from the three other erythrocytic virus infections; erythrocytic inclusion body syndrome, coho anemia, and viral erythrocytic necrosis (VEN) (see Chap. 88).

Transmission, Epidemiology, Treatment, and Control

No transmission trials have been reported. The etiologic significance of the putative virus is unknown. No methods of treatment or control are known.

PICORNALIKE VIRUS FROM ATLANTIC SALMON

SYNONYM. Atlantic salmon virus (ASV).

Host and Geographic Distribution

Preliminary reports indicate that a picornalike virus was isolated from Atlantic salmon fingerlings cultured in freshwater in Washington state (McDowell et al., 1989). Attempts to demonstrate virus replication in experimentally challenged juvenile Atlantic salmon and rainbow trout have not been successful. The virus has been isolated on only one occasion.

Clinical Signs and Pathology

The virus was initially recovered from a population of Atlantic salmon experiencing low-level, chronic mortality of unknown cause. No clinical signs were described, but histopathologic examination showed mild necrosis of the hematopoietic tissue in the kidney and focal mononuclear infiltration in the liver (McDowell et al., 1989). No mortality or clinical signs of disease have been seen in experimentally challenged Atlantic salmon or rainbow trout.

Diagnosis and Virus Isolation

Virus can be recovered from homogenates of liver, kidney, and spleen inoculated onto CHSE-214 cells—AS, EPC, and RTG-2 cells are refractory (McDowell et al., 1989). The virus replicates at 5, 10, and 15°C, little at 20°C, and not at all at 25°C. A incubation temperature of 15°C is optimum. Cytopathic effects (syncytium formation) are evident in 14 to 28 days of incubation at 15°C.

Electron micrographs of negatively stained virus show that the virion has icosahedral symmetry and is about 39.5 nm in diameter.

The relationship of this picornalike virus from Atlantic salmon to the picornalike virus from smelt (see Chap. 26) and the picornalike virus from salmonid fishes in California (see below) is unknown.

Transmission, Epidemiology, Treatment, and Control

The virus has only recently been isolated, and only once. The mechanism of transmission is unknown and as yet attempts to experimentally transmit the virus have been unsuccessful. The significance of the virus as a disease agent and its relationship to the chronic mortality are as yet unknown.

No methods of treatment or control are known. The relocation or introduction of virus-infected fish should be avoided.

PICORNALIKE VIRUS FROM SALMONID FISH IN CALIFORNIA

SYNONYMS. Cutthroat trout virus (CTV), Heenan Lake virus.

Host, Geographic Distribution, and Clinical Signs

A picornalike virus was isolated from adult brook trout, brown trout, cutthroat trout, and rainbow trout at several locations in northern California (Yun et al., 1989). Kokanee salmon can be experimentally infected, but preliminary results from laboratory challenges show that young chinook salmon do not develop detectable disease.

No clinical signs or pathologic changes are evident in the adult fish from which the virus has been isolated, and no signs of disease are seen in experimentally infected young salmon and trout (Yun et al., 1989).

Diagnosis and Virus Detection

Viral infection is detected solely by isolation of the virus in cell culture. The virus can be isolated from ovarian fluids and tissue homogenates. Samples are inoculated onto CHSE-214 cells and incubated at 10 to 15°C (Yun et al., 1989; R. P. Hedrick, unpub-

lished data). The virus replicates at 10 and 15°C, little at 20°C, and not at all at 25°C. Cytopathic effects are evident in 21 to 28 days for primary isolation and in about 7 days for subsequent passages and appear as a diffuse necrosis of the cell sheet similar to degeneration in an older cell culture.

Negatively stained preparations of virus concentrated from infected cell cultures show that the virus has icosahedral symmetry and is about 37.5 nm in diameter (Yun et al., 1989).

The relationship of this picornalike virus from salmonids in California to the picornalike virus from smelt (see Chap. 26) and the picornalike virus from Atlantic salmon (see above) is unknown.

Transmission, Epidemiology, Treatment, and Control

The virus can be transmitted horizontally by waterborne exposure. Isolation of virus from sex products suggests the potential for vertical transmission, but the virus has been isolated only occasionally from the progeny of infected adults. Both infected adults and experimentally challenged young salmonids show no clinical or pathologic changes. Thus, at present, the virus seems to have little significance as a disease agent.

No methods of treatment or control are known.

ULCERATIVE DERMAL NECROSIS

SYNONYMS. Ulcerative dermal necrosis-associated virus, UDN.

Host and Geographic Distribution

Ulcerative dermal necrosis (UDN) occurs in adult Atlantic salmon and anadromous and nonanadromous brown trout in Great Britain, Ireland, France, and Sweden.

Clinical Signs and Pathology

Lesions initially appear as small grayish areas of roughened skin or shallow ulcers, but develop to become expansive, deep ulcers (Roberts, 1972). The ulcers occur primarily on the head and adipose fin, but also on other body surfaces. Histopathologically, the disease is characterized by progressive focal cytolytic necrosis of epithelial cells. Blistering or pemphigoid degeneration of the middle layers of malpighian cells of the epidermis lead to sloughing of epidermal layers with erosion of the basal layer and the basement membrane. In affected cells, the nucleus appears granular and extensively indented and the nuclear membrane is separated. The mitochondria are enlarged, and the endoplasmic reticulum swollen. Desmosomes appear unaffected, but the normal cellular interdigitations are separated. No lesions occur in visceral organs unless secondary bacterial or fungal infection is evident.

Diagnosis and Virus Detection

Diagnosis is based on clinical signs and histopathologic examination. Virus has not been isolated in cell culture. Electron micrographs of UDN-like lesions from Atlantic salmon show spheroidal to hexagonal viruslike particles 30 to 33 nm in diameter (Lounatmaa and Janatuinen, 1978). The particles are seen free in the cytoplasm and in membrane-bound aggregates. No particles or bodies of similar size or form are seen in epidermal tissue from unaffected fish. The cytoplasmic particles are not irrefutably virus and could possibly be glycogen deposits (Lounatmaa and Janatuinen, 1978).

Transmission, Epidemiology, Treatment, and Control

Ulcerative dermal necrosis has not been transmitted experimentally, and the significance of the viruslike particles to the etiology is unknown. In anadromous species, lesions develop when the fish return to fresh water. Mortality is due to effects from secondary bacterial and fungal infections of the lesions. No methods of treatment or control are known.

LITERATURE CITED

Adair, B.M., and Ferguson, H.W. (1981) Isolation of infectious pancreatic necrosis (IPN) virus from non-salmonid fish. J. Fish Dis. 4:69–76.

Agius, C., Mangunwiryo, H., Johnson, R.H., and Smail, D.A. (1982) A more sensitive technique for isolating infectious pancreatic necrosis virus from asymptomatic carrier rainbow trout, Salmo gairdneri Richardson. J. Fish Dis. 5:285–292.

Agius, C., Richardson, A., and Walker, W. (1983) Further observations on the co-cultivation method for isolating infectious pancreatic necrosis virus from asymptomatic carrier rainbow trout, Salmo gairdneri Richardson. J. Fish Dis. 6:477–480.

Ahne, W. (1977) Some properties of an IPN-virus isolated from pike (Esox lucius). Bull. Off. Int. Epizoot. 87:417–418.

Ahne, W. (1978) Isolation and characterization of infectious pancreatic necrosis virus from pike (Esox lucius). Arch. Virol. 58:65–69.

Ahne, W. (1981) Serological techniques currently used in fish virology. Dev. Biol. Stand. 49:3–27.

Ahne, W. (1985) Viral infection cycles in pike (Esox lucius L.). Z. Angew. Ichthyol. 2:90–91.

Ahne, W. (1988) Eine neue fischkrankheit in Europa: die infectiose hamatopoetische nekrose (IHN). Tierarztl. Umsch. 43:239–242.

Ahne, W., and Negele, R.D. (1985a) Studies on the transmission of infectious pancreatic necrosis virus via eyed eggs and sexual products of salmonid fish. In: Fish and Shellfish Pathology (Ellis, A.E., ed.) Academic Press, London, pp. 261–269.

Ahne, W., and Negele, R.D. (1985b) Transmission of infectious pancreatic necrosis virus with pituitaries of fish. Fish and Shellfish Pathology (Ellis, A.E., ed.) Academic Press, London, pp. 271–275.

Ahne, W., and Thomsen, I. (1985a) Occurrence of viral hemorrhagic septicemia virus in wild whitefish Coregonus sp. Zentralbl. Veterinarmed. (B) 32:73–75.

Ahne, W., and Thomsen, I. (1985b) The existence of three different viral agents in a tumour bearing European eel (Anguilla anguilla). Zentralbl. Veterinarmed. (B) 32:228–235.

Ahne, W., Negele, R.D., and Ollenschlager, B. (1976) Vergleichende infektionsversuche mit Egtved-viren (Stamm F1) bei regenbogenforellen

(Salmo gairdneri) und goldforellen (Salmo aguabonita). Berl. Munch. Tierarztl. Wochenschr. 89:161–164.

Amend, D.F. (1970) Control of infectious hematopoietic necrosis virus disease by elevating the water temperature. J. Fish. Res. Bd. Can. 27:265–270.

Amend, D.F. (1975) Detection and transmission of infectious hematopoietic necrosis virus in rainbow trout. J. Wildlife Dis. 11:471–478.

Amend, D.F. (1976) Prevention and control of viral diseases of salmonids. J. Fish. Res. Bd. Can. 33:1059–1066.

Amend, D.F., and Chambers, V.C. (1970) Morphology of certain viruses of salmonid fishes. II. In vivo studies of infectious hematopoietic necrosis virus. J. Fish. Res. Bd. Can. 27:1385–1388.

Amend, D.F., and Nelson, J.R. (1977) Variation in the susceptibility of sockeye salmon Oncorhynchus nerka to infectious haemopoietic virus. J. Fish Biol. 11:567–573.

Amend, D.F., and Pietsch, J.P. (1972) Virucidal activity of two iodophors to salmonid viruses. J. Fish. Res. Bd. Can. 29:61–65.

Amend, D.F., and Smith L. (1974) Pathophysiology of infectious hematopoietic necrosis virus disease in rainbow trout (Salmo gairdneri): early changes in blood and aspects of the immune response after injection of IHN virus. J. Fish. Res. Bd. Can. 31:1371–1378.

Amend, D.F., and Smith, L. (1975) Pathophysiology of infectious hematopoietic necrosis virus disease in rainbow trout: hematological and blood chemical changes in moribund fish. Infect. Immun. 11:171–179.

Amend, D.F., Yasutake, W.T., and Mead, R.W. (1969) A hematopoietic virus disease of rainbow trout and sockeye salmon. Trans. Am. Fish. Soc. 98:796–804.

Amend, D.F., Yasutake, W.T., Fryer, J.L., Pilcher, K.S., and Wingfield. W.H. (1973) Infectious hematopoietic necrosis (IHN). EIFAC (Eur. Inland Fish. Advis. Comm. Tech. Pap.). Technical Paper 17, Suppl. 2:80–98.

Amend, D.F., McDowell, T., and Hedrick, R.P. (1984) Characteristics of a previously unidentified virus from channel catfish (Ictalurus punctatus). Can. J. Fish. Aquatic Sci. 41:807–811.

Amlacher, E., Ude, J., Rudolph, C., and Ernst, G. (1980) Direct electron microscopial visualization of the presumptive virus of viral haemorrhagic septicaemia (VHS) in rainbow trout Salmo gairdneri Richardson and additional histopathological and haematological observations. J. Fish Dis. 3:55–62.

Arakawa, C.K., Hursh, D.A., Lannan, C.N., Rohovec, J.S., and Winton, J.R. (1989) Preliminary characterization of a virus causing infectious anemia among stocks of salmonid fish in the western United States. In: Viruses of Lower Vertebrates (Ahne, W., and Kurstak, E., eds.) Springer-Verlag, New York, pp. 442–450.

Arkush, K.D., Bovo, G., de Kinkelin, P., Winton, J.R., Wingfield, W.H., and Hedrick, R.P. (1989) Biochemical and antigenic properties of the first isolates of infectious hematopoietic necrosis virus from salmonid fish in Europe. J. Aquatic Anim. Health 1:148–153.

Batts, W.N., and Winton, J.R. (1989) Enhnaced detection of infectious hematopoietic necrosis virus and other fish viruses by pretreatment of cell monolayers with polyethylene glycol. J. Aquatic Anim. Health 1:284–290.

Bellet, R. (1965) Viral hemorrhagic septicemia (VHS) of the rainbow trout bred in France. Ann. N.Y. Acad. Sci. 126:461–467.

Bellet, R. (1969) La necrose pancreatique virale (I.P.N.). Pisciculture Francaise 18:15–23.

Bernard, J., and de Kinkelin, P. (1989) Cloning the genes of viral haemorrhagic septicaemia of the trout. In: Viruses of Lower Vertebrates (Ahne, W., and Kurstak, E., eds.). Springer-Verlag, New York, pp. 379–387.

Besse, P., and de Kinkelin, P. (1965) La necrose pancreatique des alevins are-en-ciel (S. gairdneri). Pisciculture Francaise 2:16–19.

Billi, J.L., and Wolf, K. (1969) Quantitative comparsion of peritoneal washes and feces for detecting infectious pancreatic necrosis (IPN) virus in carrier brook trout. J. Fish. Res. Bd. Can. 26:1459–1465.

Bonami, J.R., Cousserans, F., Weppe, M., and Hill, B.J. (1983) Mortalities in hatchery reared sea bass fry associated with a birnavirus. Bull. Eur. Assoc. Fish Pathol. 3:41.

Bootland, L.M., Dobos, P., and Stevenson, R.M.W. (1990) Fry age and size effects on immersion immunization of brook trout, Salvelinus fontinalis Mitchell, against infectious pancreatic necrosis virus. J. Fish Dis. 13:113–125.

Bovo, G., Ceschia, G., Giorgetti, G., and Vanelli, M. (1984) Isolation of an IPN-like virus from adult kuruma shrimp (Penaeus japonicus). Bull. Eur. Assoc. Fish Pathol. 4:21.

Bradley, T.M., Medina, D.J., Chang, P.W., and McClain, J. (1989) Epizootic epitheliotropic disease of lake trout (Salvelinus namaycush): History and viral etiology. Dis. Aquatic Organ. 7:195–201.

Brunson, R., Yancey, J., and True, K. (1988) Polyethylene glycol use for viral assay in the diagnostic laboratory. Am. Fish. Soc. Fish Health Sect. Newsletter 16:3.

Bucke, D. (1977) Attempts to assess the occurrence of IPN in fish farms in England and Wales. Bull. Off. Int. Epizoot. 87:429–433.

Bucke, D., Finlay, J., McGregor, D., and Seagrave, C. (1979) Infectious pancreatic necrosis (IPN) virus: its occurrence in captive and wild fish England and Wales. J. Fish Dis. 2:549–553.

Bullock, G.L., Rucker, R.R., Amend, D., Wolf, K., and Stuckey, H.M. (1976) Infectious pancreatic necrosis: transmission with iodine-treated and nontreated eggs of brook trout (*Salvelinus fontinalis*). J. Fish. Res. Bd. Can. 33:1197–1198.

Burke, J., and Grischkowsky, R. (1984) An epizootic caused by infectious haematopoietic necrosis virus in an enhanced population of sockeye salmon, *Oncorhynchus nerka* (Walbaum), smolts at Hidden Creek, Alaska. J. Fish Dis. 7:421–429.

Burke, J.A., and Mulcahy, D. (1980) Plaquing procedure for infectious hematopoietic necrosis virus. Appl. Environ. Microbiol. 39:872–876.

Burke, J., and Mulcahy, D. (1983) Retention of infectious haematopoietic necrosis virus infectivity in fish tissue homogenates and fluids stored at three temperatures. J. Fish Dis. 6:543–547.

Bussereau, F., de Kinkelin, P., and Le Berre, M. (1975) Infectivity of fish rhabdoviruses for *Drosophila melanogaster*. Ann. Microbiol. 126:389–395.

Bylund, G., Valtonen, E. T., and Nienela, E. (1980) Observations on epidermal papillomata in wild and cultured Atlantic salmon *Salmo salar* in Finland. J. Fish Dis. 3:525–528.

Campbell, J.B., and Wolf, K. (1969) Plaque assay and some characteristics of Egtved virus (virus of viral hemorrhagic septicemia of rainbow trout). Can. J. Microbiol. 15:635–637.

Carlisle, J.C. (1976) A study of epithelioma in the Atlantic salmon *(S. salar)*. In: Wildlife Diseases. (Page, L.A., ed.) Plenum Press, New York, pp. 445–444.

Carlisle, J.C. (1977) An epidermal papilloma of the Atlantic salmon. II: Ultrastructure and etiology. J. Wildlife Dis. 13:235–239.

Carlisle, J.C., and Roberts, R.J. (1977) An epidermal papilloma of the Atlantic salmon. I: Epizootiology, pathology and immunology. J. Wildlife Dis. 13:230–234.

Castric, J., and Chastel, C. (1980) Isolation and characterization attempts of three viruses from European eel, *Anguilla anguilla*, preliminary results. Ann. Virol. 131E:435–448.

Castric, J., and de Kinkelin, P. (1980) Occurrence of viral haemorrhagic septicaemia in rainbow trout *Salmo gairdneri* Richardson reared in seawater. J. Fish Dis. 3:21–27.

Castric, J., and de Kinkelin, P. (1984) Experimental study of the susceptibility of two marine fish species, sea bass *(Dicentrarchus labrax)* and turbot *(Scophthalmus maximus)*, to viral hemorrhagic septicemia. Aquaculture 41:203–212.

Caswell-Reno, P., Reno, P.W., and Nicholson, B.L. (1986) Monoclonal antibodies to infectious pancreatic necrosis virus: Analysis of viral epitopes and comparison of different isolates. J. Gen. Virol. 67:2193–2205.

Caswell-Reno, P., Lipipun, V., Reno, P.W., and Nicholson, B.L. (1989) Use of a group-reactive and other monoclonal antibodies in an enzyme immunodot assay for identification and presumptive serotyping of aquatic birnaviruses. J. Clin. Microbiol. 27:1924–1929.

Chilmonczyk, S. (1980) Some aspects of trout gill structure in relation to Egtved virus infection and defence mechanisms. In: Fish Diseases. (Ahne, W., ed.) Springer Verlag, Berlin, pp. 18–22.

Chilmonczyk, S., and Monge, D. (1980) Rainbow trout *Salmo gairdneri* gill pillar cells demonstration of inert particle phagocystosis and involvement in viral infection. J. Reticuloendothel. Soc. 28:327–332.

Clark, H.F., and Soriano, E.Z. (1974) Fish rhabdovirus replication in non-piscine cell culture: new system for the study of rhabdovirus-cell interaction in which the virus and cell have different temperature optima. Infect. Immun. 10:180–188.

Conroy, D.A., and Santacana, J.A. (1980) Normal ictiosanitarias aplicables a actividades de acuicultura v afines en Latinoamerica (Ichthyosanitary regulations for aquaculture and related activities in Latin America.) Memorias Del 2. Simposio Latinoamericano de Aquaculture (Memoirs of the 2nd Latin American Symposium on Aquaculture.).

Daud, H.M., and Agius, C. (1987) Experimental infection of common carp, *Cyprinus carpio* L., by infectious pancreatic necrosis (IPN) virus. J. Fish Biol. 31 (Suppl. A):257–258.

Dea, S., and Elazhary, M.A.S.Y. (1983) Counterimmunoelectrophoresis for identification of infectious pancreatic necrosis virus after isolation in cell culture. Can. J. Fish. Aquatic Sci. 40:2200–2203.

de Kinkelin, P. (1983) Viral haemorrhagic septicemia. In: Antigens of Fish Pathogens: Development and Production for Vaccines and Serodiagnostics. (Les antigenes des micro-organismes pathogenes des poissons.) (Anderson, D.P., Dorson, M., and Dubourget, P., eds.) Collection Fondation Marcel Merieux, Lyon, France.

de Kinkelin, P., and Castric, J. (1982) An experimental study of the susceptibility of Atlantic salmon fry, *Salmo salar* L., to viral haemorrhagic septicaemia. J. Fish Dis. 5:57–65.

de Kinkelin, P., and Le Berre, M. (1974a) Necrose hematopoietique infectieuse des salmonides: production d'interferon circulant induite apres l'infection experimentale de la truite arc-en-ciel *(Salmo gairdneri)*. C.R. Seances Acad. Sci. Ser. III Sci. Vie. (Paris) 279(D):445–448.

de Kinkelin, P., Le Berre, M., and Meurillon, A. (1974b) Septicemie hemorrhagique virale: Demonstration de l'etat refractaire du saumon coho *(Oncorhynchus kisutch)*. Bull. Fr. Piscic. 253:166–176.

de Kinkelin, P., and Le Berre, M. (1977) Isolement d'un Rhabdovirus pathogene de la Truite Fario *(Salmo trutta*, L. 1766). C.R. Acad. Sci. Paris 284D:101–104.

de Kinkelin, P., and Scherrer, R. (1970) Le virus d'Egtved. I. Stabilite, developpement et structure du virus de la souche danoise F1. Ann. Rech. Vet. 1:17–30.

Department of Fisheries and Oceans. (1984) Fish health protection regulations: manual of complicance. Fish and Marine Service Miscellaneous Special Publication 31 (revised).

Desautels, D., and MacKelvie, R.M. (1975) Practical aspects of survival and destruction of infectious pancreatic necrosis virus. J. Fish. Res. Bd. Can. 32:523–531.

Diamant, A., Smail, D.A., McFarlane, L., and Thomson, A.M. (1988) An infectious pancreatic necrosis virus isolated from common dab *Limanda limanda* previously affected with X-cell disease, a disease apparently unrelated to the presence of the virus. Dis. Aquatic Organ. 4:223–227.

Dixon, P.F. (1987) Inhibition of infectious pancreatic necrosis virus infectivity by extracts of rainbow trout, *Salmo gairdneri* Richardson, tissue. J. Fish Dis. 10:371–378.

Dixon, P.F., and Hill, B.J. (1983) Inactivation of infectious pancreatic necrosis virus for vaccine use. J. Fish Dis. 6:399–409.

Dixon, P.F., and Hill, B.J. (1984) Rapid detection of fish rhabdoviruses by the enzyme-linked immunosorbent assay ELISA. Aquaculture 42:1–12.

Dorson, M. (1974) Production d'Anticorps precipitants antidinitrophenol chez les alevins de truite arc-en-ciel *(Salmo gairdneri)* immunises al'age d'un mois. Ct. R. Acad. Sci. 278(D):3151–3152.

Dorson, M. (1977) Vaccination trials of rainbow trout fry against infectious pancreatic necrosis. Bull. Off. Int. Epizoot. 87:405–406.

Dorson, M. (1983) Infectious pancreatic necrosis of salmonids: overview of current problems. In: Antigens of Fish Pathogens. (Anderson, D.P., Dorson, M.M., and Dubourget, P., eds.) Fondation Marcel Marieux, Lyon, France, pp. 7–31.

Dorson, M., and Torchy, C. (1979) Complement dependent neutralization of Egtved virus by trout antibodies. J. Fish Dis. 2:345–347.

Dorson, M., and Torchy, C. (1981) The influence of fish age and water temperature on mortalities of rainbow trout, *Salmo gairdneri* Richardson, caused by a European strain of infectious pancreatic necrosis virus. J. Fish Dis. 4:213–221.

Dorson, M., and Torchy, C. (1985) Experimental transmission of infectious pancreatic necrosis virus via the sexual products. In: Fish and Shellfish Pathology, (Ellis, A.E., ed.) Academic Press, London, pp. 251–260.

Dorson, M., de Kinkelin, P., and Torchy, C. (1975) Virus de la necrose pancreatique infectieuse: acquisition de la sensibilite au facteur neutralisant du serum de truite apres passages successifs en culture cellulaire. Ct. R. Acad. Sci. 281:1435–1438.

Dorson, M., de Kinkelin, P., Torchy, C., and Monge, D. (1987) Sensibilite du brochet *(Esox lucius)* a differents virus de salmonides (NPI, SHV, NHI) et au rhabdovirus de la perche.Bull. Fr. Peche Piscic. 307:91–101.

Duncan, I.B. (1978). Evidence for an oncovirus in swimbladder fibrosarcoma of Atlantic salmon *Salmo salar* L. J. Fish Dis. 1:127–131.

Eaton, E.D., Wingfield, W.H., and Hedrick, R.P. (1989) Prevalence and experimental transmission of the steelhead herpesvirus in salmonid fishes. Dis. Aquatic Organ. 7:23–30.

Economon, P.P. (1963) Experimental treatment of infectious pancreatic necrosis of brook trout with polyvinylpyrrolidone-iodine. Trans. Am. Fish. Soc. 92:180–182.

Economon, P.P. (1973) Polyvinylpyrrolidone-iodine as a control for infectious pancreatic necrosis (IPN) of brook trout. EIFAC (Eur. Inland Fish. Advis. Comm.) Tech. Paper 17, Suppl. 2:59–66.

Egusa, S., and Sorimachi, M. (1986) A histopathologial study of yellowtail ascites virus (YAV) infection of fingerling yellowtail, *Seriola quinqueradiata*. Fish Pathol. 21:113–121.

Elger, M., and Hentschel, H. (1983) Glomerular disease in cultured rainbow trout, *Salmo gairdneri* Richardson, suffering from presumptive chronic viral haemorrhagic septicaemia. J. Fish Dis. 6:211–229.

Elliott, D.G., and Amend, D.F. (1978) Efficacy of certain disinfectants against infectious pancreatic necrosis virus. J. Fish Biol. 12:277–286.

Ellis, A.E. (1988) Current aspects of fish vaccination. Dis. Aquatic Organ. 4:159–164.

Engelking, H.M., and Leong, J.C. (1989) The glycoprotein of infectious hematopoietic necrosis virus elicits neutralizing antibody and protective responses. Virus Res. 13:213–230.

Enzmann, P.-J. (1983) Considerations on the effectiveness of VHS-vaccination. Bull. Eur. Assoc. Fish Pathol. 3:54–55.

Enzmann, P.-J., and Konrad, M. (1985) Inapparent infections of brown trout with VHS-virus. Bull. Eur. Assoc. Fish Pathol. 5:81–82.

Enzmann, P.-J., and Konrad, M. (1990) Antibodies against VHS in whitefish of the Lake of Constance, West Germany. Bull. Eur. Assoc. Fish Pathol. 10:24.

Eskildsen, U.K., and Jorgensen, P.E.V. (1973) On the possible transfer of trout pathogenic viruses by gulls. Riv. Ital. Piscic. Ittiop. 8:104–105.

Eskildsen, U.K., and Jorgensen, P.E.V. (1974) Jodophorer som desinfektionsmiddel i dambrugene. Ferskvandsfiskeribladet 72, Argang Nr. 12:n.p.

Faisal, M., and Ahne, W. (1980) Use of immunoperoxidase technique for detection of fish virus antigens. In: Fish Diseases. (Ahne, W., ed.) Third COPRAQ Session. Springer-Verlag, New York.

Fijan, N.N., and Giorgetti, G. (1978) Infectious pancreatic necrosis: Isolation of virus from eyed eggs of rainbow trout *Salmo gairdneri* Richardson. J. Fish Dis. 1:269–270.

Finlay, J., and Hill, B.J. (1975) The use of the complement fixation test for rapid typing of infectious pancreatic necrosis virus. Aquaculture 5:305–310.

Fleury, H.J.A., Vuillaume, A., and Sochon, E. (1985) Isolation of an adeno-like virus from two cases of strawberry disease in rainbow trout. Ann. Inst. Pasteur/Virol. (Paris) 136E:223–228.

Flondro, F., Ropel, E., and Zdan, Z. (1984) Application of haematological examinations in the diagnosis of viral haemorrhagic septicaemia. Med. Vet. 40:50–54.

Follett, J.E., Thomas, J.B., and Hauck, A.K. (1987) Infectious haematopoietic necrosis virus in moribund and dead juvenile chum, *Oncorhynchus keta* (Walbaum), and chinook, *O. tshawytscha* (Walbaum), salmon and spawning adult chum salmon at an Alaskan hatchery. J. Fish Dis. 10:309–313.

Frantsi, C., and Savan, M. (1971a) Infectious pancreatic necrosis virus: Comparative frequencies of isolation from feces and organs of brook trout *(Salvelinus fontinalis)*. J. Fish. Res. Bd. Can. 28:1064–1065.

Frantsi, C., and Savan, M. (1971b) Infectious pancreatic necrosis virus—temperature and age factors in mortality. J. Wildlife Dis. 7:249–255.

Frerichs, G.N. (1989) Rhabdoviruses of fishes. In: Viruses of Lower Vertebrates. (Ahne, W., and Kurstak, E., eds.) Springer-Verlag, New York, pp. 317–332.

Fryer, J.L., Rohovec, J.S., Tebbit, G.L., McMichael, J.S., and Pilcher, K.S. (1976) Vaccination for control of infectious diseases in Pacific salmon. Fish Pathol. 10:155–164.

Fuhrmann, H., and Savvidis, G. (1984) On the occurrence of economically important viral and bacterial diseases in German fish hatcheries and the fight against them. In: The Fourth European Multicolloquim of Parasitology. (Tumbay, E., Yasarol, S., and Ozcel, M.A., eds.) Izmir, Turkey. October, 14–19, pp. 248–249. Abstract.

Fujimaki, Y., Hattori, K., Hatai, K., and Kubota, S.S. (1986) A light and electron microscopic study on yellowtail fingerlings with ascites. Fish Pathol. 21:105–111.

Georgiev, G.S., and Kamenov, I. (1980) Studies on serum proteins of trout (*S. irrideus* G.) suffering from viral hemorrhagic septicemia. Vet. Med. Nauk 16:52–57.

Gerard, J.P. (1977) Technique et resultats d'un essai de vaccination anti-SHV en pisciculture. Bull. Off. Int. Epizoot. 87:403–404.

Ghittino, P. (1965) Viral hemorrhagic septicemia (VHS) in rainbow trout in Italy. Ann. N.Y. Acad. Sci. 126:468–478.

Ghittino, P. (1968) Grave enzoozia di setticemia emorragica virale in trote fario di allevamento (*Salmo trutta*). Riv. Ital. Pisic. Ittiop. 3:17–19.

Ghittino, P. (1973) Viral hemorrhagic septicemia (VHS). EIFAC (Eur. Inland Fish. Comm.). Technical Paper 17, Suppl. 2:4–11.

Gosting, L.H., and Gould, R.W. (1981) Thermal inactivation of infectious hematopoietic necrosis and infectious pancreatic necrosis viruses. Appl. Environ. Microbiol. 41:1081–1082.

Grinnell, B., and Leong, J.C. (1979) Recovery and concentration of infectious pancreatic necrosis (IPN) virus in water. J. Fish. Res. Bd. Can. 36:1405–1408.

Grischkowsky, R.S., and Amend, D.F. (1976) Infectious hematopoietic necorsis virus: prevalence in certain Alaskan sockeye salmon, *Oncorhynchus nerka*. J. Fish. Res. Bd. Can. 33:186–188.

Hah, Y., Hong, S., Kim, M., Fryer, J.L., and Winton, J.R. (1984) Isolation of infectious pancreatic necrosis virus from goldfish (*Carassius auratus*) and chum salmon (*Oncorhynchus keta*) in Korea. Korean J. Microbiol. 22:85–90.

Halder, M., and Ahne, W. (1988) Freshwater crayfish *Astacus astacus*—a vector for infectious pancreatic necrosis virus (IPNV). Dis. Aquatic Organ. 4:205–209.

Hasobe, M., and Saneyoshi, M. (1985) On the approach to the viral chemotherapy against infectious hematopoietic necrosis virus (IHNV) in vitro and in vivo on salmonid fishes. Fish Pathol. 20:343–351.

Hattenberger-Baudouy, A.-M., Danton, M., Merle, G., Torchy, C., and de Kinkelin, P. (1989) Serological evidence of infectious hematopoietic necrosis in rainbow trout from a French outbreak of disease. J. Aquatic Anim. Health 1:126–134.

Hattori, M., Kodama, H., Ishiguro, S., Honda, A., Mikami, T., and Izawa, H. (1984) In vitro and in vivo detection of infectious pancreatic necrosis virus in fish by enzyme-linked immunosorbent assay. Am. J. Vet. Res. 45:1876–1879.

Hedrick, R.P., and Fryer, J.L. (1982) Persistent infections of salmonid cell lines with infectious pancreatic necrosis virus (IPNV): a model for the carrier state in trout. Fish Pathol. 16:163–172.

Hedrick, R.P., Fryer, J.L., Chen, S.N., and Kou, G.H. (1983a) Characteristics of four birnaviruses isolated from fish in Taiwan. Fish Pathol. 18:91–97.

Hedrick, R.P., Okamoto, N., Sano, T., and Fryer, J.L. (1983b) Biochemical characterization of eel virus European. J. Gen. Virol. 64:1421–1426.

Hedrick, R.P., Rosemark, R., Aronstein, D., Winton, J.R., McDowell, T., and Amend, D.F. (1984) Characteristics of a new reovirus from channel catfish (*Ictalurus punctatus*). J. Gen. Virol. 65:1527–1534.

Hedrick, R.P., Eaton, W.D., Fryer, J.L., Hah, Y.C., Park, J.W., and Hong, S.W. (1985) Biochemical and serological properties of birnaviruses isolated from fish in Korea. Fish Pathol. 463–468.

Hedrick, R.P., Eaton, W.D., Fryer, J.L., Groberg, W.G., Jr., and Boonyaratapalin, S. (1986a) Characteristics of a birnavirus isolated from cultured sand goby *Oxyeleotris marmoratus*. Dis. Aquatic Organ. 1:219–225.

Hedrick, R.P., McDowell, T., Rosemark, R., Aronstein, D. and Chan, L. (1986b) A comparison of four apparatuses for recovering infectious pancreatic necrosis virus from rainbow trout. Progressive Fish Culturist 48:47–51.

Hedrick, R.P., McDowell, T., Eaton, W.D., Kimura, T., and Sano, T. (1987a) Serological relationships of five herpesviruses isolated from salmonid fishes. J. Appl. Ichthyol. 3:87–92.

Hedrick, R.P., McDowell, T., Groff, J.M., and Kent, M.L. (1987b) Another erythrocytic virus from salmonid fish? Am. Fish. Soc. Fish Health Sect. Newsletter 15:2.

Hetrick, F.M., Fryer, J.L., and Knittel, M.D. (1979a) Effect of water temperature on the infection of rainbow trout *Salmo gairdneri* Richardson with infectious haematopoietic necrosis virus. J. Fish Dis. 2:253–257.

Hetrick, F.M., Knittel, M.D., and Fryer, J.L. (1979b) Increased susceptibility of rainbow trout to infectious hematopoietic necrosis virus after exposure to copper. Appl. Environ. Microbiol. 37:198–201.

Hill, B.J. (1976a) Properties of a virus isolated from the bi-valve mollusc *Tellina tenuis* (DaCosta). In: Wildlife Diseases. (Page, L.A., ed.) Plenum Press, New York, pp. 445–452.

Hill, B.J. (1976b) Molluscan viruses: Their occurrence, culture and relationships. In Proceedings of the 1st International Colloquium on Invertebrate Pathology, Kingston, Canada, pp. 25–29.

Hill, B.J. (1982) Infectious pancreatic necrosis virus and its virulence. In: Microbial Diseases of Fish. (Roberts, R.J., ed.) Academic Press, London, pp. 91–114.

Hill, B.J., and Dixon, P.F. (1977) Studies on IPN virulence and immunization. Bull. Off. Int. Epizoot. 87:425–427.

Hill, B.J., Underwood, B.O., Smale, C.J., and Brown, F. (1975) Physico-chemical and serological characterization of five rhabdoviruses infecting fish. J. Gen. Virol. 27:369–378.

Hoffman, G.L., Snieszko, S.F., and Wolf, K. (1970) Approved procedure for determining absence of viral hemorrhagic septicemia and whirling disease in certain fish and fish products. U.S. Fish and Wildlife Service Fish Disease Leaflet 9.

Hoffmann, R., Pfeil-Putzien, C., Dangschat, H., and Vogt, M. (1979) Untersuchungen zur pathogenese der viralen haemorrhagischen septikaemie (VHS) vei regenbogenforellen (*Salmo gairdneri*). Berl. Munch. Tierarztl. Wochenschr. 92:180–185.

Hofmann, W. (1971) Zur diagnostischen bedeutung der einschlu korperchen bei der hamorrhagischen virusseptikamie (HVS) der Forellen. Deut. Tierarztl. Wochenschr. 1:14–17.

Holt, R.A., and Piacentini, S. (1989) Erythrocytic inclusion body syndrome. Summary report prepared for The Pacific Northwest Fish Health Protection Committee. Oregon Department of Fish and Wildlife/Oregon State University, Corvallis.

Holt, R., and Rohovec, J. (1984) Anemia of coho salmon in Oregon. Am. Fish. Soc. Fish Health Sect. Newsletter 12:4.

Hsu, Y.-L., and Leong, J.C. (1985) A comparison of detection methods for infectious hematopoietic necrosis virus. J. Fish Dis. 8:1–12.

Hsu, Y.-L., Chen, B.-S., and Wu, J.-L. (1989a) Characteristics of a new reo-like virus isolated from landlocked salmon (*Oncorhynchus masou* Brevoort). Fish Pathol. 24:37–45.

Hsu, Y.-L., Chiang, S.-Y., Lin, S.-T., and Wu, J.-L. (1989b) The specific detection of infectious pancreatic necrosis virus in infected cells and fish by the immuno dot blot method. J. Fish. Dis. 12:561–571.

Inoue, S. (1973) Antiplasmic and antiinflammatory agents for pancreas necrosis control in fish, Inoue, Schinichi (Daiichi Seiyaku Co., Ltd.) Japan. Kokai 73 40.926 (Cl. 30 E2, 8 B3), 15 June 1973, Appl. 71 76.739. 30 Sept. 1971.

Isshiki, T., Kawai, K., and Kusuda, R. (1989) Change in incidence of yellowtail ascites virus (YAV) and anti-YAV neutralizing antibody in net-pen cultured yellowtail *Seriola quinqyeradiata*. Nippon Suisan Gakkaishi (Bull. Jpn. Soc. Sci. Fish.) 55:1305–1310.

Jorgensen, P.E.V. (1970) The survival of viral hemorrhagic septicemia (VHS) virus associated with trout eggs. Riv. Ital. Pisic. Ittiop. 5:13–14.

Jorgensen, P.E.V. (1973a) Inactivation of IPN and Egtved virus. Riv. Ital. Piscic. Ittiop. 8:107–108.

Jorgensen, P.E.V. (1973b) The nature and biological activity of IPN virus neutralizing antibodies in normal and immunized rainbow trout (*Salmo gairdneri*). Arch. Ges. Virusforsch. 42:9–20.

Jorgensen, P.E.V. (1974a)A study of viral diseases in Danish rainbow trout, their diagnosis and control. Commissioned by A/S Carl Fr. Mortensen, Bulowsvej 5 C 1870 Kobenhavn V.

Jorgensen, P.E.V. (1976) Partial resistance of rainbow trout (*Salmo gairdneri*) to viral haemorrhagic septicaemia (VHS) following exposure to non-virulent Egtved virus. Nord. Veterinarmed. 28:570–571.

Jorgensen, P.E.V. (1980) Egtved virus: the susceptibility of brown trout and rainbow trout to eight virus isolates and the significance of the findings for the VHS control. In: Fish Diseases. (Ahne, W., ed.) Third COPRAQ Session. Springer-Verlag, Berlin.

Jorgensen, P.E.V. (1982a) Egtved virus: occurrence of inapparent infections with virulent virus in free-living rainbow trout, *Salmo gairdneri* Richardson, at low temperature. J. Fish Dis. 5:251–255.

Jorgensen, P.E.V. (1982b) Egtved virus: temperature-dependent immune response of trout to infection with low-virulence virus. J. Fish Dis. 5:47–55.

Jorgensen, P.E.V., and Kehlet, N.P. (1971) Infectious pancreatic necrosis (IPN) viruses in Danish rainbow trout. Their serological and pathogenic properties. Nord. Veterinarmed. 23:568–575.

Jorgensen, P.E.V., and Meyling, A. (1972) Egtved virus: demonstration of virus antigen by the fluorescent antibody technique in tissues of rainbow trout affected by viral haemorrhagic septicaemia and in cell cultures infected with Egtved virus. Arch. Ges. Virusforsch. 36:115–122.

Kamei, Y., Yoshimizu, M., and Kimura, T. (1987) Plaque assay of *Oncorhynchus masou* virus (OMV). Fish Pathol. 22:147–152.

Kamei, Y., Yoshimizu, M., Ezura, Y., and Kimura, T. (1988) Effects of environmental water on the infectivities of infectious hematopoietic necrosis virus (IHNV) and infectious pancreatic necrosis virus (IPNV). J. Appl. Ichthyol. 4:37–47.

Kehlet, N.P. (1973) A summary of the rules, methods and results of the Danish campaign against infectious diseases of freshwater fish. EIFAC (Eur. Inland Fish. Advis. Comm.). Technical Paper 17, Suppl. 2:37–38.

Kimura, T., Yoshimizu, M., Tanaka, M., and Sannohe, H. (1981a) Studies on a new virus (OMV) from *Oncorhynchus masou*. I. Characteristics and pathogenicity. Fish Pathol. 15:143–147.

Kimura, T., Yoshimizu, M., and Tanaka, M. (1981b) Studies on a new virus (OMV) from *Oncorhynchus masou*. II. Oncogenic nature. Fish Pathol. 15:149–153.

Kimura, T., Suzuki, S., and Yoshimizu, M. (1983a) In vitro antiviral effect of 9-(2-hydroxyethoxymethyl) guanine on the fish herpesvirus, *Oncorhynchus masou* virus (OMV). Antiviral Res. 3:93–101.

Kimura, T., Suzuki, S., and Yoshimizu, M. (1983b) In vivo antiviral effect of 9-(2-hydroxyethoxymethyl) guanine on experimental infection of chum salmon (*Oncorhynchus keta*) fry with *Oncorhynchus masou* virus (OMV). Antiviral Res. 3:103–108.

Kimura, T., Yoshimizu, M., and Yasuda, H. (1984) Rapid, simple serological diagnosis of infectious pancreatic necrosis by coagglutination test using antibody-sensitized staphylococci. Fish Pathol. 19:25–33.

Klontz, G.W., Yasutake, W.T., and Parisot, T.J. (1965) Virus diseases of the Salmonidae in western United States. III. Immunopathological aspects. Ann. N.Y. Acad. Sci. 126:531–542.

Koener, J.F., and Leong, J.C. (1990) Expression of the glycoprotein gene from a fish rhabdovirus by using baculovirus vectors. J. Virol. 64:428–430.

Kruse, P., and Neukirch, M. (1989) The significance of rainbow trout brain and excretory kidney for the propagation of viral haemorrhagic septicaemia (VHS) virus. In: Viruses of Lower Vertebrates. (Ahne, W., and Kurstak, E., eds.) Springer-Verlag, New York, pp. 367–378.

Kruse, P., and Neukrich, M. (1990) Demonstration of VHS-virus antigen in the pseudobranch of rainbow trout, *Oncorhynchus mykiss*. Bull. Eur. Assoc. Fish Pathol. 10:26–27.

Kudo, S., Kurosawa, D., Kunimine, I., Nobusawa, K., and Kobayashi, S. (1973) Electron microscopic observations of the pancreas and liver in the fingerling rainbow trout with symptoms of IPN. Jpn. J. Ichthyol. 20:163–177.

Landolt, M.L., MacMillan, J.R., and Patterson, M. (1977) Detection of an intraerythrocytic virus in rainbow trout (*Salmo gairdneri*). Fish Health News 6:4–6.

LaPatra, S. (1989) The use of fish mucus in the detection of infectious hematopoietic necrosis virus (IHNV). Am. Fish. Soc. Fish Health Sect. Newsletter 17:3.

LaPatra, S.E., Roberti, K.A., Rohovec, J.S., and Fryer, J.L. (1989) Fluorescent antibody test for the rapid diagnosis of infectious hematopoietic necrosis. J. Aquatic Anim. Health 1:29–36.

Le Berre, M., de Kinkelin, P., and Metzger, A. (1977) Identification serologique des rhabdovirus des salmonides. Bull. Off. Int. Epizoot. 87:391–393.

Leek, S.L. (1985) Artificial transmission of erythrocytic virus. Am. Fish. Soc. Fish Health Sect. Newsletter 13:4.

Leek, S.L. (1987) Viral erythrocytic inclusion body syndrome (EIBS) occurring in juvenile spring chinook salmon (*Oncorhynchus tshawytscha*) reared in freshwater. Can. J. Fish. Aquatic Sci. 44:685–688.

Leintz, J.C., and Springer, J.E. (1973) Neutralization tests of infectious pancreatic necrosis virus with polyvalent antiserum. J. Wildlife Dis. 9:120–124.

Leong, J.C. (1984) Evaluation of a subunit vaccine to infectious hematopoietic necrosis (IHN) virus. Annual Report. U.S. Dept. of Energy, Bonneville Power Administration, Division of Fish and Wildlife.

Lightner, D., and Post, G. (1969) Morphological characteristics of infectious pancreatic necrosis virus in trout pancreatic tissues. J. Fish. Res. Bd. Can. 26:2247–2250.

Ljungberg, O. (1963) Report on fish diseases and inspection of fish products in Sweden. Bull. Off. Int. Epizoot. 59:111–120.

Ljungberg, O., and Jorgensen, P.E.V. (1973) Infectious pancreatic necrosis (IPN) of salmonids in Swedish fish farms. EIFAC (Eur. Inland Fish. Advis. Comm.) Tech. Paper 17, Suppl. 2:67–70.

Lorenzen, N., Olesen, N.J., and Vestergard Jorgensen, P.E. (1988) Production and characterization of monoclonal antibodies to four Egtved virus structural proteins. Dis. Aquatic Organ. 4:35–42.

Lounatmaa, K., and Janatuinen, J. (1978) Electron microscopy of an ulcerative dermal necrosis (UDN)-like salmon disease in Finland. J. Fish Dis. 1:369–375.

Lunder, T., Thorud, K., Poppe, T.T., Holt, R.A., and Rohovec, J.S. (1990) Particles similar to the virus of erythrocytic inclusion body syndrome, EIBS, detected in Atlantic salmon (*Salmo salar*) in Norway. Bull. Eur. Assoc. Fish Pathol. 10:21–23.

Macdonald, R.D., and Gower, D.A. (1981) Genomic and phenotypic divergence among three serotypes of aquatic birnaviruses (infectious pancreatic necrosis virus). Virology 114:187–195.

MacKelvie, R.M., and Artsob, H. (1969) Infectious pancreatic necrosis virus in young salmonids of the Canadian Maritime Provinces. J. Fish. Res. Bd. Can. 26:3259–3262.

MacKelvie, R.M., and Desautels, D. (1975) Fish viruses—survival and inactivation of infectious pancreatic necrosis virus. J. Fish. Res. Bd. Can. 32:1267–1273.

Maisse, G., Dorson, M., and Torchy, C. (1980) Ultraviolet inactivation of two pathogenic salmonid viruses (IPN virus and VHS virus). Bull. Fr. Piscic. 278:34–40.

Mangunwiryo, H., and Agius, C. (1987) Pathogenicity of infectious pancreatic necrosis (IPN) virus to tilapia and its immune response. J. Fish Biol. 31(Suppl. A):255–256.

Mangunwiryo, H., and Agius, C. (1988) Studies on the carrier state of infectious pancreatic necrosis virus infections in rainbow trout, *Salmo gairdneri* Richardson. J. Fish Dis. 11:125–132.

Margaritov, N. (1969) Borbata sresht virusnata hemoragichna septitsemiia po pucturvite. Ribno Stopanstvo 2:4–5.

McAllister, P.E. (1979) Fish viruses and viral infections. In: Comprehensive Virology. Vol. 14. (Fraenkel-Conrat, H., and Wagner, R.R., eds.) Plenum, New York USA.

McAllister, P.E. (1983) Infectious pancreatic necrosis (IPN) of salmonid fishes. U.S. Fish and Wildlife Service, Fish Disease Leaflet 65.

McAllister, P.E., and Herman, R.L. (1989) Epizootic mortality in hatchery-reared lake trout *Salvelinus namaycush* caused by a putative virus possibly of the herpesvirus group. Dis. Aquatic Organ. 6:113–119.

McAllister, K.W., and McAllister, P.E. (1988) Transmission of infectious pancreatic necrosis virus from carrier striped bass to brook trout. Dis. Aquatic Organ. 4:101–104.

McAllister, P.E., and Owens, W.J. (1986) Infectious pancreatic necrosis virus: protocol for a standard challenge to brook trout. Trans. Am. Fish. Soc. 115:466–470.

McAllister, P.E., and Owens, W.J. (1987) Identification of the three serotypes of viral hemorrhagic septicemia virus by immunoblot assay using antiserum to serotype F1. Bull. Eur. Assoc. Fish Pathol. 7:90–92.

McAllister, P.E., and Reyes, X. (1984) Infectious pancreatic necrosis virus: Isolation from rainbow trout, *Salmo gairdneri* Richardson, imported into Chile. J. Fish Dis. 7:319–322.

McAllister, P.E., and Schill, W.B. (1986) Immunoblot assay: a rapid and sensitive method for identification of salmonid fish viruses. J. Wildlife Dis. 22:468–474.

McAllister, P.E., Fryer, J.L., and Pilcher, K.D. (1974) Further characterization of infectious hematopoietic necrosis virus of salmonid fish (Oregon strain). Arch. Ges. Virusforsch. 44:270–279.

McAllister, P.E., Newman, M.W., Sauber, J.H., and Owens, W.J. (1984) Isolation of infectious pancreatic necrosis virus (serotype Ab) from diverse species of estuarine fish. Helgo. Meeresunters. 37:317–328.

McAllister, P.E., Owens, W.J., and Ruppenthal, T.M. (1987) Detection of infectious pancreatic necrosis virus in pelleted cell and particulate components from ovarian fluid of brook trout *Salvelinus fontinalis*. Dis. Aquatic Organ. 2:235–237.

McCain, B.B., Fryer, J.L., and Pilcher, K.S. (1971) Antigenic relationships in a group of three viruses of salmonid fish by cross neutralization. Proc. Soc. Exp. Biol. Med. 317:1042–1046.

McDowell, T., Hedrick, R.P., Kent, M.L., and Elston, R.A. (1989) Isolation of a new virus from Atlantic salmon (*Salmo salar*). Am. Fish. Soc. Fish Health Sect. Newsletter 17:7.

McIntyre, J.D., and Amend, D.F. (1978) Heritability of tolerance for infectious hematopoietic necrosis in sockeye salmon (*Oncorhynchus nerka*). Trans. Am. Fish. Soc. 107:305–308.

McKnight, I.J. (1978) Sarcoma of the swim bladder of Atlantic salmon (*Salmo salar* L.). Aquaculture 13:55–60.

McKnight, I.J., and Roberts, R.J. (1976) The pathology of infectious pancreatic necrosis. I. The sequential histopathology of the naturally occurring condition. Br. Vet. J. 132:76–85.

McMichael, J.S., Fryer, J.L., and Pilcher, K.S. (1975) Salmonid virus isolations in Oregon (U.S.A.). F.A.O. Aquaculture Bull. 5:14.

McMichael, J., Fryer, J.L., and Pilcher, K.S. (1975) An antigenic comparison of three strains of infectious pancreatic necrosis virus of salmonid fishes. Aquaculture 6:203–210.

Meier, W. (1980) La septicemie hemorragique virale (S.H.V.) chez les nonsalmonidees. La S.H.V. chez des alevins de brochets (*Esox lucius* L.): description du syndrome et son importance sur le plan epidemiologique. (Viral haemorrhagic septicaemia (V.H.S.) in non-salmonids. V.H.S. in pike fry *(Esox lucius):* description of the syndrome and its epidemiological significance. Bull. Off. Int. Epizoot. 92:1025–1029.

Meier, W., and Jorgensen, P.E.V. (1975) A rapid and specific method for the diagnosis of viral haemorrhagic septicaemia (VHS) of rainbow trout. Rev. Ital. Piscic. Ittiop. 10:11–15.

Meier, W., and Jorgensen, P.E.V. (1980) Isolation of VHS virus from pike fry *(Esox lucius)* with hemorrhagic symptoms. In: Fish Diseases. (Ahne, W., ed.) Third COPRAQ Session. Springer-Verlag, Berlin.

Meier, W., Ahne, W., and Jorgensen, P.E.V. (1986) Fish viruses: viral haemorrhagic septicaemia in white fish (*Coregonus* sp.). J. Appl. Ichthyol. 4:181–186.

Menezes, J. (1977) Septicemie hemorragique virale de la truite arc-en-ciel: Etude critique de la technique de diagnostic. Bull. Off. Int. Epizoot. 87:383–390.

Migus, D.O., and Dobos, P. (1980) Effect of ribavirin on the replication of infectious pancreatic necrosis virus in fish cell cultures. J. Gen. Virol. 47:47–57.

Miyazaki, T. (1985) A histopathological study on serious cases with viral ascites of yellowtail fingerling occurred in mie prefecture. Fish Pathol. 21:123–127.

Moewus, L. (1962) Studies on a marine parasitic *Tetrahymena* species. J. Protozool. 9(Suppl. 34).

Moewus-Knobb, L. (1965) Studies with IPN virus in marine hosts. Ann. N. Y. Acad. Sci. 126:328–342.

Mulcahy, D., and Bauersfeld, K. (1983) Effect of loading density of sockeye salmon, *Oncorhynchus nerka* (Walbaum), eggs in incubation boxes on mortality caused by infectious haematopoietic necrosis. J. Fish Dis. 6:189–193.

Mulcahy, D.M., and Fryer, J.L. (1976) Double infection of rainbow trout fry with IHN and IPN viruses. Fish Health News 5:6–6.

Mulcahy, D., and Pascho, R.J. (1984) Adsorption to fish sperm of vertically transmitted fish viruses. Science 225:333–335.

Mulcahy, D., and Pascho, R.J. (1985) Vertical transmission of infectious haematopoietic necrosis virus in sockeye salmon, *Oncorhynchus nerka* (Walbaum): Isolation of virus from dead eggs and fry. J. Fish Dis. 8:393–396.

Mulcahy, D., and Pascho, R.J. (1986) Sequential tests for infectious hematopoietic necrosis virus in individuals and populations of sockeye salmon *(Oncorhynchus nerka).* Can. J. Fish. Aquatic Sci. 43:2515–2519.

Mulcahy, D., and Wood, J. (1986) A natural epizootic of infectious haematopoietic necrosis in imported Atlantic salmon, *Salmo salar* L., reared in the enzootic region. J. Fish Dis. 9:173–175.

Mulcahy, D., Burke, J., Pascho, R., and Jenes, C.K. (1982) Pathogenesis of infectious hematopoietic necrosis virus in adult sockeye salmon *(Oncorhynchus nerka).* Can. J. Fish. Aquatic Sci. 39:1144–1149.

Mulcahy, D., Pascho, R.J., and Jenes, C.K. (1983a) Titre distribution patterns of infectious haematopoietic necrosis virus in ovarian fluids of hatchery and feral salmon populations. J. Fish Dis. 6:183–188.

Mulcahy, D., Pascho, R., and Jenes, C.K. (1983b) Mortality due to infectious hematopoietic necrosis of sockeye salmon *(Oncorhynchus nerka)* fry in streamside egg incubation boxes. Can. J. Fish. Aquatic Sci. 40:1511–1516.

Mulcahy, D., Pascho, R.J., and Jenes, C.K. (1983c) Detection of infectious haematopoietic necrosis virus in river water and demonstration of waterborne transmission. J. Fish Dis. 6:321–330.

Mulcahy, D., Jenes, C.K., and Pascho, R. (1984a) Appearance and quantification of infectious hematopoietic necrosis virus in female sockeye salmon *(Oncorhynchus nerka)* during their spawning migration. Arch. Virol. 80:171–181.

Mulcahy, D., Pascho, R., and Jenes, C.K. (1984b) Comparison of in vitro growth characteristics of ten isolates of infectious haematopoietic necrosis virus. J. Gen. Virol. 65:2199–2207.

Mulcahy, D., Pascho, R.J., and Batts, W.N. (1987) Testing of male sockeye salmon *(Oncorhynchus nerka)* and steelhead trout *(Salmo gairdneri)* for infectious hematopoietic necrosis virus. Can. J. Fish. Aquat. Sci. 44:1075–1078.

Mulcahy, D., Klaybor, D., and Batts, W.N. (1990) Isolation of infectious hematopoietic necrosis virus from a leech *(Piscicola salmositica)* and a copepod *(Salmincola* sp.), ectoparasites of sockeye salmon *Oncorhynchus nerka.* Dis. Aquatic Organ. 8:29–34.

Munro, A.L.S., and Duncan, I.B. (1977) Current problems in the study of biology of infectious pancreatic necrosis virus and the management of the disease it causes in cultivated salmonid fish. In: Aquatic Microbiology. (Skinner, F.A., and Shewan, J.M., eds.). Academic Press, London, pp. 325–337.

Munro, A.L.S., Liversidge, J., and Elson, K.G.R. (1976) The distribution and prevalence of infectious pancreatic necrosis virus in wild fish in Loch Awe. Proc. R. Soc. Edinb. Sect. B 75:223–232.

Neukirch, M. (1984) An experimental study of the entry and multiplication of viral haemorrhagic septicaemia virus in rainbow trout, *Salmo gairdneri* Richardson, after water-borne infection. J. Fish Dis. 7:231–234.

Neukirch, M., and Glass, B. (1984) Some aspects of virus shedding by

rainbow trout (*Salmo gairdneri* Rich.) after waterborne infection with viral haemorrhagic septicaemia (VHS) virus. Zentralbl. Bakteriol. Hyg. A 257:433–438.

Nicholson, B.L. (1983) Infectious hematopoietic necrosis (I.H.N.). In: Antigens of Fish Pathogens: Development and Production for Vaccines and Serodiagnostics. (Les antigenes des micro-organisms pathogenes des poissons.) (Anderson, D.P., Dorson, M., Dubourget, P., eds.) Collection Fondation Marcel Merieux, Lyon, France, p. 63.

Nicholson, B.L., and Caswell, P. (1982) Enzyme-linked immunosorbent assay for identification of infectious pancreatic necrosis virus. J. Clin. Microbiol. 16:469–472.

Nicholson, B.L., and Dexter, R. (1975) Possible interference in the isolation of IPN virus from carrier fish. J. Fish. Res. Bd. Can. 32:1437–1439.

Nishimura, T., Sasaki, H., Ushiyama, M., Inoue, K., Suzuki, Y., Ikeya, F., Tanaka, M., Suzuki, H., Kohara, M., Arai, M., Shima, N., and Sano, T. (1985) A trial of vaccination against rainbow trout fry with formalin killed IHN virus. Fish Pathol. 20:435–443.

Okamoto, N., Sano, T., Hedrick, R.P., and Fryer, J.L. (1983) Antigenic relationships of selected strains of infectious pancreatic necrosis virus and European eel virus. J. Fish Dis. 6:19–25.

Okamoto, N., Shirakura, T., and Sano, T. (1985) Precision of a plaque assay eel virus European—and infectious hematopoietic necrosis virus—RTG–2 cell systems. Fish Pathol. 19:225–230.

Olesen, N.J., and Jorgensen, P.E.V. (1982) Can and do herons serve as vectors for Egtved virus. Bull Eur. Assoc. Fish Pathol. 2:48.

Olesen, N.J., and Vestergard Jorgensen, P.E. (1986) Detection of neutralizing antibody to Egtved virus in rainbow trout *(Salmo gairdneri)* by plaque neutralization test with complement addition. J. Appl. Ichthyol. 2:33–41.

Olesen, N.J., Vestergard Jorgensen, P.E., Bloch, B., and Mellergaard, S. (1988) Isolation of an IPN-like virus belonging to the serogroup II of the aquatic birnaviruses from dab, *Limanda limanda* L. J. Fish Dis. 11:449–451.

Olson, D.P., Beleau, M.H., Busch, R.A., Roberts, S., and Krieger, R.I. (1985) Strawberry disease in rainbow trout, *Salmo gairdneri* Richardson. J. Fish. Dis. 8:103–111.

Ord, W. (1975) Resistance of chinook salmon *(Oncorhynchus tschawytscha)* fingerlings experimentally infected with viral hemorrhagic septicemia virus. Bull. Fr. Piscic. 257:149–152.

Ord, W.M., Le Berre, M., and de Kindelin, P. (1976) Viral hemorrhagic septicemia: Comparative susceptibility of rainbow trout *(Salmo gairdneri)* and hybrids (*S. gairdneri* × *Oncorhynchus kisutch*) to experimental infection. J. Fish. Res. Bd. Can. 33:1205–1208.

Osadchaya, E.F. (1981) Fish diseases caused by rhabdoviruses in the Ukraine. In: Proceedings of an International Seminar on Fish, Pathogens and Environment in European Polyculture, Szarvas, Hungary, 23–27 June 1981 (Olah, J, Molnar, K., and Jeney, Z., eds.), pp. 36–47.

Parisot, T.J., Yasutake, W.T., and Bressler, V. (1963) A new geographic and host record for infectious pancreatic necrosis. Trans. Am. Fish. Soc. 92:63–66.

Parisot, T.J., Yasutake, W.T., and Klontz, G.W. (1965) Virus diseases of the Salmonidae in western United States. I. Etiology and epizootiology. Ann. N.Y. Acad. Sci. 126:502–519.

Parsons, J.E., Busch, R.A., Thorgaard, G.H., and Scheerer, P.D. (1986) Increased resistance of triploid rainbow trout X coho salmon hybrids to infectious hematopoietic septikemia virus. Aquaculture 57:337–343.

Pelton, E. (1987) Possible horizontal transmission of EIBS. Am. Fish. Soc. Fish Health Sect. Newsletter 15:5.

Perlmutter, A., Sarot, D.A., Yu, M-L., Filazzola, R.J., and Seeley, R.J. (1973) The effect of crowding on the immune response of the blue gourami, *Trichogaster trichopterus*, to infectious pancreatic necrosis (IPN) virus. Life Sci. 13:363–375.

Peters, F., and Neukirch, M. (1986) Transmission of some fish pathogenic viruses by the heron, *Ardea cinerea.* J. Fish Dis. 9:539–544.

Pfeil, V.C., and Wiedemann, H. (1977) Virusnachweis durch indirekte immunofluoreszenz und virusanzuchtung bei experimentell erzeugter viraler haemorrhagischer septikamie (VHS) der regenbogenforelle *(Salmo gairdneri).* Dtsch. Tieraerzt. Wochenschr. 84:152–154.

Pfitzner, I. (1966) Beitrag zur atiologie der "haemorrhagischen virussepti-kaemie der regenbogenforellen."Zentralbl. Bakteriol. Parasitenk. D. Infektionskr. Hyg. Abt. I. Orig. 201:306–320.

Piacentini, S.C., Rohovec, J.S., and Fryer, J.L. (1989) Epizootiology of erythrocytic inclusion body syndrome. J. Aquatic Anim. Health 1:173–179.

Pilcher, K.S., and Fryer, J.L. (1980) The viral diseases of fish: a review through 1978. Part 1: diseases of proven viral etiology. Rev. Microbiol. 7:287–364.

Piper, D., Nicholson, B.L., and Dunn, J. (1973) Immunofluorescent study of the replication of infectious pancreatic necrosis virus in trout and Atlantic salmon cell cultures. Infect. Immun. 8:249–254.

Rasmussen, C.J. (1965) A biological study of the Egtved disease (INUL). Ann. N.Y. Acad. Sci. 126:427–460.

Reichenbach-Klinke, H. (1959) Fischkrankheiten in Bayern in den Jahren 1957 and 1958. Allg. Fishc.-ZTG. 84(125):226–228.

Reno, P.W., Darley, S., and Savan, M. (1978) Infectious pancreatic necrosis:

experimental induction of a carrier state in trout. J. Fish. Res. Brd. Can. 35:1451–1456.

Ristow, S.S., and Arnzen, J.M. (1989) Development of monoclonal antibodies that recognize a type–2 specific and a common epitope on the nucleoprotein of infectious hematopoietic necrosis virus. J. Aquatic. Anim. Health 1:119–125.

Roberts, R.J. (1972) Ulcerative dermal necrosis (UDN) of salmon (*Salmo salar* L.). Symp. Zool. Soc. Lond. 30:53–81.

Roberts, R.J., ed. (1978) Fish Pathology. Bailliere Tindall, London.

Roberts, R.J., and McKnight, I.J. (1976) The pathology of infectious pancreatic necrosis. II. Stress-mediated recurrence. Br. Vet. J. 132:209–214.

Rodak, L., Pospisil, Z., Tomanek, J., Vesely, T., Obr, T., and Valicek, L. (1988) Enzyme-linked immunosorbent assay (ELISA) detection of infectious pancreatic necrosis virus (IPNV) in culture fluids and tissue homogenates of the rainbow trout, *Salmo gairdneri* Richardson. J. Fish Dis. 11:225–235.

Rosenlund, B.D. (1977) Infectious pancreatic necrosis virus at the Willow Beach NFH, Nevada, and in rainbow trout stocked into adjacent Lake Mohave. Fish Health News 6:10.

Ross, A.J., Pelnar, J., and Rucker, R.R. (1960) A virus-like disease of chinook salmon. Trans. Am. Fish. Soc. 89:160–163.

Sano, T. (1971a) Studies on viral diseases of Japanese fishes. I. Infectious pancreatic necrosis of rainbow trout: First isolation from epizootics in Japan. Bull. Jpn. Soc. Sci. Fish. 37:495–498.

Sano, T. (1971b) Studies on viral diseases of Japanese fishes. II. Infectious pancreatic necrosis of rainbow trout: pathogenicity of the isolants. Bull Jpn. Soc. Sci. Fish. 37:499–503.

Sano, T. (1973) The current preventive approach to infectious pancreatic necrosis (IPN) in Japan. EIFAC (Eur. Inland. Fish. Advis. Comm.) Tech. Paper 17, Suppl. 2:71–75.

Sano, T. (1976) Viral diseases of cultured fishes in Japan. Fish Pathol. 10:221–226.

Sano, T., Nishimura T., Okamoto, N., Yamazaki, T., Hanada, H., and Watanabe, Y. (1977) Studies on viral diseases of Japanese fisheries. VI. Infectious hematopoietic necrosis (IHN) of salmonids in the mainland of Japan. J. Tokyo Univ. Fish. 63:81–85.

Sano, T., Okamoto, N., and Nishimura, T. (1981) A new viral epizootic of *Anguilla japonica* Temminck and Schlegel. J. Fish Dis. 4:127–139.

Sano, T., Fukuda, H., Okamoto, N., and Kaneko, F. (1983) Yamame tumor virus: Lethality and oncogenicity. Bull. Jpn. Soc. Sci. Fish. 49:1159–1163.

Savan, M., and Dobos, P. (1980). Effect of virazole on rainbow trout *Salmo gairdneri* Richardson fry infected with infectious pancreatic necrosis virus. J. Fish Dis. 3:437–440.

Schultz, C.L., McAllister, P.E., Schill, W.B., Lidgerding, B.C., and Hetrick, F.M. (1989) Detection of infectious hematopoietic necrosis virus in cell culture fluid using immunoblot assay and biotinylated monoclonal antibody. Dis. Aquatic Organ. 7:31–37.

Schutz, M., May, E.B., Kraeuter, J.N., and Hetrick, F.M. (1984) Isolation of infectious pancreatic necrosis virus from an epizootic occurring in cultured striped bass, *Morone saxatilis* (Walbaum). J. Fish Dis. 7:505–507.

Scott, J.L., Fendrick, J.L., and Leong, J.C. (1980) Growth of infectious hematopoietic necrosis virus in mosquito *Aedes albopictus* and fish cell lines. J. Biol. 38:21–29.

Seeley, R.J., Perlmutter, A., and Seeley, V.A. (1977) Inheritance and longevity of infectious pancreatic necrosis virus in the zebra fish, *Brachydanio rerio* (Hamilton-Buchanan). Appl. Environ. Microbiol. 34:50–55.

Silim, A., Elazhary, M.A.S.Y., and Lagace, A. (1982) Susceptibility of trouts of different species and origins to various isolates of infectious pancreatic necrosis virus. Can. J. Fish. Aquatic Sci. 39:1580–1584.

Sonstegard, R.A., and McDermott, L.A. (1972) Epidemiological model for passive transfer of IPNV by homeotherms. Nature 237:104–105.

Sonstegard, R.A., McDermott, L.A., and Sonstegard, K.S. (1972) Isolation of infectious pancreatic necrosis virus from white suckers (*Catostomus* [sic] *commersoni*). Nature 236:174–175.

Sorimachi, M., and Hara, T. (1985) Characteristics and pathogenicity of a virus isolated from yellowtail fingerlings showing ascites. Fish Pathol. 19:231–238.

Stephens, E.B., Newman, M.W., Zachary, A.L., and Hetrick, F.M. (1980) A viral aetiology for the annual spring epizootics of Atlantic menhaden *Brevoortia tyrannus* (Latrobe) in Chesapeake Bay. J. Fish Dis. 3:387–398.

Swanson, R.N. (1981) Use of the indirect fluorescent antibody test to study the pathogenesis of infectious pancreatic necrosis virus infection in trout. Dev. Biol. Stand. 49:71–77.

Swanson, R.N., and Gillespie, J.H. (1979) Pathogenesis of infectious pancreatic necrosis in Atlantic salmon *(Salmo salar)*. J. Fish. Res. Bd. Can. 36:587–591.

Swanson, R.N., and Gillespie, J.H. (1981) An indirect fluorescent antibody test for the rapid detection of infectious pancreatic necrosis virus in tissues. J. Fish. Dis. 4:309–315.

Swanson, R.N., and Gillespie, J.H. (1982) Isolation of infectious pancreatic necrosis virus from the blood and blood components of experimentally infected trout. Can. J. Fish. Aquatic Sci. 39:225–228.

Tack, E. (1959) Beitrage zur erforschung der forellenseuche weitere versuchsergebnisse aus der seuchenanlage wallersbach der landesanstalt fur fischerei nordrhein-westfalen. Arch. Fischereiwiss. 10:20–30.

Tesarcik, J., Cibulka, J., and Kalivoda, J. (1968) Vyskyt virove hemorrhagicke septikemie (anaemia infectiosa salmonum) u pstruhu americkych duhovych (*Parasalmo gairdnerii* Richardson 1836). Bull VUR Vodnany 3:19–26.

Toranzo, A.E., and Hetrick, F.M. (1982) Comparative stability of two salmonid viruses and poliovirus in fresh, estuarine and marine waters. J. Fish Dis. 5:223–231.

Toranzo, A.E., Barja, J.L., Lemos, M.L., and Hetrick, F. M. (1983) Stability of infectious pancreatic necrosis virus (IPNV) in untreated, filtered and autoclaved estuarine water. Bull. Eur. Assoc. Fish Pathol. 3:51–53.

Traxler, G.S., and Batts, W.N. (1989) Variation in sensitivity of two fish cell lines to rhabdovirus infection. Am. Fish. Soc. Fish Health Sect. Newsletter 17:5.

Traxler, G.S., and Rankin, J.B. (1989) An infectious hematopoietic necrosis epizootic in sockeye salmon *Oncorhynchus nerka* in Weaver Creek spawning channel, Fraser River system, B.C., Canada. Dis. Aquatic Org. 6:221–226.

Underwood, B.O., Smale, C.J., Brown, F., and Hill, B.J. (1977) Relationship of a virus from *Tellina tenuis* to infectious pancreatic necrosis virus. J. Gen. Virol. 36:93–109.

Vestergaard Jorgensen, P.E. (1973) Inactivation of IPN and Egtved virus. Riv. It. Piscic. Ittiop. 8:107–108.

Vestergard Jorgensen, P.E., and Olesen, N.J. (1987) Cod ulcus syndrome rhabdovirus is indistinguishable from the Egtved (VHS) virus. Bull. Eur. Assoc. Fish Pathol. 7:73–74.

Watanabe, R.A., Fryer, J.L., and Rohovec, J.S. (1988) Molecular filtration for recovery of waterborne viruses of fish. Appl. Environ. Microbiol. 54:1606–1609.

Watanabe, Y., Hanada, H. and Ushiyama, M. (1981) Monolayer cell cultures from marine fishes. Fish Pathol. 15:201–206.

Wechsler, S.J., McAllister, P.E., and Hetrick, F.M. (1987) Neutralizing activity against infectious pancreatic necrosis virus in striped bass, *Morone saxatilis*, from the Chesapeake Bay. J. Wildlife Dis. 23:154–155.

Wedemeyer, G.A., Nelson, N.C., and Smith, C.A. (1978) Survival of the salmonid viruses infectious hematopoietic necrosis (IHNV) and infectious pancreatic necrosis (IPNV) in ozonated, chlorinated, and untreated waters. J. Fish Res. Bd. Can. 35:875–879.

Wedemeyer, G.A., Nelson, N.C., and Yasutake, W.T. (1979) Potentials and limits for the use of ozone as a fish disease control agent. Ozone Sci. Eng. 1:295–318.

Williams, I.V., and Amend, D.F. (1976) A natural epizootic of infectious hematopoietic necrosis in fry of sockeye salmon (*Oncorhynchus nerka*) at Chilko Lake, British Columbia. J. Fish. Res. Bd. Can. 33:1564–1567.

Wingfield, W.H., Fryer, J.L., and Pilcher, K.S. (1969) Properties of the sockeye salmon virus (Oregon strain). Proc. Soc. Exp. Biol. Med. 130:1055–1059.

Winton, J.R., Lannan, C.N., Fryer, J.L., and Kimura, T. (1980) Isolation and characterization of a new reovirus from chum salmon. In: Proceedings of the North Pacific Aquaculture Symposium, Anchorage, Alaska, 18–21 August 1980; Newport, Oregon, 25–27 August 1980, pp. 359–367.

Winton, J.R., Lannan, C.N., Fryer, J.L., and Kimura, T. (1981) Isolation of a new reovirus from chum salmon in Japan. Fish Pathol. 15:155–162.

Winton, J.R., Lannan, C.N., Ransom, D.P., and Fryer, J.L. (1985) Isolation of a new virus from chinook salmon (*Oncorhynchus tshawytscha*) in Oregon U.S.A. Fish Pathol. 20:373–380.

Winton, J.R., Arakawa, C.K., Lannan, C.N., and Fryer, J.L. (1988) Neutralizing monoclonal antibodies recognize antigenic variants among isolates of infectious hematopoietic necrosis virus. Dis. Aquatic Organ. 4:199–204.

Wiren, B. (1971) Vartsjuke hos lax (*Salmo salar* L.) histologiska studier over epidermala papillom hos odlad lax. Swed. Salmon Res. Inst. Rep. LFI MEDD. 7/1971.

Wizigmann, G., Baath, C., and Hoffmann, R. (1980) Isolation of viral hemorrhagic septicemia virus from fry of rainbow trout, pike and grayling. Zentralbl. Veterinarmed. B. 27:79–81.

Wolf, K. (1966) The fish viruses. In: Advances in Virus Research. Vol. 12. (Smith, K.M., and Lauffer, M.A., eds.) Academic Press, New York, pp. 35–101.

Wolf, K. (1976) Fish viral diseases in North America, 1971–1975, and recent research of the Eastern Fish Disease Laboratory, U.S.A. Fish Pathol. 10:135–154.

Wolf, K. (1983) Biology and properties of fish and reptilian herpesviruses. In: The Herpesviruses. Vol. 2. (Roizman, B., ed.) Plenum Press, New York, pp. 319–366.

Wolf, K. (1988) Fish Viruses and Fish Viral Diseases. Cornell University Press, Ithaca, New York.

Wolf, K., and Mann, J.A. (1980) Poikilotherm vertebrate cell lines and viruses: a current listing for fishes. In Vitro 16:168–179.

Wolf, K., and Pettijohn, L.L. (1970) Infectious pancreatic necrosis virus isolated from coho salmon fingerlings. Progressive Fish Culturist 32:17–18.

Wolf, K., and Quimby, M.C. (1969) Infectious pancreatic necrosis: Clinical and immune response of adult trouts to inoculation with live virus. J. Fish. Res. Bd. Can. 26:2511–2516.

Wolf, K., and Quimby, M.C. (1971) Salmonid viruses: infectious pancreatic necrosis virus. Morphology, pathology, and serology of first European isolations. Arch. Ges. Virusforsch. 34:144–156.

Wolf, K., and Quimby, M.C. (1973) Fish viruses: buffers and methods for plaquing eight agents under normal atmosphere. Appl. Microbiol. 25:659–664.

Wolf, K., and Smith, C.E. (1981) *Herpesvirus salmonis*: pathological changes in parenterally-infected rainbow trout, *Salmo gairdneri* Richardson, fry. J. Fish Dis. 4:445–457.

Wolf, K., Snieszko, S.F., Dunbar, C.E., and Pyle, E. (1960) Virus nature of infectious pancreatic necrosis in trout. Proc. Soc. Exp. Biol. Med. 104:105–108.

Wolf, K., Quimby, M.C., and Bradford, A.D. (1963) Egg-associated transmission of IPN virus of trouts. Virology 21:317–321.

Wolf, K., Quimby, M.C., Carlson, C.P., and Bullock, G.L. (1968) Infectious pancreatic necrosis: Selection of virus-free stock from a population of carrier trout. J. Fish. Res. Bd. Can. 25:383–391.

Wolf, K., Sano, T., and Kimura, T. (1975) Herpesvirus disease of salmonids. U.S. Fish Wildlife Service Fish Disease Leaflet 44.

Wolf, K., Darlington, R.W., Taylor, W.G., Quimby, M.C., and Nagabayashi, T. (1978) *Herpesvirus salmonis*: Characterization of a new pathogen of rainbow trout. J. Virol. 27:659–666.

Wolski, S.C., Roberson B.S., and Hetrick, F.M. (1986) Monoclonal antibodies to the Sp strain of infectious pancreatic necrosis virus. Vet. Immunol. Immunopathol. 12:373–381.

Wood, E.M., Snieszko, S.F., and Yasutake, W.T. (1955) Infectious pancreatic necrosis in brook trout. A.M.A. Arch. Pathol. 60:26–28.

Yamamoto, T. (1974) Infectious pancreatic necrosis virus occurrence at a hatchery in Alberta. J. Fish. Res. Bd. Can. 31:397–402.

Yamamoto, T. (1975a) Frequency of detection and survival of infectious pancreatic necrosis virus in a carrier population of brook trout (*Salvelinus fontinalis*) in a lake. J. Fish. Res. Bd. Can. 32:568–570.

Yamamoto, T. (1975b) Infectious pancreatic necrosis (IPN) virus carriers and antibody production in a population of rainbow trout (*Salmo gairdneri*). Can. J. Microbiol. 21:1343–1347.

Yamamoto, T. (1975c) Infectious pancreatic necrosis virus and bacterial kidney disease appearing concurrently in populations of *Salmo gairdneri* and *Salvelinus fontinalis*. J. Fish. Res. Bd. Can. 32:92–95.

Yamamoto, T., and Kilistoff, J. (1979) Infectious pancreatic necrosis virus: quantification of carriers in lake populations during a six year period. J. Fish. Res. Bd. Can. 36:562–567.

Yamamoto, T., Arakawa, C.K., Batts, W.N., and Winton, J.R. (1989) Comparison of infectious hematopoietic necrosis in natural and experimental infections of spawning salmonids by infectivity and immunohistochemistry. In: Viruses of Lower Vertebrates. (Ahne, W., and Kurstak, E., eds.) Springer-Verlag, New York, pp. 411–429.

Yasutake, W.T. (1970) Comparative histopathology of epizootic salmonid virus diseases. In: A Symposium on Diseases of Fishes and Shellfishes (Snieszko, S.F., ed.). American Fisheries Society Special Publication No. 5, pp. 341–350.

Yasutake, W.T. (1978) Histopathology of yearling sockeye salmon (*Oncorhynchus nerka*) infected with infectious hematopoietic necrosis (IHN). Fish Pathol. 14:59–64.

Yasutake, W.T., and Amend, D.F. (1972) Some aspects of pathogenesis of infectious hematopoietic necrosis (IHN). J. Fish Biol. 4:261–264.

Yasutake, W.T., and Rasmussen, C.J. (1968) Histopathogenesis of experimentally induced viral hemorrhagic septicemia in fingerling rainbow trout (*Salmo gairdneri*). Bull. Off. Int. Epizoot. 69:977–984.

Yasutake, W.T., Parisot, T.J., and Klontz, G.W. (1965) Virus diseases of the Salmonidae in the western United States. II. Aspects of pathogenesis. Ann. N.Y. Acad. Sci. 126:520–530.

Yoshimizu, M., Sami, M., and Kimura, T. (1988a) Survival and inactivation of infectious hematopoietic necrosis virus (IHNV) in fertilized eggs of masu salmon *Oncorhynchus masou* and chum salmon *O. keta*. Nippon Suisan Gakkaishi 54:2089–2097.

Yoshimizu, M., Tanaka, M., and Kimura, T. (1988b) Histopathological study of tumors induced by *Oncorhynchus masou* virus (OMV) infection. Fish Pathol. 23:133–138.

Yoshimizu, M., Sami, M., and Kimura, T. (1989) Survivability of infectious hematopoietic necrosis virus in fertilized eggs of masu and chum salmon. J. Aquatic Anim. Health 1:13–20.

Yu, K-Y., MacDonald, R.D., and Moore, A.R. (1982) Replication of infectious pancreatic necrosis virus in trout leucocytes and detection of the carrier state. J. Fish Dis. 5:401–410.

Yulin, J., and Zhengqiu, L. (1987) Isolation of IPN virus from imported rainbow trout (*Salmo gairdneri*) in the P. R. China. J. Appl. Ichthyol. 3:191–192.

Yun, S., Hedrick, R.P., and Wingfield, W.H. (1989) A picorna-like virus from salmonid fishes in California. Am. Fish. Soc. Fish Health Sect. Newsletter 17:5.

Zwillenberg, L.O., Pfitzner, I., and Zwillenberg, H.H.L. (1968) Infektionsversuche mit Egtved-virus an zellkulturen und individuen der schleie (*Tinca vulgaris* Cuv.) sowie an anderen fischarten. Zentralbl. Bakteriol. Parasitenk. D. Infektionskr. Hyg. Abt. I. Orig. 208:218–226.

Chapter 39

PARASITES OF SALMONID FISHES

RICHARD A. HECKMANN

Parasites of salmonid fishes include both protozoan and metazoan forms, represented by those rarely observed in surveys (Heckmann, 1971) to those you would find in most fishes (Hoffman, 1970). These parasites can be lethal and dangerous to the host (*Myxobolus cerebralis*, *Ceratomyxa shasta*, and *Sanguinicola klamathensis*), or organisms that usually cause little damage, (*Trichophrya clarki* and *Posthodiplostomum minimum*). Salmonid fishes are intermediate hosts for helminths (*Diphyllobothrium latum*) detrimental to the definitive host, and that also serve as vectors for infectious diseases. Parasites infecting various salmonid species are presented in Tables 39–1 to 39–6.

Many studies conducted on parasites of salmonids are surveys of parasites for a particular fish species at different localities. There are many excellent books and monographs that list all parasites for a given host as well as recent articles and reviews (Hoffman, 1970; Heckmann, 1971; Heckmann and

TABLE 39–1. Parasites of Rainbow Trout

Protozoa
Ceratomyxa sp.
Chilodonella cyprini
Chloromyxum majori
C. truttae
Costia necatrix
C. pyriformis
Cryptobia borreli
C. lynchi
Cyclochaeta sp.
Hexamita salmonis
Ichthyophthirius multifiliis
Myxidium oviforme
M. minteri
Myxobolus (Myosoma)
  cerebralis
M. squamalis
Plistophora salmonae
Schizamoeba salmonis
Trichodina fultoni
Trichophyra piscium

Trematoda
Allocredium lobatum
Aponurus sp.
Bolbophorus confusus
Clinostomum marginatum
Crepidostomum cooperi
C. farionis
C. laureatum
Deropegus aspina
Diplostomum flexicaudum
D. spathaceum
Diplostomulum sp.
Discocotyle salmonis
Distomulum oregonesis
Echinochasmus milvi
Exocoitocaecum wisnienskii
Gyrodactylus elegans
Nanophyetus salmincola
Neascus sp.
Phyllodistomum sp., including
  P. lachancei
Plagioporus angusticole
Podocotyle shawi
Sanguinicola sp.
Proteocephalus sp., including
  P. ambloplitis, P. longicollis,
  P. pinguis, P. salmonidicola,
  P. tumidocollis
Schistocephalus sp.
Triaenophorus nodulous

Cestoda
Abothrium crassum
Cyathocephalus trunc
Diphyllobothrium sp.
Eubothrium salvelini
Ligula intestinalis
Phyllobothrium sp.

Hirudinea (Leeches)
Illinobdella sp.
Piscicola geometra
P. salmositica

Mollusca
Glochidia of Margaritana
  margaritifera
Pisidium sp., including P.
  variable

Gordiacea
Chorodes sp.

Crustacea
Argulus pugettensis
Ergasilus caeruleus
E. sieboldi
Lernaea cyprinacea
L. esocina
Lernaeopoda bicauliculata
Salmincola beani
S. edwardsii

Nematoda
Anisakis sp.
Ascaris acus
Ascarophis hardwood
A. skrjabini
Bulbodacnitis globo
B. occidentalis
Capillaria eupomoti
Contracaecum spiculigerum
Cucullanus globosu
C. occidentalis
C. truttae
Cystidicola farionis
C. stigmatura
Cystidicoloides harwoodi
Dacnitis truttae
Eustronglylides sp.
Goezia ascaroides
Hepaticola bakeri
Metabronema salv.
Philometra sp.
Philonema agubernaculum
P. angusticole
P. oncorhynchi
Raphidascaris acus
Rhabdochona cascadilla
R. denudata
Spinitectus gracilis
Sterliadochona tenuissima

Acanthocephala
Acanthocephalus acerbus
A. anguillae
A. jacksoni
Echinorhynchus leidyi
E. salmonis
E. truttae
Metechninorhynchus salmonis
M. truttae
Neoechinorhynchus rutili
Pomphorhynchus bulbocolli
Rhadinorhynchus sp.
Tetrahynchus sp.

Adapted from Hoffman, G.L. (1967) Parasites of North American Freshwater Fishes. University of California Press, Berkeley and Los Angeles.

Ching, 1987; Linton, 1891a; 1891b; Bangham, 1951; Scott, 1932; 1935; Cope, 1958; Heckmann and Carroll, 1985; Bailey and Margolis, 1987; Yasutake et al., 1986; Whitaker, 1985; Cone and Ryan, 1984; Li and Desser, 1985; Wier et al., 1983; Leong and Holmes, 1981;

Wootten and Smith, 1980; Margolis and Boyce, 1990; Conneely and McCarthy, 1988; Esch et al., 1988; Nagasawa et al., 1987; Mariaux, 1986; Kennedy et al., 1986; Muzzall and Peebles, 1986; Moravec et al., 1985; Vahida, 1984; McGuigan and Sommerville, 1985; Singhal et al., 1984; Muzzall, 1984; Bier et al., 1982; Rahim, 1981; Jennings and Hendrickson, 1982; Boustead, 1981; Pugachev, 1980).

Owing to their commercial importance, the salmonid fishes have received more parasite research than most other groups. Each year more and more parasitic species are described. Nevertheless, there are many parasites yet to be described for salmonid fishes in North America.

TABLE 39–2. Parasites of Brook Trout

Protozoa
Chloromyxum leydei
C. truttae
Costia pyriformis
Dactylosoma salvelini
Eimeria sp.
Epistylis sp.
Haemogregarina sp.
Henneguya fontinalis
Hexamita salmonis
Ichthyopthirius multifiliis
Leucocytozoon salvelini
Myxidium minteri
Myxobolus ovoidalis
Myxosoma cerebralis
Schizamoeba salmonis
Trichodina myakkae
Trichodina sp.
Trichophrya sp.
Trypanosoma percae canadensis
Zschokkella salvelini

Trematoda
Allocreadium lobatum
Apophallus brevis
A. imperator
Azygia angusticauda
Bolbophorus confusus
Clinostomum marginatum
Crepidostomum cooperi
Crepidostomom sp.
C14v farionis
C. fausti
C. transmarinum
Diplostomulum sp.
Iscocotyle salmonis
Gyrodactylus elegans B.
G. medius
Nanophyetus salmincola
Neascus sp.
Phyllodistomum sp., including
  P. lachancei, P. superbum
Pleurogenes sp.
Posthodiplostomum minimum
Ptychogonimus fontanus

Cestoda
Abothrium crassum
Cyathocephalus truncatus
Diphyllobothrium cordiceps
D. sebago

Diphyllobothrium sp.
Diplocotyle olrikii
Eubothrium salvelini
Ligula intestinalis
Proteocephalus sp., including
  P. arcticus, P. parallacticus,
  P. pinguis, P. Pinguis, P.
  pusillus, P. tumidicollis
Schistocephalus solidus

Nematoda
Bulbodacnitis globosa
B. scotti
Contracaecum sp., including
  C. spiculigerum
Cystidicola stigmatura
Cystidicoloides harwoodi
Hepaticola bakeri
Metabronema canadense
M. salvelini
Philonema agubernaculum
Raphidascaris laurentianus
Rhabdochona cascadilla
Rhabdochona sp., including R.
  laurentiana

Acanthocephala
Acanthocephalus anguillae
A. jacksoni
Echinorhynchus lateralis
Leptorhynchoides thecatus
L. thecatus
Neoechinorhynchus sp.,
  including N. cylindratus, N.
  rutili

Hirudinea (Leeches)
Haemopis grandis (accidental)
Macrobdella decora (accidental)
Piscicola punctata

Mollusca
Glochidia

Crustacea
Argulus canadensis
A. stizostethi
Lepeophtheirus salmonis
Salmincola edwardsii
S. salvelini

Gordiacea
Chorodes sp.

Adapted from Hoffman, G.L. (1967) Parasites of North American Freshwater Fishes. University of California Press, Berkeley and Los Angeles.

TABLE 39–3. Parasites of Cutthroat Trout in North America

Protozoa	**Digenea (Flukes)**
Costia necatrix	*Allocreadium lobatum*
C. pyriformes	*Apophallus* sp.
Haemogregarina sp.	*Clinostomum marginatum,*
Ichthyophthirius multifiliis	*C. marginatum*
Myxidium sp.	*Crepidostomum* sp., including
Myxosporidan sp.	*C. farionis, C. transmarinum*
Myxosoma sp.	*Deropegus aspina*
Octomitus sp.	*Diplostomum oregonaceum* (L)
Trichodina truttae	*D. baeri buccelentum* (L)
Trichophyra clarki	*Gyrodactylus elegans* B.
	Nanophyetus salmincola
Cestoda (Tapeworms)	*Plagioporus siliculus*
Cyathocephalus sp., including	*Podocotyle* sp.
C. truncatus	*Posthodiplostomum minimum*
Diphyllobothrium sp. (L),	(L)
including *D. cordiceps* (L),	*Sanguinicola* sp.
D. ditremum (L), *D.*	
dendriticum (L)	**Nematoda (Roundworms)**
Eubothrium salvelini	*Ascarophis globosa*
Proteocephalus sp., including	*Bulbodacnitis globosa*
P. arcticus, P. laruei, P.	*B. scotti*
primaverus, P. salmonidicola	*Capillaria* sp., including *C.*
	catenata
Acanthocephala (Spiny-	*Contracaecum* sp.
headed worms)	*Cucullanus truttae*
Echinorhynchus lateralis	*Cystidicoloides* sp., including
Neoechinorhynchus sp.,	*C. stigmatura*
including	*Eustrongylides* sp. (L)
Neoechinorhynchus rutili	*Hepaticola bakeri*
	Metabronema salvelini
Hirudinea (Leeches)	*Philometra* sp., including *P.*
Illinobdella sp.	*oncorhynchi*
Piscicola salmositica	*Rhabdochona* sp., including *R.*
	cascadilla
Crustacea (Copepods)	
Lepeophtheirus salmonis	**Mollusca (Bivalves)**
Lernaeopoda bicauliculata	Glochidia (L)
Salmincola sp., including *S.*	
edwardsii	

(L) indicates larval state.

Based on Hoffman, G.L. (1967) *Parasites of North American Freshwater Fishes.* University of California Press, Berkeley and Los Angeles.

PARASITES AS TAGS

One unique use of parasites of salmonids is as an indicator (tags) of fish migrations and origins. By understanding the biology of host-specific parasites, it is feasible to trace movements and origins of fishes, especially the anadromous salmonids. Recent studies pertaining to parasite tags include movement of sockeye salmon fry in Russian waters (Butorina and Shed'ko, 1989), use of biologic markers for mixed populations of sockeye salmon in Canada and Alaska (Wood et al., 1989), studies of salmonid biology in Japan (Urawa, 1989), and biologic tags and homing of salmon (Quinn et al., 1987).

PROTOZOA

Protozoa may cause more disease in commercial salmonid fish culture than any other type of animal parasite. When a fish is stressed, large populations of ectoparasitic protozoa may appear on its body and gills. When present in small numbers, protozoa usu-

ally produce no obvious damage except slowing fish growth, but in large numbers, they greatly impair the organs and surface structures of the fish, particularly the gills. Salmonids are infected with a great variety of protozoa, many of which have not been described or studied.

Examples of the location of protozoan parasites in the salmonid body are given in Table 39–7.

Whirling Disease

SYNONYMS. Blacktail, *Myxobolus cerebralis, Myxosoma cerebralis.*

TABLE 39–4. Parasites of Atlantic Salmon

Protozoa	*Schistocephalus dimorphis*
Chloromyxum histolyticum	*Scolex pleuronectic*
Henneguya salmonis	*S. polymorphus*
Hexamita truttae	*Stenobothrium appendiculum*
Myxicium oviforme	*Tetrabothrum minimum*
Myxosoma cerebralis	*Tetrahynchobothrium bicolor*
Trichophyra intermedia	*Tetrahynchus grossus*
	T. solidus
Trematoda	*Triaenophorus crassus*
Aphanurus balticus	*T. nodulous*
Azygia lucii	
A. tereticollis	**Nematoda**
Brachyphallus crenatus	*Agomonema capsularia*
Bucephalus polymorphus	*A. commune*
Bunocotyle cingulata	*Anisakis* sp.
Crepidostomum farionis	*Camallanus lacustris*
C. metoecus	*Contracaecum aduncum*
Derogenes varicus	*Cucullanus elegans*
Diplostomulum spathaceum	*C. serratus*
Discocotyle sagitta	*C. truttae*
D. salmonis	*Exocoitocaecum wisniewskii*
D. sybillae	*Raphidascaris acus*
Distomum appendiculatum	
D. reflexum	**Acanthocephala**
D. varicum	*Acanthocephalus anguillae*
Gyrodactyloides bychowskii	*A. lucii*
Gyrodactylus sp., including	*Bolbosoma heteracanthis*
Gyrodactylus salaris	*Echinorhynchus acus*
Hemiurus crenatus	*E. gadi*
H. levinseni	*E. inflatus*
H. lukei	*E. salmonis*
H. ocreatus	*E. truttae*
Lampritrema miescheri	*Metechinorhynchus salmonis*
(Distomum)	*Neoechinorhynchus cylindratum*
Lecithaster bothryophorus	*N. rutili*
L. confusus	*Pomphorhynchus laeve*
L. gibbus	*P. proteus*
Nanophyetus salmincola	*Pseudoechinorhynchus clavula*
Neohemiurus	
Podocotyle automon	**Crustacea**
P. simplex	*Argulus* sp.
	Lepeophtheirus pollachii
Cestoda	*L. salmonis*
Bothriocephalus osmeri	*L. stromii*
B. proboscideus	*Salmincola falculata*
B. (Schistocephalus) solidus	*S. salmonae*
Diphyllobothrium cordiceps	
D. latum	**Hirudinea (Leeches)**
D. norvegicum	*Cystobranchus (Pisicola)*
Hepatoxylon trichiuri	*respirans*
Leuckartia sp.	*Piscicola geometra*

Adapted from Hoffman, G.L. (1967) *Parasites of North American Freshwater Fishes.* University of California Press, Berkeley and Los Angeles.

TABLE 39–5. Parasites of Sockeye Salmon

Protozoa
Chloromyxum wardi
Henneguya zschokkei
Myxidium oviforme
Myxobolus neurobius
Trichophyra piscium
Trematoda
Brachyphallus crenatus
Crepidostomum farionis
Derogenes varicus
Lampritrema nipponicum
Lecithaster gibbous, L. salmonis
Podocotyle shawi
Syncoelium filiferum
Cestoda
Cyathocephalus tuncatus
Diphyllobothrium sp., including *D. ursi*
Eubothrium sp., including *E. crassum, E. salvelini*
Pelichnibothrium speciosum
Phyllobothrium sp.

Proteocephalus sp., including *P. arcticus*
Scolex pleuronectis
Triaenophorus crassus
Nematoda
Contracaecum aduncum, C. spiculigerum
Dacnitis truttae
Metabronema salvelini
Philonema oncorhynchi
Rhabdochona cascadilla
Acanthocephala
Acanthocephalus aculeatus
Bolbosoma caenoforme
Echinorhynchus gadi
Neoechinorhynchus rutili
Mollusca
Glochidia (*Anodonta*, Alaska)
Crustacea
Ergasilus auritus, E. nerkae, E. turgidus
Lernaeopoda falculata
Salmincola sp., including *S. californiensis, S. carpenteri, S. falculata*

Adapted from Hoffman, G.L. (1967) Parasites of North American Freshwater Fishes. University of California Press, Berkeley and Los Angeles.

TABLE 39–6. Parasites of Artic Grayling

Protozoa
Chloromyxum thymalli
Myxidium ventricosum
Trematoda
Ariella baikalensis
Crepidostomum sp., including *C. farionis*
Diplostomum spathaceum
Phyllodistomum conostomum
Tetracotyle intermedia
Tetraonchus alaskensis, T. borealis, T. rauschi
Cestoda
Cyathocephalus truncatus
Diphyllobothrium minus, D. strictum
Eubothrium salvelini
Proteocephalus longicollis, P. thymalli
Triaenophorus nodulous

Nematoda
Ascarophis skrjabini
Coregonema sibirica
Cucullanus truttae
Cystidicola farionis
Rhabdochona denudata
Acanthocephala
Acanthocephalus anguillae
Neoechinorhynchus rutili
Pseudoechinorhynchus clavula
Hirudinea (Leeches)
Acanthobdella peledina
Piscicola geometra
Crustacea
Salmincola baicalensis, S. carpionis

Adapted from Hoffman, G.L. (1967) Parasites of North American Freshwater Fishes. University of California Press, Berkeley and Los Angeles.

TABLE 39–7. Body Location of Protozoan Parasites (Microscopic) in Salmonid Fishes*

Gills	Blood	Intestine	Muscle	Cartilage and Bone (Histozoic)	Surface (Fins, etc.)	Kidney
Apiosoma (C) *Ichthyophthirius* (C)	*Cryptobia* (F)	*Ceratomyxa* (M)	*Henneguya* (M)	*Myxobolus* (M)	*Trichodina* (C)	Proliferative kidney disease
Ichthyobodo (F)	*Haemogregarina* (S)	*Eimeria* (S)	*Plistophora* (Mc)	*Henneguya* (M)	*Apiosoma* (F)	
Plistophora (Mc) *Schizamoeba* (A) (*Paramoeba*) *Trichodina* (C) *Trichophyra* (C)		*Hexamita* (F) *Plistophora* (Mc)			*Ichthyobodo* (F)	

This list is representative of examples and is not all inclusive.
Abbreviations: A, ameba—sarcodina; C, ciliate; F, flagellate; M, mybosporean; Mc, microsporean; S, sporozoan.

Host and Geographic Distribution

Whirling disease is one of the histozoic parasitic diseases that has been included as a notifiable or a major disease for fish health inspectors. It was first reported in Europe about 1904 and probably arrived in Pennsylvania during 1956 via frozen, processed fish. From Pennsylvania, the disease has moved across the United States, but it has not been reported in all states with salmonid populations. The original natural range of *Myxobolus (Myrosoma) cerebralis* may never be known with certainty. It has been reported in 18 countries, including Italy, USSR, Scotland, New Zealand, England, and Lebanon. It is probably in all countries with imported live or frozen salmonids or salmonid products.

All species of trout, salmon, and grayling are susceptible to whirling disease. Although *Myxobolus cerebralis* has been reported in several nonsalmonid species, there is reason to question the accuracy of those reports.

Clinical Signs and Diagnosis

The characteristic sign of the disease, from which the disease gets its name, is a frenzied, tail-chasing behavior when affected fish are frightened or trying to feed. This is due to cartilage damage in the tail region, resulting in a discurvature of the spine. In surviving fish, skeletal deformities such as blunt nose and misshapen head, jaws, and opercula occur in addition to spinal curvature. Blacktail is due to an early invasion of fingerling fish that destroys control of chromatophores on the caudal peduncle.

Cases of whirling disease or blacktail disease range from subclinical infections to acute disease with mortalities of fry and fingerlings. Some acutely infected fish may show no signs but become carriers and often suffer high mortalities. Fish with light infections show none of these symptoms, but will carry spores throughout their life.

Definitive diagnosis is based on the presence of spores in histologic sections of cartilaginous tissue from the head, gill arches, or vertebral column. Spores are ovoidal to ellipsoidal, with a piriform-shaped polar capsule at the anterior end. The sporoplasm has an iodinophilous vacuole.

Life Cycle, Transmission, and Epidemiology

Infected fishes are most commonly found in facilities with earthen ponds or raceways. Mud has been considered a requisite to condition the spores before being able to infect a host. It has been estimated that 6 months in mud are required to condition the spores. Open-water sources are also ideal for infection with *Myxobolus cerebralis*. The disease is found in native fish from streams with low stream gradients where alkalinity is typical. Water temperature is also an important factor for susceptibility.

The life cycle involves a parasitic phase and a free-living phase. A tubificid worm (*Tubifex* sp.) has recently been described as an intermediate host (Hoffmann and El-Matbouli, 1988) in the life history

of the parasite. The life cycle can be direct from fish to fish. After ingestion, the sporoplasm leaves the spore, presumably penetrates the intestine, and migrates to suitable host tissue (bone and cartilage). The sporoplasm grows into a trophozoite, the nuclei divide, and the structure produces many spores in a single cyst. Infected fish may show signs of the disease 28 weeks after exposure (Hoffman, 1976). Spore formation in infected fish takes 52 days at 17°C, 3 months at 12°C, and 4 months at 7°C (Halliday, 1973).

It has been proposed that spores are released from dead and decaying fish or shed by living fish. Shipments of fish need to be inspected for the presence of spores before being released into the environment or to the public. Freshly shed spores are not immediately infective and must spend months in mud before they develop infectivity (Hoffman and Putz, 1969).

Treatment and Control

The disease affects young fishes and has a potentially devastating effect on hatchery production. Treatment has ranged from eradication attempts with depopulation of facilities, including abandonment and burial of facility sites, to attempts to manage the pathogen. Hundreds of tons of fish have been destroyed and millions of dollars spent in attempts to eradicate the pathogen with virtually no success. These efforts have shown that enclosing open spring sources and concreting fish-rearing facilities offer protection against whirling disease. The environmentally resistant, long-lived spores make the disease virtually impossible to eradicate in the wild once it is established. Chemicals used in attempts to control whirling disease have included HTH and hydrated lime. Ultraviolet light may offer a means of treatment, although success has been variable. No effective therapy is known.

In enzootic areas, all salmonid facilities using earthen ponds or surface water should be monitored regularly for *Myxobolus cerebralis*, and at facilities where the disease exists, it can be reduced by holding fry in water known to be free of spores. Earthen ponds should be cleaned and treated or converted to concrete raceways, and contaminated stream and lake water should be filtered and/or treated with ultraviolet irradiation. Infected stock should be used carefully and only where the parasite already exists. Hot smoking of fish kills the spore. In some cases, less susceptible salmonids such as brown trout, lake trout, or coho salmon could replace rainbow trout as the cultured fish.

Ceratomysosis

SYNONYMS. Prespawn disease, salmon dropsy.

Host and Geographic Distribution

The disease was first observed in 1948 in rainbow trout spawning in the fall at Crystal Lake Hatchery,

Shasta County, California (Wales and Wolf, 1955). The etiologic agent, *Ceratomyxa shasta*, was established as a new species, the only member of the genus to parasitize freshwater fishes and the only member that is histozoic. Infected fish have been found along the northwest coast, especially from the Columbia River basin of North America in Oregon, California, Washington, British Columbia, and Idaho. The disease has been transmitted to other susceptible fish, only in certain river systems in Oregon, Washington, and California (Johnson et al., 1979). *Ceratomyxa shasta* is an important parasite in the Pacific Northwest of the United States because it not only causes losses in hatchery-reared and wild juvenile salmonids but also contributes significantly to prespawning mortality in adult salmon. It is accepted that only salmonids are susceptible to *Ceratomyxa shasta* infection. Marine fishes are known hosts for other species of *Ceratomyxa* that are found in the gallbladder and urinary bladder.

Clinical Signs and Diagnosis

Clinical signs of ceratomyxosis vary among salmonid species. Infected juvenile rainbow trout (and steelhead) become anorexic, lethargic, and darken. Ascites may distend the abdomen, the vent may be swollen and hemorrhagic, and exophthalmia is common (Schafer, 1968). Infected juvenile chinook salmon first become emaciated and may later develop large fluid-filled vesicles and renal pustules (Conrad and Decew, 1966). Other signs include nodules in the gut of adult chinook salmon and large abscesses in the musculature, liver, and spleen. The diagnosis is confirmed by the microscopic demonstration of typical spores in scrapings from the lower intestinal lumen, gallbladder, or lesions.

Internally, the intestinal tract of juvenile rainbow trout becomes swollen and hemorrhagic with a caseous pseudomembrane and mucoid intestinal contents (Conrad and Decew, 1966). The entire digestive tract, liver, gallbladder, spleen, gonads, kidney, heart, gills, and skeletal muscle may be affected (Wales and Wolf, 1955). Infected adult coho salmon show grossly thickened intestinal walls and pyloric ceca and large abscessed lesions in the body musculature (Wood, 1989).

Serologic techniques have been developed using monoclonal antibodies that react specifically with the prespore stages of the parasite, and do not cross-react with trophozoite or spore stages of other myxosporeans. Use of the monoclonal antibodies and fluorescein or enzyme conjugated secondary antibodies enables the reliable detection of early infections (Bartholomew, et al., 1989).

Spores of *Ceratomyxa shasta* are about 14 to 23 μm long and 6 to 8 μm wide at the suture line. The ends of the spores are rounded and reflected posteriorly, and the suture line is distinct. Polar capsules stained using the Ziehl-Nielsen method are red against a bluish sporoplasm. Spores can be used for a definitive diagnosis of the disease.

Trophozoites, which are rounded but variable in shape, mature to form a sporoblast that usually contains two spores. Because of the variability in size and shape of the trophozoites and their similarity to this stage in other myxosporeans, observation of trophozoites by light microscopy is not sufficient for diagnosis. Electron microscopy is an excellent method for verifying species of myxosporeans.

Pathology and Pathogenesis

Ceratomyxa shasta is capable of causing serious injury to the host and has an affinity for the intestinal tissue. It can cause high mortalities in certain strains of salmonids (Bartholomew et al., 1989). The spores can be found in other soft tissues of the host. Infected adult chinook salmon may have nodular lesions in the intestine that perforate, causing peritonitis and death.

In juvenile rainbow trout, the first sign of infection appears in the posterior intestine. The progress of the infection is temperature dependent, the first sign of infection appearing between days 12 and 18 after exposure in fish held at 12°C, and at 7 days in fish held at 18°C (Yamamoto and Sanders, 1979).

Trophozoites are first seen in the mucosa, and their appearance is followed by a strong inflammatory response in the connective tissue of the intestine. As the infection progresses, the parasite multiplies in all layers of the intestine and causes severe inflammation and desquamation of the mucosal epithelium. Trophozoites penetrate the intestinal tract, spread into the surrounding adipose and pancreatic tissues, and enter the bloodstream, which carries them to other tissues and organs. In late stages of infection, the parasite is most heavily concentrated in tissues and organs adjacent to the intestine, including the liver, kidney, pyloric ceca, and spleen. Diagnosis of the disease is sometimes delayed because the spore stage of *Ceratomyxa shasta* is not evident until the terminal stages of the infection.

Life Cycle, Transmission, and Epidemiology

Published data suggest that the parasite cannot establish itself outside of the water that contains the infective stage, and it is assumed that the parasite cannot be spread through transfer of infected fish or eggs. The life cycle of *Ceratomyxa shasta*, like many of the myxosporeans, is unknown. Natural transmission occurs when susceptible salmonids are exposed to water or sediments containing the infective stage (Schafer, 1968; Fryer and Sanders, 1970; Johnson, 1980). Neither attempts to transmit ceratomyxosis from fish to fish nor the feeding of infected tissues containing spores and trophozoites has resulted in transmission of the disease (Wales and Wolf, 1955; Schafer, 1968; Johnson, 1980). Infections have developed when susceptible fish are exposed to bottom sediments collected from a site endemic for the parasite (Fryer and Sanders, 1970).

Laboratory transmission of ceratomyxosis has been established by intraperitoneal injection and anal intubation of ascites from infected fish (Schafer, 1968;

Fryer and Sanders, 1970; Johnson et al., 1979; Bower, 1985). Establishment of infection in rainbow trout may not be dependent on ingestion of the spore (Schafer, 1968). Differential filtration of water endemic for *Ceratomyxa shasta* shows that the infective stage is larger than 14 μm.

The inability to transmit ceratomyxosis between susceptible fish has led to speculation that an intermediate host may be involved in the life cycle, somewhat similar to data recently published on the life history of *Myxobolus cerebralis*.

Natural transmission occurs only when susceptible salmonids come in contact with water containing the infective stage. A 30-minute or longer exposure to such water is necessary to initiate the disease. Fish-to-fish infection does not occur.

The incubation period, defined as the length of time from infection to death, varies with fish species and water temperature. The infection will develop only at water temperatures above 3.9°C. Deaths occur in coho salmon within 12.5 days at 23.3°C, but losses do not occur until 146 days after exposure at 9.4°C. Deaths in rainbow trout occur in 14 days at 23.3°C and 15 days at 6.7°C or colder.

Juvenile salmonids originating from waters containing the infective stage of the parasite were more resistant than strains from areas free of the infective stage (Zinn et al., 1977; Buchanan et al., 1983; Hoffmaster, 1985). The susceptibility to infection in progeny produced from crosses between resistant and susceptible coho salmon is intermediate between that of the parental stocks (Hemmingsen et al., 1986). The management implications of these studies are that relocation of salmonids from areas where *Ceratomyxa shasta* is not endemic into areas endemic for the parasite is not likely to be successful, and that these introductions may adversely affect the survival of resident resistant fish strains if interbreeding occurs.

Although juvenile salmonids from waters endemic for *Ceratomyxa shasta* are resistant to infection, ceratomyxosis remains an important cause of prespawning mortality in adults. Incidences as high as 94% have been reported (Coley et al., 1983; Sanders et al., 1970; Yasutake et al., 1986; Chapman, 1986).

There is a paucity of information available about the effects of salt water on the progress of ceratomyxosis. Although infection occurs during the freshwater phase of the fish's life cycle, it is not known whether anadromous fish are infected before they enter salt water or after they reenter fresh water. It has been reported that infections can be prevented at salt concentrations greater than 15 ppt, but while this would protect juvenile salmonids from infection in estuarine areas, the fate of fish that were infected in fresh water and then migrated into salt water has not been determined.

Experiments exposing chinook salmon to the infective stage of *Ceratomyxa shasta* found that the disease caused 100% mortality when the fish were held in either fresh water or salt water (Ching and Munday, 1984b). Similarly designed experiments with steelhead trout indicate that migration to salt water may reduce the progress of the disease, but the extent of attenuation may be masked in fish carrying high numbers of parasites (Hoffmaster et al., 1985).

Infection by *Ceratomyxa shasta* was once believed to occur only when water temperatures exceeded 10°C, accounting for the seasonal occurrence of the disease; however, later studies indicate that fish can become infected in water at temperatures as low as 4 to 6°C (Ratliff, 1983; Ching and Munday, 1984a). Although fish are infected at these lower temperatures, the progress of the disease is temperature dependent and most infections are detected later after the water warms.

Treatment and Control

The disease may be prevented in areas where it is endemic by avoiding the use of infected water supplies or by treatment of infected water with a combination of filtration followed by chlorine or ultraviolet irradiation (Sanders et al., 1972). Resistant fish stocks should be used to reduce the incidence of the disease by reducing the number of infective parasites being shed into the water (Zinn et al., 1977).

The disease can be prevented from reaching geographic regions where it does not currently occur by not transferring fish or water into these areas from locations where the disease occurs. Fish or eggs from enzootic areas should not be imported unless the fish have been inspected and certified to be free of *Ceratomyxa shasta*. There is no known effective treatment for eliminating the disease.

Ich

SYNONYM. White spot disease.

Host and Geographic Distribution

Ichthyophthirius multifiliis commonly is found on cultured salmonids and has been reported on native North American salmonids. Ich is not as dangerous in trout and salmon as it is to commercial catfishes and freshwater tropical fishes. Often the occurrence of ich in salmonids can be traced to contact with other species of fishes in the same aquatic environment. This disease organism is covered in much more detail in the chapters on parasites of catfishes (Chap. 60) and freshwater tropical fishes (Chap. 70).

Salmonids hosting *Ichthyophthirius multifiliis* will exhibit abnormal behavior such as scraping their body against the bottom or sides of the raceway or against submerged permanent objects. Fish should be isolated and tanks cleaned before the life cycle of the pathogen can be established in the immediate aquatic environment.

Trichodiniasis

To date, 90 species of *Trichodina* have been described from the gills and skin of marine and freshwater fishes in North America. Many of them have been considered as new, only because they were found in a different host or a remote geographic area. Because of this taxonomic confusion, studies of trichodinid evolution and host specificity have been often inconclusive, with several authors being unable to demonstrate any clear pattern of host preference by the parasites. However, a line of specialization toward a more exclusive niche on the host fish can be distinguished. The opportunistic parasites with a ubiquitous or wide geographic distribution are skin parasites, whereas the more specialized parasites with a clear host specificity toward a single host are found only on the gills. The opportunistic trichodinids are large species, 90 μm or more, whereas the specific parasites are small, less than 30 μm. Translocation of cyprinid and cichlid fishes for aquaculture have successfully introduced trichodinid parasites into nonendemic areas, and the more opportunistic parasites normally associated with these fishes are now also parasitizing other species. In contrast, the more specific parasites have remained associated with their original hosts. More details about these parasites are provided in the chapters on parasites of freshwater temperate fishes (Chap. 27) and freshwater tropical fishes (Chap. 70).

Hexamitiasis

Hexamitiasis is caused by a small, pear-shaped, active, flagellated parasite in the gallbladder and intestine of rainbow trout. It moves rapidly by means of long flagella. Smears of gut contents or gallbladder, in which the flagellate will show quick movement on the glass slides under magnification, are required for a definitive diagnosis. Two species of the parasite have been described: *Hexamita intestinalis* in brown trout and *Hexamita salmonis* in young trout and salmon. The piriform parasites contain two nuclei, form cysts, and can cause enteritis. More details are provided in the chapter on parasites of freshwater tropical fishes (Chap. 70).

Ichthyobodiasis

Ichthyoboda is a small, pear-shaped, ectoparasitic protozoan flagellate common on the gills of salmonids. It propels itself by means of flagella and has a major effect on fry, masking the gill surface. *Ichthyoboda* moves across the gill surface in a jerky-type movement that is useful in differentiating the organism from gill epithelial cells. Two species have been reported: *Ichthyoboda necatrix* on the epidermis of many fishes (size 5 to 18 μm × 2.5 to 7 μm) with cysts (7 to 10 μm in diameter) and *Ichthyoboda pyri-*

formis (size 9 to 14 μm × 5 to 8 μm) on the gills and skin of rainbow and brook trout. They are not detrimental to the host unless the salmonid is stressed or weakened. More information is available in the chapters on parasites of freshwater temperate fishes (Chap. 27) and freshwater tropical fishes (Chap. 70).

Cryptobiasis

Cryptobia is a biflagellated blood parasite (trypanosomelike) of salmonids with one free flagellum and the other located on the outer margin of the undulating membrane. The suspected vector and intermediate host is a fish leech. The pathogenicity is not well understood, but *Cryptobia* has been considered a serious problem in trout hatcheries in the western United States.

The protozoan blood parasites of fishes, at least those sufficiently well known to be accepted as valid taxa, are established in five genera: *Trypanosoma, Cryptobia (Trypanoplasma), Haemogregarina, Dactylosoma,* and *Babesiosoma.* The true microenvironment of these parasites in the vertebrate host is the circulatory system, in contrast to aberrant forms such as myxosporeans that may occur in the blood. The trypanosomas and cryptobiids are flagellates living in the blood plasma, whereas the hemogregarines, dactylosomes, and babesiosomes are sporozoans existing within the circulating blood cells. Many genera of hematoza occurring in other vertebrates, particularly in warm-blooded animals, have never been reported from fishes.

BABESIOSOMA. The true microenvironment of these parasites in the vertebrate host is the circulatory system, in contrast to that of aberrant forms such as myxosporeans, which may occur in the blood. The trypanosomes and cryptobiids are flagellates living in the blood plasma, whereas the hemogregarines, dactylosomes, and babesiosomes are sporozoans existing within the circulating blood cells. Many genera of hematozoa occurring in other vertebrates, particularly in warm-blooded animals, have never been reported from fishes.

Hemogregariniasis

The protozoa of the genus *Haemogregarina* parasitize erythrocytes of turtles, snakes, crocodilians, and fishes. Development proceeds with alternation of hosts. Asexual multiplication leads to the formation of numerous large merozoites, which occur in red blood cells in organ tissues of the principal host. Gametogony leads to the formation of fewer and smaller sexual forms, which occur in peripheral circulating erythrocytes. Further development through the fusion of gametes with the formation of oocysts occurs in the intestine of rhynchobdellidan leeches that have ingested blood of infected fish. The hemogregarine microgametes lack flagella, and a vestigial body is formed directly in the oocyst without spore formation. The sporozoites leave the oocyst to penetrate through the intestinal wall of the leech and via the lacunary system migrate to the proboscis, from where, during the leech's act of feeding they penetrate into the cavity of the leech proboscis and enter the vertebrate host's blood. This developmental cycle has been studied only for turtle hemogregarines. It is expected that analogous events also occur in fish hemogregarines.

The taxonomy of fish hemogregarines in salmonids has so far remained completely unelucidated. Several species described with varying degrees of accuracy have been encountered in countries of the former Soviet Union.

Milky Flesh Disease (*Henneguya* sp.)

Henneguya species, a group of parasites found in the muscle and skin of wild salmon and sea trout, are responsible for milky flesh disease. The members of this genus are characterized by tadpole-shaped cysts with two polar capsules. All are histozoic, with the vegetative stage in the form of a polysporous cyst. Vegetative stages are characterized by large, white, oval cysts attaining a size of up to 3 by 2 cm and surrounded by a thick membrane. Spores are oval, with a rounded anterior end and a tapering posterior end, which transform into the caudal processes. Piriform polar capsules are relatively small with widely divergent proximal ends. The organism is present in gills and subcutaneous muscle and connective tissues of salmonids. Additional information about this group of parasites is found in the chapters on parasites of freshwater temperate fishes (Chap. 27) and freshwater tropical fishes (Chap. 70).

Plistophoriasis

The microsporidian parasites of the genus *Plistophora* are among the smallest parasites found in salmonid fishes. These parasites invade host cells and undergo asexual division and sporogony. The infected cells usually increase in size and become enormous with enlarged host cytoplasm and nuclei. Spores are small and the membrane is a single layer with a single polar filament. Plistophoriasis can be of major economic importance in trout farms. Symptoms of infected fish are enlarged cells, tumorlike structures, lethargic host fish, and prominent cysts.

The *Plistophora* cysts, which are found in the musculature, are long, elliptical, and oriented laterally in the host. The sporonts contain an average of 16 spores, which is characteristic of this genus. The pathogenicity can be quite severe owing to the histozoic and coelozoic nature of the parasites. The myofibrils of affected skeletal muscle tissue are broken down near the large intracellular cyst masses.

Plistophora has a complex life history. The stage most readily recognized is the large number of white cysts with spores. No treatment is available. More information on this disease is provided in the chapter on parasitic diseases of freshwater tropical fishes (Chap. 70).

Coccidiosis

Freshwater coccidians have been described from Europe, Asia, and North America (Molnar and Fernando, 1974). These parasites inhabit the epithelium of the intestines and develop through a life cycle of asexual and sexual phases. Schizogony is an asexual phase of the trophozoite that encysts in the small intestine. The cyst expels merozoites that differentiate into male and female gametes. In the sexual phase (gametogony), there is a gradual process of invasion into the lining of the intestine. The zygote is passed out in the feces and, following sporulation, is taken in by another host. Spores multiply in an asexual phase (sporogony), followed by sporulation in the intestine.

Eimeria develop spores that are resistant to adverse environments. The species of *Eimeria* found in salmonids develop in epithelial cells of the intestine with sporoblasts freed in the intestine. The oocyst contains four spores with two sporozoites per spore. The pathogenicity of coccidians in salmonids is not well documented, but the rupture of large numbers of intestinal cells is postulated to be the chief mechanism of pathology caused by this parasite, and mortality is probably associated with decreased ability to absorb nutrients, blood loss, and other physiologic stresses. The damaged tissue is subject to secondary invasion by other pathogens.

Amebiasis

The amebae found on salmonids usually feed on bacteria, detritus, dead host cells, and other organic matter; only limited pathogenicity occurs. The *Schizamoeba* are very common in young hatchery trout but apparently are not pathogenic. The life cycle for the intestinal forms usually consists of a trophozoite that encysts and passes out with the feces. Salmonids are infected with amebae when cysts are ingested.

Severe gill disease, resulting in significant mortality associated with *Paramoeba pemaquidensis*, has been reported in seawater-reared coho salmon in Washington and Tasmania, Australia (Kent, 1988; Kent et al., 1988). In Washington, the disease is most prevalent in the fall, and approximately 25% mortality was observed in coho salmon at one site in the fall of 1985 (Kent, 1988). The amebae infest gill surfaces and elicit prominent epithelial hyperplasia.

Cultures have been established of the organism from coho gills, and it grows rapidly on malt-yeast extract seawater medium supplemented with *Klebsiella* bacteria. The organism can be transmitted to coho salmon held in an aquarium by exposing them to amebae from cultures. In experimental infections, *Paramoeba* organisms are consistently isolated from aquarium detritus and fish gills for 4 weeks after exposure, but the severe hyperplastic response and intense infestations seen in the field have not been replicated. This may indicate that the organisms are opportunistic pathogens that proliferate on fish gills only under certain situations that are yet to be identified.

Studies in Australia indicate that baths with formalin, copper sulfate, or malachite green are not effective, but a decrease in salinity appears to eradicate the parasite. This concurs with our in vitro observations. While optimal growth occurred at salinities between 15 and 20 ppt, growth of the amebae was greatly diminished below 10 ppt salt.

Proliferative Kidney Disease

SYNONYMS. PKX, X disease, myxosporidiosis, PKD.

Host and Geographic Distribution

Proliferative kidney disease (PKD) is caused by a recently described parasite of salmonids that is considered to be a myxosporidian (Kent and Hedrick, 1986). The disease is considered a serious problem for salmonid culture in Europe and North America (Clifton-Hadley et al., 1984; Hedrick et al., 1986). In the United States and Canada, proliferative kidney disease has been detected in Idaho, California, and Washington and in British Columbia (Smith et al., 1984; Hedrick et al., 1986).

Clinical Signs and Diagnosis

External signs of clinically ill fish may include darkened body color, bilateral exophthalmia, body swelling, and pale gills (Clifton-Hadley et al., 1984; Hedrick et al., 1984). Internally, the kidney and spleen can be swollen and have a mottled gray appearance, owing to granulomatous lesions. Diseased fish may exhibit hypoproteinemia, anemia, hypergammaglobulinemia, and heterophilia (Hoffmann and Lommel, 1984; Foott and Hedrick, 1990).

Pathology and Pathogenesis

The most consistent signs of proliferative kidney disease are exophthalmia, anemia, abdominal swelling, and renal hypertrophy. The parasitic organisms are found primarily in the kidney and may cause tubular atrophy, vasculitis, and a granulomatous nephritis. The host's response to infection can result in renal interstitial hyperplasia, renal tubular atrophy, leukocytic infiltration, and granulomatous nephritis (Ferguson and Needham, 1978). An increased number of macrophages and lymphocytes in the kidney is characteristic, and often these surround the parasites. The proliferative kidney disease organism is also frequently observed in the gills and other visceral organs, and apparently these sites become involved via the circulatory system.

The taxonomic status of the proliferative kidney disease organism has yet to be resolved. Because the organism has been observed to form pseudopodia, it has been considered an ameba (Ghittino, 1974; Ferguson and Needham, 1978). Although no spores were observed, Seagrave and others (1981) proposed that the organism might be a haplosporidan based on division by endogeny, the presence of multivesicular bodies, and electron-dense cytoplasmic inclusions reminiscent of the "haplosporosomes" of the oyster pathogens *Martellia* spp.

Life Cycle, Transmission, and Epidemiology

Proliferative kidney disease has become one of the most important diseases of cultured salmonids in Europe. In 1981, the first epidemic of the disease in North America was detected in rainbow trout from the state of Idaho. It was subsequently identified in Pacific salmon and steelhead trout in California and in Vancouver Island, B.C., Canada. The disease primarily occurs during the summer when water temperatures increase. Mortalities due to proliferative kidney disease range from 10 to 95%.

High intensities of parasites and considerable morbidity do not always correlate with mortality (Hedrick et al., 1985). Concurrent infections and adverse environmental conditions appear to exert a strong influence on the mortality rate of fish with proliferative kidney disease (Hoffmann and Dangschat, 1981).

Treatment and Control

Fish that recover from an initial infection are resistant to subsequent proliferative kidney disease outbreaks (Ferguson and Ball, 1979; Foott and Hedrick, 1987). Recent studies of proliferative kidney disease have investigated treatment of the disease using malachite green (Alderman and Clifton-Hadley, 1988), the effect of cortisol implants (Kent and Hedrick, 1987), and seasonal variation and resistance to the parasitic disease (Foott and Hedrick, 1987).

METAZOAN PARASITES

There is a wide range of multicellular parasites in salmonid fishes, and host response varies from high mortalities to essentially no response. In many cases, fish act as intermediate hosts and as vectors for the parasites. Metazoan parasites of salmonids continue to be discovered. The following are representative parasites selected for their importance or high incidence.

Examples of the location of metazoan parasites in the salmonid body are given in Table 39–8.

Gyrodactylid Flukes

Salmonids can be infected with gyrodactylid flukes. These parasites are covered in more detail in

TABLE 39–8. Body Location of Metazoan Parasites (Macroscopic) in Salmonid Fishes

Gills	Blood	Skin and Fins	Intestine	Eyes	Muscle
Gyrodactylus (MT)	*Sanguinicola* (DT)	*Gyrodactylus* (MT)	*Neoechinorhynchus* (SH)	*Diplostomum* (DT)	*Posthodiplostomum* (DT)
Dactylogyrus (MT)		*Dactylogyrus* (MT)	*Diphyllobothrium* (CL)		*Diphyllobothrium* (CL)
Sanguinicola (DT)		*Glochidia* larvae (ML)	*Eubothrium* (CA)		*Nanophyetus* (DT)
Glochidia larvae (ML)		*Illinobdella* (HL)	*Echinohynchus* (SH)		*Anisakis* (NL)
Illinobdella (HL)		*Piscicola* (HL)	*Bulbodacnitis* (NA)		
Piscicola (HL)		*Lernaea* (CC)	*Contracaecum* (NL)		
Lernaea (CC)		*Salmincola* (CC)	*Cystidicoloides* (NL)		
Salmincola (CC)		*Argulus* (CC)	*Metabronema* (NL)		
Argulus (CC)		*Ergasilus* (CC)			
Ergasilus (CC)		*Nanophyetus* (DT)			

Gallbladder	Kidney	Body Cavity	Heart	Liver	Swimbladder
Crepidostomum (DT)	*Nanophyetus* (DT)	*Ligula* (CL) *Diphyllobothrium* (CL)	*Sanguinicola* (DT) *Cotylurus* (DT)	*Crepidostomum* (DT)	*Cystidicoloides* (NL) *Cystidicola* (NL)

Abbreviations: CA, cestode adult; CC, crustacean copepod; CL, cestode larvae; DT, digenetic trematode; HL, hirudinean leech; ML, molluscan larvae; MT, monogenetic trematode; NA, nematode adult; NL, nematode larvae; SH, spiny head, acanthocephalan.

the chapters on parasites of freshwater tropical fishes (Chap. 70) and parasites of freshwater temperate fishes (Chap. 27). Direct contact between fish is not required for transmission of these parasites. Crowding of the host and contact with the bottom of the tank or pond contribute to rapid transmission.

Mortalities of host fish occur with heavy parasite loads. Mortality can extend over a period of several weeks, with a few dead fish appearing on the surface each day. One major problem of a *Gyrodactylus* infestation is secondary infection. In its feeding and attaching to the host, the parasite may damage the integument, allowing secondary infection by fungus, bacteria, or virus.

The development of epizootics of *Gyrodactylus* in hatchery ponds and holding tanks may necessitate both pond treatment and a short-term dip. However, pond treatment, appropriately timed, can avoid the necessity of treatment later when the fish are held in tanks (Lewis and Lewis, 1970). Formalin or potassium permanganate are commonly recommended for pond treatment (Allison, 1957). There is a danger of oxygen depletion associated with the use of formalin. Trichlorfon has also been used to control these parasites.

Eye Flukes

SYNONYMS. Fish eye fluke, *Diplostomum spathaceum*, *Diplostomum huronense*, diplostomatosis, diplostomatiasis.

Host and Geographic Distribution

Diplostomum spathaceum, the fish eye fluke that causes the disease diplostomatosis in salmonids, has been reported in many areas of North America and other parts of the world. The metacercariae are found throughout the world where fish and the necessary

intermediate hosts exist. Diplostomatosis has been reported in Russia, Germany, Finland, Ireland, Mexico, Italy, Africa, England, Scotland, and the United States (Hoffman, 1970; Davies, 1972). Extensive surveys have been conducted in Utah concerning incidence, life history, and pathology of the fluke (Heckmann and Palmieri, 1978). Diplostomatosis, which is due to the presence of the metacercarial stage of this parasite in fish, causes cataracts of the ocular lens and damage to the vitreous body and the retina of the eye. Diplostomatosis is considered specific to freshwater fishes. Salmon and lampreys become infected during spawning migrations into fresh water (Dogiel and Petruschewsky, 1934).

Clinical Signs and Diagnosis

Visual acuity for infected fish can be slightly hampered or lost due to worm burden. Examination of fish blinded with cataracts and containing a heavy burden of larval metacercariae usually reveals stunted growth and lack of response to visual stimuli (Palmieri et al., 1976). Fishermen consider the fluke as one of the reasons for a decrease in numbers of fish caught on artificial lures. Feeding habits are changed for infected fish because of eye flukes.

The adult worm measures 2 to 4 mm in length. The body is divided into a flat anterior portion that contains the proteolytic glands, suckers, and the holdfast organ, and the posterior portion that contains the reproductive organs. The mouth is characterized by one true sucker with a pseudosucker on each side. The ovary is generally located midway in the hindbody along with three to four testes. The eggs average 0.1 × 0.06 mm in size.

Pathology and Pathogenesis

The pathologic effects of *Diplostomum spathaceum* on the fish host are many. The first signs of an infection are usually a number of localized swellings or red patches on the fins, body, or orbital region where cercariae penetrate and cause rupture of the surface blood vessels. In certain reported cases, mass entry of cercariae through the skin or gills causes obstruction of the blood vessels in the gills, resulting in asphyxia, shock, and hypoxic damage to the nervous system.

Larvae migrate to the eye via vascular channels and the lens, and the vitreous of the eye can be heavily infected with metacercariae (Ashton et al., 1969). In older fish, chronic infections and pronounced subacute inflammatory reactions in the vitreous involving heterophils, eosinophils, and macrophages with ingested lens material occur. Generally, pathologic effects to the eye by the parasite are characterized by inflammation, vascular disturbances, exophthalmia, destruction of lens tissue, necrosis, ulceration of the cornea, and eventual loss of the lens. Secondary damage can occur through the development of *Saprolegnia* within the necrotic tissue (Palmieri et al., 1976).

Once the ultimate site is found, metacercariae penetrate the iris, retina, and lens capsule by means of anterior spines and secretions of the anterior penetration glands and encyst, causing immediate hemorrhaging of the local area. The worms may stay viable from 10 months to 2 years or longer, causing chronic blindness due to parasitic cataract, keratoglobus, herniation, and tumor formation. During this time, fish cannot feed normally, and they stop growing or die.

Cercariae only require 2 to 3 hours to reach the eye via the cardiovascular system after entry into the intermediate host (Ferguson, 1943). When the parasite penetrates the head, the fish becomes restless and shows some loss of equilibrium. Seven days are required to repair tissue damaged during cercarial penetration and migration. Cercariae not reaching the orbit of the eye in 20 to 24 hours are surrounded with monocytes, granulocytes, and phagocytes (Ratanarat-Brockelman, 1974).

Histologic examinations of infected fish show the worms to be in the vitreous body, retina, or lens. The metacercariae cause a detachment of the retina from the outer vascular and fibrous coats (choroid and sclera). Heavily infected fish (40 or more worms) are blind. Flukes found in the lens undermine lens connective tissue.

Life Cycle, Transmission, and Epidemiology

The life cycle of *Diplostomum spathaceum* includes the adult parasite that lives in the intestinal tract of a piscivorous bird. The eggs from the adult trematode are passed in fecal deposits from the definitive host. The eggs embryonate in water and release a free-swimming miracidium in 2 to 3 weeks. The miracidium has approximately 24 hours in which to locate and infect the first intermediate host, which is a species of snail. In the snail, the mother and daughter sporocysts develop in liver tissue. The daughter sporocysts release free-swimming cercariae in ap-

proximately 6 weeks after miracidial penetration of the snail.

Direct contact between the fish and the cercaria is required for penetration by the parasite. Thus, the fish must swim into an infected area, since cercariae have a limited swimming ability. Fish have a greater tendency to be infected as they move closer to the shore (Slyezynska-Jurewuz, 1959). This is due to the preferred habitat of snails. The maximum rate of infection occurs during the months of June and July, coinciding with the peak of cercarial discharge (Kamenski, 1964). Fish inhabiting the bottom area of the aquatic habitat are more vulnerable to infections.

The cercariae have from 24 to 48 hours to penetrate the second intermediate host. Fish are the most common second intermediate hosts; however, infections in amphibians, reptiles, and mammals have also been reported (Ferguson, 1943). The cercariae are not specific for points of penetration on the fish but prefer the gill region and the base of the fins (Ratanarat-Brockelman, 1974). Once the cercariae have penetrated the second intermediate host, they lose their forked tails and migrate to the lens tissue, where the metacercariae develop in 50 to 60 days (Erasmus, 1958).

When infected lens tissue is eaten by a bird, the adult fluke develops in the gut within 5 days (Oliver, 1940). Metacercariae can live in the eyes of dead fish for a number of days (Ashton et al., 1969). To date, 15 species of snails, 70 species of fishes, and 37 species of birds have been reported worldwide as hosts for *Diplostomum spathaceum* (Palmieri et al., 1976).

The life cycle of *Diplostomum spathaceum* in Utah includes two lymnaeid snails (*Lymnaea stagnalis* and *Lymnaea palustria*) as first intermediate hosts and 10 species of fishes (brown trout, brook trout, rainbow trout, cutthroat trout, largemouth bass, Utah chub, Utah sucker, redside shiner, chiselmouth sucker, and mountain sucker) as second intermediate hosts. The California gull *(Larus californicus)* and the ringbilled gull *(Larus delawarensis)* are definitive hosts.

Temperature and light seem to be the determining factors for swimming habits of the cercariae of this fluke (Haas, 1969). Cercarial movements will increase as a result of an increase in water temperature. Cercariae are phototaxic and respond to any visible wavelength of light. Phototaxis may play an important part in the orientation of the larvae (Szidat, 1924).

Snails prefer warm, clean, slow-moving water with vegetation in which to live (Macon, 1950). This was also observed for snails infected with sporocytes from the Upper Salmon River. Lymnaeidae are generally found in water with at least 15 ppm of bound carbon dioxide and with a pH of 7 or above (Pennak, 1953). These snails are known to eat both plant and animal material, but prefer vegetation when available. They live approximately 1.5 years and have been known to estivate up to 3 years (Pennak, 1953). Lymnaeids usually are found in less than 4.5 feet of water and can live without free oxygen (Cheatum, 1934). Young snails are more susceptible to miracidial penetration than older snails, which appear to have some type of resistance (Cort et al., 1957).

Public Health Significance

Diplostomum spathaceum is a strigeoid trematode with effects on the ocular lens of fish, amphibians, reptiles, birds, and mammals. Owing to the large number of intermediate (15 molluscan, 70 piscine, 3 amphibian, 1 reptilian, and 5 mammalian) and definitive (37 avian) hosts, much overlap in reporting, synonymy (23 synonyms) (McDonald, 1969), and taxonomy occurs. Two reports exist in the literature concerning infections by the metacercariae of *Diplostomum spathaceum* in the eyes of humans (Ashton et al., 1969). The first report was made by Gescheidt in 1883, who found four flukes within a cataractous ocular lens at postmortem examination of an infant. The second case was reported by Greeff in 1907, who examined the eye of a 55-year-old fisherman and concluded that the cataract was caused by a fluke similar in size and shape to those flukes reported in the ocular lenses of fish. Although these two reports are isolated, it has been suggested that the primary reason for lack of recently confirmed cases in humans is due to a total unawareness of trematode-caused cataracts in temperate climates on the part of ophthalmologists (Ashton et al., 1969).

It has been recommended that experimental infections of mammalian eyes be carried out to determine if any possible health hazard exists to fishermen and water skiers who may become exposed to the cercariae of *Diplostomum spathaceum* (Davies, 1972). Studies have reported penetration of cercariae as far as the anterior chamber of enucleated eyes of man (Lester and Freeman, 1975), and metacercariae can develop in the lens of a variety of experimentally infected vertebrate hosts, including mammals (Ferguson, 1943).

Other genera of trematodes such as *Alaria marcianae* have been researched to determine their ability to penetrate into or through the cornea, and fatal human infections in other organs due to this fluke, have been reported (Lester and Freeman, 1975).

Treatment and Control

The best method for the control of diplostomatosis is the interruption of the life cycle (Hoffman, 1970). Elimination of snails represents the best means of controlling the disease. The use of molluscicides and draining and cleaning of ponds are examples of snail control. The chemical Frescon, 0.025 ppm, was used to kill *Lymnaea* snails in a reservoir near Essex, England. No live snails were found 10 days later, and there was no lethality to trout or other aquatic invertebrates. However, snails reappeared 5 months after treatment (Crossland, 1971). It would not be economically feasible to use molluscicides for treating large bodies of water.

A second approach for snail control would be the use of predators (Hoffman, 1970). *Haplochromis*

mellandi, a snail-eating fish, was used to control the first intermediate host in the Congo. Hyperinfection of snails with Nosema sp. is another technique for controlling the disease. *Nosema* prevents larval development in the snail prior to the emergence of cercariae (Cort et al., 1960). This method of biologic control is advantageous, since *Nosema* is not lethal to the recipient snail. However, the use of this hyperparasite could prove to be pathologic to humans. Microsporidian spores of *Nosema conori* were found in a human infant at necropsy (Spraque, 1974). Firearms, nest robbing, and the use of loud speakers have unsuccessfully been used for bird control (Dietz, 1967; Frings, 1954). Ultraviolet light can be used to kill the cercariae in the water (Vlaskino, 1969). Sodium chloride, potassium permanganate, and malachite green have also been reported to control the metacercariae of *Diplostomum spathaceum* in a few isolated cases (Sassmann, 1970).

Blood Flukes

There are only three species of blood flukes known in salmonids worldwide, *Sanguinicola davisi*, *Sanguinicola klamathensis*, and *Cardicola alseae* (Evans and Heckmann, 1973). The parasites are common throughout the western part of North America. They can be established in salmonids where the optimum water temperature exists and the secondary or intermediate hosts are present.

Clinical Signs and Diagnosis

Limited hemorrhaging of infected tissues (gills, kidney, and spleen) is expressed in hosts, with slime appearing on grayish gills. Mortality is limited to extensive. *Sanguinicola* is of major importance in hatcheries receiving spring water from an "open" source. Fish infected with *Sanguinicola* become lethargic and rub the gill surface (flashing) against submerged objects.

Sanguinicola is a digenean without suckers and has nonoperculate, thin-shelled eggs. Eggs are spherical, contain a few granulated globules, and range in diameter from 17 to 27 μm, with an average of 22 μm. Immature flukes, which measure 740 to 1550 μm long by 185 to 610 μm wide, can be recovered from infected gill, kidney, and heart tissue. The adult flukes vary widely in size. The miracidium is characterized by having a darkly pigmented eyespot, which contains numerous granules and spheres.

Life Cycle, Transmission, and Epidemiology

The life cycle of these blood flukes includes transmission from snail to fish via a furcocercous cercarial stage. To be infected, the fish have to be near a snail releasing cercariae from daughter sporocysts. Cercariae presumably leave snail hosts and penetrate the fish around the pectoral and pelvic fins. They migrate via the cardiovascular system to the heart and then to other organs.

An epidemic attributed to blood flukes, eggs, and miracidia in the gills of rainbow trout and steelhead rainbow trout in California resulted in an estimated 300,000 mortalities.

Treatment and Control

The best treatment of blood fluke infection includes good hatchery management such as enclosing spring water sources and not stressing fish populations. Eliminating the snail intermediate host with molluscacides and water management would be effective. Infected fish could be treated with a suitable anthelminthic such as praziquantel, but this drug is expensive and has not been approved for use in salmonids by the FDA (Heckmann and Litchfield, 1987).

White Grub Disease

Host and Geographic Distribution

Metacercariae of the strigeoid fluke *Posthodiplostomum minimum*, the white grub, have been reported in many American helminthologic surveys of fishes. The metacercariae, first reported over a century ago, occur in abundance in many of the 100 species of North American fishes (Hoffman, 1967). It is enzootic in the United States, exclusive of alpine regions.

Clinical Signs and Diagnosis

Host reactions following cercarial penetration include petechial hemorrhage at the site of invasion, followed by congestion of surrounding venules, local edema, and an aggregation of leukocytes, particularly the phagocytic elements, at the point of entry (Spall and Summerfelt, 1969a,b).

Pathology and Pathogenesis

Metacercariae have been found in all visceral organs, but occur in abundance in the liver, spleen, kidneys, mesenteries, sinus venosus, heart, and ovaries. These parasites are generally very numerous in the liver, kidney, heart, and other viscera. Pathogenicity of the larval stage is usually due to compression or occlusion of vital organs. Death results if sufficient liver or other visceral tissues are destroyed by the metacercariae (Hunter, 1937, 1940). Wild fish with several hundreds of encysted metacercariae in the liver, sinus venosus, heart, and kidneys are often observed to suffer no obvious debilitating effects.

Life History, Transmission, and Epidemiology

The life cycle for this digenetic trematode is typical. Eggs embryonate and release miracidia that have a very short life span. The miracidia penetrate the integument of a suitable snail intermediate host and form sporocysts in the snail viscera. The daughter sporocysts release a forked tailed (furcocercous) cercaria, which seeks out the second intermediate host fish. In the piscine host, metacercaria form inside an encapsulated cyst. Nutrition of the metacercaria involves transport across the cuticle. Oral feeding is impossible because the esophagus does not begin development until 8 days after penetration and is not well developed until 17 days. Intestinal ceca also develop after 17 days (Spall and Summerfelt, 1969b). The entire life cycle, which is completed in a piscivorous bird ingesting infected fish tissue, can be completed in 3 to 4 months. The adult flukes form in the gut of a suitable bird.

Treatment and Control

Praziquantel will kill the metacercariae in fish. It can be incorporated in food or given as a bath (Heckmann and Litchfield, 1987).

Salmon Poisoning Flukes

Nanophyetus salmincola is a digenetic trematode of major hygienic importance, owing to its relationship with the neorickettsial vector for salmon poisoning in dogs. Consumption of raw salmon transmits the disease, which is 90% fatal in dogs.

Clinical Signs and Diagnosis

Signs of infection include a decrease in swimming activity, a loss of equilibrium, drifting, erratic swimming, increased respiratory rate, and vertical or horizontal tail curvature. The infection with *N. salmincola* may cause exophthalmia, prolapse of the intestine such that the anus is almost completely blocked, and may damage the fins, tail, gills, retina, and cornea of fish. In the laboratory, the growth and swimming performance of infected fish are impaired, and fish with heavy infections are killed within 24 hours after their exposure to the parasites.

Pathology and Pathogenesis

Histopathologic evidence suggests that practically every organ of the infected fish is weakened physiologically. Salmonid species, exotic to the enzootic area of the trematode, are more sensitive to the effects of the infection than are native species. Pathologic changes associated with laboratory infection include exophthalmia, papules, petechiae on the body surface and at the fin bases, orbital and muscular hemorrhages, destruction of muscle tissue, and partial renal tubule and blood vessel occlusion. The heart ventricle muscle fibers, the retina, the kidney tubules, the pancreas, and the gallbladder wall are damaged.

The metacercariae have a small, slightly flattened body. The oral sucker is large, and subterminal, and there is no prepharynx. The esophagus is short and the ceca long. The ventral sucker is nearly as large as the oral sucker, and nearly equatorial. The excretory vesicle is saccular.

Life History, Transmission, and Epidemiology

Nanophyetus salmincola requires three hosts for completion of its life cycle. The first intermediate host is *Oxytrema silicula*, a stream snail found in northwestern California, in Oregon, west of the Cascade Mountains, and in the Olympic Peninsula in Washington. The parasite develops, as far as is known, only in this snail, and thus its geographic distribution is determined by that of the snail. The second intermediate hosts are salmonid and some nonsalmonid fishes and the Pacific giant salamander, in which the parasitic cercariae encyst as metacercariae. The definitive hosts are birds and mammals that acquire the trematode by eating infected fish. The trematode is the vector for *Neorickettsia helminthoeca*, a rickettsialike organism that is the cause of "salmon poisoning," a usually fatal illness of canids.

Crepidostomum Flukes

Crepidostomum flukes are common parasites of salmonids (Doss et al., 1964). All cutthroat trout from a 1985 survey in Yellowstone Lake, Wyoming, were infected with *Crepidostomum farionis*. Adult flukes can be found in fingerling cutthroat trout, often occupying the lumen of the gallbladder (Heckmann, 1971).

The members of the genus *Crepidostomum* are characterized by an elongated, oval to subcylindrical body. The oral suckers are terminal. The esophagus is short or moderate, and the ventral sucker is in the anterior half of body. The life cycle includes the adult form in fish, oculate xiphidiocercaria in sphaeroid clams, and metacercaria in mayflies or amphipod crustaceans (Hoffman, 1967).

Diphyllobothrium Tapeworms

Host and Geographic Distribution

Diphyllobothrium cestodes are found in the liver and muscles of rainbow trout, cutthroat trout, and grayling as the plerocercoid stage. Most of the research has been done on parasites of cutthroat trout from Yellowstone Lake in Wyoming.

Clinical Signs and Diagnosis

Migrating larvae in small fish can cause much damage and even mortality. The clinical signs of infection in adult fish are generally considered inapparent; however, it is reasonable to expect that heavy infections with plerocercoids would compromise host fishes.

The plerocercoids are found in viscera or musculature and have a laterally compressed scolex with two elongate shallow bothria. The body of the worm is usually wrinkled, suggesting segmentation.

Pathology and Pathogenesis

Intact plerocercoids are encapsulated with connective tissue infiltrated with lymphocytes and macrophages. Granulomas develop around the parasite. Pancreatic tissue can be displaced in infections associated with the alimentary tract. The liver of infected fish can show general necrosis with edema, and there may be a reduction in cellularity and increased connective tissue in the spleen.

Necrotic myofibrils near encapsulated parasites are separated by edema and fatty infiltration. In general, *Diphyllobothrium cordiceps* does not appear to produce serious debilitation in cutthroat trout (Otto and Heckmann, 1984).

Nothing has been done to assess the effect of sublethal infections of this parasite on the fish from Yellowstone National Park and other localities. Quite heavy loads of plerocercoids may be carried by young, vigorous fishes without harm. However, moderate loads of plerocercoids may reduce the vitality of even the most vigorous fish (Post, 1971).

Life Cycle, Transmission, and Epidemiology

Some of the natural hosts of *Diphyllobothrium* have been delineated. Prevalence and intensity in the second intermediate hosts (fishes) and natural definitive hosts (pelicans, gulls, and bears) have been determined by various researchers (Post, 1971; Heckmann, 1971). Life cycle experiments were completed using second intermediate hosts and natural definitive hosts, as well as experimental hosts (dogs and domestic cats). Ova produced from the infected experimental hosts did not hatch. The first intermediate host for cestode-infected cutthroat trout in Yellowstone Lake, Wyoming, remains unidentified. Several aquatic zooplanktonic species in Yellowstone Lake are strongly suspected to be hosts in the life cycle. Plerocercoids of *Diphyllobothrium* sp. in Yellowstone Lake develop into adults in white pelicans, California gulls, and American mergansers (Otto and Heckmann, 1984).

In the life cycle of *Diphyllobothrium* sp., the plerocercoid encysts in the cecal wall, mesentery, or other abdominal organs. The plerocercoid continues to grow until it can break from the cyst and become free in the abdominal cavity of the fish. The plerocercoid may then migrate into the flesh and become encapsulated. Instances of plerocercoids entering the muscle have been found where part of the plerocercoid remains in the body cavity and part is in the muscle.

Public Health Concerns

The definitive hosts of these parasites feed on infected fishes containing the plerocercoids. Information on man as a definitive host for *Diphyllobothrium* continues to be published (Arh, 1960; Margolis et al., 1973; Ohbayashi et al., 1977). Some investigators have concluded, from experiments where they ingested plerocercoids and checked themselves for infections, that *Diphyllobothrium cordiceps* is not infective for man (Woodbury, 1932; Post, 1971). However, one unpublished report where adult worms were passed after ingestion of plerocercoids may indicate that human infections are possible. Plerocercoids from Yellowstone Lake cutthroat trout experimentally fed to dogs result in viable, egg-producing adult parasites (Crosby, 1970).

Treatment and Control

Treatment and control measures have not been reported.

Eubothrium Cestodes

Tapeworms of the genus *Eubothrium* are found in a variety of salmonids, both in the wild and in fish culture. The worms are adult in the salmonid intestine, the intermediate hosts being a crustacean (*Cyclops* spp.) and perch, which eat the cyclops and develop the parasite to the plerocercoid stage. Salmonids are infected by feeding on young perch. The adult tapeworm may be several centimeters in length and compressed within the intestine of the host salmonid.

Worms are of moderate size with conspicuous segmentation of the body, which is frequently masked by transverse cuticular folds. The head is trapezoidal or round, unarmed, with two distinct but not very deep bothria. The neck is frequently unmarked. There is a genital pore at the lateral sides of the segments, usually on one side of the strobila. Occasionally, there is a unilateral disposition of genital pores. There are numerous testes, lying in central parenchyma between neural trunks. The seminal duct is highly convoluted, and there is no external seminal vesicle. The cirrus is unarmed, and there is a common genital atrium present. The vitellaria lie in the medullary or the innermost layer of the cortical parenchyma. The uterus is simple, saccular or lobate, with a rudimentary aperture, usually lying ventrally. Eggs are thin-shelled, unoperculate, and embryonated on emergence from the uterus. Adult worms are found in the intestines of fish.

The adult cestode is not that common in salmonid fishes of North America. It can be treated successfully with praziquantel (Heckmann and Litchfield, 1987).

Ligula Cestodes

Adult worms and invasional plerocercoids of *Ligula* can attain enormous size. The description of the parasite includes a muscular beltlike body lacking a typical head. The function of the head is subserved by an anterior end of strobila bearing dorsal and ventral slitlike bothria. Pseudo or partial external segmentation of strobila is seen in adult worms. The neck is absent. Growth and formation of genital organs occurs in the plerocercoid stage with the rudiments of the first genital complexes differentiated simultaneously over a large area of the centroposterior part of the strobila, with processes then spreading posteriorly and anteriorly. The genital organs are numerous. The genital pores and apertures of uteri open ventrally. Numerous testes lie in a single layer in the central parenchyma closer to the dorsal surface. The bursa of the cirrus is muscular, with a well-developed external seminal vesicle. The ovaries are found in the central parenchyma, closer to the ventral surface. There is one ovary per genital complex. Numerous vitellary follicles lie in the cortical parenchyma external to the longitudinal muscles, extending in a single layer all around the strobila, or they may break off at the central line dorsally and ventrally. The eggs are oval, operculate, and unembryonated on emergence from the uterus.

The eggs develop in water. Free-swimming ciliated larvae (coracidia) hatch and enter planktonic copepod crustaceans (Cyclopoida and Calanoida) when swallowed, developing in the coelom into procercoids. Fish swallow procercoids together with copepods. Procercoids develop in the body cavity of fish into large invasive plerocercoids in 2 to 14 months. Principal growth and organogenesis of the genital system occurs in the plerocercoid phase, so that invasive plerocercoids become morphologically difficult to distinguish from adult worms. Adult worms with development amounting chiefly to production of fertilized eggs are not highly specific parasites and may develop in numerous piscivorous birds, experimentally in various birds and mammals, and in artificial environments at temperatures equaling the body temperature of warm-blooded animals (36 to 42°C). Development in a definitive host requires little time (35 to 60 hours); worms then produce eggs for 2 to 4 days and die.

Spiny-Headed Worms

SYNONYMS. Acanthocephalans, acanthocephalids, thorny-headed worms.

The members of the Acanthocephala are unusual worms with hooks on an armed proboscis that can be embedded into the host intestine, causing severe damage in the intestines of salmonids. Animals infected with high numbers of worms exhibit severe loss of weight. For correct taxonomic classification, the worms need to be relaxed in cold water and have the proboscis everted before a fixative is used.

Members of the genus *Echinorhynchus* have a proboscis that is long, cylindrical, and directed ventrad, with 9 to 26 longitudinal rows of 5 to 16 hooks each. The body is small to medium-sized with small, numerous, hypodermal nuclei. There is a lacunar system with lateral main vessels and reticular anastomoses. The eggs of these acanthocephalans are very elongated, fusiform, and have prominent bipolar prolongations of the middle shell. These worms are found in both freshwater and marine fishes. The life cycle includes a larval stage in amphipods, and no second intermediate host is involved (Hoffman, 1970).

Members of the genus *Neoechinorhynchus* include *N. rutili*, a parasite of salmonids. These acanthocephalans have a small body, and the proboscis is short and somewhat globular with hooks in six spiral rows of three. The anterior hooks are longer and stouter than others. The eggs of members of this genus are elliptical with concentric shells. The life cycle involves the eggs being shed by the adult worm in the fish intestine and then being eaten by the first intermediate host, a copepod, ostracod, amphipod, or isopod. The first larval stage, or acanthor, migrates through the intestinal wall of the crustacean, localizes in the body cavity, and becomes the next larval stage, the acanthella. Usually, there is no second intermediate host, and the fish becomes infected by eating the crustacean. Three species at least, however, use fish as a second intermediate host. One of the three species, *Leptorhynchoides thecatus*, will encyst in a fish if the larva has been in the crustacean less than 30 days, but it needs no second host if it is eaten by the fish after 30 days in the crustacean.

If acanthocephalans are numerous in the host, the damage done to the intestine by the armed proboscis may be serious. The histopathology has been studied by several authors (Hoffman, 1970). Because the life cycles are relatively simple, it is quite probable that acanthocephalans will become more important in fish culture as fisheries work increases.

Nematodes

Most adult fish nematodes reside in the intestinal tract. Filarid nematodes, however, are found in the body cavity, "cheek galleries," and caudal fin. Larval nematodes of fish may be found in almost every organ but are common in the mesenteries, liver, and musculature.

The life cycle always involves an invertebrate, usually a copepod, or insect nymph, as the first intermediate host. Many develop to adult forms in the fish host; however, some use a fish as a second intermediate host and develop to adults in the intestinal tract of piscivorous fishes, birds, and mammals.

It is thought that intestinal nematodes of fish produce little pathogenicity. However, some larval nematodes cause considerable damage in the body cavity of fish, notably *Contracaecum* sp. and *Spiroxys* sp. The large larvae of *Eustrongyloides* sp., *Anisakis* sp., and *Porrocaecum* sp. are very unsightly, and larva migrans of *Anisakis* sp. can produce an acute abdominal syndrome in humans.

One nematode genus, *Cystidicola*, occurs in the swimbladder of fish. There is no known control of these nematodes. Currently, research is being conducted toward pharmaceuticals suitable for treating salmonid nematodes (Heckmann and Litchfield, 1987).

Bulbodacnitis sp.

Members of the genus *Bulbodacnitis* are intestinal roundworms of salmonids. The key characteristics of the genus include a head with two large lateral lobes (lips), each bearing three papillae and bounding a slitlike mouth. The esophagus is muscular throughout, is dilated anteriorly to form a false buccal capsule, and is enlarged posteriorly. *Bulbodacnitis* can be differentiated from *Cucullanus* only by the presence of a tubercle on dorsal aspect of head.

The life cycle of *Bulbodacnitis* always involves an invertebrate for the first intermediate host and a fish, via the food chain, as the definitive host. Other nematodes use the fish as the second intermediate host and develop to adults in the intestinal tract of piscivorous fishes, birds, and mammals (Hoffman, 1967).

Bulbodacnitis scotti is a common parasite of the cutthroat trout in Wyoming. Adult nematodes of this species live in the intestinal tract. In contrast, larval roundworms of fish may be found in almost every organ, but they are common in the mesenteries, liver, and musculature.

Anisakis Simplex

Anisakis simplex is a common nematode found in marine fishes, especially the salmonids. Anisakiasis is a human parasitic disease caused by the digestion of raw or partially cooked seafood that has been infected with larval anisakid worms. This parasite is discussed in more detail in Chapters 81 and 89. *Anisakis* is not a serious pathogen in migrating salmonids. Pen-reared salmon have a lower incidence of anisakiasis (Deardorff and Kent, 1989).

Anisakis is a marine nematode that uses salmon, among many other marine fishes, as a second intermediate host. The first stage is spent in oceanic krill, which are eaten by salmon, where the parasite is usually found in small numbers on the surface of the liver or other viscera. Its final host is normally a porpoise, but it can invade the tissues of the seal or even man. *Anisakis* has been reported in whales.

Cystidicola sp.

The members of the genus *Cystidicola* are small (about 7 mm), white threadworms, frequently found in the swimbladder and, rarely, the esophagus of salmonids. In certain fish, very large numbers may occur, but since they are not found in the muscles and do not usually cause harmful effects, they are of little significance.

Cystidicola is a member of the family Rhabdochonidae, which is characterized by a simple mouth or one with small lips. The buccal capsule is cylindrical with a thick, chitinous wall. The esophagus is very long and divided. Males have a spirally coiled caudal extremity, and the tail is rounded at the tip. The caudal alae are narrow. There is a long row of coupled or single preanal papillae and a few simple postanal papillae. The spicules of the male are unequal and dissimilar. Female worms have a straight and blunt tail with the vulva in the middle or anterior region of the body. The uterine branches are opposed. These worms are oviparous and produce numerous, thick-shelled eggs. *Cystidicola farionis* and possibly other species have polar filaments. The life cycle involves adult worms in fish and larvae in gammarids.

Cystidicoloides sp.

Cystidicoloides is a genus of oviparous nematodes that has been reported in several species of salmonids and merits inclusion with parasites of salmonids. It has a dioecious form, which is typical for nematodes, and is found mainly in the digestive system of salmonids, where limited pathology occurs. There are also species of *Cystidicoloides* that occur in the swimbladder. The adult worms of this genus are usually parasites of fishes. Mayfly nymphs serve as intermediate hosts for *Cystidicoloides* larvae.

The worms have cuticular flanges on both sides of the body. The mouth has large lateral lips and small median lips, continuous with the lateral ones by means of cuticular folds. The whole head structure is strengthened by chitinous support, continuous with the chitinous wall of the buccal capsule. Cervical papillae are present slightly behind the lips. The buccal capsule is thick-walled and cylindrical. The esophagus consists of two parts. Male worms have a spirally coiled posterior extremity and well-developed caudal alae.

Males also have four pairs of pedunculate preanal and four pairs of pedunculate postanal papillae and a pair of large sessile papillae near the tip of the tail. The spicules of males are very unequal, and a gubernaculum is present. Female worms have a conical tail with the vulva near the junction of the anterior and middle third of the body. The uteri are divergent. These worms are oviparous, producing thick-shelled eggs, with small button-shaped structures at each end, from which arise two very delicate filaments. The eggs contain a morula when deposited.

Leeches

Leeches are segmented worms that parasitize many animals, including salmonid fishes. The leeches vary in number on the host fish; they leave the host to complete their life cycle in the summer. Suckers are characteristic at either end of their flattened to tubelike body. Leeches can swim and are also motile on the ground.

The true fish leeches belong to the family Piscicolidae, but two species of the family Glossiphoniidae (*Actinobdella triannulata* and *Placobdella pediculata*) show a strong predilection for fish. Other Glossiphoniidae are found on fish occasionally. Leeches attach periodically to a fish, take a large blood meal, and leave the fish for varying periods of time. Their life cycles have not been adequately studied. Fish host specificity is apparently lacking, although there may be exceptions. Not enough host records have been made to determine specificity, and there have been no experimental host studies.

The damage done to the fish by leeches is proportional to the number of leeches present and the amount of blood they remove. Leeches also serve as vectors of *Trypanosoma*, *Cryptobia*, and probably the blood sporozoa *Haemogregarina* and *Dactylosoma*; perhaps also bacteria and viruses.

Piscicola sp. have a body that is cylindrical at rest and usually divided at segment XIII into distinct anterior and posterior regions. The head sucker is usually distinctly marked off from body, and there are usually more than three annuli per segment. These leeches have simple eyes that may be present on the head, neck, and posterior sucker.

The margins of the body have 11 pairs of small pulsatile vesicles, which are difficult to see on preserved specimens. There are 14 annuli per segment. The body is not clearly divided into anterior and posterior regions; and the postceca are completely fused. Six pairs of testisacs are present.

Illinobdella sp. are clavate with a distinction between anterior and posterior body regions, which is more evident when the leech is in contraction. Both suckers are much smaller than the body diameter. The mouth is central in the sucker, and the stomach has six chambers. There are 14 annulate somites, and the postceca are completely fused. This genus may be congeneric with *Myxobdella*.

Molluscan Larvae

Glochidia are larval stages of bivalve mollusks that can attach on the gills of freshwater salmonids and deprive the gill surface of oxygen transfer. The larvae of most freshwater clams go through a parasitic stage on the gills or fins of freshwater salmonids (Bauer, 1987; Young et al., 1987). All salmonids in fresh water are susceptible to infection. The glochidia larvae are expelled by the parent mussel and must quickly invade the gills of a fish in order to develop further. The parasitic larvae bite off pieces of gill, which they feed upon as they enter the underlying tissues. There they are walled off by the host to form a cyst. These cysts appear as white specks on the gill filaments and may resemble trematode metacercariae. The glochidia have a thin, bivalve shell with little hooks on the inner edge.

Crustacean Parasites

There are several crustacean parasites of salmonids. They include members of the genera *Argulus*,

Lernaea, and *Ergasilus*, which are covered in more detail in Chapter 27. Salmonids are also parasitized by members of the genus *Salmincola*.

Salmincola sp. (gill maggots) are parasitic on freshwater fishes. The typical life cycle includes the hatching of free-swimming larvae, which can exist 2 days without a host. These larvae possess mouth parts that bear a peculiar filament for attachment to fish. *Salmincola* larvae force this filament into the gill tissue of the fish and attach a second maxillae to the filament. Together, these become the bulla, forming a permanent attachment to the fish. The entire larva then degenerates into a grublike parasite. The male is usually much smaller than the female. Copulation occurs 2.5 to 3 weeks after attachment. The male releases its hold on the gill and attaches to the female. After fertilization, the male dies. Each female gives rise to two batches of embryonated eggs and then dies. The entire life cycle takes about 2.5 months (Fasten, 1912; Savage, 1935; Hoffman, 1967).

The gill maggot is commonly seen on wild Atlantic salmon and sea trout. They do not affect young fish owing to the large size of the parasite. Fresh-run fish, therefore, are not infected, but once an adult fish has been in fresh water for any length of time, the parasite is usually present. It can persist on the fish when it returns to sea, so that individuals that survive to spawn again almost invariably have severe parasitic damage to their gills. Different species of *Salmincola* have been associated with gill damage in a variety of salmonid hosts.

Argulus sp. are capable of living on a variety of fish hosts. They are predominately parasites of warm, still waters, but can be a problem in trout culture in certain areas. They can easily be seen with the naked eye on any part of the body surface.

Lernaea sp. can also infect salmonids. Mature female parasites attach to the muscle of the fish by an anchor-shaped head inserted to a depth of several millimeters. This entails penetrating the skin of the fish, often at the vent, where the parasite grows its anchor and becomes readily visible.

LITERATURE CITED

Alderman, D.J., and Clifton-Hadley, R.S. (1988) Malachite green therapy of proliferative kidney disease in rainbow trout field trials. Vet. Rec. 122(5):103–106.

Allison, R. (1957) Some new results in the treatment of ponds to control some external parasites of fish. Progressive Fish Culturist 19:58–63.

Arh, I. (1960) Fish tapeworm in Eskimos in the Port Harrison area, Canada. Can. J. Public Health 51:268–271.

Ashton, N., Brown, N., and Easty, D. (1969) Trematode cataract in the freshwater fish. J. Small Anim. Pract. 10:471–178.

Bailey, R.E., and Margolis, L. (1987) Comparison of parasite fauna of juvenile sockeye salmon *Oncorhynchus nerka* from southern British Columbia, Canada, and Washington state USA lakes. Can. J. Zool. 65(2):420–431.

Bangham, R.V. (1951) Parasites of fish in the upper Snake River drainage and in Yellowstone Lake, Wyoming. Zoologica 36:213–217.

Bartholomew, J.L., Rohovec, J.S., and Fryer, J.L. (1989) Development characterization and use of monoclonal and polyclonal antibodies against the myxosporean *Ceratomyxa shasta*. J. Protozool. 36(4):397–401.

Bauer, G. (1987) The parasitic stage of the freshwater pearl mussel (*Margaritifera margaritifera L.*). II. Susceptibility of brown trout. Arch. Hydrobiol. 76(4)(Suppl. 1983):403–412.

Bier, J.W., Schwien, W.G., and Sellers, R.L, Jr. (1982) A metazoan parasite survey of fresh salmon from USA markets. Mol. Biochem. Parasitol. (Suppl.), p. 315.

Boustead, N.C. (1981) Diseases in salmon hatcheries. Fish Res. Div. Occas. Publ. 30:73–77.

Bower, S.M. (1985) *Ceratomyxa shasta* (Myxozoa: Myxosporea) in juvenile chinook salmon (*Oncorhynchus tshawytscha*): experimental transmission and natural infections in the Fraser River, British Columbia. Can. J. Zool. 63:1737–1740.

Buchanan, D.V., Sanders, J.E., Zinn, J.L., and Fryer, J.L. (1983) Relative susceptibility of four strains of summer steelhead to infection by *Ceratomyxa shasta*. Trans. Am. Fish. Soc. 112:541–543.

Butorina, T.E., and Shed'ko, M.B. (1989) On the use of parasites—indicators for differentiation of sockeye salmon fry in Lake Azabachje Kamchatka Russian SFSR USSR. Parazitologiia, 23(4):302–308.

Chapman, P.F. (1986) Occurrence of the noninfective stage of Ceratomyxa shasta in mature summer chinook salmon in the South Fork Salmon River, Idaho, USA. Progressive Fish Culturist 48(4):304–306.

Cheatum, E.P. (1934) Limnological investigations on respiration, annual migratory cycle, and other related phenomena in freshwater pulmonate snails. Am. Microsc. Soc. Trans. 53:348–407.

Ching, H.L., and Munday, D.R. (1984a) Geographic and seasonal distribution of the infectious stage of *Ceratomyxa shasta* Noble, 1950, a myxozoan salmonid pathogen in the Fraser River system. Can. J. Zool. 62:1075–1080.

Ching, H.L., and Munday, D.R. (1984b) Susceptibility of six Fraser chinook salmon stocks to *Ceratomyxa shasta* and the effects of salinity on ceratomyxosis. Can. J. Zool. 62:1081–1083.

Clifton-Hadley, R.S., Bucke, D., and Richards, R.H. (1984) Proliferative kidney disease of salmonid fish: a review. J. Fish Dis. 7:363–378.

Coley, T.C., Chacko, A.J., and Klontz, G.W. (1983) Development of a lavage technique for sampling Ceratomyxa shasta in adult salmonids. J. Fish Dis. 6(3):317–319.

Cone, D.K., and Ryan, P.M. (1984) Population sizes of metazoan parasites of brook trout Salvelinus fontinalis and Atlantic salmon salmo-salar in a small Newfoundland Lake, Canada. Can. J. Zool. 62(1):130–133.

Conneely, J.J., and McCarthy, T.K. (1988) The metazoan parasites of trout *Salmo trutta* L. in western Ireland. Pol. Arch. Hydrobiol. 35(3–4):443–460.

Conrad, J.F., and Decew, M. (1966) First report of *Ceratomyxa* in juvenile salmonids in Oregon. Progressive Fish Culturist 28:238.

Cope, O.B. (1958) Incidence of external parasites on cutthroat trout in Yellowstone Lake. Proc. Utah Acad. Sci. 35:95–100.

Cort, W.W., Hussey, K.L., and Ameel, D.J. (1957) Variations in infestations of *Diplostomum flexicaudum* (Cort and Brooks 1928) in snail intermediate hosts of different sizes. J. Parasitol. 43(2):221–234.

Cort, W.W., Hussey, K.L., and Ameel, D.J. (1960) Studies on a microsporidian hyperparasite of a strigeoid trematode. I. Prevalence and effect on the parasitized larval trematodes. Ann. Zool. Fenn. 3:317–326.

Crosby, C.W. (1970) Studies on the life cycle of *Diphyllobothrium cordiceps*. Unpublished thesis, Colorado State University, Fort Collins.

Crossland, N.O. (1971) A field trial with the Molluscide Frescon for control of *Lymnaea peregra* Muller, snail host of *Diplostomum spathaceum* Rudolfi (1819). J. Fish Biol. 3(3):279–302.

Davies, R.B. (1972) The life cycle and ecology of *Diplostomum spathaceum* Rudolfi (1891) in North Park, Colorado. Unpublished thesis, Colorado State University, Fort Collins.

Deardorff, T.L., and Kent, M.L. (1989) Prevalence of larval Anisakis simplex in pen-reared and wild-caught salmon salmonidae from Puget Sound, Washington, USA. J. Wildlife Dis. 25(3):416–419.

Dietz, R.H. (1967) Results of increasing waterfowl habitat and production by gull control. N. Am. Wildlife Nature Res. Conf. Trans. 32:316–325.

Dogiel, V., and Petruschewsky, G. (1934) Die Wirkung des Aufenthaltsortes auf die Parasitenfauna des Leches Wahrend Seiner Verschiedenen Lebensperioden. Arch. Hydrobiol. 26(4):659–673.

Doss, M.A., Roach, K.R., and Breen, V.L. (1963–1964) Trematoda and trematode diseases. In: Index-Catalogue of Medical Veterinary Zoology. U.S. Department of Agriculture, Washington, D.C.

Erasmus, D.A. (1958) Studies on the morphology, biology, and development of a strigeoid cercaria (cercaria X Baylis). Parasitology 48:312–335.

Esch, G.W., Kennedy, C.R., Bush, A.O., and Aho, J.M. (1988) Patterns in helminth communities in freshwater fish in Great Britain: alternative strategies for colonization. Parasitology 96(3):519–532.

Evans, W.A., and Heckmann, R.A. (1973) The life history of *Sanguinicola klamathensis*. Life Sci. 13:1285–1291.

Fasten, N. (1912) The brook trout disease at Wild Rose and other hatcheries. Bien. Rep. Comr. Fish. Wisconsin, pp. 12–22.

Ferguson, M.S. (1943) Development of eye flukes of fishes in the lenses of frogs, turtles, birds and mammals. J. Parasitol. 29:136–142.

Ferguson, H.W., and Ball, N.J. (1979) Epidemiological aspects of proliferative kidney disease amongst rainbow trout *Salmo gairdneri* Richardson in Northern Ireland. J. Fish Dis. 2:219–225.

Ferguson, H.W., and Needham, E.A. (1978) Proliferative kidney disease in rainbow trout *Salmo gairdneri* Richardson. J. Fish Dis. 1:91–108.

Foott, J.S., and Hedrick, R.P. (1987) Seasonal occurrence of the infectious stage of proliferative kidney disease (PKD) and resistance of rainbow trout, *Salmo gairdneri* Richardson, to reinfection. J. Fish Biol. 30:477–483.

Foott, J.S., and Hedrick, R.P. (1990) Blood parameters and immune status of rainbow trout with proliferative kidney disease. J. Aquatic Anim. Health 2:141–148.

Frings, H., Fringer, M., Cox, B., and Peissner, L. (1954) Recorded calls of herring gulls (*Larus argentatus*) as repellants and attractants. Science 121(9):121–122.

Fryer, J.L., and Sanders, J.E. (1970) Investigation of *Ceratomyxa shasta*, a protozoan parasite of salmonid fish. J. Parasitol. 56:759.

Ghittino, P. (1974) Rilievi clinici e pathologiei su un caso di Cattarata Verminosa in trotelle iridee d'allevamento. Piscicoltura Ittiopathol. X(2):59–61.

Haas, W. (1969) Reizphysiologische Untersuchungen an Cercarien von *Diplostomum spathaceum*. Z. Vergl. Physiol. 64(3):254–287.

Halliday, M.M. (1973) Studies of *Myxosoma cerebralis*: a parasite of salmonids. II. The development and pathology of Myxosoma cerebralis in experimentally infected rainbow trout (*Salmo gairdneri*) fry reared at different water temperatures. Nord. Veterinaermed. 25:349–358.

Heckmann, R.A. (1971) Parasites of cutthroat trout from Yellowstone Lake, Wyoming. Progressive Fish Culturist. 33:103–106.

Heckmann, R.A., and Carroll, T. (1985) Host-parasite studies of *Trichophrya* infesting cutthroat trout (*Salmo claki*) and longnose suckers (*Catostomus catostomus*) from Yellowstone Lake, Wyoming. Great Basin Nature 45:255–265.

Heckmann, R.A., and Ching, H.L. (1987) Parasites of the cutthroat trout, *Salmo clarki*, and longnose suckers, *Catostomus catostomus*, from Yellowstone Lake, Wyoming. Great Basin Nature 47:260–274.

Heckmann, R.A., and Litchfield, R.W. (1987) The efficacy of praziquantel (Droncit) and ivermectin in combination as a helminthicide for fish parasites. Fish Health Sect. Newslett. American Fisheries Society. 15:7.

Heckmann, R.A., and Palmieri, J.R. (1978) The eye fluke disease (diplostomatosis) in fishes from Utah. Great Basin Nature 38:473–477.

Hedrick, R.P., Kent, M.L., Rosemark, R., and Manzer, D. (1984) Occurrence of proliferative kidney disease (PKD) among Pacific salmon and steelhead trout. Bull. Europ. Assoc. Fish Pathologists 4:34–37.

Hedrick, R.P., Kent, M.L., Foott, J.S., Rosemark, R., and Manzer, D. (1985) Proliferative kidney disease (PKD) among salmonid fish in California, USA: a second look. Bull. Europ. Assoc. Fish Pathologists 5:36–38.

Hedrick, R.P., Kent, M.L., and Smith, C.E. (1986) Proliferative kidney disease in salmonid fishes. U.S. Fish and Wildlife Service Fish Disease Leaflet 74.

Hemmingsen, A.R., Holt, R.A., Ewing, R.D., and McIntyre, J.D. (1986) Susceptibility of progeny from crosses among three stocks of coho salmon *Oncorhynchus kisutch* to infection by *Ceratomyxa shasta*. Trans. Am. Fish. Soc. 115(3):492–495.

Hoffman, G.L. (1967) Parasites of North American Freshwater Fishes. University of California Press, Berkeley and Los Angeles.

Hoffman, G.L. (1970) Parasites of North American Freshwater Fishes. University of California Press, Berkeley.

Hoffman, G.L. (1976) Whirling disease of trout. U.S. Fish Wildl. Serv. Fish Dis. Leafl. No. 47. Washington, D.C.

Hoffman, G.L., and Putz, R.E. (1969) Host susceptibility and the effect of aging, freezing, heat and chemicals on spores of *Myxosoma cerebralis*. Progressive Fish Culturist 31:35–37.

Hoffmann, R., and Dangschat, H. (1981) A note on the occurrence of proliferative kidney disease in Germany. Bull. Europ. Assoc. Fish Pathologists 1:33.

Hoffmann, R.W., and El-Matbouli, M. (1988) Transmission of two species of the Genus *Myxobolus* via *Tubifex* worms in teleost fish. Proceedings of the International Fish Health Conference, Fish Health Section, American Fisheries Society; Vancouver, Canada, p. 111.

Hoffmann, R., and Lommel, R. (1984) Haematological studies in proliferative kidney disease of rainbow trout. Salmo gairdneri Richardson. J. Fish Dis. 7:323–326.

Hoffmaster, J.L., Sanders, J.E., Rohovec, J.S., Fryer, J.L., and Stevens, D.G. (1985) Geographic distribution of the myxosporean parasite, *Ceratomyxa shasta* Noble, 1950, in the Columbia River Basin, USA. J. Fish Dis. 11(1):97–100.

Hunter, G.W., III (1937) Parasitism of fishes in the lower Hudson area. In: A biological survey of the Lower Hudson Watershed. Biological Survey No. XI (1936), Suppl. to the Twenty-sixth Ann. Rept., New York State Cons. Dept., pp. 264–273.

Hunter, G.W., III (1940) Studies on the development of the Metacercaria and the nature of the cyst of *Posthodiplostomum minimum* (MacCallum, 1921) (Trematoda: Streigeidae). Trans. Am. Microsc. Soc. 59:52–63.

Jennings, M.R., and Hendrickson, G.L. (1982) Parasites of chinook salmon *Oncorhynchus tshawytscha* and coho salmon *Oncorhynchus kisutch* from the Mad River and vicinity, Humboldt County California, USA. Proc. Helminthol. Soc. Wash., 49(2):279–284.

Johnson, K.A. (1980) Host susceptibility histopathologic and transmission studies on *Ceratomyxa shasta*, a myxosporidian parasite of salmonid fish. Fish Pathol. 14(4):183–184.

Johnson, K.A., Sanders, J.E., and Fryer, J.L. (1979) *Ceratomyxa shasta* in salmonids. U.S. Fish and Wildlife Service, Fish Disease Leaflet No. 58. Washington, D.C.

Kaminskii, I.V. (1964) Diplostomatoz foreli v rybhoze "Snhodaya," TR vses inst. Geomintol. 11:194–198.

Kennedy, C.R., Laffoley, D.D., Bishop, G., Jones, P. and Taylor, M. (1986) Communities of parasites of freshwater fish of Jersey Chabnel Islands, OK. J. Fish Biol. 29(2):215–226.

Kent, M.L. (1988) *Paramoeba pemaquidensis* infestation of Coho salmon gills. International Fish Health Conference, Fish Health Section, American Fisheries Society. Vancouver, Canada, p. 116.

Kent, M.L., and Hedrick, R.P. (1986) Development of the PKX myxosporean in rainbow trout *Salmo gairdneri*. Dis. Aquatic Organ. 1(3):169–182.

Kent, M., and Hedrick, H.P. (1987) Effects of cortisol implants on the PKX myxosporean causing proliferative kidney disease in rainbow trout *Salmo-gairdneri*. J. Parasitol. 73(3):455–461.

Kent, M.L., Sawyer, T.K., and Hedrick, R.P. (1988) *Paramoeba pemaquidensis* (Sarcomastigophora: Paramoebidae) infestation of the gills of coho salmon Oncorhynchus kisutch reared in sea water. Dis. Aquatic Organ. 5(3):163–169.

Larson, O.R. (1965) *Diplostomulum* (Trematoda: Strigeoides) associated with herniations of bullhead lenses. J. Parasitol. 5(2):224–229.

LaRue, G.R., Butler, E.P., and Berkhout, P.G. (1926) Studies on the trematode family Strigeidae. Trans. Am. Microsc. Soc. 45(4):282–288.

Leong, T.S.D., and Holmes, J.C. (1981) Communities of metazoan parasites in open water fishes of Cold Lake, Alberta. J. Fish Biol. 18(6):693–713.

Lester, R.J.G., and Freeman, R.S. (1975) Penetration of vertebrate eyes by cercariae of *Alaria marcianae*. Can. J. Public Health 66:384–387.

Lewis, W.M., and Lewis, S.D. (1970) *Gyrodactylus wageneri* group, its occurrence, importance, and control in the commercial production of the Golden Shiner. In: A Symposium on Diseases of Fishes and Shellfishes. (Sniesako, S.F., ed.). Special publication No. 5, American Fisheries Society, Washington, D.C., pp. 174–177.

Li, L., and Desser, S.S. (1985) The protozoan parasites of fish from two lakes in Algonquin Park, Ontario, Canada. Can. J. Zool. 63(8):1846–1858.

Linton, E. (1891a) On two species of larval dibothria from the Yellowstone National Park. Bull. U.S. Fish Comm. 9:64–79.

Linton, E. (1891b) A contribution to the life history of *Dibothrium corcideps* Leidy, a parasite infesting trout in Yellowstone Lake. Bull. U.S. Fish Comm. 9:337–358.

Macon, T.T. (1950) Ecology of freshwater mollusca in the English Lake district. J. Anim. Ecol. 19(2):124–146.

Margolis, L., and Boyce, N.P. (1990) Helminth parasites from North Pacific anadromous Chinook salmon *Oncorhynchus tshawytscha* established in New Zealand. J. Parasitol. 76(1):133–135.

Margolis, L., Rausch, R.L., and Robertson, E. (1973) *Diphyllobothrium ursi* from man in British Columbia—first report of this tapeworm in Canada. Can. J. Public Health 64:588–589.

Mariaux, J. (1986) Helminths of fish from the Areuse River, Switzerland. Bull. Soc. Neuchatel. Sci. Nature 109:57–64.

McDonald, M. (1969) Catalogue of Heminths of Waterfowl (Anatidae). Bureau of Sport Fisheries and Wildlife. Special Scientific Report—Wildlife No. 126.

McGuigan, J.B., and Summerville, C. (1985) Studies on the effects of cage culture of fish on the parasite fauna in a lowland freshwater loch in the west of Scotland, UK. Z. Parasitenkd. 71(5):673–682.

Molnar, K., and Fernado, C.H. (1974) Some new *Eimeria* (Protozoa, Coccidia) from freshwater fishes in Ontario, Canada. Can. J. Zool. 52:413–419.

Moravec, F., Nagasawa, K., and Urawa, S. (1985) Some fish nematodes from fresh waters in Hokkaido Japan. Folia Parasitol. (Praha). 32(4):305–316.

Muzzall, P.M. (1984) Parasites of trout from 14 lotic localities in Michigan, USA. Proc. Helminth. Soc. Wash. 51(2):261–266.

Muzzall, P.M., and Peebles, C.R. (1986) Helminths of pink salmon *Oncorhynchus gorbuscha* from five tributaries of Lake Superior and Lake Huron. Can. J. Zool. 64(2):508–511.

Nagasawa K., Urawa, S., and Awakura, T. (1987) A checklist and bibliography of parasites of salmonids of Japan. Sci. Rep. Hokkaido Salmon Hatchery 41:1–76.

Ohbayashi, M., Yamaguchi, K., Kamiya, H., and Tada, Y. (1977) Studies on *Diphyllobothrium latum* in Hokkaido, with special reference to a survey of *Oncorhynchus masou*. J. Hokkaido Vet. Med. Assoc. 21:182–184.

Oliver, L. (1940) Development of *Dioplostomum flexicaudum* (Cort and Brooks) in the chicken by feeding precocious metacercariae obtained from the snail intermediate host. J. Parasitol. 26(1):85–86.

Otto, T.M., and Heckmann, R.A. (1984) Host tissue response for trout infected with *Diphyllobothrium cordiceps* larvae. Great Basin Nature 44:125–132.

Palmeiri, J.R., Heckmann, R.A., and Evans, R.S. (1976) Life cycle and incidence of *Diplostomum spathaceum* Rudolphi (1819) (Trematoda: Diplostomatidae) in Utah. Great Basin Nature 36:86–96.

Pennak, R.W. (1953) Freshwater Invertebrates of the United States. Ronald Press, New York.

Post, G. (1971) The *Diphyllobothrium* cestode in Yellowstone Lake, Wyoming. Agricultural Experiment Station, University of Wyoming, Laramie, Research Journal 41, p. 24.

Pugachev, O.N. (1980) Genesis of the parasite fauna of salmonoidea of Eurasia. Parazitologiia 14(5):403–410.

Quinn, T.P., Wood, C.C., Margolis, L., Riddell, B.E., and Hyatt, K.D. (1987) Homing in wild sockeye salmon *Oncorhynchus nerka* populations as inferred from differences in parasite prevalence and allozyme allele frequencies. Can. J. Fish. Aquatic Sci. 44(11):1963–1971.

Rahim, M.A. (1981) Occurrence of helminth parasites of brown trout in the River Alyn North Wales UK. Pak. J. Zool. 13(1–2):169–178.

Ratanarat-Brockelman, C. (1974) Migration of *Diplostomum spathaceum* (Trematoda) in fish intermediate hosts. Z. Parasitenkd. 43:123–134.

Ratliff, D.E. (1983) *Ceratomyxa shasta*: longevity, distribution, timing, and abundance of the infective stage in central Oregon. Can. J. Fish. Aquatic Sci. 40:1622–1632.

Sanders, J.E., Fryer, J.L., and Gould, R.W. (1970) Occurrence of the myxosporidian parasite, *Ceratomyxa shasta*, in salmonid fish from the Columbia River Basin and Oregon coastal streams. In: A Symposium on Diseases of Fishes and Shellfishes, (Snieszko, S.F., ed.). Special Publication No. 5, American Fisheries Society, Washington, D.C., pp. 133–141.

Sanders, J.E., Fryer, J.L., Leith, D.A., and Moore, K.D. (1972) Control of the infectious protozoan *Ceratomyxa shasta* by treating hatchery water supplies. Progressive Fish Culturist 34:13–17.

Sassmann, R. (1970) Parasiten bekaempfungin Warmwasseranlagen. Deut. Fisch. ZTG. 17(1):8–11.

Savage, J. (1935) Copepod infection of speckled trout. Trans. Am. Fish. Soc. 65:334–339.

Schafer, W.E. (1968) Studies on the epizootiology of the myxosporidan *Ceratomyxa shasta*. Noble, Ca. Fish Game 54:90–99.

Seagrave, C.P., Bucke, D., Hudson, E.B., and McGregor, D. (1981) A survey of the prevalence and distribution of proliferative kidney disease (PKD) in England and Wales. J. Fish Dis. 4:437–439.

Singhal, R.N., Jeet, S., and Davies, R.W. (1984) Ectoparasites of the freshwater food fishes of Haryana India. Proc. Ind. Acad. Sci. Anim. Sci. 93(7):663–670.

Slyezynska-Jurewuz, E. (1959) Expansion of cercariae of *Diplostomum spathaceum* Rudolfi 1819, a common parasite of fishes in the littoral zone of the Lake Polskie. Arch. Hydrobiol. 6:105–116.

Smith, C.E., Morrison, J.K., Ramsey, H.W., and Ferguson, H.W. (1984) Proliferative kidney disease: first reported outbreak in North America. J. Fish Dis. 7:207–216.

Spall, R.D., and Summerfelt, R.C. (1969a) Life cycle of the white grub, *Posthodiplostomum minimum* (MacCallum 1921: Trematoda, Diplostomatidae), and observations on host-parasite relationships of the metacer-

cariae in fish. *In:* A Symposium on Diseases of Fishes and Shellfishes. (Snieszki, S.F., ed.). Special Publication No. 5AFS, pp. 218–230.

Spall, R.D., and Summerfelt R.C. (1969b) Host-parasite relations of certain endoparasitic helminths of the channel catfish and white crappie in an Oklahoma reservoir. Bull. Wildlife Dis. Assoc. 5:48–67.

Sprague, V. (1974) *Nosema conori* N. sp. A microsporidian parasite of Man. Trans. Am. Micros. Soc. 93(3):400–403.

Szidat, L. (1924) Beitrage zur Entuicklingsgeschichte der Hostomiden. Zool. Anz. 61:249–266.

Urawa, S. (1989) Parasites as biological indicators contributing to salmonid biology. Sci. Rep. Hokkaido Salmon Hatchery (43):53–74.

Vahida, I. (1984) Parasites and parasitoses in the fish in salmonid ponds in Bosnia-Hercegovina Yugoslavia. Veterinaria (Sarajevo). 33(3):305–322.

Vlaskino, M.I. (1969) Vstoichivost'tserkarii *Diplostomum spathaceum* Rudolfi 1819, k ul'trafioletovomu izlucheniyu. Parazitologiia 3(5):420–425.

Wales, J.H., and Wolf, H. (1955) Three protozoan diseases of trout in California. Ca. Fish Game 41:183–187.

Whitaker, D.J. (1985) A parasite survey of juvenile chum salmon *Oncorhynchus keta* from the Manaimo River, Canada. Can. J. Zool. 63(12):2875–2877.

Wier, W., Mayberry, L.F., Kinzer, H.G., and Turner, P.R. (1983) Parasites of fishes in the Gila River drainage in southwestern New Mexico, USA. J Wildlife Dis. 19(1):59–60.

Wood, C.C., Rutherford, D.T., and McKinnell, S. (1989) Identification of sockeye salmon *Oncorhynchus nerka* stocks in mixed-stock fisheries in British Columbia, Canada, and southeast Alaska, USA, using biological markers. Can. J. Fish Aquatic Sci. 46(12):2108–2120.

Woodbury, L. (1932) The development of *Diphyllobothrium cordiceps* in *Pelicanus erythrohinchus*. J. Parasitol. 18(4):304–305.

Wootten, R., and Smith, J.W. (1980) Studies on the parasite fauna of juvenile Atlantic salmon, *Salmo salar* L., cultured in freshwater in eastern Scotland. Z. Parasitenkd. 63(3):221–231.

Yamamoto, T., and Sanders, J.E. (1979) Light and electron microscopic observations of sporogenesis in the myxosporidan, *Ceratomyxa shasta* (Noble, 1950). J. Fish Dis. 2:411–428.

Yasutake, W.T., McIntyre, J.D., and Hemmingsen, A.R. (1986) Parasite burdens in experimental families of Coho Salmon *Oncorhynchus kisutch*. Trans. Am. Fish Soc. 115(4):636–640.

Young, M., Purser, G.J., and Al-Mousawi, B. (1987) Infection and successful reinfection of brown trout (*Salmo trutta L.*) with glochidia of *Margaritifera margaritifera* (L.). Presented at Symposium on the Ecology of Freshwater Molluscs, Kingston, RI (USA), 29 July–3 August 1985. Am. Malacol. Union Inc. Bull. 5(1):125–128.

Zinn, J.L., Johnson, K.A., Sanders, J.E., and Fryer, J.L. (1977) Susceptibility of salmonid species and hatchery strains of chinook salmon (*Oncorhynchus tshawytscha*) to infections by *Ceratomyxa shasta*. J. Fish. Res. Bod Can. 34:933–936.

Chapter 40

NEOPLASIA IN SALMONIDS

CHARLIE E. SMITH

Fish, like other vertebrates and invertebrates, develop neoplasms. A neoplasm is an autonomously proliferating population of abnormal cells that usually retain some resemblance to the appearance and pattern of the cell type of origin. The absolute diagnosis of neoplasia rests on histologic examination, since many conditions clinically mimic neoplasia. The classification of tumors is most often based on organ systems and tissues or cells of origin, and whether or not they are benign or malignant (Wellings, 1969; Mawdsley-Thomas, 1972; Budd and Roberts, 1978;

Roberts, 1989). Classification of fish tumors is largely based on mammalian criteria. This chapter describes some of the more common tumors of domesticated and wild salmonids.

EPITHELIAL NEOPLASMS

Hepatic

Probably the most common and well-described neoplasms that have occurred in hatchery-reared salmonids are hepatic neoplasms. These reached epidemic proportions at federal, state, and private trout hatcheries in the United States in the early 1960s. The etiology of this outbreak was traced to the presence of aflatoxin-contaminated cottonseed meal being used as an ingredient in trout feeds. Both hepatic cell and bile duct cell tumors were observed; however, the former was by far the more common.

Grossly, hepatic neoplasms appear as small yellow nodules in young trout but progress into massive multinodular, sometimes cystic, tumors in adult fish. Areas of hemorrhage and necrosis are often dispersed throughout more advanced tumors (Fig. 40–1).

Histologically, early hepatocellular carcinomas occur most often as independent basophilic foci. Cells are usually intensely basophilic, mitotically active, and grouped into cords several cells thick (Fig. 40–2). Nodules may coalesce into hepatocellular carcinomas (Hendricks et al., 1984) consisting of invasive, highly anaplastic tumor cells. Metastases occur but are rare (Ashley and Halver, 1989).

Thyroid

Because of the diffuse nature of the thyroid of salmonids, it is extremely difficult to distinguish thyroid hyperplasia (goiter) from true neoplasia. Epizootic outbreaks of thyroid tumors have been reported from fish hatcheries that apparently resulted from iodine deficiency (Fig. 40–3). Thyroid tumors are now rare in hatcheries, undoubtedly because fish feeds are supplemented with iodine. In addition, thyroid tumors in fish usually regress under the influence of iodine and, therefore, should be classified as goiter (Hayes and Ferguson, 1989). Histologically, the enlarged thyroids in salmonids may be due to epithelial hyperplasia, increased colloid, or much less commonly to inflammatory infiltration.

Goiter has been reported from coho salmon captured in the Great Lakes. A survey of Lakes

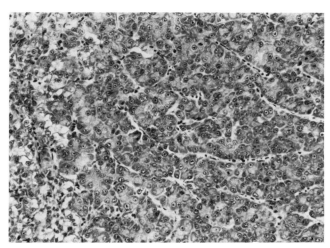

FIGURE 40–2. A well-differentiated hepatocellular carcinoma showing widened cords and basophilic hepatocytes with some normal hepatocytes on the extreme left (H&E, 400×). (Courtesy of J.D. Hendricks.)

Michigan, Ontario, and Erie suggests that the increasing frequency of overt goiter there cannot be attributed to iodine deficiency and may be related to environmental pollutants (Moccia et al., 1977).

Thymus

Thymomas are localized benign tumors of the thymus that arise from thymic epithelium and are composed primarily of epithelial cells. Lymphoid and mucus-secreting goblet cells may also be present. They occur infrequently and do not spread to other tissues. They are most common in lake trout.

Skin

While epidermal tumors are the most common neoplasms of most fishes (Wellings, 1969), they occur

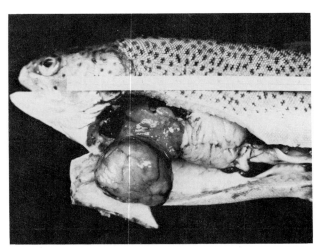

FIGURE 40–1. A massive hepatocellular carcinoma in a rainbow trout. (Courtesy of J.D. Hendricks.)

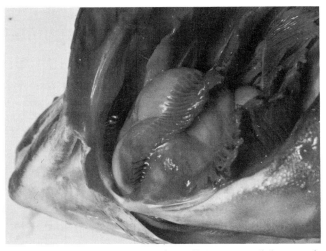

FIGURE 40–3. Thyroid tissue invading gill tissue as nodular growths in a coho salmon from the Great Lakes. (Courtesy of Michigan Department of Natural Resources.)

infrequently in most hatchery-raised and wild salmonids. An exception to this is the high incidence of papillomas and basal cell tumors in masou salmon surviving *Oncorhynchus masou* virus disease (Hayes and Ferguson, 1989), and Atlantic salmon parr where the incidence of epidermal papillomas may be as high as 50% (Roberts, 1989).

Papillomas are benign epithelial neoplasms. They may be small, rounded elevations of the skin, but are more often papillary, with a characteristic cauliflower appearance. In salmonids, many are flattened, and are sometimes referred to as hyperplastic plaques. Fibroepitheliomas are noninvasive tumors that contain both epidermal and dermal elements. Histologically, they resemble an inverted papilloma.

Squamous cell carcinomas are usually reported less frequently than papillomas. They are found mainly on the lips or in the oral cavity and may closely resemble papillomas clinically. Histologically, squamous cell carcinomas in salmonids are often transitions from papillomatous growth. Pegs of closely packed epidermal cells appear as projections through the basement membrane into the dermis, or perhaps as circumscribed nests of epidermal cells within the dermis. Invasion into underlying musculature may occur (Roberts, 1989).

MESENCHYMAL NEOPLASMS

Connective Tissue

The most common mesenchymal neoplasms in salmonids originate from fibroblasts. Benign fibromas are fairly common, whereas malignant fibrosarcomas are rare in both hatchery-raised and wild salmonids. Histologically, fibromas are usually circumscribed and encapsulated and contain mature collagenous connective tissue. Occasionally, mixtures of adipose and collagenous connective tissue can be found together, resulting in fibrolipomas (Figs. 40–4 and 40–5).

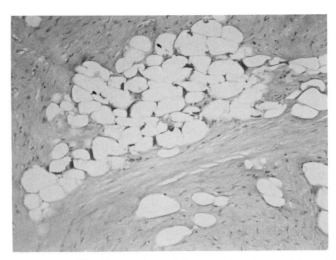

FIGURE 40–5. Fibrolipoma from a lake trout showing a mixture of dense fibrous connective tissue and adipose tissue (H&E, 175×).

Renal

Both nephroblastomas and adenocarcinomas have been diagnosed in fish. Nephroblastomas are by far the most common. Spontaneous nephroblastomas occur quite frequently in hatchery-raised trout. They are most common in fingerlings and yearlings but also occur in adults (Fig. 40–6). Histologically, nephroblastomas show large swirling masses of nephrogenic blastema and areas of epithelial differentation into well-formed tubules (Fig. 40–7). Abortive glomeruli are common.

Hematopoietic

Although primary tumors of the renal hematopoietic tissue are unknown, many widely disseminated fish lymphosarcomas have a conspicuous pres-

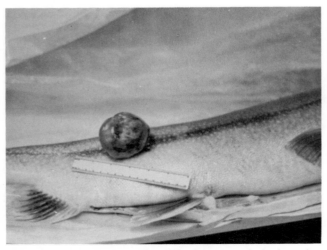

FIGURE 40–4. A large encapsulated fibrolipoma on the body surface of an adult wild lake trout.

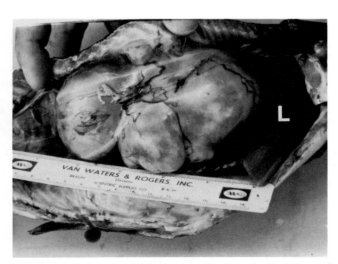

FIGURE 40–6. A large multilobed nephroblastoma in the kidney of an adult rainbow trout. The liver (L) is on the right.

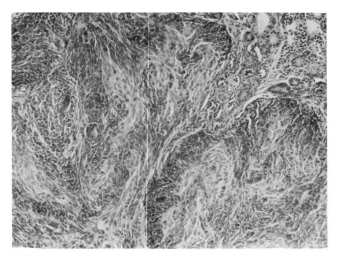

FIGURE 40–7. Nephroblastoma with large swirling masses of basophilic nephrogenic blastema interspersed among poorly differentiated, spindle-shaped tubular epithelium. Normal renal tubules are present in the upper right (H&E, 175×).

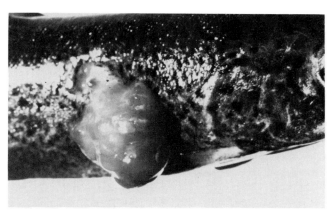

FIGURE 40–9. Hemangioma protruding from the skin of a rainbow trout.

ence in the kidney and may have originated there. Lymphoid tumors in salmonids occur with a much lower frequency than in other species such as pike. Thymic lymphosarcomas, although encountered infrequently, are probably the most common type of lymphosarcomas found in salmonids (Fig. 40–8). Quite often such tumors are leukemic and spread to other tissues, including the kidney, liver, and spleen.

Cardiovascular

Cardiac neoplasms in fish are rare. However, hemangiomas and hemangiosarcomas are relatively common and occur as spontaneoous neoplasms in salmonids. Hemangiomas are probably the most common and develop primarily in the dermis (Fig. 40–9). They are soft, highly vascular tumors. Histo-

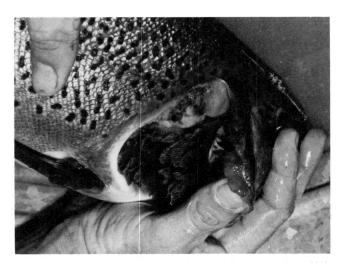

FIGURE 40–8. Large thymic tumor in a rainbow trout broodfish with malignant lymphoma.

logic features include prominent vascular spaces, growth by expansion, and few if any solid nests of endothelial cells.

Hemangiosarcomas usually originate from the subcutaneous layers or underlying musculature, but may also originate in other organs. Grossly, they may be gray to white and often contain areas of hemorrhage. They may be firm or spongy. Histologically, the tumors are composed of spindle-shaped endothelial cells, forming numerous vascular channels. The neoplastic endothelial cells demonstrate extensive nuclear pleomorphism and mitoses are common. Such tumors may be highly invasive but, like most other fish tumors, are generally not metastatic. Giant cells may be present in advanced cases.

Melanomas

Melanomas occur infrequently in salmonids, but they are the neoplasm most likely to metastasize in fish. Most originate in the dermis. Since most melanoma cells have a distinct pigment marker, it is usually quite easy to make an accurate diagnosis. However, amelanotic tumors occur. Melanomas usually are small brown or black lesions, but they can become large and invasive. Histologically, melanomas consist of interlacing bundles of spindle-shaped melanoma cells that generally are heavily laden with melanin pigment and may be highly invasive.

NEURAL NEOPLASMS

Ependymoblastomas

Ependymoblastomas in fish are considered to originate from ectodermal ependymal cells lining the ventricles and spinal canal. There is some thought that the tumors may be neurogenic (neuroblastomas), originating from paraventricular regions, and that invasion into the spinal cord is secondary (Hendricks et al., 1984). Ependymoblastomas have been reported infrequently in salmonids, and then primarily in

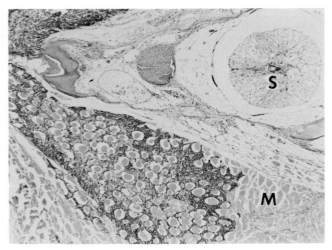

FIGURE 40–10. An ependymoblastoma with basophilic neuroblastic cells enveloping the neural canal and invading adjacent musculature. Note the spinal cord (S) and muscle (M) (H&E, 75×).

young coho salmon in hatcheries (Masahito et al., 1985). Grossly, these tumors are usually large, firm subcutaneous protruding masses that penetrate deep into the underlying musculature. Histologically, they are composed of basophilic, mitotically active, spin-

dle-shaped cells that invade and displace surrounding muscle fibers, often form rosettes, and are usually interspersed with glial fibrillar material (Fig. 40–10).

LITERATURE CITED

Ashley, L.M., and Halver, J.E. (1989) Multiple metastasis in rainbow trout. Trans. Am. Fish. Soc. 92:365–371.

Budd, J., and Roberts, R.J. (1978) Neoplasia in teleosts. In: Fish Pathology (Roberts, R.J., ed.). Bailliere Tindall, London, pp. 105–113.

Hayes, M.A., and Ferguson, H.W. (1989) Neoplasia in fish. In: Systemic Pathology of Fish: A Text and Atlas of Comparative Tissue Responses in Diseases of Teleosts (Ferguson, H.W., ed.). Iowa State University Press, Ames, pp. 230–247.

Hendricks, J.D., Meyers, T.R., and Shelton, D.W. (1984) Histologic progression of hepatic neoplasia in rainbow trout (*Salmo gairdneri*). In: Use of Small Fish in Carcinogen Testing. National Cancer Institute Monograph No. 65, Washington, D.C., pp. 321–336.

Masahito, P.T., Ishikawa, T., Yanagisawa, A., Sugana, H., and Ikeda, K. (1985) Neurogenic tumors in coho salmon (*Oncorhynchus kisutch*) reared in well water in Japan. J. Nat. Cancer Inst. 75:779–790.

Mawdsley-Thomas, L.E. (1972) Some tumors of fish. In: Diseases of Fish (Mawdsley-Thomas, L.E., ed.). Academic Press, New York, pp. 191–283.

Moccia, R.D., Leatherland, J.R., and Sonstegard, R.A. (1977) Increasing frequency of thyroid goiters in coho salmon (Oncorhynchus kisutch) in the Great Lakes. Science 198:425–426.

Roberts, R.J. (ed.) (1989) Neoplasia of teleosts. In: Fish Pathology. 2nd ed., 467 pp. Bailliere Tindall, London, pp. 153–172.

Wellings, S.R. (1969) Neoplasia and primitive vertebrate phylogeny: Echinoderms, prevertebrates, and fishes—a review. Natl. Cancer Inst. Monogr. 31:59–128.

Chapter 41

SALMONID PHARMACOLOGY AND TOXICOLOGY

DOUGLAS P. ANDERSON   FOSTER L. MAYER

Drug treatments, the presence of natural contaminants, and introduced pollutants affect many physiologic aspects of fish health (Herwig, 1979; Anderson et al., 1984; Herman and Bullock, 1986). Their degree of action depends directly or indirectly on environmental factors; therefore, when testing for the effects of drugs, chemicals, or pollutants on fishes, it is important to define the environmental conditions. For example, temperature, pH, and water hardness affect the ionic charge and solubility of drugs and toxicants (Mayer and Ellersieck, 1986). Advances in our understanding of the complex interactions of drugs and chemicals with the environment and fish physiology are occurring constantly. In addition regulations regarding these compounds

change frequently. The best avenue for keeping abreast of developments in drug use and regulation as well as the current thoughts on contaminants, pollutants, and toxicants in fish culture is careful attention to current literature reviews (Bao, 1984; Wood, 1984; Alderman, 1985; Post, 1987; Schnick, 1988).

PHARMACOLOGY

In the United States, the Food and Drug Administration (FDA) controls the use of drugs and chemicals for food fishes. Six categories are used to classify uses: (1) therapeutants—curative, (2) anesthetics, (3) disinfecting agents, (4) water-treatment compounds, (5) herbicides and algicides, and (6) fish control agents (Schnick et al., 1989). The U.S. Environmental Protection Agency (EPA) controls the release of chemicals into the environment and is, therefore, concerned about the release of pharmaceuticals and chemicals from fish farms and aquaculture facilities. The U.S. Department of Agriculture (USDA) approves bacterins and vaccines for use in food fishes. Tables 41–1 and 41–2 give a brief summary of unapproved drugs and disinfectants in common use in current fish culture as classified by application (Klontz, 1988).

Delivery Methods

Drugs are administered to salmonids by external dips, baths, flush exposures, or drip methods (Klontz, 1988). Small fish are often treated by simply holding them in a net and dipping the net into the solution in a container such as a bucket. Bath methods for salmonids are often done by holding the fish in their original raceway or pond and adding the

chemical to a known concentration, exposing the fish to a chemical of a known concentration for a limited time. A flush exposure entails adding the calculated amount of the drug to the head of the raceway and letting the current flow through at a known or regulated volume. The drip, or constant flow, method requires careful regulation of both the addition of the chemical and also the flow of the water volume. This latter method is used for treating salmonid eggs with formalin.

Drugs are also administered with the feed. They are added either at the time of manufacture or coated or mixed immediately before feeding. If individual fish can be handled economically and without damage, injection can be effective and is the most certain way of delivering a precise amount of drug.

Approved Chemicals and Drugs for Treatment in Food Fishes

Chemicals and drugs currently approved by the FDA for therapeutic treatment of salmonid diseases include oxytetracycline, sulfadimethoxine/ormeto-

TABLE 41–1. Topical Drugs (Not Approved by FDA) Used in Treating or Preventing Infectious Diseases in Salmonids

Drug or Chemical	Recommended Dosage	Duration of Exposure	Comments
Acriflavine (mixture of 3,6-diamino-10-methylacridinium chloride and 3,6-diaminoacridine)	0.5 ppt 5 ppm	20 minutes 1–2 hours	For bacterial infections on surface of eggs
Merthiolate Crystals	0.2 ppt	10 minutes	For bacterial infections on surface of eggs
Malachite green	5 ppm	Semiweekly flush	To prevent fungi on eggs (use caution). Environmental hazard
	2 ppm 1 ppm	Semiweekly flush Semiweekly or 3 days on, 3 days off for 1 hour/day	
	66 ppm 1 ppm	20-second dip 1 hour	For external fungal infections of fish For fungi, columnaris, and some protozoa
	0.1 ppm	Pond treatment	
Copper sulfate (CuSO₄)	0.5 ppt 0.5 ppm	1 minute or less Pond treatment	Toxic in soft water For external bacteria, columnaris, etc. Environmental hazard
Potassium permanganate (KMnO₄)	2.5 ppm	4 consecutive days flush	Bacterial gill disease
Diquat (algicide)	50 ppm to 250 ppm	Flush	*Columnaris*, gill disease, trichodina. Not effective in dirty water. Environmental hazard
Acetic acid (C₂H₄O₂)	250 ppm	Flush	Protozoa. *Epistylis.*
Benzalkonium chloride (quarternary ammonium compound)	2 ppm	1 hour	For external bacterial infections
Pyridylmercuric acetate	2 ppm	1 hour	For external bacteria and some parasites. Not to be used on rainbow trout. Environmental hazard
Lignasan (ethyl mercury phosphate)	1 ppm	1 hour	For external bacteria and some parasites. Sometimes toxic to rainbow trout. Environmental hazard
Furanace (nifurpirinol, furpirinol)	1–2 ppm	1 hour	*Columnaris*

TABLE 41–2. Disinfectants Used for Preparation of Ponds Holding Salmonids

Disinfectant	Recommended Dosage	Duration of Treatment	Comments
Chlorine H.T.H.	10 ppm	1 hour	To disinfect equipment, trucks
	1 ppm	24 hours	
Benzalkonium chloride (quarternary ammonium compound)	0.2 ppt	1 hour	To disinfect equipment, trucks
Live steam	Flowing	15 minutes	To disinfect equipment, trucks
Formalin (formaldehyde in water)	1%	15 minutes	To disinfect equipment, trucks

Modified from Klontz, G.W. (1988) Syllabus of Fish Health. Department of Fish and Wildlife Research, University of Idaho, Moscow, Idaho.

prim, formalin, salt (NaCl), and acetic acid. Every fish clinician must be acutely aware of recommended procedures for using these drugs, rules regulating withdrawal before marketing, and disposal of effluents containing chemicals. Since the effects of drugs vary with environmental conditions and predisposition of the individual fish, it is advised to test the drug of choice on a few fish before proceeding to treat large populations.

Oxytetracycline

Oxytetracycline (Terramycin) is approved for the treatment of furunculosis (Aeromonas salmonicida) and other bacterial infections at the dose of 50 to 75 mg/kg fish for a 10-day treatment. The drug becomes bound to the 30S ribosome of the bacterial pathogen and inhibits protein synthesis. When given through the feed, drug is absorbed through the intestine, and accumulated in the highest concentrations in the liver and muscle. While the tetracyclines are the most commonly used antibiotics in fish, a noted precaution is that oxytetracycline has been reported to have immunosuppressive effects. Avoid administering the antibiotic before or during immunization regimens (Grondel et al., 1987).

After food fish have been treated with oxytetracycline, there is a required withdrawal time of 21 days before the fish can be killed for human consumption. The drug has a high therapeutic index for salmonids and under hatchery conditions it would be difficult to feed lethal levels to them (Herman, 1969). Injection of high doses (250 mg/kg) has caused deaths in 5-g sockeye and 10-g chinook salmon (Weber and Ridgway, 1962). The stress of high doses may cause darkening and ascites in salmonids similar to what is described in carp (Schäperclaus, 1958). These antibiotics and others can persist in marine sediments, especially under anoxic conditions, which they may help create (Barinaga, 1990). The estimated half-life of oxytetracycline under such conditions is about 10 weeks (Jacobsen and Berglind, 1988). There are also concerns that antibiotic resistance to tetracycline could be transferred to human pathogens in the water column.

Sulfadimethoxine/Ormetoprim

Sulfadimethoxine/ormetoprim (Romet) is approved by the FDA for the treatment of Aeromonas

salmonicida. Sulfadimethoxine is an antagonist of dihydrofolic acid biosynthesis. Susceptible bacteria are unable to absorb dihydrofolic acid. Ormetoprim, a sequential dihydrofolic reductase blocker, potentiates the sulfonamide, since two physiologic steps are blocked. Romet 30 as a mixture is often incorporated into commercial trout feed marketed for administration to salmonids against A. salmonicida. Fish cannot be processed for market until 42 days have elapsed since the last administration. Several studies have shown that elimination of the drug may depend on environmental temperature (Alderman, 1985). Normally the drug is given in the feed at the rate of 50 mg/kg of fish/day for 5 days. The drug accumulates in the liver, kidneys, and blood (Herman and Bullock, 1986). Sulfamerazine at a dose of 33 g/100 kg biomass daily is also used to treat Renibacterium salmoninarum in carrier spawning salmonids, but this protocol is not approved for use.

Formalin

Formalin is often used in salmonid culture for the treatment of external protozoan infections or as a fungicide on eggs. A concentration of 250 ppm formalin (37% formaldehyde in water), either as a static bath or a flow-through treatment is commonly used. Formaldehyde can be carcinogenic at high doses to both fish and mammals (Takahashi et al., 1986). Clinicians and fish culturists should avoid breathing fumes or having skin contact with this commonly used chemical.

MS–222

MS–222 (tricaine methane sulfonate) is commonly used to anesthetize salmonids. There is currently a 21-day withdrawal time before marketing fish after the single use of the drug. Benzocaine, which can be used at lower concentrations, is a replacement candidate; however, it has not been approved for general use.

Iodophors

Iodophors (Betadine, Wescodyne) are used to disinfect fish facilities and work tools. Iodophors are also used for disinfecting the surface of trout and salmon eggs (Amend, 1974). There is a greater mortality in fry from eggs exposed to idophors during water hardening, and while the killing effect of the treatment is well documented in vitro against *Renibacterium salmoninarum*, it is believed that some bacteria escape by being centered in cell aggregates (Evelyn et al., 1986).

Drugs and Chemicals Not Approved for Use with Food Fishes

Many other drugs sometimes used in aquaculture and fish farming are not approved for use in salmonid culture. The U.S. Fish and Wildlife Service leaflets from the National Fisheries Research Center, Technical Information Services, Kearneysville, Wyoming 25430, is a source of information on recent developments in specific diseases and of drug registration. The following are some candidate drugs presently under investigation for efficacy and safety.

Erythromycin

Erythromycin, a macrolide antibiotic originally produced by *Streptomyces erythreus*, inhibits synthesis of bacterial protein. Currently, in the United States, the drug has a special INAD (investigational new animal drug) permit with the FDA for use in feed at 0.1 mg/kg fish weight for prespawning salmonids infected with *Renibacterium salmoninarum* (Bullock and Leek, 1986). By feeding the adults erythromycin, vertical transmission of the bacteria may be reduced. Injection of 11 mg/kg fish weight of erythromycin could reduce the mortality of the adults and increase the chances of successful spawning when these fish have to be held until ripe (Klontz, 1983). The presence of erythromycin during water hardening of eggs to prevent or reduce the numbers of *R. salmoninarum* has also been tried with varying success.

Quinolones

Quinolones, including sarafloxacin, oxolinic acid, nalidixic acid, piromidic acid, enrofloxacin, and flumequine, are synthetic drugs that interfere with nucleic acid replication in bacteria by preventing deoxyribonucleic acid (DNA) supercoiling (Fig. 41–1A–D). Oxolinic acid is registered for use in Japan and some European countries for the control of *Aeromonas salmonicida* and *Yersinia ruckeri* (Schnick, 1988). *Aeromonas salmonicida* was controlled in rainbow trout by feeding at 12 and 24 mg/kg body weight per day for 6 days during the time of challenge (Michel et al., 1981). A greater amount of information on the administration of the quinolones exists for fishes other than salmonids. These drugs are highly effective against many bacteria and have low toxicity.

Chloramine-T

Chloramine-T (sodium *p*-toluenesulfonchloramide) is a candidate compound for use in salmonids for controlling bacterial gill diseases and protozoan

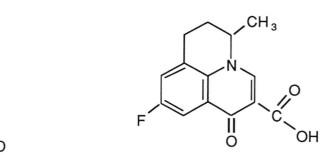

FIGURE 41–1. Quinolone antibiotics used in fish. *A.* Oxolinic acid. *B.* Nalidixic acid. *C.* Piromidic acid. *D.* Flumequine.

infections of the skin and gills. The effectiveness depends somewhat on environmental conditions, including, pH, water fecal content, and specifically temperature (Rach et al., 1988).

Malachite Green

Malachite green, *N*-[4-[[4(dimethylamino)-phenyl]phenylmethylene]-2,5-cyclohexadien-1-ylidene]-

N-methylmethanaminium chloride, long recognized by fish biologists as an effective fungicide, is also a demonstrated teratogen (Meyer and Jorgenson, 1983) (Fig. 41–2). Because of the effectiveness of malachite green in controlling external fungal infections, the drug has been given an INAD for certain species at selected hatcheries (Schnick, 1988). Malachite green also has been found effective in treating proliferative kidney disease (Clifton-Hadley and Anderman, 1988).

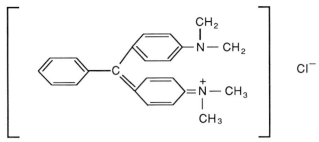

FIGURE 41–2. Malachite green.

TOXICOLOGY

Although acute toxicity tests were first reported in 1863, using the goldfish, the development of standard methods for studying toxicity in salmonids and other fishes is an intensive new area of investigation (Neff, 1985; Hunn, 1989). Acute toxicity rating scales show the marked differences in susceptibility among different animals (Table 41–3).

Sources of Toxicants

Many natural as well as human-influenced environments are disadvantageous to salmonids. As farms, manufacturing plants, and cities have grown along important migratory waterways, salmonid populations are often stressed and their numbers reduced. However, pinpointing those specific contaminants in the aquatic environment, and correlating their effects on fish populations, is often difficult. In many cases, mortalities or toxic signs may not be immediately apparent because predators eliminate the evidence. A list of pesticides, herbicides, and other possible pollutants that affect salmonids is given in Table 41–4.

The effects of toxicants are often suspected when dead fish are found in the environment. That a certain chemical caused the mortalities in the field has to be proven by careful correlation of field and laboratory tests. Sentinel fish placed in cages can be used to monitor the presence of toxicants, but a toxicant is only implicated by these tests. Further tests in the laboratory are necessary to determine specific chemical exposures and identify with certainty the chemical responsible for mortalities or sublethal toxicity.

Subacute chemical stress of fishes may be more difficult to detect and verify than mortalities. Changes in size of the fish, coloring of organs, and other physical features can indicate a toxic situation. Physiologic indicators might include changes in the hematocrit, leukocrit, or differential cell counts.

To some degree, aquatic toxicants have always been present in the environment of salmonids. Natural leaching of heavy metals from the earth into the rivers is well documented. This phenomenon can be exacerbated by mining activity (Hamilton, 1986). Also, heavy concentrations of particulate matter in aquatic environments compromise fish. This was dramatically shown by the effects of the heavy sediment load carried by rivers after the eruption of Mt. St. Helens in Washington state (Newcomb and Flagg, 1983). Lakes containing high concentrations of tannin in the water also tend to produce less plankton and fish biomass and the water may be highly acidic. The presence of natural seeps of oil is common along some coastal areas and is sometimes confused with human-caused spills.

Pollution of salmonid habitats is a serious but often repairable problem. Manufacturing plants located along rivers for the convenience of transportation and water availability can release particulate and chemical pollution. Wood-processing plant effluents are now carefully regulated in many areas to prevent high concentrations of pollutants from entering the drainage (Lindesjöö and Thulin, 1987).

TABLE 41–3. Acute Toxicity Rating Scales (ppm) for Aquatic, Avian, and Mammalian Species

Relative Toxicity	Aquatic EC or LC_{50} (mg/L)	Avian LC_{50} (mg/kg food)	Mammalian LD_{50} (mg/kg body weight)
Supertoxic	<0.01	—	<5
Extremely toxic	0.01–0.1	<40	5–50
Highly toxic	0.1–1	40–200	50–500
Moderately toxic	1–10	200–1000	500–5000
Slightly toxic	10–100	1000–5000	5000–15,000
Practically nontoxic	100–1000	>5000	>15,000
Relatively harmless	>1000	—	—

From Mayer, K.S., and Multer, E. (1984). U.S. Dept. of Interior, Fish and Wildlife Service Leaflet, Washington, D.C.

TABLE 41–4. Relative Acute Toxicities to Rainbow Trout of Pesticides, Herbicides, and Other Common Farming and Industrial Chemicals

Supertoxic (<0.01 ppm)	Extremely Toxic (0.01–0.1 ppm)	Highly Toxic (0.1–1.0 ppm)	Moderately Toxic (1–10 ppm)	Slightly Toxic (10–100 ppm)	Practically Toxic (100–1000 ppm)	Relatively Harmless (>1000 ppm)
Antimycin A	Captafol	Aldicarb	Alachlor	Acephate	Chlorowax 500C	
Aldrin	Chlordane	Benomyl	Benthiocarb	Aminocarb	Fire-trol 100	
Asinphos methyl	Chlordane-HCS-3260	Carbofuran	Carbaryl	Diflubensuron	Fire-trol 931	
DDT	Chlordecone	Chlorpyrifos-Methyl	Chlorendate Dimethyl	Merphos	Hexasinone	
Dieldrin	Chlorpyrifos	Demeton	D-D Soil	Mexicarbate	Phos-chek 25	
Endosulfan	D-*trans* Allethrin	Ethofumesate	Fumigant (EDB)	Pydraul 115E	Ureabor	
Fenvalerate	DDD	Fenthion	DEF	Silvex Acid		
Heptachlor	Dilan	MBC	Dichlobenil	2,4-D/2, 4,5-T		
Permethrin	Dinocap	Naled	Dimethoate			
Toxaphene	Fluchloralin	Ovex	Diuron			
	Leptophos	PCB (Aroclor)	Emcol AD-410			
	Lindane	Phosmet	Fenitrothion			
	Methoxychlor	Phoxim	Flamprop-Methyl			
	Phorate	Ronnel	Fluometuron			
	Profenofos	Trichlorfon	Fluridone			
	Pyrethrum		Fyrquel GT			
	Sodium pentachlorophenate		Glyphosate			
	Terbufos		Houghto-safe 1120			
	Trifluralin		Kronitex 200			
			Methomyl			
			Methyparathion			
			MON 0818			
			Neodol 25-9			
			Nitrapyrin			
			Oxamyl			
			Oxydemeton-Methyl			
			Parathion			
			Phosflex 31P			
			Phthalate Dibutyl			
			Piperonyl Butoxide			
			Ryania			
			Santicizer 154			
			Temephos			
			Tetradifon			
			2,4-D-Dodecyl/ Tetradodecylamine Salt			
			2,4-DB			

Tests performed under standard conditions at CNFRL (American Society for Testing and Materials ASTM E729-80).

Salmonids in Toxicity Testing

Relative Sensitivity

Rainbow trout is one of the four species of choice in toxicity testing, mainly because of its sensitivity. Four aquatic species are most commonly tested, daphnids, rainbow trout, fathead minnows, and bluegills. Testing sensitivity is often greatly increased by testing both daphnids and rainbow trout, since together they are more sensitive than the other two species 93% of the time and the LC_{50}s for rainbow trout are rarely significantly higher ($P \leq 0.05$) than those of fathead minnows or bluegills.

Frequency Distribution of Chemical Toxicity

Frequency distribution of the lethal concentration for 50% of the tested fish (LC_{50}) is bimodal with most species, including rainbow trout. Insecticides are mainly in the less than or equal to 1000 μg/L category, and herbicides, fungicides, industrial, and other chemicals are usually in the greater than or equal to 1000 μg/L categories (Fig. 41–3). Insecticides occurring in the lower mode are mainly botanicals and organochlorines with some carbamates and organophosphates. The higher mode consists mainly of herbicides and industrials. For rainbow trout the range of toxicities among chemicals is 9 orders of

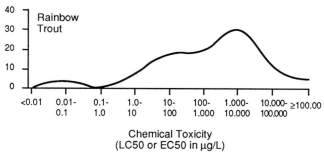

FIGURE 41–3. Toxicity distribution of 286 tests with 184 chemicals for rainbow trout (Mayer and Ellersieck, 1986). The y-axis represents the percentage frequency of LC$_{50}$s occurring within a toxicity range, and the x-axis represents the toxicity range.

magnitude. Table 41–4 lists relative acute toxicities to rainbow trout of pesticides, herbicides, and other common farming and industrial chemicals.

Life Stage and Size

Analysis of yolk-sac and swim-up fry of salmonids exposed to 11 chemicals indicates swim-up fry are most sensitive 70% of the time and yolk-sac fry 20%. Fry are generally less sensitive than yolk-sac and swim-up fry. The eyed-egg stage is often the least sensitive stage. Although eggs are generally the least susceptible stage, several exceptions exist. For example, the egg stage is more resistant than fry to two mercurials (Akiyama, 1970).

Toxicants

Heavy Metals

Heavy metals, including copper, aluminum, cadmium, and mercury, in water supplies are adverse to salmonid health. Studies have shown that salmonids held in low dilutions of copper become more susceptible to infectious diseases (Hetrick et al., 1979). These metals may make fish more susceptible by supressing the immune system (Robohm et al., 1979). Lead, copper, and cadmium are immunosuppressive when injected into brown trout (O'Neill, 1981). Studies of metallothionein concentrations in brook trout livers show this enzyme has a homeostatic function for detoxification of heavy metals (Hamilton and Mehrle, 1987).

Pesticides

The increased use of pesticides in the environment for the control of farm and forest insect infestation is the serious concern of fisheries and requires international cooperation (Food and Agriculture Organization of the United Nations, 1986). Methomyl, carbaryl, aminocarb, trichlorfon, fenitrothion, and acephate, all pesticides considered for forest use, are generally more toxic to instar daphnids, mature amphipods, and fourth instar midge larvae than salmonids (Sanders et al., 1983).

Herbicides

The increased use of herbicides in farming and intensive gardening leads to the problems of these chemicals leaching into surface and ground water, killing phytoplankton and zooplankton and depleting sources on the food chain for fish. The chemicals may also directly harm the fish themselves. Most widely used herbicides, such as glyphosate (Roundup) (Fig. 41–4) and benthiocarb (Bolero), have low to intermediate toxicities for rainbow trout. Also, the fish tend to avoid these chemicals, if possible. Fifty percent of rainbow trout exposed to 52 to 54.8 mg/L glyphosate die in 96 hours (Sullivan et al., 1982). Benthiocarb, used in rice culture, is equally toxic at exposures of 1.2 to 2.3 mg/L for these fish (Sanders and Hunn, 1982). The formation of breakdown products of many of the herbicides and pesticides remains to be fully studied. Farmers and gardeners should read labels carefully before use and take precautions against overuse because herbicide toxicity can range from extremely toxic to practically nontoxic. Also, the toxicity of different formulations of the same chemical can vary considerably.

Oncogenic Agents

The presence of tumors in fish in the wild has been reported on both the east and the west coasts of the United States (Malins et al., 1984; Myers et al., 1987; Murchelano and Wolke, 1985), and the occurrence is often linked to the presence of organic pollutants. Reports on monitoring fish health in the environment note the presence of tumors. For instance, epidermal tumors on fish are not unusual in polluted estuaries such as the New York bight (Stolen et al., 1983). Because of the environmental complexity, however, it is difficult to pinpoint the actual chemical or synergistic moeities responsible for the neoplasms. The best-documented oncogenic agent in salmonids is aflatoxin (Sinnhuber et al., 1968). Salmonids are surprisingly sensitive indicators for the presence of aflatoxins.

Other Contaminants Affecting Salmonids

Polychlorinated debenzodioxins and polychlorinated dibenzofurans are formed as trace contaminants in many commercial products. The compounds have been found in estuarine sediments, and being lipophilic, concentrate in fatty fish tissues (Mehrle and Petty, 1987). Polychlorinated biphenyls, found most commonly in electrical transformers, are less toxic. Low exposures may be actually making sal-

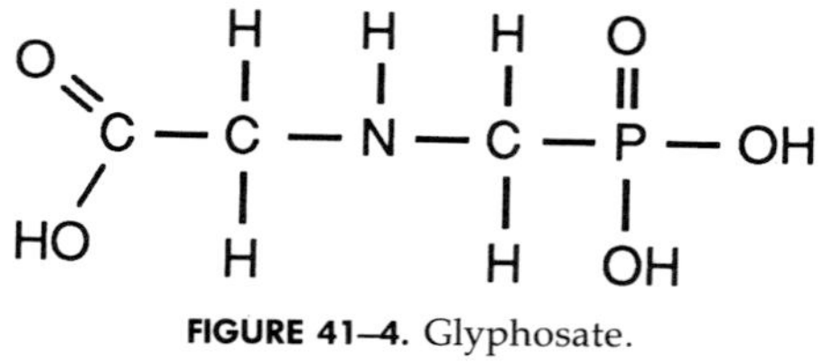

FIGURE 41–4. Glyphosate.

monids more resistant to infectious disease challenges, but higher exposures lower their resistance (Mayer et al., 1985).

Acid rain, a serious problem in industrial nations, has eroded fishing environments. The lessening of acidic aerosols by treating factory effluents has reduced this damage, but in most cases, many years are needed to restore the environment for salmonid habitation. Salmonids survive in a range of pH 5 to 9, dependent upon other environmental factors (Mayer and Schreiber, 1985).

LITERATURE CITED

Akiyama, A. (1970) Acute toxicity of two organic mercury compounds to the teleost, *Oryzias latipes*, in different stages of development. Bull. Jpn. Soc. Sci. Fishes 36:563–570.

Alderman, D.J. (1985) Fisheries chemotherapy: a review. Rec. Adv. Aquaculture 3:1–61.

Amend, D.F. (1974) Comparative toxicity of two iodophors to rainbow trout eggs. Trans. Am. Fish. Soc. 103:73–78.

Anderson, D.P., van Muiswinkel, W.B., and Roberson, B.S. (1984) Effects of chemically induced immune modulation on infectious diseases of fish. Prog. Clin. Biol. Res. 161:188–208.

Bao, D. (1984) Disease prevention and control. Some remarks on the disease therapy of freshwater fish. Aquarium 7:39–46.

Barinaga, M. (1990) Fish, money, and science in Puget Sound. Science 247:631.

Bullock, G.L., and Leek, S.L. (1986) Use of erythromycin in reducing vertical transmission of bacterial kidney disease. Vet. Hum. Toxicol. 28(Suppl. 1):18–20.

Clifton-Hadley, R.S., and Anderman, D.J. (1988) The green answer to PKD. Fish Farmer 11:18–19.

Evelyn, T.P.T., Prosperi-Porta, L., and Ketcheson, J.E. (1986) Persistence of the kidney-disease bacterium, *Renibacterium salmoninarum*, in coho salmon, *Oncorhynchus kisutch* (Walbaum), eggs treated during and after water-hardening with povidone-iodine. J. Fish Dis. 9:461–464.

Food and Agriculture Organization of the United Nations (1986). International code of conduct on the distribution and use of pesticides. Rome, Italy.

Grondel, J.L., Nouws, J.F.M., DeJong, M., Schutte, J.R., and Driessens, F. (1987) Pharmacokinetics and tissue distribution of oxytetracycline in carp, *Cyprinus carpio* L., following different routes of administration. J. Fish Dis. 10:153–163.

Hamilton, S.J. (1986) Trace elements from placer mining in Alaskan streams are toxic to young salmonids. U.S. Fish and Wildlife Service, Research Information Bulletin 86–98.

Hamilton, S.J., and Mehrle, P.M. (1987) Cadmium-saturation technique for measuring metallothionein in brook trout. Trans. Am. Fish. Soc. 116:541–550.

Herman, R.L. (1969) Oxytetracycline in fish culture—a review. In: Ten Papers on Oxytetracycline and Fish. Technical papers of the Bureau of Sport Fisheries and Wildlife, Department of the Interior, pp. 3–9.

Herman, R.L., and Bullock, G.L. (1986) Antimicrobials and fish: A review of drugs used to treat bacterial diseases of channel catfish and rainbow trout. Vet. Hum. Toxicol. 28(Suppl. 1):11–17.

Herwig, N. (1979) Handbook of Drugs and Chemicals Used in the Treatment of Fish Diseases. Charles C Thomas, Springfield, Illinois.

Hetrick, F.M., Knittel, M.D., and Fryer, J.L. (1979) Increased susceptibility of rainbow trout to infectious hematopoietic necrosis virus after exposure to copper. Appl. Environ. Microbiol. 37:198–201.

Hunn, J.B. (1989) History of acute toxicity tests with fish 1863–1867. U.S. Fish and Wildlife Service, Investigations in Fish Control 98.

Jacobsen, P., and Berglind, L. (1988) Persistence of oxytetracycline in sediments from fish farms. Aquaculture 70:365–370.

Klontz, G.W. (1983) Bacterial kidney disease in salmonids: an overview. In: Antigens of Fish Pathogens. (Anderson, D. P., Dorson, M., and Dubourget, P., eds). Fondation Marcel Merieux, Lyon, France, pp. 177–200.

Klontz, G.W. (1988) Syllabus of Fish Health. Department of Fish and Wildlife Research, University of Idaho, Moscow.

Lindesjöö, E. and Thulin, J. (1987) Fin erosion of perch (*Perca fluviatilis*) in a pulp mill effluent. Bull. Euro. Assoc. Fish Pathologists 7:11–14.

Malins, D.C., McCain, B.B., Brown, D.W., Chan, S.-L., Myers, M.S., Landahl, J.T., Prohaska, P.G., Friedman, A.J., Rhodes, L.D., Burrows, D.G., Gronlund, W.D., and Hodgins, H.O. (1984) Chemical pollutants in sediments and diseases of bottom-dwelling fish in Puget Sound, Washington. Environ. Sci. Technol. 18:705–713.

Mayer, F.L., Jr., and Ellersieck, M.R. (1986) Manual of acute toxicity: Interpretation and data base for 410 chemicals and 66 species of freshwater animals. U.S. Fish and Wildlife Service, Resource Publication 160.

Mayer, K.S., and Schreiber, R.K. (1985) Acid rain: effects on fish and wildlife. U.S. Fish and Wildlife Services Leaflet 1, Washington, D.C.

Mayer, K.S., Mayer, F.L., and Witt, A., Jr. (1985) Waste transformer oil and PCB toxicity to rainbow trout. Trans. Am. Fish. Soc. 114:869–886.

Mehrle, P., and Petty, J. (1987) Dioxin (TCDD) and furan (TCDF) toxicity to rainbow trout. U.S. Fish and Wildlife Service Research Information Bulletin 87–55.

Meyer, F.P., and Jorgenson, T.A. (1983) Teratological and other effects of malachite green on development of rainbow trout and rabbits. Trans. Am. Fish. Soc. 112:818–824.

Michel, C., Gerad, J.P., Fourbet, B., Collas, R., and Chevalier, R. (1981) Emploi de la flumequine contra la furunculose des salmonides: essais therapeutiques et perspectives pratiques. Bull. Fr. Piscicult. 277:154–162.

Murchelano, R.A., and Wolke, R.E. (1985) Epizootic carcinoma in the winter flounder, *Pseudopleuronectes americanus*. Science 228:587–589.

Myers, M.S., Rhodes, L.D., and McCain, B.B. (1987) Pathologic anatomy and patterns of occurrence of hepatic neoplasms, putative preneoplastic lesions, and other idiopathic hepatic conditions in English sole (*Parophrys vetulus*) from Puget Sound, Washington. J. Natl Cancer Inst. 78:333–363.

Neff, J.M. (1985) Use of biochemical measurements to detect pollutant-mediated damage to fish. Aquatic Toxicology and Hazard Assessment: Seventh Symposium, ASTM STP 854, R.D.

Newcomb, T.W., and Flagg, T.A. (1983) Some effects of Mt. St. Helens volcanic ash on juvenile salmon smolts. Marine Fish. Rev. 45(2):8–12.

O'Neill, J.G. (1981) The humoral immune response of *Salmo trutta* L. and *Cyprinus carpio* L. exposed to heavy metals. J. Fish Biol. 19:297–306.

Post, G. (1987) Textbook of Fish Health. 2nd ed. T.F.H. Publications, Neptune, New Jersey.

Rach, J.J., Bills, T.B., and Marking, L.L. (1988) Effects of physical and chemical factors on the toxicity of chloramine-T. U.S. Fish and Wildlife Service Research Information Bulletin 88–69.

Robohm, R.A., Brown, C., and Murchelano, R.A. (1979) Comparison of antibodies in marine fish from clean and polluted waters of the New York bight: relative levels against 36 bacteria. Appl. Environ. Microbiol. 38:248–257.

Sanders, H.O., and Hunn, J.B. (1982) Toxicity, bioconcentration and depuration of the herbicide Bolero 8EC in freshwater invertebrates and fish. Bull. Jpn. Soc. Sci. Fishes 48:1139–1143.

Sanders, H.O., Finley, M.T., and Hunn, J.B. (1983) Acute toxicity of six forest insecticides to three aquatic invertebrates and four fishes. U.S. Fish and Wildlife Service Technical Paper 110.

Schäperclaus, W. (1958) Bewahrung des Chlornitrins in der teichwirtschaftlichen Praxis und neue Versuche uber die Anwendbarkeit weiter Breitspektrum-Antibiotica bei der Bankampfung der infectiosen Bachwassersucht des Karpfens. Zeitschrift fur Fischerei, Hilfswissenschaften, VII N. F. Heft 7/8:509–628.

Schnick, R.A. (1988) The impetus to register new therapeutants for aquaculture. Progressive Fish Culturist 50:190–196.

Schnick, R.A., Meyer, F.P., and Gray, D.L. (1989) A guide to approved chemicals in fish production and fishery resource management. A cooperative publication of the U.S. Fish and Wildlife Service and the Univeristy of Arkansas, Cooperative Extension Service, Little Rock, Arkansas.

Sinnhuber, R.O., Wales, J.H., Ayres, J.L., Engebrecht, R.H., and Amend, D.L. (1968) Dietary factors and hepatoma in rainbow trout (*Salmo gairdneri*). I. Aflatoxins in vegetable protein feedstuffs. J. Natl. Cancer Inst. 41:711–718.

Stolen, J.S., Kasper, V., Gahn, T., and Lipcon, V. (1983) Monitoring environmental pollution in marine fishes by immunological technique. Biotechnology 1:1–8.

Sullivan, D.S., Hildebrand, L.D., and Sullivan, T.P. (1982) Experimental studies of rainbow trout populations exposed to field applications of Roundup herbicide. Arch. Environ. Contam. 11:93–98.

Takahashi, M., Hasegawa, R., and Furukawa, F. (1986) Effects of ethanol, potassium metabisulfite, formaldehyde and hydrogen peroxide on gastric carcinogenesis in rats after initiation with N-methyl-N-nitroso-N'-nitroguanidine. Jpn. J. Cancer Res. 77:118–124.

Weber, D.D., and Ridgway, G.J. (1962) The deposition of tetracycline drugs in bones and scales of fish and its possible use for marking. Progressive Fish Culturist 24:150–155.

Wood, J.W. (1984) Diseases of Pacific salmon their prevention and treatment. State of Washington, Department of Fisheries Hatchery Division, Olympia.

Section III

Goldfish, Koi, and Carp

MICHAEL K. STOSKOPF, *Section Editor*

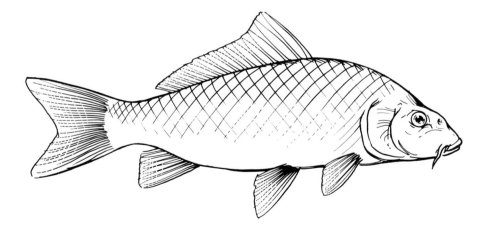

Chapter 42

CARP, KOI, AND GOLDFISH TAXONOMY AND NATURAL HISTORY

BRUCE G. HECKER

Carp, koi, and goldfish belong to the family Cyprinidae (the minnows and carps). With about 194 genera and 2070 species, it is the largest family of fishes (Nelson, 1984). Cyprinids have the widest continuous distribution of any freshwater fish family. The greatest diversity and the most advanced cyprinids occur in Southeast Asia, which is thought to be the center of origin of the family (Berra, 1981). The cyprinids' ecologic equivalents in South America are the characins, and in Australia, the rainbow fishes. Many cyprinid species have been introduced around the world, where they exist in the wild and are considered pests.

The carps are a morphologically diverse family, and species size can range from a few centimeters to over 2.5 meters. Carp, koi, and goldfish have no teeth in their jaws. Their lips are usually thin and are without plicae or papillae. The upper jaw is bordered only by the premaxilla. Fins are soft, except in a few genera where the soft rays are fused, spinelike, in the dorsal fin. There is no adipose fin. Sensory barbels around the mouth are present in some species. Scales are cycloid, covering the body. A lateral line is usually present. In breeding condition, males may intensify their coloration and some may develop tubercles on various regions of the head, body, and fins.

The cyprinids are capable of existing in a wide variety of conditions: shallow rocky riffles, quiet vegetated ponds, clear cold streams, and turbid silty rivers. They are frequently intolerant of salt water. As a largely temperate family, they are able to handle wide temperature fluctuations. Grass carp can handle 0 to 35°C over the course of the year. Most are omnivores, with some species carnivores, and others herbivores.

CARP

A larger cyprinid, carp are high-backed stout-bodied fish averaging 45 cm long and weighing an average of 5.5 kg. Exceptional fish weigh up to 26.4 kg (Scott and Crossman, 1973). Carp are distin-

guished by a long snout, triangular head, and two pairs of barbels, with the most conspicuous pair at the corners of the mouth (Fig. 42–1). Scales are large and thick, occasionally enlarged and scattered (mirror carp) or absent (leather carp). Their color is variable. Adults are usually olive-green to brown on the back, becoming yellow on the belly. The lower half of the caudal and anal fins are often colored with a reddish hue. Wild carp occasionally mutate to red and blue colors, and through selective breeding colored strains have been developed.

Native to temperate Eurasia, wild carp occur in many types of water, and over many types of substrates. Intentionally introduced into North American waters in the mid-1800s, carp are now widely distributed, even occurring in some brackish waters along the American coast. Carp are considered pests in the New World because of their habits of uprooting plant growth and stirring up the bottom while feeding, creating turbidity and siltation problems. In some areas, they are commercially fished and processed for human consumption.

Carp can hybridize with goldfish, as has happened in the Great Lakes area. Hybrids become difficult to identify, because their parental characters blend. Carp are omnivores and consume a variety of plant and animal tissues. Aquatic insects, crustaceans, annelids, and mollusks are prominent among animal foods eaten. Plant foods include weeds, tree seeds, wild rice, aquatic plants, and algae. Carp will

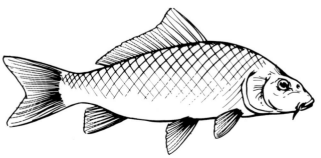

FIGURE 42–1. Common carp.

also feed by sucking up mouthfuls of bottom ooze and detritus, expelling it into the water and selecting food items (Scott and Crossman, 1973).

Spawning takes place for several weeks in spring and early summer as the water warms to about 17°C. Adults move into weedy or grassy shallows in large groups, often near the surface. They gradually form smaller groups with each female accompanied by two or three males. Spawning usually occurs on warm, sunny mornings with the fish splashing about at the water surface. At warmer temperatures, around 26°C, spawning declines and stops. Carp are a prolific species, laying from 36,000 to 2,200,000 eggs, depending on the spawner's size (Scott and Crossman, 1973). Eggs are 1 mm in diameter and are randomly deposited. They are adhesive and stick to weeds, grasses, and roots. Hatching takes place 3 to 6 days after fertilization, depending on water temperatures. Maturity in males is reached at 3 or 4 years and in females at 4 or 5 years. The normal life span of the wild carp seldom seems to exceed 20 years. Carp have keen eyesight and are a wary species, although they are well protected by their heavy scales. Predation by wild animals is mostly on the smaller younger fish.

KOI

Koi are colorful domestic mutations of the common carp, and thus are classified in the same genus and species, *Cyprinus carpio*. Similar to wild carp, the koi body is more elongate (Fig. 42–2). Carp mutations were first recorded in Persia and China around 500 B.C. By A.D. 200, they had come to Japan where they have become immensely popular. Koi presently are bred in Japan, North America, western Europe, Israel, and Singapore.

Koi can attain a maximum size of 70 to 95 cm. They are fast growing, reaching 17.5 cm at 1 year, 30 cm at 2 years, and 40 cm or more at 3 years (Caswell, 1988). Life expectancy in good environmental conditions can be as long as 60 years (James, 1985).

Breeding behavior is similar to that of the common carp. Selective crossbreedings with German carp have resulted in a line of highly metallic mutations with either no scales or very large scales. Left on their own, koi can revert to common carp morphology in two or three generations; every spawning usually results with a few ancestral throwbacks.

Like wild carp, koi are omnivorous, and in captivity are normally fed twice a day. They can be offered processed food such as flakes or, most often, pellets that are made especially for koi (see Chap. 46). Koi can be hard on plants because of their persistent rooting habits. Valuable plants should be planted in tubs, which are then placed in the pool.

Because koi are large, they need to be kept in larger water systems, preferably ponds. These ponds or pools are usually made from concrete, fiber glass, or flexible plastic liners, where the koi can be seen and judged from above, Japanese style. Kept outside in temperate climates, minimum depth should be 1.3 to 1.7 m, or 30 cm below the winter frost line in order to keep the fish in unfrozen water. A good pump, waterfall, or heater should be left on in order to keep the pond from skinning over with ice and preventing oxygenation. Basically a rugged fish, koi thrive in temperatures of 2 to 30°C. Below 7°C, koi begin to hibernate by slowing down their activity and staying low in the water column. It is not recommended to feed koi once the temperature drops below 10°C (James, 1985). The optimum temperature for koi is cool, around 16° to 24°C. These cooler temperatures provide the best coloration.

There are 14 variety classifications of koi currently recognized in most of the world; however, there are over 100 color patterns, which do not necessarily breed true. The varieties, grouped into the nonmetallic koi, and the metallic koi, are listed in Table 42–1 along with their typical color patterns. In addition to color patterns, koi are separated on the basis of scale type. In addition to the normal scales, there are pearl scales that are thickened and have a solid sparkling area in their center. Three variations of flat scales are recognized: beta-gin, where the whole surface of the scale shimmers; diamond ginrin, where the entire scale sparkles; and kado-gin, where only the edges of the scale shimmer.

In shows, koi are judged in size groups. Outside

TABLE 42–1. Koi Classifications

Nonmetallic Koi	
Kohaku	White with red markings
Taisho sanke	White with red and black
Showa sanshoku	Black with red and white
Bekko	White, red, or yellow with black markings
Utsurimono	Black with red, white, or yellow marks
Asagi	Pale blue with red belly and fins
Shusui	Asagi with doitsu scales
Koromono	White with red markings overlaid with a darker pattern
Tancho	White koi with red on head and none on body, can have black on body
Kawarimono	Any nonmetallic koi that does not fit in another category
Metallic Koi	
Hikarimono (Ogon)	Single colored
Hikari-utsurimono	Black with white, red, or yellow markings or with white and red markings
Hikarimoyo-mono	Any metallic koi that does not fit in another category
Kinginrin	Means golden silvery scales, is kohaku, Sanke, or Showa color pattern with scales in one of two forms, pearl ginrin with a solid sparkling area in center of thickened scales, or one of three variants of flat scales, beta-gin (whole surface shimmers), diamond Ginrin (sparkling all over), and kado-gin (only edges shimmer)

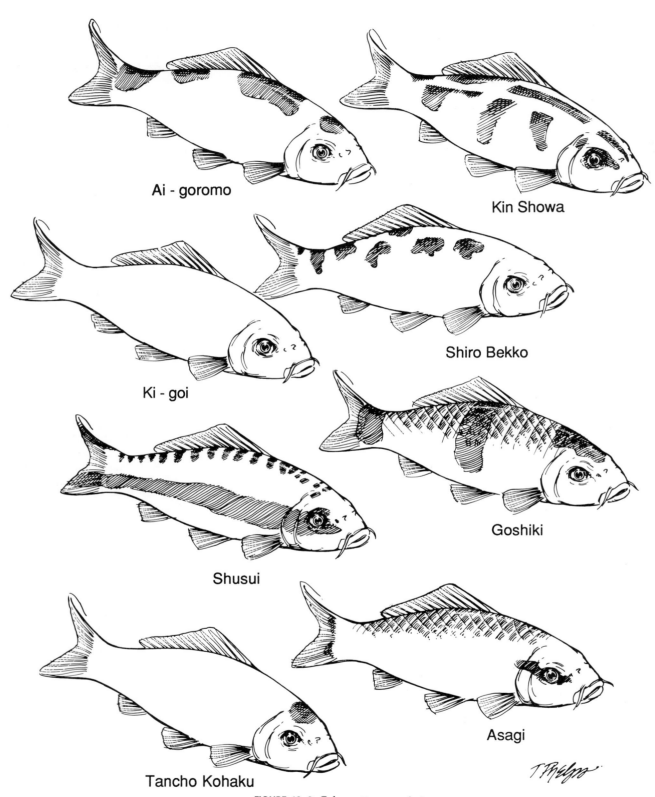

Ai - goromo

Kin Showa

Ki - goi

Shiro Bekko

Shusui

Goshiki

Tancho Kohaku

Asagi

FIGURE 42–2. Color patterns on koi.

of Japan, six size groups are judged. Group one includes young fish up to 15 cm long. Group two includes fish between 15 and 25 cm long. Subsequent groups cover 10-cm increments, up to group six which includes fish over 55 cm long.

In Japan, there are 15 size groups, starting with fish under 15 cm and proceeding by 5-cm increments to a final size group of fish over 80 cm long. Fish over 55 cm are judged separately as males or females.

Koi are judged on the criteria of shape, color, and pattern. A well-shaped koi is symmetric, with a straight backbone, fins in proportion to the body, and an abdomen more rounded than the dorsal line. The distance between the dorsal fin and the tail should be one-third the distance between first ray of the dorsal fin and the head region. If the dorsal fin is too near the tail, it is considered a serious fault. The head should be in proportion to the body and not too rounded. There should be no pits or indentations in the head and the cheeks should be solid and round. Fish are also judged for grace in movement.

The color of koi should have clarity and depth and all colors should be of even hue. White should be snow white without flecks. Red, also called "hi," should be a uniform shade and free of black or shimis specks. Bright orange is considered better than a purplish red. Round markings are favored to uneven or angular ones in most koi types. Generally, the pattern should be well balanced and consistent over the body. The borders between colors should be crisp and distinct. Overall, the skin should be lustrous and appear lacquered.

GOLDFISH

Goldfish are not koi, but descendants from the Crucian carp. Identical to Crucian carp, goldfish technically should bear the same scientific name, *Carassius carassius*, but traditionally, *Carassius auratus* has been used for goldfish since 1758 (Matsui, 1981).

Goldfish are a very popular ornamental fish in China, Japan, and North America. They first appeared in China circa A.D., 960, moving into Japan and Europe between 1500 and 1750 and then to America, where the first goldfish farm was established in Maryland in 1889 (Scott and Crossman, 1973). They are used as pond fish, aquarium fish, and bait fish. As a temperate animal, goldfish prefer cool waters, although they too can tolerate a wide temperature range. They are a hardy fish, but not as successful as carp in establishing themselves in natural waters. Most successes are in small ponds. Goldfish tolerate still, oxygen-low water with thick aquatic plant growth.

A stout fish with a short snout and a broadly triangular head, the goldfish is smaller than the carp, yet at the same length, it is a heavier fish (Fig. 42–3A–L). Total length averages from 13 to 25 cm (Scott and Crossman, 1973). The eyes are reputed to be nearsighted. The large scales are firmly attached. The

life span depends upon type and care, but can range from 5 to 20 years (Matsui, 1981). Sexual maturity is reached at about 2 years. Goldfish differ from carp by their lack of barbels, having 37 to 43 gill rakers, and pharyngeal teeth in a single row, which do not resemble molars.

Young goldfish begin life olive drab in color; the color of their Crucian carp ancestors. Between 2 and 12 months of age, adult coloring emerges. These colors vary from olive green through gold to creamy white. Occasionally, blotchy patterns appear. Color can be affected by diet, temperature, stress, and possibly lack of sunlight (Horan, 1981). High temperatures, injuries, or disease can also temporarily turn the tips of fins black; but normal color will usually reappear in a few weeks under proper conditions. When left unattended, almost all goldfish varieties will revert to a Crucian carplike form within a few generations.

Goldfish, like carp, are omnivorous. In the wild, they will eat a variety of larvae and adult aquatic insects, mollusks, crustaceans, aquatic worms, and aquatic vegetation. Aquatic plants that are eaten by goldfish include *Cambomba* and *Myriophyllum*. Goldfish normally do not eat *Vallisneria*, *Anacharis*, and *Cryptocorynes*, and these are recommended for ornamentation (Matsui, 1981). It has been stated that too much vegetable matter eaten, such as algae, can suppress the desired head growth in some goldfish varieties (Parsonson, 1983).

The preferred temperature range for goldfish is cool, 18 to 24°C. pH tolerance is wide, but 7.0 to 7.6 is best (Horan, 1981). Overwintering outside in ponds is fine, but as with koi, pools need to be below the frostline. In cold temperatures, goldfish will group together and appear inactive. Very light or no feeding is best during winter months. Metabolism and digestion slows and the food could cause intestinal problems. Uneaten food and feces can also foul the water. In summer, temperatures over 30°C can pose a problem. Dissolved oxygen levels drop with increased water temperature, and decaying organic matter and higher oxygen demand of the fish all work against the stability of the system. Increased water circulation via pumps, waterfalls, or airstones is necessary to maintain the dissolved oxygen levels. As hybrids, fancy goldfish are not particularly hardy. They expend a lot of energy with their oddly shaped bodies, requiring more oxygen than the wild variety. Water should have some hardness. Rain water or distilled water will not support goldfish. A hardness reading between 50 and 200 degrees of hardness (dH) is satisfactory (Matsui, 1981).

In general, goldfish seem to prefer environments that give them lateral movement, and they do not usually need much depth. They should not be in crowded conditions. Thick aquatic plant areas are important for environmental balance, fish cover, spawning substrate, and mineral production for these fish. In outside ponds, hornwort or *Elodea densa* are recommended choices.

Behaviorally, fancy goldfish should be observed

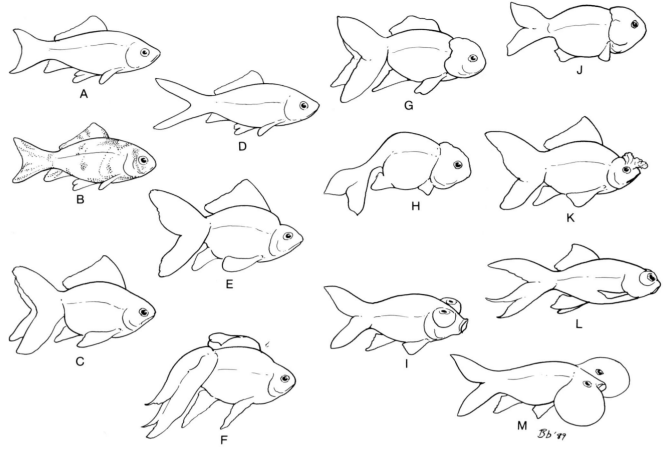

FIGURE 42–3. Breeds of goldfish. *A.* Common. *B.* Variegated. *C.* Fantail. *D.* Comet. *E.* Ryukin. *F.* Veiltail. *G.* Oranda. *H.* Ranchu. *I.* Celestial. *J.* Lionhead. *K.* Pom pom. *L.* Moor. *M.* Bubble-eye.

when healthy because of their awkward swimming styles. One needs to know what is normal and what is not. Goldfish will normally go through daily periods of inactivity and appear to rest on the bottom.

Goldfish spawning takes place as with carp. Indoors, spawning can be induced by cooling the water for a period of weeks and then warming the water back to about 21°C. They will seek warm weedy shallows in May or June. One female may be accompanied by two or more males, and mating will occur at the surface like carp, although without as much splashing. The adhesive eggs are released over submerged aquatic plants and roots and measure from 1.2 to 1.5 mm in diameter. Depending on temperature, they will hatch in 3 or more days. Young fry can feed on brine shrimp nauplii, finely sieved *Daphnia*, or similar minute infusoria.

There are approximately 30 major varieties or types of ornamental goldfish bred today. These include the Wakin, or common goldfish, Lionheads, Celestials, Bubble eyes, Telescopes, Shubunkins, Comets, Broadtails, Orandas, Ryukins and Pearlscales. They are usually classified according to head growths, dorsal fin, caudal fin and eye types. Fancy goldfish are judged on various standards such as body size and shape, fish condition, head growth, finnage, color, and swimming style.

SHINERS

Shiners are small freshwater cyprinids mostly inhabiting streams and lakes. The North American group comprises 106 species of the genus *Notropis* and one species of *Notemigonus*.

As a group, the shiners are widely distributed, spanning from the Atlantic to Pacific coasts and from Alaska and Canada in the north, to Mexico in the south. Species distribution may be local in only one watershed or stream. Most shiners avoid large turbid rivers, typically preferring clear waters. There is a great variety in habitat, ranging from pools and backwaters to flowing streams and riffles.

The body shape of shiners is elongate with large scales, a deeply forked caudal fin, and usually a darker longitudinal stripe from snout to caudal peduncle (Fig. 42–4). Size can vary. The golden shiner is the largest at 23 cm. The average adult size of shiners is about 5 cm. As a group, shiners may live 1 to 4 years, with an average longevity of 2 years.

When locally abundant, all cyprinids are used as bait. Emerald shiners are one example, but golden shiners may well be the most popular of all bait fishes in North America (Scott and Crossman, 1973). They have been successfully cultivated in ponds for many years for bait or for food for pond-cultured

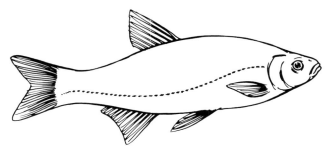

FIGURE 42–4. Golden shiner.

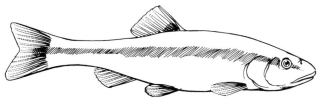

FIGURE 42–5. Chub.

bass. Golden shiners inhabit clear quiet waters and prefer shallow areas with aquatic vegetation. They are a lake rather than a river form. They swim actively, in schools, off the bottom. Golden shiners mature in 2 or 3 years, at about 7.5 cm. Life expectancy is about 5 years. They spawn between June and August. The adhesive eggs are deposited on filamentous algae or sometimes rooted aquatic vegetation. Shiners appear to be surface and midwater feeders.

CHUBS

Chubs are primarily stream- and river-dwelling fish. They are characterized by a stout body, blunt head, high back, and sometimes barbels. The size in North America ranges from 4.5 cm to 35.0 cm (Lee et al., 1980) (Fig. 42–5). Many are benthic feeders, consuming foods such as terrestrial insect larvae,

gastropods, small bivalves, crustaceans, and algae. Their life span is short, 2 to 5 years. Spawning usually occurs in spring or summer. Some construct gravel nests. They are not usually seen in aquaria.

Literature Cited

Berra, T.M. (1981) An Atlas of Distribution of the Freshwater Fish Families of the World. University of Nebraska Press, Lincoln.
Caswell, B. (1988) Articles on koi. Freshwater and Marine Aquarium Mag. R/C Modeler Corp., Sierra Madre, California.
Graham, R., and Graham, D. (1979–1981) Goldfish. Freshwater and Marine Aquarium Mag. R/C Modeler Corp., Sierra Madre, California.
Horan, J. (1981) A practical guide to keeping fancy goldfish. Freshwater and Marine Aquarium Mag. R/C Modeler Corp., Sierra Madre, California.
James, B. (1985) A Fishkeeper's Guide to Koi. Tetra Press, Morris Plains, New Jersey.
Lee, D.S., et al. (1980) Atlas of North American Freshwater Fishes. North Carolina State Museum of Natural History, Raleigh.
Matsui, Y. (1981). Goldfish Guide. 2nd ed. T.F.H. Publications, Neptune, New Jersey.
Nelson, J.S. (1984) Fishes of the World. 2nd ed. John Wiley and Sons, New York.
Parsonson, B. (1983) Some notes on goldfish nutrition. Freshwater and Marine Aquarium Mag. R/C Modeler Corp., Sierra Madre, California.
Scott, W.B., and Crossman, E.J. (1973) Freshwater fishes of Canada. Fish, Res. Bd. Can. Bull. No. 184, Ottawa.

Chapter 43

Special Anatomy and Physiology of Goldfish, Carp, and Koi

BRAD N. BOLON

Goldfish, carp, and koi are among the most popular and versatile fishes in the world. Although they exhibit their greatest diversity in Southeast Asia, these closely related cyprinids have also established

stable native populations throughout the temperate and subtropical regions of the world, including much of the United States (Courtenay and Stauffer, 1984). Goldfish and koi have been developed primarily as ornamental fish, while carp also serve food, sport, and pest control purposes (Courtenay and Stauffer, 1984).

ANATOMY

External Features

Goldfish, carp, and koi are similar in general form and physiology to prototypic pelagic fish (Penzes and Tolg, 1986). Much of the basic anatomy is covered in Chapter 1. Koi and carp are easily distinguished from goldfish by the presence of one or more pairs of barbels near their mouths as well as variations in color distribution. The stereotypic color pattern of native or wild-type fish consists of dorsal dull, green-brown scales and ventral yellow-silver scales. However, domestic goldfish, carp, and koi are multicolored. Goldfish generally have multiple colors arranged in well-defined fields with sharp margins. The margins often follow natural anatomic boundaries such as the caudal edge of the operculum or the bases of fins. In contrast, ornamental carp and koi have interdigitating, irregular patches of color. Goldfish, carp, and koi are also distinguished on the basis of structural characteristics such as local epidermal thickenings (goldfish), fin number and shape (goldfish), barbel length (carp), and eye diameter (carp) (Penzes and Tolg, 1986).

Wild members of this group have fusiform bodies with short, stiff fins, a wide caudal peduncle, and an externally symmetrical caudal fin. Adult wild goldfish average about 30 to 40 cm in length and weigh up to 1 kg, while carp range up to 20 kg, depending on the species (Sutton and Vandiver, 1986). Koi are intermediate in size and length. Domestic goldfish, carp, and koi are commonly shorter and stouter and weigh less than their wild counterparts. Common goldfish kept in aquaria are usually about 10 to 25 cm long, while pond-raised individuals may reach 30 to 40 cm. Ornamental carp and koi may reach 95 cm. Goldfish, carp, and koi usually have fusiform bodies with one slightly forked, symmetrical caudal fin and retain a full complement of proportionally sized body fins. Female fish have more rounded contours and softer bodies than males (Penzes and Tolg, 1986).

The streamlined contour of the normal pelagic fish is altered in highly inbred exotic or egg-bodied goldfishes, which have short stubby bodies with high rounded backs. Fantail and veiltail varieties have delicate, transparent caudal fins that are often duplicated, split, and/or notched. Dorsal fins are absent in some varieties. The elongated fins may exceed the body length by as much as 25% (Penzes and Tolg, 1986). Several exotic goldfish also have epidermal thickenings, or hoods, that cover the head or face. Other varieties have elevated eyes that are nestled in large fluid-filled bags (bubble-eye) or that protrude on 1 to 2 cm long, narrow, cylindrical stalks (telescope, or, if stalks are upturned, celestial). Full

expression of eye deformities and other unique features develop gradually in the young fish over 6 to 9 months (Ostrow, 1985). However, incomplete penetrance of desired variety-specific characteristics may occur. Some individuals may develop inappropriate vestigial dorsal fins or incompletely divided caudal fins. These fish should be culled from the breeding population. Egg-bodied goldfish generally mature more slowly than do flat-bodied fish (Penzes and Tolg, 1986).

Systemic Anatomy

The organ systems of goldfish, carp, and koi are similar to those in other fishes. The few added or modified organs are characteristic of most cyprinids. The skin of goldfish, carp, and koi is highly specialized (Harder, 1975; Penzes and Tolg, 1986). The bodies of adult fish are covered by about 1200 large, round (cycloid) scales arranged in reticular or mosaic formations. Epidermal club cells contain alarm substance (Schreckstoff), a pheromone that elicits a fright response in other cyprinids following damage to the skin (Nelson, 1984). Several cutaneous projections are prominent in some varieties, including minute unicellular projections, or unculi, that dot the mouth and ventral pectoral fins as well as the paired, variably sized barbels of carp and koi. Raised multicellular keratinous nodules called nuptial tubercles are found on the opercula and ventral paired fins of male goldfish during breeding season.

Skin color patterns are produced by the interaction between scale types and various pigment-filled chromophores located within the superficial dermal connective tissue (Penzes and Tolg, 1986). Metallic scales have a single solid color and high shine. Nacreous scales are dull and speckled, while matte scales are white and lusterless. Multiple shades of orange, red, yellow, silver, gray, white, brown, black, green, or, rarely, blue and lavender are possible. Beginning as relatively colorless hatchlings, young fish quickly develop a uniform dull yellow color as xanthophores mature. Colors and color patterns may change continuously for up to 2 years in some varieties (Ostrow, 1985). Adult fish may develop a single solid color. More commonly, however, two or more colors are confined to specific regions or are randomly interspersed in large, irregular patches. Colors fade to some extent during sleep or in dim light. In addition, removal of chromophores by trauma or caustic chemicals has been reported to alter adult coloration (Penzes and Tolg, 1986).

The cyprinid skeleton includes several prominent modifications (Harder, 1975; Nelson, 1984). The number and arrangement of vertebrae vary and may be used for identification. The weberian ossicles, consisting of the modified cranial four or five vertebrae, form a mobile bony bridge that connects the swim bladder to the inner ear. This bridge amplifies acoustic vibrations. Carp also have about 100 sesamoid bones, representing ossified myoseptal connective tissue. These bones anchor myofibers to redirect forces. Although these structures are composed of true bone, they are usually not considered components of the skeleton.

Muscle is the most abundant tissue in the cyprinid body (Smith, 1982; Blake, 1983). Muscle is separated into thin superficial red and intermediate pink bands and a thick, deep white layer. Goldfish, carp, and koi have moderate amounts of predominantly white muscle, most of which is located caudally. This distribution provides the slow, sustained swimming motions produced by side-to-side strokes of the caudal fin. Carp, which feed continuously, have a few more red fibers than do their cousins.

The digestive tract of goldfish, carp, and koi is generally adapted to a herbivorous diet (Harder, 1975; Smith, 1982; Penzes and Tolg, 1986). Most varieties have a protractile mouth that can extend either up or down. The narrow, tubular orifice forms a suction apparatus for inhaling floating or settled particles. Distorted craniofacial bones and muscles of blunt-headed exotic goldfish breeds alter the hydrodynamic properties of this suction apparatus and thus decrease feeding efficiency. Cyprinids lack oral dentition but instead have paired pharyngeal teeth arranged bilaterally in one to three rows. The number, size, shape, and arrangement of pharyngeal teeth are species variable and may be used for identification. The teeth grind against a thick cornified masticating plate, or carp stone, located on the roof of the pharynx. A muscular pharyngeal pad in the rostral oral cavity pushes food into the pharynx and against the teeth. The short, wide esophagus conveys crushed food to the coiled intestine. Intestine length increases with age. The intestine length of hatchlings is approximately equal to the body length, whereas that of adults is about 300% longer than the body (Harder, 1975). Goldfish and their cousins lack a true stomach, pyloric valve, and pyloric ceca. However, the cranial midgut is sometimes expanded at the junction of the esophagus and intestine, forming a pseudogaster for food storage. The liver has a constant number of true lobes and accessory lobes. The accessory lobes are molded by constant contraction of adjacent midgut coils and may thus vary slightly in shape and number between individuals (Harder, 1975). The right liver lobes enfold the gallbladder, while the left lobes enclose the spleen. Pancreatic tissue is scattered diffusely throughout the mesentery of these fish.

The cyprinid swim bladder is located in the dorsocranial retroperitoneal space (Harder, 1975; Nelson, 1984). It is divided into cranial and caudal chambers. The cranial chamber is partially elastic and can expand, while the caudal chamber is inelastic.

The gonads are located middorsally within the coelomic cavity (Harder, 1975). They may be separate or fused. Testes are usually white and fissured, whereas ovaries are pink and smooth. In carp, true ovotestes may occur in which male and female gonadal tissue is mixed in varying degrees. Such hermaphrodites have body features that are intermediate between the usual elongated male and rounded female body phenotypes. Gonads enlarge markedly during the breeding season, representing up to 30% and 70% of body weight for males and females, respectively. The ducts for sperm or egg transport are separate from and lie adjacent to the mesonephric ducts from the kidneys. The female has two caudal pores near the anal fin.

The sensory systems of goldfish, koi, and carp are similar to those of other fish. Paired nostrils are located rostrally on each side of the snout and lead to the nasal cavities, blind sacs that do not connect with the oral cavity. Taste buds are numerous in the oral mucosa and the skin surrounding the mouth, including the tips of adjacent barbels (Ostrow, 1985). Hearing depends mainly on amplification of waterborne vibrations by interactions between the stato-acoustic organ of the head, the swim bladder, and the weberian ossicles, which form a bridge between the gas-filled swim bladder and fluid-filled auditory canals. The sensitivity of the visual system is greatest in the orange spectrum, which matches the wavelength of diffuse light present in the murky, shallow aquatic habitats in which these species normally reside (Smith, 1982). Although generally less important than other sensory systems in cyprinid fish, vision is particularly poor in goldfish varieties with ocular deformities (Penzes and Tolg, 1986).

PHYSIOLOGY

Goldfish, carp, and koi are hardy fish. Mature carp, for instance, may live from one to five decades (Penzes and Tolg, 1986). Adult fish readily adapt to slowly developing environmental stressors such as decreased oxygen levels, mild pollution, overcrowding, and changing temperature by altering their behavior (Smith, 1982). Carp and common goldfish are relatively insensitive to changing temperature over the broad range of about 5°C to 37°C. Optimal growth occurs near 20°C to 23°C. In contrast, many exotic goldfish tolerate only a narrow thermal range of 14°C to 25°C. Progressively lower temperatures damage the delicate fins and hamper the immune responses. Water temperatures below about 10°C are lethal. Rapid temperature changes may be lethal to both common and exotic varieties.

Goldfish, carp, and koi grow best in systems that provide clean water of medium hardness, moderate mineral content, and low salinity (Penzes and Tolg, 1986). Space requirements vary with the variety of fish, husbandry methods, diet, breeding status, aeration, and temperature. Young goldfish (2 to 10 cm long) require about 1 to 3 L of water per individual, while adult fish need 5 to 30 L. Special breeds of goldfish may need about twice as much water per individual at any given age. Adult carp require about 300 liters of water per fish. If diet and management are adequate, less water is needed for smaller or less active fish. All cyprinids prefer diffuse light.

LITERATURE CITED

Blake, R.W. (1983) Fish Locomotion. Cambridge University Press, New York.

Courtenay, W.R., Jr., and Stauffer, J.R., Jr. (1984) Distribution, Biology and Management of Exotic Fishes. Johns Hopkins University Press, Baltimore, Maryland.

Harder, W. (1975) Anatomy of Fishes, Vols. 1 and 2. E. Schweizerbart'sche Verlagsbuchhandlung, Stuttgart, Germany.

Nelson, J.S. (1984) Fishes of the World. 2nd ed. John Wiley & Sons, New York, pp. 123–125.

Ostrow, M. (1985) Goldfish: A Complete Pet Owner's Manual. Barron's, Hauppage, New York.

Penzes, B., and Tolg, I. (1986) Goldfish and Ornamental Carp. Barron's, Hauppage, New York.

Smith, L.S. (1982) Introduction to Fish Physiology. T.F.H. Publications, Neptune, New Jersey.

Sutton, D.L., and Vandiver, V.V. (1986) Grass Carp: A Fish for Biological Management of Hydrilla and Other Aquatic Weeds in Florida. Bull. 867, Florida Agricultural Experimental Station, Gainesville, Florida.

Chapter 44

CLINICAL PATHOLOGY OF CARP, GOLDFISH, AND KOI

MICHAEL K. STOSKOPF

Routine cytology, hematology and serum chemistry techniques are applicable to carp, koi, and goldfish (Tables 44–1 to 44–3). Considerable effort remains before clinical pathology in these species can be considered as integral in medical diagnosis as it is in mammalian medicine, although certain areas have been well studied. The blood coagulation system of the carp, for example, has been well studied (Jara, 1957; Jara, 1961) and has been found to have functional homologues of all factors found in mammalian coagulation systems. Age-related changes are similar to those expected from studies in mammals and other species (Das, 1965).

The serum of carp is often yellow rather than colorless and contains a high ratio of cartotenoids to vitamin A (25:1). The serum pH can be higher (pH 7.67 [Field et al., 1943]) than mammalian or salmonid serum, and uric acid levels are low (less than 1 mg/dl). The albumin/globulin ratio is higher in carp than trout (Field et al., 1943). As in other fish, gender, age, and sexual condition can affect several parameters. Serum calcium, inorganic phosphorus, and total protein are increased in female goldfish in the breeding season or when treated with estradiol (Bailey, 1957).

SAMPLING TECHNIQUE

The method of sampling of these fish definitely affects the values obtained for certain serum enzymes. Severing the tail peduncle results in increased aspartate aminotransferase (AST), lactate dehydrogenase (LDH), and acid phosphatase levels in the serum when compared to a cardiac puncture sample (Ikeda and Ozaki, 1981). These increases are thought to be due to contamination of the sample with cellular and tissue enzymes. Alkaline phosphatase, amylase,

TABLE 44–1. Baseline Hematologic Parameters of Carp and Goldfish

Species	N	WBC (#/ml)	Het (%)	Band (%)	Mono (%)	SmLy (%)	LgLy (%)	Eos (%)	Baso (%)	Reference
						Leukocyte Indices				
Goldfish	8		29		1	70				Brenden and Huizinga (1986)
Goldfish	15	10,000	10		1	78	11			Munger (unpublished)
Goldfish (C)	100		5			92		2	0.2	Watson et al. (1963)
Goldfish			10.5		8.6	73		8	0.5	Loewenthal (1930)
Indian carp	24	6,000	16.3		0.3	61	19	2.4	1	Raizada and Singh (1982)
Mirror carp	11	34,000	1	4	1	91	3	0	1	Hines and Spira (1973)
Mirror carp	12	37,000	1	4	1	88	3	0	1	Hines and Yashouv (1970)

Abbreviations: WBC, white blood cell; Het, heterophil; Band, band cell; Mono, monocyte; SmLy, small lymphocyte; LgLy, large lymphocyte; Eos, eosinophil; Baso, basophil.

TABLE 44–2. Baseline Hematologic Parameters of Carp and Goldfish

| Species | N | Erythrocyte Indices | | | | Reference |
		RBC (mil/ml)	Hct (%)	Hb (g/dl)	Thrombocytes (1000/ml)	
Goldfish	100	2.0			51	Watson et al. (1963)
Goldfish	15	1.67	29.4		45	Munger (unpublished)
Goldfish	30	1.5	26	9.1		Brenden and Huizinga (1986)
Indian carp	24	1.2	29	7.4		Raizada and Singh (1982)
Common carp	5		32			Vars (1934)
Mirror carp	12	1.01	34.1			Hines and Yashouv (1970)
Mirror carp		1.4				Dombrowsky (1953a,b)

Abbreviations: RBC, red blood cell; Hct, hematocrit; Hb, hemoglobin.

and alanine aminotransferase (ALT) are not increased in samples from severed caudal peduncles nor are total protein values, albumin, globulin, glucose, serum urea nitrogen, cholesterol, magnesium, or creatinine (Ikeda and Ozaki, 1981). Creatine and serum inorganic phosphorus are increased (Ikeda and Ozaki, 1981).

RESPONSE TO INFECTIOUS DISEASE
(Figs. 44–1 to 44–4)

Bacterial Infection

The general response of this group of fishes to bacterial infection is a heterophilia with lymphopenia (Dombrowsky, 1953a,b). Heterophils, eosinophils, and monocytes all phagocytose bacteria (Watson et al., 1963).

Specific studies have examined the effects of infections with *Aeromonas hydrophila* in goldfish (Brenden, 1986). In these studies, a decrease in total erythrocyte numbers, hematocrit, and hemoglobin levels was apparent within 12 hours of infection by intramuscular injection of virulent bacteria. Infected

fish show a marked heterophilia and lymphopenia with a reversed ratio from baseline. Monocytosis is also seen. Serum chemistry values also change with infection. Aspartate aminotransferase peaks at approximately 24 hours postinfection with a twofold increase over baseline. Alanine aminotransferase decreases with infection. Serum urea nitrogen usually rises a small amount, but the difference is often not appreciable. Serum glucose levels elevate during the first 24 hours of infection but then rapidly return to normal in experimentally infected fish. Serum total protein may fall to about half of baseline values (Evenberg, 1986).

Protozoal Infection

Studies have been performed on mirror carp examining the effects of infection with *Ichthyophthirius multifiliis* on hematologic parameters (Hines and Spira, 1973; Reshetnikova, 1962). Infection with this ciliated protozoan results in an initial sharp lymphopenia and heterophilia with a distinct shift to the left. In the first 3 days of the infection, the ratio of lymphocytes to heterophils completely reverses from

TABLE 44–3. Baseline Serologic Parameters of Carp and Goldfish

Species	N	Urea Nitrogen (mg/dl)	Uric Acid (mg/dl)	Glucose (mg/dl)	AST* (U/L)	ALT* (U/L)	Reference
Goldfish	v†	10(3)		73(19)	900(26)	106(20)	Brenden and Huizinga (1986)
Goldfish	700			23			Young and Chavin (1963)
Common carp	19	6.3	1.4				Vars (1934)
Common carp	19	7.6	2.6	111			Field et al. (1943)

Species	N	Creatine (mg/dl)	Creatinine (mg/dl)	Total Protein (g/dl)	Albumin (g/dl)	Globulin (g/dl)	Reference
Common carp	19	2.58	0.56	4.2	2.8	0.8	Field et al. (1943)
Goldfish	17–69			3.4	2.4	0.8	Bailey (1957)

Species	N	Fibrinogen (g/dl)	Calcium (mg/dl)	Phosphorus (mg/dl)	Reference
Common carp	19	0.23	11.5	8.7	Field et al. (1943)
Goldfish	17–69		10.1	6.5	Bailey (1957)

*AST and ALT units of U/L were reported in Brenden and Huizinga (1986) from analysis made on a KDA analyzer (American Monitor Corp., Indianapolis, Indiana).
†v means N was variable with N shown in parentheses after value.

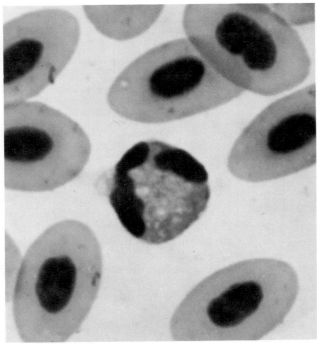

FIGURE 44-1. Blood smear from a goldfish showing a heterophil containing spindle-shaped cytoplasmic granules and a segmented nucleus (Wright-Giemsa, 1500×).

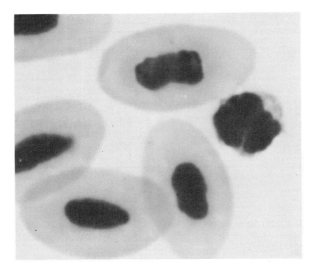

FIGURE 44-3. Blood smear from a goldfish showing a binucleate thrombocyte (Wright-Giemsa, 1500×).

baseline. The shift to the left becomes more pronounced as the infection continues. As the disease progresses, poorly staining basophilic cells can be seen. Late in the infection an increase in basophils is apparent. Except for a short duration elevation around the second day of infection, there is no appreciable increase in the total leukocyte count. Moribund fish usually have a terminal leukopenia

with this disease. The hematologic response to *I. multifiliis* does not appear to be dependent upon water temperature and progresses at much the same pace in varying water temperatures.

Metazoal Infection

Very little has been reported on the response of this group of fishes to metazoal infection. It should be expected that the responses would be similar to other fishes. One study examined the effects of fluke infection (*Dactylogyrus* spp.) on hematologic parameters (Sadkowskaya, 1958). Fluke infection resulted in a heterophilia and monocytosis with monoblasts prominent in the smear.

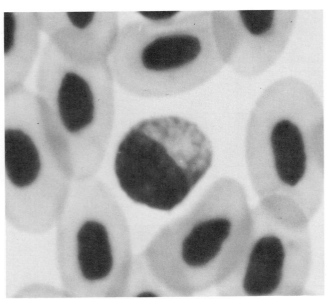

FIGURE 44-2. Blood smear from a goldfish showing a plasma cell with an eccentric nucleus and prominent Golgi apparatus (Wright-Giemsa, 1500×)

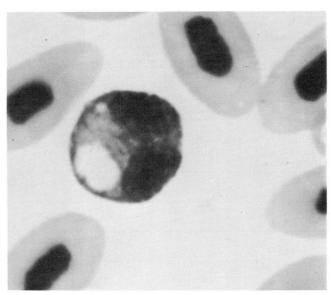

FIGURE 44-4. Blood smear from a goldfish showing a doughnut cell, apparently a member of the lymphocytic series with a large clear vacuole. This cell appears to be binucleate (Wright-Giemsa, 1500×).

RESPONSE TO NONINFECTIOUS DISEASE

Diabetes

Normal serum glucose in goldfish at 25°C is approximately 23 mg/dl with no discernible diurnal pattern of variation or changes related to photoperiod (Young and Chavin, 1963). However, goldfish can be made hypoglycemic and functionally diabetic with immersion exposure to alloxan. Fish exposed acutely rapidly develop a severe hypoglycemia that reverses completely about 3 days after exposure (Young and Chavin, 1963). Intraperitoneal injections of 200 to 300 mg/kg alloxan are also reversibly diabetogenic, but the upper dose range is also toxic (Young and Chavin, 1963).

General Stress

The general stress response of these fish is a heterophilia and lymphopenia (Hines and Spira, 1973). Mirror carp exercised for an hour show increased hematocrits and hemoglobin content, apparently caused by a combination of an increased supply of erythrocytes from the spleen, erythrocyte swelling, and water shifting out of the vasculature (Yamamoto and Itazawa, 1988).

Increased water temperature also causes an increase in hemoglobin content and hematocrit in goldfish (Koss and Houston, 1981). With increased temperature, erythrocyte sodium, chloride, and water contents increase, whereas erythrocyte potassium, magnesium, and calcium contents decrease (Koss and Houston, 1981). The only other studied effect of water parameters on the serology of these fishes is the observation that exposure to high environmental ammonia levels results in increased serum urea nitrogen and blood ammonia (Vars, 1934).

LITERATURE CITED

Bailey, R.E. (1957) The effect of estradiol on serum calcium, phosphorus and protein of goldfish. J. Exp. Zool. 136(3):455–469.

Brenden, R.A., and Huizinga, H.W. (1986) Pathophysiology of experimental *Aeromonas hydrophila* infection in goldfish, *Carassius auratus* (L.). J. Fish Dis. 9:163–167.

Das, B.C. (1965) Age-related trends in the blood chemistry and hematology of the Indian carp (*Catla catla*). Gerontologia 10:47–64.

Dombrowsky, H. (1953a) Hamatologisch-nosologishe Studien an bauchwassersuchts Kranken Karpfen (*Cyprinus carpio* L.). Biol. Zbl. 72:353–363.

Dombrowsky, H. (1953b) Untersuchungen ueber das Blut des Karpfens (*Cyprinus carpio* L.) und einiger anderer Suesswasserfischarten. Biol. Zbl. 72:182–195.

Evenberg, D., de Graaff, P., Fleuren, W., and van Muiswinkel, W.B. (1986) Blood changes in carp (*Cyprinus carpio*) induced by ulcerative *Aeromonas salmonicida* infections. Vet. Immunol. Immunopathol. 12:321–330.

Field, J.B., Elveljem, C.A., and Juday, C. (1943) A study of blood constituents of carp and trout. J. Biol. Chem. 148:261–269.

Hines, R.S., and Spira, D.T. (1973) Ichthyophthiriasis in mirror carp II. Leukocyte response. J. Fish Biol. 5:527–534.

Hines, R.S., and Yashouv, A. (1970) Differential leukocyte counts and total leukocyte and erythrocyte counts for some normal Israeli mirror carp. Bamidgeh 22:106–113.

Ikeda, Y., and Ozaki, H. (1981) The examination of tail peduncle severing blood sampling method from the aspect of observed serum constituent levels in carp (Japanese). Bull. Jpn. Soc. Sci. Fish. 47:1447–1453.

Jara, Z. (1957) The blood coagulation system in carp. Zool. Polon. 8:113–129.

Jara, Z. (1961) The mechanism of thrombinogenesis in carp (*Cyprinus carpio*). Zool. Polon. 11:101–129.

Koss, T.F., and Houston, A.H. (1981) Hemoglobin levels and red cell ionic composition in goldfish (*Carassius auratus*) exposed to constant and diurnally cycling temperatures. Can. J. Fish. Aquatic Sci. 38:1182–1188.

Loewenthal, N. (1930) Nouvelles observations sur les globules blancs du sang chez le cyprin dore (*Carassius auratus*) Arch. d'Anat. Histol. d'Embyol. 7:317–322.

Raizada, M.N., and Singh, C.P. (1982) Observations of haematological values of fresh water fish, *Cirrhinus mrigala* (Ham.). Comp. Physiol. Ecol. 7:34–36.

Reshetnikova, A. V. (1962) Changes in the blood of the carp by infection with *Ichtyophthirius*. Naucho-Tekhnicheskii Byulletin Gos NIORKh 15:71–73.

Sadkowskaya, O.D. (1958) Changes in leukocyte formula of carp blood under the influence of invasion of *Dactylogyrus extensus* (Solidus). Rob. po Helminthologii, Moscow: Academia nauk SSSR, pp. 320–321 (cited in Hines and Spira [1973]).

Vars, H.M. (1934) Blood studies on fish and turtles. J. Biol. Chem. 105:135–137.

Watson, L.J., Shechmeister, I.L., and Jackson, L.L. (1963) The hematology of goldfish, *Carassius auratus*. Cytologia 28:118–130.

Yamamoto, K., and Itazawa, Y. (1988) Erythrocyte supply from the spleen of exercised carp. Comp. Biochem. Physiol. 92A:139–144.

Young, J.E., and Chavin, W. (1963) Serum glucose levels and pancreatic islet cytology in normal and alloxan diabetic goldfish. Am. Zool. 3(4):510 (Abst. 143).

Chapter 45

ENVIRONMENTAL REQUIREMENTS AND DISEASES OF CARP, KOI, AND GOLDFISH

MICHAEL K. STOSKOPF

Carp, koi, and goldfish are found in a variety of environments. Goldfish, for example, are frequently held in small bowls or aquaria. In this habitat, many of the same concerns that arise when keeping freshwater tropical fish become important. Those concerns are covered in Chapter 65. In general, goldfish are more hardy than the freshwater tropical species and can tolerate a wider range of water parameters (Table 45–1), but attention to their needs on a more rigorous set of guidelines will not be detrimental. They are often held in ornamental ponds and are, of course, reared in production units. Food carp are production animals and are usually held in production ponds. Koi, on the other hand, are generally held in ornamental ponds. This chapter will focus on ornamental ponds.

POND DESIGN

In contrast to a production pond, which is usually rectangular and of uniform depth, ornamental ponds can take a variety of shapes and sizes. There is a strong temptation to build very intricately shaped ponds, perhaps owing to a desire to emulate, on a smaller scale, the natural shapes of river and stream-fed lakes. Unfortunately these intricate designs rarely allow for good water flow, and stagnant zones can create very serious problems (Fig. 45–1). The best pond shapes allow for good circulation and maximize surface area. Space requirements for goldfish and koi are estimated in several ways, but one rule of thumb is to provide 24 in.^{2} (150 cm^2) of surface area for each inch of fish in a system.

Surface area is important, but adequate depth is also a necessity. The depth of pond required depends very much on the local climate, but deep water (1.5 m minimum) is a necessity for maintaining healthy koi. Most experts consider ponds with areas of 2.5 m depth optimal unless the pond is in a climate where winter temperatures do not fall below 5°C

(McDowall, 1989). Deeper ponds do not have as much temperature fluctuation as shallow ponds, which is often more important than absolute water temperature. Deep ponds also provide better protection from predators such as herons, raccoons, and cats. Koi also do better if provided with the vertical swimming activity that occurs in deep ponds. In shallow ponds, optimized for viewing the fish, koi become fat and overweight (McDowall, 1989).

The natural habitat of goldfish and koi is not the crystal-clear water with unobstructed view that most pond owners achieve. These fish normally live in mud-bottomed, heavily planted areas, and benefit from consideration of their natural preference for some cover.

ESTIMATING POND VOLUME

An ability to estimate pond volumes is important, particularly when considering chemical treatments, or evaluating filtration and water-treatment

TABLE 45–1. Water Parameter Limits for Carp, Koi, and Goldfish

pH	7.0–8.5
Alkalinity	>25 ppm
Dissolved oxygen	4–10 ppm
Carbon dioxide	<5 ppm
Hydrogen sulfide	<0.3 ppm
Un-ionized ammonia	<0.01 ppm
Nitrite	<0.01 ppm
Copper	<0.01 ppm
Iron	<0.5 ppm
Phosphate	<6.0 ppm
Potassium	<2.0 ppm
Sodium	<5.0 ppm
Zinc	<0.01 ppm

Modified from Rottmann, R.W., and Shireman, J.V. (1990) Hatchery Manual for Grass Carp and other Riverine Cyprinids. Bulletin 244, Florida Cooperative Extension Service. Gainesville, Florida.

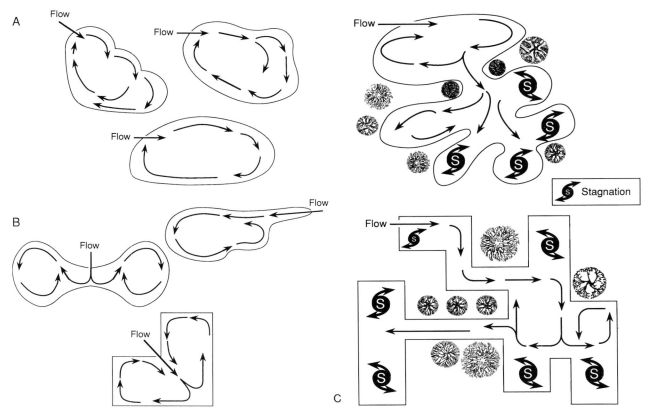

FIGURE 45–1. Schematic drawing of pond shapes and water circulation. *A.* Ponds with shapes appropriate for good circulation regardless of placement of inflow and outtake. *B.* Pond shapes that require careful placement of inflow and outtakes to provide adequate circulation. *C.* Pond shapes that produce stagnation (S) unless multiple inflow and outtake points are used.

plants. The latter are being incorporated into ornamental pond design more and more often. Unfortunately, the variety of pond shapes complicates the procedure of determining their volumes. You need to know more than just the shape and measurements of the surface area. If a pond has straight sides, calculations are relatively straightforward. The surface area is determined, and the average depth can be used to calculate the volume of the pond (Fig. 45–2A). If stepped or terraced sides are used, the pond can be broken up into two or more volumes for the calculation (Fig. 45–2B). For ponds with sloping sides, a good approximation is to determine the surface area of the pond, and the area of the bottom. These are added together, divided by two, and multiplied by the depth of the pond (Fig. 45–2C). Useful conversion factors are given in the appendices.

LINERS AND FILTERS

In contrast to production ponds, ornamental ponds are frequently lined rather than maintained with their natural dirt bottom. A common practice is to build a concrete or cinder block pond, although flexible plastic and rubber liners are very easy to install and are becoming very popular. Certain plastics should be avoided. Vinyl, particularly inexpensive grades, can be very toxic. Polythene is inexpensive, but should be avoided because of its fragility, particularly if exposed to sunlight. Butyl rubber is very long lived and excellent, but very expensive. Heavy grades (0.75 mm) will last up to 50 years (McDowall, 1989). However, butyl rubber does not conform to contours well and is easily punctured by the weight of water pressing down on poorly placed plumbing. It is also not a good choice if plants are desired.

However ponds are lined, it a serious mistake to fail to install a bottom drain (Fig. 45–3). This drain is needed to completely empty the pond for repairs or maintenance, and can be used on occasion to remove bottom detritus to the filters. Water to filters should be routinely drawn from midwater, and at least some deep water return is beneficial.

Filters are a major factor in ornamental pond success. In the past, undergravel filters were used nearly to the exclusion of any other filtration system. Recent pond technology usually eschews the undergravel filter in favor of external filtration. The purpose of the filter is not merely to keep the water clear, but more importantly to increase the carrying capacity of the pond. A client who wants to see more fish in an unfiltered pond is courting disaster unless some supplemental water filtration is installed to handle nitrogenous wastes. Sizing a filter is an art form as much as a science. Usually the adage is the

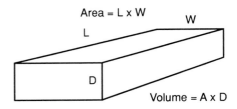

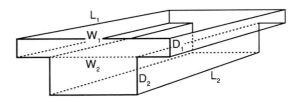

FIGURE 45–2. Estimating the volume of a pond. *A.* For a pond with straight sides, the surface area times the depth can be used to calculate volume. *B.* For a pond with terraced sides, the pond is broken up into two or more volumes for calculation. *C.* For ponds with sloping sides, the volume is approximated by adding the surface area and the bottom area and dividing by 2, then multiplying by the average depth of the pond.

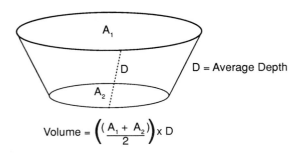

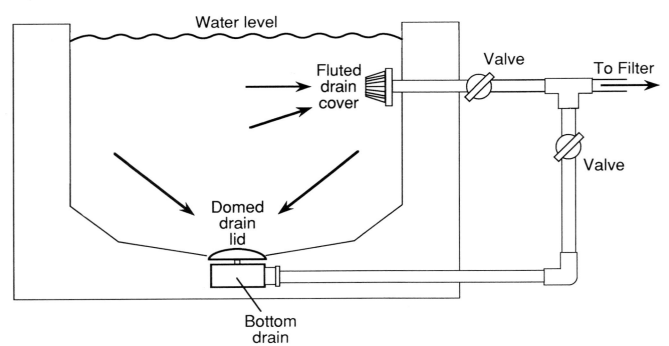

FIGURE 45–3. A schematic drawing of a properly installed bottom drain with a dome-shaped cover to direct debris, and a shielded midwater draw that routinely brings water to the pump for circulation.

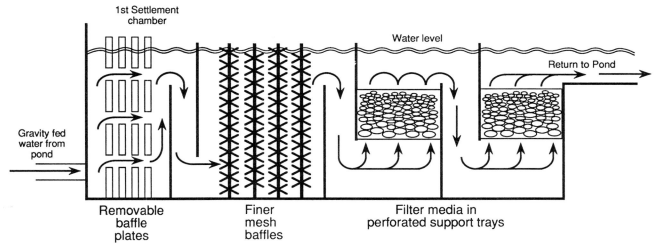

FIGURE 45–4. A schematic of a multichambered filter system that uses settling baffles and reverse flow through multiple media beds. There can be any number of chambers. Filtered water is returned to the pond by pump or gravity, depending on the design of the pond circulation system.

bigger the filter system, the better. In Japan, multichambered filters are often designed to have equal surface area with the ornamental pond (Fig. 45–4). Creative designs allow these filters to be esthetically pleasing. A more conservative design rule would be to provide filters with about one-third the surface area of the pond. They should allow a contact time of 10 to 15 minutes and be capable of turning over the entire volume of the system every 2 to 3 hours. Depths of filters need not be extreme. Media depths beyond 2 ft are usually not effective.

TEMPERATURE

Goldfish generally survive temperatures between 0 and 30°C, although fancy varieties have severe difficulties below 12°C. Koi survive in temperatures ranging from 2 to 30°C where winters are short. Long winters are a problem, however, and in far northern climes, pond koi may require some form of water heating to thrive.

Other problems with cold temperature are related to reproductive success. Egg maturation in female goldfish and koi is triggered by day lengthening. Spawning, on the other hand, is triggered by water temperatures raising above 20°C in the spring. Female koi and goldfish maintained in cold water in late spring are very stressed.

Temperature fluctuations are probably more deleterious to these fishes than absolute temperature ranges. Sudden temperature shifts greater than 1 to 3°C can trigger several problems. Eggs exposed to sudden temperature shifts often develop into fish with spinal deformities. Another problem with shifting temperature occurs with sudden warming of the water. Below about 12°C, antibody production is significantly decreased in koi and goldfish, but bacterial growth is also slowed. When water temperatures rise, bacterial growth rates increase dramati-

cally. Unfortunately there is about a week's lag time before the immune system of the fish begins to function properly. This week of vulnerability can result in high levels of infection. Problems with water temperature are most frequently detected as outbreaks of infectious diseases. Water temperatures should generally not be raised by more than 1 to 2°C per day to avoid this problem.

WATER pH

Slight daily fluctuations of pH in the range of 7.0 to 8.5 are expected and acceptable. In contrast to tropical fish systems, low pH is rarely a problem in ornamental ponds unless runoff or rain water contributes significantly to the water make-up. Alkalosis is a more common problem. Ponds with considerable amounts of plant life, particularly in the form of algae, will often fluctuate in a range of 7.0 to 11.0. In these ponds, resident fish are stressed, but usually survive. However, new fish added to such a pond frequently die shortly after introduction. Fish suffering from alkalosis may show a milkiness to their skin or mucus, and if the condition is not peracute, frayed fins are common. If the gills are examined, the epithelium will be damaged, hypertrophic, or missing depending upon the time course of the condition. When the pH of such a pond exceeds 9 on a continual basis, the pond owner should take remedial measures to lower the pH.

Another cause of highly alkaline waters is found in ponds constructed of concrete or concrete block. These materials contribute large amounts of calcium compounds and can cause pH levels to stabilize above 11. Sealing the concrete is one solution to the problem, and bituminous based paints are very popular (McDowall, 1989). Clinicians should be aware of the toxicity of cheaper compounds used to seal roofs, which are sometimes used by the frugal pond owner.

These are very toxic to fish and will usually kill all fish in the pond over a relatively short time (days to weeks). An alternative to sealing concrete is to pretreat the concrete with muriatic acid. This will probably need to be repeated two or three times before the surface layers of the concrete have been adequately leeched of alkaline compounds.

OXYGEN

Dissolved oxygen levels are the most critical requirement of mixed culture carp ponds (Jhingran and Pullin, 1988), and they are also critical in ornamental pond management. Fish exposed to low oxygen levels are usually anorexic and lethargic and spend most of their time up at the surface breathing rapidly. This is most reliably observed at dawn after a humid summer night, when oxygen levels are the lowest in the pond. Dawn is the best time to test oxygen levels because they are at their lowest.

Too much plant life in the pond contributes heavily to the depletion of oxygen at night and exacerbates the problem. This is usually unicellular algae rather than vascular plants, but it is conceivable that a pond could be so heavily planted with vascular plants that it would suffer this fate. Plants produce oxygen during photosynthesis during the day, but then use that oxygen at night, producing carbon dioxide in respiration.

The first mortalities in ponds suffering from low dissolved oxygen are usually the largest fish. These have the highest oxygen demand and are not able to move into shallow water well. Aeration of the pond is the major corrective action, although excessive use of ventures can result in supersaturation and problems with gas bubble disease.

Aeration or pumping of water is most important at night when plants are using oxygen in the water. It is also very important in the winter when plant life can deplete oxygen levels that are not restored during short days or through blocking of surface exchange by ice. Unfortunately many owners are prone to shut off their circulating pumps at these times because they do not understand the critical need and feel they can save energy and money by not running the systems at night. Obviously, just the opposite strategy should be employed.

NITROGEN COMPOUNDS

Problems with toxic nitrogen-containing compounds such as ammonia, nitrite, and nitrate are most frequently seen in the startup of a new pond, or after chemical treatment of a pond. Unfortunately, unjudicious use of chemicals in ponds can kill nitrifying bacteria and result in accumulations of toxic levels of ammonia or nitrite. After treating a pond, the water should be monitored for both ammonia and nitrite daily for at least 14 days. Problems with ammonia and nitrite will also be seen on occasion in cold weather when cold water temperatures interfere with the ability of nitrifying bacteria to process the waste. Reading ammonia and nitrite levels weekly during the winter may be a good idea in cold climates.

In contrast to oxygen depletion, nitrite or ammonia toxicity usually affects smaller fish first. These fish are seen to lie on their sides on the bottom, but swim up to the surface to feed. Un-ionized ammonia levels of 0.2 ppm can cause rapid death, and levels as low as 0.02 ppm cause severe chronic problems. Even levels as low as 1 ppb can irritate gills and cause temporary damage. Ammonia burns the gills and mucous membranes of the skin, mouth and intestines. Nervous signs are prominent as well. Nitrite toxicity interferes with oxygen uptake by the formation of methemoglobin. Affected fish respire rapidly and, if 50% or more of their hemoglobin is converted, will show brown, mud-colored gills.

The normal emergency measure would be to change water when readings of 0.1 ppm nitrite or 0.2 ppm un-ionized ammonia appear. Increased levels of ammonia or nitrite may be more difficult to ameliorate in a pond, if water changes are not possible. It is important to remember that the toxicity of ammonia increases with temperature and pH. Lowering pH can help. Also, adding salt to increase salinity can have significant benefit for spiking nitrite levels. Chloride ions compete with nitrite for transport across the gill epithelium. Adding 3 kg of table salt for every 1000 L of pond water (0.3% solution, 0.5 oz salt/gal) is beneficial when nitrite toxicity is expected.

CHLORINE

Goldfish, koi, and carp are very susceptible to chlorine. Levels of 4.0 ppm will kill them within 8 hours of exposure (Amlacher, 1970). Lower levels commonly found in drinking water of 0.2 to 0.3 ppm chlorine will kill these fish over about 20 days (Amlacher, 1970), and very low levels, even down to the range of 0.002 ppm, will cause chronic toxicity with hyperplasia of the gill epithelium. High-level exposure can cause epithelial burns of the skin, fins, and gills. Even higher level exposure causes peracute death with few signs.

New ponds filled with chlorinated water should be run with aeration for a week in sunny weather and 10 days in cloudy weather to remove chlorines before fish are added. If there is a lot of organic matter in the pond, or if the water source is disinfected with chloramines, the water should be circulated with aeration for at least 10 days and preferably 2 weeks, since chloramines are more stable than free chlorine.

PESTICIDES AND HERBICIDES

Although overall, carp, goldfish, and koi are considered among the least susceptible of fishes to

TABLE 45–2. Maximum Tolerable Levels of Pesticides for Carp (in mg/L [ppm])

DDT	0.057
Lindane	0.28
Toxaphen	0.056
Chlordane	1.16
Heptachlor	0.38
Aldrin	0.165
Dieldrin	0.067
Endrin	0.004
Thiodan	0.011
Parathion	3.5
Chlorthion	4.1
Diazinon	5.2
Malathion	29.4
Systox	15.2

From Lüdemann, D., and Neumann, H. (1960) Versuche über die akute toxische Wirkung neuzeitlicher Kontaktinsektizide auf einsömmerige Karpfen (Cyprinus carpio L.) Z. Angew. Zool. 47:11–33.

pesticides (Murty, 1986), this should not give a false sense of security (Table 45–2). Ornamental ponds are particularly prone to accidental exposures to a variety of harmful chemicals, primarily insecticides and herbicides commonly used in horticultural work. Goldfish and koi can be severely affected by these compounds when they are accidentally applied to the water or when rains wash recently applied chemicals into the pond. Goldfish are particularly susceptible to carbamates, even more so than most salmonids (Murty, 1986). In addition, pond owners are prone to try chemical treatments to combat algal growth, which obstructs their view of the fish in their ornamental ponds. Most of these treatments have an effect on the inhabiting fish and, unless very carefully applied, can result in long-term problems or even acute mortality.

PREDATORS

A major vexation of ornamental pond owners is predation (Dawes, 1989). Raccoons, cats, and fish-eating birds, never before noticed by the pond owner, will descend and rapidly decimate an unprotected population of goldfish or koi. Certainly pond design has a major impact on the problem. Deep ponds which allow fish to avoid shallows reduce predation. A stepped-edge rather than a sloping shore also helps deter predators who fish from the banks. An 18- or even 12-in. shelf does much to discourage cats and raccoons (Fig. 45–5). The amount of cover around a pond will also affect the degree of predation, although unless active measures are taken to discourage cats and raccoons, they will usually become quite bold about fishing in the open.

Once faced with a pond design and setting that cannot be easily modified, active defenses may become necessary. Recently, motion sensors that can be wired to lights and even noise-making devices have been used to detect small animals approaching a pond. This is a good solution and will convince predators to avoid the pond, but not usually before neighbors or family have grown thoroughly disgusted with being disturbed all night. Covering ponds with netting can be effective, but it is usually expensive and esthetically disastrous to a client who has the pond for the joy of looking at it.

Birds can be an even more difficult problem than terrestrial predators. Initially, pond owners are often delighted to see that they have attracted a heron to their pond. When they realize their fish are the main attraction, this joy of nature can turn quite ugly. Luckily, herons generally land on the ground and walk out into a pond. A low fence around the pond will usually deter their attacks on fish (Dawes, 1989). Kingfishers, on the other hand, are much more difficult to foil. Their arial attacks are accurate and fences have no effect. Although stringing lines across the top of the pool may make the owner feel they have accomplished something, they will rarely affect a kingfisher's kill rate. Clients with kingfisher problems should deepen their ponds or be sold on the joys of watching kingfishers.

SHIPPING

If you are providing service to a production unit or a wholesale operation, shipping and receiving fish will be a major part of the operation. Also, koi and goldfish breeders who participate in shows are often packing and transporting their fish. You should read Chapters 75 and 94 for additional information. In general, fancy goldfish and koi should be placed individually in a bag within a bag with enough water to cover their gills. The bag should be large enough to allow the fish to position itself comfortably, without being forced to bend or rub its fins against the bag.

For long transports, oxygen is much more important than water, and there should be twice as much air space in the sealed bag as water space. Once inflated with oxygen, the bag should be placed in a box, preferably insulated, and the fish should be protected as much as possible from loud noise, bright light, and temperature extremes. When transporting fish in a car, they are best placed in the trunk or on the floor of the rear of the car to avoid heater and air conditioner exhausts (McDowall, 1989).

QUARANTINE

Goldfish, koi, and carp should be quarantined before being introduced into a new environment, just as other fishes. For the homeowner with an ornamental pond or a goldfish tank, this may seem like an excessive effort, but it is not. Introduction of fish directly into a pond with other fish does not always cause a problem, but when it does, it is usually a very major and depressing one.

New fish should be held in a separate tank and water system for 4 and preferably 6 weeks. This is

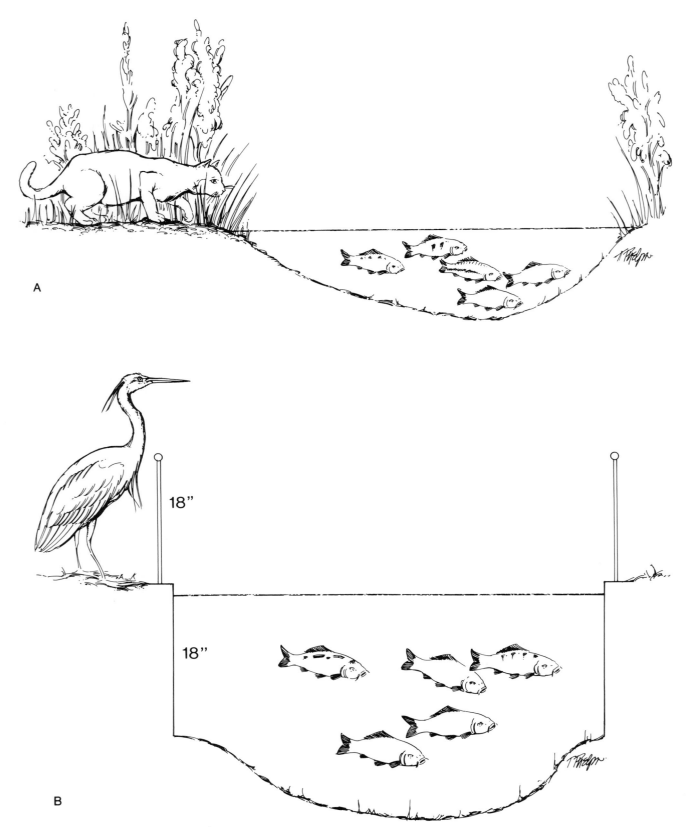

A

B

FIGURE 45–5. Designing ponds to reduce predation. *A.* A pond with shrubbery or plantings coming up to its edge invites predation. Gently sloping sides also favor the hunter. *B.* Clear areas around the pond, and stepped or terraced sides with a deep pond center, deter nonswimming predators. A short fence around the edge of the pond will further discourage herons and wading birds.

rarely done, and a 2-week quarantine will have to be accepted by veterinarians. Pond owners think they have done a very conscientious job when they have been able to wait that long before introducing fish. A major factor is probably the common problem that most quarantine systems are temporary and labor intensive and require lots of water changes. Most fish enthusiasts begin to lose enthusiasm after 2 weeks of frequent water changes.

Fish entering quarantine should be given a salt-water dip on the way into the system and, if feasible, two more saltwater baths at 3- to 5-day intervals. This will greatly reduce protozoan populations and even affect trematodes to a minor degree. On arrival, fish should also be carefully examined for the presence of external parasites visible to the naked eye, such as anchor worm and other copepods. An impression smear of the body and when appropriate a gill biopsy should also be examined. Fecal direct smear examinations can direct appropriate therapy.

GOING ON VACATION

A frequently asked question is, What should be done when a fish owner goes on vacation? Healthy, well-fed goldfish in tanks can survive 2 to 3 weeks while their owner is on vacation. Their owner should be instructed to do a partial water change a week before he or she intends to leave. No new fish should be added to the tank for at least a week and preferably several weeks before the vacation. The day before departure, the owner should change the filter

and check its operation. The tank lights should generally be left off unless there are many plants in the tank that would die. In such case, a timer should be installed to provide a day-night cycle.

It is a bad idea to overfeed fish in preparation for an upcoming holiday fast. The most common trouble with fish during a vacation is overfeeding by an inexperienced and overzealous friend or neighbor. If a fish owner is going on vacation and prefers to have a friend feed the fish, he or she should pre-measure and package the daily food rations. It is also important that owners who leave their fish unfed avoid the temptation to, in a gesture of reparation, overfeed their fish when they return from vacation. When the fish owners return, they should resume with light feedings and increase food amounts to normal over 3 days. They should also check filters and consider a partial water change.

LITERATURE CITED

Amlacher, E. (1970) Textbook of Fish Diseases. Translated by D.A. Conroy and R.L. Herman. T.F.H. Publications, Neptune, New Jersey.
Dawes, J. (1989) Book of Water Gardens. T.F.H. Publications, Neptune, New Jersey.
Jhingran, V.G., and Pullin, R.S.V. (1988) A Hatchery Manual for the Common, Chinese and Indian Major Carps. Asian Development Bank, Manila, Philippines.
McDowall, A. (ed.) (1989) The Tetra Encyclopedia of Koi. Tetra Press, Morris Plains, New Jersey.
Murty, A.S. (1986) Toxicity of Pesticides to Fish. Vol. 2. CRC Press, Boca Raton, Florida.
Rottmann, R.W., and Shireman, J.V. (1990) Hatchery Manual for Grass Carp and Other Riverine Cyprinids. Bulletin 244, Florida Cooperative Extension Service. Gainesville, Florida.

Chapter 46

NUTRITION OF KOI, CARP, AND GOLDFISH

LAURA JANE STEWART

Protein, carbohydrate, lipid, and vitamin balance is as important in the nutrition of carp, koi, and goldfish as it is in other fish groups. This chapter will emphasize the role of fat-soluble vitamins on fish nutrition (Table 46–1). More detailed coverage of protein, carbohydrates, lipids, and other nutrients can be found in Chapters 22 and 34.

VITAMINS

Vitamin A

Vitamin A has two forms (Fig. 46–1). Vitamin A_1 is found in many animal tissues as an almost colorless compound in the form of a free alcohol, retinol

TABLE 46–1. Minimum Vitamin Requirements for Growth of Young Carp (amount per kg of diet)

Vitamin A	Required
Vitamin D	Unknown
Vitamin E	Required
Vitamin K	Unknown
Thiamin	1 mg/kg diet
Riboflavin	8 mg/kg diet
Pyridoxine	6 mg/kg diet
Pantothenic acid	30–50 mg/kg diet
Niacin	28 mg/kg diet
Folic acid	Not required
Vitamin B$_{12}$	Not required
Biotin	Required
Inositol	10 mg/kg feed
Choline	4000 mg/kg feed
Vitamin C	Required

From Lovell, R.T. (1989) Nutrition and Feeding of Fish. Van Nostrand Reinhold, New York, pp. 30 and 33. © 1989, Van Nostrand Reinhold.

($C_{20}H_{30}O$), and as esters of fatty acids. Vitamin A$_2$, or retinol$_2$, has a very similar structure ($C_{20}H_{28}O$) and is found in tissues of freshwater fishes. Vitamin A is measured in international units with 1 unit being equivalent to 0.3 μg of all-*trans* retinol.

While vitamin A is not found in plants, carotenoid precursors are. Many carotenoids have vitamin A activity, including α-, β-, and γ-carotene, and cryptoxanthin. β-Carotene is one of the most plentiful carotenoids. Plants with high levels of β-carotene are often yellow to orange, such as pumpkin, cantaloupe, and carrots; or deep-green leafy plants like spinach, broccoli, or alfalfa. β-Carotene has a symmetric structure that is enzymatically split into two molecules of retinol in the liver and intestinal mucosa of fish by β-carotene 15,15'-dioxygenase. The rate of this reaction is dependent on water temperature.

Cold-water fishes cannot utilize β-carotene below 9°C (Poston et al., 1977).

The symptoms of vitamin A deficiency in various fishes are quite similar. Goldfish develop eye hemorrhages, exophthalmos, loss of scales, anorexia, and increased susceptibility to infection. Common carp fed a vitamin A– and carotene-deficient diet develop exophthalmos, deformed gill opercula, light skin color, and fin and skin hemorrhages (Aoe et al., 1968). Salmonids also develop exophthalmos and deformed gill opercula, as well as reduced growth rates, light skin color, and ascites (Lovell, 1988). Channel catfish develop exophthalmos, edema, and kidney hemorrhages (Dupree, 1970).

Vitamin D

Vitamin D, like vitamin A, is found in two forms: vitamin D$_3$, cholecalciferol ($C_{27}H_{44}O$), and vitamin D$_2$, ergocalciferol ($C_{28}H_{44}O$). The vitamin precursor for cholicalciferol, 7-dehydrocholesterol, is found in the skin of most animals, whereas the precursor for ergocalciferol, ergosterol, is found in plants (Fig. 46–2). When exposed to ultraviolet radiation these precursors are converted to vitamin D. Whereas most land animals are able to utilize both forms of the vitamin, fish utilize D$_3$ far better than D$_2$.

Vitamin D is essential in the absorption and utilization of calcium. Cholecalciferol is converted in the liver to 25-hydroxycholecalciferol, which is then carried to the kidneys and converted to 1,25-dihydroxycholecalciferol (1,25[OH]$_2$D$_3$) (Fig. 46–3). This compound, 1,25(OH)$_2$D$_3$, functions as a hormone carried to the intestinal mucosa and bone, where it induces the production of specific proteins. These in turn affect the absorption, reabsorption, and mobilization of calcium and phosphorus ions.

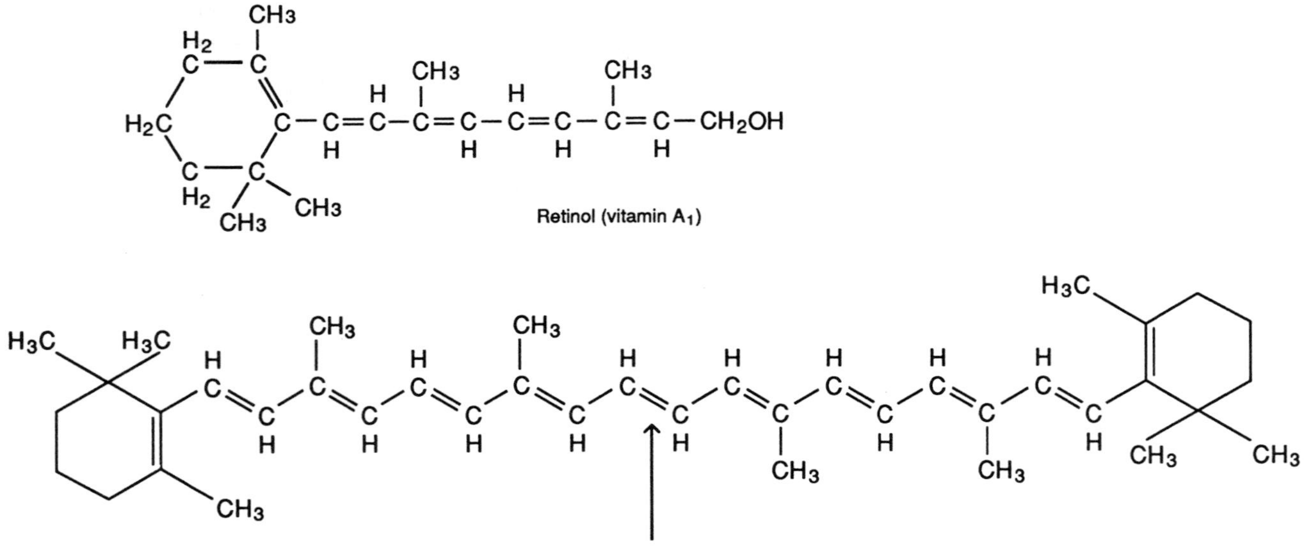

Retinol (vitamin A$_1$)

Cleavage here produces two vitamin A molecules

β-Carotene (provitamin A)

FIGURE 46–1. The structures of vitamin A$_1$ and provitamin A.

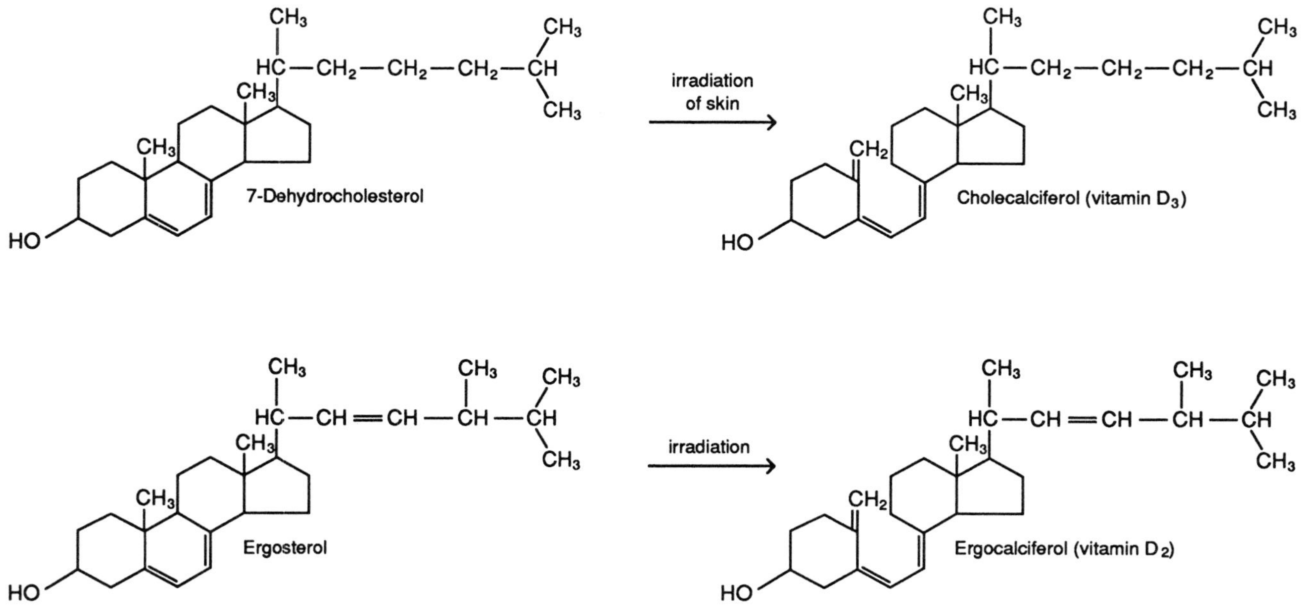

FIGURE 46–2. The conversion of ergosterol to ergocalciferol (vitamin D_2) and 7-dehydrocholesterol to cholecalciferol (vitamin D_3).

In mammals, a vitamin D deficiency results in bone malformation or rickets. The vitamin is measured in terms of its ability to prevent rickets in rats, where one IU of vitamin D activity is equal to the antirachitic effect of 0.025 μg of cholecalciferol. The symptoms of a vitamin D deficiency are less obvious in fish than in mammals. Studies in carp, koi, or goldfish are not available in the literature. In trout, symptoms include slow growth and white muscle tetany (George et al., 1979). Histologic changes in the white muscle fibers of the expaxial musculature are evident, but not in bone (Barnett et al., 1978). Catfish raised on a vitamin D–deficient diet show reduced weight gain, lower body ash, calcium, and phosphorus levels (Lovell and Li, 1978).

Natural feed products used for fish contain little to no vitamin D, with the exception of fish oils. Synthetic forms of cholecalciferol are relatively inexpensive and should be added when formulating a fish diet.

Vitamin E

When discovered in the early 1920s, vitamin E was named tocopherol from the Greek word *tokos*, which means to bear young. Vitamin E was first isolated from vegetable oils that cured infertility in rats fed milk diets. There are at least eight tocopherols that have been identified in plants, of which the most active form is *d*-α-tocopherol ($C_{29}H_{50}O_2$) (Fig. 46–4). One IU of vitamin E is equal to the biological activity of 1 mg of *d*-α-tocopherol. Vitamin E acts as an antioxidant in metabolism by preventing oxidation of unsaturated phospholipids in cellular membranes. Vitamin E is also involved in the synthesis of porphyrin and heme groups. Although all of the roles

of vitamin E are not understood, deficiency symptoms in many animals include decreased fertility of both sexes, muscular dystrophy, anemia, and hemorrhage and edema of many tissues caused by increased permeability of the capillaries.

Carp fed oxidized silkworm pupae develop Sekoke disease, which results in a loss of flesh on the back of the fish. This condition does not occur when 500 mg/kg diet of *d*-α-tocopherol acetate is added to the diet (Hashimoto et al., 1969). Fatty livers and ceroid bodies are common symptoms of vitamin E deficiency in fish (Lovell, 1988). In trout and salmon, symptoms include irregularly shaped erythrocytes, extreme anemia, susceptibility to stress, high mortality, ascites, and exudative diathesis (Poston et al., 1976). Supplementing the diet with 30 IU/kg diet is sufficient for preventing a deficiency in trout and salmon (Woodall and LaRoche, 1964; Hung et al., 1979, 1980).

If the level of polyunsaturated fats in the diet increases, the requirement for vitamin E also increases. The addition of commercial antioxidants appears to have a sparing effect on the requirement for vitamin E. Feeding 125 mg of ethoxyquin/kg of diet will prevent vitamin E deficiency symptoms in channel catfish but does not support the same level of growth as feeding 25 mg of *d*-α-tocopherol/kg diet (Lovell et al., 1984). The roles of selenium and vitamin E are also related. Increased levels of vitamin E are required if selenium is low in the diet.

Vitamin K

Vitamin K was discovered by Henrik Dam during the early 1940s. The name is derived from the word *koagulation*, since vitamin K is an essential factor

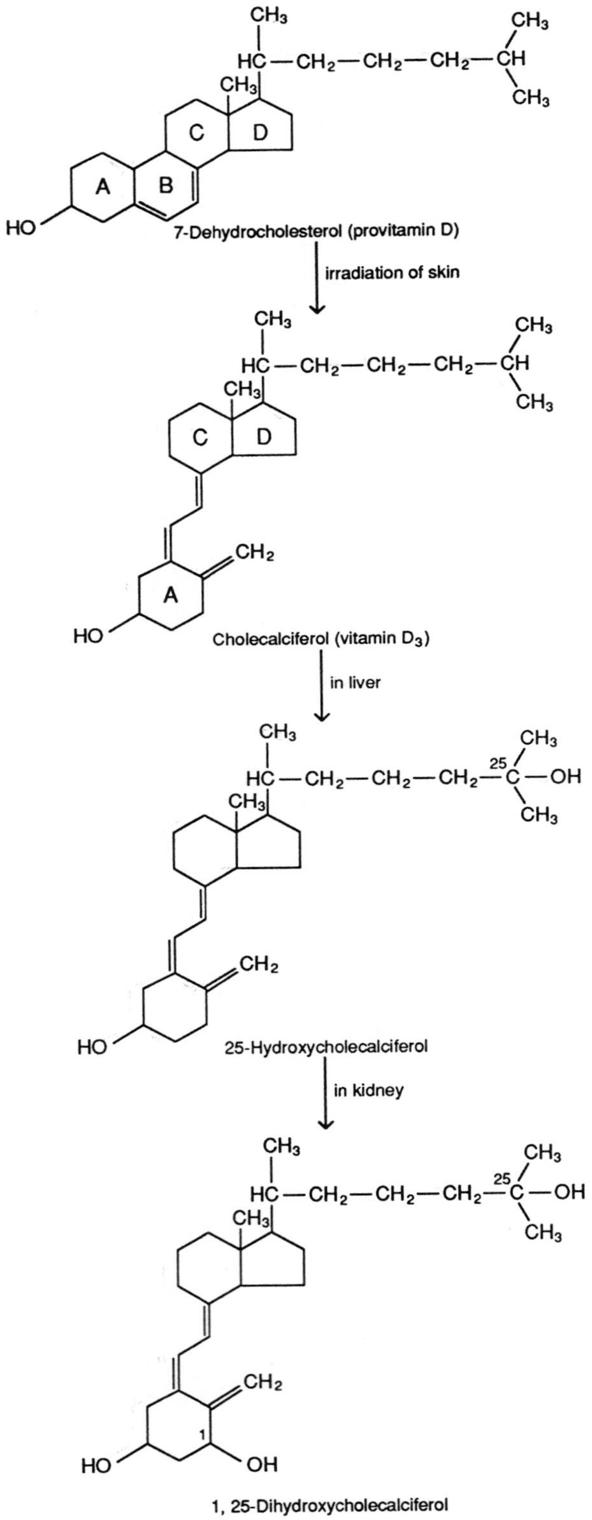

FIGURE 46–3. The conversion of 7-dehydrocholesterol to 1,25-dihydroxycholecalciferol.

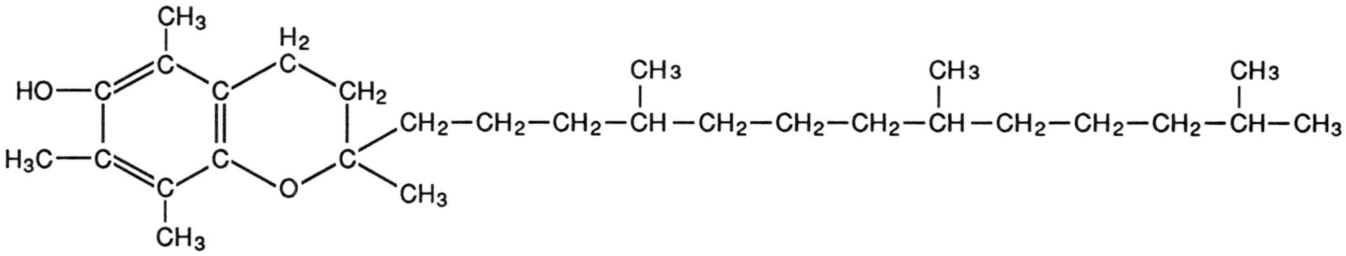

FIGURE 46–4. The structure of vitamin E.

for normal blood clotting. There are two natural forms of vitamin K: phylloquinone (K_1), found in green plants, and menaquinone (K_2) produced by the intestinal flora of animals. Vitamin K_2 is found in animal feces and fishmeal. There is a synthetic form of vitamin K, menadione (K_3), which has more vitamin activity than either of the natural forms (Fig. 46–5).

Vitamin K is just one factor in a long chain of reactions that result in the formation of blood clots (Fig. 46–6). Prothrombin, a glycoprotein, is split by the protease factor Xa in the presence of vitamin K, calcium, and a phospholipid surface to produce thrombin. Fibrinogen is then cleaved by the thrombin to produce fibrin, which then produces a fibrin clot.

It is assumed that vitamin K has other functions, since it is produced by bacteria and plants that have no blood. In metabolism, it appears to carry electrons in transport systems and oxidative phosphorylation reactions.

Prolonged blood coagulation is the only deficiency symptom identified in fish. The requirement of carp is not documented, but both trout (Poston, 1976) and channel catfish (Dupree, 1966) require vitamin K. Fingerling trout fed levels of 0.5 to 1.0 mg of menadione/kg of diet maintain normal blood coagulation. No cases are known of vitamin K toxicity in fish. In one study, 2400 mg menadione/kg diet was fed to salmonids with no adverse effects (Poston, 1971).

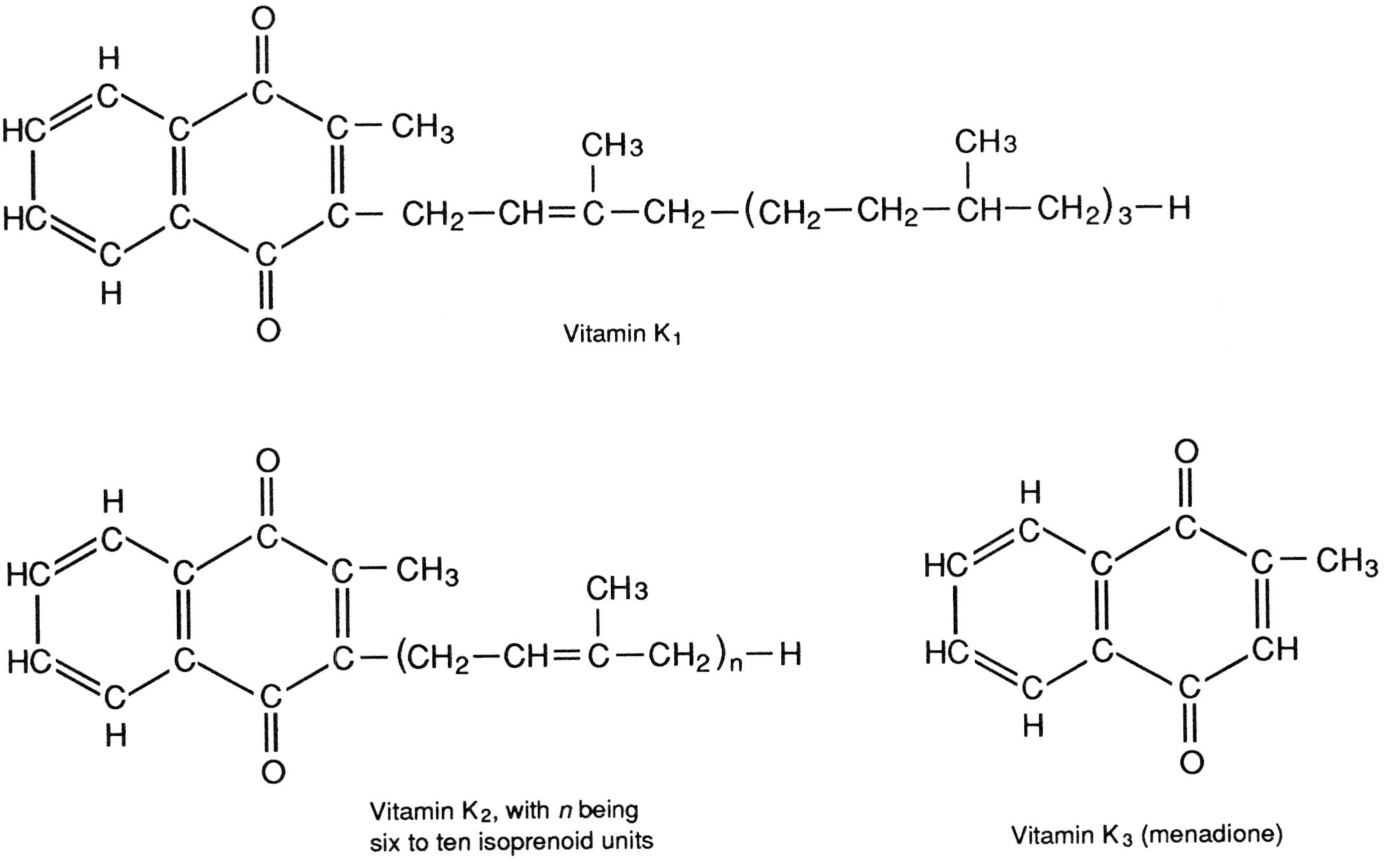

Vitamin K_1

Vitamin K_2, with n being six to ten isoprenoid units

Vitamin K_3 (menadione)

FIGURE 46–5. The structures of the three forms of vitamin K.

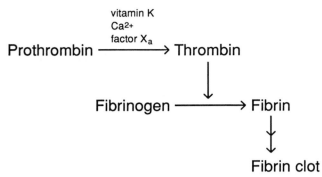

FIGURE 46–6. The role of vitamin K in fibrin clot production.

Vitamin Supplementation

Vitamins are readily destroyed when exposed to heat, air, and metals. Much of the vitamin content of feeds can be lost during processing and storage. Table 46–1 presents the minimum vitamin requirements of some species of fishes. This table does not include storage losses. Vitamin premixes should be added to the feed at an increased level to provide the minimum requirements in the face of vitamin losses due to processing and storage. Table 46–2 gives the signs of vitamin deficiency in carp.

PIGMENTATION OF FISHES

Three divergent industries, salmon fisheries, ornamental koi fanciers, and tropical fish suppliers, owe their existence to the rich colors of the fishes' skin or flesh. The bright colors are the result of deposition of pigments in the skin, eggs, gonads, milt, and muscle. Fish pigments include melanins and carotenoids. The carotenoids are responsible for the red, orange, and yellow colors so popular in koi and goldfish.

As a group, carotenoids are aliphatic, aliphatic-alicyclic, or aromatic structures composed of 5-carbon isoprene groups. There are two major subgroups of carotenoids, the carotenes and the oxycarotenoids (xanthophyls). Carotenoids are found in many plants and animals, including yellow vegetables, tomatoes, algae, mushrooms, crustaceans, peppers, and chicken.

Most carotenoids are yellow to red; however, when bound with protein they can form a variety of blues and greens. When these carotenoproteins are

TABLE 46–2. Vitamin Deficiency Signs in Carp

Vitamin	Common Carp
A	Depigmentation, twisted opercula, fin and skin hemorrhages
D	Not known
E	Muscular dystrophy, exophthalmos, renal and pancreatic degeneration, ceroid in visceral organs
K	Not known

heated, the bonds are disrupted, releasing the carotenoids. This is why blue crabs turn red when boiled. Plants and protozoa are able to synthesize carotenoids, whereas animals must consume them. In the wild, fish consume carotenoids in crustaceans, algae, plants, or other fish that consume these foods. Intensive culture of fish has made it necessary to supplement diets with carotenoids.

Pigment Metabolism of Koi and Goldfish

Unlike common carp, koi are able to metabolize dietary sources of carotenoids. Several metabolic pathways have been proposed. The conversion of dietary zeaxanthin to astaxanthin and dietary lutein to doradexanthin (4-ketolutein) has been reported (Hata and Hata, 1975a,b). A later study demonstrated that the free form of zeaxanthin is absorbed and transferred to the integument, where it is esterified and converted first to adonixanthin and then to astaxanthin (Hata and Hata, 1976a,b).

α-Doradexanthin is also present in the integument of both goldfish and koi (Fig. 46–7). Dietary lutein and zeaxanthin are converted to astaxanthin, whereas β-carotene and canthaxanthin are not (Tanaka et al., 1976). Goldfish are also able to metabolize β-carotene to astaxanthin (Rodriguez et al., 1973). Feeding 2 mg carotene/g of food produces a fourfold increase in tissue levels of astaxanthin. It is thought that β-carotene is converted to astaxanthin via isocryptoxanthin, isozeaxanthin, echinenone, 4-hydroxy–4'keto-beta-carotene, and possibly canthaxanthin and phoenicoxanthin.

Ten different carotenoids have been isolated from red koi (Matsuno et al., 1979; Matsuno and Matsutaka, 1981). These include lutein, zeaxanthin, α-doradexanthin, β-doradexanthin (4-ketozeaxanthin), astaxanthin, β-carotene, cryptoxanthin, diatoxanthin, β-carotenetriol (4-hydroxy-zeaxanthin), β-carotenetetrol, and idoxanthin. The predominance of β-carotenetriol and idoxanthin supports the hypothesis that zeaxanthin is converted to astaxanthin via the following pathway:

$$\text{zeaxanthin} \rightarrow \beta\text{-carotenetriol} \rightarrow \text{4-ketozeaxanthin} \rightarrow \text{idoxanthin} \rightarrow \text{astaxanthin}$$

After being fed test diets containing alfalfa meal, mysis, lutein, or astaxanthin, red carp produce better pigmentation with astaxanthin than with lutein (Iwahashi and Wakui, 1976). The intensity of pigmentation is proportional to the amount of carotenoids in the diet and dietary cholesterol has no influence on the uptake of carotenoids.

Many types of koi are multicolored with patterns of red, white, and black. When lutein is added to the diet, it is first absorbed in the integument in its free form, and is then esterified in the xanthophore to 4-ketolutein (Hata and Hata, 1976b). Any excess lutein remains in the integument in the free form, giving the white part a yellow color. Feeding large amounts of lutein to koi should be avoided, since

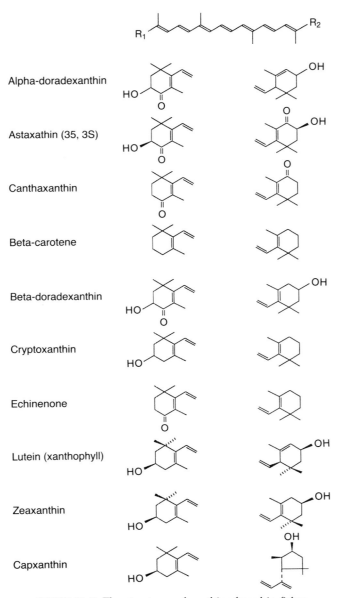

FIGURE 46–7. The structures of xanthins found in fishes.

the yellowish tones are considered undesirable among koi enthusiasts.

Pigment Supplementation of Koi

There are little to no published data concerning practical feed ingredients and feeding levels for maintaining good color in koi and goldfish. Most of the published research is written by biochemists whose primary concern is unlocking the riddles of the carotenoids' metabolic functions. More practical research is conducted by feed companies who consider the results proprietary information.

The backyard koi enthusiast will rarely have difficulty maintaining good color of their animals. The average koi pond contains filamentous blue-green algae, *Spirulina* spp., which has high levels of

β-carotene as well as echinenone, cryptoxanthin, and zeaxanthin (Choubert, 1979). Fish kept in heavily stocked ponds or tanks devoid of algae need carotenoid supplementation in the diet.

Plant and plant extracts used for pigment supplementation in the poultry industry could also be used to supplement koi diets. Marigold and squash flowers are available as whole petals or in extract form. Marigolds are very high in lutein, whereas squash blossoms contain zeaxanthin, lutein, and β-cryptoxanthin (Lee et al., 1978) (Table 46–3).

Pigmentation of Salmonids

While ornamental koi have been raised for hundreds of years, salmon fishing and farming has a far greater economic impact in both Europe and North America. Salmon flesh is highly prized for its flavor and color. It is estimated the salmon industry will purchase as much as 15,000 lb of carotenoid pigments in 1990. With a commercial price of $1000/kg of pigment, the salmon industry invests heavily each year to assure proper pigmentation of the fish (Torrissen et al., 1987).

The two primary red pigments found in salmonids are astaxanthin (3,3'dihydroxy–4,4'-diketo-beta-carotene) and canthaxanthin (4–4'diketo-beta-carotene) (Steven, 1948; Schmidt and Baker, 1969; Deufel, 1965; Satio and Regier, 1971; Hata and Hata, 1975a; Choubert, 1977; Torrissen, 1986). Other pigments found in much smaller quantities include 3-epilutein, diatoxanthin, cyantixanthin, doradexanthin, lutein, zeaxanthin, echinenone, cryptoxanthin, deepoxyneoxanthin, adonirubin, asteroidenone, and β-carotene (Schiedt et al., 1981, 1985, 1986; Sitseva, 1982; Kitahara, 1983).

Unlike koi and goldfish who convert zeaxanthin to astaxanthin (Hata and Hata, 1972, 1976), salmonid species including chum salmon, rainbow trout, and Atlantic salmon reduce astaxanthin to zeaxanthin (Hata and Hata, 1973; Kitahara, 1983; Ando, 1986). While goldfish deposit carotenoids primarily in the skin, salmonids deposit most of the metabolized carotenoids in the flesh (Hata and Hata, 1975a; Kitahara, 1983; Schiedt et al., 1985; Ando, 1986), except trout that also deposit carotenoids in chromatophores in the skin (Peterson et al., 1966; Steven, 1948, 1949).

In the wild, salmonids ingest carotenoid pigments by consuming zooplankton or fish feeding on zooplankton. Farm-raised fish are fed a source of synthetic pigment in commercially prepared feeds. The two most common sources of pigment in the salmonid industry are synthetic canthaxanthin, known as Roxanthin Red or Carophyll Red, and synthetic astaxanthin, known as Carophyll Pink. Both products are marketed by Hoffman La Roche (Basle, Switzerland) in a dry beadlet powder at a 10% concentration level. Although not yet approved as feed additives in the United States, both products are used in Canada and Europe. Astaxanthin is absorbed and deposited in the flesh of salmonids

TABLE 46–3. Carotenoid Content in Some Pigment Sources Used for Feeding Fish

Pigment Source	Carotenoid	Amount (mg/kg)
Crustaceans		
Krill (*Euphausia* spp.)	Astaxanthin	22–27
Krill (*E. pacifica*)	Astaxanthin	100–130
Krill (*Meganyctiphanes norvegica*)	Astaxanthin	46—93
Copepod (*Calanus finmarchicus*)	Astaxanthin	39–84
Red crab (*Pleuroncodes planipes*)	Astaxanthin	100–160
Crustaceans Products		
Crab (*Chinochetes opilio*), vacuum dried	"Luteinlike"	0.1
	Astaxanthin	5
	Astacene	2
Crab (*Greyon quinquedens*), freeze dried	Astaxanthin	76
Krill (*Euphausia* spp.), co-dried with oil	Astaxanthin	200
Krill oil (*Euphausia* spp.)	Astaxanthin	727
Copepod (*Calanus finmarchicus*), oil	Astaxanthin	520
Crawfish (*Procambarus clarkii*), oil extract	Astaxanthin	750
Crawfish meal (*Procambarus clarkii*)	Astaxanthin	137
Shrimp shells (*Pandalus borealis*), hand shelled	Astaxanthin	60–128
Shrimp shells (*P. borealis*), machine shelled	Astaxanthin	20–48
Shrimp shells (*P. borealis*), silaged	Astaxanthin	74
Shrimp (*P. borealis*), vacuum dried	Astaxanthin	100
Shrimp (*P. borealis*), steam dried + antioxidant	Astaxanthin	192
Shrimp oil (*P. borealis*)	Astaxanthin	1,095
Shrimp freeze dried	Astaxanthin	1,160
Fish Oils		
Capelin oil	Astaxanthin	6–94
Mackerel	Astaxanthin	6–11
Plant and Plant Products		
Marigold flowers (*Tagetes erecta*), extract	Lutein	(90%)
Squash flowers (*Curcubita marcia*), extract	Zeaxanthin	(38%)
	Leutein	(23%)
	β-Cryptoxanthin	(17%)
Paprika extract	(Capxanthin + capsorubin)	235
Algae		
Spirulina spp., spray dried	β-Carotene	434
	β-Carotene-5,6-expoxide	79
	Echinenone	118
	Cryptoxanthin	389
	Zeaxanthin	151
	Myxoxanthophyll	409
Yeast		
Rhodortorule sanneii	β-Carotene	7
	γ-Carotene	1
	Torularhodin	83
	Torulene	28
Phaffia rhodozyma	Astaxanthin	30–800
Synthetic Products		
Carophyll Red/Roxanthin Red[a]	Canthaxanthin	100,000
Carophyll Pink[a]	Astaxanthin	50,000

[a]*Hoffmann La Roche, Basle, Switzerland.*

Adapted from Torrissen, O. J., Hardy, R. W., and Shearer, K. D. (1989) Pigmentation of Salmonids—Carotenoid Deposition of Metabolism. Reviews in Aquatics Science 1(2). Reprinted with permission from Reviews in Aquatics Science. *Copyright CRC Press, Inc., Boca Raton, FL.*

more efficiently than canthaxanthin (Foss et al., 1984, 1987; Storebakken et al., 1984, 1986, 1987; Tidemann et al., 1984; Torrissen, 1987).

Owing to the high cost of synthetic pigments, the use of several natural pigments has been investigated. Crustacea and crustacean waste, including red crab, krill, crawfish, and shrimp meals, contain astaxanthin as the primary pigment. In order to produce acceptable levels of pigment in salmon, the wastes must be fed at levels ranging from 10 to 25% of the total diet (Ugletveit, 1974; Spinelli and Mahnken, 1978; Chen and Meyers, 1983; Torrissen, 1985). These levels may not be practical for commercial application, since most crustacean meals contain high levels of ash and chitin and very little protein. Oil extracts of capelin, red crab, and crawfish contain higher levels of astaxanthin; however, the availability of the astaxanthin is dependent upon the extraction process used (Ugletveit, 1974; Choubert, 1977; Spinelli and Mahnken, 1978; Chen and Meyers, 1983) (see Table 46–3).

Other natural sources of carotenoids include yeast and algae. *Phaffia rhodozyma* is a yeast containing high levels of astaxanthin and has been shown to increase carotenoid levels in rainbow trout (Johnson et al., 1977, 1980). Although blue-green algae are a good source of pigment for koi, they do not produce discernible pigmentation in rainbow trout (Choubert, 1979). The subphylum Chlorophycea does produce astaxanthin. When fed to rainbow trout at levels of 78 mg/kg food over a 7-month period, it increased tissue levels of astaxanthin from 0 to 1.2 mg/kg (Kvalheim and Knutsen, 1985). Capxanthin, the primary pigment in paprika and red peppers, has been shown to produce color in brook trout (Peterson, 1966).

Pigmentation of Warm-Water and Tropical Fishes

The pigmentation of warm-water and tropical fishes is just beginning to be studied. Unpublished studies by R.T. Lovell have found the commercial pigment Biored (Athens, Georgia) to be more effective in enhancing skin color of tilapia than astaxanthin or canthaxanthin. Astaxanthin was more effective than canthaxanthin. Biored is a commercial pigment product containing mostly capxanthin and some lutein, zeaxanthin, and cryptoxanthin.

Until recently, the bright color of tropical fishes was attributed strictly to genetics and physical cell structure. Most tropical fishes were wild caught and lived for only a short time in captivity. With improved technology, commercial suppliers are breeding more species in captivity in indoor, closed systems. As a result, some breeders are beginning to notice the colors of their captive fishes are not as vivid as wild-caught animals.

In a preliminary study also conducted by R.T. Lovell at Auburn University, cherry barbs were fed diets containing either canthaxanthin or Biored, at levels of 100 or 400 ppm of diet for 4 weeks. The skin of the barbs fed Biored was noticeably brighter than those fed canthaxanthin. The fish fed 400 ppm Biored were more vivid than those fed 100 ppm (Lovell, 1990).

LITERATURE CITED

Ando, S. (1986) Studies on the food biochemical aspects of changes in chum salmon, *Onchorynchus keta*, during spawning migration: Mechanisms of muscle deterioration and nuptial coloration. Mem. Fac. Fish. Hokkaido Univ. 33:1.

Aoe, H., Masuda, I., Mimura, T., Saito, T., and Komo, A. (1968) Requirement of young carp for vitamin A. Bull. Jpn. Soc. Fish. 34:959–964.

Barnett, B.J., Cho, C.Y., and Slinger, S.J. (1978) The requirement for vitamin D₃ and relative biopotency of dietary D₂ and D₃ in rainbow trout. J. Nutr. 109:23. (Abstr.)

Britton, G., and Goodwin, T.W. (1971) Methods in Enzymology. Academic Press, New York, pp. 654–701.

Burton, G.W., and Ihgold, K.U. (1984) Beta-carotene: an unusual type of lipid antioxidant. Science 224:569.

Chen, H. M., and Meyers, S.P. (1983) Ensilage treatment of crawfish waste for improvement of astaxanthin pigment extraction. J. Food. Sci. 48:1516.

Choubert, G. (1977) Carotenoides fixes par truite arc-en-ciel en croissance. Thesis, Diplome de Decteur de 3e Cycle. l'Universite Pierre et Marie Curie, Paris.

Choubert, G. (1979) Tentative utilization of spirulina algae as a source of carotenoid pigments for rainbow trout. Aquaculture 18:135.

Deufel, J. (1965) Pigmentierungsversuche mit canthaxanthin bei regenbogenforellen. Arch. Fisheriwiss. 16(2):125.

Dupree, H.K. (1966) Vitamins essential for growth of channel catfish, *Ictalurus punctatus*. Technical Paper No. 7, Bureau of Sport Fisheries and Wildlife, Washington, D.C.

Dupree, H.K. (1970) Dietary requirement of vitamin A acetate and beta-carotene. In: Progress in Sport Fishery Research, 1969. Resource Pub. No. 88. Bureau of Sport Fisheries and Wildlife, Washington, D.C. pp. 148–150.

Foss, P., Storebakken, T., Schiedt, K., Liaaen-Jensen, S., Austreng, E., and Streiff, K. (1984). Carotenoids in diets for salmonids. I. Pigmentation of rainbow trout with the individual optical isomers of astaxanthin in comparison with canthaxanthin. Aquaculture 41:213.

Foss, P., Storebakken, T., Austreng, E., and Liaaen-Jensen, S. (1987) Carotenoids in salmonids. V. Pigmentation of rainbow trout and sea trout with astaxanthin and astaxanthin dipalmitate in comparison with canthaxanthin. Aquaculture 65:293–305.

George, J.C., Barnett, B.J., Cho, C.Y. and Slinger, S.J. (1979). Impairment of white skeletal muscle in vitamin D₃-deficient rainbow trout. J. Nutr. 109:23. (Abstr.)

Hashimoto, Y., Okaichi, T. , Watanabe, T., Furukawa, A., and Umezu, T. (1969) Muscle dystrophy of carp due to oxidized oil and the preventative effect of vitamin E. Bull. Jpn. Soc. Sci. Fish. 32:64–69.

Hata, M., and Hata, M. (1972) Carotenoid pigments in goldfish. IV. Carotenoid metabolism. Bull. Jpn. Soc. Sci. Fish. 38(4):331.

Hata, M., and Hata, M. (1973) Studies on astaxanthin formation in some fresh-water fishes. Tohoku J. Agr. Res. 24(4):192.

Hata, M., and Hata, M. (1975a) Carotenoid pigments in rainbow trout, *Salmo gairdneri irideus*. Tohoku J. Agr. Res. 24(4):192.

Hata, M., and Hata, M. (1975b) Carotenoid metabolism in fancy red carp, *Cyprinus carpio*. I. Administration of carotenoids. Bull. Jpn. Soc. Sci. Fish. 41(6):653–655.

Hata, M., and Hata, M. (1976a) Carotenoid metabolism in fancy red carp, *Cyprinus carpio*. II. Metabolism of zeaxanthin. Bull. Jpn. Soc. Sci. Fish. 42(2):203–205.

Hata, M., and Hata, M. (1976b) Carotenoid metabolism in fancy red carp, *Cyprinus carpio*. III. Accumulation of lutein. Bull. Jpn. Soc. Sci. Fish. 44(1):83–84.

Hung, S.S.O., Cho, C.Y., and Slinger, S.J. (1979) Effect of autooxidized fish oil on the vitamin E requirement of rainbow trout fed a practical diet. J. Nutr. 109:23 (Abstr.)

Hung, S.S.O., Cho, C.Y., and Slinger, S.J. (1980) Measurement of oxidation in fish oil and its effect on Vitamin E nutrition of rainbow trout, *Salmo gairdneri*. Can. J. Fish. Aquatic Sci. 37:1248–1253.

Iwahashi, M., and Wakui, H. (1979) Intensification of color of fancy red carp with diet. Bull. Jpn. Soc. Sci. Fish. 42(12):1339–1344.

Johnson, E.A., Conklin, D.E., and Lewis, M.J. (1977) The yeast *Phaffia rhodozyma* as a dietary pigment source for salmonids and crustaceans. J. Fish. Res. Bd. Can. 34:2417.

Johnson, E.A., Villa, T.G., and Lewis, M.J. (1980) *Phaffia rhodozyma* as an astaxanthin source in salmonid diets. Aquaculture 20:123.

Kitahara, T. (1983) Behaviour of carotenoids in the chum salmon (*Oncorhynchus keta*) during anadromous migration. Comp. Biochem. Physiol. 76B:97.

Kvalheim, B., and Knutsen, G. (1985) Pigmentering av laks med astaxanthin fra mikroalger. Norsk Fiskeoppdrett 3:4.

Lee, R.G., Neamtu, G. Gh, Lee, T.C., and Simpson, K.L. (1978) Pigmentation of rainbow trout with extracts of floral parts from *Tagetes erecta* and *Curcubita maxima marcia*. Rev. Roum. Biochim. 15(4):287.

Lovell, R.T. (1988) Nutrition and Feeding of Fish. Van Nostrand Reinhold, New York.

Lovell, R. T. (1990) Personal communication.

Lovell, R.T., and Li, Y.-P. (1978) Essentiality of vitamin D in diets of channel catfish (*Ictalurus punctatus*). Trans. Am. Fish. Soc. 107:809–811.

Lovell, R.T., Miyazaki, T., and Rebegnator, S. (1984) Requirement of alpha-tocopherol by channel catfish fed diets low in polyunsaturated fatty acids. J. Nutr. 114:894–901.

Matsuno, T., and Matsutaka, H. (1981) Carotenoids of four species of crucian carp and two varieties of goldfish. Bull. Jpn. Soc. Sci. Fish. 47(1):85–88.

Matsuno, T., and Nagata, S. (1979) The occurrence of idoxanthin in fancy red carp, *Cyprinus carpio*. Bull. Japan Soc. Sci. Fish. 45(4):537.

Matsuno, T., Nagata, S., Iwahashi, M., Koike, T., and Okada, M. (1979) Intensification of color of fancy red carp with zeaxanthin and myxoxanthophyll, major carotenoid constituents of spirulina. Bull. Jpn. Soc. Sci. Fish. 45(5):627–632.

National Research Council (1983) Nutrient Requirements of Warmwater Fishes and Shellfishes. National Academy Press, Washington, D.C.

Peterson, D.H., Jager, H.K., and Savage, G.M. (1966) Natural coloration of trout using xanthophylls. Trans. Am. Fish. Soc. 95:408.

Poston, H.A. (1971) Effect of excess vitamin K on the growth, coagulation time, and hematocrit values of brook trout fingerlings. In: Fish. Res. Bull. No. 34. State of New York Conservation Department, Albany, pp. 41–42.

Poston, H.A. (1976) Relative effect of two dietary water-soluble analogues of menaquinone on coagulation and packed cell volume of blood of lake trout, *Salvelinus namaycush*. J. Fish. Res. Bd. Can. 33:1791–1793.

Poston, H.A., Combs, G.F., Jr., and Leibovitz, L. (1976) Vitamin E and selenium interrelations in the diet of Atlantic salmon (*Salmo salar*): Gross, histological and biochemical deficiency signs. J. Nutr. 106:892–904.

Poston, H.A., Riis, R.C., Rumsey, G.L., and Ketola, H.G. (1977) The effect of supplemental dietary amino acids, minerals and vitamins on salmonids fed caractogenic diets. Cornell Vet. 67:472–509.

Rodriguez, D. B., Simpson, K.L., and Chichester, C.O. (1973) The biosynthesis of astaxanthin: XVII. Intermediates in the conversion of beta-carotene. Int. J. Biochem. 4(21):213–222.

Satio, A., and Regier, L.W. (1971) Pigmentation of brook trout (*Salvelinus fontinalis*) by feeding dried crustacean waste. J. Fish. Res. Bd. Can. 28(4):509.

Schiedt, K., Leuenberger, F.J., and Vecchi, M. (1981) Natural occurrence of enantiomeric and meso-astaxanthin 5. Ex wild salmon (*Salmo salar* and *Oncorhynchus*). Helv. Chim. Acta 64:449.

Schiedt, K., Leuenberger, F.J., Vecchi, M., and Glinz, E. (1985) Absorption, retention, and metabolic transformations of carotenoids in rainbow trout, salmon, and chicken. Pure Appl. Chem. 57(5):685.

Schiedt, K., Vecchi, M., and Glinz, E. (1986) Astaxanthin and its metabolites in wild rainbow trout (*Salmo gairdneri*). Comp. Biochem. Physiol. 83B(1):9.

Schmidt, P.J., and Baker, E.G. (1969) Indirect pigmentation of salmon and trout flesh with canthaxanthin. J. Fish. Res. Bd. Can. 26(2):357.

Simpson, K.L., Katayama, T., and Chichester, C.O. (1981) Carotenoids in fish feeds. In: Carotenoids as Colorants and Vitamin A Precursors (Bauernfeind, ed.). Academic Press, New York.

Sitseva, L.V. (1982) Qualitative composition and distribution of carotenoids and vitamin A in the organs and tissues of rainbow trout (*Salmo gairdneri*). J. Ichtyol. 22(1):96.

Spinelli, J., and Mahnken, C. (1978) Carotenoid deposition in pen-reared salmonids fed diets containing oil extracts of red crab (*Pleuroncodes planipes*). Aquaculture 13:213.

Steven, D.M. (1948) Studies on animal carotenoids. 1. Carotenoids of the brown trout (*Salmo trutta* Linn.). J. Exp. Biol. 25:369.

Steven, D.M. (1949) Studies on animal carotenoids. 2. Carotenoids in the reproductive cycle of brown trout. J. Exp. Biol. 26:295.

Storebakken, T., Foss, P., Austreng, E., and S. Liaaen-Jensen, S. (1984)

Carotenoids in diets for salmonids. II. Epimerization studies with astaxanthin in Atlantic salmon. Aquaculture 44:259.

Storebakken, T., Foss, P., Huse, L., Wandsvik, A., and Lea, T.B. (1986) Carotenoids in diets for salmonids. III. Utilization of canthaxanthin from dry and wet diets by Atlantic salmon, rainbow trout, and sea trout. Aquaculture 51:245.

Storebakken, T., Foss, P., Schiedt, K., Austreng, E., Liaaen-Jensen, S., and Mainz, U. (1987) Carotenoids in diets for salmonids. IV. Pigmentation of Atlantic salmon with astaxanthin, astaxanthin dipalmitate and canthaxanthin. Aquaculture 65:279–292.

Tacon, A.G.J. (1981) Speculative review of possible carotenoid function in fish. Progressive Fish Culturist 43(4):205.

Tanaka, Y., Katayama, T., Simpson, K.L., and Chichester, C.O. (1976) The biosynthesis of astaxanthin. XIX. The distribution of alpha-doradexanthin and the metabolism of carotenoids in goldfish. Bull. Jpn. Soc. Sci. Fish. 42(8):885–891.

Tidemann, E., Raa, J., Stormo, B., and Torrissen, O. (1984) Processing and utilization of shrimp waste. In: Engineering and Food. Vol. II (McKenna, ed.). Elsevier, Amsterdam.

Torrissen, O.J. (1984) Pigmentation of salmonids—effect of carotenoids in eggs and start-feeding diets on survival and growth rate. Aquaculture 43:185.

Torrissen, O.J. (1985) Pigmentation of salmonids: factors affecting carotenoid deposition in rainbow trout (*Salmo gairdneri*). Aquaculture 46:133.

Torrissen, O.J. (1986) Pigmentation of salmonids—a comparison of astaxanthin and canthaxanthin as pigment sources for rainbow trout. Aquaculture 53:271.

Torrissen, O.J. (1987) Pigmentation of salmonids—interactions of astaxanthin and canthaxanthin on pigment deposition in rainbow trout. Aquaculture 79:363–374.

Torrissen, O.J., Hardy, R.W., and Shearer, K.D. (1987) Pigmentation of Salmonids—Carotenoid Deposition of Metabolism. Northwest and Alaska Fisheries Center, Seattle.

Ugletveit, S. (1974) Pigmentering av lakse-og orretkjott. Fisken og Havet, ser B. 9:31.

Woodall, A.N., and LaRoche, G. (1964) Nutrition of salmonid fishes XI. Iodide requirements of chinook salmon. J. Nutr. 82:475–482.

Chapter 47

CARP, KOI, AND GOLDFISH REPRODUCTION

BEVERLY A. GOVEN-DIXON

The culture of common carp is thought to be the oldest form of fish farming in the world, having been practiced in China as early as 2000 B.C. These earliest endeavors rapidly spread throughout the world, from Asia to Europe and into the Americas, where the fresh water was warm enough for carp survival. Today, however, the extent of carp farming operations is determined largely by the cultural differences in the diets of various human populations. The carp have long been culturally accepted as a valuable food fish in Eastern Europe, Asia, and Israel. However, despite experiments in carp culture in California as early as 1872, cultured carp has not created much interest in markets in the United States (McGeachin, 1986).

While common carp may not appeal to every culture's culinary taste, other members of the family have appealed to the esthetic sense. The domestic goldfish was bred in China from an orange variant of the wild goldfish more than a thousand years ago. In Japan, koi (the Japanese word for carp) arose centuries ago from selective breeding of common carp. Then, as today, numerous varieties of fancy goldfish and koi, famed for striking color patterns, are highly prized as ornamental fishes, often fetching several thousand dollars per breeding pair (Roe and Evans, 1969).

Whether for food, bait, or beauty, the selective breeding of carp has become profitable on a wide scale. At the ornamental level, in particular, the continued existence of fancy varieties is closely tied to directed breeding efforts. Even the most refined stock will regress when neglected, and individuals of neglected breeding stocks will begin to resemble the original wild-type goldfish after several generations. Close to a dozen members of the carp family are selectively bred worldwide; however, they constitute only a minor portion of the total aquaculture industry (Penzes and Tolg, 1983).

SEXUAL MATURATION

Sexual maturation occurs in male goldfish at about 2 years of age. Females reach sexual maturity slightly later, at 3 years of age. In females, the maturation process is divided into several phases, depending on ovarian development. Phase 1 lasts from hatching to the 18th or 20th month, during which the females are sexually immature. Phase 2 lasts one year, during which the fish will reach maturity, although the ovaries remain small. Phase 3 is the period between the 6th and 10th months prior to spawning, when the development of the ovary is discernible. The inactive egg cells are massed into bundles in the ovary during this stage.

Phase 4 consists of the weeks prior to spawning when the ovary is ready for reproduction. In Phase 4 all that is required is the right spawning conditions. When the fish have reached phase 4, the abdomen is round and distended with eggs. The total number of eggs that develop depends on the size of the female and her care and diet during the previous year. A well-nourished, well-developed female, 10 to 12 cm long, produces 6000 to 18,000 eggs. In smaller fish, particularly at the first spawning, only 1000 to 2000 eggs may be produced. The first four phases of ovarian development are determined largely by water temperature. Phase 4 is actually a state of readiness. Environmental conditions favorable for spawning during this stage will induce full maturation, or phase 5.

Phase 5 occurs as a result of nerve and hormonal activity. Environmental conditions such as temperature, presence of aquatic plants, fresh oxygen-rich water, and, most important, the presence of courting males trigger the hormonal development of the female into full sexual maturity and the release of eggs. This phase, in particular, is influenced by the pituitary gland, which secretes hormones, including gonadotropin, that stimulate and regulate the function of the gonads. Secreted gonadotrophin stimulates completion of egg development. The eggs detach from the ovary, fall into the body cavity, and become ready for release (Penzes and Tolg, 1983).

SPAWNING

Goldfish usually spawn in temperatures ranging from 15.5 to 25°C (60 to 85°F) with the optimal at 20°C (68°F). Spawning begins in spring and continues through summer if the fish do not become overcrowded (Stickney, 1979; McGeachin, 1986). Koi spawn in May and June in temperate regions but continue to spawn year round in the tropical regions of Indo-Malaysia (Roe and Evans, 1969). In most countries of the Indo-Pacific region, pond breeding of the common carp is conducted throughout the year. A cold snap during spawning may interrupt or delay spawning, with a substantial loss in production (Bardach et al., 1972). Once temperatures have stabilized, an additional stimulus may be natural flooding or artificial raising of pond water levels.

One of the most decisive factors in inducing the female to release her eggs is the presence of the male engaged in courting behavior. Regardless of how conducive the environment, without active male participation the females cannot mature and spawn. Just prior to spawning, the males develop secondary sexual characteristics, under the influence of hormones. Small, white tubercules, also known as pearl organs, appear on the opercula and leading rays of the fins, with particular prominence on the first ray of the pectoral fin (Matsui, 1972).

Spawning usually occurs in cycles of 2 to 5 days, beginning at dawn and continuing through midmorning. The female is induced to release her eggs by the movements of the male performing the ritual spawning dance. When the eggs contact water, a small appendage with a hole only a few microns wide (micropyle) forms on the outer cell wall of the egg. The motile sperm released by the male penetrate the micropyle to fertilize the egg. The micropyle remains open for only 30 to 60 seconds after the egg is released. If fertilization does not take place during this time, the egg can no longer accept the sperm. In addition, the sperm is only motile for 1 to 2 minutes. It has been estimated that because of these limitations, usually 30 to 40% of the spawn remains unfertilized (Penzes and Tolg, 1983).

Artificial Spawning

Recent advances in carp culture include the induction of spawning by injection of egg-maturing hormones. This technique can be used to regulate production and increase the frequency of spawning in temperate climates. Methods used to induce spawning involve the injection of pituitary gland or extracted pituitary hormones. Fresh or frozen pituitary extract is injected intraperitoneally at the axial of the pelvic fin. The extract from another goldfish of either sex is injected at 2 to 3 mg/kg of body weight. Most fish will respond to pituitary extract from other unrelated species, even animals belonging to different classes, but the common carp has thus far been shown to respond only to pituitary extract of its own species (Bardach et al., 1972). Conversely, common carp pituitary extract is most widely used to induce spawning in other fish. It maintains its potency in a dried form up to 2 years. Accepted doses of acetone-dried cyprinid pituitary for big head, black, silver, and mud carp are 2 to 3 mg/kg of body weight or the equivalent of 3 fresh ground glands per fish. Grass carp require slightly higher doses of dried extract, 3 to 4 mg/kg.

The injection of pituitary homogenates to induce ovulation is not without problems. Fish pituitary homogenates may be expensive or of unknown biologic activity and are not always readily available. The success of this method is variable, and the average percentage of induced ovulation in female carp is only 60%. In an effort to improve results, suitable reliable substitutes for pituitary tissues have been tested. For example, human chorionic gonadotropin (HCG) has been used in doses of 700 to 1000 IU/kg of body weight. HCG is potent in only a limited number of species, which include goldfish, Chinese carp, sea bass, and sea bream. Interestingly, HCG appears to have no effect on common carp, except to induce antibody production (Billard et al., 1987).

Timing is essential to successful inducement of ovulation in females. Goldfish and common carp have a natural marked ovulatory surge of gonadotropin release, lasting about 12 hours in goldfish at 20°C. Gonadotropin is the specific pituitary hormone that stimulates the release of mature eggs. To be effective in inducing ovulation in goldfish and carp, natural or synthetic hormone analogues must simulate a similar surge of gonadotropin. Gonadotropin overdose, however, can cause partial or incomplete infertility in female carp. To reduce the chance of hormone overdose, fractional injection is often used. In this procedure, one-eighth to one-tenth of the total hormone dose is injected into the females, followed by the remainder of the dose 6 to 24 hours later.

The process of artificial induction of sperm maturity or spermiation in males is often not necessary. It can be used to coordinate sexual maturity prior to hand stripping sperm. Injection of males also increases seminal plasma, providing more milt (Bardach et al., 1972). However, injection of males can cause premature release of sperm.

Once spawning has occurred, the fertilized eggs become adhesive and stick to natural or artificial vegetation. Female goldfish may release 2000 to 4000 eggs during each of several spawns. Egg development depends on the ambient water temperature. Hatching may vary from 6 to 7 days at 16°C to 3 days at 26.5°C and to as little as 48 hours at 30°C (Stickney, 1979).

Koi reach breeding size at about 12 inches in length. Like goldfish, koi attain sexual maturity at 18 to 36 months. A koi egg is smaller than the head of a pin, transparent, and adhesive. Females may deposit as many as 10,000 eggs, which are released in clutches of a few hundred at a time (Roe and Evans, 1969).

PROPAGATION

Goldfish, koi, and carp are vegetation spawners. Their eggs are deposited in shallow water either on natural living plants or artificial material, such as mats of hay, straw, or Spanish moss provided by the farmer. Usually, brood stock is treated for external parasites prior to entry into breeding ponds, which have been fertilized to stimulate plankton blooms. Breeders are stocked in ratios of 2 to 3 males per female and are fed twice the normal amount of fish meal. It is important to note that water quality should be monitored and maintained at excellent levels during the breeding season.

Three different methods are employed for the breeding and propagation of goldfish and carp. The first method, referred to as wild or free spawning, is the least demanding in terms of resources. In this method, the breeding stock is placed in ponds with suitable natural vegetation or artificial spawning mats. Some farmers lower the water level in the ponds prior to introducing the breeding stock, to encourage the growth of vegetation along the shoreline. Following spawning, the breeders are left in the pond with the fry.

The egg transfer method maintains a high stocking density of 450 to 560 kg of fish per hectare (400 to 500 lb per acre). Unlike the case with the previous method, it is crucial to keep the ponds clear of natural vegetation. Artificial spawning mats of woven wire and vegetation are placed in shoreline groupings. The water level may be raised to induce spawning, which usually begins at dawn and continues through midmorning. Egg-covered mats are removed about 9:00 a.m. and replaced. It is important that the mats are not too thick with eggs. The eggs should not touch one another because crowding may cause damage or poor ventilation, which encourages the growth of saprophytic fungi. The mats, covered with wet burlap to prevent desiccation, are placed in raceways or grow-out ponds for hatching.

In the third method, fry are transferred from ponds that have been purposely overstocked with eggs. Fine mesh nets are used to catch and transfer fry to rearing ponds. The method is most practical when uniform production and optimum pond usage are required. Using this method, fry can be stocked up to 200,000 fish per acre (Brown and Gratzek, 1980).

Fry are particularly sensitive to light and temperature changes. Too much light or a significant drop in temperature may be injurious to fish, initiating fungal and bacterial infections. It is important to provide adequate food during this stage of growth. Fry require a diet of 30 to 40% protein, which can be purchased in the form of ground powder. Rotifers, brine shrimp nauplii, and daphnia all are excellent fry foods. Fry 2 to 3 weeks old may be fed adult-type food, which may need to be ground more finely.

LITERATURE CITED

Bardach, J.E., Ryther, J.H., and McLarney, W.O. (1972) Aquaculture: The Farming and Husbandry of Freshwater and Marine Organisms. John F. Wiley & Sons, New York.
Billard, R., Bieniarz, K., Popek, W., Epler, P., Breton, B., and Alagarswami,

K. (1987) Stimulation of gonadotropin secretion and spermiation in carp by pimozide-LRH-a treatment: effects of dose and time of day. Aquaculture 62:161–170.

Brown, E.E., and Gratzek, J.B. (1980) Fish Farming Handbook. AVI Pub. Co., Inc., Westport, Connecticut.

Chang, J.P., and Peter, R.E. (1983) Effects of pimozide and DES GLY10 [D-ALA6] luteinizing hormone–releasing hormone ethylamide on serum gonadotropin concentrations, germinal vesicle migration and ovulation in female goldfish Carassius auratus. Gen. Comp. Endocrinol. 52:30–37.

Matusi, Y. (1972) Goldfish Guide. Pet Library Ltd., New York.

McGeachin, R. (1986) Carp and buffalo. In: Culture of Nonsalmonid Freshwater Fishes. (Stickney, R.R, ed.) C.R.C. Press, Inc., Chicago.

Penzes, B., and Tolg, I. (1983) Goldfish and Ornamental Carp. Barron's, Hauppauge, New York.

Roe, C.D., and Evans, A. (1969) Koi: Keeping the Fancy Carp of Japan. Petfish Publ., London.

Sokolowska, M., Peter, R.E., Nahorniak, C.S., Pan, C.H., Chang, J.P., Crim, L.W., and Weil, C. (1984) Induction of ovulation in goldfish, Carassius auratus, by pimozide and analogues of LH-RH. Aquaculture 36:71–83.

Stacey, N.E., Cook, A.F., and Peter, R.E. (1979) Ovulatory surge of gonadotropin in the goldfish, Carassius auratus. Gen. Comp. Endocrinol. 37:246–249.

Stickney, R.R. (1979) Principles of Warm Water Aquaculture. John Wiley & Sons, New York.

Weil, C., Fostier, A., Horvath, L., Marlot, S., and Berscenyi, M. (1980) Profiles of plasma gonadotropin and 17-β-estradiol in the common carp Cyprinus carpio L. as related to spawning induced by hypophysation or LH-RH treatment. Reprod. Nutr. Dev. 20:1041–1050.

Chapter 48

BACTERIAL DISEASES OF GOLDFISH, KOI, AND CARP

MICHAEL K. STOSKOPF

Goldfish, koi, and carp are susceptible to a variety of bacterial infections, most of which affect diverse fish species. The health and economic impact of bacterial infection varies but is usually severe. Some infections cause epizootic mortality, others result in chronic, low-level losses, and still others disfigure fish so they cannot be marketed. This chapter covers two major bacterial infections (Table 48–1). This group of fish is also affected by a wide variety of bacteria described in chapters describing bacterial infections of other fish groups.

BACTERIAL HEMORRHAGIC SEPTICEMIA

SYNONYMS. Motile *Aeromonas* septicemia, infectious dropsy, myoenterohepatic syndrome, redmouth, red sore, red pest, rubella, hydropigenous viral neurosis, hole in body disease, ulcer disease, pop eye.

Host and Geographical Distribution

Aeromonas hydrophila (A. formicans, A. liquefaciens; Aerobacter liquefaciens; Bacillus punctatus, B. rancida; Proteus hydrophila; Pseudomonas, P. granulata, P. hirudinis, P. hydrophila, P. melanovogenes, P. punctata) is found world wide in fresh water, and some strains tolerate brackish water. The organism appears able to affect all species of freshwater fishes.

Clinical Signs

Aeromonas hydrophila has been associated with a wide variety of clinical conditions and may be isolated in the presence of other pathogens, which confuses the clinical picture. Bacterial hemorrhagic septicemia can be peracute with few or no presenting signs. Acute cases display loss of scales, focal hemorrhages of the gills around the vent, in the mouth, and at the base of fins. Skin ulcers can develop anywhere on the body. Exophthalmia and abdominal

TABLE 48–1. Bacterial Diseases of Goldfish, Koi, and Carp*

Disease	Bacteria	Host
Bacterial hemorrhagic septicemia	*Aeromonas hydrophila*	All freshwater species
Bacterial tail rot	*Pseudomonas fluorescens*	All species

*See also sections on Flexibacter columnaris in Chapter 24; Aeromonas salmonicida in Chapter 36; and Mycobacterium spp. in Chapter 67.

distension through accumulation of ascitic fluid may be evident. Chronic cases also occur. Anemia and renal and hepatic damage are often seen.

Diagnosis

Diagnosis is based upon culture and identification of the organism. *Aeromonas hydrophila* is motile, ferments inositol and mannitol, produces hydrogen sulfide and indole, and is ornithine decarboxylase negative but oxidase positive. A differential medium is available that can determine these characteristics in a single tube (Kaper et al., 1979). Polyclonal antisera can be used in slide, tube, or macro agglutination tests, and fluorescent antibody techniques have been used in labs; however, cross-reactivity is a problem.

Culture and Identification

Nonselective media, including nutrient agar or tryptone soya agar, grow the organism. Colonies are usually cream-colored, round, raised, and shiny. At 25°C after 48 hours, they are usually 2 to 3 mm in diameter. Rimler-Shotts medium (Shotts and Rimler, 1973) is selective for the aeromonads when incubated between 20 and 25°C for 24 to 48 hours.

Speciation of the aeromonads is not well resolved. There are three motile *Aeromonas* species generally recognized, *Aeromonas hydrophila*, *Aeromonas punctata*, and *Aeromonas sobria* (Austin and Austin, 1987). Only *A. hydrophila* is considered pathogenic for fish (Leblanc et al., 1981), but some workers feel that on the basis of phenotypic, serologic, and genotypic heterogeneity, several distinct species may be lumped under a single name (Austin and Austin, 1987). This may explain the wide spectrum of pathogenicity, clinical signs, and pathology attributed to a single species of pathogenic bacteria.

Despite the potential need to divide *A. hydrophila* into several distinct organisms taxonomically, there are several stabile characteristics. The organisms are motile, gram-negative rods about 1 × 3.5 μ. They have a single polar flagellum, and in contrast to *Aeromonas salmonicida* are capable of growth at 37°C. Some strains produce brown pigments similar to *A. salmonicida*, and there is some antigenic cross-reactivity with *A. salmonicida* and *A. sobria* (Fig. 48–1) (Leblanc et al., 1981).

Transmission, Epidemiology, and Pathogenesis

There remains some controversy over whether *A. hydrophila* is a primary pathogen or merely a secondary invader. The organism is common in natural fresh water (Allen et al., 1983). Chemotaxic responses have been shown toward fish mucus in some strains (Hazen et al., 1982). While *A. hydrophila*

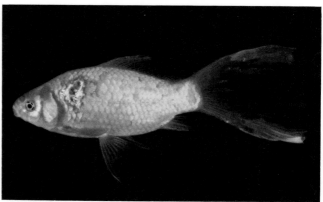

FIGURE 48–1. Goldfish infected with *Aeromonas salmonicida* typically show cutaneous ulceration. (Courtesy of W. Savage.)

may very well require environmental and other stressors to precipitate disease in fish, the organism does produce extracellular products that have enzymatic hemolytic and proteolytic activity (Austin and Austin, 1987). Hemolysis activity seems to be more closely correlated with virulence than does proteolytic activity (Lallier et al., 1984). *Aeromonas hydrophila* strains also produce enterotoxins with various modes of action.

The disease can occur in individual fish, or it can become epidemic. Mortality rates are also highly variable but can be extremely high.

Treatment and Control

Aeromonas hydrophila responds to antibiotic therapy. Oxytetracycline has been the predominant antibiotic used to treat the disease. Antibiotic resistance can develop easily in *A. hydrophila* strains. Resistance to ampicillin, chloramphenicol, erythromycin, nitrofurantoin, novobiocin, streptomycin, sulfonamides, and tetracycline all have been recorded in specific strains (Austin and Austin, 1987).

Commercial bacterins are not available yet, but considerable effort has gone into development of protective vaccination products. To date, injectable administration shows more promise and greater antibody titer production than immersion administration methods (Schachte, 1978), and heat-inactivation products are superior to formalized products (Lamers and de Haas, 1983).

BACTERIAL TAIL ROT

SYNONYMS. Bacterial fin rot, pseudomoniasis, hemorrhagic septicemia.

Host and Geographic Distribution

Pseudomonas fluorescens affects freshwater and saltwater fishes throughout the world. Published reports include outbreaks in goldfish, silver carp, bighead, tench, grass carp, black carp, golden shiner, rainbow trout, European eels, paradise fish, and other labyrinth fishes.

Clinical Signs

This disease generally presents as a septicemia. Fish may die peracutely, or they can survive for long periods with quite extensive lesions. The signs can be similar to those seen in *Aeromonas hydrophila* infections. Skin ulcers, petechiae, and erythema are often present, although tissues surrounding ulcers are usually not hemorrhagic, in contrast to an *Aeromonas* infection. Ascitic fluid may be present. Fin and/or tail erosion and degeneration are usually cardinal signs of the disease. Affected fish may continue to eat despite extensive lesions, including exposed skeletal elements. Death occurs in peracute and severely advanced cases.

Diagnosis

Diagnosis of *Pseudomonas fluorescens* infection is based on isolation of a motile, short, gram-negative rod that is cytochrome oxidase positive, and oxidative or inactive with glucose. Colonies of this organism are usually pigmented bright yellow and may be mucoid.

Pathology

Fish affected with this disease show petechiae on peritoneal and intestinal serosal surfaces and the myocardium. Melanomacrophage centers and hematopoietic tissues are depleted. Intra- and extracellular edema and capillary congestion can be extensive in areas of ulceration, much as is seen secondary to toxemia due to systemic infections in mammals. Petechiae are also found in the gills, kidneys, liver, and the lumen and submucosa of the intestines.

Culture and Identification

Pseudomonas fluorescens grows well on blood agar and nutrient agar. Incubation at 22 to 28°C for 24 to 48 hours is usually adequate (Ahne et al., 1982). It is a motile, gram-negative rod with a single polar flagellum. It produces oxidase, catalase, and arginine dihydrolase. The organism is indole negative and does not produce hydrogen sulfide, amylase, or urease. It can use citrate and ferments arabinose,

inositol, maltose, mannitol, sorbitol, sucrose, trehalose, and xylose (Austin and Austin, 1987).

Transmission, Epidemiology, and Pathogenesis

This disease is thought to be stress mediated. Water is probably the primary reservoir, and disease seems to be associated with cold water temperatures. The organism has been considered a secondary invader of damaged fish tissues but may also be a primary pathogen (Roberts and Horne, 1978). Morbidity can be variable but is often about 50%. Mortality is quite high in affected fish but can be delayed. Mortality is high in peracute outbreaks. *Pseudomonas fluorescens* releases extracellular proteases upon invasion of the fish host (Li and Flemming, 1968).

Treatment and Control

Alleviation of stress and proper water-quality maintenance help control disease due to *Pseudomonas fluorescens*. Benzalkonium chloride baths and furanace dips have been used to control early cases (Austin and Austin, 1987). No bacterins are available.

LITERATURE CITED

Ahne, W., Popp, W., and Hoffmann, R. (1982) *Pseudomonas fluorescens* as a pathogen of tench *(Tinca tinca)*. Bull. Eur. Assoc. Fish Pathologists 4:56–57.

Allen, D.A., Austin, B., and Colwell, R.R. (1983) Numerical taxonomy of bacterial isolates associated with a freshwater fishery. J. Gen. Microbiol. 129:2043–2062.

Austin, B., and Austin, D.A. (1987) Bacterial Fish Pathogens, Disease in Farmed and Wild Fish. John Wiley & Sons, New York.

Hazen, T.C., Esch, G.W., Dimock, R.V., and Mansfield, A. (1982) Chemotaxis of *Aeromonas hydrophila* to the surface mucus of fish. Curr. Microbiol. 7:371–375.

Kaper, J., Seidler, R.J., Lockman, H., and Colwell, R.R. (1979) A medium for the presumptive identification of *Aeromonas hydrophila* and Enterobacteriaceae. Appl. and Environ. Microbiol. 38:1023–1026.

Lallier, R., Bernard, F., and Lalonde, G. (1984) Difference in the extracellular products of two strains of *Aeromonas hydrophila* virulent and weakly virulent for fish. Can. J. Microbiol. 30:900–904.

Lamers, C.H.J., and de Haas, M.J.M. (1983) The development of immunological memory in carp *(Cyprinus carpio* L.) to a bacterial antigen. Dev. Comp. Immunol. 7:713–714.

Leblanc, D., Mittal, K.R., Olivier, G., and Lallier, R. (1981) Serogrouping of motile *Aeromonas* species isolated from healthy and moribund fish. Appl. Environ. Microbiol. 42:56–60.

Li, M.F., and Flemming, C. (1968) A proteolytic pseudomonad from skin lesions of rainbow trout *(Salmo gairdneri)*. I. Characteristics of the pathogenic effects and extracellular proteinase. Can. J. Microbiol. 13:405–416.

Roberts, R.J., and Horne, M.T. (1978) Bacterial meningitis in farmed rainbow trout, *Salmo gairdneri* Richardson, affected with chronic pancreatic necrosis. J. Fish Dis. 1:157–164.

Schachte, J.H. (1978) Immunization of channel catfish, *Ictalurus punctatus*, against two bacterial diseases. Marine Fish. Rev. 40:18–19.

Shotts, E.B., Jr., and Rimler, R. (1973) Medium for the isolation of *Aeromonas hydrophila*. Appl. Microbiol. 26:550–553.

Chapter 49

FUNGAL AND ALGAL DISEASES OF GOLDFISH, KOI, AND CARP

BEVERLY A. GOVEN-DIXON

Fungal and algal diseases of goldfish, koi, and carp are relatively poorly studied. These fish are susceptible to many of the same fungal and algal infections found in other freshwater fishes. Table 49–1 lists three common infections of these species.

BRANCHIOMYCOSIS

SYNONYM. Gill rot.

Host and Geographic Distribution

Branchiomycosis has long been regarded as a disease with limited geographic distribution. The "typical" outbreak reportedly occurs in eutrophic ponds or those sustaining high nitrogenous or organic loads. The disease is usually observed in 2- to 3-year-old carp during warmer water periods and is generally thought to be localized in eastern Europe. In the early 1970's, this disease was described in the Mediterranean region, including Israel (Sarig, 1971), Italy, and Switzerland. It has also been described in the eastern United States and in Japan (Egusa and Ohiwa, 1972; Wolke, 1975).

Clinical Signs

Infected fish show signs of asphyxia such as gasping. They appear weak and lethargic and often lag behind the school (Brown and Gratzek, 1988). Massive die-offs can occur with mortality in 1- to 2-year-old fish as high as 50%. Fish that do not die may recover and regenerate damaged gill tissue.

Diagnosis and Pathology

The organism typically localizes in the oxygen-rich blood vessels of the gill tissue. The nonseptate hyphae grow in the vessels, obstructing the circulation of blood through the gills, and the gills begin to lose their bright red color. Tissues become mottled with patches of brownish discoloration due to hemorrhages mixed with whitish areas of disrupted blood flow, resulting in necrotic tissue. In some cases the necrotic areas may slough off and become sites for secondary invaders such as *Saprolegnia* sp. Some authors consider a "marbled" or "rotted" appearance to be pathognomonic for acute branchiomycosis.

Culture and Identification

Two species of *Branchiomyces* have been described. *Branchiomyces sanguinis*, described in 1912, was thought to infect principally carp, while *B. demigrans* typically produces disease in pike and tench. Both fungal species produce similar disease in the gills, and fungal morphology and cultural requirements are considered to be the distinguishing criteria between the species. *Branchiomyces demigrans* has thicker hyphal walls, ranging from 0.5 to 0.7 μm, while the walls of *B. sanguinis* are 0.2 μm. *Branchiomyces demigrans* also produces slightly larger spores of 12 to 17 μm. The minor differences between these two species may not be as clear as once thought. Some question has been raised as to the existence of two separate species or merely the variation of one species in response to different hosts and environments. Further, it has been suggested that sporangia produced by *Branchiomyces* are similar to those of

TABLE 49–1. Fungal and Algal Diseases of Goldfish, Koi, and Carp*

Disease	Organism	Host
Branchiomycosis	*Branchiomyces sanguinis*	All species
Staff's disease	*Saprolegnia* spp.	Common carp
Algal gill disease	*Cladophora* spp.	Common carp

See also Chapters 25 and 37.

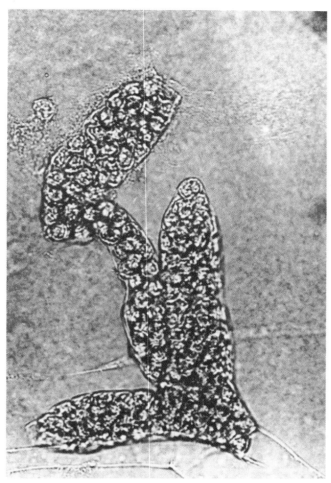

FIGURE 49–1. Wet mount of *Branchiomyces* sp. from gill. (Courtesy of Peduzzi, Meng, and Polli. From Neish, G.A., and Hughes, G.C. [1980] Diseases of Fishes: Book 6: Fungal Diseases of Fishes. [Sniezko, S.F., and Axelrod, H.R., eds.] T.F.H. Publications, Neptune, New Jersey, p. 53.)

Saprolegnia. Gill infection with *Saprolegnia* frequently mimics gill rot produced by *Branchiomyces*. The antigenic structure of *Branchiomyces* has recently been found to resemble that of *Saprolegnia*, suggesting to some researchers that the genus *Branchiomyces* may in fact belong to the family of Saprolegniaceae (Alderman, 1982). *Branchiomyces* has never been isolated from any natural source other than fish gills (Neish and Hughes, 1980).

Transmission, Epidemiology, and Pathogenesis

As in other fish, mycotic infections in goldfish, koi, and carp are also associated with stress or injury. The course of infection with *Branchiomyces* sp. is generally rapid and is thought to be exacerbated by crowding, algal blooms, water temperatures in excess of 20°C, or increased levels of un-ionized ammonia, although all cases cannot be associated with water-

quality problems. Chronic infections may be present in numerous species of fish, not reported to be involved in *Branchiomyces* epizootics.

The means of natural transmission for *Branchiomyces* is not well understood. However, two methods of infection have been proposed. It has been suggested that free-living spores may directly invade gills through damaged areas caused by poor water quality. Infection may also occur through ingestion of spores, which enter the circulation via intestinal penetration. The spores localize in areas of high oxygen tension, preferably the efferent branchial arteries, germinate within these vessels, and send long tubules into gill respiratory epithelium. The hyphae eventually displace host tissue, causing blood stoppage and swelling due to congestion and destruction of branchial tissue.

Treatment and Control

Prevention of branchiomycosis can be accomplished with management techniques that maintain good water quality. Practices that prevent the accumulation of decomposing organic matter, such as removing dead fish, decreasing feed, and increasing water flow, will enhance water quality and prevent excessive ammonia. Other methods, such as thinning out fish to prevent crowding and stress, should be practiced. Cleaning out ponds and the use of quicklime to reduce organics and increase pH between stocking are also useful in controlling fungi as well as other parasites.

STAFF'S DISEASE

SYNONYM. Saprolegniasis.

Host and Geographic Distribution

Goldfish, koi, and carp worldwide are susceptible to external infection with *Saprolegnia* sp. Staff's disease is a specific form of the fungal infection of common carp reported from Poland.

Clinical Signs

External infection by this organism appears as the typical white, "cottony" patches described in other fish. An unusual infection of *Saprolegnia* known as Staff's disease is described in carp in Poland. Staff's disease is an infection in the olfactory pits. Tufts of hyphae project from the olfactory pits to form pad-like growths between the mouth and eyes.

Diagnosis

Diagnosis is based upon identification of typical nonseptate branching hyphae (see Chapter 37).

Pathology, Culture, and Identification

See Chapter 37.

Transmission, Epidemiology, and Pathogenesis

Staff's disease occurs during the winter months in 1- to 2-year-old carp. The lowered water temperatures are thought to favor fungal development (Bauer et al., 1973).

Treatment and Control

Like other infections in fish, saprolegniasis infections are secondary to predisposing stress factors such as injury from handling or pre-existing parasitic infections, water quality (especially temperature), and malnutrition (see Chapter 37).

FUSARIUM MYCOSIS

SYNONYMS. *Fusarium culmorum*, hyphalomycosis.

Various other fungal infections have been described in carp. For example, the mortality of carp in a new earthen pond was attributed to the fungus *Fusarium culmorum*. The fish suffered from blindness and external skin infections. Beech leaves in the pond were thought to contribute to poor water quality and to provide a nutrient bed for the fungus, which was thought to be a secondary invader of the fish (Reichenbach-Klinke and Elkan, 1965).

ALGAL INFECTIONS OF CARP

Algal problems in carp culture are usually associated with uncontrolled pond blooms. For example, blooms of the phytoplankton *Chlorella* sp. and *Prymnesium parvum* have been known to interfere with carp breeding, because of the secretion of toxic algal products. On occasion, larger algae, such as the filamentous green alga *Cladophora*, have been noted on the fins and opercula of common carp (Vinyard, 1953). These reports are rare, and their significance is as yet undetermined.

LITERATURE CITED

Alderman, D.J. (1982) Fungal diseases of aquatic animals. In: Microbial Diseases of Fish. (Roberts, R.J., ed.). Academic Press, New York, pp. 189–242.

Bauer, O.N., Musselius, V.A., and Strelhov, Y.A. (1973) Diseases of Pond Fishes. Israel Program for Scientific Translations. Jerusalem, Israel.

Brown, E.E., and Gratzek, J.B. (1988) Fish Farming Handbook. AVI Pub. Co., Inc., New York.

Egusa, S., and Ohiwa, Y. (1972) Branchiomycosis of pond-cultured eels. Fish Pathol. 7:79–83 (in Japanese with English summary).

Neish, G.A., and Hughes, G.C. (1980) Fungal Disease of Fishes. (Snieszko, S.F., and Axelrod, H.R., ed.). T.F.H. Publications, Neptune, New Jersey.

Reichenbach-Klinke, H., and Elkan, E. (1965) The Principal Diseases of Lower Vertebrates, Diseases of Fishes. Academic Press Inc. Ltd., London.

Sarig, S. (1971) The Prevention and Treatment of Diseases of Warm-Water Fishes under Subtropical Conditions, with Special Emphasis on Intensive Fish Farming. In: Diseases of Fishes, Book 3 (Snieszko, S.F., and Axelrod, H.R., eds.). T.F.H. Publications, Neptune, New Jersey.

Vinyard, W.C. (1953) Epizoophyric algae from mollusks, turtles and fish in Oklahoma. Proc. Okla. Acad. Sci. 34:63–65.

Wolke, R.E. (1975) Pathology of bacterial and fungal diseases affecting fish. In: The Pathology of Fishes. (Riberlin, W.E., and Migaki, G., eds.). University of Wisconsin Press, Madison, Wisconsin.

Chapter 50

GOLDFISH, KOI, AND CARP VIRUSES

PHILIP E. MCALLISTER

Cyprinid fish are susceptible to a variety of viral infections, some of which have quite specific host range, whereas others affect diverse species (Table 50–1). Similarly, the health and economic impact of viral infection varies; some infections cause epizootic mortality, others result in chronic, low-level losses, and still others cause little mortality, but fish are disfigured and cannot be marketed. The following viral infections have been detected in cyprinid fishes.

CARP POX

SYNONYMS. Carp papillomatosis, epithelioma papulosum, fish pox, cyprinid herpesvirus I (CHV).

TABLE 50–1. Viral Diseases of Goldfish, Koi, and Carp*

Disease	Virus	Host
Carp pox	*Herpesvirus cyprini*	Barbel, bream Common carp, crucian carp, Golden ide, pike-perch Rudd, smelt, tench
Gill necrosis	Gill necrosis virus	Common carp
Unknown	Goldfish Virus-1 and -2	Goldfish
Golden shiner virus disease	Golden shiner virus	Golden shiner
Grass carp reovirus disease	Grass carp reovirus	Grass carp
Spring viremia of carp	*Rhabdovirus carpio*	Big head carp, common carp, Crucian carp, grass carp, Sheatfish
Unknown	Grass carp virus—CIVH 33/86	Grass carp

See also sections on pike fry rhabdovirus disease in Chapter 26; and infectious pancreatic necrosis in Chapter 38.

Carp pox, a benign epidermal hyperplasia, has been recognized since the Middle Ages. The disease has a variety of names, none clinically correct. The lesion is not a pock or caused by a poxvirus, nor is it a true epithelioma or papilloma (Hines et al., 1974; Nigrelli, 1952; Schlumberger and Lucke, 1948; Wolf, 1983).

Electron micrographs of carp pox lesions show a herpesviruslike particle (Schubert, 1964, 1966), and a virus designated *Herpesvirus cyprini* or cyprinid herpesvirus I has been isolated from lesions (Sano et al., 1985a,b). Although the lesions are unsightly, the disease does not cause mortality in affected fish.

Host and Geographic Distribution

Carp pox occurs principally in common carp and crucian carp but also in barbel, bream, golden ide, pike-perch, rudd, smelt, tench, carp × goldfish hybrids, and various aquarium fish (Anders and Moller, 1985; Bauer et al., 1969; Duijn, 1967; Nigrelli, 1954). The disease is recognized throughout Europe, Asia, Russia, and Israel. Despite assertions that carp pox is widespread in North America, the disease has been diagnosed only in the Great Lakes region (Sonstegard and Sonstegard, 1978) and possibly in the state of Connecticut (Nigrelli, 1948). An outbreak of carp pox occurred in golden ide imported into the state of Maryland from Europe (McAllister et al., 1985).

Clinical Signs

Carp pox lesions are superficial, milky-white to gray plaques that project 1 to 2 mm above the surface of the skin. The proliferations are smooth, but can develop a rough texture in advanced stages. The lesions gradually increase in diameter, and in severe cases fuse to cover extensive areas of the body and fins. The lesions eventually slough, and scars develop or new lesions appear. The disease is not fatal, but the growth of affected fish can be retarded, and skeletal deformations can develop. The disease rarely occurs in yearling fish or younger.

Pathology

Pathologic changes associated with carp pox are confined to the epidermis (Hines et al., 1974; Mawdesley-Thomas and Bucke, 1967; Wolf, 1983). The squamous epithelial cells become hyperplastic, and their proliferation obliterates the normal strata of the epithelium reducing the number of mucous cells. The corium and underlying structures appear normal. No significant inflammatory response is evident, and necrosis is unusual. Intracytoplasmic and intranuclear inclusions can be seen by light and fluorescence microscopy (Schubert, 1964, 1966).

Diagnosis

Carp pox is generally diagnosed based on clinical signs. Diagnosis is confirmed by isolation of the virus in cell culture and serologic identification using infectivity neutralization or fluorescent antibody assay.

Virus Isolation and Identification

Herpesvirus cyprini has been isolated from carp pox lesions taken from skin and fins of koi carp and common carp (Sano et al., 1985a,b). When lesion homogenates are inoculated onto EPC and FHM cells (see Appendix II listing fish cell line acronyms), intranuclear inclusions form, and cell lysis subsequently occurs after 2 to 3 weeks incubation at 20°C. Virus also replicates in CE–1, CE–2, and MCT cells at 15 and 20°C. No virus replication is detected at 10 or 25°C. Viral antigen can be detected in infected cells by fluorescent antibody assay after 5 days incubation at 20°C. Attempts to isolate virus from carp pox lesions using various other fish cell lines have been unsuccessful (Sonstegard and Sonstegard, 1978; McAllister et al., 1985).

Transmission

Carp pox can be transmitted to common carp and common carp × goldfish hybrids by rubbing lesion tissue against abraded epithelium and by co-habitation (Sonstegard and Sonstegard, 1978). Carp pox lesions develop in about 60 days at 10°C. Carp pox can be transmitted to common carp by intra-peritoneal injection of cell culture–grown virus (Sano et al., 1985a). When challenged fish are held at 15°C, lesions develop about 5 months after injection.

Epidemiology and Pathogenesis

The prevalence of carp pox is affected by environmental and host-associated factors. In ponds with high fish density, prevalence of the disease can be nearly double that in ponds with low fish density, and prevalence and regression of lesions varies seasonally (Hines et al., 1974; Mawdesley-Thomas and Bucke, 1967). Whether this reflects the effects of stress or the infectious character of the disease is unclear. Disease susceptibility appears influenced by genetic factors. Inbred strains of fish show higher disease prevalence than do hybrid strains (Bauer et al., 1969; Schaperclaus, 1954).

Treatment and Control

There is no effective treatment for carp pox. The following measures are recommended for prevention of the disease: segregation of diseased and healthy fish, maintenance of proper pond sanitation, elimination of conditions that promote physiologic stress, and use of selected hybrid strains of fish (Bauer et al., 1969; Hines et al., 1974; Schaperclaus, 1969).

Virus Stability

Storage temperature and suspending medium affect the stability of viral infectivity. The virus is inactivated by exposure to chloroform, ether, glycerol, sodium hypochlorite, ultraviolet irradiation, acid (pH 3), and heat (50 to 60°C for 30 to 60 minutes).

GILL NECROSIS

SYNONYMS. Gill necrosis virus, 1–LZ virus, 4–BZ virus.

Gill necrosis is a serious disease among cultured carp. The cause of the disease is uncertain, but environmental and viral etiologies have been debated. A putative iridovirus was isolated from infected carp (presumably common carp) (Popkova and Shchelkunov, 1978; Shchelkunov and Shchelkunova, 1984).

Host and Geographic Distribution

Gill necrosis is described as occurring in cultured carp, which presumptively means at least common carp. The disease is widespread in Europe and in the Soviet Union but does not occur in North America.

Clinical Signs and Pathology

Progressive clinical signs are associated with gill necrosis (Kovacs-Gayer, 1984). Initially, gills appear edematous and mildly hyperplastic with accumulating granulocytes, degeneration of epithelium, and adhesion of lamellae. Later, advanced hyperplasia, focal necrosis, hemorrhaging, and proliferation and degradation of mucous cells occur. This is followed by generalized necrosis and secondary invasion of bacteria, fungi, and parasites.

Diagnosis

Gill necrosis is generally diagnosed based on clinical signs. Although virus has been isolated from infected fish using cell culture, the significance of the virus is unproven. No serologic tests have been described.

Virus Isolation

Two virus isolations are reported. The viruses, designated 1–LZ and 4–BZ, are described as identical strains of iridovirus (Shchelkunov and Shchelkunova, 1984). They were isolated from homogenates of gill and kidney inoculated onto FHM cells and incubated at 22 and 28°C. Advanced cytopathic effects were evident in 7 to 9 days at primary isolation but in 1 to 2 days for subsequent passages. Infected cells developed enlarged nuclei with one or more intranuclear inclusions. Electron micrographs of material concentrated and purified from cell culture medium revealed iridoviruslike particles, but no virus was seen in preparations of gill tissue.

Transmission

Attempts to experimentally induce gill necrosis in carp by applying cell culture–grown virus to abraded gills and by intraperitoneal inoculation of virus have not been clearly successful (Shchelkunov and Shchelkunova, 1984). Necrotic changes characteristic of gill necrosis were observed in some fish that died in one intraperitoneally inoculated group, but clinical signs of liver degeneration were also observed. Serial passage of the putative gill necrosis virus in fish has not resulted in reproducible gill necrosis or in virus reisolation.

Treatment and Control

No specific treatment or control measures have been described. Avoiding infected fish stocks, decontaminating egg lots, using controlled water supplies, and disinfecting culture facilities and equipment are basic to controlling the disease.

GOLDFISH VIRUS-1 AND 2

SYNONYMS. GFV-1, GFV-2.

Host, Geographic Distribution, and Clinical Signs

On separate occasions, primary cultures of swimbladder cells were prepared by the same laboratory from distinct populations of commercial juvenile goldfish and wild adult goldfish from a local pond (Massachusetts). On each occasion, an iridovirus was isolated from the cultures (Berry et al., 1983). No signs of disease were evident in either group of goldfish, and the etiologic significance of the virus isolates remains unknown. The virus from the juvenile goldfish was designated goldfish virus-1 (GFV-1), and the virus from the adult goldfish was designated goldfish virus-2 (GFV-2). Both viruses replicate at 25°C in CAR and primary chicken embryo fibroblast cells. Degenerative changes in infected CAR cells include formation of an inclusion body and large vacuoles in the cytoplasm and pyknosis, convolution, and heterochromatin accumulation in the nucleus. Feulgen and acridine orange staining show that the cytoplasmic inclusion body contains double-stranded deoxyribonucleic acid (DNA). The viruses are biophysically and biologically indistinguishable and may represent isolations of the same virus, but no serologic comparisons have been reported (Berry et al., 1983).

GOLDEN SHINER VIRUS DISEASE

Host and Geographic Distribution

The golden shiner virus (GSV) was isolated during a diagnostic evaluation of several groups of golden shiners experiencing chronic, low-level mortality (Plumb et al., 1979). The virus is distributed throughout the southeastern and midwestern United States.

Clinical Signs

Affected golden shiners are lethargic and inappetant and swim near the surface unless disturbed. Severe hemorrhaging occurs in the dorsal musculature, and petechial hemorrhages become evident in the eyes, on the ventral body surface, and in the visceral fat and intestinal mucosa (Plumb et al., 1979).

Diagnosis

Golden shiner virus disease can be presumptively diagnosed by clinical signs. Confirmed diagnosis requires isolation of virus in cell culture and identification of the virus by infectivity-neutralization assay. Cross-neutralization assays indicate that golden shiner virus shares some common antigens with chum salmon virus (see Chap. 38) and catfish reovirus (see Chap. 59) but is serologically distinct (Amend et al., 1984; Hedrick et al., 1984; Schwedler and Plumb, 1980).

Virus Isolation

Golden shiner virus can be isolated from homogenates of kidney, liver, and whole viscera and from holding-tank water. Samples are inoculated onto fathead minnow cells and incubated at 30°C. Focal vacuolated syncytia with multiple intact nuclei develop in 12 to 24 hours after cell culture inoculation. Infected cells condense and detach in small masses. If the infection progresses, the entire monolayer is consumed, but if not, the foci are overgrown by normal appearing cells and virus cannot be reisolated. The optimum temperature for virus replication is 25 to 30°C (Schwedler and Plumb, 1982a). No virus replication occurs at 15 or 35°C. The virus replicates best in fathead minnow cells, but also replicates in BB, CHSE–214, grass carp kidney, goldfish kidney, silver carp kidney, and tilapia heart cell lines. The virus does not replicate in BF–2, CCO, CHH–1, or RTG–2 cell lines (Plumb et al., 1979; Winton et al., 1987).

Transmission

The virus can be transmitted experimentally by cohabitation and by intraperitoneal injection of cell culture–grown virus, but variable mortality indicates that the virus has low pathogenicity. Initially, the virus replicates in injected fish, but titers decrease during the 2 weeks after inoculation (Plumb et al., 1979).

Epidemiology and Pathogenesis

In pond culture, all age classes of fish are susceptible to infection, but the number of deaths is greatest in mature golden shiners, 5 to 6 months of age. Mortality is generally less than 5% of the total population, but losses of 75% can occur in fish held in tanks (Plumb et al., 1979). High water temperature (27 to 32°C) and crowding exacerbate disease outbreaks. Virus titer, prevalence, and duration of infection are higher in fish held at higher density (Schwedler and Plumb, 1982b).

Treatment and Control

No treatment has been described for golden shiner virus disease, and little effort has been made to control dissemination of infected fish. The chronic, generally low-level mortality does not result in severe economic loss because the disease tends to affect larger, less marketable fish. Nevertheless, the prudent fish culturist should avoid introducing the disease into a production facility. Appropriate management practices include avoiding suspect lots of fish, controlling the water supply, and disinfecting facilities, equipment, and fish eggs.

Virus Stability

The golden shiner virus is not inactivated by exposure to ether, chloroform, or pH 3. The virus remains infective after heating to 50°C for 30 minutes. No significant loss of infectivity occurs during months of storage at −70 to −80°C or at 4°C if virus is suspended in cell culture medium. All infectivity is lost in 3 days at −15°C and in 7 days at 30°C.

GRASS CARP REOVIRUS

SYNONYM. Hemorrhagic virus of grass carp.

Host and Geographic Distribution

A hemorrhagic disease of grass carp occurs in China and causes epizootic losses in cultured fry, fingerlings, and to a lesser extent yearling grass carp (Nie and Pan, 1985).

Clinical Signs and Pathology

The disease occurs when water temperatures are 25 to 30°C. Clinical signs include exophthalmia and hemorrhages on the gills and opercula, in the mouth cavity, and at the bases of the fins. Internally, hemorrhages occur in the skeletal muscle, intestinal tract, liver, kidneys, and spleen (Section of Virus Study, 1978, 1980).

Diagnosis, Virus Isolation, and Identification

A presumptive diagnosis is based on clinical signs. Virus has been isolated from affected fish using grass carp muscle, snout, and gonad cell lines (Chen and Jiang, 1983; Section of Virus Study, 1978). No serologic tests for virus identification have been described.

Transmission, Treatment, and Control

The disease can be serially transmitted to healthy grass carp by injection of cell-free filtrates prepared from infected fish tissue (Chen and Jiang, 1983; Section of Virus Study, 1978). An inactivated virus vaccine prepared from infected tissue protects fingerling grass carp when administered by injection (Nie and Pan, 1985), but the vaccine is not commercially available.

SPRING VIREMIA OF CARP

SYNONYMS. SVC, infectious dropsy, rubella, hemorrhagic septicemia, infectious ascites, *Rhabdovirus carpio*, swim bladder inflammation virus, SBI virus, 10/3 virus.

Serious losses in cultured carp are caused by infectious dropsy, which is now recognized as a complex of at least two diseases. The acute, ascitic form known as spring viremia of carp, is caused by *Rhabdovirus carpio* (Fijan et al., 1971). The chronic, ulcerative form, known as carp erythrodermatitis, is caused by a bacterium assigned to the *Aeromonas salmonicida* group (Bootsma et al., 1977). SBI virus or 10/3 virus, isolated from carp showing signs of swim bladder inflammation, is antigenically indistinguishable from *R. carpio* (Bachmann and Ahne, 1973; Hill et al., 1975; de Kinkelin and Le Berre, 1974).

Host and Geographic Distribution

Rhabdovirus carpio virus has been isolated from larvae, fry, fingerling, and adult common carp, grass carp, big head carp, crucian carp, and sheatfish fry (Fijan, 1976; Fijan et al., 1981; Pasco et al., 1987). Northern pike and the guppy are susceptible to experimental infection, but the giebel is not (Bachmann and Ahne, 1974). Other fish species may be susceptible to *R. carpio* (Bootsma and Ebregt, 1983), and the virus replicates in the fly *Drosophila melanogaster* (Bussereau et al., 1975). The disease has been diagnosed in Great Britain, most countries of eastern and western Europe, and the Middle East but not in North America (Bekesi and Szabo, 1979; Bucke and Finlay, 1979; Fijan, 1976; Hines et al., 1974).

Clinical Signs

Fish having spring viremia of carp show a variety of clinical signs (Fijan, 1972; Fijan et al., 1971). Affected fish appear dark and exophthalmic. The gills are pale, the abdomen is distended with ascites, and a thick, mucoid cast can trail from the inflamed and protruding vent. Affected fish respire weakly, are lethargic, and can display loss of equilibrium, uncoordinated swimming, muscular fibrillations, and sporadic hyperactivity. Petechiae and ecchymoses are evident in the gills and skin.

Pathology

On gross postmortem examination, peritonitis and enteritis are evident, and petechiae and ecchymoses are visible on the internal organs, brain, skeletal muscle, and the internal wall of the swimbladder. Nearly all internal organs are edematous (Rudikov et al., 1975; Negele, 1977). The cranial kidney and intestine are the first tissues macroscopically affected. Inflammatory edema and focal diapedesis can occur in the subcutaneous tissue and skeletal muscle. In the liver, hepatocytes dissociate and undergo multifocal necrobiotic changes and cytolysis. In the spleen, lymphatic and hemoblastic elements increase in number, and there is considerable reticuloendothelial hyperplasia. The pancreas shows leukocyte infiltration, inflammation, and cytolysis. In the kidneys, focal necrosis occurs in the tubular epithelium, and tubules are filled with degenerated cells. Serous fluid accumulates in the glomeruli, and the kidney hemopoietic tissue undergoes necrosis. Vascular edema and cellular infiltration occur in cardiac and brain tissue and in the intestinal membranes.

Diagnosis

Presumptive diagnosis of spring viremia of carp is based on clinical signs. The diagnosis is confirmed by isolation and serologic identification of the virus. Indirect immunoperoxidase and fluorescent antibody techniques detect viral antigen in frozen sections of liver, kidneys, and spleen (Faisal and Ahne, 1984). Detection of virus-neutralizing antibody in carp serum is used extensively to determine distribution of the virus (Hoppe and Wernery, 1985; Wizigmann et al., 1980, 1983).

Virus Isolation and Identification

Rhabdovirus carpio can be isolated from most organs and tissues (Ahne, 1978; Baudouy et al., 1980a,b; Bekesi and Csontos, 1985; Bootsma and Ebregt, 1983; Fijan et al., 1971), but liver, kidneys, and spleen yield virus with greatest consistency. Virus has not been isolated from skin.

The virus replicates well in BB, BF–2, CaPi, EPC, and FHM cells and in primary cultures of carp ovary, heart, or swimbladder (Bachmann and Ahne, 1974; Bootsma and Ebregt, 1983; Fijan et al., 1971; de Kinkelin and Le Berre, 1974; Ribeiro and Ahne, 1983). Virus replication also occurs in avian, mammalian, and reptilian cell lines (Bachmann and Ahne, 1974; Clark and Soriano, 1974). *Rhabdovirus carpio* replicates in cell culture at temperatures from 4 to 32°C. The optimum temperature for replication in fathead minnow cells is 20 to 22°C, in BHK–21 cells is 24 to 26°C,

and GL1 cells is 17 to 32°C. Neutralization, immunofluorescence, immunoperoxidase, immune precipitation, and indirect hemagglutination reactions can identify the virus (Ahne, 1981, 1982; Fijan, 1976; Hill et al., 1975, 1981; Sulimanovic, 1973). Rabbit and carp hyperimmune serum have both been used in serologic reactions.

Transmission

Rhabdovirus carpio is shed with feces and mucous casts (Ahne, 1978; Pfeil-Putzien and Baath, 1978). The gills are the site of virus entry and primary virus replication. The subsequent viremia disseminates virus to other organs and tissues (Ahne, 1977, 1978; Baudouy et al., 1980a,b). At spawning, eggs become contaminated by virus shed with sex products (Bekesi and Csontos, 1985). Disease can be transmitted experimentally by cohabitation, by intracranial and intraperitoneal injection, by intubation of virus into the intestine, and by immersion, but not by application of virus to scarified skin (Fijan, 1972; Fijan et al., 1971; Hill, 1977).

The carp louse (*Argulus foliaceus*) and the leech (*Piscicola geometra*) are mechanical vectors of *R. carpio* (Ahne, 1985; Pfeil-Putzien, 1977), but no virus replication occurs in the parasites. Similarly, the heron, *Ardea cinerea*, can serve as a mechanical vector of the virus (Peters and Neukirch, 1986). *Rhabdovirus carpio* replicates in the fly *Drosophila melanogaster* (Bussereau et al., 1975), but transmission by an insect vector has not been reported. Virus can be disseminated via contaminated hatchery equipment (Fijan, 1973).

Epidemiology and Pathogenesis

Fish of any age are susceptible to spring viremia, but the most severe losses occur in juvenile to yearling fish. The further a fish is from its physiologic thermal optimum, the more serious the disease (Baudouy et al., 1980b). At low water temperatures (<10°C), host immune response is reduced and viral replication slowed, but viral pathogenicity is not reduced and the disease becomes fatal. At temperatures between 11 and 18°C, clinical signs occur, but some fish mount an immune response and survive. At temperatures above 18°C, a durable immune response occurs, and the probability of survival increases with increasing temperature (Ahne, 1980; Fijan, 1976; Fijan et al., 1971). Interferon is produced early in infection as a protective response; however, interferon production is also directly affected by temperature (Baudouy, 1978; de Kinkelin et al., 1982).

Although cultured carp are more resistant to disease than feral carp when challenged by immersion or by intraperitoneal injection (Hill, 1977), the susceptibility of various strains of carp to viral infection has not been extensively investigated. Culture conditions that promote physiologic stress, such as crowding, excessive handling, poor water quality, malnutrition, or sudden temperature changes increase the potential for severe disease (Fijan, 1972; Stankiewicz, 1979).

Treatment and Control

Conventional carp farming methods where large, open ponds are supplied with river water make control of spring viremia of carp difficult if not impossible. Prophylactic measures such as disinfection of ponds and equipment, decontamination of eggs by iodophor treatment, and stocking ponds with fish determined to be free from the virus are more likely to be successful at smaller farms with controlled water supplies (Ahne and Held, 1980). Continuous rearing at 20 to 22°C protects fish from the disease (Fijan, 1973, 1976), but environmental-based prophylaxis is not economically feasible unless thermal effluents from power plants or geothermal sources are available.

Immunization with either infectious or inactivated virus rapidly induces protective immunity at temperatures above 20°C (Ahne, 1980; Baudouy, 1978; Fijan, 1981; Fijan and Matasin, 1980). An inactivated vaccine used in field trials (Macura et al., 1983) resulted in detectable virus-neutralizing antibody for 18 months (Tesarcik et at., 1984). Inactivated virus vaccines must be administered by intraperitoneal injection because virus uptake is inefficient by immersion (de Kinkelin et al., 1984). Fish should be immunized in the summer or autumn to prevent acute disease in the spring (Fijan et al., 1977a,b; Koelbl and Kainz, 1977). Immunization is ineffective if fish are already infected or if they are physiologically stressed (Tesarcik and Macura, 1981a,b).

Virus Stability

Rhabdovirus carpio, like the other fish rhabdoviruses, is inactivated by exposure to ether, cholorform, formalin, glycerol, diethylpyrocarbonate, ozone, sodium hypochlorite, organic iodophors, gamma and ultraviolet irradiation, extremes of pH (below pH 4 or above pH 10), and heating (60°C for 15 min). Formalin-inactivated virus remains serologically reactive for months and can be used as a positive control reagent for plate and immunoblot enzyme-linked immunosorbent assays and to vaccinate fish.

Fish rhabdoviruses are moderately stable under a variety of storage and environmental conditions. Suspension in cell culture medium containing 2 to 10% serum preserves infectivity for months to years at −20°C or colder. The viruses can also be preserved by lyophilization. The rate of virus inactivation increases as the temperature increases. In the absence of serum, the viruses are more labile to temperature and to freezing and thawing, but remain infectious in the environment for months.

GRASS CARP VIRUS CIVH 33/86

SYNONYMS. *Ctenopharyngodon idella virus Hungary* 33/86 (CIVH 33/86).

Host, Geographic Distribution, and Clinical Signs

Virus CIVH 33/86, an as yet unclassified virus, was isolated from apparently healthy 2-year-old grass carp imported into Germany from Hungary (Ahne et al., 1987). Electron micrographs of negatively stained virus show enveloped, rod to bacilliform particles, 170 nm to 220 nm in length and 50 nm to 55 nm in diameter. No clinical disease caused by this virus has been reported, and no infectivity trials have been performed.

Diagnosis, Virus Isolation, and Identification

CIVH 33/86 is isolated from homogenates of liver, kidney, and spleen inoculated onto monolayers of CAR, CLC, and FHM cells incubated at 15 to 25°C. Cell fusion followed by lysis appears 24 to 48 hours after inoculation. The optimum temperature range for viral replication is 20 to 25°C. The virus does not replicate at 10 or 28°C. CIVH 33/86 is not neutralized by antisera to the fish rhabdoviruses EVX, IHNV, PFR, SVCV, or VHSV.

LITERATURE CITED

Ahne, W. (1977) Evidence for the systemic character of *Rhabdovirus carpio* infection. Bull. Off. Int. Epizoot. 87:435–436.

Ahne, W. (1978) Uptake and multiplication of spring viraemia of carp virus in carp, *Cyprinus carpio* L. J. Fish Dis. 1:265–268.

Ahne, W. (1980) Spring viremia of carp (SVC): Studies on immunization of carp, In: Fish Diseases (W. Ahne, ed.) Third COPRAQ Session, Springer-Verlag, Berlin, p. 28.

Ahne, W. (1981) Serological techniques currently used in fish virology. Dev. Biol. Stand. 49:3–27.

Ahne, W. (1982) Comparative studies on the stability of 4 fish pathogenic viruses (VHSV, PFR, SVCV, IPNV). Zentralbl. Veterinaermed. Reihe B 29:457–476.

Ahne, W. (1985) *Argulus foliaceus* L. and *Piscicola geometra* L. as mechanical vectors of spring viraemia of carp virus (SVCV). J. Fish Dis. 8:241–242.

Ahne, W., and Held, C. (1980) Investigations of the virucidal activity of Actomar K30 on pathogenic viruses of fish. Tieraerztl. Umsch. 35:308–319.

Ahne, W., Jaing, Y., and Thomsen, I. (1987) A new virus isolated from cultured grass carp *Ctenopharyngodon idella*. Dis. Aquatic Organ. 3:181–185.

Amend, D.F., McDowell, T., and Hedrick, R.P. (1984) Characteristics of a previously unidentified virus from channel catfish *(Ictalurus punctatus)*. Can. J. Fish. Aquatic Sci. 41:807–811.

Anders, K., and Moller, H. (1985) Spawning papillomatosis of smelt, *Osmerus eperlanus* L., from the Elbe estuary. J. Fish. Dis. 8:233–235.

Bachmann, P.A., and Ahne, W. (1973) Isolation and characterization of agent causing swim bladder inflammation in carp. Nature 244:235–237.

Bachmann, P.A., and Ahne, W. (1974) Biological properties and identification of the agent causing swim bladder inflammation in carp. Arch. Gesamte. Virusforsch. 44:261–269.

Baudouy, A.M. (1978) Host virus relationships in the course of spring viremia of carp. C.R. Hebd. Seances Acad. Sci. Ser. D Sci. Nat. 286:1225–1228.

Baudouy, A.M., Danton, M., and Merle, G. (1980a) Experimental infection of susceptible carp fingerlings with spring viremia of carp virus, under wintering environmental conditions. In: Fish Diseases (W. Ahne, ed.). Fish Diseases, Third COPRAQ Session, Springer-Verlag, Berlin, pp. 23–27.

Baudouy, A.M., Danton, M., and Merle, G. (1980b) Viremie printaniere de la carpe: etude experimentale de l'infection evoluant a differentes temperatures. Ann. Virol. 131E:479–488.

Bauer, O.N., Musselius, V.A., and Strelkov, Yu.A. (1969) Diseases of pond fishes, Izdatel'stvo "Kolos" (translated from Russian). Israel Program for Scientific Translations. Jerusalem, 1973, TT–72–50070.

Bekesi, L., and Csontos, L. (1985) Isolation of spring viraemia of carp virus from asymptomatic broodstock carp, Cyprinus carpio L. J. Fish Dis. 8:471–472.

Bekesi, L., and Szabo, E. (1979) A rhabdovirus isolated from carps in Hungary. Experimental infection of carps and resistance of the virus. Acta Microbiol. Acad. Sci. Hung. 26:193–197.

Berry, E.S., Shea, T.B., and Gabliks, J. (1983) Two iridovirus isolates from Carassius auratus (L.). J. Fish Dis. 6:501–510.

Bootsma, R., and Ebregt. (1983) Spring viremia of carp. In: Antigens of Fish Pathogens (Anderson, D.P., Dorson, M., and Dubourget, P. eds.). Collection Fondation Marcel Merieux, Lyon, France, pp. 81–86.

Bootsma, R., Fijan, N., and Blommaert, J. (1977) Isolation and preliminary identification of the causative agent of carp erythrodermatitis. Vet. Arh. 47:291–302.

Bucke, D., and Finlay, J. (1979) Identification of spring viraemia in carp (Cyprinus carpio L.) in Great Britain. Vet. Rec. 104:69–71.

Bussereau, F., de Kinkelin, P., and Le Berre, M. (1975) Infectivity of fish rhabdoviruses for Drosophila melanogaster. Ann. Microbiol. 126:389–395.

Chen, Y.X., and Jiang, Y.L. (1983) Morphological and physico-chemical characterization of the hemorrhagic virus of grass carp. Mon. J. Sci. 28:1–5.

Clark, H.F., and Soriano, E.Z. (1974) Fish rhabdovirus replication in non-piscine cell culture: New system for the study of rhabdovirus-cell interaction in which the virus and cell have different temperature optima. Infect. Immun. 10:180–188.

de Kinkelin, P., and Le Berre, M. (1974) Rhabdovirus des poissons II. Proprietes in vitro du virus de la viremie printaniere de la carpe. Ann. Microbiol. 125A:113–124.

de Kinkelin, P., Dorson, P., and Hattenberger-Baudouy, A.M. (1982) Interferon synthesis in trout and carp after viral infection. Dev. Comp. Immunol. 2(Suppl.):167–174.

de Kinkelin, P., Bernard, J., and Hattenberger-Baudouy, A.M. (1984) Immunization against viral diseases occurring in cold water. Symposium on Fish Vaccination, Paris, Office International Epizooties, February 1984, pp. 167–174.

Duijn, C., van. (1967) Diseases of Fishes. Iliffe Books, London.

Faisal, M., and Ahne, W. (1984) Spring viraemia of carp virus (SVCV): comparison of immunoperoxidase, fluorescent antibody and cell culture isolation techniques for detection of antigen. J. Fish Dis. 7:57–64.

Fijan, N. (1972) Infectious dropsy in carp—a disease complex. Symp. Zool. Soc. Lond. 30:39–51.

Fijan, N. (1973) Spring viremia of carp (SVC)—a review. EIFAC (Eur. Inland Fish. Advis. Comm.). Technical Paper 17, 2(Suppl.):119–123.

Fijan, N. (1976) Diseases of cyprinids in Europe. Fish. Pathol. 10:129–134.

Fijan, N. (1981) Vaccination of fish in European pond culture: prospects and constraints. In: Proceedings of an International Seminar on Fish, Pathogens and Environment in European Polyculture (Olah, J., Molnar, K., and Jeney, Z., eds.). Szarvas, Hungary, pp. 70–81.

Fijan, N., and Matasin, Z. (1980) Spring viraemia of carp: preliminary experiments on vaccination by exposure to virus in water. Vet. Arh. 50:215–220.

Fijan, N., Petrinec, Z., Sulimanovic, D., and Zwillenberg, L.O. (1971) Isolation of the viral causative agent from the acute form of infectious dropsy of carp. Vet. Arh. 41:125–138.

Fijan, N., Petrinec, Z., Stancl, Z., Dorson, M., and Le Berre, M. (1977a) Hyperimmunization of carp with Rhabdovirus carpio. Bull. Off. Int. Epizoot. 87:439–440.

Fijan, N., Petrinec, Z., Stancl, Z., Kezic, N., and Teskeredzic, E. (1977b) Vaccination of carp against spring viraemia: comparison of intraperitoneal and peroral application of live virus to fish kept in ponds. Bull. Off. Int. Epizoot. 87:441–442.

Fijan, N., Matasin, Z., Jeney, Z., Olah, J., and Zwillenberg, L.O. (1981) Isolation of Rhabdovirus carpio from sheatfish Silurus glanis fry. In: Proceedings of an International Seminar on Fish, Pathogens and Environment in European Polyculture (Olah, J., Molnar, K., and Jeney, Z., eds.). Szarvas, Hungary, pp. 48–58.

Hedrick, R.P., Rosemark, R., Aronstein, D., Winton, J.R., McDowell, T., and Amend, D.F. (1984) Characteristics of a new reovirus from channel catfish (Ictalurus punctatus). J. Gen. Virol. 65:1527–1534.

Hill, B.J. (1977) Studies on SVC virulence and immunization. Bull. Off. Int. Epizoot. 87:455–456.

Hill, B.J., Underwood, B.O., Smale, C.J., and Brown, F. (1975) Physico-chemical and serological characterization of five rhabdoviruses infecting fish. J. Gen. Virol. 27:369–378.

Hill, B.J., Williams, R.F., and Finlay, J. (1981) Preparation of antisera against fish virus disease agents. Dev. Biol. Stand. 49:209–218.

Hines, R.S., Wohlfarth, G.W., Moav, R., and Hulata, G. (1974) Genetic differences in susceptibility to two diseases among strains of the common carp. Aquaculture 3:187–197.

Hoppe, K., and Wernery, U. (1985) Ergebnisse serologischer Untersuchungen zum Nachweis von Antikorpern gegen die Viren der infektiosen Pankreasnekrose (IPN), der viralen hamorrhagischen Septikamie (VHS) und der Fruhlingsviramie (SVC) in Schles wig-Holstein sowie deren rechtliche Auswirkungen. Deut. Tierarztl. Wochensch. 92:172–174.

Koelbl, O., and Kainz, E. (1977) The distribution of pathogens of infectious stomach dropsy in Austrian carp pond farms. Oesterr. Fisch. 30:80–83.

Kovacs-Gayer, E. (1984) Histopathological differential diagnosis of gill changes with special regard to gill necrosis. In: Fish, Pathogens and Environment in European Polyculture (Olah, J., ed.). Akadiemiai Kiado, Budapest, Hungary, pp. 219–229.

Macura, B., Tesarcik, J., and Rehulka, J. (1983) Survey of methods of specific immunoprophylaxis of carp spring viremia in Czechoslovakia. Pr. PURH Vodnany. 12:50–56.

Mawdesley-Thomas, L.E., and Bucke, D. (1967) Fish pox in the roach (Rutilus rutilus L.). Vet. Rec. 1967:56.

McAllister, P.E., Lidgerding, B.C., Herman, R.L., Hoyer, L.C., and Hankins, J. (1985) Viral diseases of fish: first report of carp pox in golden ide (Leuciscus idus) in North America. J. Wildlife Dis. 21:199–204.

Negele, R.D. (1977) Histopathological changes in some organs of experimentally infected carp fingerlings with Rhabdovirus carpio. Bull. Off. Int. Epizoot. 87:449–450.

Nie, D.S., and Pan, J.P. (1985) Diseases of grass carp (Ctenopharyngodon idellus Valenciennes, 1844) in China, a review from 1953 to 1983. Fish Pathol. 20:323–330.

Nigrelli, R. (1948) Hyperplastic epidermal disease in the bluegill sunfish, Lepomis macrochirus Rafinesque. Zoologica 33:133–137.

Nigrelli, R.F. (1952) Virus and tumors in fishes. Ann. N.Y. Acad. Sci. 54:1076–1092.

Nigrelli, R.F. (1954) Tumors and other atypical cell growths in temperate freshwater fishes of North America. Trans. Am. Fish. Soc. 83:262–298.

Pasco, L., Torchy, C., and de Kinkelin, P. (1987) Infection experimentale de l'alevin de silure (Silurus glanis L.) par le virus de la viremie printaniere de la carpe (V.P.C.). Bull. Fr. Peche Piscis 307:84–88.

Peters, F., and Neukirch, M. (1986) Transmission of some fish pathogenic viruses by the heron, Ardea cinerea. J. Fish Dis. 9:539–544.

Pfeil-Putzien, C. (1977) New results in the diagnosis of spring viraemia of carp caused by experimental transmission of Rhabdovirus carpio with carp louse (Aggulus foliaceus). Bull. Off. Int. Epizoot. 87:457 (abstract).

Pfeil-Putzien, C., and Baath, C. (1978) Demonstration of Rhabdovirus carpio infection among carp in the autumn. Berl. Munch. Tierarztl. Wochensch. 91:445–447.

Plumb, J.A., Bowser, P.R., Grizzle, J.M., and Mitchell, A.J. (1979) Fish viruses: a double-stranded RNA icosahedral virus from a North American cyprinid. J. Fish. Res. Bd. Can. 36:1390–1394.

Popkova, T.I., and Shchelkunov, I.S. (1978) Isolation of a virus from carp diseased with gill necrosis (in Russian). Rybnoe Hozyaistvo. 4:34–38.

Riberio, L., and Ahne, W. (1983) Establishment of a fish virus susceptible cell strain from pituitary of carp, Cyprinus carpio. Zentralbl. Bakteriol. Mikrobiol. Hyg. 1 Abt. Orig. A 254:441–451.

Rudikov, N.I., Grishchenko, L.I., and Lobuncov, K.A. (1975) Vesennaja virusnaja boleznej ryb. Bjulletenj Vsesojuznogo Ordena Lenina Instituta Eksperimentaljnoj Veterinarii 20:16–19.

Sano, T., Fukuda, H., and Furukawa, M. (1985a) Herpesvirus cyprini: biological and oncogenic properties. Fish Pathol. 20:381–388.

Sano, T., Fukuda, H., Furukawa, M., Hosoya, H., and Moriya, Y. (1985b) A herpesvirus isolated from carp papilloma in Japan. In: Fish and Shellfish Pathology (Ellis, A.E., ed.). Academic Press, London, pp. 307–311.

Schaperclaus, W. (1954) Fischkrankheiten. Akad. Verlag, Berlin.

Schaperclaus, W. (1969) Virusinfektionen bei fischen. In: Handbuch der Virusinfektionen bei Tieren (Rohrer, H., ed.). VEB Gustav Fischer Verlag, Jena, pp. 1067–1141.

Schlumberger, H.G., and Lucke, B. (1948) Tumors of fishes, amphibians, and reptiles. Cancer Res. 8:657–754.

Schubert, von, G. (1964) Elektronenmikroskopische untersuchungen zur pockenkrankheit des karpfens. Z. Naturforsch. 19b:675–682.

Schubert, G.H. (1966) The infective agent in carp pox. Bull. Off. Int. Epizoot. 65:1011–1022.

Schwedler, T.E., and Plumb, J.A. (1980) Fish viruses: serologic comparison of the golden shiner and infectious pancreatic necrosis viruses. J. Wildlife Dis. 16:597–599.

Schwedler, T.E., and Plumb, J.A. (1982a) In vitro growth kinetics and thermostability of the golden shiner virus. J. Wildlife Dis. 18:441–446.

Schwedler, T.E., and Plumb, J.A. (1982b) Golden shiner virus: effects of stocking density on incidence of viral infection. Progressive Fish Culturist 44:151–152.

Section of Virus Study, Third Laboratory. (1978) Studies on the causative agent of hemorrhage of the grass carp (Ctenopharyngodon idellus). Acta Hydrobiol. 6:321–329.

Section of Virus Study, Third Laboratory. (1980) Studies on the causative agent of haemorrhage of the grass carp (*Ctenopharyngodon idellus*) II. Electron microscopic observation. Acta Hydrobiol. 7:75–80.

Shchelkunov, I.S., and Shchelkunova, T.I. (1984) Results of virological studies on gill necorsis. In: Fish, Pathogens and Environment in European Polyculture (Olah, J., ed.). Akademiai Kiado, Budapest, Hungary, pp. 31–43.

Sonstegard, R.A., and Sonstegard, K.S. (1978) Herpesvirus-associated epidermal hyperplasia in fish (carp). In: Proceedings of an International Symposium Oncogenesis and Herpesviruses (de The, G., Henle, W., and Rapp, F., eds.). International Agency Res. Cancer-Sci. Publication 24, pp. 863–868.

Stankiewicz, E.B. (1979) Fish culture in water heated by thermal effluents. Gospodarka Rybna 31:11–13.

Sulimanovic, D. (1973) Immunity of carp to *Rhabdovirus carpio* and determination of antibodies by indirect hemagglutination. Vet. Arh. 43:153–161.

Tesarcik, J., and Macura, B. (1981a) Field carp vaccination against spring viremia on the fish farms of the state fisheries (I.). Bul. VURH Vodnany. 17:3–11.

Tesarcik, J., and Macura, B. (1981b) The mortality and morbidity of half-year-old and yearling carp (*Cyprinus carpio* L.) and Gudgeon (*Gobio gobio* L.) after viral and bacterial infection in spring viraemia of carp. Bul. VURH Vodnany. 17:19–23.

Tesarcik, J., Macura, B., Rehulka, J., Hrdonka, M. and Konasova, V. (1984) Summarized results of pilot vaccination of carp against spring viremia in the Czech Socialist Republic. Pr. VURH Vodnany. 13:68–74.

Winton, J.R., Lannan, C.N., Fryer, J.L., Hedrick, R.P., Meyers, T.R., Plumb, J.A., and Yamamoto, T. (1987) Morphological and biochemical properties of four members of a novel group of reoviruses isolated from aquatic animals. J. Gen. Virol. 68:353–364.

Wizigmann, G., Baath, C., and Hoffmann, R. (1980) Isolation of viral hemorrhagic septicemia virus from fry of rainbow trout, pike and grayling. Zentralbl. Veterinaermed. B. 27:79–81.

Wizigmann, G., Dangschat, H., Baath, C., and Pfeil-Putzien, C. (1983) Investigations on viral diseases in freshwater fishes in Bavaria. Tierarztl. Umschau. 38:250–258.

Wolf, K. (1983) Biology and properties of fish and reptilian herpesviruses. In: The Herpesviruses. Vol. 2 (Roizman, B., ed.). Plenum Press, New York, pp. 319–366.

Chapter 51

PARASITIC DISEASES OF GOLDFISH, KOI, AND CARP

MICHAEL K. STOSKOPF

Goldfish, koi, and carp are subject to a wide variety of parasites. Many have been covered in the chapters on parasites of freshwater temperate fishes (Chap. 27) and freshwater tropical fishes (Chap. 70). The reader is referred to those chapters for additional insight into parasites affecting this group of fishes. This chapter briefly discusses only a few parasites that are a particular concern with this group of fishes, especially goldfishes. Table 51–1 provides a listing of parasites that have been identified in common carp, goldfish, and koi in North America.

MITASPORA CYPRINI

Geographic Distribution

Infection with *Mitaspora cyprini*, called kidney bloater, is frequently observed in retail outlets and is common in goldfish kept in home aquaria.

Clinical Appearance and Diagnosis

Apparently asymptomatic fish purchased in the summer gradually bloat during the winter months. Affected fish may be severely bloated yet may live for months (Fig. 51–1). The kidneys of affected fish become massively enlarged and resemble a tumor. Diagnosis is confirmed by a wet-mount preparation of the kidneys and identification of the typical trophozoites or spores.

Pathogenesis, Transmission, and Epidemiology

Fish become infected in ponds during the summer, but clinical signs are not seen until September or October. The disease is transmitted when spores are shed from urine in the spring. It appears that infection can spread to uninfected goldfish within an aquarium. Eventually all infected fish die as renal impairment and ascites formation progresses.

Treatment and Control

Presumably, spread of infection could be prevented by isolation of sick fish. Drainage of ascitic fluid is not recommended because fluid reaccumulates immediately. Experimental injections of furosemide have not reduced the accumulation of fluids. Addition of 0.3% salt to the aquarium water may

TABLE 51–1. Parasites of Common Carp, Goldfish, and Koi in North America

Protozoa
Chilodonella cyprini
Cryptobia carassii
Cryptobia cyprini
Eimeria aurata
Glossatella minuta
Ichthyobodo necatrix
Ichthyophthirius multifiliis
Myxobolus bellus
Myxobolus dispar
Thelohanellus dogieli
Thelohanellus fuhrmanni
Trichodina domerguei
Trichodina myakkae
Trichodina reticulata
Trichodina subtilis

Trematodes
Apophallus venustus (larval)
Crepidostomum cooperi
Crepidostomum sp.
Dactylogyrus anchoratus
Dactylogyrus folax
Dactylogyrus mollis
Diplostomulum flexicaudum (larval)
Diplostomulum paradoxum
Gyrodactylus anchoratus
Gyrodactylus carassii
Gyrodactylus fairporti
Gyrodactylus gurleyi
Nanophyetus salmincola (larval)
Neodactylogyrus cryptomeres
Plagiocirrus primus

Cestodes
Archigetes iwensis
Atractolytocestus huronensis

Caryophyllaeus sp.
Corallobothrium sp.
Khawia iowensis

Nematodes
Camallanus ancylodirus
Phylometra carassii
Pomphorhynchus bulbocolli
Raphidascaris acus
Rhabdochona cascadilla
Spiroxys sp.

Acanthocephalans
Leptorhynchoides thecatus
Neoechinorhyncus rutili
Pomphorhynchus bulbocolli

Leeches
Placobdella montifera

Molluscs
Unionidae genera

Crustaceans
Argulus catostomi
Argulus flavescens
Argulus japonicus
Argulus lunatus
Argulus trilineatus
Caligus lacustris
Lernaea cyprinacea
Neoergasilus longispinosus
Paraergasilus brevidigitus
Paraergasilus longidigitus

Mites
Hydrachnellae (Hydracarina) genera (larvae)

Adapted from Hoffman, G. L. (1967) Parasites of North American Freshwater Fishes. University of California Press, Berkeley.

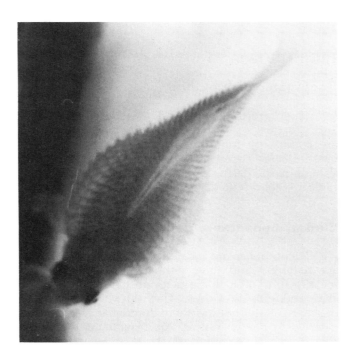

FIGURE 51–1. Severe ascites in a common goldfish with renal impairment from *Mitaspora* sp. (Courtesy of R. Floyd.)

assist the fish in osmoregulation, but clinical improvement should not be expected (Gratzek, 1988).

EIMERIA SP.

Geographic Distribution

Coccidiosis is seen most frequently in pond goldfish, but also in aquarium goldfish. It is caused by *Eimeria* sp., and occurs essentially worldwide.

Clinical Appearance and Diagnosis

Affected fish are emaciated with sunken eyes and are depressed. The contents of the intestines are fluid and yellow. Diagnosis is made by identifying oocysts in wet-mount preparations of intestinal scrapings or feces.

Pathogenesis, Transmission, and Epidemiology

This problem is most often observed in goldfish during the winter and spring under pond conditions where fish may not be fed. Immunologic responsiveness may be compromised by the colder water and poor nutrition. The disease is occasionally seen in home aquaria.

Treatment and Control

Treatment with anticoccidials in the food may be effective. Tetracyclines or monensin have been used in outbreaks. Treatment success is highly variable and depends on the nature of the outbreak.

TRICHODONIASIS

Geographic Distribution

There are three genera *Trichodina, Trichodonella,* and *Tripartiella* that have a similar appearance and are commonly found parasitizing fishes. All cultivated fish are susceptible to trichodoniasis, but goldfish are particularly susceptible. There is no apparent limit to geographic distribution.

Clinical Appearance and Diagnosis

Trichodinids are ciliated, circular parasites that are flattened and have denticular rings. They are usually 40 to 60 μ in diameter and are found on the skin and gills of fishes. They move in a distinct manner, often rotating their denticular ring continuously. In a wet mount, the organisms are dome shaped when viewed from the side. Heavy infesta-

tions cause respiratory distress and skin ulcers. Affected fish produce excess mucus and develop a white cast to the skin. The infestation can be entirely limited to the gills. This is often the case in koi. *Trichodina* organisms are larger than *Trichodonella* or *Tripartiella* and have complete rings of cilia. Many individual species have been described.

Pathogenesis, Transmission, and Epidemiology

These parasites are commonly found on the skin and gills of pond-reared fish, especially if the water has a high organic load. These organisms multiply by binary fission and do not produce resting spores. They do survive off of a host and can be introduced to aquaria with plants or substrates.

The smaller *Trichodonella* and *Tripartiella* species appear to inflict more injury to gills through their tendency to attach firmly to gill epithelium. Trichodinids are rarely a problem in home aquaria, since water changes associated with shipping and transportation will often effect a cure. It is common to observe *Trichodina* infestations in wholesale or retail establishments. Infestations are usually very light and apparently do not affect the host fish.

Treatment and Control

Removal of fish to fresh water will often effect a cure. Otherwise, treatments with formaldehyde baths or salt baths have been effective. Prevention centers around maintaining good water quality in the tank or pond.

DACTYLOGYRIDIASIS

Geographic Distribution

Goldfish can be heavily infested with dactylogyrid, or gill, flukes. Pond-reared fish and imported fish commonly have infections.

Clinical Appearance and Diagnosis

Fish in ponds or the wild rarely exhibit clinical signs. The development of clinical signs is associated with crowding where the probability of transmission is greatly enhanced. Consequently, clinical disease is more common in aquaria and holding vats. Clinical signs include rapid respiratory movements, clamped fins, flashing, or rubbing. Fish may also become inactive and sit at the bottom of the aquarium. Death can be caused by heavy infestations. Diagnosis can be confirmed by biopsies of the gills where worms are readily apparent if present. Dactylogyrid flukes are recognized by a four-pointed anterior end, a sucker near the anterior end, and four anterior eye spots. The caudal end has a fixation apparatus, or haptor, that consists of one or two large hooks surrounded by up to 16 smaller hooklets. The worms are approximately 400 μ long and have both testes and ovaries.

Pathologic Effects and Pathogenesis

Dactylogyrid flukes are usually found on the gills, but can be found on the body. If present in sufficient numbers, they can cause hyperplasia, destruction of gill epithelium, and clubbing of gill filaments, which can lead to asphyxiation.

Life Cycle, Transmission, and Epidemiology

Dactylogyrid flukes reproduce by mutual fertilization followed by release of eggs, which develop off of the host. Eggs from some species hatch into ciliated forms as early as 60 hours after being released. Other species require 4 to 5 days before hatching. The ciliated larvae attack suitable hosts, lose their cilia, and develop into adult trematodes. Transmission is greatly enhanced by overcrowding of fish. The parasite load per fish in a single aquarium, even within a single host species, can be quite variable. Immunocompetence may play a role in this variability.

Treatment and Control

Specific treatments include long-duration exposure to formaldehyde or short-term baths. Saltwater baths have also been used. Organophosphates are used, but it appears that extended use of organophosphates may develop resistant strains of flukes (Goven et al., 1980). Praziquantel will effectively remove monogenetic trematodes from gills and body surfaces when administered as a bath.

Control centers around careful quarantine and treatment of infected fish before they are placed in a tank. Latent infections can occur with clinical disease flaring in times of suboptimal environmental conditions.

LERNAEA SP.

SYNONYM. Anchor worms.

Geographic Distribution

Lernaea infestations are very common in koi and goldfish from production ponds. *Argulus*, or fish lice, infestations also are most common in goldfish production ponds.

Clinical Appearance and Diagnosis

Lernaea are elongated copepods, the females of which have an anchor-shaped head that is embedded in the host flesh for attachment. The presence of adult parasites is diagnostic. Larval stages are free-swimming and have a typical crustacean form with segmented body and legs. Only the females penetrate the host fish to form typical "anchor worms." The smaller males enter into permanent copulation with the females. At the time of initial penetration by female parasites, affected fish show irritation and localized hemorrhagic reactions at the point of entry. These areas may become secondarily infected with bacteria.

Pathologic Effects and Pathogenesis

Mortalities occur with heavy infestations of *Lernaea*, and secondary infections are common at the site of attachment.

Life Cycle, Transmission, and Epidemiology

Free-swimming immature forms of *Lernaea* sp. feed on superficial mucus and debris, undergoing a number of molts while differentiating into smaller males and larger females. When the parasites reach maturity, copulation occurs, and the females penetrate the skin of the host fish. The females develop large egg sacs that retain up to 700 eggs until hatching. The life cycle is temperature dependent and can take as little as 15 days at 30°C. Free-swimming and preadult stages can live up to 4 days without a host. Crowded conditions favor transmission of the parasite.

Treatment and Control

Extraction with forceps is commonly used to treat *Lernaea* infestations of aquarium or display fishes. It is important to be careful to avoid breaking the parasite during the procedure. An incision in the skin is usually required for successful removal of the entire head of the parasite, which may be deeply imbedded in reactive connective tissue. Extraction can be followed by local treatment with cotton swabs permeated with a suitable disinfectant (iodine, acriflavine, alcohol). Antibiotic treatment may accelerate healing of lesions. Infested aquaria can be treated with organophosphate, which will kill free-living juvenile forms. Dimulin, a chitin synthesis inhibitor, has been used successfully as a pond treatment or an aquarium water treatment. This treatment must be repeated every week for 4 to 6 weeks to achieve eradication. Quarantine for anchor worms should be at least 15 days at 30°C and longer at lower temperatures. Skin smears should be examined to look for preparasitic forms, since it can take up to several months between penetration and development of grossly visible parasites. Water, live food, plants, or other material should be stored for more than 4 days without contact with the potential host to avoid introduction of the parasite. Adequate ultraviolet light sterilization and filtration reduce the potential of spread of an infestation in a multiaquarium system.

LITERATURE CITED

Goven, B.A., Gilbert, J.P., and Gratzek, J.B. (1980) Apparent drug resistance to the organophosphate dimethyl (2,2,2-trichloro-1-hydroxyethyl) phosphonate by mongenetic trematodes. J. Wildlife Dis. 16(3):343–346.

Gratzek, J.B. (1988) Parasites associated with ornamental fish. Vet. Clin. North Am., Small Anim. Pract. 18(2):375–400.

Hoffman, G.L. (1967) Parasites of North American Freshwater Fishes. University of California Press, Berkeley.

Chapter 52

GOLDFISH, KOI, AND CARP NEOPLASIA

ERIC B. MAY

Tumors or neoplastic diseases of goldfish, koi, (Fig. 52–1), and carp are well represented in the literature, particularly those affecting the goldfish, where culture and use as ornamentals began more than 4000 years ago. Information on predisposing factors, such as environmental, genetic, and nutritional conditions, remains lacking for this group. There is little doubt that viruses (Roberts, 1978) and environmental contaminants are involved (Brown et al., 1973). A unique feature of this group is their longevity, particularly the koi. Goldfish and carp are also well adapted to environments that are suboptimal to other species of fishes. Part of this adaptation involves the ability to detoxify and repair damage caused by potentially toxic and carcinogenic agents (Bend and Foureman, 1984). A list of tumors reported in this fish group is given in Table 52–1.

Reported tumors among goldfish, koi, and carp appear to be concentrated in the nervous system. This is probably a reflection of interest on the part of the investigators and does not reflect actual distribution or incidence. Predisposing factors such as carcinogenic compounds, viruses, irritants, oncogenes, and parasites all have been reported for this group and should be considered potential sources for tumor induction. Inbreeding, particularly among the goldfish and koi, exists and should be considered as a potential problem.

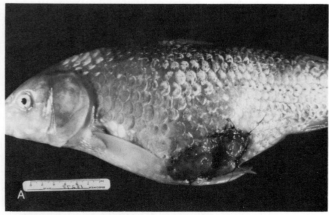
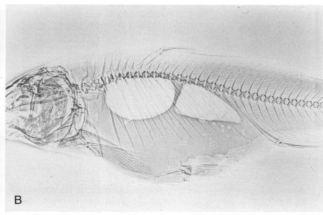

FIGURE 52–1. Hepatocelluar tumor in a koi. *A.* Gross appearance with tumor eroding the abdominal wall. *B.* Xeroradiograph of the same patient. (Courtesy of M. Stoskopf.)

TABLE 52–1. Neoplasias Reported in Goldfish, Koi, and Carp

Site/Neoplasia	Fish	References
Nervous System		
Neuroepithelioma	Carp	Harshbarger, 1979
	Goldfish	Ishikawa et al., 1978a
Medulloepithelioma	Goldfish	Lahav and Albert, 1978
Chordoma (induced)	Goldfish	Levy, 1962
Schwannoma	Goldfish	Picchi, 1932
Neurilemoma	Carp	Harshbarger, 1977
	Goldfish	Nakatsukasa, 1973
Neurilemal sarcoma	Carp	Harshbarger, 1983
Esthesioneuroepithelioma	Goldfish	Harshbarger, 1978
Melanophoroma	Goldfish	Harshbarger, 1979
Erythrophoroma	Carp	Harshbarger, 1981
	Goldfish	Ishikawa et al., 1978b
Chondroblastoma	Carp	Harshbarger, 1983
	Goldfish	Etoh et al., 1983
Cardiovascular System		
Fibrous histiocytoma	Koi	Harshbarger, 1983
Mesothelioma	Carp	Harshbarger, 1983
Gastrointestinal System		
Pancreatic acinar cell carcinoma	Goldfish	Otte, 1964
Hepatocellular tumor*	Koi	Stoskopf, personal communication
Urinary System		
Fibrous histiocytoma	Carp	Weis and Einzinger, 1978
	Crucian carp	Konishi et al., 1982
Carcinoma of bladder	Goldfish	Plehn, 1909
Endocrine System		
Pituitary chromophobe adenoma	Carp × goldfish	Down, 1984
Thyroid adenoma	Carp	Nigrelli, 1952
	Goldfish	Nigrelli, 1952
	Koi	Nigrelli, 1952
Reproductive System		
Adenomatous epizootic testicular tumor	Carp × Goldfish	Sonstegard, 1977
Musculoskeletal System		
None reported		
Integumentary System		
None reported		
Respiratory System		
None reported		

*See Figure 52–1.

LITERATURE CITED

Bend, J.R., and Foureman, C.L. (1984) Variation of hepatic aryl hydrocarbon hydroxylase (AHH) and 7-ethoxyresorufin O-deethylase (7-ERD) activities in marine fish from Maine: Evidence that monoxygenase activities of only a few species are induced by environmental exposure to polycyclic aromatic hydrocarbon (PAH)-type compounds. Marine Environ. Res. 14:405–406.

Brown, E.R., Hasdra, J.J., Keith, L., Greenspan, I., Kwapinski, J., and Beamer, P. (1973) Frequency of fish tumors found in a polluted watershed as compared to nonpolluted Canadian waters. Cancer Res. 33:189–198.

Down, N.E. (1984) Studies on the reproductive biology of gonadal tumour-bearing carp-goldfish hybrids. Ph.D. Thesis Dissertation, University of Guelph, Guelph, Ontario, Canada.

Etoh, H., Hyodo-Taguchi, Y., and Aoki, K. (1983) Incidence of chromatoblastomas in aging goldfish. J. Natl. Cancer Inst. 70:523–528.

Harshbarger, J.C. (1977) RTLA supplement. Registry of Tumors in Lower Animals. Smithsonian Inst., Washington, D.C.

Harshbarger, J.C. (1978) RTLA supplement. Registry of Tumors in Lower Animals. Smithsonian Inst., Washington, D.C.

Harshbarger, J.C. (1979) RTLA supplement. Registry of Tumors in Lower Animals. Smithsonian Inst., Washington, D.C.

Harshbarger, J.C. (1981) RTLA supplement. Registry of Tumors in Lower Animals. Smithsonian Inst., Washington, D.C.

Harshbarger, J.C. (1983) RTLA supplement. Registry of Tumors in Lower Animals. Smithsonian Inst., Washington, D.C.

Ishikawa, T., Masahito, P., and Takayma, S. (1978a) Olfactory neuroepithelioma in a domestic carp (*Cyprinus carpio*). Cancer Res. 38:3954–3959.

Ishikawa, T., Masahito, P., Matsumoto, J., et al. (1978b) Morphologic and biochemical characterization of erythrophoromas in goldfish (*Carassius auratus*). J. Natl. Cancer Inst. 61:1461–1470.

Konishi, Y., Maruyama, H., Mii, Y., et al. (1982) Malignant fibrous histiocytomas induced by 4-(hydroxyamino)quinoline 1-oxide. J. Natl. Cancer Inst. 68:859.

Lahav, M., and Albert, D.M. (1978) Medulloepithelioma of the ciliary body in the goldfish (*Carassius auratus*). Vet. Pathol. 15:208–212.

Levy, B.M. (1962) Experimental induction of tumor-like lesion of the notochord of fish. Cancer Res. 22:441–442.

Nakatsukasa, Y. (1973) A case of neurilemmoma developed in a hibuna *Carassius auratus*. Jpn. J. Ichthyol. 20:182–184.

Nigrelli, R.F. (1952) Spontaneous neoplasms in fishes. VI. Thyroid tumors in marine fishes. Zoologica 37:185–189.

Otte, E. (1964) Eine Bosartige Neubildung in der Basschhole eines Goldfisches (*Carassius auratus*). Wein. Tieraerztl. Monatsschr. 51:485–488.

Picchi, L. (1932) Di un non commune tumore di un pesce (neurinoma). Seperimentale 86:128–130.

Plehn, M. (1909) Uber einige bie Fishchen Beobachtete Geschwulste und Geschwulstartige Bildunged. Ber. Bayer Biol. Verssta 2:55–76.

Roberts, R.J. (ed.) (1978) Fish Pathology. Bailliere Tindall, London.

Sonstegard, R.A. (1978) Environmental and carcinogenesis studies in fishes of the Great Lakes and North America. Ann. N.Y. Acad. Sci. 298:261–269.

Stoskopf, M.K. (1990) Personal communication, unreported cases, NAIB.

Weiss, S.W., and Einzinger, F.M. (1978) Malignant fibrous histiocytoma: an analysis of 200 cases. Cancer 41:2250–2267.

SECTION IV

CATFISHES

MARSHALL H. BELEAU, *Section Editor*

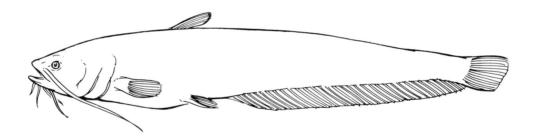

Chapter 53

TAXONOMY AND NATURAL HISTORY OF CATFISHES

MARSHALL H. BELEAU

The catfishes of the world are represented by at least 2000 species in over 25 families within the order Siluriformes, which has been known from the Paleocene epoch. The family Diplomystidae, from South America, comprises the most primitive of the living species. Catfishes are found in commercial fisheries, sport fisheries, and aquaculture, as ornamental fish, and on endangered species lists. Most catfishes are strictly freshwater species, although two families contain saltwater species. Over half of the known species of catfishes are native to South America, but representatives of the Siluriformes are found worldwide.

One of the largest catfishes is the sheatfish from Europe (maximum recorded 5 m, 330 kg) (Fig. 53–1). Many catfishes have a maximum length of less than 12 cm (Nelson, 1984). The families Loricariidae and Callichthyidae include the South American armored catfishes, which are sometimes used as ornamental fish (Bond, 1979). The genus *Vandallia*, from Brazil, includes small parasitic catfish that are attracted to the nitrogenous waste from gill cavities of larger fish (Fig. 53–2). They may mistakenly enter the urinary openings of mammals, including man (Halsted, 1967; Nelson, 1984). The African electric catfish has specialized electroplaques capable of producing a strong, stunning electric current (Keynes et al., 1961). Another African family, the Mochokidae, contains the upside-down catfish, a species that habitually swims with its belly to the water surface. *Clarius* spp. are air-breathing fish equipped with arborescent accessory breathing apparatuses in their gill chamber, which allows them to estuate and maintain themselves buried in the mud for several months over the dry season. Catfishes, like cyprinid fishes, have a weberian apparatus, an anatomic modification that consists of fusion of the first four or five vertebrae and associated small ossicles that allows the swimbladder to serve as a resonator in sound reception.

A catfish that is grabbed or restrained typically lashes back and forth, usually with dorsal and pectoral spines locked in erect position. The sea catfishes are particularly adept at this defensive maneuver. Injuries due to puncture wounds from the serrated spines produce immediate and intense pain, but most such injuries are not dangerous. As a safety precaution, fish diagnosticians will often use rongeurs to remove the spines prior to necropsy procedures. Several catfish families, including those kept as aquarium fish, contain species that are venomous. These fish may have venom glands in the skin sheathing the dorsal and pectoral spines or may have axillary venom glands that supply secretions to the exterior of the pectoral spines. An Indo-Pacific family, the Plotosidae, are the most dangerous of the venomous catfishes (Russell, 1969).

The catfishes are nonmigratory and relatively slow swimmers. Most are nocturnal and tend to live in protected habitats. Catfishes are generally considered omnivorous, opportunistic bottom feeders. Juveniles feed mainly on invertebrates, and piscivory becomes more pronounced with age. Catfishes are easily identified by their smooth scaleless bodies and elongate fleshy barbels on the maxillary, nasal, and chin regions. The dorsal and pectoral fins are frequently armed with single strong, sometimes serrated, spines. Usually an adipose fin is present and bands of numerous bristlelike teeth on the jaws. Annual spawning occurs in the spring or summer with the eggs typically guarded by the male. In the

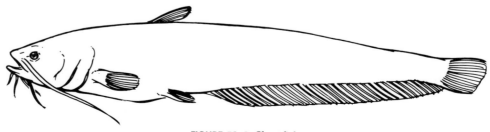

FIGURE 53–1. Sheatfish.

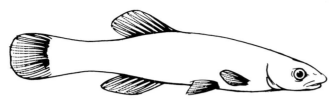

FIGURE 53–2. *Vandallia* sp. catfish.

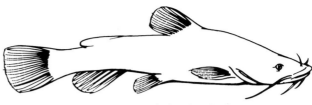

FIGURE 53–4. Flathead catfish.

freshwater family Ictaluridae, the eggs are laid in a nest as a gelatinous mass and are protected by the male. In the saltwater family Ariidae, the eggs are incubated within the mouth of the male, and the young may reach 10 cm before leaving paternal shelter.

Chemical communication among the ictalurid catfishes, and perhaps other sensory stimuli, affect social behavior. The channel catfish possesses an acute olfactory sense, and the social interactions of bullheads are mediated by pheromones or other substances. In natural situations, ictalurids can live together peacefully, since the social status of individuals within the group and displacement of hierarchy as well as amicable or agonistic behavior are, at least partially, chemically communicated (Todd, 1971; Todd et al., 1968).

Several freshwater catfishes are especially favored as a table delicacy. Among these, the channel catfish is the most popular and has become the most important commercially cultured fish in the United States (Fig. 53–3). The blue catfish, a larger but similar species, and the flathead catfish (Fig. 53–4) are the most favored of the commercial wild-caught species. The bullhead, or mudcat catfishes are frequently plentiful in turbid ponds and creeks, but they are less popular owing to their small size. The diminutive and secretive catfishes known as madtoms are usually inhabitants of the rocks and gravel bottoms of flowing water, especially the riffles and shoals of clearer streams and rivers. Being relatively small, they are not considered sport or food fish. The African catfish is gaining importance in aquaculture, especially in Israel and South Africa.

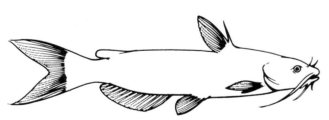

FIGURE 53–3. Channel catfish.

LITERATURE CITED

Bond, C.E. (1979) Class Osteichthyes—Bony fishes. In: Biology of Fishes, W.B. Saunders, Philadelphia, pp. 134–210.

Brinn, J.E., Jr. (1971) The pancreatic islet cells of the channel catfish. *Ictalurus punctatus.* Anat. Rec. 169:284.

Halsted, B. W. (1967) Poisonous and Venomous Marine Animals of the World. Vol. 2. U.S. Government Printing Office, Washington, D.C.

Keynes, R.D., Bennett, M.V.L., and H. Grundfest, H. (1961) Studies on the morphology and electrophysiology of electric organs. II. Electrophysiology of the electric organ of *Malapterurus electricus.* In: Bioelectrogenesis (Chagas, C., and Paes de Carvalho, A., eds.). American Elsevier, New York, pp. 102–112.

Nelson, J.S. (1984) Fishes of the World. John Wiley and Sons, New York.

Russell, F.E. (1969) Poisons and venoms. In: Fish Physiology, Vol. 3 (Hoar, W.S., and Randall, D.J., eds.) Academic Press, New York, pp. 401–449.

Todd, J.H. (1971) The chemical languages of fishes. Sci. Am. 224(5):98–108.

Todd, J.H., Atema, J., and Bardach, J.E. (1968) Chemical communication in social behavior of a fish, the yellow bullhead *(Ictalurus matalis).* Science 158:672–673.

Chapter 54

SPECIAL ANATOMY AND PHYSIOLOGY OF CATFISHES

MARSHALL H. BELEAU

By definition, anatomic and physiologic adaptations of catfishes make them distinct from other species. Some of these characteristics are noteworthy in order to differentiate normal from pathologic change, to know when special procedures or handling techniques may be necessary, and to give a proper description of the anatomic presentation during necropsy procedures. General anatomy is addressed in Chapter 1.

Depending on age, sex, season, aquatic environment, and geographic location, the external appearance of the channel catfish can be variable. Most of the ventral surface is white except in mature males during spawning when it may turn gray. The sides and dorsum grade into a grayish blue. Old individuals may be completely black on the dorsum and fish from clearer water tend to be lighter in color. Young channel catfish typically have small round to irregular dark spots distributed on the lateral body surface, which are usually lost with age. The white underside, mildly depressed body shape, and lack of scales make skin tattooing for individual identification quite easy.

The dorsal and ventrolateral pectoral fins, with associated hard rays (spines) that can be locked into erect position, and smooth skin covered by a mucous slime layer can present a challenge for physically handling live fish. With moderate-sized individuals, a cotton-gloved hand placed palm to skull anterior to the dorsal spine, with thumb and index finger in the opposite axillary regions, will usually prevent injury.

Sexual differentiation using external morphologic characteristics can usually be accomplished only in mature individuals (Fig. 54–1). The task is also much easier during spawning season. The genital area is between the anus and anterior base of the anal fin. The male has a common urogenital pore at the top of a small fleshy papilla. The female has an anterior genital pore and separate posterior urinary pore sometimes bordered by small lateral skin folds. As males mature, their broad muscular head and dark underside aid in differentiation. Mature females during spawning will have a full distended abdomen as eggs develop in the body cavity.

The lateral line runs longitudinally from the head to the caudal fin and presents a good landmark for blood sampling from the dorsal aorta as it approximates the internal position of the vertebral column. A hypodermic needle of adequate length can be inserted midway between the lateral line and ventral midline in the posterior third of the body and angled toward the lower vertebral column to reach the dorsal aorta. Unlike other species, blood sampling from heart puncture by ventrodorsal needle insertion directly into the heart is not possible as it is protected ventrally by a heavy pectoral girdle. Access to the carotid sinus, medial to the dorsal insertion of the third gill arch, provides an additional sampling site.

The digestive system of channel catfish is typical of omnivorous fishes. Pyloric ceca are not present; the stomach is highly expandable and the intestine is not clearly differentiated into regions. The swimbladder is derived from the foregut, and is physostomous with the pneumatic duct connecting the midventral bladder to the right side of the esophagus near the stomach (Grizzle and Rogers, 1976). The anterior chamber of the swimbladder is in direct contact with the skin below the weberian apparatus. The large liver varies from yellow-brown to dark red. A common bile duct connects the gallbladder to the intestine ventral to the esophagus. Thymic tissue is

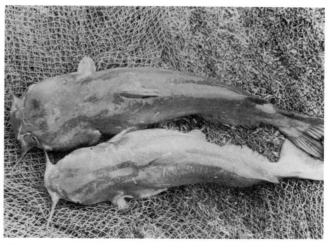

FIGURE 54–1. Sexual dimorphism in channel catfish. The top fish is a male, and the lower fish is a female. (Courtesy of P. R. Bowser.)

located in the posterior portion of the dorsal wall of the pharynx and is not grossly visible. The endocrine pancreas consists of scattered white nodules (Brockman bodies) in the mesenteries between the spleen and liver, and exocrine pancreatic tissue is located within the liver and occasionally the spleen. The endocrine pancreas contains three cell types: aldehyde fuchsin–positive B cells, ponceau and PTAH–positive A cells, and argyrophilic, light green–positive D cells (Brinn, 1971). The channel catfish is unique in that the D cells numerically constitute a major portion of the islet cells.

The ultimobranchial gland in channel catfish is located in the transverse septum between the heart and liver, and is not grossly visible. The paired glands are a source of calcitonin that regulates calcium levels. In the walking catfish, glucagon activates ultimobranchial cells to induce hypocalcemia similar to mammals (Srivastav et al., 1987). In channel catfish, thyroid tissue is also not grossly visible and is located in the ventral head region along the ventral aorta and afferent brachial arteries. Other parts of the endocrine system are relatively similar to other fish species.

The kidney of channel catfish is divided into a completely separate cranial hemopoietic, endocrine portion, and caudal excretory portion. The cranial portion is located cranial to the swimbladder and is composed of intermingled interrenal, chromaffin, and hemopoietic tissues easily distinguished in histologic sections. The caudal nephronic kidney is located caudal to the swimbladder and is U-shaped on the cranial end. On histologic examination it is not unusual to find cranial kidney cell types in the caudal kidney, and vice versa.

Respiration in channel catfish and the anatomic structure of the gills are typical of other teleosts. Of note, however, when fresh gills are examined under the light microscope, the lamellae appear much thicker and the edges are more rounded than salmonid gills. The African catfish provides for aerial respiration with its elaborate treelike modified gills arising from the upper ends of the gill arches. The additional respiratory capacity explains why they can tolerate extremely high fish densities per unit water volume and unit volume water exchange. For example, in Thailand, annual pond production of 80,000 kg/hectare has been achieved with air-breathing catfish (Panayotou et al., 1982).

The musculature of the relatively sedentary channel catfish is essentially all white muscle and does not contain the dark, highly vascularized lateral superficial muscles typical of more pelagic fishes. Aside from the weberian apparatus previously mentioned, the skeletal system is not remarkable from other teleosts. However, from a diagnostic perspective, the location of a fossa on the midline of the frontal bone of the skull is important. Part of normal microbiologic diagnostic procedures in catfish is to take cultures with a sterile microbiologic loop from the brain. This is especially true when *Edwardsiella ictaluri* is the suspected pathogen. This procedure is accomplished by incising the disinfected skin with a scalpel, directly on the midline at the posterior level of the eyes, and inserting a loop directly in line with the vertebral column to a point one-third the distance to the dorsal spine.

The scaleless nonkeratinized epidermis of the channel catfish is composed of stratified squamous epithelium containing goblet cells, alarm substance cells, the lateral line, and an enormous number of taste buds. The alarm substance cells are large (usually 50 to 60 μ) with a centrally located double nucleus (Grizzle and Rodgers, 1976). These cells never extend to the epithelial surface and the "fright substance" that they contain is only released during injury (Pfeiffer, 1963). The cranial innervated taste buds are found over the entire external surface as well as in the mouth, pharynx, and anterior esophagus. They have a characteristic flask shape with centrally located nuclei near the base. The acutely sensitive cutaneous taste system of the channel catfish is truly remarkable in that the fish will detect, process, and behaviorally respond to enantiomers of amino acids (L- and D-alanine) at levels of 10^{-9} molar (Brand et al., 1987; Kanwal et al., 1987). The ability to study both biochemical and electrophysiologic taste responses to the same stimuli is one unique advantage of the channel catfish animal model (Holland and Teeter, 1981), and also helps explain why oral therapeutic compounds offered in feed are sometimes rejected by the fish.

LITERATURE CITED

Brand, J.G., Bryant, B.P., Cagan, R.H., and Kalinoski, D.L. (1987) Biochemical studies of taste sensation. XIII. Enantiomeric specificity of alanine taste receptor sites in catfish, *Ictalurus punctatus*. Brain Res. 416:119–128.

Brinn, J.E., Jr. (1971) The pancreatic islet cells of the channel catfish, *Ictalurus punctatus*. Anat. Rec. 169:284.

Grizzle, J.M., and Rogers, W.A. (1976) Anatomy and Histology of the Channel Catfish. Auburn University Agricultural Experiment Station, Alabama.

Holland, K.N., and Teeter, J.H. (1981) Behavior and cardiac reflex assays of the chemosensory acuity of channel catfish to amino acids. Physiol. Behav. 27:699–707.

Kanwal, J.S., Hidaka, I., and Caprio, J. (1987) Taste responses to amino acids from facial nerve branches innervating oral and extra-oral taste buds in the channel catfish, *Ictalurus punctatus*. Brain Res. 406:105–112.

Panayotou, T., Wattanutchariya, S., Isvilanonda, S., and Tokbrisna, R. (1982) The Economics of Catfish Farming in Central Thailand. International Center for Living Aquatic Resources Management (ICLARM), Manila.

Pfeiffer, W. (1963) The fright reaction in North American Fish. Can. J. Zool. 41:69–77.

Srivastav, S.P., Swarup, K., and Srivastav, A.K. (1987) Ultimobranchial gland of male *Claras batrachus* in response to glucagon treatment. Zoo. Anz. 218:389–393.

Chapter 55

CLINICAL PATHOLOGY OF CATFISHES

RUTH FRANCIS-FLOYD

SAMPLE COLLECTION

Blood samples can be readily collected from channel catfish larger than 100 g and are accessible in smaller fish, although sacrifice of the individual may be necessary. Anesthesia is recommended when handling fish larger than 1 kg. Channel catfish are easily bled from the caudal vein (Fig. 55–1) (Campbell and Murru, 1990). Blood can also be collected by cardiac puncture, or by severing the caudal peduncle in small fish.

Serum samples tolerate prolonged storage well. Catfish serum stored for 240 days at –72°C principally shows a loss of triglycerides, and increases in lactate dehydrogenase (LDH) and alkaline phosphatase. Electrolyte values, liver enzymes, total protein, and glucose are unaffected as long as the sample is not allowed to dehydrate (Bentick-Smith et al., 1987). Tissue contamination of serum samples results in mild increases in urea, cholesterol, triglycerides, total bilirubin, and alanine transaminase along with a massive increase in lactic dehydrogenase (Bentick-Smith et al., 1987).

Care must be taken to avoid premature clotting of samples. In the author's experience, the best way of avoiding premature clotting is to collect the sample quickly (less than 1 minute) and immediately mix it gently with the anticoagulant. Blood collected from

small fish or from a very low pressure flow should be double-checked for small clots before releasing the fish.

HEMATOLOGY

Channel catfish are the most widely studied member of the catfish family. Baseline data are available for normal erythrocyte (Table 55–1), leukocyte (Table 55–2), and serum chemistry (Tables 55–3 to 55–5) parameters. Limited data available for other catfishes are also presented in these tables. Variability in parameters reported by different authors may be due to technical, environmental, or individual variation between study groups.

Erythrocytes

Erythrocytes are the predominant cell in blood smears taken from normal catfishes (Fig. 55–2). Immature erythrocytes of channel catfish are larger and rounder than mature cells, the nucleus is more centrally located, and the cytoplasm stains more blue with Wright-Giemsa (Grizzle and Rogers, 1976). Staining smears with brilliant crystal blue helps visualization of the reticular network of reticulocytes (Grizzle and Rogers, 1976). Smudge cells are commonly encountered in blood smears from channel catfish blood. These cells may represent old or particularly fragile erythrocytes (Yuki, 1960). This common artifact can be minimized by immobilizing cells in an isotonic agarose solution prior to fixing or staining (Ellsaesser et al., 1984).

Leukocytes

Lymphocytes and thrombocytes are the most commonly encountered leukocytes in the peripheral blood of channel catfish (Ellsaesser et al., 1985). Lymphocytes from channel catfish are small, 5 to 11 μm in diameter, round, have a large basophilic

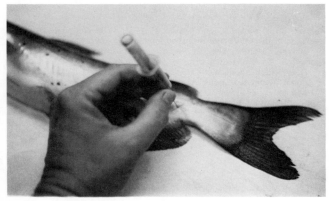

FIGURE 55–1. Blood collection from the caudal vein of a channel catfish. (Courtesy of P. Reed.)

498

TABLE 55–1. Baseline Hematologic Parameters of Catfishes

Species	N	Total RBC (million/ml)	Hct (%)	Hgb (gm/dl)	Thrombocytes #/ml	References
			Erythrocyte Indices			
Black bullhead				10.1–11.3		Black, 1955
Blue catfish	2	1.6	31.0	6.9		Brader et al., 1982
Brown bullhead				6.6		Hawes, 1959
Channel catfish	35	2.4	40 (N = 142)		68,000	Grizzle and Rogers, 1976
	28–51	1.6	22.7	4.0	15,000	Breazile et al., 1982
	9	1.7	39.3	8.4		Brader et al., 1982
Isher catfish	25	1.55	31.6	14.6		Kori-Siakpere, 1985
Mud barbel catfish		2.1	28.9	5.8		Hattingh, 1972
Stinging catfish	10	2.6	34.5	8		Murad and Mustafa, 1988
Stripped dwarf catfish		2.9	25.4			Natarajan, 1981
Walking catfish	20	4.5	47.5	9.8		Sharma and Shandilya, 1982
Yellow bullhead				9.7		Smith et al., 1952

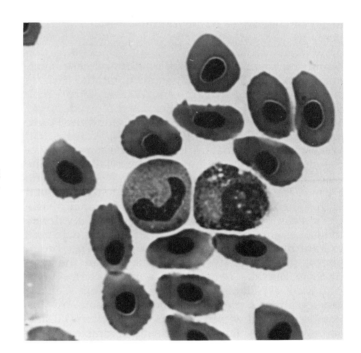

FIGURE 55–2. A hemoblast, mature erythrocytes, and a heterophil from the peripheral blood of a channel catfish (Giemsa, 1000×). (Courtesy of M. Stoskopf.)

TABLE 55–2. Baseline Hematologic Parameters of Catfishes

Species	N	WBC (/ml)	Heterophils (%)	Monocytes (%)	Lymphocytes (%)	Eosinophils (%)	References
				Leukocyte Indices			
Channel catfish			5		94		Grizzle and Rogers, 1976
	20	28,100	15		85		Breazile et al., 1972
	98*		5	3	92		Ellsaesser et al., 1985
	51*		4	2	94		Ellsaesser et al., 1983
Stinging catfish	20	30,000	11	3.5	79.5	5.5	Murad and Mustafa, 1988
Walking catfish	20	21,000	33	5	small = 50 large = 2.5	8.5	Sharma and Shandilya, 1982

Data presented in this table have been pooled from data presented in the original text of cited reference.

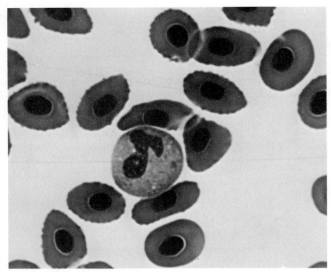

FIGURE 55–3. A heterophil from the peripheral blood of a channel catfish (Giemsa, 1000×). (Courtesy of M. Stoskopf.)

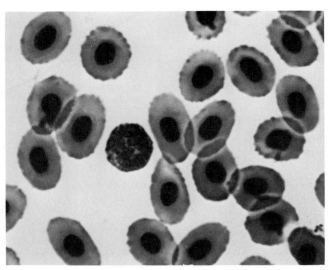

FIGURE 55–4. A typical small lymphocyte from the peripheral blood of a channel catfish (Giemsa, 1000×). (Courtesy of M. Stoskopf.)

staining nucleus and a small amount of peripheral, nongranular cytoplasm that stains light blue (Grizzle and Rogers, 1976; Williams and Warner, 1976) (Figs. 55–3 and 55–4). Thrombocytes are involved in the clotting process. The cells are either round, fusiform, or elongate (Grizzle and Rogers, 1976; Williams and Warner, 1976). Variation in cell shape may be associated with cellular maturity or be related in some way to the clotting process (Grizzle and Rogers, 1976; Ellis, 1977). In channel catfish blood smears stained with Wright-Giemsa, thrombocytes are small, basophilic cells that have a large nucleus and moderate to sparse amounts of cytoplasm that stains pale pink to light blue (Grizzle and Rogers, 1976). The thrombocyte nucleus stains more densely than the lymphocyte nucleus resulting in a more compact appearance (Williams and Warner, 1976). Cellular identification is greatly enhanced if smears are prepared and fixed within 2 hours of collection (Ellsaesser et al., 1985). Rapid processing minimizes loss of cytoplasmic projections and increased rounding of thrombocytes.

Basophils have not been reported in peripheral blood smears of channel catfish (Grizzle and Rogers, 1976; Ellis, 1977; Ellsaesser et al., 1985). Eosinophils occur occasionally and are 7 to 10 μm in diameter.

Their cytoplasm contains large, eosinophilic granules (Grizzle and Rogers, 1976). Heterophils and monocytes are the largest leukocytes found in the peripheral blood of channel catfish (Ellsaesser et al., 1985). Heterophils measure 8 to 13 μm in diameter and contain coarse cytoplasmic granules (Grizzle and Rogers, 1976; Williams and Warner, 1976). Nuclei of channel catfish heterophils are only occasionally lobulated (Ellsaesser et al., 1985). Both channel catfish heterophils and monocytes are phagocytic (Finco-Kent and Thune, 1987).

Discontinuous density Percoll gradient techniques have been used to separate leukocytes from channel catfish blood for research (Waterstrat et al., 1988). Blood is diluted with two or three parts calcium and magnesium-free Hank's balanced salt solution, and centrifuged at 300 G for 20 minutes. Greater dilution improves the purity of the sample, but decreases yield. Monocytes (up to 50% pure) are separated at the 1.060 to 1.065 G/ml interface. Lymphocytes (60 to 70% pure) are separated at the 1.065 to 1.070 G/ml interface, and heterophils (60 to 75% pure) are separated at the 1.070 to 1.080 G/ml interface. This procedure results in 95% or greater viability of cells; however, the efficiency of the procedure is reduced by lipemia.

TABLE 55–3. Baseline Serum Chemistry of Catfishes

Species	N	Urea Nitrogen (mg/dl)	Uric Acid (mg/dl)	Creatinine (mg/dl)	Total Protein (gm/dl)	Albumin (gm/dl)	References
Channel catfish	300–648	2.6	1.6	0.5	2.2	0.5	Bentick-Smith et al., 1987
	21				4.0		Breazile et al., 1972
		1.4	1.3	1.8	4.5	0.8	Warner and Williams, 1972
Isher catfish	25				3.27		Kori-Siakpere, 1985
Mud barbel catfish	—				4.1		Hattingh, 1972

TABLE 55–4. Baseline Serum Chemistry of Catfishes

Species	N	Glucose (mg/dl)	Cholesterol (mg/dl)	Triglycerides (mg/dl)	AST (U/L)	ALT (U/L)	Alk Pos (U/L)	LDH (U/L)	Amylase (U/L)	References
Channel catfish	300–648	64.5	152	199	95	17.5	20	172	54	Bentick-Smith et al., 1987
	—	77.8	212		143		45	319		Warner and Williams, 1977
Isher catfish	25	104.41								Kori-Siakpere, 1985
Mud barbel catfish		36.5								Hattingh, 1972

SERUM CHEMISTRY

Serum chemistry reference values (Tables 55–3 to 55–5) have been reported for channel catfish (Bentick-Smith et al., 1987). Seasonal declines in serum potassium and glucose occur during fall and winter months, possibly secondary to declines in metabolic rate and feeding activity that occur as water temperature drops (Bentick-Smith et al., 1987). Serum cortisol also increases in channel catfish in the fall and winter (Ainsworth et al., 1985).

SEROLOGY

Serology is used as a diagnostic and research tool for two economically important diseases of channel catfish, channel catfish virus disease and enteric septicemia of catfish. Seasonal variation in channel catfish virus titer is reported in adult channel catfish that survived an epizootic (Bowser and Munson, 1986). Although fish were not individually identified, a greater number of animals had high titers during summer and fall.

Comparisons of fluorescent antibody techniques with enzyme immunoassay for detection of *Edwardsiella ictaluri* and *E. tarda* in channel catfish show both techniques to be fast, efficient, and relatively easy to perform (Rogers, 1981). The principal disadvantage of fluorescent antibody techniques is the expense of a fluorescent microscope.

EFFECTS OF TECHNIQUES

Comparisons of three techniques for accuracy of hemoglobin determination in blood from channel catfish indicate that the oxyhemoglobin method is the most accurate, and therefore the method of choice. Correction factors exist for use with the cyanomethemoglobin method and the acid hematin hemoglobin method (Larsen, 1964). The correction factor reported for the cyanomethemoglobin method is:

$$0.68 + (1.01 \times \text{C-M Hb value})$$

where C-M Hb value is the numerical value obtained from the cyanomethemoglobin method. The correction factor provided for acid hematin hemoglobin is:

$$0.193 + (0.86 \times \text{A-H Hb value})$$

where A-H Hb value is the numerical value obtained by acid hematin hemoglobin determination (Larsen, 1964).

Handling

The effects of sampling stress on hematologic parameters have been studied in rainbow trout (Railo et al., 1985). Changes in blood parameters are observed within 1 minute of handling. Changes observed in the sample collected following handling included increases in packed cell volume, plasma potassium, and plasma chloride; and decreases in plasma sodium and blood pH (acidosis). Rapid increases in serum cortisol are also reported following handling of channel catfish (Ainsworth et al., 1985). Increases in cortisol have also been associated with confinement of channel catfish (Strange, 1980; Limsuwan et al., 1983; Ainsworth et al., 1985). Catfish held in a net for 10 minutes in one experiment had cortisol levels of 30.86 μg/dl compared to baseline concentrations of 5.6 μg/dl (Ainsworth et al., 1985).

Transport

The effect of controlled, 15-minute, transport on hematologic parameters and immune function in channel catfish has been evaluated (Ellsaesser and Clem, 1986). Fish were bled prior to stress and 18 to 24 hours poststress. No change in hematocrit was observed in transported fish; however, there were

TABLE 55–5. Baseline Serum Chemistry of Catfishes

Species	N	Sodium (mM/L)	Chloride (mM/L)	Potassium (mM/L)	Inorganic Phosphorus (mg/dl)	Calcium (mg/dl)	Magnesium (mg/dl)	Total Bilirubin	References
Channel catfish	300–648	139	131	3.6	9.5	13.5	4.1		Bentick-Smith et al., 1987
		137	97	2.1	16.2	9.2		0.4	Warner and Williams, 1977
Isher catfish	25	153	145	3.4		0.9	0.2		Kori-Siakpere, 1985

dramatic changes in leukocytes characterized by a 47% loss of circulating leukocytes, with the lymphocytes being the principal cells involved. A heterophilia accompanies the leukocytopenia and lymphopenia. These changes are not observed in fish bled at 0 and 18 hours but not transported. Immune function in transported fish has been measured by testing mitogen responsiveness. The immune system of transported fish shuts down, and B and T cells remaining in the circulation are incapable of responding to antigenic stimulation. At least 2 weeks are required for acclimation of fish following transport. Channel catfish with more than 4% circulating heterophils should be excluded from experiments (Ellsaesser and Clem, 1986).

Restraint

Catfishes can be restrained manually or chemically or can be temporarily stunned by a blow to the head. It is very difficult to manually restrain fish larger than 1 to 2 kg. Some type of anesthetic should always be provided if fish are to be bled by cardiac puncture or by severing the caudal peduncle. Manual restraint may be considered a form of acute stress, so hematologic changes might be similar to those mentioned under handling. However, fish bled at 18-hour intervals and not transported do not exhibit the stress response observed in fish transported for 15 minutes (Ellsaesser and Clem, 1986).

The effects of three different restraint methods on erythrocyte, leukocyte, and thrombocyte counts in the crussian carp and rainbow trout have been studied (Hoffmann et al., 1982). The methods tested include tricaine methane sulfonate (MS-222, 0.007% solution), trichlor-butanol (0.09% solution), and a blow to the head. In all cases, leukocyte count was less affected by restraint procedures than red cell or thrombocyte counts. Anesthesia with tricaine methane sulfonate has the least effect on peripheral blood cell counts (Hoffmann et al., 1982).

The percent methemoglobin in channel catfish anesthetized with 40 mg/L tricaine methane sulfonate increases in the absence of environmental nitrite (Huey and Beitinger, 1982). An artificial increase in hematocrit occurs in stored blood samples from rainbow trout anesthetized using tricaine methane sulfonate (Korcock et al., 1988). Channel catfish sedated with 3 mg/L etomidate and restrained for 10 minutes in a net have decreased plasma cortisol levels compared to unanesthetized controls, and plasma glucose does not increase, although hyperchloremia is observed (Limsuwan et al., 1983). The mild decrease in cortisol levels is not dramatic, but is still detectable 23 days after the anesthesia (Brown et al., 1986). Increases in serum cortisol are seen with handling and blood sample collection in unanesthetized channel catfish and those treated with flunixin meglumide (Brown et al., 1986). The increase peaks after 30 minutes and decreases to near baseline levels during the next 24 hours. Little change from baseline cortisol

values is observed in fish anesthetized with tricaine methane sulfonate.

Feeding

Fasting channel catfish for 24 hours prior to blood sample collection has no effect on serum chemistry enzyme values (Bentick-Smith et al., 1987). Fasting fish does, however, minimize lipemia, which can affect some serum chemistry parameters (Bentick-Smith et al., 1987).

Stocking Density

There is no consistent effect of stocking density on serum chemistry parameters (Bentick-Smith et al., 1987). However, increased serum cortisol concentrations often correlate with increased stocking densities (Ainsworth et al., 1985).

Seasonal Changes

No seasonal variation in red blood cell count, hematocrit, or differential white blood cell count is observed in channel catfish sampled from production ponds during summer and winter months (Ellsaesser et al., 1985). Seasonal decreases in plasma potassium and plasma glucose occur during fall and winter months in pond-reared channel catfish (Bentick-Smith et al., 1987). A seasonal increase in serum cortisol has been observed September through December in channel catfish from commercial production ponds (Ainsworth et al., 1985).

RESPONSE TO INFECTIOUS DISEASES

Clinical pathologic responses to infectious diseases have not been well studied. Effects of viral and fungal diseases on blood or serum parameters have not been reported in catfishes.

Bacterial Diseases

Channel catfish experimentally infected with *Edwardsiella ictaluri* develop a moderate normocytic normochromic anemia (hematocrit 19.53 ± 1.90%) after 96 hours compared to 25.60 ± 1.60% in control fish (Areechon and Plumb, 1983). Infected fish also develop a moderate leukopenia (WBC 85.8 ± 4.32 x 10^3 cells/mm^3 after 96 hours compared to 123.0 ± 4.30 x 10^3 cells/mm^3 in control fish). Decreases in total protein, plasma glucose (Areechon and Plumb, 1983), and corticosteroid (Cooper et al., 1984) are reported in channel catfish experimentally infected with *Edwardsiella ictaluri*.

A marked increase in circulating heterophils and a concurrent marked decrease in circulating lymphocytes occurs in channel catfish infected with *Aeromonas* sp. and *Flexibacter columnaris* (Ellsaesser et al., 1985). Inflammatory cells invade peripheral tissues following infection of channel catfish with *Flexibacter columnaris* and *Corynebacterium* sp. (Marks et al., 1980). Small lymphocytes and mononuclear cells are observed in the affected area 12 hours postinfection, and within 72 hours, almost all bacteria are phagocytized by mononuclear cells.

Parasitic Diseases

Little information is available on hematologic or serum chemistry changes occurring in catfishes infected with parasitic diseases. Circulating heterophils increase and lymphocytes decrease in channel catfish infected with *Icthyopthirius multifiliis* (Ellsaesser et al., 1985). Hematocrit, hemoglobin, and total erythrocyte counts decrease and total leukocyte counts and erythrocyte sedimentation rates increase in stinging catfish parasitized by the digenetic trematodes (*Diplostomulum* sp.) (Murad and Mustafa, 1988).

RESPONSE TO NONINFECTIOUS DISEASES

Water Quality

Channel catfish exposed to hypoxic conditions for 10 minutes become acidotic and develop an increase in plasma osmolality and hematocrit (Kirk, 1974). Acidosis, evidenced by a decrease in blood pH and an increase in blood lactate, is transient and largely resolves within 12 hours. Transient increases in plasma sodium and potassium and decreases in chloride may be noted (Kirk, 1974).

The effect of environmental temperature on erythrocyte and leukocyte indices in channel catfish from laboratory aquaria and production ponds has been studied (Ellsaesser et al., 1985). No significant difference has been detected in packed cell volume, hemoglobin, total erythrocyte counts, or differential leukocyte counts attributable to environmental temperature.

Plasma cortisol and plasma glucose of channel catfish maintained at 10°C are higher than those of fish maintained at 20 or 30°C (Strange, 1980). Fish acclimated to 10°C for 4 weeks in one study had cortisol concentrations of 53 ± 6 ng/ml compared to 20 ± 4 ng/ml and 20 ± 5 ng/ml in fish housed at 20 and 30°C, respectively. Plasma glucose in catfish held at 10°C was 0.45 ± 0.06 mg/ml compared to 20 ± 0.05 mg/ml and 0.27 ± 0.04 mg/ml in fish acclimated to 20 and 30°C, respectively. The higher plasma glucose observed at 10°C is possibly a consequence of the apparent elevation in cortisol (Strange, 1980).

Channel catfish exposed to a total ammonia nitrogen of 2.5 mg/L at pH levels of 7 and 8, resulting in exposure to toxic un-ionized ammonia concentrations of 0.106 and 1.025 mg/L, do not show changes in blood pH, hematocrit, plasma protein, or plasma chloride (Tomasso et al., 1980). At higher un-ionized ammonia concentrations, plasma sodium is decreased (117.1 ± 5.8 mEq/L) compared to controls (147.2 ± 7.5 mEq/L). An increase in hematocrit of channel catfish correlates with exposure to lethal concentrations of un-ionized ammonia (Sheehan and Lewis, 1986). Because there is no change in plasma osmolality or red blood cell diameter, the increased hematocrit may be caused by isotonic dehydration, which could result in increased toxicity because of increased concentrations of ammonia in the blood.

Plasma corticosteroids increase in channel catfish exposed to ammonia (Tomasso et al., 1981). Plasma corticosteroid concentrations of 1.3 ± 0.1 µg/100 ml increase to more than 10 µg/100 ml, then begin to decline when catfish are exposed to 200 mg/L total ammonia nitrogen at pH 6.9 to 7.1 (Tomasso et al., 1981). Plasma corticosteroid concentrations are significantly greater in channel catfish exposed to ammonia at pH of 7.6 than at a pH of 7.0 (Tomasso et al., 1981).

Of the water-quality parameters routinely monitored in the production of channel catfish, nitrite has the most profound effect on hematology. Nitrite causes methemoglobinemia in catfish (Konikoff, 1975). Exposure to 5 mg/L nitrite results in 50% methemoglobinemia within 6 hours, 80% methemoglobinemia within 12 hours, and 90% methemoglobinemia within 24 hours (Huey et al., 1980). Channel catfish seem able to tolerate 90% methemoglobinemia for short periods until they are disturbed. Increased activity results in piping, erratic swimming, and rapid death (Huey et al., 1980). Methemoglobin levels return to normal levels within 24 hours when fish exposed to nitrites are placed in clean water (Huey et al., 1980). Methemoglobin levels in catfish that have not been exposed to nitrite can be as low as 2.2 ± 0.4% (Huey and Beittinger, 1982) and as high as 13% (Huey et al., 1980). Methemoglobin levels of 20.7 ± 1.9, 59.8 ± 1.9, and 77.4 ± 1.4 are reported in channel catfish exposed for 24 hours to 1.0, 2.5, and 5.0 mg/L NO_2, respectively (Tomasso et al., 1979).

The percent methemoglobin present in affected fish depends on the molar ratio of chloride to nitrite (Schwedler and Tucker, 1983). A molar ratio of 16 to 1 chloride to nitrite is sufficient to suppress methemoglin formation (Tomasso et al., 1979). Channel catfish exposed to 5 mg/L nitrite for 5 hours develop methemoglobinemia (42.5 ± 3.8%); however, the condition resolves within 24 hours if fish are moved to water containing 5 mg/L NO_2 plus 250 mg/L NaCl (Tomasso et al., 1979). A molar ratio of 3 to 1 chloride to nitrite is adequate to prevent acute mortalities caused by sudden elevations in nitrite (Bowser et al., 1983). Percent methemoglobin formation can also be decreased by feeding increased levels of dietary ascorbic acid (Wise et al., 1988). The percent methemoglobin is reported to be reduced in channel catfish infected with *E. ictaluri* (Tucker et al., 1984). It is postulated that disruptions in monovalent anion balance in diseased fish result in decreased plasma concentrations of nitrite, and consequently, decreased percent methemoglobin. The percent methemoglobin is reduced in fish exposed to nitrite and tricaine methane sulfonate compared to those exposed to nitrite alone (Huey and Beittinger, 1982), but fish exposed to tricaine methane sulfonate alone show higher methemoglobin percentages than control fish.

Chronic exposure to sublethal nitrite concentrations results in anemia (Tucker et al., 1989). Channel catfish exposed to 2.88 mg/L nitrite for 21 days develop a moderate anemia of 18% hematocrit. The anemia may result from decreased erythrocyte life span brought about by excessive energy drain on the cell by the methemoglobin reductase system. The effects of methemoglobinemia and anemia were additive and result in a marked decrease in functional hemoglobin.

Exposure to 5 mg/L nitrite results in a continuous rise in plasma corticosteroids over 24 hours (Tomasso et al., 1981). Significant increases in plasma corticosteroids are not observed in channel catfish concurrently exposed to 5 mg/L and 303 mg/L chloride.

Nutrition

There is no difference in hematocrit or erythrocyte fragility when fingerling or adult catfishes are fed diets with different levels of vitamin E (36 mg/kg; 66 mg/kg; 72 mg/kg or 144 mg/kg) (Jarboe et al., 1989).

A diet-related anemia has been reported in pond-reared channel catfish in the southeastern United States. Twenty-nine field cases are reported in which hematocrits of moribund catfish were 0 to 5% (Klar et al., 1986). Fish in 27 of the affected ponds recovered following a change in feed to a different brand. Fish in the remaining two ponds responded to the change in feed after treatment for an infectious disease that was confounding recovery. Moderate anemia was produced in channel catfish fry by feeding suspect rations for 69 days under laboratory conditions. Following a change in feed the fry recovered and hematocrits returned to normal ranges (28.8 ± 3.7%) after 90 days. Attempts to reproduce the condition in larger fish have not been successful.

Pesticides

The effects of pesticides on various hematologic parameters in catfishes are not well known. Red blood cell count was reduced by half in albino *Clarias* sp. exposed to carbon tetrachloride (Sharma and Gupta, 1982). Affected fish also exhibited a reduction in hemoglobin content disproportional to the loss of cells. Total white cell count in these fish was not significantly altered. Lymphocytes were markedly increased in the differential white blood cell count with an apparent decrease in eosinophils and heterophils.

Plasma T_4 decreases in stinging catfish following exposure to malathion (Yadav and Singh, 1986). Concurrently the T_3/T_4 ratio is elevated.

Concentrations of specific chemicals in serum of sick fish can aid in the diagnosis of toxicosis. Evaluated serum concentrations of endrin, toxaphene, and DDT can be detected in moribund channel catfish and brown bullhead catfish following pesticide-induced fish kills. Pesticide concentrations in the serum of control animals range from nondetectable to 0.02 µg/g endrin, nondetectable to 0.10 µg/g toxaphene, and up to 0.10 µg/g DDT (Plumb and Richburg, 1977). Endrin concentrations in moribund channel catfish average 0.29 µg/g with a high value of 1.80 µg/g. Moribund brown bullhead catfish have had serum endrin concentrations of 2.4 µg/g. Toxaphene concentrations in moribund channel catfish average 1.71 µg/g. Serum DDT levels averaging 0.10 µg/g have been detected in moribund channel catfish. Higher concentrations of DDT have been observed in brown bullhead serum (0.53 µg/g) (Plumb and Richburg, 1977). Residual-fat soluble pesticides, particularly endrin, may be released as fat reserves are mobilized during winter months when feeding activity is reduced (Plumb and Richburg, 1977). In the spring, feeding activity increases and serum concentrations of pesticides decrease.

LITERATURE CITED

Ainsworth, A.J., Bowser, P.R., and Beleau, M.H. (1985) Serum cortisol levels in channel catfish from production ponds. Progressive Fish Culturist 47:176–181.

Areechon, N., and Plumb, J.A. (1983) Pathogenesis of *Edwardsiella ictaluri* in channel catfish, *Ictalurus punctatus*. J. World Mariculture Soc. 14:249–260.

Bentick-Smith, J., Beleau, M.H., Waterstrat, P.R., Tucker, C.S., Stiles, F., Bowser, P.R., and Brown, L.A. (1987) Biochemical reference ranges for commercially reared channel catfish. Progressive Fish Culturist 49:108–114.

Black, E.C. (1955) Blood levels of hemoglobin and lactic acid in some freshwater fishes following exercise. J. Fish Res. Bd. Can. 12(6):917–929.

Bowser, P.R., and Munson, A.D. (1986) Seasonal variation in channel catfish virus antibody titers in adult channel catfish. Progressive Fish Culturist 48:198–199.

Bowser, P.R., Falls, W.W., Van Zandt, J., Collier, N., and Phillips, J.D. (1983) Methemoglobinemia in channel catfish: Methods of prevention. Progressive Fish Culturist 45:154–158.

Brader, J.D., Freeze, T.M., and Goetz, F.W. (1982) Hematological values of blue and channel catfish from two Kentucky lakes. Trans. Ky. Acad. Sci. 43(1–2):4–9.

Breazile, J.E., Zinn, L.L., Yauk, J.C., Mass, H.J., and Wollscheid, J. (1982) A study of haematological profiles of channel catfish, *Ictalurus punctatus* (Rafinesque). J. Fish Biol. 21:305–309.

Brown, L.A., Ainsworth, A.J., Beleau, M.H., Bentick-Smith, J., Francis-Floyd, R., Waterstrat, P.R., and Freund, J. (1986) The effects of tricaine methanesulphonate, flunixin meglumide and metomidate on serum cortisol in channel catfish (*Ictalurus punctatus* Rafinesque). Proc. Int. Assoc. Aquatic Anim. Med. 1(3):33–38.

Campbell, T.W., and Murru, F. (1990) An introduction to fish hematology. Compend. Contin. Educ. Pract. Vet. 12(4):525–532.

Cooper, J.L., David, S.N., and Beadles, J.K. (1984) The effect of *Edwardsiella ictaluri* infection on plasma corticosterone in channel catfish (*Ictalurus punctatus*). Ak. Acad. Sci. 38:33–36.

Ellsaesser, C., and Clem, L.W. (1986) Hematological and immunological changes in channel catfish stressed by handling and transport. J. Fish. Biol. 28:511–521.

Ellsaesser, C., Miller, N., Lobb, C.J., and and Clem, L.W. (1984) A new method for the cytochemical staining of cells immobilized in agarose. Histochemistry 80:559–562.

Ellsaesser, C.F., Miller, N.W., Cuchens, M.A., Lobb, C.J., Clem, L.W. (1985) Analysis of channel catfish peripheral blood leucocytes by brightfield microscopy and flow cytometry. Trans. Am. Fish. Soc. 114:279–285.

Ellis, A.E. (1977) The leukocytes of fish: a review. J. Fish. Biol. 11:453–491.

Finco-Kent, D., and Thune, R.L. (1987) Phagocytosis by catfish neutrophils. J. Fish Biol. 31:41–49.

Grizzle, J.M., and Rogers, W.A. (1976) Anatomy and Histology of the Channel Catfish. Auburn University Agricultural Experiment Station, Alabama, pp. 15–18.

Hattingh, J. (1972) Observations on the blood physiology of five South African freshwater fish. J. Fish Biol. 4:555–563.

Hawes, T. (1959) Some Aspects of the Hematology of Two Species of Catfish in Relation to Their Habitat. Ph.D. Dissertation, Purdue University, Card #59–1661. University Microfilms Inc., Ann Arbor, Michigan.

Hoffmann, R., Lommel, R., and Reidel, M. (1982) Influence of different anesthetics and bleeding methods on hematological values in fish. Arch. Fisch. Wiss. 33:91–103.

Huey, D.W., and Beittinger, T.L. (1982) Methemoglobin levels in channel catfish, Ictalurus punctatus, exposed to nitrite and tricaine methanesulfonate. Can. J. Fisheries Aquat. Sci. 39(4):643–645.

Huey, D.W., Simco, B.A., and Criswell, D.W. (1980) Nitrite-induced methemoglobin formation in channel catfish. Trans. Am. Fish. Soc. 109:558–562.

Jarboe, H.H., Robinette, H.R., and Bowser, P.R. (1989) Effect of selected vitamin E supplementations of channel catfish production feeds. Progressive Fish Culturist 51:91–94.

Kirk, W.L. (1974) The effects of hypoxia on certain blood and tissue electrolytes of channel catfish, Ictalurus punctatus (Rafinesque). Tran. Am. Fish. Soc. 103:593–600.

Klar, G.T., Hanson, L.A., and Brown, S.W. (1986) Diet-related anemia in channel catfish: case history and laboratory induction. Progressive Fish Culturist 48:60–64.

Konikoff, M. (1975) Toxicity of nitrite to channel catfish. Progressive Fish Culturist 37:96–98.

Korcock, D.E., Houston, A.H., and Gray, J.D. (1988) Effects of sampling conditions on selected blood variables of rainbow trout, Salmo gairdneri Richardson. J. Fish Biol. 33:319–330.

Kori-Siakpere, O. (1985) Haematological characteristics of Clarias isheriensis Sydenham. J. Fish Biol. 27:259–263.

Larsen, H.N. (1964) Comparison of various methods of hemoglobin determination on catfish blood. Progressive Fish Culturist 26(1):11–15.

Limsuwan, C., Limsuwan, J., Grizzle, J.M., and Plumb, J.A. (1983) Stress response and blood characteristics of channel catfish (Ictalurus punctatus) after anesthesia with etomidate. Can. J. Fish Aquatic Sci. 40:2105–2112.

Marks, J.E., Lewis, D.H., and Trevino, G.S. (1980) Mixed infection in columnaris disease of fish. J. Am. Vet. Med. Assoc. 177(9):811–814.

Murad, A., and Mustafa, S. (1988) Blood parameters of catfish, Heteropneustes fossilis (bloch), parasitized by metacercariae of Diplostomulum sp. J. Fish Dis. 11:365–368.

Natarajan, G.M. (1981) Some blood parameters in two air-breathing fishes of South India. Comp. Physiol. Ecol. 6(3):133–135.

Plumb, J.A., and Richburg, R.W. (1977) Pesticide levels in sera of moribund channel catfish from a continuous winter mortality. Trans. Am. Fish Soc. 106:185–188.

Railo, E., Nakinmaa, M., and Soivio, A. (1985) Effect of sampling on blood parameters in rainbow trout (Salmo gairdneri Richardson). J. Fish Biol. 26:725–732.

Rogers, W.A. (1981) Serological detection of two species of Edwardsiella infecting catfish. International Symposium on Fish Biologics: Serodiagnostics and Vaccines. Dev. Biol. Stand. 49:169–172.

Schwedler, T.E., and Tucker, C.S. (1983) Empirical relationship between percent methemoglobin in channel catfish and dissolved nitrite and chloride in ponds. Trans. Am. Fish. Soc. 112:117–119.

Sharma, R.C., and Gupta, N. (1982) Carbon tetrachloride induced hematological alterations in Clarias batrachus L. J. Environ. Biol. 3(3):127–131.

Sharma, R.K., and Shandilya, S. (1982) Observations on the haematological values of some fresh water teleosts. Comp. Physiol. Ecol. 7(2):124–126.

Sheehan, R.J., and Lewis, W.M. (1986) Influences of pH and ammonia salts on ammonia toxicity and water balance in young channel catfish. Trans. Am. Fish. Soc. 115:891–899.

Smith, C.G., Lewis, W.M., and Kaplan, H.M. (1952) Comparative morphologic and physiologic study of fish blood. Progressive Fish Culturist 14(4):169–172.

Strange, R.J. (1980) Acclimation temperature influences cortisol and glucose concentrations in stressed channel catfish. Trans. Am. Fish. Soc. 109:298–303.

Tomasso, J.R., Simco, B.A., and Davis, K.B. (1979) Chloride inhibition of nitrite-induced methemoglobinemia in channel catfish (Ictalurus punctatus). J. Fish. Res. Bd. Can. 36:1141–1144.

Tomasso, J.R., Goudie, C.A., Simco, B.A., and Davis, K.B. (1980) Effects of environmental pH and calcium on ammonia toxicity in channel catfish. Trans. Am. Fish. Soc. 109:229–234.

Tomasso, J.R., Davis, K.B., and Simco, B.A. (1981) Plasma corticosteroid dynamics in channel catfish (Ictalurus punctatus) exposed to ammonia and nitrite. Can. J. Fish Aquatic Sci. 38:1106–1112.

Tucker, C.S., and Schwedler, T.E. (1983) Acclimation of channel catfish (Ictalurus punctatus) to nitrite. Bull. Environ. Contam. Toxicol. 30:516–521.

Tucker, C.S., MacMillan, J.R., and Schwedler, T.E. (1984) Influence of Edwardsiella ictaluri septicemia on nitrite-induced methemoglobinemia in channel catfish (Ictalurus punctatus). Bull. Environ. Contam. Toxicol. 32:669–673.

Tucker, C.S., Francis-Floyd, R., and Beleau, M.H. (1989) Nitrite-induced anemia in channel catfish, Ictalurus punctatus Rafinesque. Bull. Environ. Contam. Toxicol. 43:295–301.

Warner, M.C., and Williams, R.W. (1977) Comparison between serum values of pond and intensive raceway cultured channel catfish, Ictalurus punctatus. J. Fish Biol. 11:385–395.

Waterstrat, P.R., Ainsworth, A.J., and Capley, G. (1988) Use of a discontinuous Percoll gradient technique for the separation of channel catfish, Ictalurus punctatus (Rafinesque), peripheral blood leukocytes. J. Fish Dis. 11:289–294.

Williams, R.W., and Warner, M.C. (1976) Some observations on the stained blood cellular elements of channel catfish, Ictalurus punctatus. J. Fish Biol. 9:491–497.

Wise, D.J., Tomasso, J.R., and Brandt, T.M. (1988) Ascorbic acid inhibition of nitrite-induced methemoglobinemia in channel catfish. Progressive Fish Culturist 50:77–80.

Yadav, A.K., and Singh, T.P. (1986) Effect of pesticide on circulating thyroid hormone levels in the freshwater catfish, Heteropneustes fossilis (Bloch). Environ. Res. 39(1):136–142.

Yuki, R. (1960) Blood cell constituents in fish IV on "the nuclear shadow" found on blood smear preparations. Bull. Jpn. Soc. Sci. Fish 26:490–495.

Chapter 56

Environmental Diseases of Catfishes

RUTH FRANCIS-FLOYD

Environmental conditions can be a direct cause of fish mortality or can contribute to mortality by predisposing fish to opportunistic infections. Water quality is discussed in detail in Chapter 13. This chapter specifically addresses environmental conditions that contribute to disease and mortality of channel catfish. Information presented here has been limited to naturally occurring compounds. The clinical significance of the pond environment for channel catfish is reviewed extensively in the literature (Noga and Francis-Floyd, 1991; Boyd, 1979; Tucker, 1985).

OXYGEN

In pond culture, photosynthesis by algae is the most important source of oxygen (Boyd, 1973). Other sources of dissolved oxygen include agitation, caused by wind and wave action, and least significant, direct diffusion of atmospheric oxygen into the pond. The need for supplemental or emergency aeration is closely related to stocking density and feeding rate (Cole and Boyd, 1986). Supplemental aeration should be available if fish are stocked at densities greater than 2500 to 3000 kg/hectare (Tucker and Boyd, 1978).

Commercial production units often hire personnel specifically for oxygen management. During warm weather, dissolved oxygen concentrations are monitored in each pond throughout the night and during the day as needed. Oxygen meters, aeration equipment, and trained personnel are readily available. In contrast, recreational pond owners are often poorly informed about oxygen management and aeration techniques. These individuals may invest in equipment that is not designed for emergency aeration, or they may design and build their own system. Some home-built systems are quite functional, others are not. Misconceptions about aeration and pond management are often confounded by improper stocking and excessive crowding (Boyd, 1979; Tucker, 1985).

Low levels of dissolved oxygen can be a direct cause of mortality or can contribute to outbreaks of infectious disease. In general, the minimum acceptable concentration of dissolved oxygen for channel catfish is 5 mg/L (Tucker, 1985). Catfish can tolerate lower concentrations of dissolved oxygen as long as

the period of exposure is not excessive. Physiologic effects of hypoxia have been reviewed (Schwedler et al., 1985). Dissolved oxygen concentrations less than 1.0 mg/L are lethal if exposure is prolonged (Tucker, 1985). Sublethal exposure to hypoxia can contribute to secondary bacterial infections (Snieszko, 1974; Plumb et al., 1976). Also sterile, necrotic lesions in the musculature of channel catfish following oxygen depletion have been reported (Plumb et al., 1976). Such lesions may contribute to carcass condemnation.

Excessive concentrations of dissolved oxygen can also cause catfish mortality. The etiology and physiology of gas bubble disease has been well studied (Weitkamp and Katz, 1980; Bouck, 1980; and Schwedler et al., 1985). Fish affected may exhibit exophthalmia and distension of the abdomen (Weitkamp and Katz, 1980; Bowser et al., 1983a; Schwedler et al., 1985), and gas bubbles may be observed within the capillaries of fresh gill biopsies. Confirmation of the diagnosis requires determination of the total gas pressure of the water (Weitkamp and Katz, 1980; Schwedler et al., 1985). To correct clinical disease, aerate the water to release excess gases to the atmosphere.

TEMPERATURE

Channel catfish are eurythermic animals capable of tolerating a wide range of temperatures. Commercial production ponds may ice over in the winter, and water temperatures can reach 35°C in the summer. Although catfish may be able to survive exposure to these temperature extremes, their optimal environmental temperature is closer to 28 to 30°C.

Temperature changes dramatically influence the immune system of poikilotherms (Finn and Nielson, 1971; Avtalion et al., 1973). Low (15.4°C) and fluctuating (15.4 to 26.9°C in 24 hours) water temperatures have a detrimental effect on the immune response of channel catfish (Collins et al., 1976). A temperature decrease from 27 to 22°C temporarily eliminated the ability of channel catfish T cells to respond to mitogenic stimulation and greatly slowed the response of B cells (Clem et al., 1984). Many infectious diseases of channel catfish are seasonal,

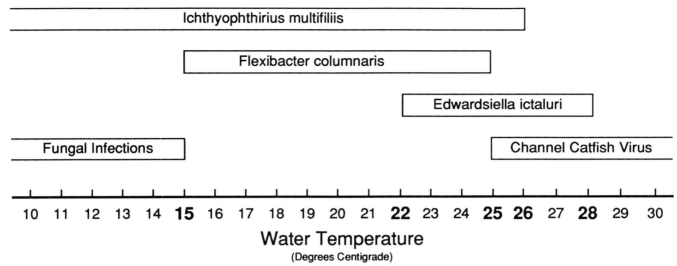

FIGURE 56–1. Temperature-dependent diseases of catfishes. Several infectious diseases of catfishes have been associated with specific water temperatures.

occurring primarily in the spring and the fall (Meyer, 1970; MacMillan, 1985). This predilection to disease during periods of environmental transition (i.e., summer to winter) may be attributed, in part, to the adverse effect of fluctuating water temperature on the immune system.

Three important diseases of channel catfish are temperature dependent (Fig. 56–1). Heavy mortality from the bacterial disease enteric septicemia of catfish, caused by *Edwardsiella ictaluri,* usually occurs in the temperature range 22 to 28°C (Francis-Floyd et al., 1987). Mortality from channel catfish virus disease is most severe at water temperatures of 25°C or greater (Plumb, 1973; Wolf, 1988). The parasitic disease caused by *Ichthyophthirius multifiliis* is usually a problem at water temperatures below 26°C. Treatment of *Ichthyophthirius multifiliis* infection is closely correlated with water temperature. At cooler temperatures, the life cycle is prolonged and treatment intervals must be extended (Post, 1987).

A few other diseases have a predilection for certain temperature ranges. For example, *Flexibacter columnaris,* the bacterial agent that causes "saddle-back disease," is most likely to cause disease at water temperatures in the range of 15 to 25°C (MacMillan, 1985). External fungal diseases are more prevalent at temperatures less than 15°C (MacMillan, 1985).

Another disease that may be temperature related is "winter mortality syndrome," a poorly understood phenomenon observed during the winter months in commercial catfish ponds. Affected fish exhibit endophthalmia, depigmentation, and loss of mucus. Secondary infections with bacteria and external fungi are common (MacMillan, 1985). The disease is managed by decreasing stocking densities in late fall to decrease carrying capacities during the winter. Catfish are also fed when they will eat in an effort to improve the nutritional plane during the winter.

Sudden temperature changes or thermal shock can be fatal. When fish are handled, it is important to "temper" them when moving from one container to another. Water temperature differences greater than 3°C should be avoided (Schwedler et al., 1985). Water temperatures should be adjusted slowly; 1°C per 2 minutes is an acceptable rate of temperature change when tempering catfish (Schwedler et al., 1985).

CARBON DIOXIDE AND pH

Diurnal fluctuations in carbon dioxide and pH are interrelated and can be dramatic during any given 24-hour period. At dawn, carbon dioxide is high and pH is low. Carbon dioxide is usually not a cause of clinical problems per se; however, high concentrations of carbon dioxide can exacerbate hypoxia caused by low concentrations of dissolved oxygen, both of which are common in the early morning hours (Tucker, 1985; Schwedler et al., 1985).

pH is dynamic and changes from hour to hour in a catfish pond. Low pH occurs in the morning when carbon dioxide concentrations are highest, and high pH occurs late in the afternoon when the carbon dioxide concentrations are lowest (Tucker, 1985) (Fig. 56–2). The magnitude of change depends on several factors, including phytoplankton blooms and the buffering capacity of the water. Channel catfish are able to survive exposure to pH extremes as low as 4 and as high as 10 (Swingle, 1961; Tucker, 1985). For optimum health, however, pH should remain in the range of 6.5 to 9.0 (Swingle, 1961; Tucker, 1985). A diurnal pH fluctuation within this range is common within catfish ponds and is acceptable for rearing fish.

Excessively low pH can be caused by acidic soils and low alkalinity. Liming the pond with agricultural limestone ($CaCO_3$) is often beneficial. An alkalinity

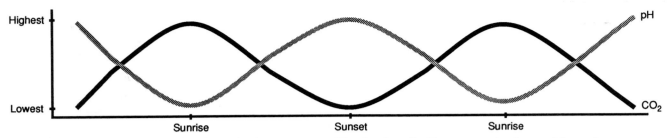

FIGURE 56–2. The relationship between water pH and carbon dioxide concentration in a catfish pond.

of 100 mg/L to 200 mg/L is ideal. Excessively high pH can be caused by very dense algal blooms or by improper application of hydrated lime ($Ca[OH]_2$, or quick lime) to a pond. Hydrated lime is a sterilant that should never be placed in a pond containing live fish. It rapidly drives the pH up to around 11 and will kill everything in the pond. Unfortunately, recreational pond owners occasionally misunderstand the term "lime the pond" and use the more accessible hydrated lime with devastating results. If hydrated lime is used improperly in a catfish pond, the pond should not be restocked until the pH returns to an acceptable level.

The most clinically significant aspect of pH may be its effect on ammonia toxicity (Tucker, 1985). The equilibrium between ionic ammonium (NH_4^+) and ammonia (NH_3) favors the toxic un-ionized fraction (NH_3) at high pH. Therefore, if ammonia-nitrogen is present in a pond, it will be most toxic late in the afternoon when pH is highest. Fish dying from ammonia toxicity often do not show behavioral signs of stress until late in the day.

AMMONIA

Ammonia is the principal nitrogen waste product produced by catfishes. Ammonia excretion occurs across the gill membrane (Schwedler et al., 1985). Excessive concentrations of ammonia can cause acute mortality or contribute to chronic disease caused by opportunistic pathogens in the environment (Walters and Plumb, 1980).

High levels of ammonia are frequently associated with high stocking densities (Tucker et al., 1979; Tucker et al., 1984a). Growth rate, stocking density, and feeding rate are all closely related. The objectives of the pond owner should be carefully considered before making recommendations concerning stocking. The recreational pond owner will not want to be bothered with intensive pond management. Under these conditions, a low stocking density (1853 to 2470 fish per hectare), and a maximum feeding rate of 34 kg of feed per hectare per day is suggested (Busch, 1985). Commercial producers are usually prepared to manage ponds intensively and consequently stock (and feed) at much higher rates. Feeding rates of 90 to 112 kg/hectare/day are not unusual in the catfish production ponds of Mississippi (Busch,

1985). An average feeding rate of 75 kg of feed per hectare per day results in a daily increase in total ammonia nitrogen of about 0.25 mg/L/day (Tucker, 1985). Most nitrogen is eliminated from the aquatic environment by volatilization (Weiler, 1979) or is utilized by phytoplankton (Tucker et al., 1984a). A minor accumulation of nitrogen may occur in heavily stocked ponds resulting in higher total ammonia nitrogen levels during late summer and early fall (Tucker et al., 1979).

Toxic ammonia levels will be noticed late in the afternoon when pH is highest. Fish can be observed skittering on the surface and dying if toxic un-ionized ammonia (NH_3) concentrations approach 2 mg/L (Noga and Francis-Floyd, 1991). There is no easy practical remedy for an ammonia crisis in a catfish pond. Water exchange rates available for commercial catfish ponds are usually insufficient to improve water quality, although flushing a pond can provide a localized haven during an ammonia crisis (McGee and Boyd, 1983). Prevention of ammonia accumulation in heavily stocked catfish ponds may not be possible, but measuring total ammonia nitrogen every 10 to 14 days should alert the manager to an impending problem before fish actually begin to die. An observed increase should stimulate a review of managerial practices, including daily feeding rates. Fish should not be fed more than they will eat, and if the problem is severe, food should be withheld for a few days. Fish will not eat when highly stressed by an accumulation of ammonia. As the problem is resolved, the fish should be closely observed for 1 to 2 weeks as they may contract an opportunistic bacterial infection (Walters and Plumb, 1980; Tucker et al., 1984a).

NITRITE

Nitrite is formed by the oxidation of ammonia by nitrifying bacteria (*Nitrosomonas* sp.). In channel catfish, nitrite can function as an acute toxin causing direct mortality from methemoglobin formation (Lewis and Morris, 1986; Konikoff, 1975; Tucker and Schwedler, 1983a) or can contribute to anemia following chronic exposure (Tucker et al., 1988). Sublethal nitrite exposure can contribute to outbreaks of bacterial disease (Hanson and Grizzle, 1985) and, conversely, active bacterial disease may affect the response of the fish to the environmental disease (Tucker et al., 1984b). Catfish exposed to nitrite under laboratory conditions are less tolerant of high water temperatures (Watenpaugh et al., 1985).

The clinical significance of nitrite concentrations in catfish ponds is closely correlated with chloride concentrations (Schwedler and Tucker, 1983). Chloride is believed to minimize methemoglobin formation in catfish exposed to nitrite by competing with nitrite ion transport across the gill membrane (Tomasso et al., 1979). A chloride to nitrite ratio (wt:wt) of 3:1 protects catfish from acute mortality caused by methemoglobinemia due to nitrite exposure (Bowser et al., 1983b). This ratio may not, however, protect naive fish from lethal methemoglobin formation following acute exposure to high levels of nitrite (Tucker and Schwedler, 1983b). More recent work suggests that a chloride to nitrite ratio of 5:1 is preferable because it prevents anemia as a sequela to sublethal nitrite exposure (Tucker et al., 1988).

The amount of chloride needed to protect fish can be calculated with the following formula:

$$\text{Chloride Needed (mg/L)} = (5 \times [NO_2]) - [Cl^-]$$

where $[NO_2]$ is the concentration of nitrite (mg/L) and $[Cl^-]$ is the concentration of chloride (mg/L). Both can be measured with a water-quality testing kit. Once the concentration of chloride needed (CLN) is known, the amount of salt to be added can be calculated if the pond volume (PV) is known.

$$\text{Salt Needed (lb)} = \text{PV (Acre Ft.)} \times 4.54 \text{ CLN (mg/L)}$$

Addition of salt to a pond containing catfish dying of methemoglobinemia results in almost immediate correction of the problem, and fish should begin to feed within 24 hours. It is always a good practice to correct methemoglobinemia before treating infectious diseases, which may be present concurrently.

Increased concentrations of dietary ascorbic acid prior to nitrite exposure result in decreased methemoglobin formation (Wise et al., 1988). The protection provided by ascorbic acid, however, is less than that provided by increased water chloride concentrations.

ALKALINITY AND HARDNESS

Total alkalinity and total hardness are closely related. Both are measured as milligrams per liter $CaCO_3$. Total water hardness can be considered less specific than total alkalinity.

The principal clinical significance of alkalinity relates to its effect on copper toxicity. Copper sulfate is approved for use as an algicide in channel catfish ponds (Schnick et al., 1986). It also is an effective chemical for control of protozoan infections. The principal disadvantage of copper sulfate is the toxicity of the cupric ion (Cu^{2+}) (Cardeilhac and Whitaker, 1988). The cupric ion combines with CO_3^{2-}, and in water of moderate alkalinity (100 to 250 mg $CaCO_3$/L), the resultant salt allows safe use of $CuSO_4$. In water with very low alkalinity (less than 50 mg $CaCO_3$/L), there is insufficient carbonate present to adequately protect fish from the toxic cupric ion. In water with high alkalinity (more than 250 mg $CaCO_3$/L), the copper ion is tied up as an insoluble salt ($CuCO_3$) and precipitates out of solution, thereby preventing any therapeutic effect.

Total water hardness can impact survivability of catfish fry in hatcheries. Impaired growth and survival of catfish fry reared in water with total hardness less than 5 mg/L has been observed (Tucker, 1987). Calcium chloride can be used to increase calcium content in hatchery water. A minimum total hardness of 10 mg/L is recommended (Tucker, 1987).

HYDROGEN SULFIDE

Hydrogen sulfide can be quite toxic to catfish and is commonly formed during anaerobic processes in the hypolimnion of fish ponds. Despite its common occurrence in benthic aquatic environments, it is rarely a cause of fish kills because it is rapidly oxidized in the presence of oxygen (Schwedler et al., 1985). Accumulations of hydrogen sulfide in catfish ponds can be prevented by avoiding pond stratification. Excess hydrogen sulfide can be removed from a pond by aeration or by the addition of potassium permanganate (Schwedler et al., 1985).

ALGAL TOXINS

Phytoplankton blooms are natural events in catfish ponds that have a tremendous influence on water quality. During late summer, blue-green species are often predominant (Tucker et al., 1984a). Some species of blue-green algae have been associated with fish kills under natural and experimental conditions (Phillips et al., 1985). Decomposition of heavy algal blooms can cause very low levels of dissolved oxygen; however, toxic principles produced by certain species of blue-green algae may also contribute to fish mortality. Blue-green algae, particularly members of the genera *Microcystis* and *Anabaena*, are known to produce toxins under certain poorly understood environmental conditions. The frequency and significance of toxin production in catfish ponds is unknown. A case in which large amounts of *Microcystis* sp. were found in the gut of channel catfish fingerlings showing signs of neurotoxicity and limited mortality has been reported (Schwedler et al., 1985). The author has been involved in two cases of acute mortality of channel catfish where the involvement of algal toxins was suspected but never proved. The potential role of these toxins in catfish culture is poorly understood and deserving of further study.

OFF-FLAVOR

Off-flavor is not a pathologic condition but an esthetic and economic one. Affected fish develop various unacceptable flavors or odors, which are detected during cooking. This condition makes the fish nonsaleable. In commercial processing plants, fish are routinely checked for flavor for several weeks prior to harvest, as well as immediately prior to being unloaded at the plant. Those which are unacceptable are rejected. Off-flavor is frequently caused by natural processes. For example, certain species of blue-green algae and Actinomycete bacteria are known to produce compounds that are absorbed by catfish and which contribute to off-flavor (Lovell and Sackey, 1973; Armstrong et al., 1986). In many cases, fish will spontaneously lose the objectionable flavor characteristics within 3 to 6 weeks. Occasionally, however, a pond of fish may remain off-flavor and, therefore, nonsaleable, for prolonged periods of time (i.e., longer than 12 to 18 months). This creates a major liability for the producer, and a considerable research effort is currently being directed at solving this problem.

LITERATURE CITED

Armstrong, M.S., Boyd, C.E., and Lovell, R.T. (1986) Environmental factors affecting flavor of channel catfish from production ponds. Progressive Fish Culturist 48:113–119.

Avtalion, R.R., Wojdani, A., Malik, Z., Shahrabani, R., and Duczyminer, M. (1973) Influence of environmental temperature on the immune response in fish. Current topics. In: Microbiology and Immunology (Aber, W. and Haas, R., eds.). Springer-Verlag, Berlin, pp 1–35.

Bouck, G.R. (1980) Etiology of gas-bubble disease. Trans. Am. Fish. Soc. 109:703–707.

Bowser, P.R., Toal, R., Robinette, H.R., and Brunson, M.W. (1983a) Coelomic distention in channel catfish fingerlings. Progressive Fish Culturist 45:208–209.

Bowser, P.R., Falls, W.W., VanZandt, J., Collier, N., and Phillips, J.D. (1983b) Methemoglobinemia in channel catfish: methods of prevention. Progressive Fish Culturist 45:154–158.

Boyd, C.E. (1973) Summer algal communities and primary productivity in fish ponds. Hydrobiologia 41:357–390.

Boyd, C.E. (1979) Water Quality in Warm Water Fish Ponds. Auburn University, Auburn.

Busch, R.L. (1985) Channel catfish culture in ponds. In: Channel Catfish Culture (Tucker, C. S., ed.). Elsevier, Amsterdam, pp. 13–84.

Cardeilhac, P.T., and Whitaker, B.R. (1988) Copper treatments: uses and precautions. In: Tropical Fish Medicine (Stoskopf, M.K., ed.). Vet. Clin. North Am., Small Anim. Pract. 18:435–448.

Clem, L.W., Faulmann, E., Miller, N.W., Ellsaesser, C., Lobb, C.J., and Cuchens, M.A. (1984) Temperature-mediated processes in teleost immunity: differential effects of in vitro and in vivo temperatures on mitogenic responses of channel catfish lymphocytes. Dev. Comp. Immunol. 8:313–322.

Cole, B.A., and Boyd, C.E. (1986) Feeding rate, water quality, and channel catfish production in ponds. Progressive Fish Culturist 48:25–29.

Collins, M.T., Dawe, D.C. and Gratzek, J.B. (1976) Immune response of channel catfish under different environmental conditions. J. Am. Vet. Med. Assoc. 169:991–994.

Finn, J.P., and Nielsen, N.O. (1971) The effect of temperature on the inflammatory response of rainbow trout. J. Pathol. 105:257–268.

Francis-Floyd, R., Beleau, M.H., Waterstrat, P.R., and Bowser, P.R. (1987) Effect of water temperature on the clinical outcome of infection with Edwardsiella ictaluri in channel catfish. J. Am. Vet. Med. Assoc. 191:1413–1416.

Hanson, L.A., and Grizzle, J.M. (1985) Nitrite-induced predisposition of channel catfish to bacterial diseases. Progressive Fish Culturist 47:98–101.

Konikoff, M. (1975) Toxicity of nitrite to channel catfish. Progressive Fish Culturist 37:96–98.

Lewis, W.M., and Morris, D.P. (1986) Toxicity of nitrite to fish: a review. Trans. Am. Fish. Soc. 115:183–195.

Lovell, R.T., and Sackey, L.A. (1973) Absorption by channel catfish of earth-musty flavor compounds synthesized by cultures of blue-green algae. Trans. Am. Fish. Soc. 102:774–777.

MacMillan, J.R. (1985) Infectious diseases. In: Channel Catfish Culture (Tucker, C.S., ed.). Elsevier, Amsterdam, pp. 405–496.

McGee, M.V., and Boyd, C.E. (1983) Evaluation of the influence of water exchange in channel catfish ponds. Trans. Am. Fish. Soc. 112:557–560.

Meyer, F.P. (1970) Seasonal fluctuations in the incidence of disease on fish farms. In: Diseases of Fish and Shellfish (Snieszko, S.F., ed.). American Fisheries Society, Special Publication No. 5, Washington, D.C., pp. 21–29.

Noga, E.J., and Francis-Floyd, R. (1991) Medical management of channel catfish. I: the environment. Compend. Contin. Ed. Pract. Vet. 13.

Phillips, M.J., Roberts, R.J., Stewart, J.A. and Codd, G.A. (1985) The toxicity of the cyanobacterium Microcystis aeruginosa to rainbow trout, Salmo gairdneri Richardson. J. Fish Dis. 8:339–344.

Plumb, J.A. (1973) Effects of temperature on mortality of fingerling channel catfish (Ictalurus punctatus) experimentally infected with channel catfish virus. J. Fish. Res. Bd. Can. 30:568–570.

Plumb, J.A., Grizzle, J.M., and de Figueiredo, J. (1976) Necrosis and bacterial infection in channel catfish (Ictalurus punctatus) following hypoxia. J. Wildlife Dis. 12:247–253.

Post, G.W. (1987) Textbook of Fish Health, 2nd ed. T.F.H. Publications, Neptune City, New Jersey, pp. 182–185.

Schnick, R.A., Meyer, F.P. and Walsh, D.F. (1986) Status of fishery chemicals in 1985. Progressive Fish Culturist 48:1–17.

Schwedler, T.E., and Tucker, C.S. (1983) Empirical relationship between percent methemoglobinemia in channel catfish and dissolved nitrite and chloride in ponds. Trans. Am. Fish. Soc. 112:117–119.

Schwedler, T.E., Tucker, C.S., and Beleau, M.H. (1985) Noninfectious diseases. In: Channel Catfish Culture (Tucker, C.S., ed,). Elsevier, Amsterdam, pp. 497–541.

Snieszko, S.F. (1974) The effects of environmental stress on outbreaks of infectious diseases of fish. J. Fish Biol. 6:197–208.

Swingle, H.S. (1961) Relationship of pH of pond waters to their suitability for fish culture. Proc. Pacific Sci. Cong. 9(1957);10:72–75.

Tomasso, J.R., Simco, B.A., and Davis, K.B. (1979) Chloride inhibition of nitrite-induced methemoglobinemia in channel catfish (Ictalurus punctatus). J. Fish. Res. Bd. Can. 36:1141–1144.

Tucker, C.S. (1985) Water quality. In: Channel Catfish Culture (Tucker, C.S., ed.). Elsevier, Amsterdam, pp. 135–227.

Tucker, C.S. (1987) Calcium Needed for Catfish Egg Hatching and Fry Survival. Mississippi Cooperative Extension Service Ref. #87–2, pp. 1–2.

Tucker, C.S., and Boyd, C.E. (1978) Consequences of periodic applications of copper sulfate and simazine for phytoplankton control in catfish ponds. Trans. Am. Fish. Soc. 107:316–320.

Tucker, C.S., and Schwedler, T.E. (1983a) Variability of percent methemoglobin in pond populations of nitrite-exposed channel catfish. Progressive Fish Culturist 45:108–110.

Tucker, C.E., and Schwedler, T.E. (1983b) Acclimation of channel catfish (Ictalurus punctatus) to nitrite. Bull. Environ. Contam. Toxicol. 30:516–521.

Tucker, C.S., Boyd, C.E., and McCoy, E.W. (1979) Effects of feeding rate on water quality, production of channel catfish, and economic returns. Trans. Am. Fish. Soc. 108:389–396.

Tucker, C.S., Lloyd, S.W., and Busch, R.L. (1984a) Relationships between phytoplankton periodicity and the concentrations of total and un-ionized ammonia in channel catfish ponds. Hydrobiologia 111:75–79.

Tucker, C.S., MacMillan, J.R., and Schwedler, T.E. (1984b) Influence of Edwardsiella ictaluri septicemia on nitrite-induced methemoglobinemia in channel catfish (Ictalurus punctatus). Bull. Environ. Contam. Toxicol. 32:669–673.

Tucker, C.S., Francis-Floyd, R., and Beleau, M.H. (1988) Nitrite-induced anemia in channel catfish, Ictalurus punctatus Rafinesque. Bull. Environ. Contam. Toxicol. 43:295–301.

Walters, G.R., and Plumb, J.A. (1980) Environmental stress and bacterial infections in channel catfish, Ictalurus punctatus Rafinesque. J. Fish Biol. 17:177–185.

Watenpaugh, D.E., Beitinger, T.L., and Huey, D.W. (1985) Temperature tolerance of nitrite-exposed channel catfish. Trans. Am. Fish. Soc. 114:274–278.

Weiler, R.G. (1979) Rates of loss of ammonia from water to atmosphere. J. Fish. Res. Bd. Can. 36:685–689.

Weitkamp, D.E., and Katz, M. (1980) A review of dissolved gas supersaturation literature. Trans. Am. Fish. Soc. 109:659–702.

Wise, D.J., Tomasso, J.R., and Brandt, T.M. (1988) Ascorbic acid inhibition of nitrite-induced methemoglobinemia in channel catfish. Progressive Fish Culturist 50:77–80.

Wolf, K. (1988) Fish Viruses and Fish Viral Diseases. Cornell University Press, Ithaca, New York, pp. 21–42.

Chapter 57

BACTERIAL DISEASES OF CATFISHES

RONALD L. THUNE

Bacteria are the most significant disease agents in commercial catfish culture. For 3 years, from 1987 to 1989, bacteria were identified as the primary or secondary cause in 85% (7183 of 8395) of the cases submitted to diagnostic labs in Alabama, Louisiana, and Mississippi. Although the economic impact of these infections varies, depending on the species of bacteria, the vast majority of total disease losses in the catfish industry are caused by bacteria (Table 57–1).

Although each bacterial disease of catfishes will be treated separately in the following chapter, it is important to note that mixed causes are common in catfish epidemics. For example, in a study evaluating the effectiveness of a selective media for the isolation of *Flexibacter columnaris* from diseased channel catfish in 99 natural epidemics, *Edwardsiella ictaluri* was the sole etiology in 29 cases, a motile aeromonad in 8 cases, and *Flexibacter columnaris* in 7 cases. Fifty-one of 99 cases involved multiple causes, with the most common combinations being *Edwardsiella ictaluri* with *Flexibacter columnaris* (18 cases) and a motile aeromonad with *Flexibacter columnaris* (17 cases). In seven cases, all three of the major catfish bacterial species were isolated. Clinical evaluation of catfish epidemics must consider this tendency, and antibiotic sensitivities need to be determined for all pertinent isolates.

ENTERIC SEPTICEMIA OF CATFISHES

SYNONYMS. Edwardsiellosis, *Edwardsiella ictaluri* septicemia.

Host and Geographic Distribution

Enteric septicemia of catfishes is a relatively new disease in commercial catfish culture, having first been described in 1976 (Hawke, 1979). Owing to extensive transfer of fish nationwide and the highly infectious nature of the causative bacteria, enteric septicemia of catfishes has rapidly become the most devastating disease problem affecting the commercial catfish industry. It is responsible for millions of dollars in losses and treatment costs annually. Although the causative agent, *Edwardsiella ictaluri*, has been described from walking catfish, white catfish, and brown bullheads, as well as some species of freshwater tropical fish (Plumb and Sanchez, 1983; Waltman et al., 1985; Humphrey et al., 1986), the bacteria is fairly host specific for the channel catfish. It is nonpathogenic for several warmwater fish species, although the bacteria can be isolated from the peritoneal cavity, kidney, and liver of some nonictalurid species for several days postinoculation. The European catfish is susceptible to *Edwardsiella ictaluri* after injection, but 100 times the infective dose for channel catfish is necessary, and typical clinical signs are not observed (Plumb and Hilge, 1987). Recent reports from California surprisingly indicate that chinook salmon and rainbow trout are extremely sensitive to this infection. Fish challenged by immersion exhibit greater mortality than even channel catfish (Baxa and Hedrick, 1989). However, no natural epizootics have been reported in salmonids.

Geographically, *Edwardsiella ictaluri* has caused epizootics throughout the channel catfish–producing areas of the United States, including all of the south-

TABLE 57–1. Bacterial Diseases of Catfishes

Disease	Bacteria	Host
Enteric septicemia of catfishes	*Edwardsiella ictaluri*	Channel catfish, walking catfish, brown bullheads, rosy barb, danio, chinook salmon, rainbow trout
Columnaris disease	*Flexibacter columnaris*	All freshwater species
Motile aeromonad septicemia	*Aeromonas hydrophila*	All freshwater species
Emphysematous putrefactive disease of catfish	*Edwardsiella tarda*	Channel catfish, eels, carp, goldfish, largemouth bass, brown bullheads, mullet, chinook salmon, striped bass, tilapia, and flounder

eastern states, Idaho, Indiana, Colorado, Maryland, Arizona, and California. In addition, *Edwardsiella ictaluri* was identified in a group of tropical fish (rosy barbs) being shipped from Singapore to Australia, and has been reported in walking catfish in Thailand.

Clinical Signs

Clinical manifestations of enteric septicemia in channel catfish vary considerably, but generally resemble those of other gram-negative septicemias in fish. Infected fish hang tail-down at the surface or spin and spiral rapidly in circles. Gross external signs are occasionally absent in acute cases, but include petechial hemorrhages, particularly around the mouth and on the ventral surface (Fig. 57–1); raised or open ulcers on the midline of the frontal bone between the eyes (Fig. 57–2); cutaneous, ulcerative, white lesions on the lateral and dorsal aspects of the head and body; and bilateral exophthalmia and ascites. Gross internal signs include bloody or occasionally clear yellow ascitic fluid accumulations; swollen kidneys, liver, and spleen; and a mottled liver (Fig. 57–3) with either pale, necrotic areas in a darker red liver or hemorrhagic areas in a pale liver. Petechial hemorrhage in the musculature, adipose tissue, inner walls of the peritoneal cavity, and intestine are also seen.

Diagnosis, Culture, and Identification

The etiologic agent of enteric septicemia of catfishes, *Edwardsiella ictaluri*, can be presumptively identified on isolation by establishing the presence of pinpoint colonies on blood agar after incubation for 24 hours at 30°C and determining them to be gram-negative, cytochrome oxidase–negative organisms that ferment glucose and produce an alkaline/

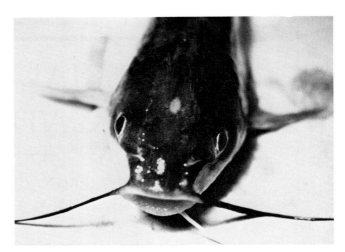

FIGURE 57–2. Typical cranial ulcer associated with *Edwardsiella ictaluri* infections in channel catfish.

acid reaction with gas and no H_2S in triple-sugar–iron agar. *Edwardsiella ictaluri* is indole negative and motile at 25°C but not at 37°C. Immunologic techniques such as fluorescent antibody are also useful for confirming a diagnosis because *Edwardsiella ictaluri* strains are serologically homogeneous. Complete biochemical and morphologic characteristics have been described (Hawke et al., 1981; Waltman et al., 1986). A selective medium for the isolation of *Edwardsiella ictaluri* has been recently described (Shotts and Waltman, 1990).

Transmission, Epidemiology, and Pathogenesis

Enteric septicemia of catfishes is generally an acute disease. Epidemics often occur with little or no warning. Premonitory signs include reduced feeding activity or low-grade mortality. Prompt treatment is critical to effective control. The incidence of enteric

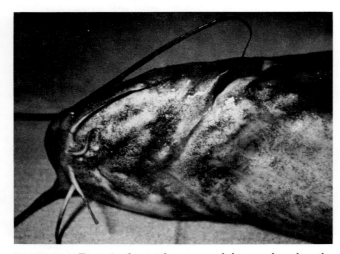

FIGURE 57–1. Extensive hemorrhage around the mouth and on the ventral surface of a channel catfish infected with *Edwardsiella ictaluri*.

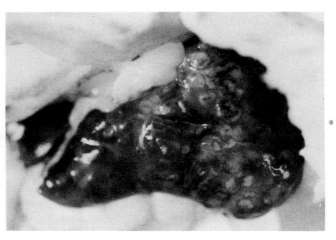

FIGURE 57–3. Liver from a channel catfish that died of an *Edwardsiella ictaluri* infection. (Courtesy of R. Floyd and M. Beleau.)

septicemia is highly correlated with water temperature. Peak disease levels occur between 22 and 28°C (Francis-Floyd, 1987). Although epidemics occasionally occur outside of this temperature range, the disease presentation is more chronic in nature and mortality rates are low. During the season of high-risk temperatures, April through May in south Louisiana, to May through June in Mississippi and Arkansas, a rapid response to suspected epidemics is important in mounting effective control measures.

Treatment and Control

At present, the only treatments available for enteric septicemia are oxytetracycline in a sinking pellet and ormetoprim and sulfadimethoxine in a floating pellet. Catfish farmers report variable treatment success with either of these compounds, with the degree of success probably depending on the promptness with which the treatment is applied. Detection of fish with enteric septicemia indicates the need for an immediate application of oral antibiotics, especially if the temperatures are just entering the high-risk temperature window (i.e., about 28°C in the fall when temperatures are falling and about 22°C in the spring when they are rising). However, contributions to mortality and poor feeding responses caused by the presence of external protozoans and/or concomitant *Flexibacter columnaris* or *Aeromonas hydrophila* infections can also affect antibiotic treatment success. Occasionally, a bath treatment with copper sulfate or potassium permanganate is used in these cases to reduce the external parasite load. However, copper sulfate baths increase the susceptibility of channel catfish to enteric septicemia, so a permanganate bath is preferable. Antibiotic feed treatment should be initiated immediately after the pond treatment, or if possible, the day prior to pond treatment, if limited feeding activity is observed. Since there is a risk that the pond treatment will exacerbate the enteric septicemia, this course of treatment should only be undertaken when fish are off feed or feeding poorly, and a complete diagnosis of the situation has indicated high levels of external protozoa and/or *Flexibacter columnaris* are present.

Bacterins for the prevention of enteric septicemia are not currently available, but research indicates this approach may be feasible in the near future. The bacteria appears to be serologically homogeneous, with 20 of 20 isolates of unreported origin reacting to antiserum prepared against formalin-killed whole cells (Rogers, 1981). Additional studies with *Edwardsiella ictaluri* lipopolysaccharide have indicated that strains are cross-reactive. Further, both the lipopolysaccharide fraction and whole cells are protective following intraperitoneal injection, and immersion or a combination of immersion and oral vaccination may be effective in reducing enteric septicemia losses (Thune et al., 1988). In a field experiment, fingerling channel catfish vaccinated against enteric septicemia in February using either sonicated or whole cell vaccine preparations, either by intraperitoneal injection or immersion, reduced mortalities following challenge in March (Plumb et al., 1986). Mortality in fish vaccinated by immersion in the sonicated preparation was 11.8%, whereas mortalities in fish immersed in whole cells, injected with whole cells, or injected with sonicate were 24.6, 57.9, and 41.7%, respectively. However, fingerlings are most susceptible to enteric septicemia, and the majority of losses occur during their first exposure when temperatures conducive to the disease occur in the fall of their first year. Fish vaccinated by immersion with a whole-cell preparation in the hatchery just prior to stocking (7 to 10 days posthatching) and fed an oral booster just prior to the enteric septicemia temperature window in the fall, realize a 5.5% mortality following laboratory challenge (Thune et al., 1988). Mortalities in fish vaccinated by a single immersion and nonvaccinated controls were 32 and 47%, respectively, with the same challenge.

COLUMNARIS DISEASE

SYNONYMS. *Flexibacter columnaris, Cytophaga columnaris, Bacillus columnaris.*

Host and Geographic Distribution

Columnaris disease, caused by the gliding bacterium *Flexibacter columnaris*, was first described by Davis in 1922. Davis gave a microscopic description of the bacteria and named it *Bacillus columnaris*, based on the columnar arrangements of the cells in wet mounts. Columnaris disease is common throughout the world, affecting virtually all species of freshwater fishes, and is the second most common bacterial problem in commercial catfish culture systems.

Clinical Signs

Externally, columnaris disease can affect both the skin and gills. Skin lesions usually begin as irregular areas of epidermal loss, causing the lesion to lose its natural "sheen" and coloration (Fig. 57–4). Infections frequently begin on the fins, which eventually become frayed and ragged. Initial lesions can progress to areas of extensive ulceration with penetration of the dermis and underlying musculature. *Aeromonas hydrophila* is commonly present in advanced lesions and probably contributes to the pathology. In the gills, the infection appears as irregular areas of light to dark brown discoloration and necrosis (Fig. 57–5). The most severe infections can affect almost all of the gill arches.

Diagnosis, Culture, and Identification

Characteristic long, slender, flexing bacteria observed in wet mounts of skin scrapings and gill

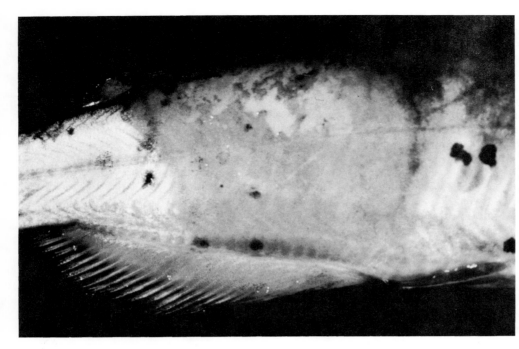

FIGURE 57–4. Epithelial loss on a channel catfish due to *Flexibacter columnaris*. Also apparent in the center of the primary lesion is an early lesion associated with a secondary motile aeromonad.

clippings of infected fish are usually considered diagnostic for external columnaris disease because of the difficulty of isolation (Fig. 57–6). If wet mounts are allowed to stand for a few minutes, the bacteria will orient closely to mucus and tissue debris, producing characteristic "haystacks." Isolation of *Flexibacter columnaris* from external lesions can be difficult, requiring the use of low-agar, low-nutrient media (Anacker and Ordal, 1955). It is important that freshly prepared media be used because sufficient surface moisture must be present for the bacteria to spread and grow. Since systemic columnaris disease occurs routinely, cultures of the liver and kidney should

also be taken. However, growth of *Flexibacter columnaris* on routine Ordal's or cytophaga media is often inhibited by even scant growth of other fish pathogens in mixed infections, so selective media should be used. A modification of the medium of Fijan (1969) containing 5 μg/ml of neomycin and 200 U/ml of polymyxin B has been effective in increasing the detection of internal columnaris in mixed bacterial infections of channel catfish by a factor of 7 (Hawke and Thune, 1989). The media of Hsu and Shotts is also effective, but is more complex and difficult to make.

The taxonomy of the gliding bacteria has always

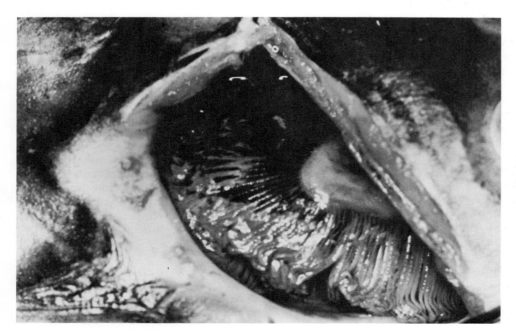

FIGURE 57–5. Columnaris disease in the gills of a channel catfish demonstrating extensive necrosis of the primary lamellae.

been controversial. Recently, all yellow pigmented, gliding bacteria that colonize fish were placed in the order Cytophagales, genus *Cytophaga*, in *Bergey's Manual* (Reichenbach, 1989). Although several species are described as fish pathogens, the predominant species in catfish culture, *Flexibacter columnaris*, was renamed *Cytophaga columnaris;* however, this suggested change has not withstood challenge. The older, established name *Flexibacter columnaris* will be used throughout this text.

The typical *Flexibacter columnaris* causing disease in channel catfish is a long, thin (4 to 8 μm by 0.5 to 0.7 μm) gram-negative rod that is motile by a gliding or flexing action. On Anacher and Ordal's (1955) or other appropriate media, typical colonies are rough, rhizoid growths that produce a gold-yellow pigment. Colonies tend to adhere to the agar and can be difficult to transfer. In young cultures, individual cells take on the long, thin, flexing shape characteristic of cells in necropsy wet mounts. However, they become short, almost coccoid, nonmotile rods in older cultures, and occasionally, coiled, isolated, and branched cells can be observed.

Transmission, Epidemiology, and Pathogenesis

In vitro, *Flexibacter columnaris* will grow from 25 to 30°C (Reichenbach, 1989), but causes disease in catfish primarily in the range of 25 to 32°C. Epidemics also occur in water temperatures below 25°C, even as low as 15°C, but mortalities are generally significantly less than in warmer temperatures. It is possible that these cold-water isolates are a different species. This temperature relationship correlates to the late spring and early fall seasonality of *Flexibacter columnaris* clinical cases.

Flexibacter columnaris can persist in water for up to 32 days when the hardness is 50 ppm $CaCO_3$ or more, but a hardness of 10 ppm $CaCO_3$ reduces viability considerably (Fijan, 1968). The addition of organic carbon to the system increases the survival of *Flexibacter columnaris* in hard but not soft water. This fits clinical observations that columnaris disease is favored in systems with high organic loads.

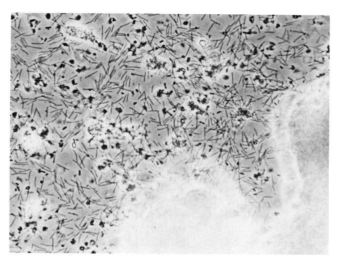

FIGURE 57–6. *Flexibacter columnaris* in a wet mount of a skin scraping from a channel catfish.

Crowded conditions, handling, and low dissolved oxygen also favor the development of columnaris infections, especially in water with a high organic load at temperatures above 20°C. Lesions generally develop in 24 to 48 hours following handling, followed by death at 48 to 72 hours if not treated. At lower temperatures secondary fungal infections may be present on the columnaris lesions, which may persist even if the columnaris becomes inapparent.

Treatment and Control

The treatment of choice for control of columnaris epidemics depends on the state of the infection. For a purely external infection, which is generally the case when diagnosis is made early, a bath treatment with potassium permanganate at 2 mg/L above the permanganate demand of the water is usually thought to be effective; however, some investigators feel that this therapy can exacerbate lesions (Fig. 57–7) (Tucker, 1989). However, if the infection is systemic, antibiotic therapy with either oxytetracycline or ormetoprim and sulfadimethoxine is indicated. In situations in which the bacteria are both external and

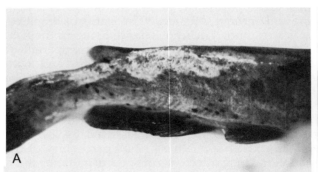
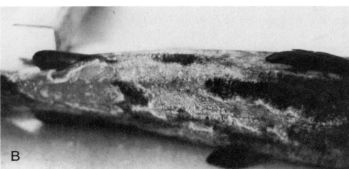

FIGURE 57–7. *A.* Channel catfish with skin lesions infected with *Flexibacter columnaris* and *Aeromonas hydrophila. B.* The same fish following treatment with a potassium permanganate bath. (Courtesy of P. Reed.)

internal, antibiotic therapy alone will often control the infection, unless the epidemic has progressed to a stage where feeding activity is poor. In this case, a potassium permanganate treatment, followed immediately by antibiotic therapy, is indicated.

An important consideration in using antibiotic therapy to control columnaris disease is the antibiotic sensitivity of the strain in question. Since *Flexibacter columnaris* will not grow on Mueller-Hinton-IH agar, some laboratories have used the media of Anacher and Ordal (1955) for antibiotic sensitivity testing. However, these media contain sulfonamide inhibitors and should not be used to determine sensitivity to potentiated sulfonamides (Fijan and Voorhees, 1969). A dilute Mueller-Hinton medium (3 g Mueller-Hinton broth and 9 g agar per liter) supplemented with 5% fetal calf serum should be used. This medium is effective in determining resistance/sensitivity patterns, but interpretation of zone diameters relative to zone diameters on standard Mueller-Hinton-IH agar is difficult because the reduced agar content affects diffusion rates.

Immunotherapy is a possible method for reducing losses to *Flexibacter columnaris* in channel catfish. Although extensive serologic studies on isolates from catfish have not been done, studies on 325 strains from fish in the Pacific Northwest and one from Texas indicate that four serologic groups exist, but that all strains possess a common antigen. High agglutinating antibody titers against *Flexibacter columnaris* in channel catfish have been induced following subcutaneous and intraperitoneal injections, but these titers have not been evaluated with challenge (Schachte and Mora, 1973). Rainbow trout have been protected when given continuous oral doses of a heat-killed *Flexibacter columnaris* antigen (Fujihara and Nakatani, 1971). Pooled serum samples from vaccinated fish had an average agglutinating titer of 1:168 compared to 1:17 in control fish. The effectiveness of a *Flexibacter columnaris* bacteria in commercial catfish production remains to be investigated.

MOTILE AEROMONAD SEPTICEMIA

SYNONYMS. Ulcer disease, aeromoniasis.

Sanarelli (1891) originally called the causative organism of motile aeromonad septicemia (MAS) *Bacillus hydrophilus fuscus*. Later it was referred to as *Bacillus hydrophilas* (Chester, 1901) and *Proteus hydrophilas*. Subsequently, the causative bacteria has been referred to as *Pseudomonas fermentus*, *Flavobacterium fermentus*, *Proteus melanovogenes*, and *Pseudomonas hydrophila*. Snieszko (1957) proposed dividing the group into three species: *Aeromonas hydrophila*, *Aeromonas punctata*, and *Aeromonas liquefaciens* with the fish pathogenic strains generally identified as *Aeromonas liquefaciens*. Schubert (1967) felt that there was enough biochemical similarity to establish the genus, but limited species distinction to *Aeromonas hydrophila* and *Aeromonas punctata* with various subspecies and biotypes. Later, three subspecies of *Aeromonas hydro-*

phila, including *Aeromonas hydrophila hydrophila*, *Aeromonas hydrophila anaerogenes*, and *Aeromonas punctata*, including *Aeromonas punctata punctata* and *Aeromonas punctata caviae* were defined (Schubert, 1974). The current edition of *Bergey's Manual* lists *Aeromonas hydrophila*, *Aeromonas sobria*, and *Aeromonas caviae* as the motile members of the genus *Aeromonas*. Generally, the motile aeromonad species isolated from catfish are *Aeromonas sobria* and *Aeromonas hydrophila*.

Host and Geographic Distribution

The motile aeromonads represent a phenotypically and genotypically heterogeneous group of gram-negative bacteria that are essentially ubiquitous in aquatic environments. Sanarelli (1891) published the first report of disease presumably caused by members of this taxon, but it has been speculated that disease caused by motile aeromonads was probably common in Europe during the Middle Ages (Otte, 1963). These organisms have been implicated in causing disease in many cold- and warm-blooded species, including humans (Newman, 1982; Popoff, 1984). In channel catfish, motile aeromonad septicemia is the third most common bacterial disease, and motile aeromonads are common secondary invaders.

Diagnosis and Identification

The motile aeromonads are gram-negative rods, approximately 0.5 by 1.0 μm, with a single, polar flagellum. They are facultative anaerobes, fermenting a variable array of carbohydrates with the formation of acid and/or gas. The cytochrome oxidase reaction is positive, and they are insensitive to the vibriostatic compound 0/129 (2,4,diamino-67-disopropylpteridine). The genus *Aeromonas* has a Mol % G + C ratio of 57 to 63. Species identification is based on the biochemical properties (Popoff and Veron, 1976; Popoff, 1984).

Clinical Signs

Clinically, the motile aeromonads in channel catfish are opportunistic pathogens that can occur in acute and chronic situations. The status of the infection is a result of a delicate balance between the fish, the pathogen, and the environment. Inapparent or subclinical infections are often present, and both *Aeromonas hydrophila* and *Aeromonas sobria* can be routinely isolated from the intestinal tract of healthy fish (MacMillan, 1985), from pond water (Hazen et al., 1978) and from clinical specimens. Chronic motile aeromonad septicemia is characterized by low-level mortalities, with a relatively small percentage of the population being affected. Affected fish often exhibit extensive external pathology ranging from frayed fins (Fig. 57–8) and shallow, hemorrhagic, or grayish

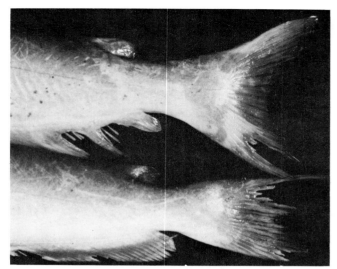

FIGURE 57–8. Frayed fins associated with a motile aeromonad infection in a channel catfish.

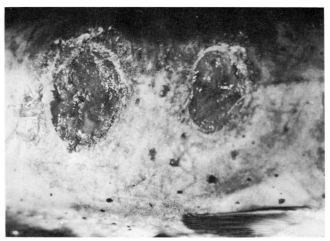

FIGURE 57–9. Shallow, hemorrhagic ulcers on the flank of a channel catfish with a motile aeromonad septicemia.

ulcers (Fig. 57–9) to extensive necrotic lesions of the skin and underlying musculature (Fig. 57–10). Bacteria may be confined to the external lesions, but can usually be isolated from the internal organs, especially in advanced cases. Acute disease is characterized by significant mortality, with a greater percentage of the population being affected. External signs of disease are generally less severe, with pectechial hemorrhage or ecchymoses most common. Internally the bacteria can be readily isolated from the blood and internal organs. Gross internal pathology may include serosanguinous ascites, enteric hyperemia, a soft and swollen liver and kidney, splenomegaly, and hemorrhage. In addition, the intestine may be flaccid and filled with bloody fluid or a yellowish material. Histologically, the bacteria cause extensive congestion, tissue necrosis, and hemorrhage.

Transmission, Epidemiology, and Pathogenesis

Two principal factors of the host-pathogen-environment interaction contribute to the acute/chronic status of motile aeromonad infections. Although consideration of these factors applies to other diseases, the opportunistic nature and heterogeneity of the motile aeromonad group makes the interaction of primary interest.

The first factor to consider is stress-mediated predisposition to infection. Although the very nature of catfish ponds, with excessive crowding and high feeding rates, is conducive to the spread of infectious disease, outbreaks of motile aeromonad septicemia most commonly occur following shipping/handling, suboptimal oxygen stress, nitrite-induced methemoglobinemia, application of chemical treatments, rapid changes in temperature, or as a result of stress induced by infection with other bacteria or infestations with internal or external parasites.

The second important factor to consider in evaluating the status of an *Aeromonas* epidemic is the virulence of the *Aeromonas* strain, which is quite variable (de Figueirido and Plumb, 1977; Lallier et al., 1980; Thune et al., 1986; Chabot and Thune, 1991). Several factors have been suggested to play roles in strain virulence in motile aeromonads, including extracellular enzymes, extracellular toxins, and surface characteristics.

Motile aeromonads release a variety of biologically active enzymes or toxins into culture media, and channel catfish injected intraperitoneally with crude extracellular products from cell-free supernatants of cultures grown in a chemically defined media (Riddle et al., 1981) display many of the clinical signs of motile aeromonad septicemia (Thune et al., 1982b). This indicates that these extracellular enzymes play a significant role in the pathogenesis of the disease. Studies have demonstrated a hemolysin and several proteases as the primary extracellular enzymes contributing to this effect in channel catfish (Thune et al., 1982a,b; Thune et al., 1986). However, there is a

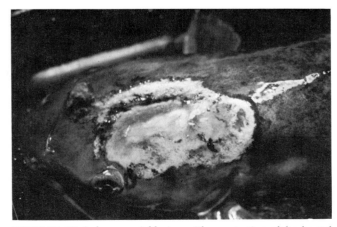

FIGURE 57–10. A deep cranial lesion with penetration of the frontal bone exposing underlying neural tissue in a chronic manifestation of motile aeromonad septicemia.

lack of correlation between virulence and the differential production of significant quantities of these enzymes (Thune et al., 1986; Chabot and Thune, 1991). Field studies have demonstrated that strains freshly isolated from moribund channel catfish produce only insignificant amounts of these enzymes (Ford and Thune, 1991).

Surface characteristics of the motile aeromonads have also been correlated with virulence. The most virulent strains of *Aeromonas hydrophila* in rainbow trout share a common O-antigen, do not agglutinate in acriflavin, settle after boiling, and are resistant to the bacteriocidal action of normal mammalian serum (Mittal et al., 1980). Studies in channel catfish have indicated that motile aeromonad strains require a crystalline S-layer coating to induce mortality in fish challenged by intraperitoneal or intramuscular injection. In addition, field studies of fresh isolates from moribund fish indicate that the S-layer is present in all isolates in which an aeromonad is the primary agent (Ford and Thune, 1991).

Treatment and Control

Clinical decisions for managing or treating an aeromonad epidemic should consider both environmental and pathogen related factors. Generally, *Aeromonas* infections are much easier to control than enteric septicemia or columnaris disease, but at times the cost of treatment may exceed the benefits. The recent history of the fish pertaining to potential stressors, along with mortality data and feeding activity, should influence any decision to deliver an antibiotic feed. Although current practice does not include rapid screening techniques for evaluating differential strain virulence, future efforts to define and evaluate motile aeromonad virulence factors may assist clinicians in evaluating the risk of a particular *Aeromonas* strain.

Decisions to treat fish affected by aeromonads must also consider current or potential infections with other bacteria or protozoa. For example, heavy branchial infestations with external protozoa may act as a predisposing stressor, and chemical treatment to reduce the parasite load may also control the aeromonad. On the other hand, the chemical treatment may stress the fish enough to cause a shift from chronic to acute motile aeromonad septicemia.

Although minimizing stress is a key to control of aeromoniasis, stress is an inherent part of intensive fish culture and cannot always be controlled. In instances where aeromoniasis is causing significant mortality, antibiotic therapy can be particularly helpful if delivered quickly at the onset of an epidemic. However, many epidemics will resolve themselves without treatment. The degree of stress and the mortality pattern must be carefully evaluated. Occasionally, the prophylactic use of antibiotics has been recommended for the control of motile aeromonas septicemia, especially following a known stress such as low dissolved oxygen or handling. There are two

major drawbacks to this approach. First, antibiotic-resistant strains of the motile aeromonads are well documented (Aoki and Egusa, 1971; Shotts, 1976; MacMillan, 1985), and the prevalence of resistant strains increases with increasing use of antibiotics. Second, the cost of the treatment often exceeds the benefit.

At present, vaccination against motile aeromonad septicemia is not practical because of the heterogeneous nature of the cell wall antigenic determinants. Although protection from challenge has been demonstrated in carp (Schaperclaus, 1954; Baba et al., 1988), rainbow trout (Post, 1966), and channel catfish (Thune, 1980), protection is generally limited to the homologous strain. Since lipopolysaccharide heterogeneity precludes traditional vaccination approaches, the use of extracellular products such as the proteases and hemolysins and proteins of the crystalline S-layer is being examined.

EMPHYSEMATOUS PUTREFACTIVE DISEASE

Host and Geographic Distribution

Emphysematous putrefactive disease of catfish (EPDC), caused by *Edwardsiella tarda*, was first described by Meyer and Bulloch (1973). The disease is currently implicated in less than 1% of all bacterial diseases in catfish.

Clinical Signs

Classic clinical signs range from small cutaneous lesions measuring 3 to 5 mm in diameter to large, gas-filled, malodorous, necrotic lesions in the muscle (Meyer and Bulloch, 1973). The initial lesions may resemble catfish spine wounds but actually appear to develop from fistulae deeper in the muscle (Meyer, 1975). The course of classic emphysematous putrefactive disease is chronic, with incidence in ponds seldom exceeding 5%. Secondary or concurrent infections with *Aeromonas* or *Flexibacter* are common and can increase mortality rates. However, the most common manifestation of *Edwardsiella tarda* in catfish is generalized septicemia rather than the classic emphysematous putrefactive disease.

Diagnosis, Culture, and Identification

Edwardsiella tarda, as a member of the Enterobacteriaceae, is a gram-negative, oxidase-negative rod approximately 0.5 to 0.75 μm by 1.25 μm in size. The organism grows well on most media, with no requirement for serum or blood, although double-strength *Salmonella-Shigella* broth can be used for specific isolation of *Edwardsiella tarda* from environmental samples (Wyatt et al., 1979). *Edwardsiella tarda* differs from *Edwardsiella ictaluri* in that it produces H₂S in triple-sugar–iron agar and is indole positive.

Transmission, Epidemiology, and Pathogenesis

Edwardsiella tarda can be isolated from normal catfish carcasses, pond water samples, and pond mud samples (Wyatt et al., 1979). In addition, 100% of frogs, turtles, and crawfish sampled from catfish ponds in one study carried *Edwardsiella tarda*. The prevalence of *Edwardsiella tarda* in pond water increases dramatically during the warmer summer months, probably because of increased water temperatures, higher organic loads due to heavier feeding rates, or possibly because of increases in the number of amphibians in the pond. This increase in pond water numbers correlates closely with the epidemiology of the disease, with epidemics most numerous when water temperature exceeds 30°C and when high levels of organic matter are present in the water (Meyer and Bulloch, 1973).

Treatment and Control

Once an epidemic is initiated, antibiotic therapy is indicated. Resistance to oxytetracycline is common. Some control of emphysematous putrefactive disease can be achieved by optimizing water quality, particularly in broodfish ponds where classic, chronic disease is most commonly seen. Optimal conditions of water quality with minimal organic loading can be achieved by limiting the broodfish standing crop to a maximum of 1350 kg/hectare and feeding rates to a maximum of 1% of the standing crop per day.

LITERATURE CITED

Anacker, R.L., and Ordal, E.J. (1955) Study of a bacteriophage infecting the myxobacterium *Chondrococcus columnaris*. J. Bacteriol. 70:738–740.

Aoki, T., and Egusa, S. (1971) Drug sensitivity of *Aeromonas liquefaciens* isolated from freshwater fishes. Bull. Jpn. Soc. Sci. Fish. 37:176–185.

Baba, T., Imamura, J., Izawa, K., and Ikeda, K. (1988) Immune protection in carp, *Cyprinus carpio* L., after immunization with *Aeromonas hydrophila* crude lipopolysaccharide. J. Fish Dis. 11:237–244.

Baxa, D.V., and Hedrick, R.P. (1989) Two more species are susceptible to experimental infections with *Edwardsiella ictaluri*. Fish Health Sect. Am. Fish. Soc. Newslett. 17(1):4.

Bergey, D.H., Harrison, H.C., Breed, R.S., Hammer, B.W., and Huntoon, F.M. (1923) Bergey's Manual of Determinative Bacteriology. Williams & Wilkins, Baltimore.

Bullock, G.L., Hsu, T.C., and Shotts, E.B. (1986) Columnaris disease of fishes. Fish disease leaflet 72. U.S. Fish and Wildlife Service, Washington, D.C.

Chabot, D.J., and Thune, R.L. (1991) Proteases of the *Aeromonas hydrophila* complex: identification, characterization, and relation to virulence in channel catfish. J. Fish Dis. (in press).

Chester, F.D. (1901) Manual of Determinative Bacteriology. Macmillan, New York.

Davis, H.S. (1922) A new bacterial disease of freshwater fish. U.S. Bur. Fish. Bull. 38:261–280.

de Figueirido, J., and Plumb, J.P. (1977) Virulence of different isolates of *Aeromonas hydrophila* in channel catfish. Aquaculture 11:349–354.

Dooley, J.S., and Trust, T.J. (1988) Surface protein composition of *Aeromonas hydrophila* virulent for fish: identification of an S-layer protein. J. Bacteriol. 170:499–506.

Dooley, J.S., Lallier, R., and Trust, T.J. (1986) Surface antigens of virulent strains of *Aeromonas hydrophila*. Vet. Immunol. Immunopathol. 12:339–334.

Fijan, N.N. (1968) The survival of *Chondrococcus columnaris* in waters of different quality. III. Symposium de la Commission de l'Office International des Epizooties pour l'Etude des Maladies des Poissons. Stockholm, Sweden.

Fijan, N.N. (1969) Antibiotic additives for the isolation of *Chondrococcus columnaris* from fish. Appl. Microbiol. 17(2):333–334.

Fijan, N.N., and Voorhees, P.R. (1969) Drug sensitivity of *Chondrococcus columnaris*. Vet. Arh. 39:259–267.

Ford, L.A., and Thune, R.L. (1991) S-layer positive motile aeromonads isolated from channel catfish. J. Wildlife Dis. 27:557–561.

Francis-Floyd, R., Beleau, M.H., Waterstrat, P.R., and Bowser, P.R. (1987) Effect of water temperature on the clinical outcome of infection with *Edwardsiella ictaluri* in channel catfish. J. Am. Vet. Med. Assoc. 191:1413–1416.

Fujihara, M.P., and Nakatani, R.E. (1971) Antibody production and immune responses of rainbow trout and coho salmon to *Chondrococcus columnaris*. J. Fish. Res. Bd. Can. 28(9):1253–1258.

Hawke, J.P. (1979) A bacterium associated with disease of pond cultured channel catfish, *Ictalurus punctatus*. J. Fish. Res. Bd. Can. 36:1508–1512.

Hawke, J.P., and Thune, R.L. (1988) Evaluation of a medium for the selective isolation of *Flexibacter columnaris* from diseased channel catfish (abs.). Proceedings International Fish Health Meeting, Vancouver, B.C., Canada.

Hawke, J.P., McWhorter, A.C., Steigerwalt, A.G., and Brenner, D.J. (1981) *Edwardsiella ictaluri* sp. nov., the causative agent of enteric septicemia of catfish. Int. J. Syst. Bacteriol. 31(4):396–400.

Hazen, T.C., Fliermans, R.P., Hirsch, R.P., and Esch, G.W. (1978) Prevalence and distribution of *Aeromonas hydrophila* in the United States. Appl. Environ. Microbiol. 36(5):731–738.

Humphrey, J.D., Lancaster, C., Gudkovs, N., and McDonald, W. (1986) Exotic bacterial pathogens *Edwardsiella tarda* and *Edwardsiella ictaluri* from imported ornamental fish *Betta splendens* and *Puntius conchonius*, respectively: Isolation and quarantine significance. Aust. Vet. J. 63:369–370.

Lallier, R., Boulanger, Y., and Olivier, G. (1980) Difference in virulence of *Aeromonas hydrophila* and *Aeromonas sobria* in rainbow trout. Progressive Fish Culturist 42:199–200.

MacMillan, J.R. (1985) Infectious diseases. In: Channel Catfish Culture (Tucker, C.S., ed.). Elsevier, Holland.

Meyer, F.P. (1975) The pathology of the major diseases of catfish. In: The Pathology of Fishes (Ribelin, W.E., and Migaki, G., eds.). University of Wisconsin Press, Madison, pp. 275–286.

Meyer, F.P., and Bulloch, G.L. (1973) *Edwardsiella tarda*, a new pathogen of channel catfish (*Ictalurus punctatus*). Appl. Microbiol. 25(1):151–156.

Mittal, K.R., Lalonde, G., LeBlanc, D., Olivier, G., and Lallier, R. (1980) *Aeromonas hydrophila* in rainbow trout: relation between virulence and surface characteristics. Can. J. Microbiol. 26:1501–1503.

Newman, S.G. (1982) *Aeromonas hydrophila*: A review with emphasis on its role in fish disease. In: Antigens of Fish Pathogens: Development and Production for Vaccines and Serodiagnostics (Anderson et al., eds.). Association Corporative des Etudiants en Medecine de Lyons, France, pp. 87–118.

Ordal, E.J., and Rucker, R.R. (1944) Pathogenic myxobacteria. Proc. Soc. Exp. Biol. Med. 56:15–18.

Otte, E. (1963) Die heutigan asichten uber die atiologie der infektiosen Bauchwassersucht der Karpfen. Wein. Tierartzl. Monatsschr. 50:995–1005.

Plumb, J.A., and Hilge, V. (1987) Susceptibility of European catfish (*Siluris glanis*) to *Edwardsiella ictaluri*. J. Appl. Ichthyol. 3:45–48.

Plumb, J.A., and Sanchez, D.J. (1983) Susceptibility of five species of fish to *Edwardsiella ictaluri*. J. Fish Dis. 6:261–266.

Plumb, J.A., Wise, M.L., and Rogers, W.A. (1986) Modulary effects of temperature on antibody response and specific resistance to challenge of channel catfish, *Ictalurus punctatus*, immunized against *Edwardsiella ictaluri*. Vet. Immunol. Immunopathol. 12:297–304.

Popoff, M. (1984) Aeromonas. In: Bergey's Manual of Systematic Bacteriology. Vol. 1 (Holt, J.G., ed.). Williams & Wilkins, Baltimore, pp. 545–548.

Popoff, M., and Veron, M. (1976) A taxonomic study of the *Aeromonas hydrophila–Aeromonas punctata* group. J. Gen. Microbiol. 94:11–12.

Popoff, M., and Veron, M. (1981) *Aeromonas sobria* sp. nov. In: Validation of the publication of new names and new combinations previously effectively published outside the IJSB. List No. 6. Int. J. Syst. Bacteriol. 31:215.

Post, G. (1966) Response of rainbow trout (*Salmo gairdneri*) to antigens of *Aeromonas hydrophila*. J. Fish. Res. Bd. Can. 23:1487–1494.

Reichenbach, H. (1989) Cytophagales. In: Bergey's Manual of Systematic Bacteriology. Vol. 3. (Holt, J.G., ed.). Williams & Wilkins, Baltimore.

Riddle, L.M., Graham, T.E, Amborski, R.L., and Hugh-Jones, M. (1981) Production of hemolysin and protease by *Aeromonas hydrophila* in a chemically defined medium. Dev. Biol. Stand. 49:125–133.

Rogers, W.A. (1981) Serological detection of two species of *Edwardsiella* infecting fish. In: Developments in Biological Standardization. Vol. 49:

Fish Biologics: Serodiagnostics and Vaccines. S. Karger, Basel, Switzerland.

Sanarelli, G. (1891) Ueber einen mikro-organismus des wassers, welches fur thiere mit vernderlicher und constanter temperatur pathogen ist. Zentbl. Bakt. Parasit. Kde. 9:193–199.

Schachte, J.H., and Mora, E.C. (1973) Production of agglutinating antibodies in the channel catfish (Ictalurus punctatus) against Chondrococcus columnaris. J. Fish. Res. Bd. Can. 30:116–118.

Schaperclaus, W. (1954) Die verhtung der ingectiosen Bauchwassersucht des karpens duch Imorfuns und Behandling arot Medikamenten. Deutsch. Fisch. Ztg. 1:102–108.

Schubert, R.H.W. (1967) The taxonomy and nomenclature of the genus Aeromonas. Part I. Suggestions on the taxonomy and nomenclature of the aerogenic Aeromonas species. Int. J. Syst. Bacteriol. 17:23–37.

Schubert, R.H.W. (1974) Aeromonas. In: Bergey's Manual of Determinative Bacteriology. 8th ed. Williams & Wilkins, Baltimore, pp. 345–348.

Shaw, D.H., and Hodder, H.J. (1978) Lipopolysaccharides of the motile aeromonads: core oligosaccharide analysis as an aid to taxonomic classification. Can. J. Microbiol. 24:864–868.

Shotts, E.B., and Waltman, W.D. (1990) A medium for the selective isolation Edwardsiella ictaluri. J. Wildlife Dis. 26(2):214–218.

Shotts, E.B., Vanderwork, V.L., and Cambell, L.N. (1976) Occurrence of R factors associated with Aeromonas hydrophila isolates from aquarium fish and waters. J. Fish. Res. Bd. Can. 33:736–740.

Snieszko, S.F. (1957) Aeromonas. In: Bergey's Manual of Determinative Bacteriology. 7th ed. Williams & Wilkins, Baltimore, pp. 189–193.

Thune, R.L. (1980) Immunization of Channel Catfish (Ictalurus punctatus) Against Aeromonas Hydrophila via Hyperosmotic Infiltration. Ph.D. Thesis. Auburn University, Auburn.

Thune, R.L., Graham, T.E., Riddle, L.M., and Amborski, R.L. (1982a) Extracellular products and endotoxin from Aeromonas hydrophila: effect on age–0 channel catfish. Trans. Am. Fish. Soc. 111:404–408.

Thune, R.L., Graham, T.E., Riddle, L.M., and Amborski, R.L. (1982b) Extracellular proteases from Aeromonas hydrophila: partial purification and effects on age–0 channel catfish. Trans. Am. Fish. Soc. 111:749–754.

Thune, R.L., Johnson, M.C., Graham, T.E., and Amborski, R.L. (1986) Aeromonas hydrophila β-hemolysin: Purification and examination of its role in virulence in channel catfish. J. Fish Dis. 9:55–61.

Thune, R.L., Hawke, J.P., Johnson, M., and Busch, R. (1988) Enteric septicemia of catfish vaccination studies (Abstract). Proceedings of the International Fish Health Meeting, Vancouver, B.C., Canada, p. 36.

Tucker, C.S. (1989) Method for estimating potassium permanganate treatment rates for channel catfish in ponds. Progressive Fish Culturist 51:24–26.

Waltman, W.D., Shotts, E.B., and Blazer, V.S. (1985) Recovery of Edwardsiella ictaluri from danio (Danio devario). Aquaculture 46:63–66.

Waltman, W.D., Shotts, E.B., and Hsu, T.C. (1986) Biochemical characteristics of Edwardsiella ictaluri. Appl. Environ. Microbiol. 51(1):101–104.

Wyatt, L.E., Nichelson, R., and Vanderzant, C. (1979) Edwardsiella tarda in freshwater catfish and their environment. Appl. Environ. Microbiol. 38(4):710–714.

Chapter 58

FUNGAL DISEASES OF CATFISHES

MICHAEL K. STOSKOPF

There are surprisingly few reports of fungal diseases in catfishes (Table 58–1). Catfishes are probably susceptible to a variety of fungal infections that have yet to be reported in the literature. Responses of catfishes to fungal organisms are not significantly different from those of other fish species to those organisms that have been reported to affect catfishes.

EXOPHIALIOSIS

SYNONYM. Fungal ulcer disease.

Host and Geographic Distribution

A single epizootic caused by *Exophiala pisciphila* in channel catfish has been reported in the literature. This outbreak occurred in a pond in Alabama (Fijan, 1969). Other species of catfishes are probably also susceptible.

Clinical Signs, Pathology, and Diagnosis

Clinical signs are dominated by the presence of round or irregular skin ulcers, 2 to 15 mm in diam-

TABLE 58–1. Fungal Diseases of Catfishes*

Disease	Organism	Host
Exophialiosis	*Exophiala pisciphila*	Channel catfish, white catfish, bluegill, and several other species
Branchiomycosis	*Branchiomyces* spp.	Black bullhead and other species
Saprolegniasis	*Saprolegnia* spp.	Brown bullhead and other species

*See also Chapters 25, 49, 68, and 79.

eter. Upon gross examination, soft nodules of varying size are evident in the abdominal organs. Histologically, acute nonproliferative responses and chronic proliferative granulomatous responses can be found to hyphae. Diagnosis is based upon culture and identification of the organism. No serologic tests are available.

Culture and Identification

The organism can be cultured from the nodular lesions in abdominal organs. Potato-dextrose, cereal, or V-8 juice agar can be used to culture *E. pisciphila*, but it does not grow well on Sabouraud's agar. Colonies are black or gray and reach 25 to 28 mm in diameter in 14 days at 25°C. Incubation at 37°C results in no growth. *Exophiala pisciphila* is a yellow-brown hypomycete with aseptate conidia.

Transmission, Epidemiology, Treatment, and Control

The disease has not been well studied in catfishes. Intraperitoneal injection of suspensions of organisms cultured from the outbreak in channel catfish have resulted in experimental infections in channel catfish, white catfish, and bluegill. These fish began to die 13 days after injection and all injected animals died within 1 month (Fijan, 1969).

LITERATURE CITED

Fijan, N. (1969) Systemic mycosis in channel catfish. Bull. Wildlife Dis. Assoc. 5:109–110.

Chapter 59

CATFISH VIRUSES

RONALD L. THUNE

Catfish are undoubtedly affected by numerous viruses yet to be characterized. The intensive nature of production culture of channel catfish in the United States has resulted in the identification and characterization of virus diseases affecting that species. Essentially all viral research on catfish has been on diseases of the channel catfish. This chapter discusses two viral diseases affecting channel catfish (Table 59–1).

CHANNEL CATFISH VIRUS DISEASE

Host and Geographic Distribution

Channel catfish virus disease (CCVD) was initially found throughout the catfish industry in the southeastern United States, but has subsequently been isolated in almost every area with commercial catfish development. The principal host is the channel catfish, although low-grade mortalities have been induced in blue catfish and hybrid blue × channel catfish by injection, but not by natural routes of infection (Plumb and Chappel, 1978). Different strains of channel catfish have different mortality rates when injected with live virus (Plumb et al., 1975).

Clinical Signs

Clinically, channel catfish virus disease manifests primarily in fry and fingerlings less than 10 cm long. External signs include erratic swimming, petechial hemorrhage at the base of the fins and throughout the skin, severe exophthalmia and abdominal swelling (Fig. 59–1). Gills are often pale, sometimes with petechiae. Fish often swim in a head-high posture at the surface, and at the edges of the pond.

TABLE 59–1. Viral Diseases of Channel Catfish

Disease	Virus	Host
Channel catfish disease	Channel catfish herpesvirus	Channel catfish, blue catfish, channel × blue hybrids
Unknown	Channel catfish reovirus	Channel catfish

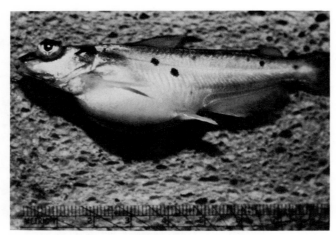

FIGURE 59–1. Fingerling channel catfish showing the abdominal distention and exophthalmia characteristic of channel catfish virus infection. (Courtesy of the Southeastern Cooperative Fish Disease Laboratory, Auburn University, Alabama.)

Pathology

Affected fish have generalized petechial hemorrhage in the musculature. The liver and kidney are pale and the spleen enlarged and congested. The abdominal cavity usually contains a clear yellow ascitic fluid. Histologically, renal lesions include necrosis of hematopoietic tissue, tubules and occasionally glomeruli. Macrophages invade the hematopoietic tissue. Hepatic edema, necrosis, and congestion are usually evident. Intestinal edema with focal areas of macrophage invasion is common. Splenic congestion and hemorrhage, occasionally with mild necrosis of hematopoietic tissue, is seen.

Diagnosis, Culture, and Identification

Channel catfish virus is an α herpesvirus. It is enveloped, 90 to 100 μm in diameter, and has icosahedral symmetry. Replication of the viral deoxyribonucleic acid (DNA) occurs in the nucleus, and the envelope is obtained by budding through nuclear, intercytoplasmic, and outer cell membranes. Channel catfish virus epizootics are currently diagnosed by culturing filtered tissue extracts on susceptible cells lines such as channel catfish ovary or brown bullhead cells and examining them at 24 and 48 hours for the characteristic fusion produced by viral infection (Fig. 59–2). Positive identification is provided by serum neutralization procedures if desired. An indirect fluorescent antibody technique can be used to detect viral antigen in tissue and primary cell cultures (Plumb et al., 1981). A recombinant DNA technology using a channel catfish virus probe with a sensitivity limit of detection of one viral DNA per cell has been developed (Wise and Boyle, 1985).

Usually virus can only be isolated from fish with active infections during an epizootic. The preferred sample for virus isolation is a live, freshly dead, or moribund fish. The kidney is the primary organ affected and yields maximum infectious viral particles. It is the tissue of choice when attempting isolation, although a pool of tissue from several internal organs is often used. Skeletal muscle yields very low virus numbers and only in latter stages of the infection.

Virus will persist in iced fish for up to 14 days, but with a loss of about 90% of infectivity. Fish stored at −20°C maintain up to 50% infectivity after storage for 100 days (Plumb et al., 1973). Channel catfish virus has been isolated from healthy adult broodfish using a leukocyte coculture procedure enhanced by immunosuppression of the fish with dexamethasone (Bowser et al., 1985).

Transmission, Epidemiology, and Pathogenesis

Transmission of channel catfish virus occurs both horizontally and vertically. The exact mode of transmission is unknown, but the virus is easily transmitted from fish to fish during an epizootic. Probably the infection progresses from entry through the branchial and intestinal epithelium. In experiments in which the virus was inoculated intraperitoneally, virus appeared in the kidney within 24 to 48 hours and was subsequently isolated from the intestine and liver at 72 to 96 hours and finally from the brain at 96 to 120 hours postexposure (Plumb, 1971).

Channel catfish virus disease is primarily a disease of fry and fingerlings. Fish older than 1 year or longer than 10 to 15 cm are not susceptible to experimental challenge. Larger fish are not at risk in natural conditions, although the virus has been isolated from moribund broodfish under severe winter conditions (Bowser et al., 1985). Mortality rates are directly related to water temperature, with the most severe losses occurring in water temperatures greater

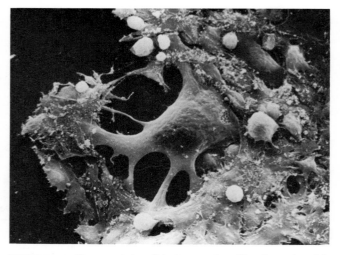

FIGURE 59–2. Characteristic cell fusion produced by channel catfish virus in channel catfish ovary cells at 24 hours incubation.

than 28°C. The rate of development of clinical disease is also directly related to water temperature, with clinical signs developing in 32 to 72 hours at 30°C, whereas at 20°C the incubation period is 10 days.

A majority of commercial channel catfish carry channel catfish virus DNA in a latent state (Wise et al., 1985). The carrier state does not correlate with channel catfish virus disease history or serum-neutralizing activity. Concurrent infections with bacterial pathogens such as *Aeromonas hydrophila, Edwardsiella ictaluri,* and *Flexibacter columnaris* are common in commercial production units and it is often difficult to establish a primary cause. It has been postulated that the high mortalities seen in commercial situations are not due solely to virus but are the result of concurrent infections and water-quality problems (McConnell and Austen, 1978).

Early work with channel catfish virus disease supplied circumstantial evidence for vertical transmission of the virus from adults to fry via the reproductive products. Epizootics in fry and fingerlings usually correlate with the use of broodfish with detectable levels of serum-neutralizing activity. Channel catfish virus DNA probe studies on fry from the mating of two virus-positive fish showed all offspring to be positive for channel catfish virus DNA, indicating vertical transmission (Wise et al., 1985).

Treatment and Control

There is no effective treatment for channel catfish virus disease once an epizootic begins, making prevention the only effective means of managing the disease. One possibility, given the situation of vertical transmission, is to use virus-free broodfish. However, the widespread presence of the channel catfish virus in commercial catfish operations probably precludes this approach. Losses resulting from channel catfish virus disease can be minimized or eliminated by following some simple management practices that will also benefit the fish farmer by reducing bacterial and protozoan problems.

The development of channel catfish virus disease is strongly stress associated, with conditions of low dissolved oxygen and high water temperatures favoring disease development.This is especially true when fish are crowded or handled during periods of poor water quality. Sanitation should be maintained by ensuring proper water flow and circulation, and by removing eggshell debris and wasted feed daily. Fish should be fed a nutritionally complete fry starter with a minimum of 50% protein. If disease risk is suspected, stocking densities should be less than 100,000/acre and feeding rates should be held under 75 lb/acre, especially during periods of high water temperature. Handling of susceptible fingerlings at temperatures greater than 25°C increases the risk of disease, and as a general rule, harvesting and handling of fingerlings should be conducted when water temperatures are less than 20°C. Maintenance of adequate dissolved oxygen levels using supplemental aeration will also reduce the risk of losses to channel catfish virus.

CHANNEL CATFISH REOVIRUS

Host and Geographic Distribution

Channel catfish reovirus (CCRV, CRV) was isolated from fish undergoing chronic mortality in southern California (Amend et al., 1984). To date, there are no reports of this virus elsewhere in the world and significant epizootics have not been described.

Clinical Signs, Diagnosis, and Pathology

The only signs of channel catfish reovirus are moderate mortality (Wolf, 1988). Hyperplasia of gill lamellae and gill epithelial fusion can be seen in affected fish. Diagnosis must be made by viral isolation.

Antisera to channel catfish reovirus does not neutralize the virus but does partially neutralize two other fish reoviruses, golden shiner virus and Chum salmon virus, indicating that channel catfish reovirus is probably a third serotype of a novel group of reoviruses from fish (Wolf, 1988).

Channel catfish reovirus induces extensive fusion in channel catfish ovary cells incubated at 26°C. It also replicates in BB and CHSE-214 cell lines, but with only minimal cytopathic effect. Purified virions are double-shelled icosahedral capsids with an average diameter of 75 μm and a genome composed of double-stranded RNA in 11 segments, placing the virus in the reovirus group.

Transmission, Epidemiology, Treatment, and Control

Nothing is known about the transmission or epidemiology of this virus. No treatment or control measures are known.

LITERATURE CITED

Amend, D.F., McDowell, T., and Hedrick, R.P. (1984) Characteristics of a previously unidentified virus from channel catfish *(Ictalurus punctatus).* Can. J. Fish. Aquatic Sci. 41:807–811.
Bowser, P.R., Munson, A.D., Jarboe, H.H., Francis-Floyd, R., and Waterstrat, P.R. (1985) Isolation of channel catfish virus from channel catfish, *Ictalurus punctatus* (Rafinesque), brood stock. J. Fish Dis. 8:557–561.
McConnell, S. and Austen, J.D. (1978) Serologic screening of channel catfish virus. Marine Fish. Rev. 40:30–32.
Plumb, J.A. (1971) Tissue distribution of channel catfish virus. J. Wildlife Dis. 7:213–216.
Plumb, J.A. (1973) Survival of channel catfish virus in chilled, frozen and decomposing channel catfish. Progressive Fish Culturist 35:170–172.
Plumb, J.A., and Chappel, J. (1978) Susceptibility of blue catfish to channel catfish virus. Proc. Ann. Conf. Southeast. Assoc. Fish Wildlife Agenc. 32:680–685.
Plumb, J.A., Green, J.A., Smitherman, R.O., and Pardue, G.B. (1975) Channel catfish virus experiments with different strains of channel catfish. Trans. Am. Fish. Soc. 104:140–143.

Plumb, J. A., Thune, R.L., and Klesius, P.H. (1981) Detection of channel catfish virus in adult fish. Dev. Biol. Stand. 49:29–34.

Wise, J.A., and Boyle, J.A. (1985) Detection of channel catfish virus in channel catfish, *Ictalurus punctatus* (Rafinesque): use of a nucleic acid probe. J. Fish Dis. 8:417–424.

Wise, J.A., Bowser, P.R., and Boyle, J.A. (1985) Detection of channel catfish virus in a symptomatic adult channel catfish, *Ictalurus punctatus* (Rafinesque). J. Fish. Dis. 8:485–493.

Wolf, K. (1988) Fish Viruses and Fish Viral Diseases. Cornell University Press, Ithaca, New York.

Chapter 60

PARASITES OF CATFISHES

RONALD L. THUNE

Protozoa are the most significant parasitic organisms affecting commercially raised catfishes, accounting for nearly all fish losses associated with parasitic agents. Some protozoa do not cause significant pathology and do not derive nutritional benefit from the host. These ectocommensals utilize the host only for attachment and derive their nutrition from the pond water. There is still some controversy relative to the commensal/parasitic status of some external protozoa found on catfishes. The protozoa listed in Table 60–1 are significant problems in commercial catfish culture.

PROLIFERATIVE GILL DISEASE

SYNONYM. Hamburger gill disease.

Host and Geographic Distribution

Proliferative gill disease is a serious parasitic problem that has been described only in channel catfish. It has been reported throughout the catfish-growing regions of the southeastern United States and California.

TABLE 60–1. Protozoa Found in Catfishes

Myxospora
  Proliferative gill disease organism
  Henneguya

Ciliophora
  Ambiphrya
  Apiosoma
  Chilodonella
  Ichthyophthirius
  Trichodina
  Trichophrya

Sarcomastigophora
  Ichthyobodo

Clinical Signs and Diagnosis

Fish infested with proliferative gill disease become anorexic early in the development of the disease. Affected fish are extremely listless and exhibit increased susceptibility to moderately low dissolved oxygen levels. The principal external sign is massive degeneration of the primary lamellae of the gills (Fig. 60–1). Proliferative gill disease can be presumptively diagnosed by observation of pale, swollen, clubbed, and broken gill lamellae (Fig. 60–2). In early stages, where filament breakage and loss has not occurred, microscopic examination of wet mounts will generally reveal focal areas of clearing of the cartilaginous support rod of the lamella. Although this cartilaginous necrosis is a strong indicator that the proliferative gill disease organism is present, microscopic examination of histologic sections for the character-

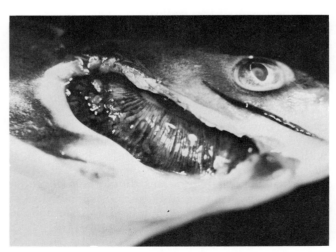

FIGURE 60–1. A channel catfish with severe degeneration of the primary lamellae resulting from an infestation with proliferative gill disease.

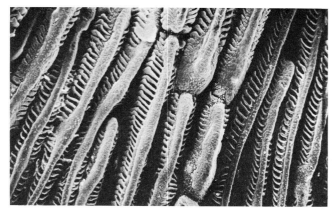

FIGURE 60–2. An electron micrograph of a channel catfish gill lamella affected by proliferative gill disease.

istic cyst is often required for confirmation. Cysts are usually not visible in necropsy wet mounts unless samples are examined from live fish within a few minutes of excision.

Pathologic Effects and Pathogenesis

In early stages of proliferative gill disease the gill lamellae appear pale and swollen, progressing to a state where filament breakage and loss are apparent. Light microscopy of early infections reveals extensive epithelial hyperplasia that in combination with infiltrating inflammatory cells, results in occlusion of the lamellar troughs. As the infestation progresses, severely swollen nodules that contain characteristic parasitic cysts become apparent (Fig. 60–3). Moderate to severe cartilaginous necrosis, along with hydropic degeneration and liquefactive necrosis of cells within the nodules, is characteristic. Necrosis of the cartilaginous support rod ultimately results in breakage and loss of the lamella. Histochemical stains and ultra-

structural examination of infested tissue demonstrate intense concentrations of neutrophils surrounding the parasite (Fig. 60–4), and there is a significant heterophilia in the circulating blood. Although the primary pathology of proliferate gill disease is in the gills, cysts have been detected in the liver, cranial and caudal kidney, spleen, and brain. An extrasporogonic stage of a myxosporidian has been described in the circulating blood of fish from an epidemic of proliferative gill disease, but the possibility of a concurrent infection could not be ruled out (Groff et al., 1989). Severe inflammatory responses to the cysts in tissues other than the gills are not apparent. In fish that survive, the final stage of infection is characterized by an absence of cysts in the gills and chondroplasia associated with regeneration of the lamellae.

Life Cycle, Transmission, and Epidemiology

Clinically, proliferative gill disease has occurred at temperatures from 14 to 26°C, but predominantly from 16 to 20°C. After experimental exposure to sediments from ponds with ongoing epidemics at temperatures above 16°C, fish develop clinical disease (MacMillan et al., 1989). Clinical data to date suggest that the occurrence of proliferative gill disease is associated with new ponds, and that recurrence in previously affected ponds is rare and generally occurs only in ponds that have been drained and refilled. All sizes of fish are affected by proliferative gill disease, with mortality rates ranging from less than 1% to greater than 90%.

The etiology of proliferative gill disease is currently controversial, although it is almost certainly a myxosporidian. Initial reports implicated *Henneguya*

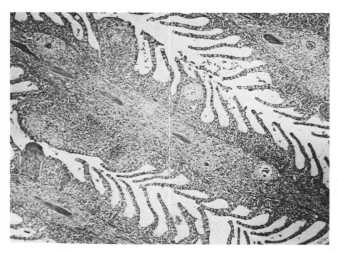

FIGURE 60–3. A thin section of channel catfish gill lamellae showing the intense proliferative response and characteristic cysts of proliferative gill disease.

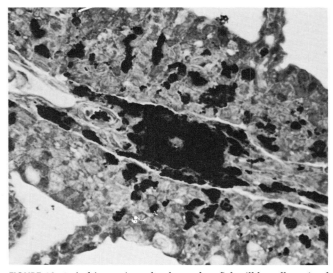

FIGURE 60–4. A thin section of a channel catfish gill lamella stained for heterophils with Sudan black B. Note the intense concentration of black-stained heterophils and the central proliferative gill disease cyst.

sp. (Bowser and Conroy, 1985; Haskins et al., 1985), but this was most likely due to concurrent infections. Ultrastructural studies have noted distinct differences in the development of the progressive gill disease organism and *Henneguya* sp. Also, transmission studies conducted by exposing specific pathogen–free catfish to pond water or mud from ponds experiencing epidemics did not result in the production of mature *Henneguya* sp. spores (MacMillan et al., 1989). The occurrence of a bloodborne form that appeared to be a *Sphaerospora* sp. in catfish with clinical progressive gill disease, and the presence of possible mature sphaerospores from wet mounts of kidney has been noted (Groff et al., 1989). There are similarities between the progressive gill disease organism induced experimentally and the myxosporidians associated with gill sphaerosporosis and swimbladder inflammation in carp (MacMillan et al., 1989). When the lack of information about mature spore development, the lack of recurrence in affected ponds, and the acute nature of the inflammatory response are considered, it is possible that the channel catfish are not the normal host for the parasite.

The mode of transmission of the proliferative gill disease organism is unknown, but as a myxosporidian parasite it is most likely an oral route. A myxosporidian similar to *Guyenotia* has been observed in tubifex worms from ponds with ongoing epidemics (Burtle, 1989), so it is possible that the organism has a life cycle similar to that proposed for *Myxosoma cerebralis* in trout. However, to date, infection trials with infected worms have not been successful.

Treatment and Control

Management options to reduce losses are limited. Harvesting and marketing all market-size fish is a common practice in affected ponds with a high percentage of harvestable fish. Maintenance of high dissolved oxygen and low un-ionized ammonia levels are of benefit, especially with less severe infestations and lower mortality rates. Suggestions to pump water from unaffected ponds have been made based on anecdotal data, but the effectiveness of this procedure is unproven. When no action of any kind was taken to mitigate losses, 14 of 33 outbreaks in Louisiana resolved themselves with less than 10% mortality. This is similar to the success rate attributed to pumping. However, in practice, pumping water is unlikely to do harm and may help maintain water quality. Suggestions to apply chemical treatments are controversial and efficacy is unproven. There are some indications that mortality may actually be increased as a result of drug toxicity. There is currently no known therapeutant that can be safely and successfully administered to treat progressive gill disease.

HENNEGUYA INFESTATION

SYNONYMS. Myxosporidiosis, blister disease, adipose fin disease.

Clinical Signs and Diagnosis

Henneguya is a common myxosporidian parasite of channel catfish, although it rarely causes extensive mortality. The forms of *Henneguya* that are found on the skin appear as white cysts or as white amorphous masses. Gill forms can be present as a visible cyst but are generally inapparent to the naked eye. Microscopic diagnosis of *Henneguya* is made by examining wet mounts of gill biopsies or cysts for characteristic elongated spores with two polar capsules and a pair of extended tails.

Pathology and Pathogenesis

There are six species of *Henneguya* currently recognized in catfish, with speciation dependent on the location of the cyst and several spore characteristics, including total length (Minchew, 1977). Three of these species occur on the body and three on the gills. *Henneguya diversis* causes formation of gross cutaneous masses. *Henneguya pellis* forms small cutaneous blisters on the skin and is called the blister form (Fig. 60–5). *Henneguya adiposa* occurs as a small rice grain–sized cyst in the adipose fin.

The three species found in the gill are *Henneguya exilis, Henneguya longicauda,* and *Henneguya postexilis.* These three species cause three distinct forms of disease in catfish gills: a visible cyst form, an intralamellar (intracapillary) form, and an interlamellar form (McCraren et al., 1975; Minchew, 1977; Current and Janovy, 1978). There is some confusion in the literature concerning which parasitic species causes which form, but it is thought that *Henneguya exilis* causes the visible form, with cyst sizes up to 1 mm (Minchew, 1977). *Henneguya postexilis* or *Henneguya longicauda* can apparently both cause either intralamellar or interlamellar forms of disease, depending on whether the initial site of infection is within the blood sinuses of the lamellae or within the connective tissue. Regardless of the parasitic species involved, the most severe pathology is associated with the interlamellar form, which can cause almost complete occlusion of the lamellar troughs (see Fig. 60–5) and

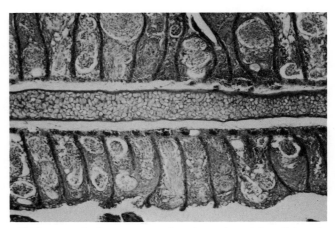

FIGURE 60–5. A thin section of a channel catfish gill lamella demonstrating extensive occlusion of the lamellar troughs associated with an interlamellar infestation with *Henneguya* sp.

result in significant mortality (McCraren et al., 1975; Current and Janovy, 1978).

Grossly, *Henneguya postexilis* and *Henneguya longicauda* are inapparent except in severe infestations, in which case the gills may have a pale white cast. Differentiation of the three gill species in wet mounts is based on spore lengths (*Henneguya exilis*, 52 μm; *Henneguya postexilis*, 70 μm; and *Henneguya longicauda*, 108 μm).

Treatment and Control

There is no treatment for *Henneguya* sp. infestations. In cases of moderate or severe interlamellar disease, supplemental aeration can give relief, particularly when moderately low dissolved oxygen is a problem.

ECTOCOMMENSAL PROTOZOANS

Clinical Signs and Diagnosis

Catfish exhibiting respiratory distress when dissolved oxygen concentrations are marginal (2 to 3 ppm) may be harboring significant protozoan infestations. The presence of ectocommensal protozoa on catfishes is determined by microscopic examination of skin scrapings and gill clippings from moribund or freshly dead fish, preferably under a phase contrast microscope. Samples must be fresh because these organisms detach and become free-swimming soon after the death of the host. Individual parasites are identified by their distinctive physical features.

Trichophrya sp. are characterized by a lack of cilia on mature stages and by asexual reproduction by budding. *Trichophrya* sp. have distinctive feeding tentacles on a rounded, orange to brown body (Fig. 60–6). These organisms can be overlooked, particularly in old specimens, because the tentacles may be

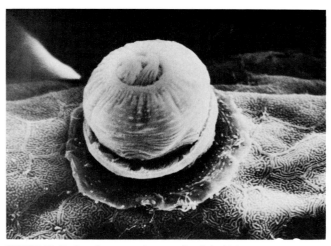

FIGURE 60–7. An electron micrograph of *Ambiphrya* sp. on the gill of a channel catfish. Note the oral and medial rings of cilia and the large basal attachment disc.

retracted. Careful examination of the gills will reveal the orange-brown rounded organisms in lamellar troughs.

Several species of *Trichodina*, including *Trichodina discoidea* and *Trichodina vallata* (Wellborn, 1967), have been described on catfishes. Speciation on wet mounts is difficult and generally not done. Differences in pathogenesis between species has not been reported. *Trichodina* organisms are generally observed moving over the surface of the gills or skin in fresh preparations, but they are capable of attaching to the epithelium using the adoral region as an adhesive disk (Lom, 1973).

Ambiphrya ameiuri and *Apiosoma* sp. are very similar peritrichous ciliates commonly found attached to the gill epithelium of commercial channel catfish. They have cylindrical bodies with enlarged attachment disks and medial and oral rings of cilia (Fig. 60–7). Although the two genera can be distinguished by the ribbon-shaped macronucleus in *Ambiphrya* and the compact, lobular one in *Apiosoma* (Wellborn and Rogers, 1966), the distinction apparently has no clinical consequence.

Both *Ambiphrya* and *Apiosoma* are considered ectocommensal and do not penetrate the host epithelium to assist attachment or derive any nutrients from the host (Fitzgerald et al., 1982). However, since both organisms are bacteriovores, the high levels of organic matter that results in extremely high bacterial concentrations in catfish pond water are conducive to heavy proliferation of these protozoa (Thompson et al., 1947).

Pathology and Pathogenesis

Excessive numbers of ectocommensal protozoa on the gill epithelium results in occlusion of the respiratory epithelium, disruption of the laminar flow of water through the gills, and irritation-induced mucus production that together greatly reduce res-

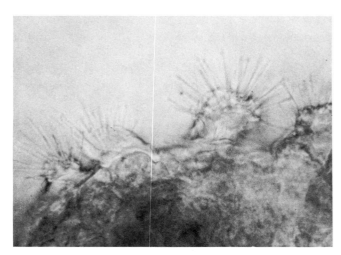

FIGURE 60–6. *Trichophrya* sp. attached to channel catfish gill epithelium showing the distinctive tentacled appearance of the parasite.

piratory efficiency and can result in significant mortality. In less severe situations, these organisms reduce catfish feeding activity and retard growth.

Life Cycle, Transmission, and Epidemiology

Ectocommensal protozoa on catfish have direct life cycles, reproducing on the host by simple cell division. The sessile forms are transmitted from fish to fish via motile dispersal forms that can either be produced by budding, as in *Trichophrya*, or by detachment of the trophozoite and subsequent transformation into a motile form.

The nutrient-rich conditions of catfish ponds are conducive to blooms of plankton and microorganisms that are the primary food of ectocommensal protozoa. In combination with the effects of poor water quality on the general health and activity of catfish in commercial ponds, the nutrient-rich conditions can result in extremely high levels of these organisms on the gill surface.

Often more severe bacterial or viral disease problems are associated with increased numbers of ectocommensal protozoa. It is sometimes difficult to determine whether the protozoa have proliferated on a host weakened by the concomitant infectious disease or vice-versa. In this case, it may be helpful to evaluate protozoan loads on apparently healthy individuals.

Treatment and Control

Owing to its efficacy and low cost, the most common treatment for ectocommensal protozoa on catfish is copper sulfate at a rate equal to the alkalinity of the pond water divided by 100 and expressed in milligrams per liter. For example, in a pond with an alkalinity of 150, copper sulfate should be added at a rate of 0.15 mg/L (150/100 = 0.15). However, since copper sulfate is also a potent algicide, precautions should be taken in anticipation of an algal die-off and subsequent oxygen depletion. Also, chemical treatment to control protozoa will often exacerbate bacterial infections and should be avoided in cases of mixed etiology unless the fish are off feed and will not accept antibiotic-treated feed.

One approach to controlling ectocommensal protozoa is to anticipate potential problems in early spring, and to have fish checked and treated if protozoan loads are high prior to the development of pond temperatures conducive to bacterial or viral disease.

Formalin (125 to 250 mg/L) is occasionally used to treat protozoa on fingerling and stocker-size catfish in short-duration baths in holding or hauling tanks prior to shipping or restocking. Formalin is rarely used in catfish ponds because of the expense and the negative effect on dissolved oxygen concentrations.

CHILODONELLA INFESTATION

Clinical Signs and Diagnosis

Chilodonella is a round to heart-shaped ciliate with a flattened body and several rows of ventral and dorsal cilia that can be seen in wet mounts of gill and skin preparations. Two species have been described that can be distinguished by the number and arrangement of the ciliary rows: *Chilodonella hexasticha* and *Chilodonella cyprini*. *Chilodonella hexasticha* has 9 to 15 left ciliary rows and 8 to 13 right rows. *Chilodonella cyprini* has 5 to 8 left ciliary rows and 6 to 10 right rows (Kazubski and Migala, 1974; Wiles et al., 1985).

Pathologic Effects and Pathogenesis

Chilodonella sp. can elicit pronounced responses in the gills and skin of infested fish, suggesting that they may feed directly on epithelial cells (Wiles et al., 1985). Attachment to the gill surface either by a coagulated substance on the host cell surface or by ventral cilia has been described (Paperna and Van As, 1983; Wiles et al., 1985).

Life Cycle, Transmission, and Epidemiology

Both species of *Chilodonella* appear to be obligate parasites, with transmission occurring by fish to fish contact (Van Dujin, 1967; Mawdesley-Thomas and Jolly, 1967; Hoffman, 1979). The clinical implications of speciation are not clear, but *Chilodonella cyprini* usually infects the gills and skin of young hosts and *Chilodonella hexasticha* is found on the gills of older fish only (Wiles et al., 1985). Although *Chilodonella* infestations in catfishes occur primarily in cool water, *Chilodonella hexasticha* can cause mortality at 21°C (Rogers, 1979).

Treatment and Control

Treatment and control of *Chilodonella* is the same as for the ectocommensal protozoa.

ICHTHYOBODO INFESTATION

Ichthyobodo, previously known as *Costia*, is a genus of small tear-shaped parasites, about the size of a red blood cell, that attaches to the skin and gills of catfish (Fig. 60-8). On microscopic examination, *Ichthyobodo* may be difficult to diagnose because of its small size. Best success is achieved when fresh specimens are available and the characteristic "flickering" movement of the parasite is visible. *Ichthyobodo* detaches from a dead host rather quickly, and it is

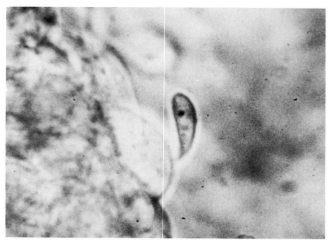

FIGURE 60–8. *Ichthyobodo* sp. attached to a channel catfish gill epithelial cell. (Courtesy of the Southeastern Cooperative Fish Disease Laboratory, Auburn University, Alabama.)

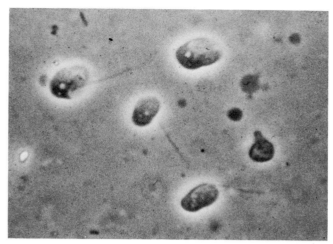

FIGURE 60–9. Flagellated, free-swimming forms of *Ichthyobodo* sp.

not uncommon to primarily observe free-swimming forms (Fig. 60–9).

Ichthyobodo is an obligate parasite that extends small tubules into the host cell for both attachment and feeding purposes (Schubert, 1966; Robertson et al., 1981). Affected fish often exhibit a blue to gray film caused by excess mucus production in the areas where the parasite is attached.

Ichthyobodo has a direct life cycle. The parasite is discussed in detail in Chapter 70. The free-swimming stage is destructive. *Ichthyobodo* infestations occur primarily in the cooler months of the year. Mortality can range from chronic to acute depending on the level of parasitism and the pond water–quality conditions. Treatment and control are the same as for the ectocommensal protozoa.

ICHTHYOPHTHIRIUS MULTIFILIIS INFESTATION

Clinical Signs and Diagnosis

Ichthyophthiriasis is a serious parasitic disease of catfishes. The disease is covered in detail in Chapter 70.

Contrary to the other ectoprotozoa of catfishes, *Ichthyophthirius multifiliis* has an indirect life cycle. The adult stage or trophont develops within the epithelium of the skin or gills where it actively feeds on host fluids and tissue (Beckert and Allison, 1964). After several days residence on the catfish, the mature parasite exits by rupturing the overlying host epithelial cells. The life cycle of the parasite on catfish is identical to the cycle on tropical freshwater fishes. Temperature plays an important role in the development of *Ichthyophthirius multifiliis* infestations. At 21 to 24°C, the life cycle takes 3 to 4 days, but takes 10 to 14 days at 15°C and up to 5 weeks at 10°C (Meyer, 1974). In addition, the maximum number of

theronts produced per trophont is 2.5 times greater at 24 than at 21°C in 5 days (Ewing et al., 1986).

Early detection and treatment of an *Ichthyophthirius* infestation is critical to successful control because the parasite burden can increase very rapidly, and the mortality rate is directly proportional to the number of trophonts infecting the fish (McCallum, 1985).

Any treatment currently available for use against *Ichthyophthirius multifiliis* is not effective against encysted parasites on the fish. Therefore, multiple treatments are required. In catfishes, three or four copper sulfate treatments are recommended at 2- to 5-day intervals, depending on the water temperature. At higher ambient temperatures (21 to 24°C) treatments should be applied every other day. At 15°C, a 3- to 4-day interval is more appropriate because of the slower development of the parasite.

LITERATURE CITED

Beckert, H., and Allison, R. (1964) Some host responses of white catfish to *Ichthyophthirius multifiliis*, Fouquet. Proceedings from the Eighteenth Annual Conference, Southeastern Association of Game and Fish Commissioners 18:1–3.

Bowser, P.R., and Conroy, J.D. (1985) Histopathology of gill lesions in channel catfish associated with *Henneguya*. J. Wildlife Dis. 21(2):177–179.

Burtle, G.J., Harrison, L.R., and Styer, E.L. (1989) Discovery of a Triactinomyxid, *Guyenotia* sp., in tubifex worms from ponds with catfish showing granulomatous branchitis (PGD) (Abstract). Proceedings of the Joint Meeting of the Fish Health Section of the American Fisheries Society and the Eastern Fish Health Workshop, July 17–20, Annapolis, Maryland, p. 19.

Current, W.L., and Janovy, J. (1978) Comparative study of the ultrastructure of interlamellar and intralamellar types of *Henneguya exilis* Kudo from channel catfish. J. Protozool. 25:56–65.

Duhamel, G.E., Kent, M.L., Dybdal, N.O., and Hedrick, R.P. (1986) *Henneguya exilis* Kudo associated with granulomatous branchitis of channel catfish *Ictalurus punctatus* (Rafinesque). Vet. Pathol. 23:354–361.

Ewing, M.S., and Kocan, K.M. (1986) *Ichthyophthirius multifiliis* (Ciliophora) development in gill epithelium. J. Protozool. 33(3):369–374.

Ewing, M.S., and Kocan, K.M. (1987) *Ichthyophthirius multifiliis* (Ciliophora) exit from gill epithelium. J. Protozool. 34(3):309–312.

Ewing, M.S., Lynn, M.E., and Kocan, K.M. (1986) Critical periods in development of *Ichthyophthirius multifiliis* (Ciliophora) populations. J. Protozool. 33(3):388–391.

Ewing, M.S., Ewing, S.A., and Kocan, K.M. (1988) *Ichthyophthirius multifiliis* (Ciliophora): Population studies suggest reproduction in host epithelium. J. Protozool. 35(4):549–552.

Fitzgerald, M.E.C., Simco, B.A., and Coons, L.B. (1982) Ultrastructure of the peritrich ciliate *Ambiphrya ameiuri* and its attachment to the gills of the catfish *Ictalurus punctatus*. J. Protozool. 29(2):213–217.

Groff, J.M., McDowell, T., and Hedrick, R.P. (1989) Sphaerospores observed in the kidney of channel catfish *(Ictalurus punctatus).* Fish Health Sect. Am. Fish. Soc. Newslett. 17(1):5.

Haskins, C., Torrans, L., and Lowell, F. (1985) A sporozoan induced proliferative gill disease in channel catfish. Arkansas Farm Research March–April:6.

Hoffman, G.L., Kazubski, S.L., Mitchell, A.J., and Smith, C.E. (1979) *Chilodonella hexasticha* (Kiernik, 1909) (Protozoa: Ciliata) from North American warmwater fish. J. Fish Dis. 2:153–157.

Kazubski, S.L., and Migala, K. (1974) Studies on the distinctness of *Chilodonella cyprini* (Moroff) and *C. hexasticha* (Kiernik) (Chlamydodontidae, Gymnostomatida), ciliate parasites of fishes. Acta Protozool. 13:9–39.

Kudo, R.R. (1977) Protozoology. Charles C Thomas, Springfield, Illinois.

Lom, J. (1973) The adhesive disc of *Trichodonella* epizootica—Ultrastructure and injury to the host tissue. Folia Parasitol. (Praha) 20:193–202.

MacMillan, J.R., Wilson, C., and Thiyagarajah, A. (1989) Experimental induction of proliferative gill disease in specific-pathogen–free channel catfish. J Aquatic Anim. Health 1(4):245–254.

Mawdesley-Thomas, L.E., and Jolly, D.W. (1967) Diseases of fish. II. The goldfish *(Carassuis auratus).* J. Small Anim. Pract. 8:533–541.

McCallum, H.I. (1985) Population effects of parasite survival on host death: experimental studies of the interaction of *Ichthyophthirius multifiliis* and its fish host. Parasitology 90:529–547.

McCraren, J.P., Landolt, M.L., Hoffman, G.L., and Meyer, F.P. (1975) Variation in response of channel catfish to *Henneguya* sp. infections (Protozoa: Myxosporidea). J. Wildlife Dis. 11:2–7.

Meyer, F.P. (1974) Parasites of freshwater fishes; II, Protozoa 3. *Ichthyophthirius multifiliis.* Fish Disease Leaflet 2, United States Department of the Interior, Fish and Wildlife Service, Washington, D.C.

Minchew, C.D. (1977) Five new species of *Henneguya* (Protozoa: Myxosporida) from ictalurid fishes. J. Protozool. 24:213–220.

Paperna, I., and Van As, J.G. (1983) The pathology of *Chilodonella hexasticha* (Kiernik). Infections in cichlid fishes. J. Fish Biol. 23:441–450.

Robertson, D.A., Roberts, R.J., and Bullock, A.M. (1981) Pathogenesis and autoradiographic studies of the epidermis of salmonids infested with *Ichthyobodo necator* (Henneguy, 1983). J. Fish Dis. 4:113–125.

Rogers, W.A. (1979) Protozoan parasites. In: Principal Diseases of Farm Raised Catfish. (Plumb, J.A., ed.). Southern Cooperative Research Series No. 225, Alabama Agricultural Experiment Station, Auburn University, Auburn, pp. 28–37.

Schubert, G. (1966) Zur ultracytologie von *Costia necatrix* Leclerq, unter besonderer berucksichtigung des kinetoplast-mitochondrions. Z. Parasitenkunde 27:271–286.

Thompson, S., Kirkgaard, D., and Jahn, T.J. (1947) *Scyphidia ameiuri,* N. Sp., a peritrichous ciliate from the gills of the bullhead, *Ameiurus melas melas.* Trans. Am. Microsc. Soc. 66:315–317.

van Dujin, C. (1967) Diseases of Fish. Iliffe Books, London.

Wellborn, T.L. (1967) *Trichodina* (Ciliata: Urcerlariidae) of freshwater fishes of the southeastern United States. J. Protozool. 14:399–412.

Wellborn, T.L., and Rogers, W.A. (1966) A key to the common parasitic protozoans of North American fishes. Fisheries Bulletin No. 4, Auburn University Agricultural Experiment Station, Auburn, Alabama.

Wiles, M., Cone, D.K., and Odense, P.H. (1985) Studies on *Chilodonella cyprini* and *C. hexasticha* (Protozoa: Ciliata) by scanning electron microscopy. Can. J. Zool. 63:2483–2487.

Chapter 61

NEOPLASIAS OF CATFISHES

MARSHALL H. BELEAU

TABLE 61–1. Neoplasms Reported in Catfishes

Neoplasm/Location	Fish	References
Nervous System		
None reported		
Cardiovascular System		
Lymphosarcoma	Channel catfish	Bowser et al., 1985
Gastrointestinal System		
Hepatoma	Brown bullhead	Dawe et al., 1964
Urinary System		
Renal adenoma	Brown bullhead	Schlumberger and Lucké, 1948
Endocrine System		
None reported		
Reproductive System		
None reported		
Musculoskeletal System and Connective Tissue		
Leiomyoma	Indian catfish	Sarkar et al., 1955
Osteogenic fibroma	Attu catfish	Sarkar and Dutta-Chaudhuri, 1958
Lipoma	Channel catfish	McCoy et al., 1985
Integumentary System		
Melanoma	Armored catfish	Cohen, 1965
Papilloma	Yellow bullhead	Harshbarger, 1973
	Brown bullhead	Steeves, 1969
Squamous cell carcinoma	Brown bullhead	Harshbarger and Baumann, 1988
	Black bullhead	Harshbarger and Baumann, 1988
Epidermoid carcinoma	Brown bullhead	Lucké and Schlumberger, 1941

Catfishes are not known for their overt predisposition to neoplastic disorders. There has been only one report of tumors in catfish implicating environmental contamination: a transplantable epithelioma, sometimes invasive, occurred on the lips and buccal cavity of 166 brown bullheads from heavily polluted waters near Philadelphia (Lucké and Schlumberger, 1941). The early lesions consisted of a focal zone of intense hyperemia of the skin followed by epidermal thickening and finally by the development of epidermoid carcinoma. Autotransplants and homotransplants to the anterior chamber of the eye, and autotransplants to the cornea, were successful. The authors suggested the possible role of pollution in the etiology. The only other report of a large number of tumors in catfishes was 23 multiple leiomyomas occurring on the fins of Indian catfish (Sarkar et al., 1955).

Table 61–1 lists neoplasms reported in catfishes.

LITERATURE CITED

Bowser, P.R., McCoy, C.P., and MacMillan, J.R. (1985) A lymphoproliferative disorder in a channel catfish, *Ictalurus punctatus* (Rafinesque). J. Fish Dis. 8:465–469.

Cohen, S. (1965) Malignant melanoma of the eye of a catfish, *Corydoras juli*. Copeia 1965:382–383.

Dawe, C.J., Stanton, M.F., and Schwartz, F.J. (1964) Hepatic neoplasms in native bottom-feeding fish of Deep Creek Lake, Maryland. Cancer Res. 24:1194–1201.

Harshbarger, J. (1973) Activities Report. Registry of Tumors of Lower Animals. Museum of Natural History, Smithsonian Institution, Washington, D.C.

Harshbarger, J. (1988) Activities Report. Registry of Tumors of Lower Animals. Museum of Natural History, Smithsonian Institution, Washington, D.C.

Lucké, B., and Schlumberger, H.G. (1941) Transplantable epithelioma of the lip and mouth of catfish. I. Pathology. J. Exp. Med. 74:397–408.

McCoy, C.P., Bowser, P.R., Steeby, J.A., Beleau, M.H., and Schwedler, T.E. (1985) Lipoma in channel catfish (*Ictalurus punctatus* Rafinesque). J. Wildlife Dis. 21:74–76.

Sarkar, H.L., and Dutta-Chaudhuri, R. (1958) On the occurrence of osteogenic fibroma on the pre-maxilla of an Indian catfish, *Wallago attu* (Bloch and Schneider). Gann 49:65–68.

Sarkar, H.L., Kapoor, B.G., and Dutta-Chaudhuri, R. (1955) A study of leiomyoma, a mesenchymal tumour on the fins of an Indian catfish, *Mystus* (Osteobagrus) *seenghala* (Sykes). Growth 19:257–262.

Schlumberger, H.G., and Lucké, B. (1948) Tumors of fishes, amphibians, and reptiles. Cancer Res. 8:647–712.

Steeves, H.R. (1969) An epithelial papilloma of the brown bullhead, *Ictalurus nebulosus*. Natl. Cancer Inst. Monogr. 31:215–218.

SECTION V

FRESHWATER TROPICAL

FISHES

MICHAEL K. STOSKOPF, *Section Editor*

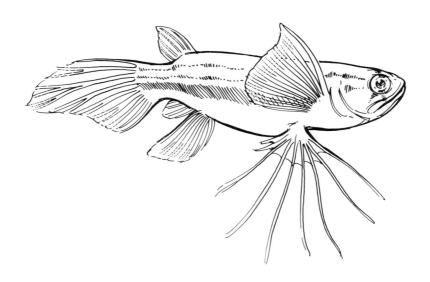

Chapter 62

TAXONOMY AND NATURAL HISTORY OF FRESHWATER TROPICAL FISHES

MICHAEL K. STOSKOPF

The diversity of species of tropical freshwater fishes is daunting (Axelrod et al., 1980; Mondadori, 1977; Riehl and Baensch, 1987; Studer, 1986). There are 15 families of catfishes displayed in home aquaria alone. This chapter gives a brief overview of 25 families that contain members frequently held in captivity. Common names are used throughout. The exact taxonomy of many of these fishes remains in flux, with some species having dozens of Latin synonyms. The most recent scientific nomenclature for each species mentioned can be found in Appendix VI.

BARBS AND RASBORAS (CYPRINIDAE)

This family is extremely large and diverse. It includes the barbs and rasboras, among other popular aquarium fishes. Examples of the family include the rosy barb (Fig. 62–1), which is a peaceful, undemanding fish from India, and the redtailed black shark (Fig. 62–2), actually a rasbora. The rosy barb prefers cooler, slightly acid water and requires some open swimming room in the tank.

The Siamese algae eater from Thailand is another peaceful member of the Cyprinidae; however, this fish will fight with other members of its own species. It prefers slightly acid, warm water. It is considered the best algae eater in an aquarium and is very common in hobbyists' tanks. The Siamese algae eater also eats planaria and other nematodes in addition to algae. It does not eat vascular plants.

BONY-TONGUED FISHES (OSTEOGLOSSIDAE)

This family of fishes includes four genera and six species. They all are quite large fish. The most commonly held in captivity are the arowanas (Fig. 62–3). These are large predatory fish that grow rapidly. They can be kept only with fish larger than themselves. They tend to swim in open areas near the surface. Arowanas can breathe air using their swimbladders as a respiratory organ. The arowanas are jumpers and should be kept only in covered tanks.

FRESHWATER BUTTERFLYFISHES (PANTODONTIDAE)

There is only a single species of freshwater butterflyfish; it is found in a limited region of the Niger delta and Ethiopian River in Zaire (Fig. 62–4). This fish has an accessory respiratory organ and does

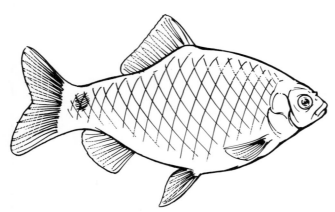

FIGURE 62–1. Rosy barb.

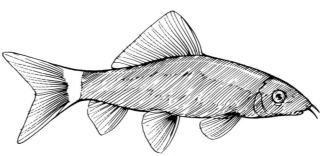

FIGURE 62–2. Red-tailed black shark.

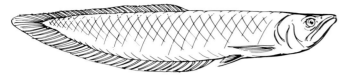

FIGURE 62–3. Arowana.

well in a shallow tank. It is generally intolerant of other surface fishes. Floating plants are important to its well-being in captivity. It is a good jumper, and tanks should be kept covered.

CATFISHES

The catfishes include 15 families of fishes. The aquaculturally important ones are covered in Section V. The common nomenclature for these families is confusing. Two separate families are called the armored catfishes. The family Loricariidae, usually referred to as armored or armor-plated catfishes, includes the popular "plecostomus" fishes and other algae eaters commonly found in home aquaria. The family Callichthyidae is also called the armored catfishes. This family includes the genus *Corydoras*, the popular large-headed, short-bodied, bottom-dwelling catfishes seen in almost every home tank (Fig. 62–5). Unfortunately, the genus *Corydoras* is also often referred to as the armored catfish, adding to the confusion. There are over 140 species in the genus *Corydoras*, about 10 of which are reared in captivity in production ponds, and another 20 or so are commercially available through collection in South America. In nature, the *Corydoras* species are schooling fish. Many species may be found together in joint schools in the wild. This group prefers slightly acid water with a fine gravel or sand bottom.

Other families of catfishes commonly kept in aquaria include the banjo catfishes (Aspredinidae), two families called naked catfishes (Bagridae and Mochocidae), the glass catfishes (Schilbeidae), thorny catfishes (Doradidae), and true catfishes (Siluridae). Most catfishes kept in aquaria are peaceful, but some

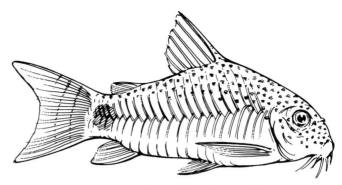

FIGURE 62–5. Spotted *Corydoras* catfish.

of the naked catfishes can be highly aggressive and will kill other smaller fish in the tank.

CICHLIDS (CICHLIDAE)

There are about 160 genera and more than 900 species of cichlids. The taxonomy is currently under revision, particularly with the large genus *Haplochromis*. The three largest genera are *Haplochromis*, *Cichlasoma*, and *Tilapia*. Most cichlids are small to medium-sized fish with a perchlike body (Fig. 62–6). The family is distinguished from the true perches and sunfishes by having one nostril on each side of the head. Cichlids have a single dorsal fin that is usually hard-rayed cranially and soft-rayed caudally. The lateral line of cichlids is usually divided into two distinct parts. Some species of cichlids, such as the freshwater angelfishes, are markedly laterally compressed.

Cichlids inhabit widely varied habitats, including salt water, soda lakes, and high-temperature waters (104°F). Members of the family are found in Central and South America, Africa, and parts of Asia. The approximately 200 American species range from southern Texas through Central America, Cuba, Haiti, and south to Argentina. In Asia, cichlids are found only in southern India and Sri Lanka as a single genus with three species. The most commonly held Asian cichlid is the chromide cichlid, a peaceful fish adapted to fresh and brackish water. In nature, the chromide cichlid is found in pairs. It prefers a

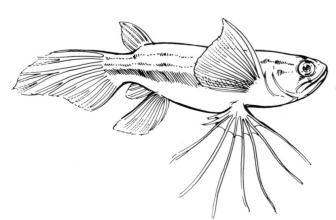

FIGURE 62–4. Freshwater butterflyfish.

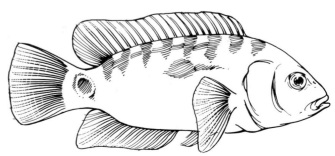

FIGURE 62–6. Jack Dempsey, a commonly kept cichlid species.

sandy bottom with a heavy growth of plants. African cichlids are distributed across the continent, with the exception of the northwest and southern tip of Africa. There are about 700 species of African cichlids.

COMB-TOOTHED BLENNIES (BLENNIIDAE)

This group of fishes has no swimbladder. They have elongated bodies and are either covered with small scales or are naked, having no scales. They are usually found in coastal waters, although some species inhabit fresh water and a few species can leave the water for brief forays on land. The blennies are territorial and usually burrow. It is best to hold only a single species in a tank. Breeding programs require three or four females to each male.

ELECTRIC EEL (ELECTROPHORIDAE)

There is only one species of electric eel. It has the typical eel shape, lacking dorsal and pelvic fins. It has a small tail fin that merges with the anal fin in a single line. Younger electric eels snap and fight. Larger specimens are more peaceful. It helps if electric eels destined for display together are raised together. Electric eels are nocturnal. They do best in a single-species tank with medium-sized gravel and acid water (pH 6). They have not been bred in captivity.

ELEPHANT-NOSED FISHES, OR MORMYRIDS (MORMYRIDAE)

The elephant-nosed fishes, or mormyrids, have a distinctive, comical appearance with their mouth extended like a nose or an elephant's trunk (Fig. 62–7). The protruding "trunk" is actually an extension of the mandible and sometimes also the rostrum. It is used as a sensory organ for weak electric signals. The mormyrids have a weak electric organ near their caudal peduncle. Peter's elephant-nosed fish is a nocturnal fish that is territorial and will harass weaker members of its own species. It prefers a heavily planted tank with darkness, caves to hide in, and a soft sandy bottom for burrowing. This species becomes nervous and increases its electric pulse rate

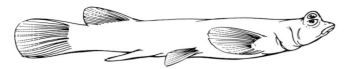

FIGURE 62–8. Four-eyes.

when water quality goes bad. For this reason, this species has been considered for biological waste water–treatment monitoring.

FOUR-EYES (ANABLEPIDAE)

This family has a single genus and three species, characterized by large protruding eyes that are each divided into two anterior chambers (Fig. 62–8). The dorsal anterior chamber is used for observing above the water surface, and the ventral chamber provides simultaneous focused vision below the water surface. These fish are surface dwellers that do best in shallow tanks with fine gravel or sand bottoms. They normally live in and thrive best in brackish water. All three species are good jumpers, and it is important to have a well-covered tank.

KILLIFISHES AND EGG-LAYING TOOTHCARPS (CYPRINODONTIDAE)

The killifishes and egg-laying toothcarp deserve much more coverage than they can receive here. They are very diverse and interesting fishes, with more than 450 species, with representatives from every continent except Antarctica and Australia. Most killifishes are tropical. They can be freshwater, estuarine, or marine. They are characterized by distinctive round scales and a lateral line system that is usually restricted to the area around the head (Fig. 62–9). Representative freshwater tropical species include the rivulus, medaka, and lyretail panchax.

KNIFEFISHES (APTERONOTIDAE, GYMNOTIDAE, RHAMPHICHTHYIDAE, AND NOTOPTERIDAE)

There are four families of knifefishes, including the speckled knifefish. The speckled knifefishes (Ap-

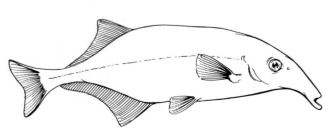

FIGURE 62–7. Elephantnose fish, a typical mormyrid.

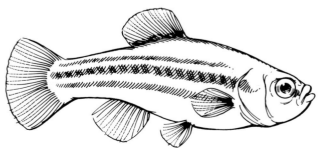

FIGURE 62–9. Cuban killifish.

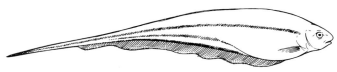

FIGURE 62–10. Green knifefish.

teronotidae) have an elongated, laterally flattened, tapered body, a small caudal peduncle, and distinct caudal fin. The anal opening of these fishes is found under the chin, anterior in the abdomen. These South American fish can be aggressive but are generally timid and prefer a dark aquarium with lots of hiding places. They require a fine gravel or sand bottom. Speckled knifefish grow very rapidly to over a foot long. They are sensitive to water quality problems.

The Central and South American knifefishes (Gymnotidae) are anatomically very similar to the speckled knifefish, but lack a caudal peduncle or fin. They are scaleless or very finely scaled. The banded knifefish, a member of this family, is aggressive with others of its own species, but peaceful with larger tank mates. Like other knifefishes, it prefers to have plenty of hiding places in the tank and is a nocturnal fish. Newly acquired banded knifefish may initially stand on their head for a period as a result of swimbladder damage during capture.

The American knifefishes (Rhamphichthyidae) also lack caudal fins and have a very delicate appearance (Fig. 62–10). In contrast to members of the Gymnotidae, the American knifefishes lack teeth or have only small ones. These are gentle fish that prefer to hide in dense plantings. They can be held in community tanks with fish of similar size.

The African knifefishes and featherbacks (Notopteridae) have the same laterally compressed elongated bodies of the other knifefishes. They are generally larger species found in the fresh water of Africa and Asia. Members of this family usually have only anal and pectoral fins. As young fish, the African knifefish school, but as they become adults they seek isolation from conspecifics. They are peaceful to tank mates and prefer dense vegetation with a central swimming space. They are nocturnal and prefer soft, slightly acid water. They have the remarkable ability to make bell sounds by expressing air from their swimbladder. The Asian knifefish is distinguished by the presence of a discrete and distinct dorsal fin. These fish are also solitary and are intolerant of other species; therefore, they must be kept alone. They also are nocturnal.

LABYRINTH FISHES (ANABANTIDAE, BELONTIIDAE, HELOSTOMATIIDAE, AND OSPHRONEMIDAE)

There are four families of labyrinth fishes, grouped together here for their possession of adaptations, that allow them to breathe air. The climbing perches (Anabantidae) are found throughout the world. The type species, the climbing bass or climbing perch, is aggressive and not suited to community tanks. It is an extremely hardy species that prefers a large shallow tank with floating plants. It is a good jumper, and aquaria must be kept covered. These fish were one of the first species kept in captivity. Climbing bass can travel on land using their pectoral fins for propulsion and may even climb trees. In high-humidity areas, they can survive up to 2 days out of water. They will also dig into mud to survive dry seasons.

The most popular family of aquarium fish among the labyrinth fishes is the Belontiidae, which includes the paradisefish, bettas, and most of the gouramis. Paradisefish are extremely hardy and tolerate wide variation in water temperature and quality. They prefer a densely planted aquarium, and only young fish are suitable for a community tank with fish larger than themselves. Adult paradisefish are highly territorial and must be kept alone. This species has a long history as an aquarium fish and was brought to Europe just after the goldfish. It is a combative fish that destroys plantings. Paradise fish will eradicate planaria in infested tanks, as they find them a delicacy. Covered tanks are a necessity because this species jumps.

The betta, or Siamese fighting fish, from Thailand is another member of the Belontiidae (Fig. 62–11). The males of this species are highly decorative with long and brightly colored fins. They are so bellicose that they are routinely kept in their own individual container. Bettas should never be kept in less than a liter of water. They are sensitive to temperature changes, contrary to popular belief.

The majority of the gouramis also belong to the family Belontiidae (Fig. 62–12). These are Asian fishes that prefer heavy vegetation with room to swim. They do better in soft, slightly acid water and are peaceful additions to community tanks. They are very popular with home aquarists.

The kissing gourami is the only member of the Helostomatiidae maintained in captivity. It is found in Thailand and Java. It is a browser that eats vege-

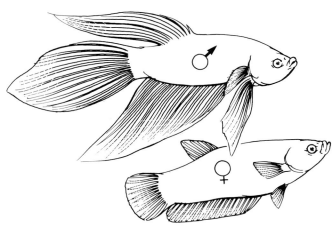

FIGURE 62–11. Sexual dimorphism in Siamese fighting fish.

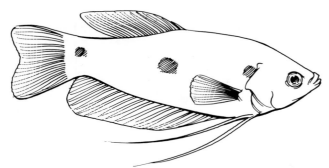

FIGURE 62–12. Three-spot gourami.

tation and algae. Kissing gouramis are tolerant fish that prefer soft water. The "kissing" behavior that gives them their name is actually a display of aggression. The giant, or common, gourami is also the only member of its family (Osphronemidae) maintained in captivity. This is an important food fish in China. In aquaria it is usually kept alone or with larger fish in a community tank. The term *giant* may be misleading. The fish rarely exceed 4 in. in length. They prefer a well-planted tank and soft slightly acid water.

LOACHES (COBITIDAE)

The loaches are popular, eel-like fishes commonly sold for home aquaria. The clown loach is a diurnal, active fish from Indonesia. It is prone to infection with *Ichthyophthirius multifiliis*. The Kuhlli loach (sometimes mistakenly referred to as the coolie loach) (Fig. 62–13) is a nocturnal fish from Thailand that hides during the day. This fish requires a soft sand or loam bottom heavily planted to provide lots of roots for the fish to hide in. The Kuhlli loach prefers slightly acid (pH 6), soft water.

RAINBOWFISHES (MELANOTAENIIDAE)

Rainbow fishes are found in eastern Australia. They are peaceful, active, schooling fish with long, oval, laterally compressed bodies. They can have problems with water that is too soft.

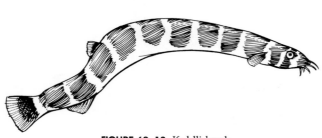

FIGURE 62–13. Kuhlli loach.

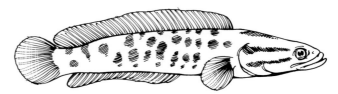

FIGURE 62–14. Green snakehead.

SILVERSIDES (ATHERINIDAE)

Most silversides species are found in flat coastal regions, although a few species have been acclimated to fresh water and are held in home aquaria. The group is distinguished by two widely separated dorsal fins, and the location of the pectoral fins high and very cranial on body. The Madagascar rainbow fish (not to be confused with the rainbowfishes of the Melanotaeniidae) is a member of this family that comes from mountain streams in Madagascar. It is a peaceful, schooling fish that needs open room for swimming and prefers hard neutral water. It should be kept only in schools, and not as single or paired specimens. It requires frequent water changes.

SLEEPER GOBIES (ELEOTRIDAE)

Sleeper gobies are brackish water species but can adapt to fresh water. They have an elongated body, normally with no lateral line. Their ctenoid scales are distinctive. The marbled sleeper, or sand, goby is a predatory nocturnal fish that must be able to hide and burrow. It prefers dim light, heavy plantings, and hard water.

SNAKEHEADS (CHANNIDAE)

The snakeheads grow quite large but are commonly held by hobbyists as young fish (Fig. 62–14). They have an elongated body, which is round cranially and laterally compressed caudally. They have a large mouth that can be opened wide to accept large prey. The nostrils have tube extensions that are

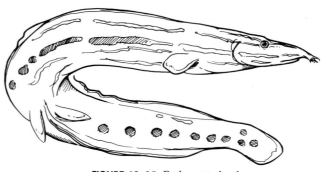

FIGURE 62–15. Red spotted eel.

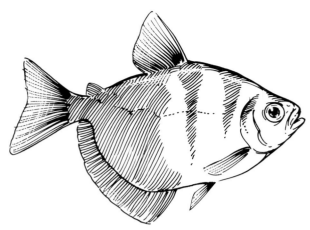

FIGURE 62–16. Black tetra.

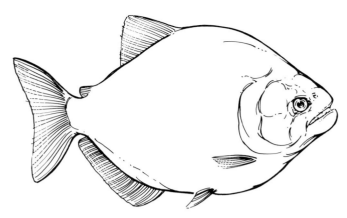

FIGURE 62–17. Red-bellied piranha.

characteristic. These fishes are predatory and are best kept alone in heavily planted tanks with fine sand bottoms. They require warm water (79 to 82°F). Snakeheads are excellent jumpers, so a well covered tank is a necessity.

SPINY EELS (MASTACEMBELIDAE)

Spiny eels are found in fresh and brackish waters of Southeast Asia and tropical Africa. As the name implies, they are eel-shaped and have a prehensile projection of their rostrum with their nostrils enclosed in extended tubes on each side of the rostrum. Spiny eels do better in slightly brackish water. They are difficult to train to take flake food. Fire eels are also members of this family (Fig. 62–15). Fire eels should be kept alone or with larger fish. They are nocturnal predators that do best in tanks with soft sand bottoms for burrowing and multiple hiding caves. They thrive in tanks with lots of aeration and where floating plants reduce the amount of light reaching the bottom. They are very prone to traumatic injury and ciliate infestations.

TETRAS, OR CHARACINS (CHARACIDAE)

Over 1000 species of tetras and their relatives have been identified in South America alone, and 200 more in Africa. Many more species are probably yet to be discovered. The family is characterized by having an adipose dorsal fin and toothed jaws (Fig.

62–16). In many species in this family, the sex of the fish can be told by looking for "characin hooks," small hooklike processes or spines on the anal fin or projecting from the ventral caudal peduncle of the males.

The tetras, or characins, are divided into 14 suborders and include such widely diverse species as the neon tetra and the red-bellied piranha (Fig. 62–17). The vast majority are schooling fishes and should be kept in schools in tanks with adequate swimming room. The family includes both carnivorous and herbivorous species. Most members of this family are peaceful and are excellent in community tanks. Of course, the piranhas are an exception. Piranhas are schooling species and do best in groups. Young piranhas raised as individual fish do not integrate well into established schools. Unexpectedly perhaps, fish raised alone survive well when introduced to an established school but gradually kill off the entire school one by one. This has been postulated to be due to failure of the fish raised alone to recognize and respond to subtle behavioral signals used to control aggression within the school. Adult piranhas raised as single specimens should never be introduced to a functioning piranha school.

LITERATURE CITED

Axelrod, H.R., Emmens, C.W., Burgess, W.E., Pronek, N., and Axelrod, G.S. (1980) Exotic Tropical Fishes. Expanded Looseleaf Edition. T.F.H. Publications, Neptune, New Jersey.

Mondadori, A. (ed.) (1977) Simon & Schuster's Complete Guide to Freshwater and Marine Aquarium Fishes. Simon & Schuster. New York.

Riehl, R., and Baensch, H.A. (1987) Aquarium Atlas. Baensch Publishing, Melle, Germany.

Studer, P. (1986) Nasse Welt. Friedrich Reinhardt Verlag, Basel, Switzerland.

Chapter 63

SPECIAL ANATOMY AND PHYSIOLOGY OF FRESHWATER TROPICAL FISHES

BRAD N. BOLON

Structural diversity among species that occupy similar environmental niches is perhaps greatest among freshwater tropical fishes (Bone and Marshall, 1982). Numerous adaptations permit life in the shallow, stagnant swamps and gently flowing rivers that are commonly found in equatorial regions. Although the degree of diversity precludes excessive generalization, some broad trends in anatomic specialization may be identified among the various families of freshwater tropical fishes.

The anatomic characteristics of freshwater tropical fishes are often remarkable. Most species have tapered bodies in which gently curved dorsal and ventral surfaces form an elliptical profile. Hatchetfish, however, have straight backs and prominent keels that define a triangular profile (Fig. 63–1), whereas the discus are roughly spherical. Lateral compression is usual in surface dwellers, whereas bottom-dwelling species are often flattened dorsoventrally (Moyle and Cech, 1982). Most species are small, rarely exceeding 30 cm in length (Nelson, 1984). Small size confers several advantages, notably increased mobility, more rapid maturity, and greater population density. Reduced size also enables many species to fill small, oxygen- and nutrient-poor habitats, which are unavailable to larger cousins. A few species from each group of freshwater tropical fish, however, reach adult lengths of 1 to 2 m.

External sexual dimorphism exists in some species. Females may have soft, rounded bodies and longer fins than males, while the anal fins of the males of some livebearering species are modified to form intromittent organs called gonopodia, which aid in internal fertilization (Migdalski and Fichter, 1976).

Modifications of the axial skeleton among freshwater tropical fish species are often pronounced, and many can be used for identification (Nelson, 1984). The number and arrangement of bones in the skull, vertebral column, and pectoral and pelvic girdles are extremely variable (Harder, 1975). For example, the cranial four to five vertebrae of barbs and danios (both cyprinids) as well as loaches are modified to produce weberian ossicles, a mobile bony bridge connecting the swim bladder and the inner ear. This bridge transduces air movements in the swim bladder into fluid vibrations in the auditory canals. Barbs, danios, loaches, and killifishes also have abdominal pelvic girdles. In contrast, the pelvic girdles of cichlids such as angelfish and discus are usually located in the cervical or cranial thoracic regions. The pelvic girdle is vestigial or absent in those species that have reduced or missing pelvic fins (e.g., eels). Most freshwater tropical species have a full complement of fins, and some have an adipose fin (characins, some loaches). Fins may be short or long with spiny or soft rays (or both) supporting the same fin. Eels, however, have an elongated anal fin with 140 to 260 rays but lack dorsal, pelvic, and caudal fins. This special fin arrangement allows eels to move forward, backward, up, and down with almost equal facility. The pelvic fin of livebearers (e.g., guppies, mollies, platys) is modified to produce an intromittent organ for use in fertilization (Fig. 63–2).

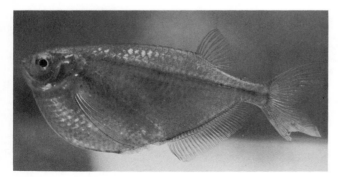

FIGURE 63–1. The hatchetfish is laterally compressed, with a straight back and prominent keel, giving it a triangular profile (Courtesy of M. Stoskopf).

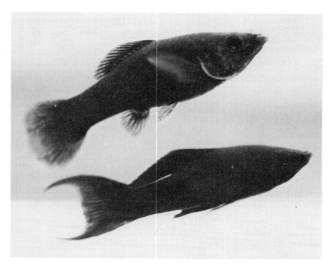

FIGURE 63–2. Livebearers such as the black mollie are relatively easy to sex. The pelvic fin of the male *(below)* is modified into a gonopodium, whereas that of the female *(above)* is a typical rounded fin (Courtesy of M. Stoskopf).

Muscle is the most abundant tissue in most fishes (Blake, 1983). Muscle is separated into thin superficial red and intermediate pink bands and a thick, deep white layer. Freshwater tropical fishes have modest amounts of predominantly white muscle, most of which is located caudally. This distribution provides the slow, sustained swimming motions produced by side-to-side strokes of the caudal fin. The remarkably narrow cichlids, which use pectoral fin rowing motions for low-speed propulsion, and the serpentine eels have little muscle mass. In contrast, hatchetfish, another extremely compressed family, have abundant white muscle located in a prominent thoracic keel, which allows them to make short flights out of the water and often the tank. Red muscle fibers represent only 5% to 15% of the muscle tissue in most freshwater tropical fishes (Bone and Marshall, 1982).

The axial muscles on each side of the caudal peduncle of mormyrids and eels are modified to produce electric organs (Harder, 1975). The electrocytes are short, flattened, plump fibers that contain myofibrils but no sarcoplasmic reticulum. The electrocytes are arranged in parallel columns, which are visible grossly; the number of electrocytes per column may vary from 200 (most mormyrids) to 6000 (eels). The fibers are surrounded by gelatinous matrix and usually connected to conduct current in series. A few eels also have accessory electric organs in the head. The electric organs are innervated by ventral spinal nerve roots. The weak electric organs of mormyrids and most eels aid in communication, navigation, and foraging, but the strong fields generated by larger eels are capable of stunning or even killing prey.

Freshwater tropical fishes have digestive systems adapted to many different diets (Harder, 1975; Smith, 1982). Small species usually consume invertebrates or algae, while larger species are carnivores or bottom scavengers. Most tropical fishes are surface feeders with terminal protractile mouths, which can extend either up or down. In contrast, many tetras and killifishes have terminal to supraterminal, nonprotractile mouths, whereas loaches have subterminal mouths. In many mormyrids, the mouth is a small orifice at the tip of a long flexible trunk, but other mormyrids have blunt mouths with jutting upper or lower jaws. The narrow, tubular orifice is a suction apparatus for inhaling food particles and, in some species, for maintaining position as a holdfast organ. Many species have sharp jaw teeth, ranging in size from small (killifishes) to large and serrated (piranha). Barbs, danios, and loaches lack oral dentition, having instead paired pharyngeal teeth, and some species with oral dentition also have pharyngeal teeth (Harder, 1975). Many characins have specialized gill rakers and blind, sac-like epibranchial organs for trapping prey, which range in size from plankton to small fish.

The intestinal arrangement is also highly variable, even in closely related species. Carnivorous fish usually have elongated stomachs containing abundant enzymes and acid that empty into relatively short, straight intestines. In contrast, herbivores and omnivores (e.g., cyprinids, loaches, killifishes) often lack true stomachs and have elongated, supercoiled intestines. Many agastric fish have saccular dilatations of the caudal esophagus (pseudogaster) for food storage, but these organs lack a gastric mucosa and do not produce acid or digestive enzymes. The presence of pyloric valves and ceca as well as the arrangement of the intestinal loops is highly variable and often species specific. The anus may be located anywhere from the head to tail. Pancreatic tissue is usually scattered diffusely throughout the mesentery in barbs, danios, loaches, and killifishes but is incorporated into the liver to form a hepatopancreas in angelfish, discus, and other cichlids.

Most freshwater tropical fishes respire by means of internal gills. The gill filaments are supported by cartilaginous rods of variable thickness and are protected externally by a bony operculum. Gill lamellae of active fishes are more numerous and thinner than those of sluggish species (Lagler et al., 1977). Many species with reduced gills have accessory respiratory organs (Harder, 1975). These accessory organs may be produced by dorsal extensions of one or more gill arches or from vascular pharyngeal diverticula. Loaches absorb oxygen from the vascular hindgut after swallowing air bubbles (Migdalski and Fichter, 1976), and some eels absorb oxygen through the skin (Moyle and Cech, 1982).

The heart of freshwater tropical fish species is located in the cranial thorax deep to the operculum. Heart size and structure are variable. The mixed arteriovenous circulation of the prototypic fish is present in all species except lungfish. One or more blind diverticula that project down and forward from the ventral surface of the bulbus arteriosus in mormyrids may help to dampen the pulse waves produced by pumping blood (Harder, 1975). Peripheral movement of blood in the dorsal aorta may be aided by movement of the spinal column during swimming. The aorta is closely applied to the ventral surface of the vertebrae and partially encloses the ventral intervertebral ligament, which is distorted by vertebral flexion and thus impinges on the aortic lumen to increase arterial pressure (Harder, 1975). Both hepatic and renal portal systems are present in most species. Depending on the species, the hepatic portal system may consist of a single large vessel or many small vessels (Harder, 1975). The lymphatic system consists of well-defined ducts and sinuses but no lymph nodes. Some species (e.g., eels) have muscular subvertebral lymphatic dilatations ("lymph hearts") in the caudal peduncle. Lymph hearts develop from blind dilatations of the distal portion of the caudal vein. Contraction of these flat, two-chambered sacs forces lymph to circulate.

The gonads are located middorsally within the coelomic cavity (Harder, 1975). They may be separate or fused. Testes are usually white and fissured, while ovaries are pink and smooth. Gonads enlarge markedly during the breeding season. Most species of freshwater tropical fish have separate ducts for sperm or egg transport, which lie adjacent to the mesonephric ducts from the kidneys.

The skin of freshwater tropical fishes is highly specialized (Harder, 1975). Most surface-dwelling species have multiple colors that often include brilliant shades of green, blue, red, orange, and yellow. Color patterns often include broad bands and patches of black and silver. Bright colors may be limited to only one sex, which is usually, but not always, the male. The degree of color varies between members of the same species owing to differences in the background colors of the water and soil (Migdalski and Fichter, 1976). In contrast, bottom dwellers usually have dull, mottled skin. Several cutaneous projections are prominent in some species, including minute unicellular projections (unculi) that dot the mouth and ventral pectoral fins as well as the multiple pairs of variably sized sensory barbels of loaches and some mormyrids. Many loaches also have an erectile spine located near the eye.

The sensory systems of freshwater tropical fishes are similar to those of other fishes. The lateral line of many species may be reduced, being discontinuous or absent in the trunk (Moyle and Cech, 1982). In most species, paired nostrils located on each side of the snout enter a blind nasal cavity and do not connect with the oral cavity. Many cichlids such as angelfish and discus can channel water into the oral cavity via a palatal orifice. Taste buds are numerous in the oral mucosa and the skin surrounding the mouth, including the barbels of loaches (Bone and Marshall, 1982). Hearing in fishes depends mainly on amplification of vibrations by otoliths and is relatively poor. However, in some gouramis and mormyrids, diverticula from the swim bladder extend into the head and directly abut the endolymphatic canals of the inner ear to directly transmit vibrations. Discus, tetras, and barbs are diurnal and have large eyes with greatest sensitivity in the orange light wavelengths. This matches the wavelength of diffuse light present in murky, shallow aquatic habitats (Smith, 1982). Nocturnal loaches and eels have small eyes. Most fish have eyes that provide partially independent lateral visual fields, but hatchetfish have tubular eyes that allow binocular dorsal or forward vision.

LITERATURE CITED

Blake, R.W. (1983) Fish Locomotion. Cambridge University Press, New York.

Bone, Q., and Marshall, N.B. (1982) Biology of Fishes. Chapman & Hall, New York.

Courtenay, W.R., Jr., and Stauffer, J.R., Jr. (1984) Distribution, Biology and Management of Exotic Fishes. Johns Hopkins University Press, Baltimore, Maryland.

Harder, W. (1975) Anatomy of Fishes. Vols. 1 and 2. E. Schweizerbart'sche Verlagsbuchhandlung, Stuttgart, Germany.

Lagler, K.F., Bardach, J.E., Miller, R.R., and May Passino, D.R. (1977) Ichthyology. 2nd ed. John Wiley & Sons, New York.

Migdalski, E.C., and Fichter, G.S. (1976) The Fresh and Salt Water Fishes of the World. Greenwich House, New York.

Moyle, P.B., and Cech, J.J., Jr. (1982) Fishes: An Introduction to Ichthyology. Prentice-Hall, Inc., Englewood Cliffs, New Jersey.

Nelson, J.S. (1984) Fishes of the World. 2nd ed. John Wiley & Sons, New York.

Smith, L.S. (1982) Introduction to Fish Physiology. T.F.H. Publications, Neptune, New Jersey.

Chapter 64

CLINICAL PATHOLOGY OF FRESHWATER TROPICAL FISHES

MICHAEL K. STOSKOPF

The amount of information available on the clinical pathology of freshwater tropical fishes is embarrassingly little. Despite a long history in captivity, little is known about the hematologic and cytologic parameters of the many species kept by hobbyists. Certainly the small size of many species is a factor in this deficit, but with modern microtechniques in plasma and hematologic analysis there is considerable room for development of reliable diagnostic tests for disease in freshwater tropical fishes.

Baseline hematologic parameters of freshwater tropical fishes leukocyte indices are given in Tables 64–1 and 64–2.

SAMPLING TECHNIQUE

Cytologic and hematologic sampling techniques for these fishes are similar to those used in other species. For hematologic work-ups of very small fish it is necessary to sacrifice the patient. Blood is best obtained by viewing the euthanatized patient under loupes or a dissecting microscope. Glass Pasteur pipettes can be drawn out to very fine capillary diameters in a flame and used to draw the blood from a cardiac puncture through the carefully opened opercular wall. This yields more blood than would severing the caudal peduncle. The capillary pipettes can be heparinized and the heparin allowed to dry before use to provide plasma, which has a better yield than serum from such small samples.

Cytologic samples from the skin of small species are more akin to taking a whole body impression. If fish are intended to survive, they must be handled very gently. There is no scraping motion involved. The fish is simply laid upon the slide and then dumped off back into the water. A coverslip is applied to the slide, and it is examined as a wet mount.

Gill biopsy is relatively simple in larger species of tropical fish (greater than 4 cm) but can be very difficult to perform without damaging smaller fish. For small species, a gill swab is a more common approach in patients intended to survive. A microswab designed for bacterial culture of the avian oropharynx can be used. Whether to wet the swab with carrying medium or to use it dry has not yet been definitively decided. Different clinicians prefer each method. Once the swab has been inserted into the opercular cavity and withdrawn, the tip of the swab is rolled on or touched to a slide or agar plate.

RESPONSE TO INFECTIOUS DISEASES

There are very few published data on the baseline clinical pathologic parameters of freshwater tropical species and much less information from con-

TABLE 64–1. Baseline Hematologic Parameters of Freshwater Tropical Fishes Leukocyte Indices

Species	N	Total WBC (thousand/ml)	Hetero. (%)	Band (%)	Mono. (%)	Small Lymph. (%)	Large Lymph. (%)	Eosino. (%)	Baso. (%)	References
Green snakehead*	20	26.0	40			42	1	17		Sharma and Shandilya, 1982
Green snakehead	10	13.0								Raizada and Singh, 1981

*In lab 1 week, possibly not feeding.
Hetero., heterophils; Band, band forms; Mono., monocytes; Lymph., lymphocytes; Eosino., eosinophils; Baso., basophils.

TABLE 64–2. Baseline Hematologic Parameters of Freshwater Tropical Fishes Erythrocyte Indices

Species	N	Total RBC (million/ml)	Hematocrit (%)	Hemoglobin (g/dl)	Thrombocytes (thousand/ml)	References
Brown snakehead	Unknown	3.8	30	9.1		Natarajan, 1981
Green snakehead	10	3.31	49	15.0		Raizada and Singh, 1981
Green snakehead*	20	2.25	40.5	11.0	6.0	Sharma and Shandilya, 1982

*In lab 1 week, possibly not feeding.

trolled studies looking at response to infections and other diseases. It is, therefore, necessary to assume that these fishes respond in a similar manner to the better-studied aquaculture species. Unfortunately, this is not as simple as it sounds, since the expected variation between animals with widely different lifestyles is apparent in fish clinical pathology. Empirically, in uncontrolled clinical cases with freshwater tropical fishes, bacterial infections have generally resulted in a leukocytosis, often with a heterophilia. However, on occasion, cases that appear in every other way to be due to bacterial septicemia demonstrate a pronounced leukopenia. Lymphopenias with viral infections remain a theoretic consideration in the ornamental freshwater tropical species. Clinically diagnosed protozoal infections seem to cause a variety of patterns, including a leukocytosis due to lymphocytosis.

RESPONSE TO NONINFECTIOUS DISEASES

Heavy Metal Toxicity

The response of freshwater tropical species to noninfectious diseases has been better studied, particularly in the area of heavy metal toxicity. Chronic sublethal cadmium exposure in rosy barbs results in cytoplasmic vacuolation of erythrocytes, hypochromia, basophilic stippling, and extrusion of erythrocyte nuclei. Anemia with a decreased total erythrocyte count, hemoglobin content, and hematocrit is seen, along with a distinct thrombocytopenia and a lymphocytosis due to increased numbers of circulating small lymphocytes. Cadmium exposure also results in a basophilia, monocytosis, and heteropenia (Gill and Pant, 1985).

Exposure of the Asian knifefish to mercuric chloride for periods of 15, 30, 45, and 60 days results in increased serum lactate and glucose levels as well as increased serum concentrations of aspartate aminotransferase (AST) and alanine aminotransferase (ALT). Serum cholesterol also decreases with exposure to mercury (Verma et al., 1986).

General Stress

The response of freshwater tropical aquarium species to stress has been studied to some extent.

Adrenocorticotropic hormone injections into intact male sailfin mollies being held at 25°C resulted in a distinct leukocytosis 4 hours after injection, indicating that the hematologic stress reaction of these fishes is mediated by the pituitary-adrenal axis (Ball and Slicher, 1962).

Stress due to cold shock caused by immersion into ice water for 2 minutes results in an initial leukopenia 1 hour after immersion. This is followed by a significant secondary leukocytosis 4 hours after immersion, with the leukocyte count falling back below normal again 6 hours after exposure to the ice bath. Blocking cortisol synthesis with etomidate blocks the response of tropical fishes to cold shock. Etomidate blocks 11-hydroxylation in the synthesis of cortisol in mammals and may have a similar effect on fish. Hypophysectomy alters the response to cold shock. Hypophysectomized fish have an abnormally low baseline leukocyte count. When cold shocked, hypophysectomized sailfin mollies do show an additional leukopenia 1 hour after the exposure to cold, indicating that the leukopenia is not mediated by the pituitary.

Starvation

Starvation has a predictable impact upon tropical fishes. With increasing duration of starvation, a gradual decline in total erythrocyte count is observed, as well as a decrease in hematocrit and hemoglobin content. Four weeks of starvation of otherwise healthy fish can result in a drop in erythrocyte parameters to about two-thirds of baseline levels. In the meantime, the total leukocyte count will drop to about half of baseline after 2 weeks of starvation and remain stable until another drop is seen at about 5 weeks of starvation. At the 5-week mark, the erythrocyte parameters also show a second sudden drop (Raizada and Singh, 1981). The absolute baseline values for the erythrocyte parameters in different species of fishes vary. The most apparent variation is with the obligate air-breathing fish, which invariably have higher hematocrits, erythrocyte counts, and hemoglobin content (Natarajan, 1981).

LITERATURE CITED

Ball, J.N., and Slicher, A.M. (1962) Influence of hypophysectomy and an adrenocortical inhibitor (SU–4885) on the stress-response of the white blood cells in the teleost fish, *Mollienesia latipinna*. Nature 196:1331–1332.

Gill, T.S., and Pant, J.C. (1985) Erythrocytic and leukocytic responses to cadmium poisoning in a freshwater fish, *Puntius conchonius* (Ham). Environ. Res. 36(2):327–337.

Lockwood, A.P.M. (1961) Ringer solutions and some notes on the physiological basis of their ionic composition. Comp. Biochem. Physiol. 2:241–289.

Natarajan, G.M. (1981) Some blood parameters in two air-breathing fishes of south India. Comp. Physiol. Ecol. 6(3):133–135.

Planas, J., and Gras, J. (1957) Estudio sobra las proteinas plasmaticas de peces de aqua dulce (*Barbus fluviatilis,* Cuv. et *Leuciscus cephalus,* L.) Rev. Espan. Fisiol. 13(1):17–24.

Raizada, M.N., and Singh, C.P. (1981) Effect of starvation on the blood of *Ophiocephalus punctatus* (Bloch). Experientia 37:1206–1207.

Sharma, R.K., and Shandilya, S. (1982) Observations on the haematological values of some fresh water teleosts. Comp. Physiol. Ecol. 7(2):124–126.

Verma, S.R., Chand, R., and Tonk, I.P. (1986) Mercuric chloride–induced physiological dysfunction in *Notopterus notopterus.* Environ. Res. 39(2):442–447.

Chapter 65

ENVIRONMENTAL REQUIREMENTS OF FRESHWATER TROPICAL FISHES

MICHAEL K. STOSKOPF

Nearly 80% of the freshwater tropical fish sold in the United States for home aquaria are reared in captivity, many in large production pond operations. Environmental requirements and diseases in production tropical fish facilities are sometimes distinct from the problems faced in the home aquarium, but other times they are very similar. Most of the literature focuses on the home aquarium, and unfortunately tropical fish producers have been left to fend off disease problems with little assistance from the medical community. Luckily, the physiologic responses of tropical fishes to environmental problems in any environment are essentially the same as those of temperate fishes, with slightly altered thresholds. This chapter covers common environmental concerns and *faux pas* of hobbyists maintaining tropical fish in their homes and offices and touches briefly on some concerns in production and research facilities.

GENERAL CONSIDERATIONS

Water Sources

As with all fish, the source of the water is paramount in preventing environmental diseases. This is discussed in some detail in Chapter 13. Specific problems arise when home aquarists seek to use their home water sources for tropical fishes.

Few home owners test their water sources routinely. This should be done, regardless of whether the source is a well or municipal water. Nitrate, phosphate, and copper levels should be determined before the water is used for fish. If this has not been done, it behooves the clinician who suspects a possible environmental problem to check the possibility of an incompatible water source.

Frequently home water supplies are not adequate for the maintenance of healthy fish. Plumbing with copper pipes can result in toxic accumulations of copper ions in aquaria. In this situation, fish owners should be cautioned to avoid using water from their hot water systems. This water is usually more heavily laden with copper than is the cold water system simply because water sits in the hot water pipes for such longer periods between use. Flushing of toilets and drinking or ice-making equipment cause cold-water systems to turn over their volume much more frequently. Even so, fish owners who live in single family dwellings should allow the water to run for at least 3 minutes before collecting any for use in fish tanks. This will usually purge the system of any water that has been sitting in the pipes.

Another point of caution must be considered if a client uses bacteriostatic filters on his or her well. These filters use silver ions as their bacteriostatic agent. Unfortunately, silver is much more toxic to fishes than even copper.

If the home water supply is poor, it will be well worth the expense to use distilled or spring water for the aquarium. While this might seem expensive, it is often the most economical solution to poor-quality water if only one or two moderate-sized aquaria are involved. A more serious hobbyist with several tanks, or a significantly large one, should be encouraged to install a water treatment device. Membrane-based reverse osmosis units can be used to improve many types of water problems, but demineralization plants, which use exchange resins, provide water that is of better overall quality. A unit capable of processing 5 gallons per day is adequate for an aquarium up to about 350 gallons (Thiel, 1989). Activated carbon filters can also be used to remove copper, other trace metals, and, to some degree, nitrates. These filters should use fairly large-grain carbon (25 μm or larger) to avoid constant problems with clogging. Charcoal filters, like the demineralization resins, must be periodically changed. While this is routinely handled by a service for water softeners, the home owner will need to monitor the carbon filters and/or to change the media on a prescheduled basis.

Water Changes

The world is full of advice on water changes for freshwater tropical fishes. The only real agreement is that they should be done and that they must involve removing some water from a tank or system before new water is added. A good schedule of maintenance usually involves removing particulate matter from filters weekly, to avoid any undesirable reverse exchange of compounds removed by the filters.

Except when disaster is impending, and major water changes are indicated, frequent small water changes are preferable. Not only do they maintain a more constant environment, but they are also less onerous to the person making the change. Large water changes, made at less frequent intervals, usually involve a fairly major production. This can often lead to procrastination and eventually environmental problems. Changing 4% of the water weekly or 2% every 3 days is superior to changing 20% of the water each month. For a client with a 20-gallon tank decorated with an average amount of gravel and rocks, a 2% change requires dipping out just over 1 quart of water (2 pints) and replacing it.

Laboratory systems for freshwater tropical fishes should be designed with automatic water changers. These are relatively inexpensive and simple to install. A daily change of 0.75% of the water volume in the system is usually sufficient.

Temperature

The change in water temperature experienced in most tropical streams is minimal. High-altitude streams, which show the most variation, usually are stable between 15 and 20°C (59 to 68°F). The diurnal variation in shallow streams (less than 30 cm deep) is less than 3°C. Therefore, it is appropriate that freshwater tropical fish be maintained at relatively constant temperatures.

The rule of thumb for heaters is 2 to 4 watts per gallon, depending on the normal temperature of the room where the aquarium is kept. Selection of too small a heater will result in the inability to maintain temperature. On the other hand, too large a heater runs the risk of rapid disaster if the thermostat fails and the heater begins to overheat the water. Multiple smaller heaters work well together in larger tanks or systems. In any event, it is always wise to have a back-up heater in case of a malfunction. Otherwise, you may be reduced to making warm water changes in an emergency situation. Most temperature changes should be made no faster than at the rate of 1 to 2°C per hour.

Water Monitoring

The complexities of monitoring freshwater systems are usually grossly exaggerated. The major issues of water chemistry are relatively straightforward, and relatively few parameters are routinely monitored. A few simple tests generally keep aquarists and their fishes out of trouble. Aside from temperature, pH is the most frequently measured parameter. This can be accomplished with pH papers or an electronic pH meter. The latter gives a digital read-out that is convenient and is usually accurate to the 0.1 pH point. That level of accuracy is probably not necessary for this application, but certainly 0.25 pH point would be of value. Most freshwater tropical fishes prefer the pH to be between 6.0 and 7.5. If the water has appropriate hardness and alkalinity, pH is not a very volatile parameter, and measurements every week or two are more than sufficient to detect trends.

Dissolved oxygen is not usually measured in freshwater systems. This does not mean that oxygen problems cannot develop. Heavily planted tanks can experience oxygen depletions very similar to those experienced in ponds if the water temperature is allowed to rise and inadequate aeration is provided. This might occur if air pumps are unplugged at night because of their noise. Routinely, however, oxygen depletion is not a major problem in aerated fish tanks.

Carbon dioxide is not routinely monitored either, but it plays an important role in the water chemistry of a system. Carbon dioxide is forty times more soluble in water than oxygen. About 0.2% of dissolved carbon dioxide is routinely converted to carbonic acid through a variety of reactions, and the carbonic acid causes the pH of the water to fall. If insufficient carbon dioxide is present in the water, carbonate formation is favored as the equilibrium between calcium carbonate and calcium bicarbonate is shifted to the less soluble calcium carbonate. When water has an acid pH (below pH 6), free carbon dioxide is favored and carbonate formation is negligible. In neutral to slightly alkaline water (pH 7 to 8), the reaction to form soluble bicarbonate from carbonic acid predominates, while in alkaline water (over pH 9) there is little if any dissolved carbon dioxide available to drive the formation of bicarbonate via carbonic acid and prevent the formation of calcium bicarbonate. This has an obvious impact on the parameter known as water hardness.

Water hardness, the calcium and magnesium salt content of the water, is often used to manage water for freshwater tropical fishes. Certain fishes are naturally found in relatively soft water (discus), whereas others require very hard water to survive (African cichlids). When total hardness is measured, the cationic calcium and magnesium ions in the water are determined. It is important to know that two major calcium salts contribute to hardness. Hardness attributable to calcium bicarbonate is removed if the water is boiled. Hardness due to calcium sulfate, on the other hand, is permanent and remains after boiling. Together, these two salts and the magnesium salts represent the TOTAL HARDNESS of the water (Table 65–1). One degree of total hardness (dH) is defined as equal to 10 mg of calcium or magnesium oxide per liter of water (10 ppm). The total hardness of the water can have direct effects on fish, plants, and even nitrification bacteria. Most freshwater fishes do best in water between 3 and 10 degrees of total hardness. The cichlids from Lake Tanganyika and Malawi in Africa are major exceptions and require a total hardness in excess of 10 to thrive.

Water hardness can be confusing because there is a second measurement commonly referred to as the carbonate hardness of the water. Degree of carbonate hardness is usually abbreviated dKH, using the K instead of a C because the primary work with the parameter has been established in Germany. When carbonate hardness is measured, the anions are quantified rather than the cations. This is an important distinction, because carbonate hardness can be a higher value than total hardness. This can be a confusing distinction for many aquarists. When carbonate hardness is measured, sodium, potassium, and other cations can contribute to the hardness in addition to calcium and magnesium. Most freshwater tropical fishes thrive best with a carbonate hardness between 2 and 8 dKH.

Adjusting Water Parameters

Reducing Hardness

The most effective rapid remedy is to institute water changes with distilled or deionized water. Installation of a water softener is indicated if the condition is a chronic problem and large water volumes are required. Water can also be filtered through peat to reduce hardness, but the effects on pH must be monitored.

TABLE 65–1. Water Total Hardness (dH)

	dH
Very soft water	0–4
Soft water	4–8
Slightly hard water	8–12
Moderately hard water	12–18
Hard water	18–30
Very hard water	Over 30

Increasing Hardness

Water that is too soft can be corrected by performing water changes with hard water. If this is not available, calcium or magnesium sulfate can be added to the water. Water for changes can also be filtered through marble chips or coral sand to increase hardness.

Lowering pH

In areas where water is too alkaline, filtration through peat will acidify water for changes. It will also remove calcium and magnesium, softening the water. Addition of hydrochloric acid is routinely used to lower pH in tanks.

Increasing pH

In closed-system aquaria, the pH of the water tends to fall with the addition of fish wastes and the activity of nitrifying bacteria. The usual corrective measure is partial water changes with more alkaline water. Alternatively, if the local waters are acid, sodium bicarbonate can be added to the system to provide some buffer capacity. This is probably a better solution than the use of sodium hydroxide solutions to raise the pH, although this has been used successfully with no apparent detriment to the fish. The use of sodium hydroxide does not affect the buffering capacity of the water and therefore is not a very long-term solution. Another approach to the problem is to aerate the water vigorously to expel carbon dioxide. This will increase the pH of the water but may affect the ability of aquatic plants to survive.

Reduction of Nitrogenous Wastes

Rapidly removing nitrite, nitrate, or ammonia waste products from an aquarium system is usually accomplished with water changes. There is no more rapid way of effectively reducing these levels. Reducing the amount of food fed can greatly help reduce the accumulation of these wastes in the water and help ameliorate an acute problem. Planting the tank or using an algae filter can reduce nitrate levels, but, more commonly, it merely slows the accumulation of nitrate. Carbon filters and zeolite filters can be used to remove nitrogenous wastes, although these filters are very prone to leak or re-exchange nitrogenous compounds if not monitored carefully. Zeolite is seeing more use recently because of its ability to be recharged with brine solutions and reused.

Tanks and Containers

Location of Tanks

Aquaria for freshwater tropical fishes should be located where temperature fluctuations can be minimized. In the home, they should not be placed above or below heating or air-conditioning vents. Windows and direct sunlight should also be avoided, not only because of the problem with rapid algae growth but also because sunlight can rapidly overheat a tank. Few fish can tolerate temperatures above 30°C (85°F) for any prolonged period (Riehl and Baensch, 1987).

Aquaria should be located where maintenance will be relatively trouble-free. There must be adequate room above a tank to allow the use of nets or tools that reach the bottom of the tank. A rule for designing research tanks is that there should be unobstructed space above the tank equal to or greater than the depth of the tank. Tanks should be close to water sources and drains, to facilitate water changes.

Aquarium Size and Substrates

Larger tanks are actually easier to maintain. Unfortunately, beginning aquarists are usually convinced to start small and see whether they like the hobby before investing too heavily in aquaria. They are then saddled with very volatile systems that require very close attention. In a large tank or system, dilutional effects allow for a relatively slow or modest change to occur when a problem arises. The amount of ammonia production that will increase a 10-gallon tank's ammonia level to very serious levels (10 ppm) will increase a 30-gallon tank's ammonia level to only 3.3 ppm, still a problem, but not nearly so devastating. All in all, larger tanks and systems give the aquarist more leeway for error, and the minimal starter tank should be 20 gallons.

The configuration of a tank can be important (Fig. 65–1). For example, catfishes and labyrinth fishes prefer broad, long tanks that are relatively shallow. This is particularly important for obligate air breathers, which can spend a great deal of energy going from the bottom of a deep tank to the surface just to breathe (Riehl and Baensch, 1987). Tetras and danios also prefer long tanks with considerable swimming room. These can be deep without compromising the fish. Angelfish do well in tall deep tanks and tend to use the vertical dimension of the water column. From the standpoint of fish health, wider tanks are always preferred over narrower tanks, since narrower tanks of the same volume are higher and have less surface area for gas exchange.

Substrates for freshwater tanks are varied and can be the cause of serious health problems if sand, gravel, or rocks containing toxic minerals are used. Calcareous gravel will cause hard water and may be

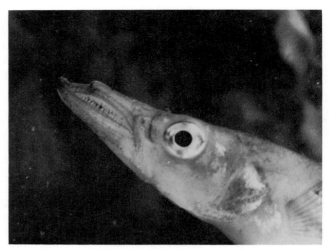

FIGURE 65–1. A piketop minnow with a broken upper jaw. This is a common sequela in a tank that is too small for the individual or is improperly configured. (Courtesy of T. Wenzel.)

very appropriate if local water is soft and an aquarist wants to maintain cichlids. To test gravel to see whether it is calcareous, simply place a drop of hydrochloric acid on a piece of the gravel. If it foams, it is calcareous. Since calcareous gravels should usually be avoided in freshwater systems, marble chips, dolomite, and coral sands should not be used. More appropriate substrates are coarse silicate sands, silicate gravel, quartz gravel, basalt chips, or washed river gravel. Many aquarists want to supplement their aquatic plants with soil. Simple addition of soil to a tank should be avoided at all costs. However, garden loam can be pressed into pellets and baked at 350°F for 1 hour for safe use in aquaria. The pellets should be pressed into the gravel near the plant so that none of the pellets are exposed above the gravel.

Light

Light is an important part of the aquarium environment. It is also a controversial one. Unfortunately, direct sunlight, which would seem to be ideal, is not. It provides too much heat energy and can rapidly thermally load a small aquarium. The controversy over intensity and spectrum of light required for an aquarium continues to rage. There are few data to evaluate regarding the light requirements of fishes. Most of the studies have naturally examined the requirements of plants. The optimal spectrum of light also remains in controversy. Suffice it to say that no deleterious effects of actinic or high ultraviolet content spectra have been documented in this group of fishes.

It is fairly well agreed that a day-night cycle is important and that 12 hours of daylight is a good starting point for equatorial species. Intensity is an interesting problem. Intensity of light can be measured in many ways, but most appropriate for clinical purposes is the amount of light delivered to a place in the tank. This is measured in LUX, a unit of intensity related to the foot candle. Bright midday sun in areas near the equator delivers about 75,000 LUX to the surface of a stream. Most aquatic plants thrive on 9500 LUX in nature. In an aquarium, surface plants do well with 2400 LUX or more. Midwater plants can survive in light as low as 300 LUX, and some very low light species of plants such as the cryptocorynes can grow in only 75 LUX.

To measure LUX delivered to an aquarium, it is not necessary to purchase a dedicated instrument. It can be done quite simply with a photographic light meter or a single-lens reflex camera with through-the-lens metering (Table 65–2). There are several approaches to the measurement. One can put a hand-held meter in a sealed plastic bag and submerge the meter to the place in the tank you wish to measure. This is more difficult than it might seem, since reading the meter through the bag and the aquarium while maintaining alignment of the meter with the light source without blocking the light can be difficult.

It is also possible to estimate LUX from outside the tank. One way is to angle the camera or meter toward the light source, to detect the light passing through the water column and the glass of the tank. Alternatively, a mirror can be placed in the tank at roughly a 45-degree angle to the light source and the meter. Light reflecting off the mirror is measured. Any of these methods is suitable for estimating the light delivery to a tank within the accuracy that is needed to assess the situation.

Starting a Filter in a New Tank

What should be a relatively simple process, rarely is. When the budding aquarist buys his fish tank, he rarely has the patience to wait for the biological filter to establish itself before he begins to load the system with his chosen fishes. Unfortunately, there are no real short cuts to this process. It will take between 4 and 6 weeks, and with even the most aggressive manipulation of the process, it will not go any faster. Products on the market to speed filter starting include freeze-dried bacteria and enzymes. These can help, but they will not give miraculous, near-instant start-ups. Raising the tank temperature can help a bit. However, unfortunately when the temperature is returned to something a fish can tolerate, many bacteria are usually lost, and the net result is not as dramatic as the theoretical calculations of bacterial reproduction rates would suggest.

Seeding a new tank with fresh gravel from an established biological filter does help. To see significant effects, tanks need to be seeded with about 1 L of established filter substrate for each 10 gallons of water in the new system. Experiments with frozen filter media and freeze-dried filter media have not been particularly successful. If this form of seeding a tank filter is used, it is important to know the source of the seed material. It is very easy to transfer disease organisms and strains of bacteria resistant to antibiotics with this practice. The long and the short of it is, even with seeding heavily from an established filter bed, it takes about 4 to 5 weeks to cycle a new system and achieve effective biofiltration.

Vacations

One of the major advantages of fish as pets is that they can tolerate several days of inattention with few effects. They can be left over a weekend and can even go 2 weeks or more without food if they are in good condition and the aquarium is well maintained. A week prior to leaving on vacation a client should clean the tank gravel and filters and replace between 20% and 30% of the water. The algae growing on the sides of the tank should be left, to allow fish to graze during the vacation. The day before leaving, fish owners should check the filter and, if they desire, load an automated feeder. It may be safer to leave the fish without feed. This is particularly true if inexperienced friends are being left in charge of the tank. The risk of overfeeding is much more serious than the risk of starvation. It is advisable to preweigh and package the daily rations if the tank will be left with a tank sitter.

ENVIRONMENTAL DISEASES

Acidosis

Fish suffering from acidosis due to low water pH swim in darting movements and jump as if trying to leave the water. Respiration rates may be high, and gasping at the surface can be observed. The jerky movements as fish dart through the tank are quite dramatic. Fish may gasp for air and then die in a normal swimming position. Occasionally, affected fish will be seen to swim in circles or to "shimmy" in position. A sudden raising of the scales can also be associated with this condition.

TABLE 65–2. Converting Photographic Light Meter Readings to LUX*

f Stop	Shutter Speed	LUX	
2.8	2	19	
2.8	1	38	
2.8	1/2	75	low-light plants
2.8	1/4	150	
2.8	1/8	300	mid-tank plants
2.8	1/15	600	
2.8	1/30	1200	
2.8	1/60	2400	surface plants
2.8	1/125	4800	
2.8	1/250	9500	plants in nature
4	1/250	19000	
5.6	1/250	38000	
8	1/250	75000	bright sunlight

*Camera or meter set to ASA 50 or 18 DIN (Deutsche Industrie Norm).

Fish exposed to more chronic conditions will develop excess mucus and skin inflammation, which is often reported as a milkiness. Gill epithelium erodes, and gill hemorrhages are common. Hemorrhages on the skin may also occur; however, more often, the fish is reported in excellent condition. Affected fish show very bright colors, and owners are sometimes dismayed that their fish is finally showing very good color and then is found dead on the bottom, in normal posture, still with excellent color. This is very mysterious to most owners, who often suspect malicious poisoning or some other toxic episode.

Alkalosis

Fish suffering from alkalosis have pale gills and frequently show areas of skin erosion and elevated mucus production. Early signs are usually limited to a bluish-white turbidity of the skin, sometimes with fin necrosis. Necrosis of the gills is usually appreciated only at postmortem examination.

Ammonia Toxicity

Ammonia, as a major excretory product of fishes, is always a potential environmental disease. Ammonia is extremely irritating to mucous membranes. Fish exposed to ammonia may show dyspnea, irregular breathing, or, as exposure continues, spasticity with extended fins. Just prior to death fish exhibit tetany. Gill damage from ammonia results in hyperplasia, aneurysms, telangiectasis, and corrosion of gill epithelium. Decreasing the pH of a tank will reduce the amount of ionized ammonia, which is the most toxic form. Partial water changes to reduce ammonia levels and acidification of the tank are warranted when high ammonia readings are obtained, even if fish are showing few or no clinical signs. Individual fish may benefit from a vinegar dip.

Carbon Dioxide Toxicity

Carbon dioxide toxicity is relatively rare, but it does occur. Usually, high levels of dissolved carbon dioxide are the result of anaerobic metabolism on the part of bacteria in the tank. They can also be the result of malfunctions in carbon dioxide injection systems, which are popular with aquarists who seek to stimulate luxuriant plant growth. These systems usually consist of pressurized carbon dioxide cylinders with a sensing regulatory valve. Fish affected by hypercapnia often appear to be dead, lying on their sides at the bottom of the tank. Their respiration is very slow, and they may be mistaken for dead. Raising the pH is beneficial, although the primary treatment is to increase aeration to drive off excessive carbon dioxide. It is also important to detect the source of the carbon dioxide and correct the underlying problem.

Chlorine Toxicity

Chlorine is an ever present concern when aquarists are using city water supplies. Levels of 0.1 ppm, which are common in city drinking water supplies, are fatal to most species of tropical fishes. Fish exposed to chlorine lose color and develop nonspecific signs of respiratory difficulty as a result of damage to their gill epithelium. The pattern of mortalities differs with the level of exposure. If a tank is exposed to high levels of chlorine (0.5 ppm or higher), the usual pattern is complete mortality over a short period. A more usual scenario is lower-level intermittent exposure from improper processing of water for changes. When this occurs, the variability in species and individual susceptibility results in a pattern of sporadic losses. At postmortem examination, nonspecific branchial epithelial hyperplasia is commonly the only finding. Occasionally fish affected by chlorine exhibit sunken eyes. The history is very important in the diagnosis of this disease. There is no suitable treatment for chronic damage due to chlorine exposure. The obvious course is to eliminate further exposure. Immediate application of sodium thiosulfate to the tank will reduce chlorine to chloride extremely rapidly and is the best remedial action when there has been an accidental exposure.

Detergents

Detergents are toxic to fish. They destroy the mucus that forms a major protective barrier to external pathogens and osmotic challenges. There are three classes of detergents, anionic, nonionic, and cationic. Anionic detergents are most common in household applications. They are often sulfonated or phosphorylated hydrocarbons, which can cause epithelial irritation. Nonionic detergents are less irritating to human skin but can still have severe effects on fish gill epithelium. Cationic detergents include the quaternary ammonium disinfectants. These compounds are frequently used to treat external infections in fish. They are toxic. They are readily absorbed and interfere with several functions at the cellular level. They also break down into compounds that will induce methemoglobinemia. Fish poisoned with exposure to these detergents are usually found dead. If high doses were present, corrosive skin lesions may be apparent. No antidote is known for the systemic effects of these compounds. It is safest to avoid the use of disinfectants when cleaning fish tanks, implements, or tank substrates or to use only compounds that can be readily rendered harmless, such as chlorine, which can be neutralized with sodium thiosulfate.

Heavy Metal Toxicity

In general, heavy metals tend to break down the mucus coat of tropical fishes. They also damage the gill epithelium. Each heavy metal has different specific toxic effects on fish. Copper can be lethal at concentrations as low as 0.1 ppm, depending on other water chemistry parameters. Clinical signs are usually evident only a day or two after initial exposure. Copper is much more toxic when dissolved oxygen levels are low. Fish affected by copper may show abnormal behavior, anorexia, edema, disorientation, and protruding scales. Frequently fish become extremely colorful just before death when suffering from copper toxicity. This is due to a relaxation of the chromatophores. Zinc is also very toxic to fish. It is more toxic in soft water, as it will usually precipitate out as a carbonate in hard water. This is similar to the behavior of copper in hard water. Zinc and copper toxicity are additive. Mercury toxicity can also result in disorientation, edema, and rapid death.

Treatment of heavy metal toxicity centers on removing the exposure. There has been very little evaluation of the use of chelating agents or specific antidotes to treat fish. This needs further investigation, particularly for copper toxicity, which is unfortunately quite common as a sequela to misguided therapy.

Hydrogen Sulfide Toxicity

Anaerobic bacteria frequently generate toxic amounts of hydrogen sulfide, which can cause severe problems in an aquarium system. This happens when water circulation is impeded by clogged substrates or filter media. An early warning sign of impending problems is a sudden increase in algal growth, which further clogs substrates. The physiologic impact of hydrogen sulfide is to interfere with oxygen binding by hemoglobin, as well as direct damage to the central nervous system. The exposure limit for hydrogen sulfide is less than 10 ppm. The most common clinical signalment is sudden death; however, fish exposed to lower levels may be observed in respiratory distress, gasping for air at the surface. The gills of affected fish are cyanotic, with a violet color.

It is possible for fish to be exposed to very low levels of hydrogen sulfide for longer periods of time. These fish will be irritable, will lose weight, and may have equilibrium problems. The best treatment is prevention. Dirt and debris should not be allowed to block filter media or gravel, and gravel should be cleaned frequently. Switching to a coarser gravel may be beneficial.

Clinical cases should be removed from exposure by transfer to another water system. Increasing aeration of the tank may drive off residual dissolved hydrogen sulfide in the water. Sodium nitrite has been recommended as an antidote, to increase the formation of sulfmethemoglobin and remove sulfide from tissues. This treatment should be done with extreme care because of the toxicity of nitrite to fishes. Baths in 0.1 ppm sodium nitrite can be used judiciously. Pyridoxine baths (25 mg/L) have been suggested as a treatment, with pyridoxine acting as a sulfide acceptor.

Hyperthermia

Fishes exposed to water temperatures above their thermal range usually show signs of hyperactivity, swimming rapidly and sometimes breathing more rapidly than normal. If the condition is not corrected, blood vessels in the fins, skin, and subcutis engorge and then rupture, causing the formation of hemorrhagic streaks visible to the naked eye. Affected fish die within a very short time.

The exact cause of death in fish exposed to high temperatures is unknown. Oxygen deficiency has been postulated as one mechanism, based on the decreased solubility of oxygen at higher temperatures, but the disease seems to have a more complex pathogenesis. Osmotic stresses are thought to play a major role (Allanson and Nobel, 1964). The mechanism appears to be due to the loss of the ability to maintain serum ion and protein concentrations, which is remarkably similar to that seen in hypothermia. The addition of sodium, magnesium, and calcium to the water increases the resistance of many fishes to high temperatures.

Fish exposed to high water temperatures should be returned to normal temperatures immediately, but gradually. A temperature decrease rate of 2 to 3°F per hour is appropriate if fish are within 15°F of their optimal temperature. If they are above that and still surviving, an immediate reduction of 5°F is warranted, followed by a more gradual decline. Addition of 0.5 to 1.0% (5 to 10 g/L) sodium chloride to the water apparently improves survival.

Hypothermia

Fish affected by hypothermia are listless and pale and may have clamped fins. They will often show slow nonprogressive swimming in place, sometimes with rapid movement of their pectoral fins, sometimes referred to as "whirring." They may rock from side to side or shimmy in the water. If the problem is not corrected, fish may develop an equilibrium deficit, and pectoral fins will be held stiff out from the body.

If the onset of hypothermia was sudden, marked decreases in serum total protein, sodium, and chloride may be seen owing to osmoregulatory collapse and acute renal failure (Allanson et al., 1971). Allowed to progress, this response to low temperatures will produce shock and even intravascular hemolysis

(Reichenbach-Klinke and Elkan, 1965). Addition of 0.5% (5 g/L) sodium chloride to the water can reduce the osmotic effects of hypothermia (Allanson et al., 1971). The other major physiological effect is seen in even mild degrees of hypothermia—immuno-suppression, both humoral and cellular, which can leave fish vulnerable to infectious diseases (Wede-meyer et al., 1976).

Nicotine

Mysterious losses of fish can sometimes be traced to exposure to nicotine. Smoke is rapidly absorbed into water. Exposure to a smoky room for an hour is usually lethal to guppies, which are fatally affected by low doses of nicotine. As little as 10 ppm will kill a guppy within 5 minutes (Emmens, 1978; Reichenbach-Klinke and Elken, 1965). Blowing smoke into the water will kill fish within 3 to 5 minutes. Affected fish exhibit stiff, rigid pectoral fins, sometimes clamped tightly to their sides. They are pale and may rise and then sink to the bottom as their pectoral fins spasm. In peracute cases, muscular spasms are apparent prior to death. Lower doses can result in deaths over several days or weeks. Even lower doses cause infertility, abortion, and malfor-mation of young. Nicotine toxicity should be sus-pected whenever a client smokes. Nicotine is so toxic that one notable case was identified in an apartment of a nonsmoker where there was no separation of air handling in the apartment building. Neighbors of the client did smoke. The problem was resolved successfully by placing the air pump for the aquarium outdoors on the balcony.

Nitrite Toxicity

Nitrite is a natural product of nitrification in biological filters. In normal situations it is rapidly converted to nitrate by heterotrophic bacteria. How-ever, during initial start-up of new filter systems or after treatments that have compromised the integrity of the biofilter, nitrite can accumulate in a system. Exposure to nitrite results in methemoglobinemia in fish. Fish with greater than 50% methemoglobinemia will exhibit muddy-colored gills and will be in severe respiratory difficulty. Fish may be seen to hang in the water, vertical, head up, about 2 inches off the bottom. This may be followed by convulsions, coma, and respiratory paralysis. Addition of sodium chlo-ride to the water will reduce the impact of dissolved nitrite by competing for absorption across the gills. Chloride levels of 100 ppm are protective but will not affect nitrite that has already been absorbed. Fish showing muddy membranes may respond to meth-ylene blue baths.

Oxygen Deficit

Oxygen deficit can occur for a variety of reasons, including the effects of decaying food in the tank;

the presence of too many plants, which use too much oxygen during the dark cycle of respiration; and elevated water temperatures, which reduce the sol-ubility of oxygen in the water. Species requirements for oxygen vary considerably, and it is common that all fish in a tank do not succumb at once. Signs of oxygen deficit mimic many other problems in which respiration is compromised. Fish gather at the sur-face, breathe rapidly, and may break the surface gulping for air. The treatment is to restore dissolved oxygen levels. This may require reducing water tem-peratures and increasing aeration.

Pesticides

Freshwater tropical fishes encounter pesticides when precautions are not taken during home exter-minations. Flea and tick bombs used to fumigate homes can cause serious problems for home aquar-ium fish. Before the pesticide bombs are set off, clients should disconnect the air pumps serving their tanks. They may want to seal the pumps in a plastic bag. The top of the fish tank should also be sealed with plastic wrap. It helps if the tank is not com-pletely filled to the top. One to two inches of air space over the water surface will allow a well-bal-anced tank to be left sealed for several hours. Most fumigation schemes are complete within 4 hours. The client should return to the house as soon as the fumigation is complete, air out the house, and then open the top of the tank. The plastic should be discarded. The air pump should not be reactivated until the house has been aired out thoroughly, and the odor of the pesticide is gone. If it is necessary to start the pump sooner, it can be placed outside to take in uncontaminated air.

Another means by which pesticides find their way into fish tanks is with the injudicious use of hand-held spray cans or pump bottles used to erad-icate ants, wasps, or other insects or to treat plants with scale or mites. Pyrethrins, the active ingredient of many of these preparations, are particularly toxic to fishes.

The signs of pesticide intoxication in fishes vary with the specific toxic compound involved, although autonomic dysfunction is common. Jerking or trem-bling movements, convulsions, and coma can be seen. Larger fish can be injected with atropine, and atropine baths may have an effect if they are admin-istered early in the course of organophosphate or chlorinated hydrocarbon toxicity.

Phenol Toxicity

Phenols are introduced into aquaria through the unwise selection of creosoted driftwood or the use of phenol-based household disinfectants to clean tanks, substrates, or decorations. Phenols are very toxic to tropical fishes. They cause severe corrosive damage to gills, skin, and intestinal mucosa. They are also hepatotoxic. Affected fish show restlessness, aimless swimming, and increased respiratory rates. Increased swimming, followed shortly by spastic staggering and death, will be seen with exposures to concentrations as low as 5 ppm. Recovery is possible only if the problem is noticed very shortly after exposure. Treatment is based on removal of further exposure. Treatment for methemoglobinemia with a methylene blue bath may be of some value.

Potassium Permanganate Toxicity

Potassium permanganate solutions are often recommended to disinfect plants, ornaments, or substrates destined for aquaria. The recommended protocol is to soak the object in a 10-ppm solution for 30 minutes and then to rinse it thoroughly in water before placing it into a tank. Potassium permanganate is quite toxic. It is a caustic alkali that severely irritates mucous membranes and skin on contact. Corrosion is the most common clinical sign. Emergency treatment for an accidental exposure is to rinse off the exposed fish. A dip into evaporated milk, followed by a rinse, will inactivate the permanganate. The prognosis for exposure to potassium permanganate is poor. Deaths due to severe gill compromise may be delayed for weeks.

Supersaturation

Supersaturation, which results in a syndrome called gas bubble disease, can be the result of abnormal accumulations of any gas in aquarium water. Contrary to popular opinion, oxygen is not the most frequent offender. Nitrogen supersaturation is actually more common. Affected fish show bubbles of gas under the skin of the fins, body, and mouth. The most severe problems occur in internal tissues with the least blood supply. Gas bubble formation in capillary beds causes ischemia and tissue necrosis. Cavitation of the heart due to the formation of bubbles by blood turbulence can result in severe reduction of venous pressure and can cause acute death.

Causes of supersaturation include accumulations of oxygen due to heavy plant and algal growth, and too much exposure to light. Correct this by reducing the exposure to sunlight or shortening the day cycle. Cavitating pumps can also supersaturate the water. Care should be taken to make sure that feed lines are full of water and that no leaks allow gas into the influent side of the pump. Excessive aeration from airstones does not usually cause this syndrome. Usually, excessive bubbling simply displaces other gases from water open to the atmosphere.

LITERATURE CITED

Allanson, B.R., and Nobel, R.G. (1964) The tolerance of *Tilapia mossambica* (Peters) to high temperature. Trans. Am. Fish. Soc. 93:323–332.

Allanson, B.R., Bok, A., and Van Wyk, N.I. (1971)The influence of exposure to low temperature on *Tilapia mossambica* Peters (Cichlidae). II. Changes in serum osmolarity, sodium and chloride ion concentrations. J. Fish Biol. 3:181–185.

Amlacher, E. (1970) Textbook of Fish Diseases. Trans Conroy, D.A., and Herman, R.L. T.F.H. Publications, Neptune, New Jersey.

Emmens, C.W. (1978) Diseases of Aquarium Fish. Proc. 36. Post Graduate Committee in Veterinary Science. University of Sydney, Sydney, Australia, p. 175–185.

Reichenbach-Klinke, H., and Elkan, E. (1965) The Principal Diseases of Lower Vertebrates: Diseases of Fishes. Academic Press, New York.

Riehl, R., and Baensch, H.A. (1987) Aquarium Atlas. Mergus-Verlag, Melle, Germany.

Thiel, A.J. (1989) Advanced Reef Keeping. Aardvark Press, Bridgeport, Connecticut.

Wedemeyer, G.A., Meyer, F.P., and Smith, L. (1976) Environmental Stress and Fish Diseases. T.F.H. Publications, Neptune, New Jersey.

Chapter 66

REPRODUCTION OF FRESHWATER TROPICAL FISHES

RUTH FRANCIS-FLOYD   JEROME V. SHIREMAN

The mode of reproduction of freshwater tropical fishes is the most commonly used criterion for general classification. Fishes are either live-bearers or egg-layers. This fundamental division influences many aspects of husbandry and reproductive management. Commercial farms tend to specialize in live-bearers or egg-layers, and the requirements for each are different enough that a live-bearer farm cannot be readily adapted to production of egg layers and vice versa.

Issues to consider prior to initiating a freshwater tropical fish–breeding program (Axelrod, 1980) include breeding seasonability, water-quality characteristics of natural spawning sites, and preferred spawning habitats. Courtship and spawning rituals, parental care mechanisms, reproductive life span, and the presence or absence of secondary sex characteristics all are important factors. Re-creation of natural spawning conditions is necessary for spawning many species in captivity.

LIVE-BEARERS

Most live-bearing aquarium fishes are in the family Poeciliidae, which includes the guppies, mollies, and platyfishes. Live-bearing freshwater species from other families include the foureyes, the North American cavefish, the halfbeaks, and gars (Marshall, 1970; Jacobs, 1971). All freshwater tropical live-bearers are native to the American continent except members of the halfbeak family that are native to Southeast Asia (Jacobs, 1971).

Fertilization is internal for live-bearing fishes. The anal fin of the male is modified as a copulatory organ called the gonopodium. The structure of the gonopodium varies considerably between the various phylogenetic groups (Jacobs, 1971). In guppies and mollies, the gonopodium is frequently an elaborate structure involving modifications of the third, fourth, and fifth finrays of the anal fin. Other fishes have simpler modifications of the gonopodium (Jacobs, 1971).

Spawning behavior usually includes a short period of ventrum to ventrum contact between male and female fish. The male deposits a sperm bundle, called a spermatophore, into the genital opening of the female. The sperm deposited internally is retained in longitudinal folds within the female and, in most species, it retains its viability long enough to fertilize eggs for several successive pregnancies.

In truly ovoviviparous fishes, the fertilized eggs remain within the ovarian tract of the female until ready to hatch. Each developing embryo has its own individual yolk sac within its egg. Some species such as the dwarf topminnow have developed placentalike structures that allow some transfer of products between the maternal vasculature and the developing embryo (Marshall, 1970). Gestation varies between species but averages 4 to 6 weeks, usually depending on water temperature and the condition and age of the female. Once parturition is initiated, it may continue for several hours or even several days in some species. In dwarf topminnows, the female may continue to give birth for several weeks. The number of fry resulting from any one pregnancy in live-bearing species is small compared to that in egg-layers. The number of fry in any one brood most commonly ranges between 5 and 150 individuals (Jacobs, 1971).

One of the most popular live-bearing aquarium fishes is the guppy (Axelrod, 1980). These fish are hardy and breed readily in home aquaria. Pregnancy is evidenced by a darkening in the posterior abdomen of the female. Gestation is 4 to 6 weeks at water temperatures of 23 to 28°C (Van Ramshorst, 1981). Gravid females should be placed in small, well-planted tanks. The female may eat her own young, so she should be removed from the nursery as soon as possible postpartum (Axelrod, 1980). A brood will average 20 to 100 fry, and these will reach sexual maturity at about 6 months of age (Van Ramshorst, 1981). Separation of male and female juveniles as soon as secondary sex characteristics are noticed is necessary if selective breeding is desired. Females are larger and less colorful than males. Males can be identified by the modification of the anal fin into a gonopodium.

The black molly is a popular relative of the guppy. Reproduction in the two species is similar; however, in the black molly, gestation is slightly longer, 8 to 10 weeks, and brood size may be a little smaller, averaging 20 to 80 fry per pregnancy (Van Ramshorst, 1981). Ideal water temperature for breeding black mollies is 20 to 24°C (Jacobs, 1971).

Two other popular live-bearers from the family Poeciliidae are the swordtail and the platyfishes. These fishes can also be easily bred in the home aquarium. Gestation is 4 to 6 weeks at 26°C. The number of fry produced varies but is often in the range of 10 to 50 young (Van Ramshorst, 1981). These species are less aggressive toward their offspring than guppies or mollies, but it is still recommended to remove the female after parturition (Van Ramshorst, 1981). If she is not removed, the tank should be heavily planted to provide the young fish with hiding areas. Females should be housed separately from males during the immediate postpartum period if possible (Axelrod, 1980).

EGG-LAYERS

Most species of freshwater tropical fishes are oviparous. Popular examples include the cichlids, characins, and anabenids. Sexual dimorphism is marked in some species, with the male being brightly colored. A well-recognized example is the Siamese fighting fish. Males of this species are large and brightly colored and have long, flowing fins. Females are small, comparatively nondescript, with very modest finnage. A variety of reproductive strategies have evolved within the egg-laying group. Representative species are discussed below.

African Cichlids

Most popular species of African cichlids are mouth-brooders. These include species from both Lake Malawi and Lake Tanganika. Some species are monogamous, and both parents participate in fry rearing (Loiselle, 1985). Other mouth-brooders are polygamous, and parental care is provided exclusively by the female. Some species from Lake Tanganyika and Lake Malawi are categorized as aterritorial polygamists (Loiselle, 1985). Females of these species may spawn in different locations in a tank, and the males compete for the chance to fertilize the sporadically released eggs. More commonly, small territories are established by males on a temporary basis. This system is exhibited by many Rift Lake cichlids (Loiselle, 1985). Less commonly, males will establish permanent territories and attempt to attract females by behaviorial displays and site selection. This strategy is exhibited by the Diagramma and frontosa cichlids from Lake Tanganyika. Following spawning, mouth-brooding females pick up eggs in the buccal cavity and elicit fertilization from the male in a number of ways (Loiselle, 1985). In many instances, fertilization occurs within the buccal cavity of the female. The female may then seclude herself from other fish and refuse food. Distention of the buccal-pharyngeal region may be noticeable. Females may be able to rear fry in a community tank, but it is recommended that they be placed in a separate tank during gestation (Loiselle, 1985). The time required for incubation of eggs is temperature dependent; however, many species of Tanganyikan and Malawi cichlids incubate eggs for approximately 3 weeks (85°F). Some species will abandon fry following hatching, whereas others continue to provide parental care (Loiselle, 1985). Fry are usually precocious and large enough to accept brine shrimp nauplii as a first food (Loiselle, 1985).

Angelfishes

Angelfishes form breeding pairs prior to spawning. Although breeding pairs can be purchased, it is generally more cost effective to place a number of large fish together in a 20-gal or larger tank and allow them to form their own pairs. Pair formation is evidenced by courtship behavior, including lip-locks, pushing against each other, and establishment of a territory from which other fish are excluded. Paired fish can be removed from the larger tank and placed in a 10-gal tank for spawning. The spawning tank can be planted with broad-leafed plants such as Amazon sword plants, or a slate can be placed in a bare tank at an angle of approximately 30 degrees from the vertical (Fig. 66–1). A typical slate measures 24.5 cm long, 6.5 cm wide, and 0.5 cm thick.

Prior to spawning, the pair will clean the slate. The female approaches the slate with the ovipositor extended and lays a single row of eggs. The male

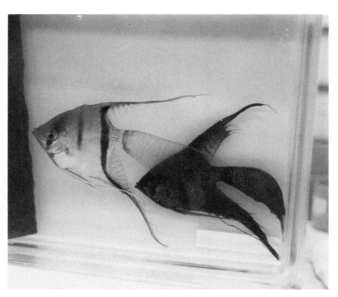

FIGURE 66–1. Angelfish examining an angled spawning slate. (Courtesy of P. Reed.)

approaches the slate behind the female and fertilizes the eggs. Following spawning, the slate may be left in the tank and the fry reared by the parents, or the slate can be removed to a hatching jar and the fry reared artificially. If the eggs are left with the parents, the adults will circulate water around the attached eggs by fanning them. Parents must be well fed to minimize cannibalism of newly hatched fry. For this reason, fry are raised in separate containers in most commercial hatcheries. Slates can be placed in 1-gal hatching jars supplied with a small airstone for gentle aeration and water circulation (Fig. 66–2). The slate should be positioned so that eggs are on the bottom of the slate. This avoids accumulation of debris and minimizes fungal or bacterial invasion.

Angelfish eggs hatch in 3 days at water temperatures of 28 to 29°C. Fry sink to the bottom of the hatching jar until the yolk sac is absorbed in 48 to 96 hours. Following absorption of the yolk sac, food can be offered to developing fry. Chicken egg yolk is an excellent first food for swim-up fry, fry that have resorbed their own yolk. A chicken egg can be hard-boiled and the yolk separated and frozen. A fine cloud of egg yolk should be offered two to three times a day. After 3 days, young angelfish should be able to accept decapsulated or newly hatched brine shrimp. Early feeding success is dependent upon availability of food items of an appropriate size and in sufficient abundance that fry frequently contact food particles during random swimming.

Barbs

In general, the barbs spawn in groups in heavily planted tanks. No parental care is provided, and adult fish should be removed after spawning. Brine shrimp is appropriate as a first food for swim-up fry (Axelrod, 1980).

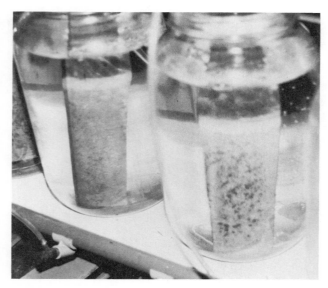

FIGURE 66–2. Aerated hatching jars with slates bearing freshwater angelfish eggs.

Discus

The discus are flat-bodied cichlids from the Amazon. They reproduce in a fashion very similar to that described for angelfishes. Several pairs may be maintained in a 40-gal or larger spawning tank. Clay flower pots are an excellent substrate for egg deposition and can be stacked so that a flower pot with eggs adhered to it can be removed, leaving a fresh pot underneath. This decreases distress exhibited by parents following removal of eggs. Eggs can be hatched artificially using a system similar to that used for angelfishes. In nature, the discus provide excellent parental care, and fry feed on a mucoid substance secreted by the female fish (Wattley, 1985).

Siamese Fighting Fish

Siamese fighting fish are bubble nest builders. Males and females must be housed separately until ready to spawn. A transparent divider allows visualization of behavioral displays (Axelrod, 1980). Foliage or similar protection should be available to allow the female to escape from the aggressive male during the actual breeding. The male constructs an elaborate bubble nest by expelling air from its mouth. When the female is introduced, the two fish will fight. During copulation the male will encircle and squeeze the female's body until eggs are expelled. The male will then swim down, pick the eggs up, and deposit them in the bubble nest (Axelrod, 1980). Spawning may continue for up to 24 hours. The female should be removed as soon as spawning has been completed. Eggs will hatch within 48 hours. Sac-fry occasionally sink to the bottom of the tank but are returned to the bubble nest by the male. The male continues to care for the fry for up to 10 days, but then he must be removed or he may eat them (Axelrod, 1980).

INDUCED SPAWNING

Hormone spawning of freshwater tropical fishes is a relatively recent technique. This technique will become extremely important in the ornamental fish trade. Many species currently collected only from the wild are candidates for induced spawning and subsequent culture. Hormone injections coupled with manipulation of photoperiod and water temperature should allow the spawning of many ornamental species throughout the year (Shireman et al., 1978).

Broodstock Conditioning

Broodfish selection and conditioning are the most important considerations for successful results. In many cases, broodfish are collected from the wild and induced to spawn. Some species, however, are more domesticated, and breeders are selected for their conformation, growth, or color. The quality of the broodfish determines egg quality. Nutrition and good water quality are important for proper conditioning. Eggs are actually being formed before spawning. Smaller ornamental fishes may actually form eggs 1 to 2 months prior to maturity. No matter what fish species is to be spawned, the broodfish must be fed a suitable diet and stressed as little as possible.

Spawning in natural situations results because of environmental cues that may include water level, suitable substrate, the presence of vegetation, water temperature, or day length. These cues are transmitted through external receptors to the hypothalamic-pituitary axis, which produces hormones to initiate and finalize the reproductive process.

Environmental cues that cause fish to reproduce are often not present in the hatchery or laboratory; therefore, fish are induced to spawn using hormone injections. Not all fish respond identically to the same hormones or combination of hormones. However, human chorionic gonadotropin (HCG), carp pituitary, or synthetic LH-RH analogue (LRH-A) will induce mature fish of most species to spawn. Dopamine blockers are sometimes used in combination with LRH-A in fish that do not respond to LRH-A alone. These hormones will not cause eggs to mature but will trigger the release of eggs if they are in an advanced stage of development (Rottmann and Shireman, 1988a).

Prior to injection, the female should be checked to determine egg maturity. Females can be lightly anesthetized with tricaine methanesulfonate prior to the egg-sampling procedure. A small-diameter polyethylene tube, attached to a syringe, is carefully inserted into the oviduct to remove an egg sample (Fig. 66–3). Once the tube is placed properly in the

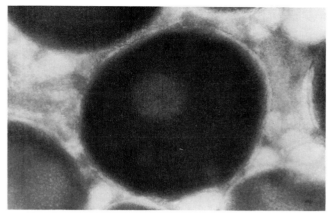

FIGURE 66–4. Immature oocyte of a clown loach. When the oocyte is mature, indicating that the female is a viable candidate for induced spawning, the nucleus migrates to the periphery of the oocyte and is fully polarized. (Courtesy of R. Whiteford.)

oviduct, gentle aspiration can be applied (Rottmann and Shireman, 1988a). The eggs can then be examined under a microscope to determine the location of the nucleus. If the nucleus is located near the periphery of the egg (Fig. 66–4), the egg is ripe, and the fish should be injected (Rottmann and Shireman, 1990).

Hormone Doses

Human chorionic gonadotropin is measured in international units (IU). The total recommended dose for small ornamental fishes is 60 IU/kg, divided into two injections (Rottmann and Shireman, 1988a). Carp pituitary is available in a dried powder form and can be used in conjunction with HCG. Two injections of a mixture of 20 IU/cc of HCG and 5 mg of dried carp pituitary are given. The first injection (0.02 cc/50 g body weight) is followed after 6 hours by a second injection (0.13 cc/50 g body weight). Both injections are given intramuscularly at the base of the dorsal fin behind the last ray, where there are no scales (Fig. 66–5).

LRH-A(des-GLY[10] [D-Ala[6]]LRH ethylamide) is available in 1- and 5-mg vials. It is water soluble and should be mixed with sterile water. The recommended dosage is 10 µg/kg of fish. The injection can be given in one or two doses, depending upon the species. It has been our experience that two doses are best. The first injection (2 µg/kg) is followed 6 hours later by a second injection (8 µg/kg). If the fish does not respond to LRH-A injections, use of a dopamine blocker may be indicated in the next series. Reserpine or haloperidol are most commonly used. These should be administered at the time of the first injection of LRH-A. Reserpine is given at a dosage of 50 mg/kg fish, or haloperidol can be used at a dosage of 0.5 mg/kg (Rottmann and Shireman, 1988a, 1990).

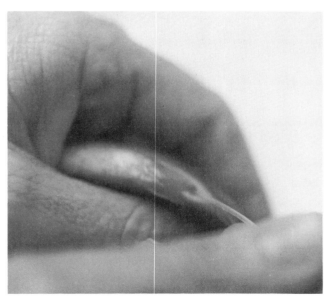

FIGURE 66–3. A small polyethylene tube inserted into the oviduct of a clown loach for obtaining a sample of eggs for staging. (Courtesy of P. Reed.)

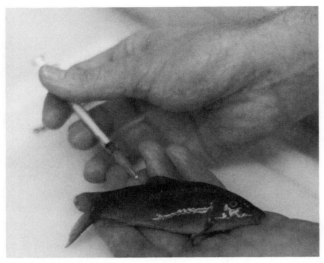

FIGURE 66–5. An intramuscular injection of HCG is given at the base of the dorsal fin of a clown loach. (Courtesy of P. Reed.)

Spawning

Most egg layers can be spawned in a tank or aquarium following injection. Ovulation and subsequent fertilization by the male take place in the container. Often this method works best when a large number of spawners are placed in the container.

Hand stripping can also be used. If hand stripping is to be done, males and females must be housed separately during the postinjection period. Females should be checked at least 1 hour prior to the earliest predicted time of ovulation and every hour thereafter. Ovulation of rainbow sharks and redtail black sharks usually occurs about 6 hours after the second injection (Shireman and Gildae, 1989). The female is ready to strip when eggs flow freely from the vent during gentle manipulation of the abdomen. Prior to stripping, the female should be gently dried to avoid water dripping onto the eggs. Eggs can be stripped into a small dry bowl by gently squeezing her abdomen. A male can then be netted, carefully dried, and milt stripped onto the eggs. Eggs and sperm are carefully mixed in the absence of water. This procedure is generally referred to as dry fertilization. Finally, a small amount of water, sufficient to cover the eggs, is added to the bowl. This activates the sperm, which have approximately 1 minute to penetrate the oocyte before sperm activity ceases. Fertilized eggs can be placed into hatching jars for incubation (Rottmann and Shireman, 1988b). Following incubation, fry are reared according to the needs of the species.

LITERATURE CITED

Axelrod, H.R. (1980) Breeding Aquarium Fishes. T.F.H. Publications, Neptune, New Jersey.

Campton, D.E., and Busack, C.A. (1989) Simple procedure for decapsulating and hatching cysts of brine shrimp (*Artemia* spp.). Progressive Fish Culturist 51:176–179.

Goldstein, R.J. (1971) Anabantoids: Gouramis and Related Fishes. T.F.H. Publications, Neptune, New Jersey.

Jacobs, K. (1971) Live-Bearing Aquarium Fishes. T.F.H. Publications, Neptune, New Jersey.

Loiselle, P.V. (1985) The Cichlid Aquarium. Tetra Press, Morris Plains, New Jersey.

Marshall, N.B. (1970) The Life Of Fishes. Universe Books, New York.

Rottmann, R.W., and Shireman, J.V. (1988a) Hormone Spawning of Tropical Aquarium Fish. Florida Cooperative Extension Service, Bulletin 246, University of Florida, Gainesville, Florida.

Rottmann, R.W., and Shireman, J.V. (1988b) Hatching jar that is inexpensive and simple to assemble. Progressive Fish Culturist 50:57–58.

Rottmann, R.W., and Shireman, J.V. (1990) Hatchery Manual for Grass Carp and Other Riverine Cyprinids. Florida Cooperative Extension Service, Bulletin 244, University of Florida, Gainesville, Florida.

Shireman, J.V., and Gildae, J.A. (1989) Induced spawning of rainbow sharks (*Labeo erythrurus*) and redtail black sharks (*L. bicolor*). Progressive Fish Culturist 51:104–108.

Shireman, J.V., Colle, D.E., and Rottmann, R.W. (1978) Manipulation of temperature and photoperiod for inducing maturation in grass carp. In: Culture of Exotic Fishes Symposium Proceedings (Smitherman, R.O., Shelton, W.L., Grover, J.H., (eds.). Fish Culture Section, American Fisheries Society, Auburn, Alabama, pp 156–184.

Van Ramshorst, J.D. (1981) Aquarium Encyclopedia of Tropical Freshwater Fish. HP Books, Tucson, Arizona.

Wattley, J. (1985) Handbook Of Discus. T.F.H. Publications, Neptune, New Jersey.

Chapter 67

BACTERIAL DISEASES OF FRESHWATER TROPICAL FISHES

MICHAEL K. STOSKOPF

Freshwater tropical fishes are susceptible to a wide variety of bacterial pathogens. Regrettably, relatively few studies have examined these diseases in detail. This is unfortunate, since misdiagnosis of bacterial diseases and inappropriate use of antibacterial drugs is pervasive in the freshwater tropical fish industry and is the cause of many treatment failures. Culture and drug sensitivity testing are underutilized in this group of patients and should be considered mandatory in cases of suspected bacterial-caused morbidity. Four bacterial diseases affecting freshwater tropical fishes listed in Table 67–1 are the focus of this chapter. This group of fishes is affected by other bacteria covered in Chapters 24, 48, 57, and 78.

MYCOBACTERIOSIS

SYNONYMS. Fish tuberculosis, piscine tuberculosis, acid-fast disease, granuloma disease. *Mycobacterium anabanti* and *Mycobacterium platypoecilus* are obsolete synonyms of *Mycobacterium marinum* (Van Duijin, 1981); *Mycobacterium salmoniphilum* is an archaic synonym of *Mycobacterium fortuitum*; *Mycobacterium piscium* is in doubt taxonomically and is not currently accepted as a species.

Host and Geographic Distribution

Mycobacteriosis is worldwide in distribution. All fish species should be considered susceptible; however, certain species figure more prominently in the literature. Of the tropical freshwater species, the anabaenids, labyrinth air breathers, gouramis, and neon tetras are affected. Carp, goldfish, and koi are also affected. The disease is economically important in anadromous fishes, since it causes premature mortality in infected salmon.

Clinical Signs

Mycobacteriosis is a chronic progressive disease. It may take years for it to develop into a clinically apparent illness. Clinical manifestations of mycobacteriosis in fish include lethargy, anorexia, fin and scale loss, exophthalmia, emaciation, skin inflammation and ulceration, edema, peritonitis, and nodules in muscles that may deform the fish.

Pathology and Diagnosis

Postmortem examination usually reveals gray or white nodules in the liver, kidney, heart, or spleen.

TABLE 67–1. Bacterial Diseases of Freshwater Tropical Fishes*

Disease	Organism	Host
Mycobacteriosis	*Mycobacterium marinum* *Mycobacterium fortuitum* *Mycobacterium piscium*	All species of freshwater and marine fishes
Nocardiosis	*Nocardia* spp. *Nocardia asteroides*	Giant gourami Neon tetra Salmonids
	Nocardia seriolae	Yellowtail
Mollie granuloma	*Flavobacterium* spp.	Black mollies
Bacterial neurotoxicosis	*Flavobacterium piscicida*	All species

*See also sections on Flexibacter columnaris in Chapter 24; Aeromonas hydrophila and Pseudomonas fluorescens (Figs. 67–1 to 67–3) in Chapter 48; Edwardsiella spp. in Chapter 57; and Streptococcus spp. and Vibrio spp. in Chapter 78.

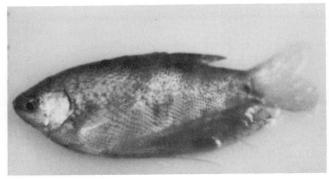

FIGURE 67–1. Freshwater tropical fishes are highly susceptible to *Aeromonas hydrophila*. The diseases caused by the organism vary with the species and individual affected. This gold gourami has a skin ulcer due to *Aeromonas hydrophila* infection. (See Chap. 48.) (Courtesy of P. Reed.)

Skeletal involvement may result in deformities. Diagnosis is usually based on clinical signs and the presence of acid-fast bacteria in tissue sections or smears. Culture of the organism is considered definitive.

Culture and Identification

The mycobacterial species that infect fish are classed in Runyon group IV. They can be cultured successfully on standard tryptone soy agar and brain and heart infusion agar (Arakawa and Fryer, 1984). More commonly, more specialized media, including Petragnani, Lowenstein-Jensen, Middlebrook 7H10, and Dorset egg media, are used for isolation (Austin and Austin, 1987). Whether fish can be infected with other species of *Mycobacterium*, including *Mycobacterium tuberculosis*, is controversial. Most references refer to experiments conducted in 1897 at a French tuberculosis sanitarium (Bataillon and Terre, 1897), but these experiments were not conclusive. An interesting note about a related human pathogen is the

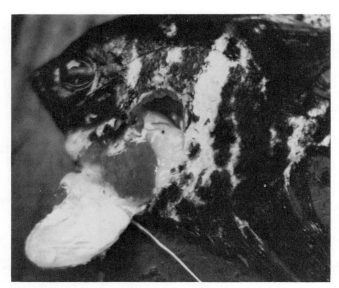

FIGURE 67–2. This angelfish with an *Aeromonas hydrophila* septicemia shows a typical mottled liver. (Courtesy of R. Floyd.)

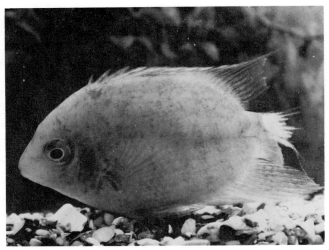

FIGURE 67–3. *Pseudomonas fluorescens* is commonly cultured from tail rot lesions, although mixed bacterial infections are also common in lesions, such as those shown here in a discus. (Courtesy of R. Floyd.)

apparently successful experimental infection of perch with *M. leprae* (Chaussinand and Besse, 1951).

Mycobacteria are gram-positive, pleomorphic rods that are acid-fast and nonmotile. They form cream-colored to yellow colonies on solid media. The optimum temperature for culture varies with the species and apparently the strain of the bacterium; however, 25°C is generally considered optimum for isolating mycobacteria from fish. Differential characteristics of *Mycobacterium fortuitum* and *M. marinum* are shown in Table 67–2.

Transmission and Epidemiology

The methods of transmission of mycobacteria are not well established. Transmission may be from ingestion of contaminated food (Nigrelli and Vogel, 1963; Dulin, 1979). Transovarian transmission has been established in Mexican platyfish and other viviparous fishes (Conroy, 1966). Vertical transmission through eggs is not thought to occur in ovoviviparous fishes (Ross and Johnson, 1962).

These organisms are widespread in most bodies of water. In Oregon as many as 26% of hatchery salmonids have been found to be infected (Arakawa and Fryer, 1984). Infection rates can be quite high in

TABLE 67–2. Differential Characteristics of *Mycobacterium fortuitum* and *M. marinum*

	M. fortuitum	*M. marinum*
Nitrate reduction	+	−
Tween 80 degradation	+/−	+
Nicotinamidase production	−	+
Pyrazinamidase production	−	+

From Runyon, E. H., et al. (1974) Genus I. Mycobacterium Lehmann and Neumann 1896, 363. In: Bergey's Manual of Determinative Bacteriology. 8th ed. (Buchannan, R. E., and Gibbons, N. E., eds.). Williams & Wilkins, Baltimore, pp. 682–701. © 1974, the Williams & Wilkins Co., Baltimore.

contaminated freshwater tropical fish production facilities. The aquatic environment is considered the reservoir. *Mycobacterium marinum* has been cultured from swimming pools, beaches, natural streams, estuaries, tropical fish tanks, and city tap water. Human epidemics of granulomatous skin disease have occurred from swimming in infected water. This mode of human infection is much more common than infections from exposure to infected tropical fish tanks. Granulomas from *M. marinum* usually occur at sites of minor skin abrasions that become apparent 2 to 3 weeks after exposure.

Treatment and Control

In general, mycobacteria that infect fish are highly resistant to typical antimycobacterial drugs. They are almost uniformly resistant to isoniazid. Treatments have been described with chloramine-B or -T, cyclosporine, doxycycline, ethambutol, ethionamide, isoniazid, kanamycin, minocycline, penicillin, rifampin, streptomycin, sulfonamides, and tetracycline (Austin and Austin, 1987). Multiple drug therapy is generally more successful than single drug therapy. The drug combination of choice is probably doxycycline and rifampin.

No bacterins are available for prevention of the infection. Control measures center around avoidance of overcrowding and poor water conditions, removal of affected fish, and effective quarantines for periods of 4 weeks or more.

NOCARDIOSIS

Host and Geographic Distribution

Nocardiosis, due to *Nocardia asteroides*, was first reported in neon tetras reared in Argentina (Conroy, 1963). That organism was pathogenic to threespot gouramis and paradise fish, but not goldfish. The disease has also been reported in hatchery-reared rainbow trout in West Virginia (Snieszko et al., 1964), chinook salmon (Wolke and Meade, 1974) and cultured yellowtail in Japan (Kusuda and Nakagawa, 1978). Most recently, the disease has been reported to be due to a new species of *Nocardia* in giant gourami farms in Japan (Kitao et al, 1989).

Clinical Signs

In the enzootics in the Japanese giant gourami farms, typical external signs included sloughed scales, exophthalmia, and opaque eyes. In the original outbreak in neon tetras, the clinical signs included skin ulcers, listlessness, anorexia, and emaciation. In other outbreaks of nocardiosis, it is difficult to differentiate the syndrome from mycobacteriosis. Affected fish are sluggish and may have faded colors. Exophthalmia, fin and tail rot, abdominal distention, emaciation, surface hemorrhages, and surface ulcers may

be present. Occasionally, small white spots due to granuloma formation in the dermis, muscle, gills, and internal organs are seen. Anemia can be a component of the disease.

Culture and Diagnosis

The major difficulty is to differentiate this disease from mycobacteriosis. Immunofluorescence techniques can be used to identify the agent, as can chemical reactions of lipids extracted from isolated bacteria. Otherwise culture of the organism is required for a diagnosis. *Nocardia* spp. have variable incubation temperature requirements and can be grown on Sabouraud's dextrose agar and blood agar, although if infection is suspected, *Cytophaga* agar or Lowenstein-Jensen medium is advised. Colonies are generally small, round, and dry.

Pathology

Affected fish have numerous creamy-white nodules in the gills, spleen, kidney, and liver. Occasionally nodules are found in the swimbladder, stomach, and other organs. The lesions are granulomatous with acid-fast organisms often evidenced in the centers.

Transmission, Epidemiology, and Pathogenesis

Nocardia spp. occur in fresh water and soil. The organism remains viable in clean sea water for only a few days, but polluted water extends viability markedly (Kariya et al., 1968). Infected animals are thought to serve as a reservoir of infection. Experimental attempts to infect rainbow trout through ingestion or injection of isolated organisms have failed (Snieszko et al., 1964).

Treatment and Control

Vaccines investigated to date have not been effective. Some success with chemotherapy using sulfonamides has been reported (Van Duijin, 1981).

MOLLIE GRANULOMA

SYNONYMS. Mollie popeye, Mollie madness.

Host and Geographic Distribution

A *Flavobacterium*-caused granulomatous disease occurs in black mollies. It has not been described in other species and has been reported in the literature only once (Kluge, 1965).

Clinical Signs

Clinical signs of this disease include disorientation, bilateral and unilateral exophthalmia, and occasionally firm nodules in the musculature that are palpable externally.

Pathology and Diagnosis

The disease is characterized by disseminated granulomas in all internal organs. The brain, meninges, optic nerve, orbit, and retina may be affected. The granulomatous panophthalmitis in this disease is similar to what is seen in nocardiosis and mycobacterial infections. Granulomas of the choroid are common. Multinucleate giant cells are rarely found in the granulomas. Diagnosis is based upon culture and identification of the organism. No serodiagnostic tests are available.

Culture and Identification

The organism can be cultured on *Cytophaga* agar as well as a variety of other media. Colonies are pigmented yellow to orange, and are usually mucoid. The bacteria are gram-negative pleomorphic rods with a polar flagellum.

Transmission and Epidemiology

Transmission is thought to be by direct contact. Waterborne transmission cannot be eliminated as a possibility. Little is known about predisposing factors in the disease. The disease has been experimentally induced in black mollies using inoculation of organisms isolated from naturally occurring infections (Kluge, 1965).

Treatment and Control

Control measures center upon avoiding the introduction of infected fish. No bacterins are available. Although treatment with tetracyclines might have efficacy based on in vitro sensitivity testing, the granulomatous nature of the response may preclude effective delivery of drug to the disease organism.

FLAVOBACTERIUM NEUROTOXICOSIS

SYNONYMS. Bacterial toxicosis, *Flavobacterium* spp., *Flavobacterium piscicida, Pseudomonas piscicida.*

Host and Geographic Distribution

Flavobacterium neurotoxicosis appears to affect any fish exposed to the endotoxin produced by the bacteria. There is considerable confusion over the taxonomy of the organism, with some workers placing it in the genus *Pseudomonas* and others not specifying its taxonomy. The putative organism is common in marine water as well as fresh water and is probably essentially worldwide in distribution.

Clinical Signs

The clinical signs of this disease include aimless swimming, loss of equilibrium, convulsions, paralysis, and death (Meyer et al., 1959).

Pathology and Diagnosis

Diagnosis is relatively nonspecific and is based upon appropriate clinical signs along with culture and identification of the organism. No serologic or immunologic diagnostic tests are available. The mortality experienced is acute and significant pathologic changes may be difficult to identify (Bein, 1954).

Culture and Identification

The taxonomic status of *Flavobacterium* is at best uncertain. *Flavobacterium piscicida* is not listed in *Bergey's Manual of Systemic Bacteriology* (Holmes et al., 1984), and there is controversy over its actual existence. Other *Flavobacterium* species, including *F. branchiophila* and *F. balustinum,* have been reported, but again the taxonomy is poorly defined. The disease organism in question in this disease is a gram-negative, motile, pleomorphic rod that produces yellow or orange water-soluble pigment. It produces arginine dihydrolase but not β-galactosidase. It does not produce acid from glucose or lactose but will with inositol and rhamnose. It has also been placed in the *Pseudomonas* genus by some investigators (Buck et al., 1963).

Transmission and Epidemiology

These organisms apparently occur in large numbers in both marine and fresh water (Allen et al., 1983; Austin, 1982; Meyer, 1959). In marine systems, they have been found associated with red tide conditions and may contribute to fish mortality. Direct transmission from fish to fish via water is considered likely. The neuromuscular endotoxin produced by the organism is potent and considered responsible for the pathogenesis of the disease.

Treatment and Control

Treatment and control measures are not well established for this disease. Tetracyclines are apparently effective as a control measure against this disease organism (Acuigrup, 1980; Farkas, 1985), but no treatment for the neurotoxicosis caused by exposure to the endotoxin is known. It should be a relatively rare event in a well-managed aquarium.

LITERATURE CITED

Acuigrup (1980) Flavobacteriosis in coho salmon *(Oncorhynchus kisutch)*. In: Fish Diseases (Ahne, W., ed.). Third COPRAQ-Session, Springer-Verlag, Berlin, pp. 212–217 (cited in Austin and Austin, 1987).

Allen, D.A., Austin, B., and Colwell, R.R. (1983) Numerical taxonomy of bacterial isolates associated with a freshwater fishery. J. Gen. Microbiol. 129:2043–2062.

Arakawa, C.K., and Fryer, J.L. (1984) Isolation and characterization of a new subspecies of *Mycobacterium chelonei* infectious for salmonid fish. Helgolander Meeresuntersucheungen 37:329–342.

Austin, B. (1982) Taxonomy of bacteria isolated from a coastal, marine fishrearing unit. J. Appl. Bacteriol. 53:253–268.

Austin, B., and Austin, D.A. (1987) Bacterial Fish Pathogens. John Wiley & Sons, New York.

Bataillon, E., and Terre, L. (1897) Un nouveau type de tuberculose. C.R. Soc. Biol. 49:446–449.

Bein, S.J. (1954) A study of certain chromogenic bacteria isolated from "red-tide" water with a description of a new species. Bull. Mar. Sci. in the Gulf and Caribbean 4:110–119.

Buck, J.D., Meyers, S.P., and Leifson, E. (1963) *Pseudomonas (Flavobacterium) piscicida* Bein Comb. nov. J. Bacteriol. 86:1125–1126.

Chaussinand, R., and Besse, P. (1951) Inoculation de bacille de Hansen et du bacille de Stefansky a la perche arc en ciel. Rev. Brasil. Leprol. 19:4–7.

Conroy, D.A. (1963) The study of tuberculosis-like condition in neon tetras *(Hyphessobrycon innesi)*. I. Symptoms of the disease and preliminary description of the organism isolated. Microbiol. Espan. 16:47–54.

Conroy, D.A. (1966) Observaciones sobre casos Espontaneous de tuberculosis ictica. Microbiol. Espan. 19:93–113.

Dulin, M.P. (1979) A review of tuberculosis (mycobacteriosis) in fish. Vet. Med./Small Anim. Clinician May: 735–737.

Farkas, J. (1985) Filamentous *Flavobacterium* sp. isolated from fish with gill diseases in cold water. Aquaculture 44:1–10.

Holmes, B., Owen, R.J., and McMeekin, T.A. (1984) Genus *Flavobacterium* Bergey, Harrison, Breed, Hammer and Huntoon 1923, 97. In: Bergey's Manual of Systematic Bacteriology. Vol. 1 (Krieg, N.R., ed.). Williams & Wilkins, Baltimore, pp. 353–361.

Kariya, T., Kubota, S., Nakamura, Y., and Kira, K. (1968) Nocardial infection in cultured yellowtail *(Seriola quinquiradiata* and *S. purpurascens)*. I. Bacteriological study. Fish Pathol. 3:16–23.

Kitao, T., Ruangpan, L., and Fukudome, M. (1989) Isolation and classification of a *Nocardia* species from diseased giant gourami osphronemus goramy. J. Aquatic Anim. Health 1:154–162.

Kluge, J.P. (1965) A granulomatous disease of fish produced by flavobacteria. Pathol. Vet. 2:545–552.

Kusuda, R., and Nakagawa, A. (1978) Nocardial infection of cultured yellowtail. Fish Pathol. 13:25–31.

Meyer, S.P., Baslow, M.H., Bein, S.J., and Mark, C.E. (1959) Studies on *Flavobacterium piscicida* Bein. 1. Growth, toxicity and ecological consideration. J. Bacteriol. 78:225–230.

Nigrelli, R.F., and Vogel, H. (1963) Spontaneous tuberculosis in fishes and in other cold-blooded vertebrates with special reference to *Mycobacterium fortuitum* Cruz from fish and human lesions. Zoologica 48(9):130–143.

Ross, A.J., and Johnson, H.E. (1962) Studies of transmission of mycobacterial infections of chinook salmon. Progressive Fish Culturist 24:147–149.

Runyon, E.H., Wayne, L.G., and Kubica, G.P. (1974) Genus I. Mycobacterium Lehmann and Neumann 1896, 363. In: Bergey's Manual of Determinative Bacteriology. 8th ed. (Buchannan, R.E., and Gibbons, N.E., (eds.). Williams & Wilkins, Baltimore, pp 682–701.

Snieszko, S.F., Bullock, G.L., Dunbar, C.E., and Pettijohn, L.L. (1964) Nocardial infection in hatchery-reared fingerling rainbow trout *(Salmo gairdneri)*. J. Bacteriol. 88:1809–1810.

Van Duijin, C. (1981) Tuberculosis in fishes. J. Small Anim. Pract. 22:391–411.

Wolke, R.E., and Meade, T.L. (1974) Nocardiosis in chinook salmon. J. Wildlife Dis. 10:150–154.

Chapter 68

FUNGAL AND ALGAL DISEASES OF FRESHWATER TROPICAL FISHES

BEVERLY A. GOVEN-DIXON

Fungal disease in freshwater tropical fishes is associated with adverse environmental conditions. Infection, whether occurring in isolated individuals or in epidemic proportions, is preceded by some environmental insult that disrupts host homeostasis. The diseases are listed in Table 68–1.

SAPROLEGNIASIS

SYNONYMS. Skin fungus, cotton tuft disease.

Host and Geographic Distribution

In ornamental fishes, the fancy varieties, particularly long-finned fishes, are most subject to infection because of a greater frequency of damage to fins. Integumental damage coupled with adverse water conditions, in particular lower water temperatures, initiates hyphal growth, leading to dermal necrosis (Amlacher, 1970).

Most of these infections have been attributed to members of the family Saprolegniaceae, which in-

TABLE 68–1. Fungal and Algal Diseases of Freshwater Tropical Fishes*

Disease	Organism	Host
Saprolegniasis	*Saprolegnia, Calyptralegnia, Achlya, Aphanomyces, Dictyuchus, Leptolegnia, Pythiopsis,* and *Thraustotheca*	All freshwater species
Ichthyophoniasis	*Ichthyophonus hoferi*	Cichlids, anabaenids, guppies, majority of freshwater and marine species
Algal skin disease	*Mucophilus cyprini*	Kissing gouramis, swordtails
Algal toxicity	*Prymnesium parvum*	All freshwater species

*See also Chapters 25, 37, and 79.

cludes the genera *Saprolegnia, Calyptralegnia, Achlya, Aphanomyces, Dictyuchus, Leptolegnia, Pythiopsis,* and *Thraustotheca.* These genera are considered to be saprophytic "water molds" and are normal, ubiquitous components of freshwater ecosystems (Neish and Hughes, 1980). They appear able to infect most species of fish as secondary invaders.

Clinical Signs

The term *saprolegniasis* refers to a cotton-like growth of fungi adherent to skin or gills. Although the condition is primarily a problem of freshwater fish, some species may affect fish in low-salinity waters (Wolke, 1975). Spores of *Saprolegnia* spp. are usually present on the skin of fish but are prevented from germinating by healthy skin and antibody-containing mucus (Reichenbach-Klinke, 1973). It has been noted that alkaline water from ponds where concrete was not matured affects mucus and increases susceptibility to fungal infection (van Duijin, 1967). When these normal defenses are damaged, the spores germinate, grow into the skin, and form the hyphal mat consisting of grayish-white to brown layers.

The characteristic gross lesion consists of a focal epidermal erosion with a cotton-like mass randomly distributed on the surface. The cottony appearance is seen only when the fish are in the water. Once they are taken out of water the mass collapses, resembling a ball of wet cotton.

Diagnosis and Pathology

Microscopically, the mycelial mass is weakly eosinophilic overlying a zone of necrotic epithelium. The hyphae are cenocytic and slightly branched (Fig. 68–1). In early lesions, scales may be lifted away from the body wall, exposing a pale area with peripheral erythema. As the infection advances, ulceration occurs with the exposure of underlying musculature. Individual hyphae extend into the dermis and, in far advanced cases, into the muscle fibers. A slight inflammatory response is generated with lymphocytic and macrophagic infiltration. No systemic involvement has been reported (Wolke, 1975). Toxin production has not been reported. Damage can be directly related to tissue necrosis in the area of the hyphae. The infection is usually chronic. Death is due to impaired osmoregulation and the inability to maintain body-fluid balance (Neish and Hughes, 1980). *Saprolegnia* occasionally infects gills and eyes and is opportunistic in eyes that are already damaged.

Culture and Identification

Saprolegnia spp. are among the easiest fungi to isolate and cultivate in the laboratory. Samples can be plated directly onto medium containing GYS-tellurite or YpSs-tellurite (Emerson YpSs, Difco) to prevent bacterial contamination (Wolke, 1975). Antibiotics, such as penicillin and streptomycin at 0.5 g/L of agar, will also reduce bacterial growth (Alderman, 1982).

Alternatively, pieces of infected fish tissue can be placed in sterile water with "bait" such as sterile dead flies, split boiled wheat, hemp seed, or corn kernels. Within 2 or 3 days at room temperature, fungal growth will occur on the "bait" by asexual reproduction. Sexual reproduction usually can be observed in 5 to 7 days, and cultures can be transferred to diagnostic media.

In vitro sexual reproduction is stimulated by media containing peptone, glucose, and maltose. The sexual stages consist of a small clavate or pyriform anteridium and a spherical oogonium. Oogonia may develop parthenogenetically (Krause, 1960). During the sexual cycle, the antheridium approaches the oogonium, forming a process that penetrates the oogonium through pores in its walls. Nuclei of the antheridium fertilize the egg, forming a zygote. After fusion, double membranes form around the zygote, or oospore. Several golden-brown oospores are formed per fusion.

The genus *Saprolegnia* is characterized by the production of biflagellate motile zoospores, which function in asexual reproduction and dispersal. Zoospores are produced from specialized hyphae that form long, cylindrical zoosporangia approximately 180 to 350 μm by 20 to 24 μm. Two types of zoospores are formed, a primary pie-shaped spore with flagella inserted into the top of the spore, and a secondary bean-shaped spore that is a stronger swimmer (Davis, 1953). Asexual reproduction is also carried

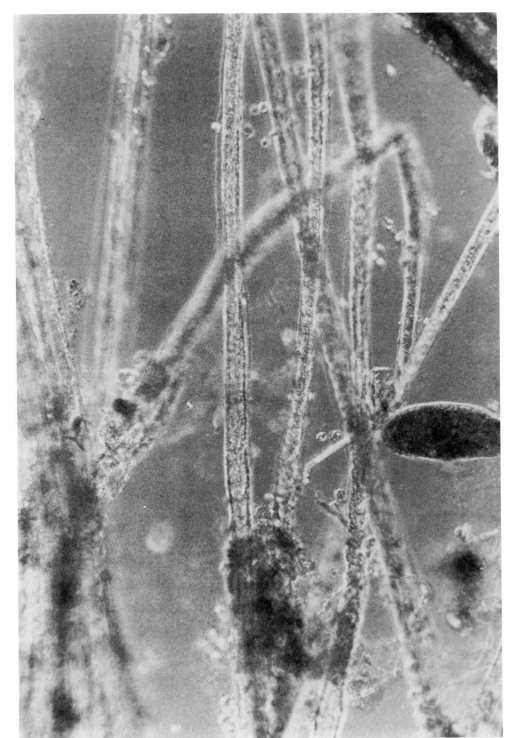

FIGURE 68–1. Wet mount of *Saprolegnia* sp. from a surface lesion (400×).

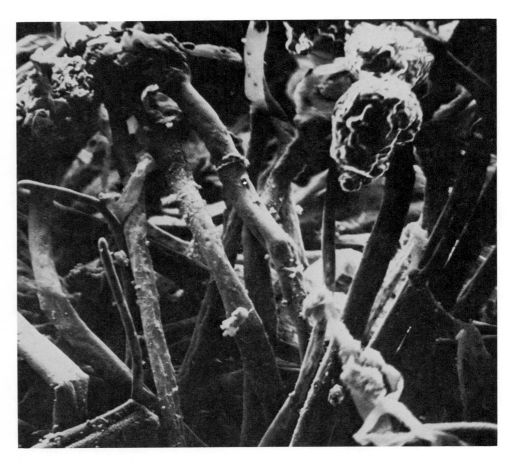

FIGURE 68–2. A scanning electron micrograph of *Saprolegnia* sp. from a skin infection (375×). (Courtesy of B. Contreras.)

out by means of chlamydospores (chlamydoconidia). These spores form chains of up to 4 mm long, with as many as 20 spores per chain. The chlamydospores give rise to either hyphae or the biflagellate zoospores.

Transmission, Epidemiology, and Pathogenesis

The Saprolegniaceae, worldwide in distribution, are reported to infect both fish and fish eggs. The predominant genus in terms of frequency of isolation is the genus *Saprolegnia*. Infection with *Saprolegnia* spp., as with many other mycotic infections, is contingent upon certain predisposing factors. This disease is generally considered as an opportunistic secondary invasion following injury. However, once the infection is established, the lesions usually continue to enlarge and may cause death. Fish are more likely to be infected through injuries produced by spawning, handling, or prior parasitic infection. Other stress factors such as malnutrition and water temperature may also predispose to fungal infection with *Saprolegnia* spp. It has also been noted that the pesticide DDT appears to stimulate the growth of *Saprolegnia* (Jones, 1976).

Saprolegnia spp. thrive in poorly maintained, badly aerated tanks, on unconsumed food, dead fish, and dead eggs (Reichenbach-Klinke and Elkan, 1965). Normally, abundant vegetative growth is produced in the form of hyphae. Zoospores cannot infect fish eggs, but hyphae can colonize dead eggs, producing an abundant mycelial mat. Live eggs then die of respiratory obstruction as hyphae inhibit the entry of oxygenated water (Hoffman, 1967; Bauer et al., 1973).

The degree of virulence of Saprolegniaceae varies with the fungal species and host susceptibility. Vishniac and Nigrelli (1957) were able to infect platys with 16 species in seven genera of the Saprolegniales following scale removal. Infection was thought to occur only secondarily following trauma; however, *Saprolegnia parasitica* and *S. ferax* are highly virulent and are known to be primary pathogens capable of causing infections without the presence of preceding bacterial or viral disease. Virulence varies greatly and may be specific to certain pathogenic strains.

The virulence of various strains is thought to correlate with the production of a chymotrypsin-like proteolytic enzyme that provides the capacity to go from a saprophytic to a necrotrophic mode of nutrition (Neish and Hughes, 1980). The hormonal status of fish may also contribute to susceptibility. A direct correlation between increased plasma corticosteroid and susceptibility to infection has been observed (Roth, 1972).

High levels of estradiol, progesterone, and thyroid-stimulating hormone related to spawning induce an increase in pituitary-intrarenal activity and corticosteroid release. In these circumstances, *Saprolegnia* may act as a primary pathogen. These steroids reduce the immune response, causing impairment of antibody formation and suppression of reactive tissue inflammation.

Treatment and Control

Saprolegnia infections of eggs can be minimized by reduction of organic material in the water and dips in antifungal medications. Several treatments are recommended in the literature, including formalin or malachite green baths or dips (Brown and Gratzek, 1980; van Duijn, 1967). Both treatments present some human and environmental health hazards.

Infected fish have been routinely treated in a variety of ways, including copper sulfate baths, zinc-free malachite green baths, and potassium permanganate baths. Localized wounds can be swabbed with 10% povidone-iodine or tincture of Mercurochrome (merbromin). Raising the tank temperature to between 27° and 28°C, with increased aeration, may be beneficial. Sodium chloride baths are as effective as other chemotherapeutic treatments.

ICHTHYOPHONIASIS

SYNONYMS. *Ichthyophonus hoferi*, Traumelkrankeit, *Basidiobolus*, *Ichthyosporidium*.

Host and Geographic Distribution

Ichthyophonus hoferi is generally considered to be a fungal disease of marine fish. However, at one time it was held responsible for half of the total losses in ornamental fish worldwide (Geisler, 1963). More recently, evidence has shown that many of those cases attributed to *I. hoferi* were misidentified piscine mycobacteriosis that, like *Ichthyophonus*, elicits a chronic granulomatous response. *Ichthyophonus hoferi* is now considered fairly rare in aquarium fish, although a tropical form of the disease differing from the salmonid form has been described. The disease also occurs in carp, trout, and salmon.

Clinical Signs

Infected fish become lethargic. Infection of the brain results in loss of equilibrium, exophthalmos, and staggering movements. Liver infection may cause skin pallor and thrombosis of blood vessels. Perhaps the strangest case of infection was a report of sex reversal in guppies whose ovaries were affected by this fungus (Reichenbach-Klinke and Elkan, 1965).

Diagnosis

Diagnosis is commonly made by examination of wet mounts of kidney or other tissues. The fungus is generally seen in the form of variably sized (10 to 100 μm) spherical bodies with hyphal germ tubes. The wide variation in morphology makes it very likely that more than one pathogenic organism is being interpreted as *I. hoferi*. No serologic tests are available.

Pathology

Generally the pathology associated with *I. hoferi* is that of typical eosinophil-laden granulomas. In tropical fishes, the predominant feature is a degenerate cyst consisting of a concentrically laminated, melanin-pigmented capsule. Long germinative tubular hyphae fail to develop (Neish and Hughes, 1980). Brain, gills, skin, and gonads are most notably affected. In anabantids, this organism has been observed to penetrate through muscle to the hypodermis and break through to the exterior of the fish, causing bleeding ulcerations. Tumor-like changes in the skin have also been noted. In cichlids, skin lesions and bone damage occur.

Culture and Identification

The organism can be cultured on the surface of Sabouraud's dextrose medium slants supplemented with 1% bovine serum. Germination and growth is seen 7 to 10 days after inoculation at an optimum temperature of 10°C. Growth occurs in a temperature range of 3° to 20°C. Identification of this organism is controversial. There is reasonable evidence that there may be more than one species of fungus involved. The differing development of the forms affecting salmonids and the forms affecting aquarium fishes has been attributed to differing environmental factors or to the presence of two distinct species. Reichenbach-Klinke (1973) showed that a fungus isolated from discus fish did not differ from *Ichthyophonus* described from salmonids and herring.

Transmission, Epidemiology, Pathogenesis, Treatment, and Control

Ichthyophoniasis is not highly contagious, and infection is rare if fish are kept under good conditions (Reichenbach-Klinke, 1973). The mechanisms of infection are speculative. Infection is thought to occur through ingestion of cyst material, which is dissolved in the digestive process. The released infective stage germinates, invades the intestine epithelium, penetrates into the blood vessels, and is distributed to numerous organs (Reichenbach-Klinke and Elkan, 1965). There is no known treatment for *Ichthyophonus hoferi* infection.

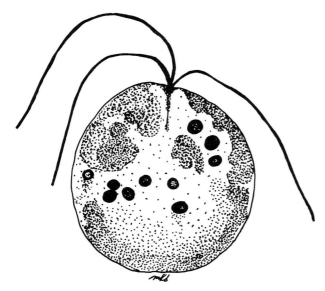

FIGURE 68–3. The phytoflagellate *Prymnesium parvum* (4000×). (Courtesy of M. Stoskopf.)

ALGAL INFECTIONS IN FRESHWATER TROPICAL FISHES

Algal problems in freshwater tropical fishes held in aquarium systems are rare. Mortalities in kissing gouramis and swordtails have been attributed to *Mucophilus cyprini,* which occurs in the skin and gills of fish (Hoffman et al., 1960). The majority of problems relating to algae in these species of fish occur in production ponds as a result of phytoplankton blooms that result in oxygen depletion. These blooms are associated with recent pond fertilization, increases in organic matter, or pollution. Algal mats can shade deeper water, causing decreased photosynthesis and decreased oxygen levels. Areas of low oxygen saturation may eventually become anaerobic, resulting in the production of hydrogen sulfide, methane, and ammonia. Decaying algae also provide food for subsequent bacterial blooms.

Occasionally, lesions will be evident in fish that are directly related to algal invasions of tissues. Sometimes algal cysts or cells are evident in gills, the eye orbit, or the viscera. Other algae produce toxins that are protein decomposition products liberated by dead cells or by-products of photosynthesis. Some algal by-products are neurotoxins that cause erratic swimming, convulsions, and death in fish. One organism in particular, *Prymnesium parvum* (Fig. 68–3), produces the ichthyotoxin prymnesin, which is known to cause extensive fish mortalities. Prymne-

sin, which is produced during algal reproduction, causes a loss of selective membrane permeability, interfering with normal gill osmoregulation (Wedemeyer et al., 1976; Schubert, 1974).

Algal growth and control in pond culture needs to be dealt with in terms of preventative maintenance. While it is true that algae are required as the basis of the food chain in ponds, too much growth can result in severe problems. Algal control can easily be facilitated with numerous chemical treatments, including copper sulfate, diquat, and simazine. If growth gets out of control, application of these substances may only exacerbate the problem. Large amounts of dying algae further decrease available oxygen supplies, and encourage bacterial and fungal growth. A continual monitoring and controlled growth program rather than a last-ditch shotgun approach is necessary for healthy and productive ponds.

LITERATURE CITED

Alderman, D.J. (1982) Fungal diseases of aquatic animals. In: Microbial Diseases of Fish. (Roberts, R.J., ed.). Academic Press, New York, pp. 189–242.

Amlacher, E. (1970) Textbook of Fish Diseases. (Conroy, D.A., and Herman, R.L., trans.). T.F.H. Publications, Neptune, New Jersey.

Bauer, O.N., Musselivs, V.A., and Strelhov, Y.A. (1973) Diseases of Pond Fishes. Israel Program for Scientific Translations, Jerusalem, Israel.

Brown, E.E., and Gratzek, J.B. (1980) Fish Farming Handbook. AVI Pub. Co., Inc., Westport, Connecticut.

Davis, H.S. (1953) Culture and Diseases of Game Fishes. University of California Press, Berkeley, California.

Geisler, R. (1963) Aquarium Fish Diseases. T.F.H. Publications, Neptune, New Jersey.

Hoffman, G.L. (1967) Parasites of North American Freshwater Fishes. University of California Press, Berkeley and Los Angeles, California.

Hoffman, G., Bishop, H., and Dunbar, C.E. (1960) Algal parasites in fish. Progressive Fish Culturist 22:180.

Jones, G.E.B. (ed.) (1976) Recent Advances in Aquatic Mycology. John Wiley & Sons, New York.

Krause, R. (1960) Untersuchungen Uber Den Einfluss Der Aussenfaktoren Auf Die Bildung Der Oogonien Bei *Saprolegnia ferax* (Gruith) Thuret. Arch. Microbiol. 36:373–386.

Neish, G.A., and Hughes, G.C. (1980) Diseases of Fishes, Book 6: Fungal Diseases of Fishes. (Snieszko, S., and Axelrod, H.R., eds.). T.F.H. Publications, Neptune, New Jersey.

Reichenbach-Klinke, H.H. (1973) Fish Pathology. T.F.H. Publications, Neptune, New Jersey.

Reichenbach-Klinke, H.H., and Elkan, E. (1965) The Principal Diseases of Lower Vertebrates: Diseases of Fishes. Academic Press Inc. Ltd., London, United Kingdom.

Roth, R.R. (1972) Some factors contributing to the development of fungus infections in freshwater fish. J. Wildl. Dis. 8:24–28.

Schubert, G. (1974) Cure and Recognize Aquarium Fish Diseases. T.F.H. Publications, Neptune, New Jersey.

van Duijin, C. (1967) Diseases of Fishes. Charles C Thomas, Springfield, Illinois.

Vishniac, J.F., and Nigrelli, R.F. (1957) The ability of Saprolegniaceae to parasitize platyfish. Zoologica 43:131.

Wedemeyer, G.A., Meyer, F.P., and Smith, L. (1976) Diseases of Fishes, Book 5: Environmental Stress and Fish Disease. (Snieszko, S., and Axelrod, H.R., eds.). T.F.H. Publications, Neptune, New Jersey.

Wolke, R.E. (1975) Pathology of bacterial and fungal diseases affecting fish. In: Pathology of Fishes. (Ribelin, W.E., and Migaki, G., eds.). University of Wisconsin Press, Madison, Wisconsin, pp. 33–116.

Chapter 69

FRESHWATER TROPICAL FISH VIRUSES

PHILIP E. McALLISTER

Knowledge of the viruses of freshwater tropical fishes is limited because research interest has focused on the intensively cultured food and sport fishes. Some of the freshwater tropical fish viruses are unique, whereas others are part of well-established taxonomic groupings of fish viruses. The viruses listed in Table 69–1 have been detected in freshwater tropical fishes.

RAMIREZ' DWARF CICHLID VIRUS

SYNONYMS. Cichlid virus, cichlid blood disease.

Host and Geographic Distribution

Leibovitz and Riis (1980) reported an acute disease of putative viral etiology in young adult (3 to 5 cm long) Ramirez' dwarf cichlids imported into the United States from South America.

Clinical Signs

Affected fish are inappetent and pale and show respiratory distress, uncoordinated swimming, and transitory scoliosis. Hemorrhages occur in the skin and in the iris of the eye. As the disease progresses, fish become emaciated and lethargic and die.

Pathology

The internal organs are pale and displaced to the anterior of the body cavity. The spleen is enlarged three to four times normal, and the liver and kidneys are shrunken. The intestine is devoid of food but contains a clear, mucoid fluid. Degenerative changes are seen in the liver, kidneys, spleen, pancreas, intestine, and eyes. Extensive focal necrosis and occasional petechial hemorrhages occur in affected organs. Numerous inclusions are seen in spleen cells early in the infection, whereas late in the infection, spleen cells contain only remnants of nuclear membrane and a single, eosinophilic cytoplasmic inclusion.

Diagnosis and Virus Detection

Diagnosis is based on clinical signs and pathology. The virus has not been isolated in cell culture, and no serologic tests have been developed for virus identification. Electron micrographs of spleen cells show cytoplasmic arrays of viruslike particles, 110 to 130 nm in diameter, early in the infection. No viruslike particles are seen in the eosinophilic inclusions found late in the infection.

Transmission, Epidemiology, and Pathogenesis

Although controlled transmission trials have not been performed, empirical evidence indicates that the disease runs its course in 3 to 4 weeks with 100% morbidity and 40 to 80% mortality.

Treatment and Control

Methods for the treatment and control of the disease are unknown. The prudent fish culturist quarantines feral fish until their health status is determined.

XIPHOPHORUS SP. HYBRID MELANOMA PAPOVAVIRUS AND *XIPHOPHORUS* SP. HYBRID NEUROBLASTOMA RETROVIRUSES

Certain platy × swordtail hybrids develop neoplasms spontaneously or after exposure to carcinogens or mutagens. Neoplastic and nonneoplastic cells from all of these fish appear to contain the cellular homology of the avian sarcoma virus oncogene (Barnekow et al., 1982; Schartl et al., 1982).

Because this "tumor gene" might be related to a spore virus, tumor-bearing fish were treated with 5-bromo–2'-deoxyuridine to induce the production of viral particles (Kollinger et al., 1979). When examined by electron microscopy, papovaviruslike particles

569

TABLE 69–1. Viral Diseases of Freshwater Tropical Fishes*

Disease	Virus	Host
Cichlid blood eye disease	Ramirez' dwarf cichlid virus	Ramirez' dwarf cichlid
Melanoma	*Xiphophorus* sp. hybrid melanoma papovavirus	*Xiphophorus* sp.
Neuroblastoma	*Xiphophorus* sp. hybrid neuroblastoma retroviruses	*Xiphophorus* sp.
Skin ulcerative disease	Snakehead rhabdovirus	Striped snakehead Swamp eel
Deep angelfish disease	Deep angelfish herpesvirus	Deep angelfish
Chromide cichlid anemia	Chromide cichlid iridovirus	Chromide cichlid

*See also sections on Lymphocystis (Fig. 69–1) and Rio Grande perch rhabdovirus in Chapter 26; infectious pancreatic necrosis in Chapter 38; and carp pox, goldfish virus-1 and goldfish virus-2, and spring viremia of carp in Chapter 50.

were seen in treated melanomas, and retroviruslike particles were seen in treated neuroblastoma tissue.

Melanomas contain an unenveloped particle, 40 to 50 nm in diameter, seen in large concentrations in the cytoplasm, in intercellular spaces, and in membrane-bound aggregates and crystalline arrays of particles, 25 to 30 nm in diameter, in the nucleus. The morphology, size, and arrangement resembled polyoma-type papovaviruses, and the two particles may be alternative forms of the same virus (Kollinger et al., 1979). No virus has been isolated in cell culture, and the etiologic significance of the virus to the tumor is unknown.

The neuroblastomas induced by exposure to *N*-methyl-*N*-nitrosourea showed retroviruslike particles randomly distributed in the cytoplasm of tumor cells. The virions were enveloped, measured about 100 nm in diameter, and contained a somewhat electron-lucent core. Two morphologic types of retrovirus were seen, a type B particle with an eccentric core and a type C particle with a centrally located core

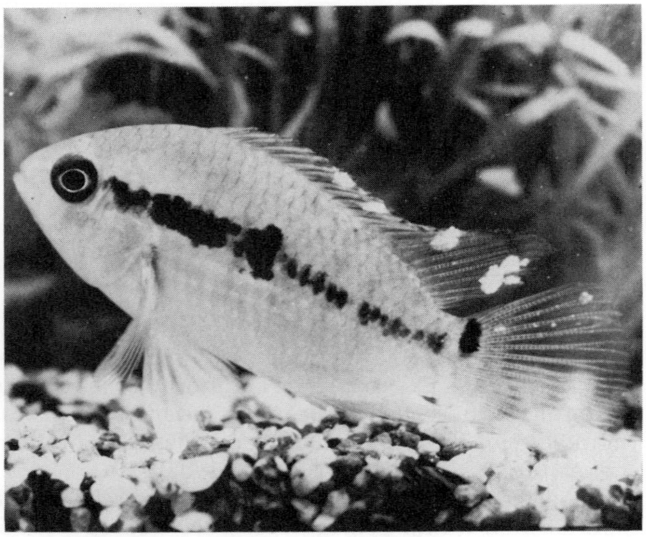

(Kollinger et al., 1979). The type B particles were found mostly in intracellular vacuoles. Neither particle was seen in normal tissue or untreated tumor tissue, and the viruslike particles seen in the neuroblastoma tissue were morphologically distinct from those seen in the melanoma tissue. No virus has been isolated, and the etiologic significance of the viruses to the tumor is unknown.

STRIPED SNAKEHEAD SKIN ULCERATIVE DISEASE

SYNONYMS. Snakehead ulcerative disease, striped snakehead ulcerative rhabdovirus, snakehead rhabdovirus infection, ulcerative rhabdovirus.

Host and Geographic Distribution

Skin ulcerative disease occurs in many species of feral and pond-cultured freshwater fishes in Southeast Asia. In this instance, virus was recovered from striped snakehead and swamp eel taken from various locations in Burma and Thailand (Ahne et al., 1988; Frerichs et al., 1986). Two virus isolations have been reported, but the isolates appear to be very similar, if not identical.

Clinical Signs, Pathology, and Diagnosis

Affected fish have large, deep ulcerations of the skin on the head and body. The ulcers heal, but underlying tissues are partly destroyed. Skin ulcerative disease, in a generic sense, can be diagnosed by gross clinical signs. However, the case of skin ulcerative disease described here can be diagnosed only by isolation of virus in cell culture and its identification using specific immune serum.

Virus Isolation

Samples of liver, kidney, and spleen were taken from striped snakeheads and freshwater eels show-

FIGURE 69–1. White lesions on the fins of a cichlid typical of lymphocystis virus infection. (This virus is covered in detail in Chapters 26 and 80.) It also affects freshwater tropical fishes. (Courtesy of T. Wenzel.)

ing skin ulcerations. Filtered tissue homogenates were inoculated onto susceptible cells and incubated at 25 to 28°C. Cytopathic effects (cell rounding, detachment, and lysis) appear 3 to 14 days after inoculation (Frerichs et al., 1986, 1989). The snakehead rhabdovirus replicates in AS, BF–2, FHM, several snakehead cell lines, and a cell line from perch and from common carp, but not in CHSE–214, EPC, RTG–2, and cell lines from Nile tilapia and grass carp (Ahne et al., 1988; Frerichs et al., 1989). The snakehead rhabdovirus is serologically distinct from infectious hematopoietic necrosis and viral hemorrhagic septicemia rhabdoviruses (see Chap. 38); from American eel and European eel rhabdoviruses (see Chap. 26); from perch and pike fry rhabdoviruses (see Chap. 26); and *Rhabdovirus carpio* (see Chap. 50) (Ahne et al., 1988; Frericks et al., 1989).

Transmission, Epidemiology, Pathogenesis, Treatment, and Control

The etiologic significance of the snakehead rhabdovirus (striped snakehead ulcerative virus, ulcerative rhabdovirus) remains uncertain (Frerichs, 1989). In Thailand, outbreaks of skin ulcerative disease occur in the cooler months of the year. Some speculate that outbreaks of the disease are precipitated by physiologic stress caused by adverse environmental conditions, such as low water temperature and pollution (Frericks et al., 1986). No methods for treatment or control of skin ulcerative disease have been described. The snakehead rhabdovirus is relatively temperature stable in cell culture medium from 15 to 35°C at pH 5 to 7, but stability is poor in saline solutions and water (Frerichs, 1989). The virus is inactivated by acid (pH 3), heat (56°C), and chloroform (Ahne et al., 1988).

DEEP ANGELFISH DISEASE

SYNONYMS. Deep angelfish herpesvirus infection, angelfish herpesvirus infection.

HOST AND GEOGRAPHIC DISTRIBUTION

Adult deep angelfish were imported to Denmark from the Amazon River basin (South America) and for several months cohabitated with locally bred adult scalare angelfish without incident. Following an aquarium modification, the deep angelfish were found moribund. Herpesviruslike particles were seen in electron micrographs of tissue from the deep angelfish. The scalare angelfish appeared healthy and were not examined. This viral infection in deep angelfish has been documented only once (Mellergaard and Bloch, 1988).

Clinical Signs and Pathology

Affected deep angelfish show loss of equilibrium and hang quiescent at the water surface or swim in a spiral manner. The gills are pale. Sometimes diffuse, ulcerative hemorrhages occur on the body surface. Internally, the liver and spleen are enlarged.

Histopathologic examination of spleen shows varying degrees of edema and necrosis of the splenic stroma. Splenic sinusoids are dilated and contain variable numbers of erythrocytes and macrophages. Hypertrophic, desquamated reticuloendothelial cells collect in the lumen of sinusoids. The pathology is suggestive of severe hemolytic anemia (Mellergaard and Bloch, 1988).

Diagnosis and Virus Detection

The viral infection is diagnosed by electron microscopic examination of thin-sectioned spleen tissue. Viral nucleocapsids are about 100 nm in diameter and contain an electron-dense, irregularly shaped core about 55 nm in diameter. The nucleocapsids are seen in the nucleus of spleen cells and occasionally in the nucleus, cytoplasm, and cytoplasmic vacuoles of macrophages and monocytes. The enveloped herpesviruslike particles measure about 135 nm in diameter (Mellergaard and Bloch, 1988).

Transmission, Epidemiology, and Pathogenesis

Empirical evidence suggests that the imported feral deep angelfish possibly harbored a latent herpesvirus infection that was activated by stress. The disease outbreak occurred 2 days after decorative manipulations within the aquarium, suggesting that once the virus is activated, the infection and subsequent clinical disease progress rather rapidly. The virus-carrier status of the "local" scalare angelfish is unknown, but the fish were described as healthy, based on behavior and absence of clinical signs.

Treatment and Control

No specific methods for the treatment or control of the infection are known. Fish of uncertain health status should be quarantined until their health status is determined.

CHROMIDE CICHLID ANEMIA

SYNONYM. Chromide cichlid iridovirus infection.

Host and Geographic Distribution

Young adult chromide cichlids were imported from Singapore (Malaysia). The fish were held in brackish water, and some began to die. Several of the live fish were taken for diagnostic evaluation, and iridoviruslike particles were seen in electron micrographs of tissue sections (Armstrong and Ferguson, 1989).

Clinical Signs and Pathology

Affected fish appear pale and are thin and weak, suggesting that the fish do not feed well. The gills and internal organs appear pale, but hyperemia is sometimes seen in the serosal vessels of the stomach and intestine.

Histopathologic examination shows replacement of the hematopoietic interstitial tissue of the kidney by a mixed array of hypertrophic cells. The heterogeneity of the hypertrophic cells seems to be the result of the progressive change of blastlike cells to ballooned cells. The blastlike cells have a slightly enlarged nucleus that contains large amphophilic inclusion bodies. In the "ballooned" cells, the nuclear membrane is indistinct, and the cytoplasm is granular, containing small refractile eosinophilic bodies (Armstrong and Ferguson, 1989). The hypertrophic cells are seen in the blood vessels of the brain, eye, gills, intestine, heart, liver, spleen, and swimbladder. Concentrations of ballooned cells in the lamina propria of the intestine are associated with focal congestion and hemorrhage.

Diagnosis and Virus Detection

The infection is diagnosed by correlating clinical signs, pathologic changes, and detection of iridoviruslike particles in the species of concern. The iridolike virus has been detected by electron microscopy but has not been isolated in cell culture.

Electron microscopic examination of tissue from the gill, intestine, and kidney shows cytoplasmic accumulations of iridoviruslike particles in hypertrophic cells. The particles are 180 to 200 nm in diameter and have an electron-dense central core (Armstrong and Ferguson, 1989).

Transmission, Epidemiology, Treatment, and Control

At present, little concerning the mechanisms and course of infection is known for this virus, or if indeed the virus seen in the electron micrographs is the etiologic agent of disease. It is not clear whether the fish were carrying the virus at the time of importation, or if they became infected in their new environment.

No methods of treatment or control of the infection are known. Prudent fish management practice dictates that fish of unknown health status should be quarantined until their health status is established.

LITERATURE CITED

Ahne, E., Jorgensen, P.E.V., Olesen, N. J., and Wattanavijarn, W. (1988) Serological examination of a rhabdovirus isolated from snakehead (Ophiocephalus striatus) in Thailand with ulcerative syndrome. J. Appl. Ichthyol. 4:194–196.

Armstrong, R.D., and Ferguson, H.W. (1989) Systemic viral disease of the chromide cichlid Etroplus maculatus. Dis. Aquatic Organ. 7:155–157.

Barnekow, A., Schartl, M., Anders, F., and Bauer, H. (1982) Identification of a fish protein associated with a kinase activity and related to the Rous sarcoma virus transforming protein. Cancer Res. 42:2429–2433.

Frericks, G.N. (1989) Stability of snakehead (Ophiocephalus striatus) rhabdovirus under different environmental conditions. J. Appl. Ichthyol. 5:122–126.

Frericks, G.N., Millar, S.D., and Roberts, R.J. (1986) Ulcerative rhabdovirus in fish in South-East Asia. Nature 322:216.

Frericks, G.N., Hill, B.J., and Way, K. (1989) Ulcerative disease rhabdovirus: cell-line susceptibility and serological comparison with other fish rhabdoviruses. J. Fish Dis. 12:51–56.

Kollinger, G., Schwab, M., and Anders, F. (1979) Virus-like particles induced by bromodeoxyuridine in melanoma and neuroblastoma of Xiphophorus. Cancer Res. Clin. Oncol. 95:239–246.

Leibovitz, L., and Riis, R.C. (1980) A viral disease of aquarium fish. J. Am. Vet. Med. Assoc. 177:414–416.

Mellergaard, S., and Bloch, B. (1988) Herpesvirus-like particles in angelfish, Pterophyllum altum. Dis. Aquatic Organ. 5:151–155.

Schartl, M., Barnekow, A., Bauer, H., and Anders, F. (1982) Correlations of inheritance and expression between a tumor gene and the cellular homologue of the Rous sarcoma virus transforming gene in xiphophorus. Cancer Res. 42:4222–4227.

Chapter 70

PARASITES ASSOCIATED WITH FRESHWATER TROPICAL FISHES

JOHN B. GRATZEK

APPROACH TO DIAGNOSIS

History

When establishing a diagnosis of parasitism in freshwater tropical fishes, other problems must be excluded by taking a careful history. Poor husbandry practices often promote or exacerbate parasitic problems. Poor water quality can affect normal defenses and promote multiplication of a parasite. Overcrowding, inadequate filtration, and inattention to tank hygiene create an ideal situation for the propagation of fish parasites.

Clinical evidence strongly suggests that fish in a good plane of nutrition can withstand moderate parasite loads better than fish on poor diets. Most advanced aquarists feed a variety of foods, including live foods, to their fish. This should be established early in taking the history, because aquarists may feed live invertebrates such as *Cyclops, Daphnia,* and tubifex worms that may carry the intermediate stages of nematodes, tapeworms, and sporozoans.

Probably the most common source of introduction of parasites into an aquarium is the failure to quarantine fish or to use proper quarantine procedures. It is important to determine whether newly added fish were quarantined, the length of the quarantine period, and whether they were medicated during that period. If they were medicated, it is important to establish the type of drug used, the dose, and the treatment period. Overtreatment, with subsequent damage to gill epithelium, is common.

Examination

Many parasites of freshwater tropical fishes induce similar lesions and/or behaviors. Skin lesions include excessive mucus, ulceration, petechiae, white spots, or white discolorations, which may be restricted to fins or particular areas of the body. Behavior changes in severe cases of gill parasitism generally include depression during which fish lay motionless at the bottom of the aquarium. Opercula

may be flared, and opercular movements increased, indicating respiratory distress. In less severe cases, fish may swim in twisting motions, scraping gills on solid objects. This is called flashing. Fish affected with these parasites usually exhibit reduced feeding or complete anorexia.

Biopsies can and should be done. Clients involved in breeding ornamental fish normally expect full diagnostic services including biopsies. Biopsies are usually limited to recovering samples for wet mount examination from light scrapings or impressions of affected areas of skin and fins, but gill biopsies can also be extremely useful. Biopsy procedures and anesthesia are covered in chapters in the General Medicine section of this volume.

It is common for clinicians treating aquarium fishes to receive cases submitted fixed in formaldehyde. External parasites of these fishes are likely to be found in the sediment of the fixative and can be concentrated by centrifugation for wet mount examination.

EPIDEMIOLOGIC CONSIDERATIONS

Carriers

Freshwater tropical fishes may carry a parasite or populations of several classes of parasites without apparent signs of disease. In nature, it is a rare fish that is free from parasites. Carrier fish may, in fact, have developed a degree of immunity to a particular parasite. Many carriers are mature fish and, when they are introduced into a group of uninfected fishes, will initiate an enzootic within the aquarium without showing any signs of disease themselves. This is probably the most common way in which parasites are introduced into aquatic systems.

Factors Affecting Transmissibility

Many parasites infecting fish can be transmitted by direct extension through the water. Crowding fish will increase the chances of contact between parasites and potential hosts. Additionally, crowding will lead to changes in the organic load of the water, which promotes parasitism by enhancing the microenvironment for the parasite. It has been well established that ciliates of the genus *Trichodina* disappear from fish if fresh water is introduced into the fish culture system.

Many fish parasites require an intermediate host. Nematode eggs passed from fish are frequently ingested by free-living invertebrates such as *Daphnia* and *Cyclops*, which are, in turn, eaten by fish. If these intermediates are not found in the aquarium, transmission is impossible. Another example would be digenetic trematodes, for which a variety of wild-caught or pond-reared ornamental fish serve as the secondary intermediate host. These fish are dead-end hosts for the parasite in an aquarium environment, and no direct transmission to other fishes can occur.

Since fish will eat other dead fish in an aquarium, failure to remove dead fish enhances the spread of sporozoan parasites, including Coccidia and the causative agent of neon tetra disease, *Plistophora hyphressobryconis.*

Factors Affecting Clinical Severity

Young fish are more susceptible to parasites than are mature fish. This may be because fewer parasites are required to inflict compromising damage to a small patient as opposed to a larger one. Alternatively, mature fish may have developed specific immunity by response to previous subclinical infections or through exposure to antigens of nonpathogenic commensal organisms encountered in an aquatic system.

Environmental factors may enhance the clinical severity of parasitism, especially those involving the gills. Any water-quality change that can affect the efficiency of the gills can exacerbate a parasitic infestation. It is also well known that various parasites appear to be temperature dependent. The common ciliate protozoan parasite *Ichthyophthirius multifiliis* is predominantly associated with colder seasons.

Immunity most likely plays an important role in the relative resistance of fish to parasitic disease. Fish have been shown to be resistant to *Ichthyophthirius multifiliis* after surviving an infection (Hines and Spira, 1974). There is good evidence that fish will develop resistance to monogenetic trematodes (Scott and Robinson, 1984). The role of various stress situations in the suppression of the immune system has been postulated. Bacterial diseases following stress situations are well documented, but attempts to quantitatively reproduce stress situations under laboratory conditions have often failed.

Nutritional problems have long been associated with parasitism in mammals. It has been suggested that deficiencies in vitamin E will reduce macrophage activity in trout (Blazer and Wolke, 1984), but similar experiments have not been done with tropical aquarium species. From clinical experience it is apparent that fish fed a high-quality diet and kept in good water are less likely to develop a clinically apparent illness from parasites.

Mixed infestations are common and may influence the severity of the clinical disease. Fish debilitated with a massive infestation of metacercariae or nematodes are frequently the first to die in an epidemic caused by common external protozoans such as *Chilodonella cyprinii.*

QUARANTINE CONSIDERATIONS FOR PARASITIC DISEASES

Sooner or later aquarists with large investments in fish realize that the introduction of new fish into a breeding colony without quarantine will lead to problems. Apparently healthy fish can introduce many parasites into aquaria. Quarantining fish for 14 to 21 days avoids many problems.

Fish in quarantine must be held in an aquarium with good water and filtration that maintains appropriate pH and nitrogen waste product levels. Flow-through systems are ideal, but not always practical for clients. Frequently changing water to avoid ammonia and nitrite build-up is one approach to managing a single quarantine tank that can be successful. This is really only a modification of a flow-through system with the water changes coming in boluses, at intervals. Water should be tested for pH, ammonia, and nitrites periodically. Ammonia toxicity can be reduced using ammonia-adsorbing clays in filters and by maintaining the pH near neutral, in addition to frequent water changes. If the water change method is being used, it is important to avoid stress by making sure that the temperature of the water does not fluctuate over a few degrees Fahrenheit when making a water change. Dechlorination of water for changes can be accomplished by the addition of two drops of 13% sodium thiosulfate solution per gallon of new water prior to the change. Nitrite levels usually begin to rise in a tank after 3 to 5 days, and water changes should be performed accordingly.

The quarantine should extend for at least 21 days, although 14 days is better than nothing. During this period, water changes alone will serve to rid fish of parasites by dilution and minimizing reinfection. In some cases, fish will die for known or unknown causes, and the clients may blame the deaths on the quarantine procedure. This emphasizes the importance of maintaining and testing for good water quality.

Net and Tool Disinfection

Net and implement disinfection becomes a major problem in wholesale, retail, or any facility where multiple tanks are used. Indiscriminate use of nets between aquaria should be avoided, since they can be a source of spread of parasites.

Air-drying kills many parasites, but spores and cyst forms such as reported with *Ichthyobodo necatrix* can withstand drying. The problem in establishments with many tanks is that air-drying necessitates many nets.

Chlorine is not recommended as a disinfectant, because it destroys netting. Quaternary ammonia compounds can be used, following the dilution instructions for general disinfection. It is very important to rinse nets and implements in clear water after disinfection with these compounds, since there can be a carry-over problem resulting in toxicity to sensitive fish. This is particularly true in smaller aquaria.

Formaldehyde can be used at 75 to 100 ppm (3 to 4 ml of 37% formaldehyde) per 10 gallons of water. Formaldehyde is a good all-purpose parasiticide. Aquarists should be careful to avoid skin contact with the formalin and nets, and tools should be rinsed.

Potassium permanganate is an oxidizing compound that can be used at 100 ppm by adding 1 g to 5 gallons of water. This disinfectant has the disadvantage that it stains. Nets and tools should be rinsed well.

Povidone-iodines can be used, following the directions for general disinfection. Freshwater rinses should remove all of the disinfectant before nets or tools are placed in a tank.

Chemotherapeutic Prophylaxis

Although quarantine can be done without the routine administration of parasiticides, the author feels the incidence of parasitism in freshwater tropical fishes is high enough to warrant routine medication of fish during quarantine. Diagnostic testing, biopsy, and necropsy sampling of individuals from large groups can help to direct quarantine therapy, but the following recommendations are made for a routine parasite quarantine for freshwater tropical fishes.

All parasitic conditions are not readily treatable, and even when the best available medications are used some parasites cannot be eradicated without the risk of killing the fish during quarantine. From a clinical approach, one can attempt to rid fish of known, highly infectious problems that are readily treatable and are primary agents of disease.

The suggestions provided in the following disease summaries are based on the availability of drugs to the veterinary practitioner, the efficacy of the drug for a broad spectrum of parasites, and the safety of the drug. The adage "Know your fish, the chemical, and the water" refers to the fact that some fish are more sensitive to medication than others. For example, some species of ornamental catfish such as members of the *Corydoras* genus do not tolerate salt. The effective therapeutic dose of a drug can also be altered by the pH of the water. For example, organophosphates tend to degrade more quickly at a higher pH. Safety can be maximized by using correct dosages and treatment times. The reader is referred to the drug tables in the appendix of this volume for doses for the chemotherapeutic agents mentioned.

ICHTHYOPHTHIRIUS MULTIFILIIS

SYNONYMS. Ich, white spot disease.

Geographic Distribution

Ichthyophthirius multifiliis has a worldwide distribution and affects all freshwater fishes. Under aquarium conditions, it is particularly virulent.

Clinical Appearance and Diagnosis

Ich is one disease that is readily identified by most aquarists. Predominant signs include small white spots over the body. In some cases, infestation is limited to the gills. A diagnosis can be confirmed by microscopic examination of biopsy material from skin or gills. Theronts appear round to oval and may be from 30 to 1000 μm in diameter (Fig. 70–1). The organism moves slowly by means of cilia observable with a high-power objective. The motion is typically a rolling motion where the parasite rotates across the epithelial surface. The horseshoe-shaped nucleus is often visible and aids in identification. *Ichthyophthirius multifiliis* is one of the few fish parasites with cilia surrounding the entire organism. The free-swimming infective ciliated theronts are usually pear-shaped, actively motile, and about 30 to 45 μm in diameter.

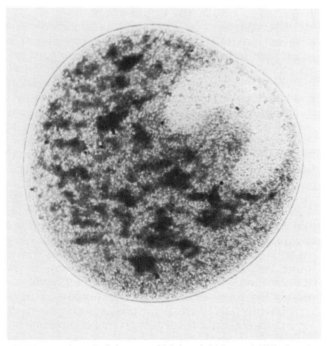

FIGURE 70–1. A typical theront of *Ichthyophthirius multifiliis* showing the horseshoe-shaped nucleus characteristic of the organism. (Courtesy of M. Stoskopf.)

Pathogenesis, Life Cycle, Transmission, and Epidemiology

These parasites have a complex life cycle that includes stages on the host as well as in the environment. The white spot observed on the affected fish is called the trophont. It is the encysted feeding stage. Eventually, the trophont enlarges, breaks through the epithelium, and drops to the bottom of the aquarium, where it attaches to any object, such as gravel or tubing. At this point the organism is referred to as a tomont. The time taken for development on the fish is very temperature dependent and requires 3 to 4 days at 22°C, up to 11 days at 15°C, and nearly 30 days at 10°C.

The tomont attached to bottom substrates or plants begins to undergo mitosis shortly after attachment. Within 18 to 21 hours at 23°C to 25°C, this mitosis will result in hundreds of ciliated theronts that are released into the water. Theronts actively swim and, on encountering a host fish, attach and actively penetrate skin and gill epithelium, where they enlarge until they are visible as a white spot. Free-swimming newly excysted ciliated theronts have only about 48 hours in which to find a host before they die. The disease is usually observed several days after introducing new fish to an aquarium.

Treatment and Control

Medicants available do not penetrate the encysted trophonts. All treatment is directed towards preventing reinfection of fish by free-swimming trophonts. Formaldehyde or malachite green or both is also used to rid aquaria of the trophonts.

Formaldehyde at 25 ppm (1 ml/10 gallons) is an excellent treatment method. Three treatments are recommended on alternate days. Water changes of up to 75% should be done 4 to 8 hours after treatments. Malachite green and formaldehyde–malachite green mixtures have also been used successfully. It is important to remember that activated carbon should be removed from filters during treatment and that air stems supplying lift stack on undergravel filters should be removed from the aquarium to avoid pulling any medicants through undergravel filters.

In addition to chemotherapy, management adjustments serve to control infestations. Elevating water temperatures several degrees Celsius over normal aquarium temperatures for 5 to 7 days will tend to limit the infection by adversely affecting the heat-sensitive theronts as well as by enhancing the immune response of the host. Heavy filtration with diatomaceous earth or membrane filters will also reduce the number of circulating theronts. Further, transferring fish to clean hospital aquaria every day for 7 days will limit the infection by keeping one step ahead of theront reinfestation. In home aquaria where medicants might harm plants, removal of theronts can be done by making heavy daily water changes. When water changes are made with a distended-end siphon tube, developing theronts in cysts attached to the surface gravel are more likely to be removed. This method, while efficacious, may stress fish excessively unless attention is paid to temperature and pH regulation. Alternatively, fish can be treated in a separate aquarium equipped with a heater and filter. Parasites in the main aquarium eventually die for lack of a host. To ensure that all theronts are eliminated in the main tank, at least one complete water change, along with removing debris from the gravel, should be done. Elevating the temperature several degrees Celsius over normal temperatures will accelerate the death of theronts.

ICHTHYOBODO NECATRIX

SYNONYMS. *Costia necatrix, Costia,* costiasis.

Geographic Distribution

This organism has been reported from a wide variety of aquarium fishes around the world. It infects various trout, channel catfish, and goldfish in addition to freshwater tropical fishes. There is no marine counterpart known, but similar organisms have been found on haddock off the coast of Nova Scotia (Morrison and Cone, 1986).

Clinical Appearance and Diagnosis

Fish affected with *Ichthyobodo* are frequently depressed and show respiratory distress. They often are anorectic. A whitish film from excess mucus production is frequently observed on the surface of the body. Some fish die without visible external signs. Diagnosis is confirmed by microscopic examination of wet mounts of skin or gills. The organisms are actively motile, small (7 to 15 μm long), and somewhat comma shaped (Fig. 70–2). They can be seen as free-swimming forms or attached to cells by their flagella. When attached, the parasites move in a characteristic circular fashion.

Pathologic Effects and Pathogenesis

The *Ichthyobodo* organism feeds directly on epithelial cells by penetrating with its gullet. The parasite can destroy gill and skin epithelium.

Life Cycle, Transmission, and Epidemiology

These flagellates reproduce by simple binary fission. Transmission appears to be by direct contact or exposure to water that has held infected fish within several hours. The disease is found in both

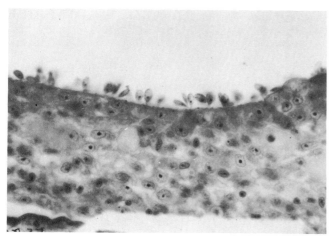

FIGURE 70–2. A typically comma-shaped *Ichthyobodo* organism attached to an epithelial surface. (Courtesy of H. S. Davis and G. L. Hoffman.)

winter and summer months but is more serious in warmer water. Infestations are seen most frequently in fish that have recently been shipped from a primary producer. The disease is a major problem for wholesalers and retailers. It is relatively rare in established home aquaria, because affected fish are unsuitable for sale. The organism survives only an hour or so off the fish host.

Treatment and Control

This parasite is susceptible to common antiprotozoal therapies. We suggest one treatment of 25 ppm of formaldehyde followed by a water change of up to 75% in 4 to 8 hours. This treatment approach will kill attached parasites, as well as those in the water column.

CHILODONELLA CYPRINII

SYNONYMS. None.

Geographic Distribution

As with other protozoan parasites of freshwater tropical fishes, there seem to be no discernible geographic limitations. Infections are common in cultured food fish species, goldfish, and many species of freshwater tropical ornamental fishes. A saltwater counterpart, *Brooklynella horridus,* is occasionally seen in marine fishes.

Clinical Appearance and Diagnosis

The principal signs of *Chilodonella* infestation are respiratory distress, clamped fins, and depression. Excessive mucus production is also common. Death can be sudden with minimal external signs of disease. Examination of the gills of infected fish will reveal heavy loads of oval, flattened organisms, with a shape suggestive of a valentine heart (Fig. 70–3). Cilia appear in rows. The organism is approximately 50 to 70 μm in diameter. The organism moves with a characteristic, slow circular movement and appears to glide. Organisms begin to die within minutes of preparation of the wet mounts. Dead organisms are round with a granular cytoplasm and a distinct oval macronucleus that is about one-third the length of the parasite.

Pathogenesis, Transmission, and Epidemiology

Infestations with *Chilodonella* are infrequently seen in home aquaria, since infestation is usually initially encountered by wholesalers and retailers. At that level, the disease is a severe and common problem. The organism feeds by pinocytosis after contacting epithelial cells, where it feeds on the cytoplasmic contents. It reproduces by simple binary fission and does not form any resting spore stage. It cannot survive more than a few hours off a host.

Treatment and Control

This parasite is susceptible to commonly used parasiticides. Again, 25 ppm of formaldehyde, followed by a water change in 4 to 8 hours, will kill parasites on the fish, as well as in the water. This is

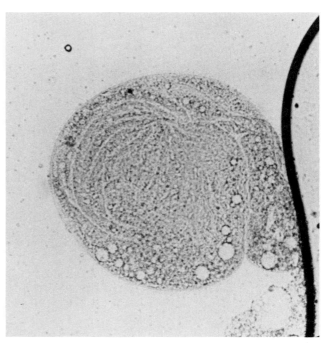

FIGURE 70–3. *Chilodonella* sp. in a fresh smear (1000×). (Courtesy of M. Stoskopf.)

one parasite that responds well to 0.3% salt added to water (about 12 g/gallon), in which case parasites on the fish and in the water are killed.

TRICHODONIASIS

SYNONYMS. None.

Geographic Distribution

There are three genera, *Trichodina*, *Trichodonella*, and *Tripartiella*, that have similar appearances and are commonly found parasitizing fishes (Fig. 70–4). All cultivated fish are susceptible, including pond-reared tropicals, goldfish, channel catfish, and trout. There is no apparent limit to geographic distribution. A marine counterpart to *Trichodonella* has been seen infesting gills.

Clinical Appearance and Diagnosis

Trichodinids are ciliated, circular parasites that are flattened and have denticular rings. They are usually 40 to 60 μm in diameter and are found on the skin and gills of fishes. They move in a distinct manner, often rotating their denticular ring continuously. In a wet mount, the organisms are dome shaped when viewed from the side. Heavy infestations cause respiratory distress and skin ulcers, and in some fish species these parasites have been reported to infect the urinary bladder and oviducts. Affected fish may show hypermucus production in the form of a white cast to the skin, or the infestation may be entirely limited to the gills. This is often the case in koi or striped bass. *Trichodina* organisms are larger than *Trichodonella* or *Tripartiella* and have complete rings of cilia. Many individual species have been described.

Pathogenesis, Transmission, and Epidemiology

These parasites are commonly found on the skin and gills of pond-reared fish, especially if the water has a high organic load. These organisms multiply by binary fission and do not produce resting spores. They do survive well off a host and can be introduced to aquaria with plants or substrates.

The smaller *Trichodonella* and *Tripartiella* species appear to inflict more injury to gills through their tendency to attach firmly to gill epithelium. Trichodinids are rarely a problem in home aquaria, since water changes associated with shipping and transportation will often effect a cure. It is common to observe *Trichodina* infestations in wholesale or retail establishments. Infestations are usually very light and apparently do not affect the host fish. Goldfish are particularly commonly infested.

Treatment and Control

Removal of fish to fresh water will often effect a cure. Otherwise, treatments with formaldehyde baths or salt baths have been effective. Prevention centers on maintaining good water quality in the tank or pond.

TETRAHYMENA PYRIFORMIS

SYNONYM. Guppy killer.

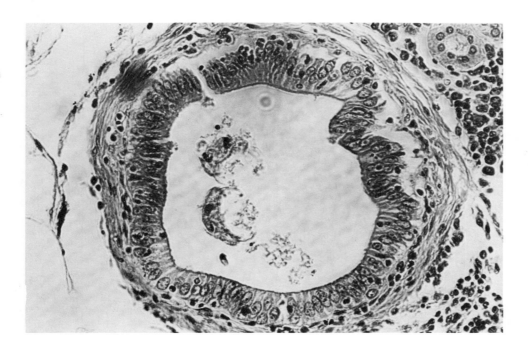

FIGURE 70–4. Trichodinids in the renal duct of an ornamental killifish. (H & E, 400×). (Courtesy of M. Stoskopf.)

Geographic Distribution

Tetrahymena pyriformis is a free-living ciliated protozoan infusorian that occasionally becomes parasitic. It has worldwide distribution and affects a wide range of hosts, particularly live-bearing fishes, cichlids, and various tetra species. The dwarf cichlid appears particularly susceptible.

Clinical Appearance and Diagnosis

Systemic cases show signs of necrosis and hemorrhagic areas on the skin. Occasionally tissues surrounding the eye are invaded, resulting in exophthalmus. Diagnosis is confirmed by wet-mount preparations showing hundreds of actively motile, pear-shaped ciliated parasites approximately 60 by 100 μm.

Pathogenesis, Transmission, and Epidemiology

As mentioned, *Tetrahymena pyriformis* is usually a free-living organism (Fig. 70–5). It occasionally becomes parasitic. It is possible that various strains of *Tetrahymena* have a potential for being more virulent, especially when the water is high in organic content and fish are immunologically depressed. In systemic cases, foci of parasites are found in the kidneys, brain, or muscles. In these cases, the parasites are frequently found within capillaries or the gills. The organism can routinely be found in decaying food in any aquarium and is considered to be a secondary or tertiary invader of lesions initiated by other parasites or bacteria.

Treatment and Control

Control seems to center on maintaining excellent water quality and removing uneaten food. Treatment of the disease is discouraging. Baths with external parasiticides such as formalin may reduce external parasites but have no effect on internal parasites. Maintaining good water quality and nutrition is the best approach to this disease.

HETEROPOLARIA COLISARUM

SYNONYMS. *Epistylis,* red sore disease.

Geographic Distribution

Heteropolaria colisarum is an epistylid parasite that has been associated with a variety of North American fishes (Fig. 70–6). Goldfish and many species of bottom-dwelling fish, such as ornamental catfish, are affected. It has been isolated from the skin of giant gouramis. The organism is frequently isolated from any species of fish coming from organically enriched water. It can also be found living on vegetation or crustaceans and presents a problem when it grows on fish eggs in production ponds. It is also discussed in Chapter 27.

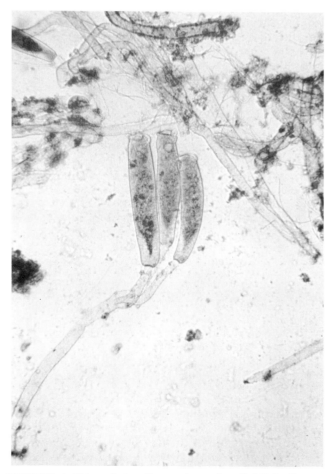

FIGURE 70–6. *Heteropolaria colisarum,* formerly called *Epistylis,* seen in a fresh smear from the skin of an infected bluegill. (Courtesy of G. L. Hoffman.)

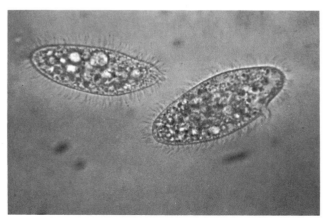

FIGURE 70–5. Two *Tetrahymena* organisms, probably *Tetrahymena corlissi,* which cause the disease commonly referred to as guppy killer disease. (Courtesy of J. Camper and G. L. Hoffman.)

Clinical Appearance and Diagnosis

Frequently, the parasite is seen as a white area or white tuft on the surface of the fish body or fins. Such fish may show no other signs. The organism has also been found in ulcerated areas from which *Aeromonas hydrophila* has been isolated. Diagnosis is confirmed by wet-mount preparations of affected areas showing bell-shaped ciliated organisms on stalks. Apical cilia are present. The body of the organism will be seen to contract periodically from an elongated form to a ball-shaped form. The stalk tends to coil during the contraction phase. Clinicians should be aware that other sessile protozoa of the genera *Scyphidia* and *Glossatella* present with similar signs and morphology. Clinically, the approach to control and therapy has been similar, and differentiation of these organisms has not been considered of major importance. However, this may change as more aggressive therapies are developed.

Pathogenesis, Transmission, and Epidemiology

It is not known whether this organism is a primary parasite or an opportunistic invader. It appears to survive well in the absence of a host if there is sufficient organic material in the water to provide nutrients. Fish often show no signs other than the characteristic white tufts that are often in areas that experience frequent mild trauma.

Treatment and Control

In aquaria, the problem is best avoided by regular cleaning of gravel and avoiding overfeeding. Treatment can be accomplished by swabbing the affected area with tincture of iodine or povidone-iodine solutions. A single treatment in a 1.5% salt bath for 3 hours has controlled the disease (Foissner et al., 1985). Formaldehyde treatments can also be used. Infected eggs can be salvaged with dips in iodophor solutions.

HEXAMITA SP.

SYNONYMS. *Octomitus*, discus parasite, *Spironucleus*, "hole in the head" disease.

Geographic Distribution

Hexamita sp. are flagellated protozoans found in the gastrointestinal tract of a wide variety of fishes. They frequently infect discus. *Spironucleus* may be a distinct organism from *Hexamita*, as it is longer and possibly more sinuous, but for practical purposes, both organisms appear to cause similar clinical responses.

Clinical Appearance and Diagnosis

These parasites are about the size of erythrocytes and are very motile. In wet mounts, they move similarly to the trichomonad parasites of mammals. They are pear shaped and about 5 to 12 μm long. The eight flagella are usually not easily seen. In many fishes, including trout, goldfish, and many freshwater tropical species, infections are inapparent. However, in angelfish, discus, and gouramis, the disease is characterized by poor condition, inappetence, unthriftiness, weight loss, and death. Fish may show excessive nervousness and sometimes hyperemia of the cloaca. Diagnosis is made by observing highly motile flagellates in feces or, if a fish is available for necropsy, by massive infestations in the intestines. Organisms can also be found in the liver, gallbladder, and kidney.

A disease frequently seen in discus, angelfish, red oscars, and other cichlids has been associated with the presence of a *Hexamita* sp. A direct causal relationship has not been established. This disease is characterized by erosions of the epithelium and underlying muscles, which can extend to the bones of the skull. The lesions are progressive and can cover a large percentage of the head. The lateral line is also a preferred site for these lesions.

Pathogenesis, Transmission, and Epidemiology

Hexamitiasis can be seen at the producer, wholesaler, retailer, or home aquarist level. Infestations in adult breeding angelfish result in lowered hatchability of eggs or death in young fry shortly after hatching. Since *Hexamita* sp. can be kept alive in laboratory media, we assume that it is an inhabitant of aquaria where organic material has been allowed to accumulate. A cyst form has been described and may play a role in transmission. Direct contact spread in crowded tanks is certainly an important route of transmission.

The relationship between *Hexamita* organisms and the "hole in the head" syndrome is not well established. Scanning electron micrographs of lesions have not been conclusive. Empirical observations relate the condition to poor nutrition, dirty aquaria, and the use of activated carbon as well as the presence of flagellates in the lesions. The observation by cichlid breeders that deletion of activated carbon from filter systems seems to avoid the problem is interesting and deserves controlled investigation.

Treatment and Control

Maintenance of good water with regular cleaning of the aquarium gravel and water changes seems to be important in preventing hexamitiasis. Transferring fish to larger tanks and implementing frequent water changes alone can be curative. Improved nutrition, with supplementation of vitamin C, has been reported to improve the condition. A single metronidazole bath (5 ppm) is effective in treating classic hexamitiasis. The drug appears to be absorbed via skin or gills and is nontoxic at doses up to 20 ppm. It does not appear to affect biological filters, but as a precaution, filtration should not be exposed to the drug. Massive doses of metronidazole received mixed reviews in anecdotal reports of treating the "hole in the head" syndrome.

PLISTOPHORA HYPHRESSOBRYCONIS

SYNONYMS. Microsporidiosis, neon tetra disease, black holes.

Geographic Distribution

Plistophora hyphressobryconis is a microsporidian parasite of freshwater tropical fishes. The common name, "neon tetra disease," is misleading, as the disease affects a variety of angelfish, barbs, rasboras, and tetras.

Clinical Appearance and Diagnosis

Signs of the disease include the appearance of whitened areas in the musculature, which result in aberrant swimming motions and the apparent loss of color in neon tetras. In angelfish, the parasite can cause muscle necrosis, which results in an uneven, undulating appearance to the body surface. In white angelfish, strongly localized melanophore responses have given the disease the name of "black holes." Diagnosis is confirmed by examining impression smears or wet mounts of muscles from the affected area and observing pansporoblasts filled with spores containing one polar capsule (Fig. 70–7). Mycobacteriosis is an important consideration in the differential diagnosis, as mycobacterial granulomas can be seen in these species of fish and may be mistaken for pansporoblasts in the living fish.

Pathogenesis, Life Cycle, Transmission, and Epidemiology

The life cycle of *Plistophora hyphressobryconis* is primarily intracellular with the end result being the production of spores. The course of the disease in groups of infected neon tetras is invariably fatal. Moribund fish are frequently bloated, but this appears to be attributable to a variety of bacterial secondary invaders. Mycobacterial infections are also common in neon tetras, and concomitant infections are common. The disease in mature angelfish is a chronic one, resulting in deformities of the musculature and low mortality.

Treatment and Control

Treatment attempts have been discouraging. Claims of cures by individuals using either formaldehyde or nalidixic acid have not been substantiated in controlled experiments. The author's experience suggests that the mortality rate in a group of infected fish is initially high. Remaining fish appear healthy but will die over a period of weeks, suggesting a gradual extension of the parasite within the body.

Disease within an aquarium system can be limited by removing dying fish before they are cannibalized. Periodic cleaning of gravel would serve to

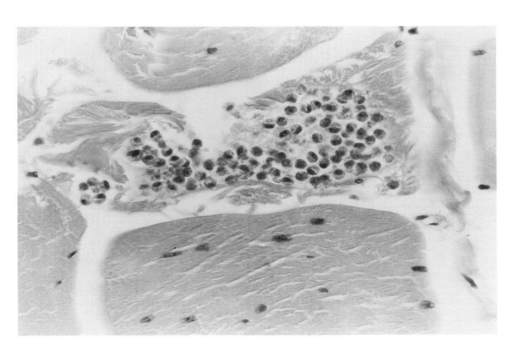

FIGURE 70–7. A microsporidian pansporoblast filled with spores that has essentially replaced a skeletal muscle bundle. (H & E, 400×). (Courtesy of M. Stoskopf.)

remove any spores that may have accumulated. In ponds, control can be approached by draining and disinfecting them.

MYXOSPORIDIOSIS

GENERA. *Henneguya, Myxidium, Mitraspora.*

Geographic Distribution

Many genera of myxosporidia are found in freshwater tropical fishes. They are found worldwide, infecting a wide variety of fish species. *Henneguya* is frequently found on the gills of wild-caught *Corydoras* and on the dorsal fins of *Leporinus* (Fig. 70–8).

Clinical Appearance and Diagnosis

Myxobolus can cause nodules on the skin and gills. These can be few or numerous and vary in size from microscopic to several millimeters in diameter. They do not appear to affect the fish except in appearance. *Henneguya* and *Myxidium* are also found

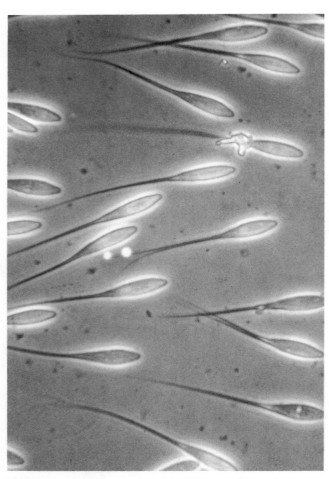

FIGURE 70–8. Spores of *Henneguya exilis* released from large cysts on the gills of a channel catfish (400×). (Courtesy of G. Hoffman.)

as white cysts on body surfaces and gills. Diagnosis is based on examination of wet mounts or histologic sections of affected areas and identification of typical spores containing two polar capsules. Spores are classified according to genus, based on the position of the polar capsules within the spores. *Henneguya* spores have two caudal processes that are distinctive for the genus.

Pathogenesis, Life Cycle, Transmission, and Epidemiology

Nodules from myxosporidian infestations are common, largely incidental findings in routine post-mortem examinations of wild-caught freshwater tropical fish. The parasites seem to cause no harm except in distortions of appearance. Cysts associated with *Henneguya* infestations frequently disappear in time. Presumably, spores are released into the aquarium. It does not appear that these infections spread readily in aquaria. It is possible that an intermediate host is required that is not normally found in aquaria.

Treatment and Control

Cysts can be lanced and treated with local application of antiseptics if they are objectionable. Treated fish should be isolated during recovery. Chemotherapeutic approaches to these parasites are disappointingly ineffective.

CRYPTOSPORIDIOSIS

SYNONYMS. None.

Geographic Distribution

A *Cryptosporidium*-like organism has been isolated from freshwater angelfish.

Clinical Appearance and Diagnosis

Affected fish were anorectic, regurgitating food, and passing feces that contained undigested food. They lost condition and eventually died. *Cryptosporidium*-like organisms were identified in the feces and from intestinal scrapings of affected fish.

Life Cycle, Transmission, and Epidemiology

The single identified outbreak was widespread in an angelfish hatchery. Otherwise, nothing is known about the life cycle, transmission, or epidemiology of this parasite. It is possible that many unexplained deaths seen in angelfish may eventually prove to be infections with *Cryptosporidium*.

Treatment and Control

No treatment or control measures have been developed for this disease.

OODINIUM SP.

SYNONYMS. Velvet, gold dust disease, rust disease, coral fish disease.

Geographic Distribution

There are three or four species of this genus that have been associated with disease in freshwater, brackish, and marine fish from around the world.

Clinical Appearance and Diagnosis

The organism is a dinoflagellate that can vary in size from 40 to 100 μm (Fig. 70–9). It is found on skin and gill biopsy material and contains chlorophyll, which imparts a color to the parasite. The principal sign of infestation is the observation of a fine dusty effect on the skin of the fish. Directing the beam of a flashlight on the dorsal aspect of the fish in a darkened room enhances visualization of this effect. On microscopic examination of wet mounts of skin or gills, pear-shaped cysts attached to the underlying tissues will be seen. The organisms are not motile. Within the cysts are the mature dinospores, which are flagellated and actively motile.

Pathogenesis, Life Cycle, Transmission, and Epidemiology

This infestation is less common than in previous years. It can become endemic in a retail shop, but its presence is generally due to failure of the store owners to clean and disinfect aquaria between shipments of new fish. The life cycle is reminiscent of *Ichthyophthirius*, since a parasitic stage attaches to the fish, matures, drops off the host, and eventually undergoes excystation, releasing motile infective forms. The visible cysts seen on wet mounts from infected fish contain maturing dinospores, which are eventually released some time after the cyst drops off the fish and settles on the bottom. The dinospores are actively motile flagellates that seek out and infect a new host. Newly excysted dinospores survive 12 to 14 hours without a host. The entire cycle takes up to 10 days.

Treatment and Control

The organisms responsible for this disease are relatively salt tolerant. They do respond to formaldehyde treatments. Malachite green has been used. Reinfection is a common problem and may be associated with the parasite's ability to colonize the intestine. Copper is used to treat marine fish affected with the disease.

DACTYLOGYRIDIASIS

SYNONYM. Gill flukes.

Geographic Distribution

Dactylogyrid flukes are common in aquarium fish and can infest species of all major fish groups (Fig. 70–10). Pond-reared fish such as goldfish can be heavily infested. Infections in imported and domestic tank-reared angelfish and discus are common.

Clinical Appearance and Diagnosis

Fish in ponds or the wild rarely exhibit clinical signs. The development of clinical signs is associated

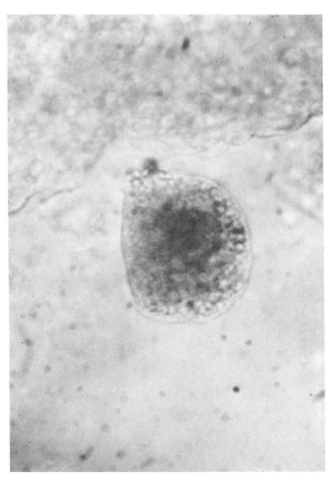

FIGURE 70–9. *Oodinium* sp. (Courtesy of F. Meyer and G. L. Hoffman.)

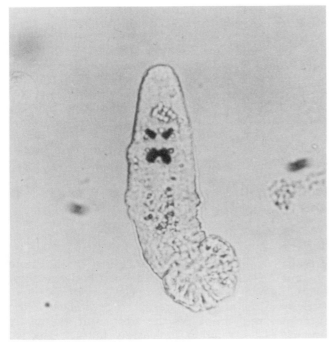

FIGURE 70–10. *Dactylogyrus* sp. from a fresh smear (40×). (Courtesy of M. Stoskopf.)

with crowding, when the probability of transmission is greatly enhanced. Consequently, clinical disease is more common in aquaria and holding vats. Clinical signs include rapid respiratory movements, clamped fins, flashing, and rubbing. Fish may also become inactive and sit at the bottom of the aquarium. Death may be caused by heavy infestations. Diagnosis can be confirmed by biopsies of the gills where worms are readily apparent if present. Dactylogyrid flukes are recognized by a four-pointed anterior end, a sucker near the anterior end, and four anterior eye spots. The caudal end has a fixation apparatus, or haptor, that consists of one or two large hooks surrounded by up to 16 smaller hooklets. The worms are approximately 400 μm long and have both testes and ovaries.

Pathologic Effects and Pathogenesis

Of the many genera of monogenetic trematodes that infest freshwater tropical fishes, the species of the genus *Dactylogyrus* are the most important. They are usually found on the gills but can be found on the body. If present in sufficient numbers, they can cause hyperplasia, destruction of gill epithelium, and clubbing of gill filaments, which can lead to asphyxiation.

Life Cycle, Transmission, and Epidemiology

Dactylogyrid flukes reproduce by mutual fertilization followed by release of eggs that develop off the host. Eggs from some species hatch into ciliated forms as early as 60 hours after being released. Other species require 4 to 5 days before hatching. The ciliated larvae attack suitable hosts, lose their cilia, and develop into adult trematodes. Transmission is greatly enhanced by overcrowding of fish. The parasite load per fish in a single aquarium, even within a single host species, can be quite variable. Immunocompetence may play a role in this variability.

Treatment and Control

Specific treatments include long-duration exposure to formaldehyde or short-term baths. Saltwater baths have also been used. Organophosphates are used for freshwater fishes, but it appears that extended use of organophosphates may develop resistant strains of flukes (Goven et al., 1980). Praziquantel will effectively remove monogenetic trematodes from gills and body surfaces when administered in aquaria at 3 ppm or as a bath at 6 ppm. Low levels of formaldehyde (25 ppm) are effective.

Control centers on careful quarantine and treatment of infected fish before they are placed in a tank. Latent infections can occur, with clinical disease flaring in times of suboptimal environmental conditions.

GYRODACTYLIDIASIS

SYNONYM. Skin flukes.

Geographic Distribution

Many species of the genus *Gyrodactylus* have been described (Fig. 70–11). They infect a broad range of hosts, including most freshwater tropical fishes maintained in aquaria. Their distribution as a genus is most likely worldwide.

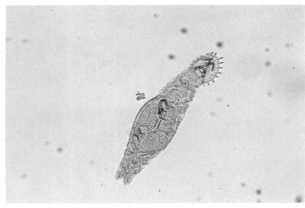

FIGURE 70–11. *Gyrodactylus* sp. from a goldfish (100×, Picromount). (Courtesy of G. Hoffman.)

Clinical Appearance and Diagnosis

Inapparent infections are common. The parasites feed on blood and epithelium by scraping and sucking. Lesions can include localized hemorrhagic areas, excessive mucus, and localized ulcerations. Infected fish may have a ragged-appearing tail from localized hyperplasia and necrosis and loss of epithelial cells on the fins.

Gyrodactylid trematodes are usually found on the skin but may occasionally be found on the gills. They can be up to 0.8 mm long with two points at the anterior end. An anterior sucker is present, but no eye spots. An attachment organ (haptor) with two large hooks, surrounded by up to 16 hooklets, is located at the caudal end.

Pathogenesis, Transmission, and Epidemiology

Secondary infections with bacteria (*Aeromonas, Flexibacter*) are common. *Aeromonas hydrophila* has been isolated from gyrodactylids removed from goldfish, suggesting that the worms may actively transmit bacteria. Gyrodactylids are viviparous, and embryos with prominent hooks are commonly seen in adult parasites.

Treatment and Control

Praziquantel at 3 ppm in aquarium water will effectively remove gyrodactylid trematodes. Older treatments include addition of formaldehyde to aquaria at 25 ppm, saltwater baths (2.5 to 3%), and organophosphate baths. Extended use of organophosphates can result in development of resistant trematodes (Goven et al., 1980). Since these worms are live-bearing flukes, the problem of drug-resistant ova is not a problem. Single treatments can clear the infection.

DIGENETIC TREMATODES

SYNONYMS. Flukes, grubs.

IMPORTANT GENERA. *Neascus, Clinostomum, Diplostomulum,* and members of the family Heterophyidae.

Geographic Distribution

Many genera of digenetic trematodes have been described, and many unidentified species exist. Tropical freshwater fishes frequently serve as secondary intermediate hosts with encysted stages in tissues (Fig. 70–12) but are rarely the final hosts with adult forms of the parasite within the intestine. Members of the Heterophyidae are frequently found encysted

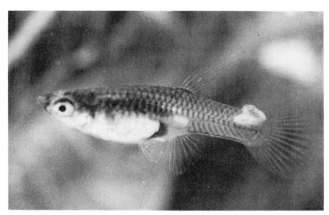

FIGURE 70–12. Encysted metacercaria of digenetic trematodes on the caudal peduncle of a guppy. (Courtesy of T. Wenzel.)

as metacercariae in the gills of fish raised in Florida. Similar parasites are seen on fish from Malaysia.

Clinical Appearance and Diagnosis

Larval forms referred to as *Neascus* are frequently seen in freshwater tropical fish as round black spots (2 to 3 mm) in the skin. The black spots represent a melanophore reaction that surrounds the encysted metacercaria. Silver dollar fish are frequently infested with *Neascus* metacercariae. Many people mistake the small black spots for normal coloring or genetic variations.

Larvae of *Clinostomum* sp. are commonly called "grubs" and may be white to yellow. Severely infected fish are not marketed, but cysts may occasionally be seen on fish in retail stores. In these cases, the fish is not suitable for sale until the parasite is removed by simple excision. In many cases, grubs may be found within the body cavity and deeply embedded in the musculature, where they escape clinical detection. Heavy infections with grubs may result in stunted fish.

Diplostomulum larvae, commonly called "eye flukes," are found in the lens of fish. The resulting opacity of the lens is often called "white eye" by aquarists. These fish are frequently blind.

Members of the family Heterophyidae can cause massive infestations in freshwater tropical fishes. These result in extensive proliferation of gill cartilage and destruction of secondary lamellae. Infested fish die when handled and frequently fail to survive shipment.

Pathogenesis, Life Cycle, Transmission, and Epidemiology

The majority of the time, the definitive host for these parasites is a fish-eating bird that sheds parasite eggs into the water. These eggs eventually form ciliated miracidia, which penetrate specific species of snails. After asexual development in snails, procercaria are released that penetrate fish and develop into metacercariae in enclosed cysts.

A wide variety of birds serve as final host for mature *Diplostomulum* sp. The problem is rarely seen in retail outlets, as affected fish are usually culled by the wholesaler or producer.

Treatment and Control

Elimination of the snail intermediate hosts *(pleurocerca sp.)* or controlling access of birds to ponds will control infestations. Unfortunately, snail control is very difficult, since they can distance themselves from a chemical either by burrowing in mud or by closing their opercula. Chemotherapy has not been successful, with the possible exception of praziquantel baths (Heckmann, 1985). Surgical excision of cysts can be accomplished if the parasites are readily accessible near the surface of the fish's body. Fish with *Diplostomulum* larvae in the lens of the eye have not been treated successfully.

TURBELLARIANS

SYNONYMS. Flatworms, *Planaria*, white worms.

Geographic Distribution

These worms are found worldwide in both freshwater and saltwater systems. They are not generally true parasites but can startle aquarists and make a dramatic appearance as they occur in swarms crawling on the aquarium glass as well as on fish.

Clinical Appearance and Diagnosis

Turbellarians are occasionally seen as free-living pests in an aquarium. They are small, white worms that may be up to 5 mm long. Under the microscope, many species exhibit two eye spots. Turbellarians lodge on fish, particularly those that prefer the bottom of the aquarium. Affected fish do not usually show signs, although the pests may cause some hyperactivity and general discomfort in affected fish.

Life Cycle, Transmission, and Epidemiology

Turbellarians develop where organic matter accumulates from overfeeding fish and failure to clean the gravel. They are not usually parasitic but may cause irritation when they bloom in large numbers and settle on fish. Some marine forms have been incriminated in fish mortalities, but controlled experimental studies have not confirmed the hazard.

Treatment and Control

These worms can be controlled in most cases by reducing the amount of feed being delivered, prompt removal of excess feed, and regular cleaning of gravel with a distended-end siphon hose. Long-term formalin baths followed by a water change and gravel cleaning have been used to rid an aquarium of these pests.

CESTODES

SYNONYMS. Tapes, tapeworms.

Clinical Significance

Cestodes, like the digenetic trematodes, rarely affect ornamental fishes as adult worms. However, wild-caught ornamental fish frequently serve as secondary intermediate hosts. In such cases, encysted larvae are found on necropsy. The presence of these worms is usually silent. Occasionally, poor growth or emaciation will be blamed on their presence. Praziquantel as a bath may kill larval forms (Moser et al., 1986). Experiments done by the author indicate that 3 ppm of praziquantel in aquarium water will rid fish of tapeworms.

NEMATODES

SYNONYMS. Round worms, red worms, stomach worms, gut worms.

GENERA. There are a number of genera of nematodes associated with freshwater tropical fishes. Larval forms of *Eustrongyloides* spp. and adult forms of *Capillaria* sp. and *Camallanus* sp. affect a wide variety of freshwater tropical fishes.

Clinical Significance

Adult or larval nematodes can be found in ornamental fishes within the lumen of the intestine, as free migratory forms in the peritoneal cavity, or as encysted forms in internal organs or musculature. Larval *Eustrongyloides* sp. are usually found encysted in the muscles or peritoneum of the fish and cause no harm or clinical signs. These are found as red worms at postmortem examination. Occasionally, cysts located close to the skin are confused with neoplasias.

Infections by camallanids are usually initially noticed by aquarists who complain of a red worm that protrudes from the anus of the fish. Live-bearing fishes such as guppies and swordtails seem to be most frequently infected.

Capillaria are frequently found in freshwater tropical fishes, but their clinical significance is difficult to determine. They are usually found at post-mortem examination, although ornamental-fish farmers believe that they can be a problem, reducing reproductive potential and growth rates. Diagnosis can be made by finding typical capillarid ova in fecal flotations of detritus or feces taken from the bottom of the tank.

Life Cycle, Transmission, and Epidemiology

The life cycle of these worms usually involves an intermediate host such as an aquatic insect that harbors the larval stage of the nematode. Feeding of live foods may allow continuance of infestations, which would otherwise be self-limiting in an aquarium environment.

Treatment and Control

Adult nematodes can be treated with common nematocides in the food. Fenbendazole is a good candidate for control of *Camallanus* sp. The drug can be mixed with commercial food enhanced with cod liver oil and bound with gelatin. Preparations such as Panacur can be used in food at the rate of 0.25% (250 ppm). Since fish may not accept medicated food immediately, but most will begin feeding after a few days, Panacur (equine formulation contains 100 mg of active drug per ml) can be used at 2 ppm in aquarium water. This treatment should be repeated three times at weekly intervals. Carbon filters should be removed, and avoid passing medication through undergravel beds. Make a partial water change 2 to 3 days after treatment, then resume filtration. Since fish are quick to refuse medicated food, withholding food for a few days prior to feeding medicated food may be beneficial. Piperazine in food is also effective against some intestinal nematodes.

Ivermectin as a bath has been successfully used to treat nematodes (Heckmann, 1985); however, toxicity is high, and its use should be avoided. Migratory forms of nematodes cannot be treated, and clients should avoid feeding insect larvae or free-swimming copepods to their fish, as these may carry immature stages of nematodes.

ACANTHOCEPHALANS

SYNONYM. Thorny-headed worms.

Clinical Significance

Acanthocephalans can be a problem in wild freshwater or marine fishes. The incidence in ornamental freshwater tropical fish is low. Usually the parasite load per fish is very low, generally one or two parasites. Wild-caught ornamental fish can serve as an intermediate host when the final host is either a bird or a larger fish. The presence of the intermediate forms in low numbers does not appear to affect fish. Diagnosis is usually a postmortem one. There is no effective treatment established.

COPEPODS, BRANCHIURANS, AND ISOPODS

SYNONYMS. Anchor worm *(Lernaea)*, fish lice *(Argulus)*, fish bears (isopods).
IMPORTANT GENERA. *Lernaea, Ergasilus, Argulus, Livoneca.*

Geographic Distribution

The various members of this large group of crustacean parasites are found around the world. They infest a wide variety of species. *Lernaea* infestations are very common in koi and goldfish from production ponds, but any species can be affected. *Argulus* infestations are also most common in goldfish production ponds but can occur in a wide variety of fish species as well as amphibians. Ergasilids are occasionally found in ornamental fish production ponds but are rarely a problem in commercial outlets or home aquaria. Parasitic isopods *(Livoneca)* are rare in freshwater tropical species but are usually spectacular when they are found. There are over 400 species of parasitic isopods, and most parasitize marine fishes.

Clinical Appearance and Diagnosis

Lernaea, commonly called anchor worms, are elongated copepods that attach to the skin of the fish. Several species are described, but all females have a head that has a classic anchor shape and is embedded in the host flesh for attachment. The presence of adult parasites is diagnostic. Larval stages are free-swimming and have a typical crustacean form with segmented bodies and legs. Only the fertilized female copepods penetrate the host fish to form typical "anchor worms." At the time of initial penetration by female parasites, affected fish show irritation and localized hemorrhagic reactions at the point of entry. These areas may become secondarily infected with bacteria.

Ergasilus are parasitic copepods that resemble anchor worms. They are found firmly attached to the gills of fish by specialized prehensile hooks. Under the microscope these parasites appear multicolored.

Argulus are easily identified. They are approximately 5 to 8 mm long and are flat with prominent eyes, sucking discs, and a stiletto mouthpart. These parasites can move about the host. They are transparent and tend to take on the color of the fish they parasitize. Affected fish scratch against rocks and substrates and show irritation. They may develop skin ulcers where the parasites feed, and secondary bacterial infections are common.

Isopods are segmented with several pairs of legs. They are usually between 1 and 2 cm long as adults. *Livoneca* parasites generally burrow into the gill or buccal cavity but may excavate and live in a cavity in the lateral musculature. One species, *Livoneca symmetrica*, can be a particular problem in freshwater tropical fishes.

Pathologic Effects and Pathogenesis

Heavy infestations of *Lernaea* can be fatal. The site of penetration of the female parasites is often secondarily infected by bacteria or fungi or both.

Argulus sp. feed by piercing the host with their stiletto mouth parts. It is thought that the parasite elaborates toxic substances during feeding, which are responsible for the severe local reaction surrounding the area of feeding. As the parasites suck blood and tissue fluids, they leave a focal hemorrhagic area that frequently becomes an ulcer, possibly as a result of secondary invading bacteria. It has been suggested that argulids may carry these bacteria in addition to parasites such as trypanosomes. Wounds are also frequently infected with fungi.

Life Cycle, Transmission, and Epidemiology

Young free-swimming forms of *Lernaea* sp. feed on superficial mucus and debris, undergoing a number of molts while growing and differentiating into smaller males and larger females. When the parasites reach maturity, copulation occurs, and the females penetrate the skin of the host fish. The females develop large egg sacs that retain up to 700 eggs until hatching. The life cycle is temperature dependent and can take as little as 15 days at 30°C. Free-swimming and pre-adult stages can live up to 4 days without a host. Crowded conditions favor transmission of the parasite.

Mature *Argulus* deposit up to 400 eggs on substrates under pond conditions. Upon hatching, which takes about 4 weeks at temperatures common for freshwater tropical species, microscopic early stages lacking a sucking disc actively seek a host. Sexual maturity develops after parasitizing the fish for 5 to 6 weeks. Development is also temperature dependent and can vary from 40 to 100 days. *Argulus* infections build up dramatically in crowded conditions. Slow-moving waters also favor massive infestations.

Most isopods are protandrous hermaphrodites, developing first as males and later changing into

TABLE 70–1. Representative Parasites of Freshwater Tropical Fishes

	Hosts	Location in Host	Method of Infection	Prevalence	References
Sarcomastigophora					
Cryptobia	Killifishes, other freshwater tropical fishes	Blood	Leech vector Copepod vector (?)	Common	Gratzek, 1988
Ichthyobodo	Guppies, platys, tropical mouth-breeders, swordtails, other fishes	Skin, gills	Direct contact with free-swimming larvae	Common	Walliker, 1966 Hoffman, 1967 Schubert, 1968 Tavolga and Nigrelli, 1947
Oodinium	Guppies, mollies, platys, swordtails, tropical mouth-breeders, danios, other fishes	Skin, gills	Direct contact with free-swimming larvae	Common	van Duijn, 1967 Hoffman, 1967 Walliker, 1966
Hexamita	Cichlids, oscars, most fishes	Intestine, lateral line	Ingestion of cyst	Common	van Duijn, 1967
Ciliata					
Ichthyophthirius	All freshwater fishes	Skin, gills	Direct	Very common	Gratzek, 1988
Chilodonella	Goldfish, many freshwater tropical fishes	Gills, skin	Direct	Common	Gratzek, 1988
Tetrahymena	Dwarf cichlid, other cichlids, live-bearers, tetras	Skin, eye, systemic	Direct		Gratzek, 1988
Trichodina	All cultivated fishes	Gills, skin	Direct	Common	Gratzek, 1988
Trichodonella	All cultivated fishes	Gills, skin	Direct	Common	Gratzek, 1988
Tripartiella	All cultivated fishes	Gills, skin	Direct	Common	Gratzek, 1988
Scyphidia	Bottom-dwelling fishes	Skin, fins	Direct	Uncommon	
Glossatella	Bottom-dwelling fishes	Skin, fins	Direct	Uncommon	
Heteropolaria	Giant gouramis, bottom-dwelling fishes	Skin, fins	Direct	Common	
Apicomplexa					
Cryptosporidium	Freshwater angelfish	Intestines	Unknown	Unknown	
Eimeria	Many freshwater tropical fishes	Intestines	Ingestion of oocysts	Common	

TABLE 70–1. Representative Parasites of Freshwater Tropical Fishes *Continued*

	Hosts	Location in Host	Method of Infection	Prevalence	References
Microspora					
Plistophora	Tetras, swordtails, other fishes	Muscle	Ingestion of spores	Uncommon	van Duijn, 1967
Myxozoa					
Henneguya	Corydoras catfishes, other freshwater tropical fishes	Gills, skin	Possible intermediate host	Common	
Myxidium	Freshwater tropical fishes	Gills, skin	Possible intermediate host		
Mitraspora	Goldfishes	Kidneys	Direct	Common	
Monogenea					
Dactylogyrus	All freshwater tropical fishes	Gills	Direct	Common	
Gyrodactylus	Guppies, all freshwater tropical fishes	Skin, gills	Direct	Common	Hoffman, 1967 Hoffman and Putz, 1964
Urocleidoides	Guppies	Gills	Direct	Common	Hoffman, 1967
Digenea					
Posthodiplostomum	Mollies	Mesentery, kidneys, spleen, liver, pericardium	Snail intermediate host	Common	Hoffman, 1958
Macroderoides	Mollies	Muscle	Snail intermediate host	Uncommon	Hoffman, 1967
Paramacroderoides	Mollies	Muscle	Snail intermediate host	Uncommon	Hoffman, 1967
Ascotyle	Mollies	Conus arteriosus, mesentery, viscera muscle, gills, intestinal wall, liver	Snail intermediate host	Common in gills; otherwise, uncommon	Hoffman, 1967
Neascus	Silver dollar, many freshwater fishes	Skin, muscle	Snail intermediate host	Common	Hoffman, 1967
Clinostomum	All cultivated freshwater fishes	Body cavity, muscle	Snail intermediate host	Common	Hoffman, 1967
Diplostomulum	Many freshwater tropical fishes	Eye lens	Snail intermediate host	Common	Hoffman, 1967
Cestoda					
Haplobothrium	Guppies	Liver	Invertebrate intermediate host	Common	Hoffman, 1967
Nematoda					
Eustrongyloides	Guppies, freshwater tropical fishes	Encysted in muscles, peritoneum	Aquatic insect intermediate host	Common	
Capillaria	Most freshwater tropical fishes	Intestines	Aquatic insect intermediate host	Common	
Camallanus	Live-bearers	Colon, intestines	Aquatic insect intermediate host	Common	
Acanthocephala					
Acanthocephalus	Australian native fishes	Intestines, abdominal cavity	Crustacean intermediate host	Rare	
Copepoda					
Lernaea	African tropical mouth-breeders	Gills, fins, skin	Direct	Common	Flynn, 1973 Hoffman, 1967
Ergasilus	Tropical mouth-breeders	Gills	Direct	Common	Hoffman, 1967
Branchiura					
Argulus	Various freshwater tropical fishes, goldfish, amphibians	Skin	Direct contact	Uncommon	Flynn, 1973
Isopoda					
Livoneca	Various freshwater tropical fishes	Mouth, gills	Water-borne	Rare	Flynn, 1973
Mollusca					
Glochidia	Pond-reared tropical fishes	Fins, mouth	Water-borne	Uncommon	Hoffman, 1967

females. Females attach on a host and inhibit the development of other attached parasites so they remain males. Often, the large female is found in the mouth, and the males in the gill cavity.

Treatment and Control

Lernaea sp. infecting aquarium fishes are usually removed by extraction using forceps, being careful to avoid breaking the parasite. Extraction can be followed by local treatment with cotton swabs permeated with a suitable disinfectant (iodine, acriflavine, alcohol). Antibiotic treatment may accelerate healing of lesions. Infested aquaria can be treated with organophosphate, which will kill free-living juvenile forms. Dimulin, a chitin synthesis inhibitor, has been used successfully at 1 to 2 ppm as a pond treatment and an aquarium water treatment. This treatment must be repeated twice at a 7- to 10-day interval to achieve eradication. Quarantine for anchor worms should be at least 15 days at 30°C and longer at lower temperatures. Treatment during quarantine is recommended. Water, live food, plants, or other material from infected ponds should be stored for more than 4 days without contact with a potential host to avoid introduction of the parasite. Adequate ultraviolet light sterilization and filtration reduce the potential of spread of an infestation in a multiaquaria system.

Ergasilus sp. are too small to be removed mechanically. Infested production ponds are usually treated with organophosphates or dimulin.

Argulus survive for up to 14 days without access to a host. They are generally treated with organophosphates when large numbers of fish are infected. They can be removed manually with a forceps when few fish are involved. Live food should be held for at least 15 days before feeding to ensure that no early stages of argulids are included. Beware of rocks or plants from infested sources. Mosquito fish have been used as a biological control in ornamental ponds.

Praziquantel baths will kill larval forms of *Livoneca symmetrica* (Moser et al., 1986). However, simple removal with forceps can be done, since the parasite is easily seen and is loosely attached to the fish.

LITERATURE CITED

Blazer, V.S., and Wolke, R.E. (1984) Effect of diet on the immune response of rainbow trout (*Salmo gairdneri*). Can. J. Fish. Aquat. Sci. 41(8):1244–1247.

Flynn, R.J. (1973) Parasites of Laboratory Animals. Iowa State University Press, Ames, Iowa.

Foissner, W., Hoffman, G.L., and Mitchell, A.J. (1985) *Heteropolaria colisarum* Foissner & Schubert, 1977 (Protozoa: Epistylididae) of North American freshwater fishes. J. Fish Dis. 8:145–160.

Goven, B.A., Gilbert, J.P., and Gratzek, J.B. (1980) Apparent drug resistance to the organophosphate dimethyl (2,2,2-trichloro-1-hydroxyethyl) phosphonate by mongenetic trematodes. J. Wildl. Dis. 16(3):343–346.

Gratzek, J.B. (1988) Parasites associated with ornamental fish. Vet. Clin. North Am. [Small Anim. Pract.] 18(2):375–400.

Heckmann, R. (1985) Ivermectin efficacy trials for nematodes parasitic to fish. Fish Health Section/American Fisheries Society, 13(1):6.

Hines, R.S., and Spira, D.T. (1974) Ichthyophthiriasis in the mirror carp Cyprinus carpio (L.) V. Acquired immunity. J. Fish Biol. 6:373–378.

Hoffman, G.L. (1958) Experimental studies on the cercaria and metacercaria of strigeoid trematode *Posthodiplostomum minumum*. Exp. Parasitol. 7:23–50.

Hoffman, G.L. (1967) Parasites of North American Freshwater Fishes. Univ. California Press, Berkeley, California.

Hoffman, G.L., and Putz, R.E. (1964) Studies on *Gyrodactylus macrochiri* n. sp. (Trematoda: Monogenea) from *Lepomis macrochirus*. Proc. Helminthol. Soc. Washington, DC 31:76–82.

Morrison, C.M., and Cone, D.K. (1986) A possible marine form of *Ichthyobodo* sp. on haddock, *Melanogrammus aeglefinus* (L.), in the northwest Atlantic Ocean. J. Fish Dis. 9:141–142.

Moser, M., Sakanari, J., and Heckmann, R. (1986) The effects of praziquantel on various larval and adult parasites from freshwater and marine snails and fish. J. Parasitol. 72(1):175–176.

Schubert, G. (1968) The injurious effects of *Costia necatrix*. Bull. Office Int. Epizootiol. 69:1171–78.

Scott, M.E., and Robinson, M.A. (1984) Challenge infections of *Gyrodactylus bullatarudis* (Monogenea) on guppies, *Poecilia reticulata* (Peters), following treatment. J. Fish Biol. 24:581–586.

Tavolga, W.N., and Nigrelli, R.F. (1947) Studies on *Costia necatrix* (Henneguya*). Trans. Am. Microscop. Soc. 66:366–78.

van Duijn, C. (1967) Diseases of Fishes. 2nd ed. Iliffe Books, London, U.K.

Walliker, D. (1966) The management and diseases of fish: III. Protozoal diseases of fish with special reference to those encountered in aquaria. J. Small Anim. Pract. 7:779–807.

Chapter 71

NEOPLASIAS OF FRESHWATER TROPICAL FISHES

ERIC B. MAY

Tumors or neoplastic diseases of freshwater tropical fish have been poorly represented in the literature, with the exception of the Japanese medaka (Hawkins et al., 1986; Nakazawa et al., 1985) and the swordtail (Schwab et al., 1979; Li and Baldwin, 1944). Tumors often require considerable time to develop following exposure to carcinogenic agents (Farber and Cameron, 1980). Also, the hobbyist often does not have access to diagnostic services, and many of the freshwater tropical species are relatively short-

lived. The likelihood of these fishes dying of other diseases is greater than that they will develop tumors. Equally important is the lack of reporting of tumors in these fishes. The cumulative result is a paucity of information on tumors of ornamentals. Because both the swordtail and the medaka (Fig. 71–1) are highly regarded as models for tumor and aquatic toxicologic research, information on these two genera is much more available.

Equally problematic is information on predispos-

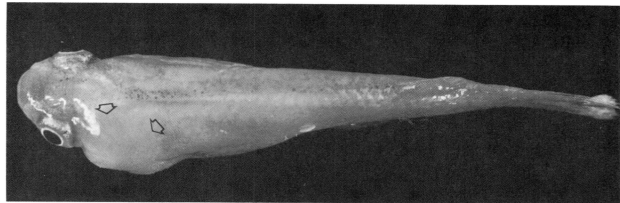

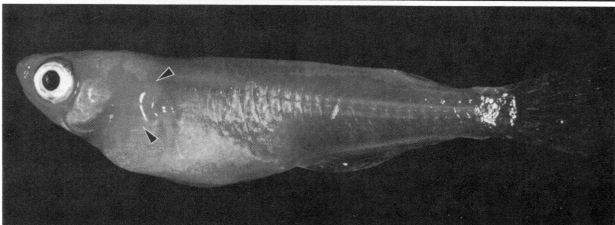

FIGURE 71–1. Japanese medaka with lymphoma. *A.* Dorsal view showing the tumor (arrows) protruding from the lateral aspect of the head. *B.* Lateral view of the same fish. (From Okihiro, M.S., and Hinton, D.E. [1989] Lymphoma in medaka, *Oryzias latipes*. Dis. Aquatic Organ. 7:79—87.)

TABLE 71–1. Neoplasias Reported in Freshwater Tropical Fishes

Site/Neoplasia	Fish	References
Nervous System		
Retinoblastoma	Green swordtail	Harshbarger, 1978
Neuroblastoma	Swordtail hybrid	Schwab et al., 1979
Medulloepithelioma	Medaka	Hawkins et al., 1986
Melanoma	Platyfish	Ghadially and Gordon, 1974
	Guppy × black molly	Ghadially and Gordon, 1974
	Variable platyfish	MacIntyre and Baker-Chohen, 1961
Cardiovascular System		
Hemangioma	Oscar	Harshbarger, 1978
Lymphoblastic lymphoma	Medaka	Smith et al., 1936
Malignant fibrous histiocytoma	Medaka	Smith et al., 1936
Gastrointestinal System		
Cholangioma	Rivulus	Park and Kim, 1984
Cholangiocarcinoma	Danio	Stanton, 1965, 1966
	Guppy	Simon and Lapid, 1984
Hepatocellular adenoma	Medaka	Nakazawa et al., 1985
Urinary System		
None reported		
Endocrine System		
Pituitary chromophobe adenoma	Guppy	Stok, 1953
Thyroid adenoma	Common in many species	Baker 1959; Hoover, 1984
Reproductive System		
Seminoma	African lungfish	Masahito et al., 1984
Sertoli cell tumor	Platyfish	Li and Baldwin, 1944
Leydig cell tumor	Swordtail	Li and Baldwin, 1944
Musculoskeletal System		
Chondroma	Jewelfish	Schlumberger and Lucke, 1948
Integumentary System		
None Reported		
Respiratory System		
None Reported		

ing factors. Although environmental, genetic, and nutritional factors are known to be involved in predisposing fish to tumors (Mix, 1985), except for a few instances, specific reference to freshwater tropical fishes is lacking. The neoplasias reported in these species are listed in Table 71–1.

In the platyfish and black molly, genetics appears to play a large part in development of melanomas (Ghadially and Gordon, 1974; MacIntyre and

Baker-Chohen, 1961). To date, no intracranial tumors have been reported even though all of the cell types known to develop tumors are present. Tumors of the cardiovascular system are too few to make any assessment of predisposing conditions. Although little is known about the incidence of tumors in freshwater tropicals, our general state of knowledge regarding tumors in teleosts is good. Predisposing factors such as carcinogenic compounds, viruses, irritants, oncogenes, and parasites all have been reported in teleosts and should be considered potential sources for tumor induction in tropicals.

LITERATURE CITED

Baker, K.F.(1959) Renal and other heterotopic thyroid tissue in fishes. In: Symposium on Comparative Endocrinology (Gorbman, A., ed.). John Wiley & Sons, New York.

Farber, E., and Cameron, R.G. (1980) The sequential analysis of cancer development. Adv. Cancer Res. 31:125–226.

Ghadially, F.N., and Gordon, M.D. (1974) A localized melanoma in a hybrid fish *Lebistes × Mollienisia*. Cancer Res. 17:597–599.

Ghadially, F.N., and Whiteley, H.J. (1951) An invasive red-pigmented tumor (erythrophoroma) in a red male platyfish (*Platypoecilus maculatus* var *rubra*). Br. J. Cancer 5:405–408.

Harshbarger, J.C. (1978) RTLA Supplement. Registry of Tumors in Lower Animals. Smithsonian Institution, Washington, D.C.

Hawkins, W.E., Fournie, J.W., and Overstreet, R.M. (1986) Intraocular neoplasms induced by methylazoxymethanol acetate in Japanese medaka (*Oryzias latipes*). J. Natl. Cancer Inst. 76:453–465.

Hinton, K.E., Walker, E.R., Pinkstaff, C.A., and Zuchelkowski, E.M. (1984) Morphological survey of teleost organs important in carcinogenesis with attention to fixation. Natl. Cancer Inst. Monogr. 65:291–320.

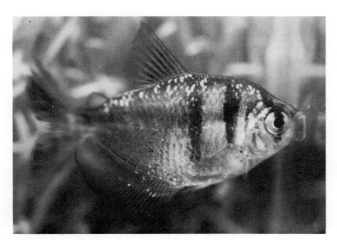

FIGURE 71–2. Black tetra with an unclassified tumor of the lower lip. (Courtesy of T. Wenzel.)

Hoover, K.L. (1984) Hyperplastic thyroid lesions in fish. Natl. Cancer Inst. Monogr. 65:275–289.

Levine, M., and Gordon, M. (1962) Ocular tumors with exophthalmia in xiphophorin fishes. Cancer Res. 6:197–204.

Li, H.H., and Baldwin, F.M. (1944) Testicular tumors in the teleost (*Xiphophorus helleri*) receiving sesame oil. Proc. Soc. Exp. Biol. Med. 57:165–167.

MacIntyre, P.A., and Baker-Chohen, K.F. (1961) Melanoma, renal thyroid tumor and reticulo-endothelial hyperplasia in a nonhybrid platyfish. Zoologica 46:125–131.

Masahito, P., Ishikawa, T., and Takayama, S. (1984) Spontaneous spermatocytic seminoma in African lungfish. J. Fish Dis. 7:169–172.

Mix, M.C. (1985) Cancerous diseases in aquatic animals and their association with environmental pollutants: a critical review of the literature. American Petroleum Institute, College Station, Texas.

Nakazawa, T., Hamaguchi, S., and Kyono-Hamaguchi, Y. (1985) Histochemistry of liver tumors induced by diethylnitrosamine and differential sex susceptibility to carcinogenesis in *Oryzias latipes*. J. Natl. Cancer Inst. 75:567–573.

Park, E.H., and Kim, D.S. (1984) Hepatocarcinogenicity of diethylnitrosamine to the self-fertilizing hermaphroditic fish *Rivulus marmoratus*. J. Natl. Cancer Inst. 73:871–876.

Schlumberger, H.G., and Lucke, B. (1948) Tumors of fishes, amphibians, and reptiles. Cancer Res. 8:657–754.

Schwab, M., Kollinger, G., and Hass, J. (1979) Genetic basis of susceptibility for neuroblastoma following treatment with *N*-methyl-*N*-nitrosourea and X-rays in *Xiphophorus*. Cancer Res. 39:519–526.

Simon, K., and Lapid, K. (1984) Carcinogenesis studies on guppies. Natl. Cancer Inst. Monograph 65:71–81.

Smith, G.M., Coates, C.W., and Strong, L.C. (1936) Neoplastic diseases in small tropical fishes. Zoologica N.Y. 21:219–224.

Stanton, M.F. (1965) Diethylnitrosamine-induced hepatic degeneration and neoplasia in the aquarium fish, *Brachydanio rerio*. J. Natl. Cancer Inst. 34:117–130.

Stanton, M.F. (1966) Hepatic neoplasms of aquarium fish exposed to *Cycas carcinalis*. Fed. Proc. 25:661.

Stok, A. (1953) Tumors of fishes. II. Chromophobe adenoma of the pituitary gland in the viviparous cyproinodone, *Lebistes reticulatus*. Proc. Ned. Acad. Wet. (C), 56:34–38.

Chapter 72

FRESHWATER TROPICAL FISH PHARMACOLOGY

MICHAEL K. STOSKOPF

In the arena of tropical fish medicine, the doses for most commonly used drugs are truly empirical (Stoskopf, 1988). This is likely to remain true for a considerable time because of the lack of funding available for carefully controlled research in this important field. In the meantime, practicing clinicians are forced to rely on anecdotal and incomplete information. The requirements for extrapolation are great, and unfortunately there is abundant misinformation based on incomplete observations. The rules for extrapolations in fish pharmacology seem to be essentially the same ones used in mammalian veterinary pharmacology. They will at least serve well until careful research and the experience of trained veterinarians treating fishes on the basis of confirmed diagnoses show a need to modify them.

Freshwater tropical fishes will respond to a wide range of chemotherapeutants, including, but by no means limited to, antibacterial drugs (Amlacher 1970; Bassleer, 1983; Herwig, 1979; Kuhns, 1981; Reichenbach-Klinke, 1965; Stoskopf, 1988; Van Duijn, 1973). None of the drugs mentioned in this chapter have U.S. Food and Drug Administration approval for use in tropical fishes and all treatments mentioned technically represent extra label use. While the risk of drugs entering the human food supply through treatment of ornamental tropical fishes is infinitesimally small, clinicians should consider the risks of direct exposure of fish owners or the environment to chemotherapeutic agents when prescribing a course of therapy.

ROUTES OF DELIVERY

Every practitioner is familiar with the available routes for delivery of medications to mammals. The same routes are available for fish with only minor modifications. Drugs can be given orally (PO), intramuscularly (IM), intraperitoneally (IP), intravenously (IV) or topically as baths or dips. Selection of the proper route depends on the environmental situation, the species and condition of the patient, and the drug being delivered. Failure to consider any of these factors can result in unsatisfactory treatment.

Intravenous Administration

The small size of most tropical fish precludes effective intravenous dosage. In some larger fish the intravenous route might be feasible on an anesthetized patient using veins in the mouth. Caudal veins commonly used for venipuncture to obtain blood samples are generally not suitable. In most small species, these procedures involve a blind puncture into a network of small venules and arterioles that contribute to the pooled blood sample. Perivascular escape of drugs is effectively unavoidable in those situations. Cannulation of small vessels in the mouth is possible on anesthetized patients of reasonable size, but the procedure requires microsurgical skills and equipment as well as the physiologic impact of anesthesia.

Intraperitoneal Administration

This route of administration is the most common substitute for the intravenous route. It is practical if the drug selected is nonirritating and capable of crossing endothelial barriers. It may not be practical in situations involving very large numbers of fish. This is rarely a limiting factor in treating the fish of home hobbyists but becomes a very real problem when working in large aquaria. It is particularly useful in treating critically ill patients who require rapid drug distribution to optimize their chances of survival.

The procedure is relatively safe and simple even in very small fish. Once the abdomen is located and defined, an appropriately small needle (22- to 30-gauge, depending on the size of the fish), is inserted under the scales in the caudoventral aspect of the abdomen, directed craniodorsad. A controlled insertion through the skin and muscle to a depth approximating the wall of the abdomen will rarely cause complications. Bowel is generally not penetrated and moves away from the sharp needle. The posterior ventral site of insertion minimizes the chance of injuring the liver, spleen, or kidney.

For very flighty and nervous fish, anesthesia is necessary and most practitioners will have greater success if they use minimal sedation in all fish to facilitate their efforts. This route can be used without anesthesia or sedation by experienced practitioners. If handled properly, most fish will tolerate the procedure remarkably calmly. Injection volume is not generally a major concern when injecting antibiotics at appropriate doses for the fish's body weight; however, fluid administration can require some common sense and consideration of the total volume of the coelomic cavity.

Here a short word on asepsis might be appropriate. Although surface disinfection of injection sites is impractical in fish medicine owing to the fish's essential mucous covering and wet environment, fish are susceptible to iatrogenic infections. Care to avoid introducing infection is important. Use sterile syringes and needles and observe all practices to reduce cross-infection between patients or contamination of multidose drug containers in fish practice as you would in mammalian practice.

Intramuscular Administration

There is considerable controversy among fish practitioners over the efficacy and appropriateness of this route of administration. My own experience has led me to believe that it is extremely useful, and I use it routinely for a wide selection of drugs, which distribute well from mammalian muscle.

Intramuscular injections are generally administered into the dorsal muscle mass under the dorsal fin. A site roughly halfway between the lateral line and the dorsal fin is usually selected and the needle directed cranially under scales as in the IP injection. If appropriate doses are being used, concern about injection volume is rarely necessary, although if dilutions are made from stock drugs, I try to limit injections to 1 to 2 µl per g body weight. In very small fishes, microliter syringes and 30-gauge needles are a necessity.

Intramuscular injection eliminates any risk of abdominal organ injury and is more readily administered without use of sedatives or anesthetics. In situations in which your technical staff or the client will be administering the drug, an IM injection is less intimidating. Also, for certain drugs the apparent increase in distribution time from muscle as opposed to coelomic distribution is clinically useful. For example, intramuscular administration of steroids such as dexamethasone empirically seems to allow less frequent dose intervals, reducing the number of times a critically ill fish must be handled. Considerably more kinetics research must be done before the issue of IM injections is resolved, but it appears to be a viable route for many drugs in many situations in which relatively few fish require treatment.

Objections to the use of the IM route include the belief that fish muscle is less well vascularized than mammalian muscle. This would lead to poor distribution of drugs, formation of sterile abscesses, and increased local impact of irritating drugs. In practical application, however, this does not seem to be the case when drugs are properly selected and administered. Many drugs are rapidly distributed from fish muscle and the concept of poor vascularity is highly questionable. Sterile abscessation and traumatic injury to fish injected IM is no more common than in routine mammalian practice. A second objection is based on the fact that drugs will leak out of the needle tract after injection. This does occur, but it can be minimized by proper manipulation of the needle. A slight twist to the needle during withdrawal will help close the tract. Partial reinsertion of the needle before complete withdrawal also helps prevent drug loss.

Oral Administration

If fish are still eating when they are presented for treatment, oral administration is usually the route of choice. This is particularly true in production systems where large numbers of fish must be medicated. It also holds for the situation of the home aquarist who will have to administer daily treatments. Exceptions to this general statement include the delivery of drugs intended for systemic treatment that will not be absorbed intact through the digestive system such as aminoglycosides. Drugs being delivered to individual fish which require very critical dosage control is another exception.

A variety of flake foods are available commercially that have antibiotics incorporated into them. Other drugs can be sprayed lightly over plain flake foods, which are then redried and fed. This should be done in a chemical fume hood. If larger food will be eaten by the fish being treated, drugs can be injected into the food and fed. The practice of soaking food in drugs before feeding is less precise, and is generally not very successful using water-soluble drugs. Lipophilic drugs, on the other hand, will reach appreciable levels in fat-containing foods and will remain in the food a reasonable time before being leached out into the water.

Fish who feed solely on live foods can be medicated by exposing the food animals to drug prior to their use. This is an art. Very little is known about the kinetics of drugs in such complicated situations. The trick is to obtain useful levels of drug in the feed animal without killing it and making it unacceptable to the patient. Much of the controversy over effective doses of drugs fed in this manner can be attributed to the difficulty of accomplishing this. Much more work needs to be done in this area of drug kinetics.

In general, oral delivery offers the advantages of relatively discrete drug delivery compared to baths and dips and extreme ease of administration. Disadvantages include all of those practitioners are familiar with from mammalian medicine, and in particular the possibility of causing patients to refuse unpalatable feed. Medication in feed is of little value unless the feed is eaten. I generally try to err on the side of complete drug delivery by reducing the amount of food offered initially, making sure that all medicated feed is taken. If aggression problems appear or the fish are not receiving adequate calories, their diet can easily be supplemented with unmedicated food immediately after the treated food is eaten.

The dose interval can also present a problem. If a fish feeds normally every third day but needs drug delivery at least daily, effective levels will not be reached unless the feeding schedule is modified. This is not a trivial problem. Increased tank aggression may become serious if small daily feeds are substituted for large periodic feeds. On the other hand, satiation may make feeding normal amounts of food daily quite unworkable. Satiated fish will not take drugged food and deprived fish, even though receiving the same total amount of food in many small feedings, may seriously injure or kill each other in aggression. In these cases, which usually involve large carnivorous fish, compromises in drug delivery may be necessary.

Topical Administration

Four basic forms of topical treatment must be considered in any chapter on fish therapeutics. These include the direct localized topical administration, short-duration dips, longer-duration baths, and tank treatments. Each has its advantages and disadvantages.

Tank Treatments

Fish owners and most practitioners will be most familiar with this type of treatment. It is probably the most frequently used method of treating small tropical fish. In this treatment, drug is put directly into the aquarium or pond where the fish lives. The entire environment is saturated with drug, it is hoped at a level that will produce effective systemic or topical effects in the affected fish. Its advantages are apparent, including ease of administration, since fish need not be handled, and the extension of the treatment to the environmental substrates, potentially successfully destroying pathogenic organisms not yet on the fish.

It is my least favorite method of treatment and one I avoid if at all possible. The disadvantages usually outweigh the advantages. Achieving safe but therapeutic levels of most drugs with this type of treatment is difficult, if not impossible. Drugs tend to bind to substrates and organic debris in the tank with alarming lack of predictability. Biologic filtration can be severely affected by some drugs, resulting in major water-quality complications (see Antibacterial Treatments below) (Levine and Meade, 1976). Also plants and invertebrate inhabitants may be very seriously affected at otherwise therapeutic doses.

The basic problem of therapeutic index is complicated because efficacy must now be weighed against safety in a whole array of organisms ranging from bacteria to other species of fishes. Therefore, most commonly prescribed doses for this type of therapy error on the side of safety. Most people find it objectionable to kill all of their plants and destroy their filter beds during a treatment. As a result, achievement of therapeutic levels is very rare, but the opportunity to produce resistant organisms is not. Even the apparent advantage of ease of administration is misleading, since usually any advantage is negated by extensive clean-up and reset-up efforts after the treatment is completed. In most situations, another form of drug delivery is preferable to tank treatment.

Long-Duration Baths and Dips

An excellent alternative to tank treatments when many fish are affected and not feeding is the use of a long-term bath or a dip. These treatments require handling the fish but have the major advantages of sparing the environment from damage and increasing the predictability of drug delivery. To carry out these treatments, another container is required that can be filled with a known volume of water from the tank where the fish to be treated are housed. Drug is added to this separate container and the patients are then exposed to it for varying periods of time.

The distinction between dips and baths is arbitrary, but I generally consider treatments lasting no more than 15 minutes as dips and longer exposures as baths. The length of exposure should be based on the time required to reach therapeutic levels, but in practice this really is not known for most drugs. The length of exposure is actually more often based on the ability of the fish to tolerate the treatment. Even so, the variations in species susceptibility and individual condition make it imperative that fish be observed for signs of stress during treatment. If the treatment seems to be compromising the fish, they can be removed immediately and returned to their untreated tank.

Short-Duration Dips

Short dips are often employed in the hope of achieving systemic levels of a drug. This is a questionable goal with most drugs, but the final analysis of the ability of this type of administration to achieve therapeutic systemic levels must wait for kinetic studies. Some drugs are absorbed across gill and other mucous membranes, but the degree of systemic effect as opposed to local topical effects is very hard to judge. It is best to consider short dips of 1 second to 1 minute to be purely topical administrations. They can be very effective in removing external parasites but should not be expected to be effective in disseminated systemic disease.

Direct Topical Application

This very valuable method of treatment is often forgotten in fish medicine, but localized application of antiseptics, antibiotics, steroids, and dressings can be very beneficial. The most common use of this application is to cauterize or disinfect a localized lesion. A fish is netted, positioned, and localized lesions are quickly painted with povidone-iodine, quaternary ammonium compounds, or other dilute disinfectants using a cotton swab. It is important to move quickly and the whole procedure should not take longer than about 30 seconds before the fish is rinsed off in a container of water and replaced in its tank. Otherwise, severe tissue necrosis and burns can be caused by leaving the disinfectant in place too long on the first tissues painted. This type of treatment works well to reduce infection and promote healing in localized diseases. It is also quite useful as an adjunct to systemic therapy.

Other drugs besides disinfectants can be applied locally to lesions. Surprisingly, short applications of topical steroids and antibiotics are remarkably effective in treating ulcers and sores. I have found Panolog (Solvay, Princeton, New Jersey) particularly useful for treating wounds, and particularly ulcerated corneas and corneal edema (Fig. 72–1). This type of application is not nearly so difficult or ridiculous as it might seem. Many fish rapidly become conditioned to the treatment and with careful handling they are easily subdued without damage. In other fish, I find the treatment important enough to use repeated sedations to accomplish my ends.

To treat an ulcerated eye with Panolog, the patient is carefully caught with a soft net or plastic bag. It is brought to the surface and held on its side with the lower operculum and mouth under the water so it can breathe. A drop of Panolog is applied to the eye and the fish gently floated in position for 30 seconds to 1 minute. This is apparently long enough for appreciable drug to be absorbed across the cornea. Then the fish is released from the net to the tank, the Panolog washes off and floats on the surface, where it can be removed with a dry paper towel. Daily applications in this manner in conjunction with oral antibiotics improve the chances of successful treatment. My own crude clinical evaluations suggest that this type of combined treatment succeeds nearly 75% of the time if the eye is still intact when treatment is initiated. This is a considerable improvement over simple administration of oral antibiotics alone (25 to 40% success) or no treatment at all (less than 10% success).

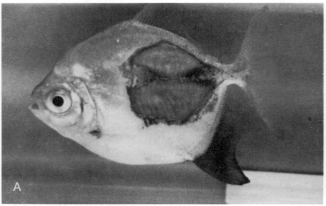 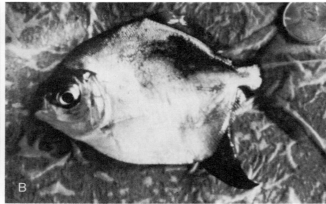

FIGURE 72–1. *A.* Silver dollar with skin ulcerations due to *Flexibacter columnaris*. *B.* Same fish following treatment with Panolog ointment. (Courtesy of R. Floyd.)

DRUGS AND DOSES

Antibacterial Treatments

Bacteria can cause primary disease in fish or become secondary complications to other problems. In either case, treatment with antibacterial drugs is common and frequently contributes to the positive outcome of a case. Interpretation of the need for antibacterial therapy can be based on a variety of factors and the selection of appropriate drugs is fairly complex. The need for culture, identification, and sensitivity testing is a given. Other factors to consider are an antibiotic's kinetics for a specific route of delivery, its interactions with other drugs or environmental molecules, and certainly any deleterious side effects. Unfortunately as mentioned earlier, none of these data are very complete for fish. Kinetics studies of antibacterial antibiotics in fish have been done, but most of these studies examine food fish (catfishes and trout) (Setser, 1985; Snieszko and Friddle, 1951; Willford, 1967). Where these studies have contributed to the recommended dose given in Appendix V, there is a comment, but the majority of drugs remain unstudied. Information does exist for human and other mammal species and should be considered in lieu of specific fish-related data. It can be used as an extrapolation point if no other information is available.

My own experience suggests that underdosing or delivery failure is a more common cause of therapeutic failure with antibacterial drugs than overdosing or drug toxicity. There are exceptions of course. The most difficult to identify are delayed toxicity effects such as renal damage due to improper aminoglycoside administration. These cases may recover dramatically from their initial disease, only to succumb as much as a year later with severe tubular damage in the kidneys. Apparently the major excretion functions of the gills of fish allow them to survive relatively long times with extensive kidney damage. I prefer oral or injectable routes of delivery over baths and dips because I feel I have better control of dosing.

The potential for developing resistant strains of organisms causes me to rely heavily on a single drug for treatments initiated before culture and sensitivity results are available (Trust and Chipman, 1974; Wolf and Snieszko, 1964). If antibiotic sensitivity reports begin to show resistance to one drug, I switch my initial drug of choice. I have not used sulfas or trimethoprim extensively. There is some concern about their potential toxicity to various fish (Wood et al., 1957), but recent extensive use in catfishes seems to have allayed many of these concerns. Nevertheless, I hold them in reserve along with aminoglycosides and nitrofuran-based drugs. The nitrofurans apparently have very consistent dose-response effects on fish pathogens (Nusbaum and Shotts, 1981). I do not use some of the drugs listed in Appendix V. Acriflavin, for example, has been

abused enough that resistant strains are very common. Carbenicillin results in fish refusing medicated food and a very severe malodorous problem in the tank water.

Species-specific differences are not well documented for any antibiotics in fish. This is not surprising, considering the wide variety of fish treated. Species variations do exist. Scaleless species are generally more susceptible to topical treatments and dips than scaled species. Some of the algae-eating species seem to be particularly susceptible to dyes and chemical baths. When administering antibiotics it is important that the patients be monitored carefully for signs of toxicity or improvement of the condition so doses can be adjusted. Successful dosing is usually rewarded with noticeable clinical improvement within 2 or 3 days.

Antibiotic resistance and incomplete therapy are very real problems in fish medicine (Stoskopf, 1984; Watanabe et al., 1971). Even though improvement is noted early in treatment, it is very advisable to continue treatment for a minimum period of a week. I generally expect to maintain successful antibiotic treatments for 10 days to 2 weeks, much as I would if treating a mammalian patient. This helps avoid relapses and seems to decrease the number of resistant organisms created. The current state of the art in dosage timing is basically no different than judging mammalian treatments.

Effects of Antibacterial Treatments on Biologic Filters

The impact of drugs and chemicals on the bacteria used in biologic filters has long been a controversial subject. It is a good idea to avoid exposing filter beds to antibiotics and other chemicals for a number of reasons, which include loss of bacterial populations and filter efficiency and development of resistant bacterial strains. However, in some situations there may be no practical alternative to treating a system with its biologic filter in place. Also, remember that when feeding or injecting antibiotics, small amounts are going to be excreted unchanged from the fish, and there is no way to avoid some exposure of biologic filtration beds to drugs. The published experiments looking at the effects of fish chemotherapeutants on nitrification rates have disagreed dramatically (Table 72–1).

One cause of the confusion may be the variable of the population dynamics of the filter bacteria at the time of exposure and its relationship to the timing of bacterial population recovery. Drugs can affect the efficiency of nitrification by individual bacteria. When this happens the effects can be uniform across a population or certain strains of bacteria may be more significantly affected. In this situation the resistance patterns of the bacterial populations making up the filter will have a major impact on the effect of a given drug on nitrification. The extreme case of affecting nitrification ability is when a drug causes the death

TABLE 72–1. The Effects of Chemotheraputic Agents on Nitrification

Agent	Dose (mg/L)	Inhibition	References
Chloramphenicol	50	Critical	Levine and Meade, 1976
Chlortetracycline	10	Critical	Levine and Meade, 1976
Copper sulfate	5	None	Levine and Meade, 1976
Erythromycin	50	Critical	Collins et al., 1976
Formaldehyde	15	Moderate	Levine and Meade, 1976
Malachite green	0.5	Slight	Levine and Meade, 1976
Methylene blue	1	Critical	Levine and Meade, 1976
Nifurpirinol	1	Moderate	Levine and Meade, 1976
Oxytetracycline	50	None	Collins et al., 1976
Sulfadiazine	25	Critical	Levine and Meade, 1976
Sulfamerazine	50	None	Collins et al., 1976
Sulfanilamide	25	Critical	Levine and Meade, 1976

of a bacterium. Here again, the individual resistance patterns of bacteria will affect the impact of a given drug. In addition, if a given drug kills a set percentage of the bacteria important for nitrification in a filter, the effect on nitrification will be amplified if the drug is applied at a time when the population is small and the growth rate has not yet entered logarithmic phase (Fig. 72–2). Usually at this time the balance of bacterial biomass to available nitrogen for nutrition has not yet plateaued. Given a stabilized temperature and bacterial reproductive rate, it will take much longer to reach a suitable plateau population of bacteria in a newly started biologic filter than in an established, heavily populated one.

An example may help to clarify the problem. In a system with enough fish wastes being added daily to feed 10 million bacteria in the biologic filter, levels of toxic nitrogenous wastes will remain very low as long as there are approximately 10 million or more bacteria produced or living in the filter bed each day. The doubling rate of the bacteria is directly related to water temperature, and if that is held steady in our example, it is easy to see how the relationship between the total population of the filter bed and the nutrient load affects the impact of a bacterial mortality rate. When food is limiting, only enough additional bacteria will survive as can be supported by the additional available nitrogen wastes. In our hypothetical system, the longer the filter has been established, the smaller the percentage of the population required to handle the daily additional waste input equivalent to feeding 10 million bacteria (see Fig. 72–2A).

Now consider a drug that will kill 50% of the bacteria in the filter bed with a single treatment. If the drug is applied to the bed when there are 4 million bacteria, only 2 million organisms will remain. This leaves a deficit of nitrogen fixation equivalent to the nitrogen required to feed 8 million organisms, which will cause deteriorating water quality. Had the drug not been added, the system would have reached equilibrium in 3 days (see Fig. 72–2A), but with the drug's impact, the time to equilibrium has been doubled to 6 days (see Fig. 72–2B), and during that time, fish are exposed to higher levels of

nitrogen wastes. On the other hand, if the drug is applied to the system after it has reached equilibrium, for example, when the bacterial population has reached 79 million (see Fig. 72–2C), equilibrium will be reachieved in less than 48 hours. The larger the bacterial population, the more rapid the recovery.

Antifungal Treatments

Primary fungal diseases are uncommon in freshwater tropical fishes. Examine the environmental conditions associated with outbreaks of these diseases carefully. Without remedying the underlying cause, therapy will not be successful. I am not aware of any kinetics studies of antifungal drugs in tropical fish, and the doses listed in the Appendix V are purely empirical. I eschew the popular dye malachite green because of its toxic and mutagenic potential (Fig. 72–3) (Meyer and Jorgenson, 1983; Alderman, 1985).

Antiprotozoan Treatments

The plethora of protozoan diseases that can plague fish is truly remarkable to a veterinarian grounded in mammalian medicine in a temperate climate. Fish are subject to every type of protozoan infection known, and most of these can remain in inapparent carrier states until stressful situations depress the host response, allowing uncontrolled proliferation of the parasites. Ciliated protozoa are frequently the cause of problems. The damage protozoa can inflict can be devastating. Identification of the offending organism is crucial to any attempt at therapy, and some knowledge of the pathogenesis and life-cycle involved is very important.

Successful therapeutic regimens against protozoa are scarce. Again, I eschew acriflavin and the majority of the chemical dyes, although other authors recommend them. I have not had good luck with quinine or other antimalarials as baths or orally administered. Other authors recommend these drugs as baths (Van Duijn, 1973). I rely heavily on saltwater baths, acetic acid dips, and formalin baths for freshwater species. Formalin baths must be used judiciously. Copper therapy is particularly unamenable to home treatments in freshwater systems, since it must be monitored very carefully and very low levels can be toxic. Oral medication with metronidazole seems to have considerable promise, and tetracycline or sulfa administration has been beneficial in cases that have not progressed too far. They seem to serve as excellent adjuncts to baths and dips.

Antitrematode Therapy

Freshwater tropical fishes are subject to parasitism by a variety of trematodes. The concept from mammalian medicine of trematodes having host spe-

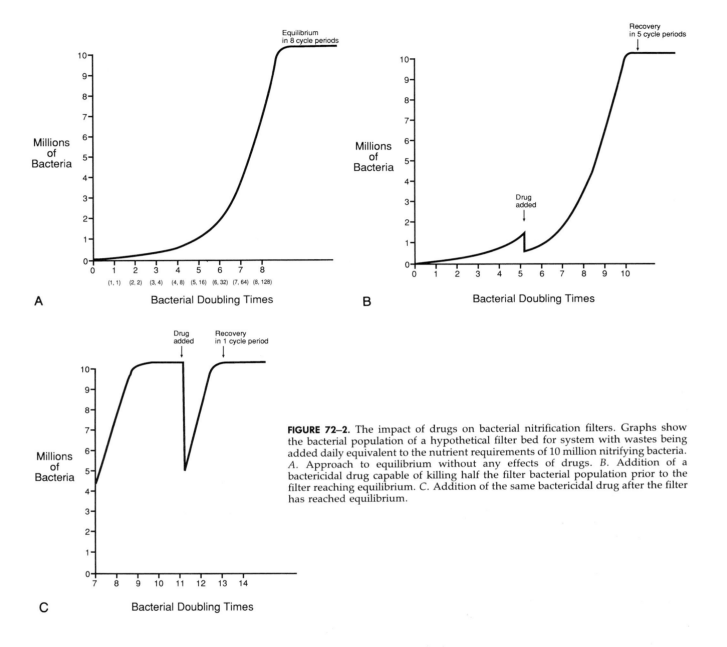

FIGURE 72–2. The impact of drugs on bacterial nitrification filters. Graphs show the bacterial population of a hypothetical filter bed for system with wastes being added daily equivalent to the nutrient requirements of 10 million nitrifying bacteria. *A.* Approach to equilibrium without any effects of drugs. *B.* Addition of a bactericidal drug capable of killing half the filter bacterial population prior to the filter reaching equilibrium. *C.* Addition of the same bactericidal drug after the filter has reached equilibrium.

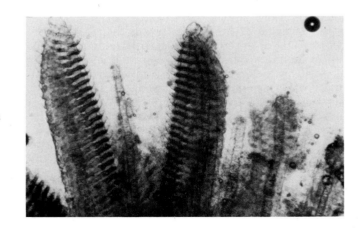

FIGURE 72–3. Gills of a clown loach damaged by treatment with malachite green. (Courtesy of R. Floyd.)

cies specificity may be misleading in fish medicine, but without careful speciation of the parasites we remove from these fishes, the question remains open. It is common for trematode blooms to affect more than one species of fish in a system. It is also common for some species of fish in the same tank to be unaffected.

Just as with protozoan infections, it is important to have some understanding of the life cycle of the trematode you are trying to eradicate. The difference between monogenetic (no intermediate host) and digenetic (obligate intermediate host) life cycles can have serious implications on the success of your therapeutic and eradication efforts.

To treat external or gill parasites in freshwater fishes, I rely on saltwater dips, formalin baths, acetic acid dips, or praziquantel baths. These seem effective at the dose given in Appendix V, but success has not been uniform. I treat internal trematode parasitisms with oral praziquantel. The dose in Appendix V is remarkably small and was originally taken from the literature (Schmahl and Mehlhorn, 1985). It may be reasonable to increase this dose as the treatment is not uniformly successful in treating body and gill flukes. I prefer to avoid trichlorfon because of its toxicity, but I have used it with success on occasion. Trichlorfon, also known under the trade name Masoten, should be handled and measured in a fume hood, wearing gloves. The dose is given for active ingredient, since preparations vary in the amount of binder used. I do not treat large established tanks with trichlorfon. Instead, I set up a treatment tank with minimal substrates. Lower doses may be necessary to treat fish in acidic environments, since the environmental breakdown of the drug is so much slower. After the treatment, the fish are removed and the water discarded after bringing the pH to 11 with sodium hydroxide.

Antinematode Treatments

Fish are affected by a wide variety of nematodes. Intestinal and gastric parasitism is the most common form encountered, but nematodes can also be found in the vascular system, gonads, swimbladder, or subcutaneous tissues. Treating these conditions in fishes is very similar to treating mammals. Oral administration of antihelminthics is the treatment of choice. The dose required to clear a nematode infestation depends heavily on the species of nematode as well as the drug. The response to therapy for many of these infestations appears to be excellent, but the clinician must be aware of the possibility of incomplete cures where female nematodes cease producing eggs for a time but are not killed. For example, levamisole used in prolonged (up to 6 hours) baths at concentrations up to 5 mg/L kills only about half of the load of swimbladder worms (*Anguillicola crassus*) and reduces egg production, but in 3 weeks, numbers of eggs and larvae begin to rise and reach pretreatment levels in about 7 weeks (Hartmann, 1989).

Anticestode Therapy

Cestodes use fish as both primary and intermediate hosts, similar to the situation with trematodes. Treatment of encysted forms is difficult and not well studied. Gastrointestinal forms can generally be controlled with therapy. Praziquantel appears to be efficacious.

Anticrustacean Therapy

For the most part, crustacean parasites are external parasites of fish. They are found on the body surface, in the mouth, or on the gills. There are, however, forms which can be found internally. These are usually described as oddities, having burrowed into any organ, including the heart. The therapies listed are primarily directed against external parasites. Occasionally one or two large copepods will be observed on a single fish. In such a case, anesthesia and manual removal of the parasites may be the treatment of choice. The bath treatments all have their various hazards referred to previously. The potential value of ivermectin in these cases requires further evaluation. There are obvious species differences, but many fish appear to develop neurologic signs before marked reductions in parasite loads occur. Diflubenzuron (Dimulin, Uniroyal) is a chitin-synthesis inhibitor that has been used in gypsy moth control. This compound has been used successfully to control anchorworm infestations and may possibly provide effective control of other crustacean parasites of freshwater tropical fishes. It has been used as a long-duration bath, and its effectiveness seems to vary significantly in different water systems. Motile naupulii are rapidly killed at 0.04 ppm levels, but adults are more resistant. The treatment must be repeated at least three times at approximately 4-week intervals to be effective.

Antihirudinean Therapy

Infestations of leeches can severely compromise affected freshwater fishes, but this is more frequently a problem in newly imported fish and usually larger species. Acetic acid dips are often effective (Van Roekel, 1929). More aggressive therapy can use Masoten baths. This is not a common problem.

EMERGENCY AND OTHER DRUGS

I have tried clinically, and found useful on an empirical basis, a number of drugs with various pharmacologic actions other than eradication of an infectious organism. Many of these drugs I have used only infrequently. These are listed along with their empirical doses in Appendix V.

LITERATURE CITED

Alderman, D.J. (1985) Malachite green: a review. J. Fish Dis. 8:289–298.

Amlacher, E. (1970) Textbook of Fish Disease. T.F.H. Publications, Neptune, New Jersey.

Bassleer, G. (1983) Wegwijs in Visziekten. Thieme & Cie, Zutphen, Netherlands.

Collins, M.T., Gratzek, J., Dawe, D., and Nemetz, T. (1976) Effects of antibacterial agents on nitrification in an aquatic recirculating system. J. Fish. Res. Bd. Can. 33:215–218.

Hartmann, F. (1989) Investigations on the effectiveness of Levamisol as a medication against the eel parasite *Anquillicola crassus* (Nematoda). Dis. Aquatic Organ. 7:185–190.

Herwig, N. (1979) Handbook of Drugs and Chemicals Used in the Treatment of Fish Diseases. Charles C Thomas, Springfield, Illinois.

Kuhns, J. (1981) FISHDRUG/TXT: a computer generated bibliographic index of the drugs and chemicals used in treating fish diseases. Aquariculture 2(1):4–18; 2(2):29–43; 2(3):45–58.

Levine, G., and Meade, T.L. (1976) The Effects of Disease Treatment on Nitrification in Closed System Aquaculture. Proceedings of the 7th. Annual Management of World Mariculture Society, pp. 483–493.

Meyer, F.P., and Jorgenson, T.A. (1983) Teratological and other effects of malachite green on development of rainbow trout and rabbits. Trans. Am. Fish. Soc. 112:818–824.

Nusbaum, K.E., and Shotts, E.B. (1981) Action of selected antibiotics on four common bacteria associated with disease of fish. J. Fish Dis. 4:397–484.

Reichenbach-Klinke, H.H. (1965) Fish Pathology (English translation). T.F.H. Publications, Neptune, New Jersey.

Schmahl, G., and Mehlhorn, H. (1985) Treatment of fish parasites. 1. Praziquantel effective against Monogenea (*Dactylogyrus vastator*, *Dactylogyrus extensus*, *Diplozoon paradoxum*). Z. Parasitenkunde 71:727–737.

Schnick, R.A., Meyer, F.P., and Gray, D.L. (1985) A Guide to Approved Chemicals in Fish Production and Fishery Resource Management. University of Arkansas and U.S. Fish and Wildlife Service.

Setser, M.D. (1985) Pharmacokinetics of gentamicin in channel catfish (*Ictalurus punctatus*). Am. J. Vet. Res. 46(12):2558–2561.

Snieszko, S.F., and Friddle, S.B. (1951) Tissue levels of various sulfonamides in trout. Trans. Am. Fish. Soc. 80:240–250.

Stoskopf, M.K. (1984) Antibiotic therapy for fish. Proc. Am. Assoc. Zoo Vet. 29–30.

Trust, T.J., and Chipman, D.C. (1974) Evaluation of aquarium antibiotic formulations. Antimicrob. Agents Chemother. 5(4):379–395.

Van Duijn, C. (1973) Diseases of Fishes. 3rd ed. Charles C Thomas, Springfield, Illinois.

Van Roekel, H. (1929) Acetic acid as a control agent for cyclochaeta and gyrodactylus in hatchery trout. Ca. Fish Game 15(3):230–233.

Watanabe, T., Aoki, T., Ogata, Y., and Egusa, S. (1971) R Factors related to fish culturing. Ann. N.Y. Acad. Sci. 182:383–410.

Willford, W.A. (1967) Toxicity of 22 therapeutic compounds to six fishes. Investigations in Fish Control, BSFW, FWS, U.S. Department of the Interior, Washington, D.C. No. 18., pp 1–10.

Wolf, K., and Snieszko, S.F. (1964) The use of antibiotics and other antimicrobials in therapy of diseases of fishes. Antimicrob. Agents Chemother. 3:597–603.

Wood, E.M., Yasutake, W.T., and Snieszko, S.F. (1957) Sulfonamide toxicity in brook trout. Trans. Am Fish Soc. 84:155–160.

SECTION VI

MARINE TROPICAL FISHES

MICHAEL K. STOSKOPF, *Section Editor*

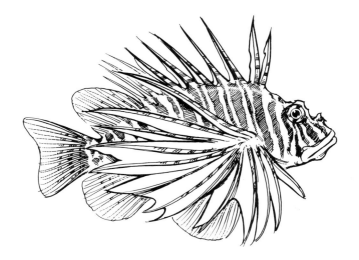

Chapter 73

Taxonomy and Natural History of Marine Tropical Fishes

MICHAEL K. STOSKOPF

The wide variety of marine tropical fishes can be extremely daunting. The strategies for survival on tropical reefs and other marine tropical environments are diverse and often extremely specialized. Only a limited number of these adaptations are suitable for captive conditions. Whole volumes are devoted to the natural history and taxonomy of individual families within this group, but even a cursory knowledge of the basic characteristics of the more commonly held families can help the clinician evaluate the potential health impact of ecologic adaptations or social and individual behaviors (Axelrod et al., 1981).

BASSLETS (GRAMMIDAE)

Several basslets are commonly kept by private aquarists. In large public facilities, they are most commonly displayed in smaller reef and invertebrate displays where their bright colors are better appreciated. The royal gramma, recently renamed the fairy basslet, is a Caribbean fish prized by aquarists (Fig. 73–1). It is easy to care for and peaceful, although it often hides by sitting upside down on the underside of an overhang or a floating piece of material. The fairy basslet grows to about 3 inches and is recognized by its brilliant purple head and cranial body, and bright yellow to yellow-orange caudal body. There is a black spot on the dorsal fin and the body colors do not continue on the fins to differentiate

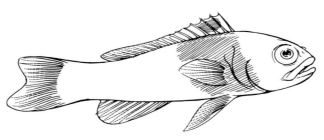

FIGURE 73–1. Fairy basslet.

this fish from the royal dottyback, an Indo-Pacific fish with different temperament.

The fairy basslet, like the swissguard basslet, another commonly kept fish, lives a life closely associated with coral. The swissguard basslet, also from the Caribbean, is horizontally striped with dark, centered, orange stripes, and has black tips fringed in light blue on the second dorsal, anal, and caudal fins. It grows to be a little over 3 inches. The swissguard tends to hide continually, although it can become quite tame over time and will come out of its hiding places in coral heads to feed.

BATFISHES (PLATACIDAE)

The batfishes are rapid-growing, delicate fish that do not do well in community tanks. The orbiculate batfish, from the Red Sea and Indo-Pacific, is prized by aquarists for its personality. They become quite tame. Orbiculate batfish must usually be kept alone to avoid having their fins bitten by tank mates, and they rapidly outgrow smaller tanks. Adults require at least 100 gals. In their native habitat, these fish school.

BLOWFISHES (TETRAODONTIDAE)

The blowfishes, or true puffers, are able to inflate themselves with air or water. They are better known for their toxicity when eaten than for their use as aquarium fish. They can have significant levels of tetrodotoxin, which is particularly concentrated in their ovary. They are deadly to eat unless every trace of the ovary is removed. Some taxonomists divide this family into four separate families, but recent work indicates that they are one family. Most blowfishes reach between 0.25 and 0.5 ms in length and are too large for home aquaria. They are shallow-water fish and are seen singly and in groups. There are two genera of freshwater blowfishes, one with a single species in the rivers of South America, and the other with a single African species and several Asian species. The blowfishes do not poison a tank as is popularly believed, but they can carry protozoan parasites and remain asymptomatic, making them a health risk in community tanks.

BUTTERFLYFISHES (CHAETODONTIDAE)

This is a large family of laterally compressed fishes (Fig. 73–2). The butterflyfishes do not get very large, and may have very specialized food requirements. Some may specialize on specific species of coral. The butterflyfishes are usually not aggressive, although they are usually left alone by other fishes.

ANGELFISHES (POMACANTHIDAE)

Angelfishes have heavier bodies and grow much larger than the butterflyfishes (Fig. 73–3). Marine angelfishes are significantly herbivorous, and need lots of vegetable matter in their diets. The gray angelfish, found from the West Indies to New Jersey, is frequently held by hobbyists as a juvenile, but adults are too large for most systems other than large public aquaria. The juvenile gray angel is almost identical to the juvenile French angel. The differences are relatively slight. Juvenile French angelfish have a median yellow band on the forehead that usually stops at the base of the upper lip, but this is not a reliable identification mark. Usually the juvenile French angelfish has more yellow on its face than a juvenile gray angelfish. More reliable is the difference in the shape of the black spot in the middle of the tail in these two species. In the French angelfish the spot is large and nearly round and occupies almost the entire tail. The juvenile gray angelfish has a yellow tail fin with a vertically elongated black spot in the middle. Adult gray angelfish are quite large and are light gray. French angelfish adults are dark gray with yellow edges on their scales. Both species are found on shallow reefs, near growths of sponges, which are part of their natural diets.

The emperor angelfish is a smaller angelfish that is popular in hobby aquaria. The young fish is dark blue with concentric white rings. Adults have 28 horizontal lines. These fish are found in pairs or as solitary fish, near caves or ledges. They make a distinct clicking sound when disturbed.

DAMSELFISHES (POMACENTRIDAE)

The Damselfish family also includes the very popular clownfishes. Damselfishes are hardy and brightly colored. They are indiscriminate eaters and territorial. They fight less when there are several of them rather than one or two. The clownfishes are also very popular with their commensal relationship to anemones (Fig. 73–4). The clownfishes have been commercially spawned in captivity, greatly reducing the pressure for wild fish in this popular family.

FILEFISHES (BALISTIDAE)

The filefishes resemble the triggerfishes, having a large dorsal spine (Fig. 73–5). They are often sold to hobbyists as small, 1-inch fish that are easily caught in schools in open waters in the Gulf Stream. Unfortunately they grow very large and can rapidly outgrow their aquaria. They are peaceful vegetarians that are very hardy and live for many years when provided with the proper environment. They have very abrasive skin, and need lots of vegetable matter in their diet.

FROGFISHES (ANTENNARIIDAE)

The frogfishes, sometimes called anglerfishes, are hardy and survive well in captivity, but unfortunately they also eat most anything they can reach, including each other (Fig. 73–6). They require live foods and are ravenous feeders. A small 3-inch specimen may eat 2 to 3 inches of food fish each day. There are nearly 60 different tropical species. Some can inflate their body to float among weeds near the water surface. These fish must be kept alone in a tank or they eat everything in the tank.

GOATFISHES (MULLIDAE)

The goatfishes are sometimes kept as small specimens in private aquaria but rapidly become too large for most hobby tanks (Fig. 73–7). They are more frequently seen in public aquaria and do well in large community tanks. These fish are somewhat nervous and tend to dig in bottom substrates. They feed on the bottom and have characteristic barbels on their chin that they rake through the bottom to find food. Goatfishes are peaceful fish, normally found in large schools working along sandy bottoms. They survive as individual specimens but seem to do better if maintained as a school.

GOBIES (GOBIDAE)

The most popular species of gobies kept in captivity are small thin fish that are generally peaceful (Fig. 73–8). There are a wide variety of gobies with differing body morphology. Many are bottom dwellers, although other species are found living in coral heads and small holes and crevices in rocks. Some, but not all, members of this family are cleaner fishes, setting up stations and eating the parasites on other fish. The neon goby and sharknose goby are two cleaner species. The neon goby has a brilliant light blue horizontal stripe the length of its body. It is a West Indian species frequently associated with

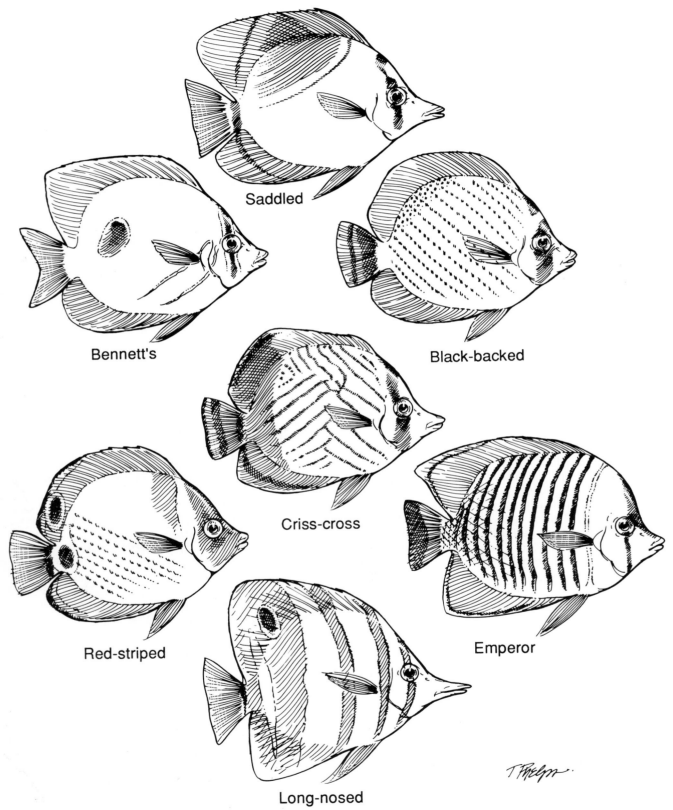

Saddled

Bennett's

Black-backed

Criss-cross

Red-striped

Emperor

Long-nosed

FIGURE 73–2. Butterflyfishes showing different color patterns.

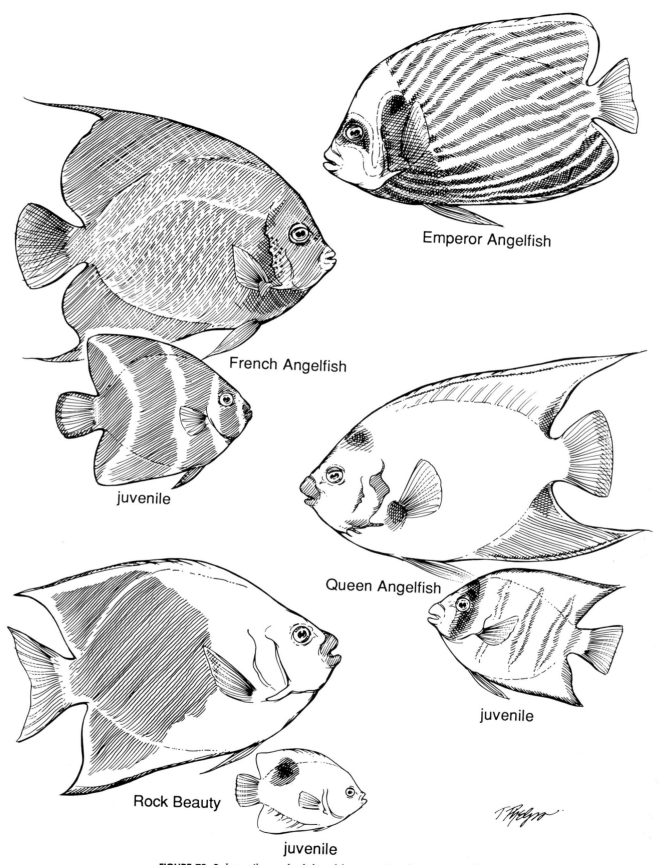

Emperor Angelfish

French Angelfish

juvenile

Queen Angelfish

juvenile

Rock Beauty

juvenile

FIGURE 73–3. Juveniles and adults of four species of marine angelfish.

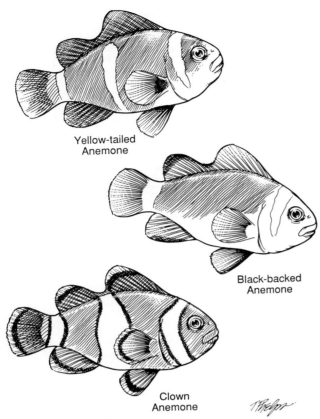

FIGURE 73—4. Three different clownfishes, commonly referred to as anemonefishes, can be differentiated by their color patterns.

Yellow-tailed
Anemone

Black-backed
Anemone

Clown
Anemone

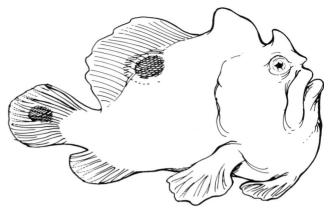

FIGURE 73—6. Frogfish.

red coral. The Catalina goby is bright orange and has five or six vertical blue stripes on the cranial half of its body. These fish are found off the coast of Catalina Island, offshore of Los Angeles, California. The water there is colder than that maintained in tropical aquaria, and the fish are found down to 100 m depth. Although they will survive in a warm-water aquarium, the practice is questionable. These are cleaner gobies.

GROUPERS (SERRANIDAE)

The groupers are large fish (Fig. 73–9). Some species become immense. They tend to hide in dark

holes and caves and are generally not good aquarium fish for hobby tanks. In large public display facilities, large individuals of the giant species are held to demonstrate the huge potential for growth in fishes. Groupers have relatively large mouths and take prey with a powerful and sudden oral suction. The red grouper, sometimes called the miniatus grouper, is a beautiful Indo-Pacific fish that is sometimes kept by hobbyists alone in their own large tank. They require live food to remain healthy and will eat anything up to half their own size. They are not active and spend most of their time hiding or laying on the bottom. They are nocturnal.

This group also includes the hamlets. The mutton hamlet is perhaps most commonly seen in private aquaria. It is a bright, red, western Atlantic species, although most specimens fade rapidly in captivity from poor management and inadequate carotenes in the diet. The mutton hamlet grows to nearly 10 inches and requires hiding places. The hamlets, like the groupers, can become pets and are very trainable. They will eat any fish small enough to swallow whole.

HAWKFISHES (CIRRHITIDAE)

This group of fishes is not very active and is found only occasionally in aquaria. The redspotted

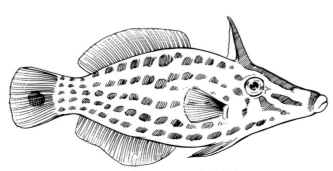

FIGURE 73—5. Orange spotted filefish.

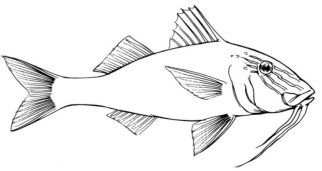

FIGURE 73—7. Yellow goatfish.

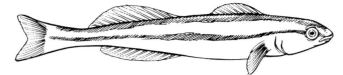

FIGURE 73–8. Neon goby.

hawkfish is a tropical Atlantic species that is not really a coral reef dweller (Fig. 73–10). It has broad vertical brown stripes on a white body and the head is speckled with small brilliant red dots. It grows to about 3.5 inches. In aquaria this hawkfish is hardy and stays close to the bottom, avoiding interaction with other fishes for the most part. They are sometimes called curlyfins.

Other hawkfish species are from the Indo-Pacific. Their name comes from the way they sit on coral heads or outcroppings and then swoop down on prey. These fish do better with coral ledges or rocks for perching. In the wild they eat small fish and crustaceans. The spotted hawkfish has blotchy spots, which more or less form into vertical bands. Their color varies with locality. In nature they are usually associated with red organ-pipe corals. The arch-eyed hawkfish is found in Hawaii and has a dark body with a white, horizontal stripe on the upper half of its body, from behind the head to the caudal peduncle. It gets its name from an orange arching line that loops behind its eye.

LIONFISHES, SCORPIONFISHES, OR ZEBRAFISHES (SCORPAENIDAE)

Despite the lacy, delicate appearance of the fins and striping of these fish, they are hardy predators, which catch their prey with venomous dorsal spines (Fig. 73–11). There are several species, all Indo-Pacific. The spotted lionfish and the turkeyfish are most commonly seen in captivity. They can be maintained in a community tank with other large fish if kept adequately fed. In nature they are nocturnal and tend to hide in the daytime in grottos and caves.

Their venom is a protein that can be denatured with heat. The severity of the sting varies with the species of the fish, as well as the sensitivity of the

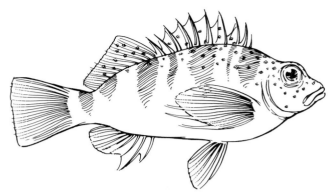

FIGURE 73–10. Redspotted hawkfish.

person stung. Although most stings by this fish are not life-threatening, merely excruciatingly painful, a physician should be consulted. Certainly precautions should always be taken to avoid direct contact with the venom spines in the fins of these fish.

The diet of these fishes in the wild consists mainly of crustaceans and some small fishes, although in captivity they are maintained primarily on a fish diet. They can be trained to take dead food. They would probably benefit from more shrimp and crab in their diet than is currently the common practice.

MOORISH IDOL (ZANCLIDAE)

The moorish idol is the only species in this family (Fig. 73–12). There were once thought to be two species, one with spines in front of the eye. Actually, these spines are found only in juvenile fish and are shed when the fish reaches maturity. The moorish idol is a delicate laterally compressed fish with a long trailing dorsal fin process. It is a difficult fish to keep, primarily because it is reluctant to feed. It is nevertheless very attractive to aquarists because of its dramatic body and fin shape and its coloration.

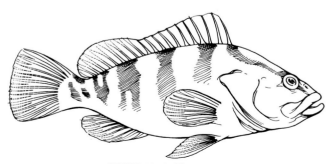

FIGURE 73–9. Nassau grouper.

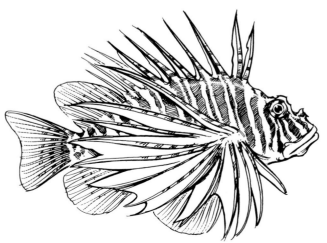

FIGURE 73–11. Lionfish.

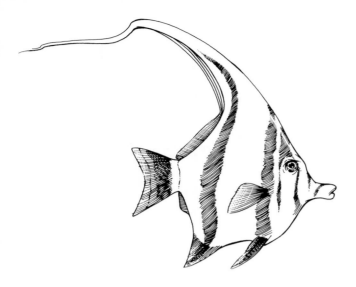

FIGURE 73–12. Moorish idol.

PARROTFISHES (SCARIDAE)

The parrotfishes are related to the wrasses but can be more territorial. These fish are adapted to eating bites of hard coral to extract the algae and coral for food. They can be kept in very large community tanks in commercial aquaria but generally grow too large for the private aquarist to maintain. These colorful reef dwellers have mouths that resemble the beaks of parrots. They have an interesting behavior of exuding a cocoon of mucus at night when they bed down in the reef. This large bubble of mucus completely surrounds the fish. It is thought that the bubble serves as an early-warning device, since if it is disturbed, the sleeping fish darts out and away from harm. The parrotfishes are difficult to maintain for prolonged periods in captivity. They tend to lose color and condition with time. Nutrition may be the limiting factor.

PORCUPINEFISHES (DIODONTIDAE)

The porcupinefishes, sometimes also called balloonfishes, have many erectile spines and may also release a poison when startled, which can affect fish in the same system. These fish frequent reefs, canals, and mangrove creeks. They prefer crustaceans, sea urchins, and mollusks to fish but will survive on fish diets. They become very tame and are not overly aggressive, but they can inflict a painful bite if provoked. Their normal response to harassment is to take in air or water and expand their body to erect their spines.

SEA HORSES AND PIPEFISHES (SYNGNATHIDAE)

Members of this family are sometimes mistaken for invertebrates because of their hard exoskeleton-like skin; however, they are true fishes. They are shy eaters and do not compete well with other fishes for food. They are usually best kept in a system where there is no food competition. The most common problem with these fishes is the inability of the aquarist to reliably deliver the required live foods throughout the year. The northern or Atlantic sea horse is a resident of cooler waters than those maintained in most private tanks (Fig. 73–13). They are voracious feeders and require large amounts of live food. They do not tolerate long periods of fasting well. Sea horses must be provided with thin branch-

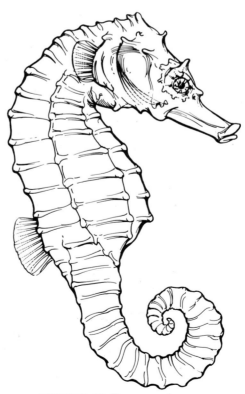

FIGURE 73–13. Pygmy sea horse.

ing tank furniture to which they can comfortably anchor themselves or they will become exhausted from constant swimming.

SHARPNOSE PUFFERS (CANTHIGASTERIDAE)

This family of fishes looks much like the trunkfishes, but without the hard body wall. They inflate themselves when disturbed. The common sharpnose puffer from Caribbean waters is found very commonly in hobby tanks. It is not very colorful but is easily maintained and entertaining. They normally feed on seagrass, sponges, crustaceans, and mollusks as well as sea urchins, starfish, hydroids, and algae. They grow to about 4.5 inches. Sharpnose puffers can inflict a painful bite with their hard, beaklike mouth. They also produce typical croaking sounds when removed from the water.

The Red Sea sharpnose puffer is not limited to the Red Sea and is also found in the Indo-Pacific. They have a pattern of lines and spots and are more colorful than the Caribbean species. They are also fairly common in aquaria. The Indo-Pacific sharpnose puffer is banded and as a young fish has round blue and orange dots on the sides. These fade normally as the fish matures. This puffer requires warmer waters (80°F) than the other sharpnose puffers and is a shallow-water fish.

SQUIRRELFISHES AND SOLDIERFISHES (HOLOCENTRIDAE)

The squirrelfishes are large-eyed nocturnal predatory species that tend to be easily startled (Fig. 73–14). They prefer to hide in crevices and small holes in the reef during the day. They must have this cover in an aquarium. They are voracious eaters, but feedings should be timed to accommodate their nocturnal ways. They will eat anything they can take in their mouths and are not safe with smaller fish. Although they are fairly hardy in captivity, they grow too large for home aquaria, and their nocturnal habits make them relatively difficult to enjoy. They are commonly displayed in public aquaria in large reef exhibits.

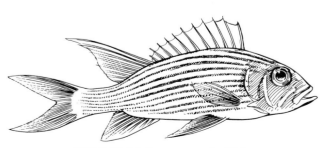

FIGURE 73–14. Common squirrelfish.

TANGS AND SURGEONS (ACANTHURIDAE)

The members of this family are primarily vegetarians (Fig. 73–15). They are peaceful fish but can become aggressive toward smaller fish in a small system. The yellow tang is perhaps the brightest colored member of the family. It is an Indo-Pacific fish that is commonly found in Hawaii. It thrives on green algal mats and is somewhat more delicate than some of the other tangs. The powder-blue surgeon is a popular aquarium species because it is so hardy. It is a voracious eater from the Indo-Pacific.

The striped surgeon, also from the Caribbean, is a popular aquarium fish. This species has three color phases. It begins life as a bright yellow fish with a barely noticeable blue edge on the dorsal fin. As it reaches about 8 months of age, blue rims appear prominently on the dorsal and anal fins. The yellow color begins to fade, until as an adult the only yellow is a striping on the fins. The body has a delicate striped pattern of blues.

The blue tang is another Caribbean species that is very similar to the striped surgeon. The body of the blue tang is rounder than that of the striped surgeon, and the yellow on the fins of the adult is solid rather than striped. Most easily identified, though, is the blue iris of the blue tang as opposed to the yellow-gold iris of the striped surgeon.

TRIGGERFISHES (BALISTIDAE)

The triggerfishes are aggressive, particularly as they get older. They have a large, hinged dorsal spine, which is referred to as the trigger, and very sharp teeth (Fig. 73–16). They can inflict a painful bite. They seem to delight in tearing up their tank and have been known to bite electric lines and be electrocuted.

The whitelined triggerfish, or humuhumu lei, is very common in aquaria. This abundant Hawaiian fish grows to 8 or 9 inches and becomes very tame in captivity. They require adequate shelter and hiding areas to thrive in captivity. The queen triggerfish, from the Caribbean, is perhaps a rival for the title of most common captive triggerfish. This fish is easily collected and relatively inexpensive. It is aggressive and can be dangerous, although they can be tamed. They usually attack other fishes in the tank and end up being kept alone. The clown triggerfish is a rarer fish, but it is kept in many public aquaria because of its spectacular color patterns.

TRUNKFISHES (OSTRACIIDAE)

This family includes the Australian spotted trunkfish, the spotted boxfish of the Indo-Pacific,

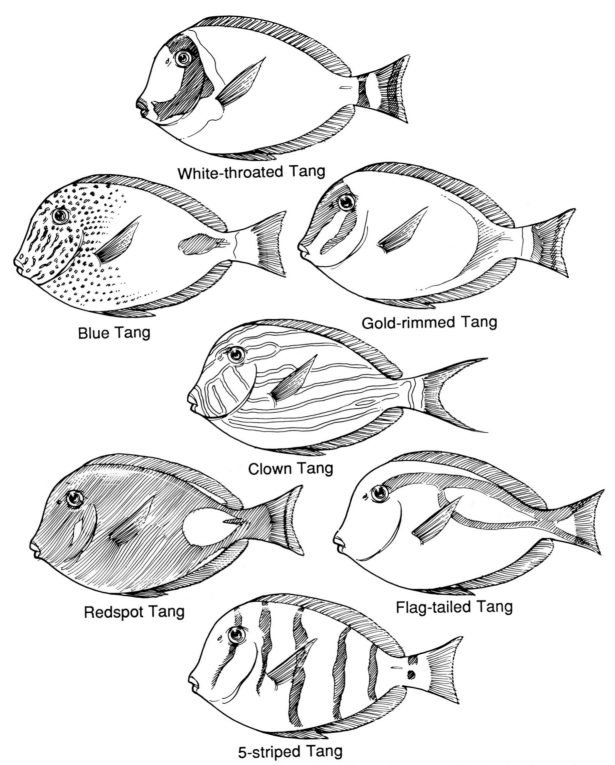

White-throated Tang

Blue Tang

Gold-rimmed Tang

Clown Tang

Redspot Tang

Flag-tailed Tang

5-striped Tang

FIGURE 73–15. Many tangs have similar body configurations but widely differing color patterns. The five-striped tang, also commonly called the convict tang, has a narrower face and more pronounced dorsal fin than shown.

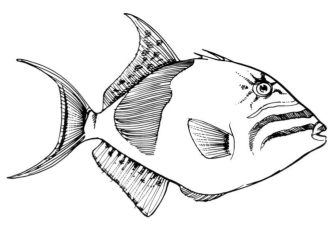

FIGURE 73–16. Clown triggerfish.

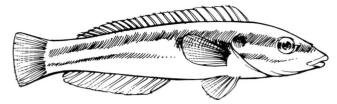

FIGURE 73–18. Rainbow wrasse.

WRASSES (LABRIDAE)

The wrasses are a diverse and large group of long thin fish that have unusual reproductive strategies (Fig. 73–18). Many burrow into the sand and require this substrate to survive in aquaria. Some wrasses are considered cleaner wrasses and are accepted by other fish when they feed on ectoparasites. Some species of wrasses grow quite large and are not suitable in aquaria as adults. The dottybacks mentioned above under the basslets are wrasses. Many species are shy and tend to hide much of the time. Many other species of wrasses can be quite aggressive.

COMPATIBILITY

The commonly maintained marine tropical fishes have been divided into groups based upon behavioral attributes that have major impacts on their ability to get along with other fishes (Kingsford, 1979). Of

and the Caribbean cowfish and spotted trunkfish. Members have a very hard exoskeleton of bony plates under the dermis. They have very angular bodies and are slow swimmers. Little is known about their habits in the wild. They are very unique and interesting fish, and hobby aquarists are drawn to their strange appearance. These fish may release toxins into the tank when they are startled or stressed and poison other fish.

The spotted boxfish has been well studied in regard to the release of toxins (Thompson, 1964) (Fig. 73–17). When startled, the fish releases large amounts of foamy mucus from the folds of skin at the junction of the trunk and the caudal peduncle, and at the base of the fins and from their mouths. This mucus is toxic when injected into fish or mice or when eaten by humans. The signs of intoxication in other fish exposed to the toxin in the water include irritability followed by gasping, then stupor with a decreased respiratory rate. This is followed by a loss of equilibrium and locomotor control, and finally convulsions and death. The toxin is water-soluble, heat-stable, and acid- and alkali-resistant, but it is detoxified with exposure to strong bases, including potassium hydroxide. The toxin is found only in live animals and is toxic to the spotted boxfish itself if injected.

TABLE 73–1. Compatibility Groupings for Marine Tropical Fishes Based on Feeding Behavior

Rapid Eaters	Slow Eaters
Angelfishes	Anemonefishes
Damselfishes	Basslets
Groupers	Blennies
Squirrelfishes	Cardinalfishes
Triggerfishes	Catfishes
	Croakers
Gluttons	Filefishes
Grunts	Goatfishes
Snappers	Moonfishes
	Parrotfishes
Cannot Compete Well for Food	Scats
Except with Conspecifics	Trunkfishes
Sea Horses	Wrasses
Pipefishes	Butterflyfishes
Jawfishes	Hawkfishes
Mandarins	Porcupinefishes
Psychedelic fish	Puffers
Razorfishes	Rabbitfishes
Sweetlips	Surgeonfishes
Moorish idol	Eels
Batfishes	Gobies
	Squirrelfishes

Modified from Kingsford, E. (1979) Marine Aquarium Compatibility Guide. Palmetto Publishing Company, St. Petersburg, Florida.

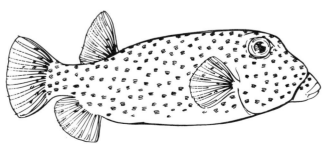

FIGURE 73–17. Spotted boxfish.

TABLE 73–2. Compatibility Groupings for Marine Tropical Fishes Based on Territoriality

Not Territorial	Tolerate Other Species of Same Group	Territorial
Blennies	Anemonefishes	Damselfishes
Cardinalfishes	Basslets	Groupers
Catfishes	Butterflyfishes	
Croakers	Hawkfishes	**Very Aggressive**
Filefishes	Eels	Angelfishes
Goatfishes	Gobies	Triggerfishes
Moonfishes		
Parrotfishes		**Cannibals, Eat Anything Smaller Than Themselves**
Scats		Anglerfishes
Squirrelfishes		Frogfishes
Trunkfishes		Scorpionfishes
Wrasses		

Modified from Kingsford, E. (1979) Marine Aquarium Compatibility Guide. Palmetto Publishing Company, St. Petersburg, Florida.

course, individual variations occur, and compatibility is a complex issue affected by the size of the system, the mix of the fishes in the system, and even the order in which they are introduced into the system. Nevertheless, it is useful to have some idea of the behavioral traits of the various marine tropical fishes. The modification of the groupings developed by Kingsford presented in Table 73–1 and Table 73–2 can be used to evaluate potential incompatibilities that may underlie clinical problems.

LITERATURE CITED

Axelrod, H.R., Burgess, W.E., and Emmens, C.W. (1981) Exotic Marine Fishes, Looseleaf Edition. T.F.H. Publications, Neptune, New Jersey.

Kingsford, E. (1979) Marine Aquarium Compatibility Guide. Palmetto Publishing Company, St. Petersburg, Florida.

Thompson, D.A. (1964) Ostracitoxin: an ichthyotoxic stress secretion of the boxfish, *Ostracion lentiginosus.* Science 146:244–245.

Chapter 74

CLINICAL PATHOLOGY OF MARINE TROPICAL FISHES

MICHAEL K. STOSKOPF

HEMATOLOGY

The lack of standard methods and the survey approach to fish hematology has resulted in little baseline information of value for clinicians interested in the diagnosis of diseases. This is particularly true for the marine tropical species. There remains a vast void for the eager hematologist to fill, that of developing a foundation for the clinical evaluation of blood and serum in these fishes. I have found no well-controlled studies of the effect of specific diseases or toxicoses on the hematology or serology of these fishes. At this point, the clinician will have to make do with a compilation of impressions from survey projects.

Certainly, the relatively small size of many of the marine tropicals held in home aquaria makes hematologic and serologic assessment difficult. This is complicated by a tendency for the blood from many of the popular display species to clot readily. It is imperative to use an anticoagulant-coated syringe and needle for sampling the parrotfishes and butterflyfishes. Coating the needle with anticoagulant may not be necessary in the large angelfishes, the squirrelfishes, and the soldierfishes. Also, it is extremely common for fragile erythrocytes to rupture in the process of sample collection and preparation. This complicates the interpretation of the blood smear for the differential leukocyte count and makes a total erythrocyte count very difficult to assess.

The use of bovine serum albumin to stabilize the erythrocyte membrane in the preparation of a differential slide has been a large boon to clinicians interested in these fish. The techniques described in the

TABLE 74–1. Serum Protein Values in Marine Tropical Fishes

Species	N	Total Protein	Albumin	Globulin
French grunt	3	3.2 ± 0.2	0.7 ± 0.3	2.3 ± 0.1
Blue tang	5	2.9 ± 0.7	0.6 ± 0.2	2.3 ± 0.6

general chapter on clinical pathology (Chap. 9) work very well to eliminate the large numbers of "smudge cells" that normally plague these samples.

The dimensions of the erythrocytes vary widely in the diverse species that make up this group. They are quite large in the moray eels and are quite small in the hogfish and wrasses. The general rule that slower moving, more sedentary fish tend to have larger erythrocytes (Dawson, 1933) tends to hold true to an extent for this broad group (Saunders, 1966), but it is certainly an oversimplification. For example, members of the butterfly group tend to have large erythrocytes.

Another complication to evaluating the erythrocyte indices is the apparent increase in the red blood cell count that accompanies exposure to low oxygen levels. A relatively rapid response to hypoxia (less than 1 hour), puts a large number of immature erythrocytes into circulation. Hemogregarine infection has been associated with elevated erythrocyte counts in a wild schoolmaster (Saunders, 1966).

The hematocrit of marine tropical fishes that are failing to adapt to captivity is quite frequently lower than that of animals caught in the wild or well adapted to their captive situation. This may be because they fail to compete for food, or it may have a more complex mechanism. Hemoglobin values almost invariably follow the hematocrit, which is a good index of the erythrocyte count. The total protein will also be low in these fish (Table 74–1).

Total leukocyte counts in marine tropical fishes are apparently responsive to all of the same influences that affect the counts in terrestrial mammals. Unfortunately, there is little available in the way of baseline values, and the variation between species is considerable (Table 74–2). Total leukocyte counts of wild redband parrotfish range between 3500 and 12,000 cells/mm³ of blood, whereas wild four-eyed butterflyfish have normal baseline counts of between 12,000 and 20,000 cells/mm³.

The lymphocyte is the most common leukocyte in the blood of most reef fishes (Table 74–3). The vast majority are small mature lymphocytes in healthy fish. Occasionally, large immature lympho-

cytes are seen. It is important to distinguish the small lymphocyte from the thrombocyte in most reef species. Usually, the nuclear chromatin of the lymphocyte is less dense than that of the thrombocyte. In many species, particularly the parrotfishes, the mature thrombocytes have distinct terminal processes, but younger thrombocytes can be quite rounded, and, occasionally, small lymphocytes will extend pseudopods that can be mistaken for terminal processes. The differentiation between thrombocytes and small lymphocytes is very important if an interpretable hemogram is to be obtained.

Monocytes occur in reef fishes, but may be misinterpreted as large lymphocytes. There is considerable disagreement about the nomenclature of the monocyte. Some workers refer to circulating macrophages (Klontz, 1972), and the main survey of marine reef fishes uses the term *hemoblast* (Saunders, 1966), but in order to maintain compatibility with hematologic nomenclature used in all other vertebrates, the term *monocyte* is preferable. Any evidence of phagocytosis should be considered a marker for a monocyte. Fish monocytes are histochemically similar to mammalian monocytes, and often contain fine cytoplasmic granules that are PAS- and acid phosphatase–positive. They are present in small numbers in many reef fish species.

Other mononuclear leukocyte types can be identified in marine tropical fishes. These include occasional plasma cells, which display the typical eccentric nucleus with a distinct light-staining halo in the cytoplasm. These cells are usually counted with the lymphocytes. Another cell type, the "ring cell," has been described in the balloonfishes (Saunders, 1966). This unusual cell has a distinctly peripheral, dark, flattened nucleus, and appears to contain a round mass that stains deep pink with no granules. There is some question whether this cell should be considered a variant of granulocytic cells, but no intermediate forms of the cell have been identified to assist in identifying the lineage of the cell.

Heterophils are not a predominant cell in reef-dwelling species. With the exception of the moray eels and some damselfishes, they make up a third or less of the total leukocyte count. The nucleus of the heterophil may be slightly indented or highly segmented with typical lobed morphology. They are distinguished by their lightly staining granules, which obscure much of the nucleus. It is common to observe degranulated granulocytes that must be recognized by their nuclear morphology.

Eosinophilic granulocytes are present in low

TABLE 74–2. Total Leukocyte Counts and Erythrocyte Parameters of Marine Tropical Fishes

Species	N	Total Leukocyte	Total Erythrocyte	Hematocrit	Hemoglobin	Total Protein
French grunt	8	9006 ± 3259	3.59 ± 0.39	37.1 ± 6.2	10.7 ± 1.6	3.2 ± 0.2
Blue tang	8	13,100 ± 6355	2.84 ± 0.52	35.0 ± 11.5	8.2 ± 1.5	2.9 ± 0.7
Four-eyed butterflyfish	5	16,400 ± 3150	2.53 ± 1.0			
Redband parrotfish	10	7,095 ± 4384	1.63 ± 0.48			

TABLE 74–3. Differential Leukocyte Counts in Marine Tropical Fishes

Species	N	Percent				
		Heterophil	Lymphocyte	Monocyte	Eosinophil	Basophil
Family Acanthuridae						
Blue tang	10	22	76	2	0	0
Family Balistidae						
Tail-light filefish	10	31	59	9	0	0
Family Carangidae						
Horse-eye jack	5	23	69	7	1	0
Family Chaetodontidae						
Queen angelfish	10	26	60	13	1	0
Rock beauty	10	34	64	2	0	0
Banded butterflyfish	10	27	60	5	8	0
Four-eyed butterflyfish	10	18	51	27	4	0
Family Elopidae						
Ladyfish	3	12	73	3	12	0
Family Ephippidae						
Glassy sweeper	6	16	81	3	0	0
Family Holocentridae						
Blackbar soldierfish	10	19	51	5	25	0
Common squirrelfish	10	18	57	13	3	9
Longjaw squirrelfish	10	23	58	10	1	8
Family Labridae						
Bluehead wrasse	5	20	77	3	0	0
Family Lutjanidae						
Schoolmaster	10	19	76	5	0	0
Lane snapper	10	20	72	8	0	0
Yellow snapper	10	10	79	7	4	0
Family Muraenidae						
Green moray eel	2	10	85	0	4	0
Purple mouth moray eel	3	49	49	2	0	0
Family Pomadasyidae						
Blue striped grunt	10	13	77	8	2	0
French grunt	10	7	77	15	1	0
Tomtate	10	14	79	5	1	0
Family Pomcentridae						
Beau gregory	10	10	87	3	0	0
Atlantic yellowtail damsel	10	46	49	5	0	0
Sargent major	10	28	66	5	0	0
Family Scaridae						
Princess parrotfish	10	34	63	2	1	0
Rainbow parrotfish	10	13	76	9	2	0
Redtail parrotfish	10	18	72	8	2	0
Stoplight parrotfish	10	16	69	12	3	0
Striped parrotfish	10	10	84	5	1	0
Family Scombridae						
Wahoo	5	12	86	1	1	0
Family Serranidae						
Graysby	10	30	66	2	1	0
Red hind	10	19	67	7	7	0
Family Sparidae						
Jolthead porgy	10	8	84	1	7	0
Sea bream	10	7	70	11	12	0
Family Sphyraenidae						
Barracuda	10	8	84	8	0	0

Adapted from Saunders, D.C. (1966) Differential blood cell counts of 121 species of marine fishes of Puerto Rico. Trans. Am. Microsc. Soc. 85(3):427–449.

TABLE 74–4. Serum Electrolyte Values in Marine Tropical Fishes

Species	N	Na	Cl	K	Ca	PO₄
French grunt	5	191 ± 1.4	148.9 ± 2.8	2.8 ± 0.5	11.7 ± 0.5	4.8 ± 0.4
Blue tang	7	224 ± 28.1	166.4 ± 18.9	2.9 ± 1.0	14.0 ± 1.7	10.9 ± 3.4

numbers in most reef fishes. They are roughly the same size as the heterophilic granulocytes of a given species. The nucleus of the eosinophil is usually less lobated than that of the heterophil. The eosinophilic granules are round and fairly large. They stain bright red with Romanovsky stains.

Basophilic granulocytes occur infrequently in most reef species. They have been reported in significant numbers in wild squirrelfishes (Saunders, 1966), but this does not seem to be a consistent feature with captive animals. They are easily recognized by their round, dark staining, cytoplasmic granules, which may or may not obscure the nucleus of the cell. Often basophils of marine tropical fishes will contain only a few, large, cytoplasmic granules.

SERUM CHEMISTRY

Marine reef fishes drink seawater and must, therefore, eliminate a large salt burden. Sodium and chloride are excreted by the chloride cells of the gills. Elevated serum sodium and chloride levels (Table 74–4) are often indicative of gill disease. Another indication of gill disease would be rising serum uric acid levels (Table 74–5), since uric acid is excreted primarily by the gills.

Magnesium and sulfate are also accumulated by drinking salt water. These ions are eliminated by the kidney of marine tropical fishes. Increased serum levels of magnesium and sulfate are indicative of kidney disease. Unfortunately, most commercial laboratories do not assay these ions routinely. Serum magnesium levels generally run around 9 mEq/L or less (Stoskopf, 1987). Baseline levels for serum sulfate in marine tropical fishes are not available. Rising

TABLE 74–5. Serum Nitrogen Parameters in Marine Tropical Fishes

Species	N	BUN	Creatinine	Uric Acid
French grunt	7	7.0 ± 1.7	0.2 ± 0.1	0.5 ± 0.3
Blue tang	8	9.0 ± 4.2	1.9 ± 1.2	1.3 ± 1.1

TABLE 74–6. Serum Enzymes and Liver Indices in Marine Tropical Fishes

Species	N	AST	ALT	Total Bilirubin
French grunt	4	30.0 ± 4.6	2.5 ± 1.5	0.00 ± 0.0
Blue tang	6	19.2 ± 13.9	5.5 ± 1.4	0.08 ± 0.07

serum creatinine levels are also indicative of renal problems. Creatinine is excreted unchanged by the kidney and serum levels are normally in the range of 0.5 to 2.0 mg/dl (Stoskopf, 1988).

Most urea in fish is produced by the liver, but its major route of excretion is the gills. An elevated BUN is indicative of gill disease, not kidney dysfunction. A falling BUN is indicative of starvation, among other conditions (Stoskopf, 1987).

Ammonia is the main excretory product of marine tropical reef fishes. It is excreted by the gills through passive diffusion and in exchange for sodium. Serum ammonia concentrations increase after feeding; however, excretion remains relatively constant. This results in serum ammonia spikes approximately 4 hours after feeding. Serum ammonia spikes are also seen after rapid swimming episodes. This variability because of normal activity makes serum ammonia a poor diagnostic tool. Levels in fasted, calm fish are between 0.3 and 5.5 mg/dl.

LITERATURE CITED

Dawson, A.B. (1933) The relative numbers of immature erythrocytes in the circulating blood of several species of marine fishes. Biol. Bull. 64:33–43.

Klontz, G.W. (1972) Haematological techniques and immune response in rainbow trout. In: Diseases of Fish. (Mawdesley-Thomas, L.E., ed.) Symposium of the Zoological Society of London, No. 30. Academic Press, New York, pp 89–99.

Saunders, D.C. (1966) Differential blood cell counts of 121 species of marine fishes of Puerto Rico. Trans. Am. Microsc. Soc. 85(3):427–449.

Stoskopf, M.K. (1987) Basic physiology. In: Workshop on Marine Tropical Fish. (Stoskopf, M.K., and Citino, S., eds.) Aquatic Diagnostic Press, Baltimore, Maryland, pp. 13–19.

Stoskopf, M.K. (1988) Avian and piscean hematology and serology. Proceedings of the Fifth Annual Veterinary Medical Forum. Am. Coll. Vet. Intern. Med. 5:608–611.

Chapter 75

Environmental Requirements of Marine Tropical Fishes

MICHAEL K. STOSKOPF

Seawater systems used to maintain marine tropical fishes are of two basic types, those that use natural seawater and those that use artificial salt mixtures. Each has advantages and disadvantages. Source information is important in both systems, but possibly more so in those systems using natural seawater.

NATURAL SEAWATER

Natural seawater systems usually take water from either a subsand or a direct water intake. Subsand abstraction takes the water from deep wells in beach sand, after it has been filtered through large depths of sand. This has the advantage of filtering out almost all living organisms before the water enters the intake pipes, reducing the incidence of fouling and clogging. The water is essentially sterile. It is also devoid of oxygen and frequently quite cold (depending on locale). It is necessary to aerate this water and in many cases to heat it before use. It is not generally necessary to treat it in other ways if the sand bed is good.

Water taken directly from the sea does carry all of the life to be found in the sea of source. This has the obvious disadvantage of allowing fouling of intake pipes and all of the concomitant maintenance involved. It also allows the system to supply microscopic foods that are not otherwise readily available for invertebrates and certain types of small fish. This type of water must usually be subjected to settling and possibly additional filtration before use.

ARTIFICIAL SEAWATER

Artificial seawater systems are becoming more common as aquaria are built in areas with marginal or no seawater availability. Artificial seawater is usually produced by using city drinking water. This water is pretreated to remove disinfectants such as chlorine, chloramines, or bromine added by city water departments to ensure low bacteria counts in drinking water. Water-treatment plants also occasionally add copper to reduce algal growth in reservoirs or processing systems. These additions can result in copper levels that would be toxic to invertebrates, and even fish, if allowed to go into the final water make-up for a marine system. To remove these additives, water for use in an aquarium system is usually preprocessed through large filters charged with activated charcoal. The media in these filters must be monitored and changed on a regular basis before they begin to leak toxic chemicals. Disposal of the spent exchange media should also be considered carefully, as it can contain high levels of metals and organic toxicants accumulated from the trace amounts in the drinking water. The reader is also referred to the chapter on freshwater tropical fish environmental requirements for a discussion of other precautions that may affect water quality in smaller home systems (Chap. 65). The bulk of these concerns are also valid for marine water make-up.

To make artificial seawater, pretreated fresh water is then mixed with a variety of salts (Table 75–1). This can be done on the basis of a recipe, or more commonly the premixed salts are purchased from commercial firms that produce them for aquaria. It is important to realize that quality control is important regardless of the source of salts. Commercial salt mixes may or may not be adequate, depending upon the application. They tend to be low in expensive trace ions such as gold and are also usually low in calcium and somewhat high in sodium, iron, and magnesium (Table 75–2).

Water Additives

A number of water additives are available for artificial seawater systems. Several brands of trace element additives are marketed on the basis of replacing elements that are depleted through metabolic processes of the animals and plants living in the tank. These are probably not needed if adequate

TABLE 75–1. Average Ionic Composition of Seawater

Element	Molar	μg/L	Element	Molar	μg/L
H	55	1.1×10^8	Cd	1×10^{-9}	1×10^{-1}
O	55	8.8×10^8	Co	8×10^{-10}	5×10^{-2}
Cl	5.46×10^{-1}	18.8×10^6	Ge	6.9×10^{-10}	5×10^{-2}
Na	4.68×10^{-1}	10.77×10^6	Be	6.3×10^{-10}	5.6×10^{-3}
Mg	5.32×10^{-2}	12.9×10^5	W	5×10^{-10}	1×10^{-1}
S	2.82×10^{-2}	9.05×10^5	Ga	4.3×10^{-10}	3×10^{-2}
N	1.07×10^{-2}	1.5×10^5	Ag	4×10^{-10}	4×10^{-2}
Ca	1.02×10^{-2}	4.12×10^5	Xe	3.8×10^{-10}	5×10^{-2}
K	1.02×10^{-2}	3.8×10^5	Zr	3.3×10^{-10}	3×10^{-2}
C	2.3×10^{-3}	2.8×10^4	Pb	2×10^{-10}	3×10^{-2}
Br	8.4×10^{-4}	6.7×10^4	Hg	1.5×10^{-10}	3×10^{-2}
B	4.1×10^{-4}	4.44×10^3	Bi	1×10^{-10}	2×10^{-2}
Sr	9.1×10^{-5}	8×10^4	Ce	1×10^{-10}	1×10^{-3}
Si	7.1×10^{-5}	2×10^6	Nb	1×10^{-10}	1×10^{-2}
F	6.8×10^{-5}	1.3×10^3	Sn	8.4×10^{-11}	1×10^{-2}
Li	2.6×10^{-5}	1.8×10^2	Tl	5×10^{-11}	1×10^{-2}
P	2×10^{-6}	60	Hf	4×10^{-11}	7×10^{-3}
Rb	1.4×10^{-6}	1.2×10^2	Th	4×10^{-11}	1×10^{-2}
I	5×10^{-7}	60	Au	2×10^{-11}	4×10^{-3}
Ba	1.5×10^{-7}	2	La	2×10^{-11}	3×10^{-3}
Ar	1.1×10^{-7}	4.3	Re	2×10^{-11}	4×10^{-3}
Mo	1×10^{-7}	10	Nd	1.9×10^{-11}	3×10^{-3}
Zn	7.6×10^{-8}	4.9	Y	1.5×10^{-11}	1.3×10^{-3}
Al	7.4×10^{-8}	2	Sc	1.3×10^{-11}	6×10^{-4}
As	5×10^{-8}	3.7	Ta	1×10^{-11}	2×10^{-3}
V	5×10^{-8}	2.5	Dy	6×10^{-12}	9×10^{-4}
Fe	3.5×10^{-8}	2	Yb	5×10^{-12}	8×10^{-4}
Ni	2.8×10^{-8}	1.7	Er	4×10^{-12}	8×10^{-4}
Ti	2.0×10^{-8}	1	Gd	4×10^{-12}	7×10^{-4}
U	1.4×10^{-8}	3.2	Pr	4×10^{-12}	6×10^{-4}
Cu	8×10^{-9}	5×10^{-1}	Sm	3×10^{-12}	5×10^{-4}
Ne	7×10^{-9}	1.2×10^{-1}	Ho	1×10^{-12}	2×10^{-4}
Cr	5.7×10^{-9}	3×10^{-1}	Eu	9×10^{-13}	1×10^{-5}
Mn	3.6×10^{-9}	2×10^{-1}	Lu	9×10^{-13}	2×10^{-4}
Cs	3×10^{-9}	4×10^{-1}	Tb	9×10^{-13}	1×10^{-5}
Se	2.5×10^{-9}	2×10^{-1}	In	8×10^{-13}	1×10^{-4}
Kr	2.4×10^{-9}	2×10^{-1}	Tm	8×10^{-13}	2×10^{-4}
Sb	2×10^{-9}	2.4×10^{-1}	Ra	3×10^{-16}	7×10^{-8}
He	1.7×10^{-9}	6.8×10^{-3}	Pa	2×10^{-16}	5×10^{-8}
Unknown: Pm, Po, Ac, Fr, Pt, Ir, Os, Tc, Ru, Rh, Pd, Te			Rn	2.7×10^{-21}	6×10^{-13}

Adapted from Spotte, S. (1979) Seawater Aquariums: The Captive Environment. John Wiley & Sons, New York. Copyright © 1979, John Wiley & Sons, Inc. Reprinted by permission of John Wiley & Sons, Inc.

TABLE 75–2. Natural Levels of Dissolved Metals in Seawater

Metal	Concentration (μg/L [ppb])
Ag	0.3
Al	3.0
As	3.0
Cd	0.03
Co	0.5
Cr	0.05
Cu	2.0
Fe	10.0
Hg	0.03
Mn	2.0
Mo	10.0
Ni	2.0
Pb	0.03
Sb	0.3
Se	4.0
Sn	3.0
V	2.0
Zn	10.0

After Johnston (1977) Marine Pollution. Academic Press, New York.

water changes are made; however, foam fractionators will preferentially remove iron, manganese, and vitamins in addition to proteins (Thiel, 1989a), and compensation may be needed if this filtration technology is employed. It is particularly important to avoid oversupplementation with trace element mixes. Many of these elements can build up to toxic levels very easily. In addition to trace elements, some products market the addition of vitamins, particularly vitamin B_{12} and biotin to marine salt mixes. The effectiveness of this is very questionable. Certainly, if ozonation is used as a water disinfection process, all of the added vitamins will be destroyed. Also on the market are "fertilizers" that are marketed to assist in the maintenance of macroalgae, which many hobbyists find very attractive. The use of these products is questionable. Those that supply manganese, iron, and other trace elements may be acceptable, but under no circumstances should products that contain nitrates or phosphates be added to a tank. Also iron levels should be maintained in the range of 0.05 to 0.1 ppm (Thiel, 1989a).

TABLE 75–3. Maintenance Ranges for Marine Aquaria

Parameter	Range
Ammonia	0.0–0.05 ppm
Calcium Hardness	60–80 ppm
Carbonate Hardness	5.35–6.54 mEq/L
	15–18 dKH (German)
Conductivity	51,000–53,000 microsiemens
Copper (routine)	0.00–0.05 ppm
(therapy)*	0.13–0.20 ppm
Iron	0.1–0.5 ppm
Nitrate	Up to 20.0 ppm
Nitrite	00.0–0.1 ppm
Oxygen, Dissolved	5.5 to Saturation
	Prefer over 7 mg/L
pH	7.9–8.4
Phosphate	0.1–0.2 ppm total PO_4
Redox Potential	350–390 mv
Salinity	27.5–32 ppt
Specific Gravity	1.022–1.025
Temperature	23–26° C
	74–79° F

Therapeutic value only on prescribed basis in tanks under treatment. Otherwise the copper levels should be less than 0.05 ppm.

MONITORING WATER

Water monitoring in marine systems is as vital a component of maintaining healthy fish as it is in freshwater systems (Table 75–3). The degree of monitoring any system, and particularly a marine system, is dictated by economic reality, since it can become quite labor-intensive and involved. No matter how many water tests are run, they are of no value unless they are interpreted and integrated to assist in a water-management plan. This is vital whether the system is a closed system that continually recycles the same water, or a flow-through system obtaining fresh seawater on a continuous basis.

Temperature

No matter how restricted the budget, there are some parameters that should be taken and used to aid in the management of the health of the system. Water temperature requires only a simple thermometer and little technical expertise to achieve repeatable readings. Temperature fluctuations in marine systems can be very important in predicting the timing of disease outbreaks due to protozoans, as well as viral and bacterial disease epidemics. Small fluctuations in temperature in either direction can be enough additional physiologic stress on fish maintained in otherwise marginal conditions to precipitate disease outbreaks a few days after the insult. Temperature can also provide keys to activity levels, feeding intensities, and other signs important in fish diagnostics. For tropical species, a stable temperature of 75 to 76°F is a good goal.

Salinity and Specific Gravity

Specific gravity, sometimes improperly referred to as salinity, is another easily obtained parameter important to the proper management of a marine system. Specific gravity refers to the ratio of the density of seawater to an equal volume of distilled water at 4°C (Spotte, 1979). As a ratio, it has no units. Salinity is a measure of the total dissolved material in a kilogram of water when all carbonate has been converted to oxide, all bromine and iodine replaced by chlorine, and all organic matter completely oxidized (Spotte, 1979). This is a difficult determination to accomplish directly and is therefore usually calculated from a determination of specific gravity. Specific gravity in turn is usually derived either from a determination of water density using a floating bulb hydrometer, or determination of refractive index with a refractometer. The hydrometer bulb is a relatively inexpensive instrument but sometimes is more cumbersome to use. Few hobbyists will want to invest several hundred dollars in a hand-held refractometer, but practicing veterinarians usually have one they use for urinalysis. The same instrument can be used to double check hydrometer readings of clients (Fig. 75–1).

The addition of 1 g of salts to 1 kg of water (1 ppt) increases the water density by about 0.0008 (Spotte, 1979), and this is the rough relationship between salinity readings and specific gravity values. Professional aquarists tend to use salinity in parts per thousand when examining the salt concentration of their systems, but many hobbyists have learned their craft using specific gravity values. Multiplying salinity readings in parts per thousand by 0.0008 and adding 1.0 gives a good approximation of specific gravity. Subtracting one from a specific gravity reading and multiplying by 1250 approximates salinity readings in parts per thousand.

Determination of salinity is important in interpreting the osmotic burden of fish, particularly those with superficial wounds. For all fish, it is important to keep the salinity in a range tolerable to that

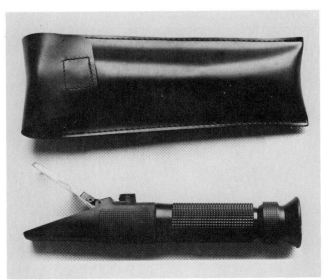

FIGURE 75–1. A temperature-correcting refractometer suitable for determining specific gravity in a marine tank.

species. Reef fishes are often quite tolerant of relatively rapid salinity changes in nature, particularly after large rainstorms or long dry spells. Pelagic fishes are very much less tolerant of salinity manipulations or fluctuations. Salinity measurements are needed for readjusting salinities after osmotic treatments as well as in routine tank monitoring.

Hydrogen Ion Concentration (pH)

Next on the list of relatively inexpensive and unspecialized tests is pH. The hydrogen ion concentration of water is vital to the survival of fish. This reading is particularly important in recirculating systems, where after a period of time the buffering capacity of the water is diminished and the pH will begin to fall from the constant addition of acidic waste products from the fishes and the biologic filters. This drop can be adjusted some with the use of sodium bicarbonate, which adds carbonate buffering capacity to the water. Unfortunately at the pH levels of normal marine waters (8.0 to 8.3), the carbonate buffering system is not particularly efficient. Its optimal buffering power lies in the area of pH 11. For this reason, eventually water changes will be required to supplement the buffering capacity of the protein and phosphate buffers that operate more efficiently at pH 8.

A number of devices are available for measuring pH. Papers are very inexpensive but labor intensive. Hand-held meters with pH probes can be obtained for as little as $40 up to $80 (Fig. 75–2). These are accurate and reasonably precise. Bench-top models can cost as little as $100 and up to several thousands of dollars. With the inexpensive machines available,

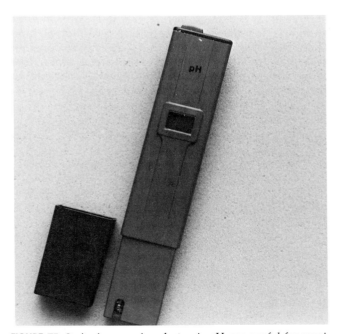

FIGURE 75–2. An inexpensive electronic pH pen useful for monitoring the hydrogen ion content of a home aquarium.

there is no excuse for not being able to monitor pH on a regular basis.

Nitrogen

Monitoring the nitrogen cycle is more difficult than some of the other monitoring, but it is certainly a valuable tool in evaluating the success of a filtration system. Ammonia is present in water in both ionized and un-ionized forms. The un-ionized form is the most toxic form for fish. Ammonia can be detected by a variety of kits that use colorimeteric means to determine ammonia concentration. Professional aquarists and marine chemists usually prefer to use an ion-specific probe, such as the Orion model 901 microprocessor ion analyzer with an Orion ammonia probe spiked for low-level readings with sodium nitrate, over more laborious bench methods.

Home hobbyists are frequently sold ammonia test kits when they first buy their marine aquaria. They are told to test ammonia daily or on some other fairly frequent schedule, a practice which may be useful in the initial setting-up stages of a system, but that yields little in well-maintained and long-established tanks. Other than during the breaking in of a new tank, or with the addition of new animals to an established one, routine measurement of ammonia levels by the hobbyists should probably be reserved for those with a strong interest in chemistry. The readings will almost always be zero in a balanced tank, and intermittent testing is unlikely to detect transient spikes in ammonia. Most aquarists will be better off using the time to look into their tank, observing the fish carefully and taking inventory, rather than trying to detect a dead fish or invertebrate through increasing water ammonia levels.

Nitrite, the breakdown product of ammonia in the metabolism of *Nitrosomonas* bacteria, is highly toxic to fish because of its ability to convert hemoglobin to methemoglobin. In large facilities, nitrite is usually determined with an automated spectrophotometric method using the methods outlined in *Standard Methods for Examination of Water and Waste Water*. Kits are also available that can determine this parameter colorimetrically. Much like ammonia testing, determination of water nitrite levels is primarily an exercise for the initial start up of a new tank or filter bed. The elevations of nitrite are usually even more transient than those of ammonia. If a hobbyist is inclined toward chemistry and water testing, determining nitrite levels may give an indication of impending problems, but again, the time probably could be better used to observe and carefully evaluate the animals in the tank or to perform routine water changes.

Nitrate is the least toxic step in the nitrogen cycle, being produced from nitrite by *Nitrobacter* bacteria. Fish can tolerate higher levels of nitrate than other nitrogenous waste products, but the build-up of nitrates will contribute to the declining pH as well as supply nutrients for excessive algae growth.

Nitrate levels can be read with a specific ion probe, such as the Orion model 901 equipped with an Orion nitrate probe spiked for saltwater readings. Kits are also available for colorimetric and spectrophotometric determinations. Nitrates build slowly in any closed system and are usually reduced only by water changes. Measuring nitrate levels can give an aquarist an idea of how effective their water-change routine is and may help identify the need for water changes in well-established systems. It does not need to be determined frequently, as the build-up is usually fairly slow. Monthly determinations are probably adequate in most stable situations.

Dissolved Oxygen

Dissolved oxygen is a much more volatile parameter than most people imagine. It can be affected by system flow, filtration, and temperature. Dissolved oxygen determinations are most commonly obtained with a dissolved oxygen meter (Fig. 75–3). A wide variety of these exist, the least expensive costing about $300. Titration methods exist and are available in kits for hobbyists, but rarely do hobbyists monitor this parameter. This is unfortunate because many of the rather mysterious problems that are observed in marine systems are associated with sudden or gradual loss of dissolved oxygen. A reasonably reliable dissolved oxygen meter is probably a good investment for any clinician involved in marine tropical fish medicine.

Other Parameters

Recently redox potential has been touted as a useful parameter to monitor in marine tanks. Small battery-operated redox meters are readily available for $40 or $50 (Fig. 75–4). With more experience, this may become a standard parameter to watch. It is

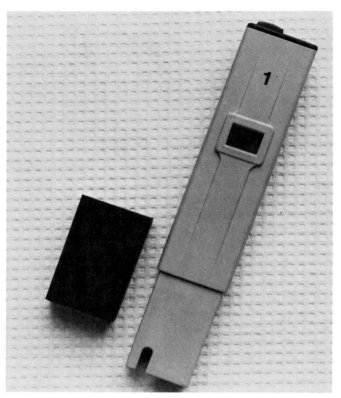

FIGURE 75–4. A hand-held redox meter for monitoring the cycling of newly established tanks or filters.

easier to obtain than ammonia and nitrite levels, and can be used to monitor the cycling of new systems.

Copper determinations are a must if copper therapy is employed. The margin of safety in copper administration is low and dosages must be confirmed by true readings and adjusted. Spectrophotometric methods are generally used in large aquaria, but hobbyists are usually forced to use colorimeteric methods that are very insensitive and not all that accurate. This is a service that you might consider providing for clients, since systems are available that allow you to run copper levels on any spectrophotometer with an adjustable wavelength.

HUSBANDRY AND RECORDS

Most clients will have their own ideas about the frequency of husbandry activities, but you may find yourself in a position to advise on such basic questions. Aquarists should remove dead material as soon as it is seen. Mechanical filters should optimally be cleaned weekly. Synthetic ion-absorption filters (Poly filters) should be changed every 4 to 5 weeks to avoid problems with leaking of toxins.

Many clients overtest and overmonitor their marine systems. In an established tank with no problems, weekly monitoring and careful record keeping is adequate. Monitoring is of relatively little value unless the values are recorded.

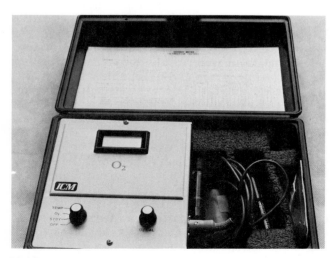

FIGURE 75–3. A dissolved oxygen meter suitable for home or clinical use.

CYCLING NEWLY SET-UP FILTERS

Biological filters are a tremendous boon to aquarium management, but they do require careful attention when starting up a new tank or system. It is necessary to build up the number of nitrifying bacteria present in the filter to a level where they can use all of the ammonia and nitrite produced in the system. This takes time. There are a number of ways to speed the process along, but even the most aggressive takes 4 to 5 weeks before the system has completely cycled. Clients may need some advice in this area, since few hobbyists are well schooled in starting up a new system.

For marine systems that will include both invertebrates and fin fishes, the following method for cycling a tank is a modification of one recommended by experienced marine aquarists (Thiel, 1989a). It uses "live rock" (rock collected from underwater that houses a grab-bag mixture of marine life) and starter enzymes (commercially available tank starter enzymes). The environmental impact of using live rock is a concern, and it should be emphasized that similar results can be achieved using other sources of "seed starter," such as gravel from established tanks. The timing and amounts of material used will be similar to those advised by Thiel's method.

To use Thiel's live rock method, the client should add up to 0.1 kg of "live rock" per liter of water in the system after carefully rinsing the rock in a bucket of marine salt water and removing any stone crabs, bristle worms, or small toadfishes that might damage future inhabitants of the tank. Caution your clients to discard the water and sediment. Even though they may be tempted to conserve the water, it is not worth the impact of the sediment on the tank.

When the rock is added, the tank water will cloud up for a day or two but will clear as the tank water circulates. Then, if they wish, the client can add the enzymes, using the recommendations of the manufacturer. About 12 hours after adding the enzymes, baseline ammonia, nitrate, carbonate hardness, and pH readings should be taken. At this point, the tank owner is usually very dismayed because if too much of the enzyme is added, a very unpleasant smell develops. There is no alternative to waiting it out. If water is changed during the start-up cycle, it will delay the cycle time significantly. Also, protein skimmers and ozonation devices should not be run until the tank has finished cycling.

The tank, with its "live rock" and no fish will now begin to cycle. The first event of note will be about 5 days after the enzymes are added when the pH will begin to fall. It may bottom out as low as 7.6, but no adjustment is necessary unless the carbonate hardness drops below 8 dKH. If that occurs, the carbonate hardness should be slowly adjusted up at a rate of about 1 dKH/day to help stabilize the pH.

The first ammonia peak will occur on day 10, 11, or 12. As long as the carbonate hardness is above 12, the pH will take care of itself. After day 10,

testing for ammonia and nitrite should be done daily. The nitrite spike will be sudden and may be missed unless testing is done daily. When nitrite and ammonia levels return to zero after the first cycle, the client can add more rock, up to another 0.1 kg/L, but no fish. Most enzyme companies suggest adding a second dose of enzymes, although this is not particularly critical to the length of time it takes the tank to cycle. If a second batch of enzymes is added, the tank may have a white haze for several days, which will be self-limiting, as will most occurrences of small white planaria, which are sometimes seen crawling on the aquarium glass. If enzymes are added the second time, only half as much should be used as the first time. The second cycle will take 10 to 14 days.

If your client has the equipment to monitor redox potential in the tank, initial values will be between 230 and 240 mV and will rapidly drop to 90 or 100 before beginning a slow climb. The first cycle ends with redox values between 200 and 250 mV. The second cycle is accompanied by a large drop to between 90 and 100 mV again. When the redox potential has returned to baseline values, the tank is ready for initial introductions of larger animals. Usually, it is best to add invertebrates first, adding two at a time, waiting at least 4 days between additions. Two weeks after the invertebrates have been introduced, fish can be placed in the tank using the same rules.

It is possible to cycle tanks other ways. If your client does not want invertebrates in the tank, hardy fishes such as damsels and wrasses should be used. For starting, 1 cm of fish for every 10 to 25 L (1 inch of fish for every 7 to 15 gal) is appropriate. Enzymes can be used. When ammonia and nitrite return to zero after the first cycle, add more fish at a rate of 1 cm of fish per 25 L (1 inch of fish per 15 gal), bringing the total to no more than 1 cm of fish per 8 L (1 inch of fish per 5 gal).

Cycling with both fish and invertebrates in the tank at the same time is not advisable. The complexities in this method make it very difficult to accomplish without problems. Tanks can be cycled without any fish or invertebrates, using only ammonium chloride to feed the tank. This takes a bit longer (6 weeks), but again the minimum time for any process is 4 to 5 weeks. Enzymes shorten the start up, but only by perhaps a week. It is important to take the tank through two cycles before building up populations, and there is no way of stabilizing a biological filter bed faster.

LIGHTING

There are many opinions about the absolutely optimal scheme for lighting a marine tank, but all aquarists agree that light is a critical component of the marine environment and that proper lighting is very important to the health and well-being of marine tropical reef species.

Intensity

There are several parameters of light that must be considered when evaluating the lighting of an aquarium system. Intensity, or the amount of light being delivered, is important. Bulb intensity is usually listed in lumens, which measures the output of the bulb as opposed to watts, which measures the energy consumption of the bulb. The rule of thumb of 1 W/L of seawater to deliver appropriate lumens to a tank is useful, but in an aquarium system it is more important to know the amount of light reaching the plants and animals in the tank than the amount of light produced by a bulb or the energy consumed in producing it. Footcandles or LUX are units that evaluate the amount of light available at a given distance from a light source. One lumen of light on a square meter of surface equals 1 LUX. With the higher intensities of light required in aquarium systems, it is more convenient to work with the metric LUX rather than the footcandles (1 ftc equals 1 lumen on a square foot surface). To convert footcandles to LUX, multiply by 0.0929. LUX meters are available and can be used to measure the light being delivered to a point in a tank. You can also use your single-lens reflex camera as described in Chapter 65.

Although it is often a good goal to try to reproduce natural light conditions, it is not feasible to try and duplicate the extremely high light levels found over natural coral reefs at midday. Problems of heat dissipation and power consumption in addition to bulb design make this very impractical. Unfortunately, only a few studies have provided much insight into how much compromise from natural conditions is allowable. Corals and macroalgae appear to require up to 16,000 LUX for several hours each day (Thiel, 1989a,b). LUX are not necessarily cumulative, and the strategy of delivering less intense light for longer periods of time each day does not work (Thiel, 1988, 1989a).

Spectrum

Intensity cannot be completely divorced from considerations of spectrum. The ability of light to pass through seawater is related to the wavelength of the light. The blue end of the spectrum penetrates marine water much deeper than the red or yellow wavelengths of light. For pure intensity, halogen quartz halide lamps give off many lumens, but tungsten, mercury, and sodium vapor quartz halides are too yellow and deliver comparatively fewer LUX.

Although spectral output of a bulb is usually discussed in terms of wavelengths of light emitted, a convenient way of characterizing the light spectrum given off by a bulb is the use of color temperature in degrees Kelvin. A high color temperature bulb, one with high degrees Kelvin, has a lot of blue in its spectrum. Cool bulbs, such as cool white fluorescent bulbs, are high-Kelvin bulbs. Actinic blue lights, which give the best depth penetration, are approximately 5000° K, and come as close to simulating noontime sun in tropical reef regions as any bulb. The rule of thumb is that the higher the Kelvin rating the better, although this remains to be examined in detail. True colors are rendered better and fish and corals seem to thrive better with a spectrum that has more blue wavelengths capable of penetrating the water to greater depths.

Mercury vapor bulbs are usually in the range of 3700° K. Phosphorus-coated plant growth bulbs that give off a reddish light are around 3300° K. Attempts to use cheaper lights found in other applications usually result in too yellow of a light for good penetration of the water. Another factor that must be considered when selecting lights is the longevity of the bulb, or the time it will provide its entire spectrum. Regular fluorescent bulbs generally provide reasonably full spectra for up to 6 months. High-output fluorescent tubes last about 9 months, and metal halide lamps maintain their spectrum for 3 to 4 years (Thiel, 1989a).

Periodicity

The importance of periodicity has been discussed in Chapter 8. As mentioned above, attempts to deliver cumulative LUX are doomed to disappointment. Most marine tropical systems should be maintained on 12 hours light and 12 hours dark. The importance of providing staged illumination varies with the species being maintained, but it is difficult to go wrong with a well-designed crepuscular period. This is facilitated in systems in which several light sources are used to achieve adequate LUX and an appropriate spectrum.

TABLE 75–4. Instrumentation Sources

Gilford Instrument Labs Inc Oberlin, OH 44074 (216) 774-1041
Hach Chemicals Loveland, CO (303) 669-3050
La Motte Chemicals P.O. Box 329 Chestertown, MD 21260 (301) 778-3100
Orion Research Inc 840 Memorial Drive Cambridge, MA 02139 (617) 864-5400
YSI Yellow Springs Instrument Co. P.O. Box 279 Yellow Springs, OH 45387 (513) 767-7241

LITERATURE CITED

A.P.H.A. (1980) Standard Methods for the Examination of Water and Wastewater, 15th ed. American Public Health Association, Washington, D.C.

Brewer, P.G. (1975) Minor elements in sea water. In: Chemical Oceanography. 2nd ed. Vol. 1 (Riley, J.P., and Skirrow, G., eds.). Academic Press, New York, pp 415–496.

Spotte, S. (1979) Seawater Aquariums: The Captive Environment. John Wiley & Sons, New York.

Thiel, A.J. (1988) The Marine Fish and Invert Reef Aquarium. Aardvark Press, Bridgeport, Connecticut.

Thiel, A.J. (1989a) Advanced Reef Keeping. Aardvark Press, Bridgeport, Connecticut.

Thiel, A.J. (1989b) Small Reef Aquarium Basics. Aardvark Press, Bridgeport, Connecticut.

Chapter 76

MARINE TROPICAL FISH NUTRITION

MICHAEL K. STOSKOPF

A long chapter on the nutrition of marine tropical fishes would be begging the point at this stage of our knowledge. Although nutrient requirements have been determined for commonly cultured fishes such as carp and salmonids, little is known about the nutrients and nutrient balances required for marine tropical fishes. These animals obviously represent a diverse array of adaptations both behaviorally and nutritionally. They are also subject to seasonal demands and different nutritional requirements at different stages of development. This makes the job of providing balanced and complete diets to mixed tanks very difficult and perhaps more a matter of luck and art than of science.

Providing adequate calories is usually the first concern when feeding marine tropical fishes. This is rarely figured on the cost basis used for commercial aquacultural fishes, but rather on the availability and palatability of feed. Calorie provision is almost always evaluated by visual evaluation of the appearance of the fish and its apparent growth rate. Overfeeding is a more frequent problem than providing too few calories and leads to a number of serious problems both in the fish and the water system. On the other hand, caloric deficits can become a real problem if the rule of thumb, "Do Not Overfeed," is taken too seriously, particularly for small species with high metabolic requirements.

Emaciated fish develop sunken bellies followed by loss of dorsal musculature causing them to look dished-in above the lateral line (Fig. 76–1). The most common cause of inadequate calories is competition in the tank from other more aggressive fish. Heavy parasitism can also increase the energy requirements of a fish, making an otherwise acceptable feeding level deficient in maintenance calories. Of course, underfeeding can be a cause as well. This happens most often in species such as sea horses and pipefishes that are essentially obligate feeders on live foods. When local supplies of live brine shrimp are interrupted, these fish may suffer serious consequences. Feeding a food of too low calorie density is rarely the cause of a problem, as most foods normally fed to marine fish are calorie-dense. Calorie limiting is much more common than bulk limiting (Tytler and Calow, 1985).

The problems that calorie limiting cause in the nutrition of marine fishes are many, and they are rarely considered by aquarists. These include the very real potential for dietary insufficiencies in essential nutrients, including amino acids, fatty acids, and of course vitamins and minerals. Since the requirements of the many different marine tropical fish species maintained are not known, we are required to base most of our effort on observing for signs of deficiency and correcting problems rather than preventing them with properly calculated and supplemented diets. Hopefully this will change in the future.

We do have some rules of thumb generated from work with primarily freshwater fishes. Many fishes require dietary sources of ω-3 fatty acids (linolenic family). Many fishes require arginine, histidine, leucine, isoleucine, lysine, methionine, phenylalanine, tyrosine, tryptophan, and valine as exogenous essential amino acids (Lovell, 1989). Many also require exogenous vitamin A, vitamin K, vitamin E, niacin, pyridoxine, and vitamin B_1 among others.

First, to examine the problem of fatty acid deficiencies, the signs usually occur in older fish, which

A

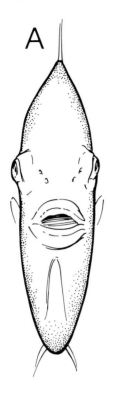

B

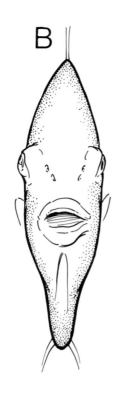

C

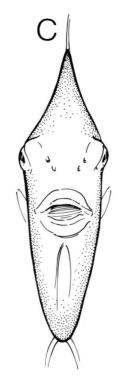

FIGURE 76–1. Judging body condition in laterally compressed fishes. *A.* Good body condition. *B.* Good body condition, but recently not feeding. *C.* Emaciated, with long-term energy deficit, but actively eating.

lose color, become pale, and exhibit poor growth rates despite adequate calories. The fish may become listless and anoretic, and low-level mortalities may occur if the condition is severe enough. Anemia is a common hematologic sign. At postmortem examination, fish suffering from an ω-3 fatty acid deficiency will have pale membranes, lack fat in the pyloric ceca, and possibly exhibit a shrunken air bladder. The most characteristic sign, although certainly far from pathognomonic, is a loss of color. Histopathology is more useful in approaching a diagnosis Necrosis and myolysis of skeletal muscle will be evident, especially in the trunk dorsolateral muscles. Spaces between muscles will be infiltrated with fat. Foamy macrophages proliferate and are laden with lipofuchsins in the melanomacrophage centers, meninges, and heart. Pancreatic necrosis and degeneration may also be evident.

Causes of ω-3 fatty acid deficiencies include the feeding of foods deficient in them (river smelt, some invertebrate feeds) and the feeding of improperly stored feeds. Feeds held too long or at improper temperatures will lose ω-3 fatty acids through autooxidation.

Amino acid deficiencies are also difficult to diagnose. They may not be fatal for a long time, and at postmortem they may be complicated with a variety of infectious problems, making the underlying nutritional problem difficult, if not impossible, to identify. Again, clinical signs are generally manifest in older fish and are relatively nonspecific, including inadequate growth rates or reproductive failures (Halver, 1972). In colorful reef fishes, colors may fade. Blue fish that begin to pale may be showing

signs of tyrosine deficiency. Tyrosine is required for the production of the melanins used to create the brilliant blue colorations (Fig. 76–2). While discoloration may be the only apparent sign of problems, tyrosine is also needed in the synthesis of epinephrine and norepinephrine, as well as thyroxine. Deficiencies can result in nervous and endocrine imbalances. Mammalian blood is high in tyrosine, and bloodmeal can be supplemented to combat these problems.

Fading yellow colors are another matter. They are generally carotenoid based, although some yellows and oranges are part of the tyrosine metabolic pathway. Supplementation with carotenoids, including vitamin A, can be beneficial. Other vitamin deficiencies in marine tropical fishes mimic the signs and symptoms in freshwater fishes. The role of carotenoids in fish coloration is discussed in more detail in Chapter 46.

Water-soluble B vitamin deficiencies are common in situations in which frozen fish are fed as a major portion of the diet and improper thawing techniques are employed. Thawing in water is particularly ill advised, since it tends to leach nearly all of the water-soluble vitamins from the food even before it is placed in the tank. Antioxidant vitamins such as vitamin C and vitamin E can be depleted below adequate levels by prolonged storage, even when frozen, since the continual oxidative pressure on the lipids in the frozen fish continues to occur. These vitamins can become used up, blocking oxidative chain reactions in polyunsaturated fats, which are common in fishes. Tropical fish species would not be expected to be as susceptible to vitamin E prob-

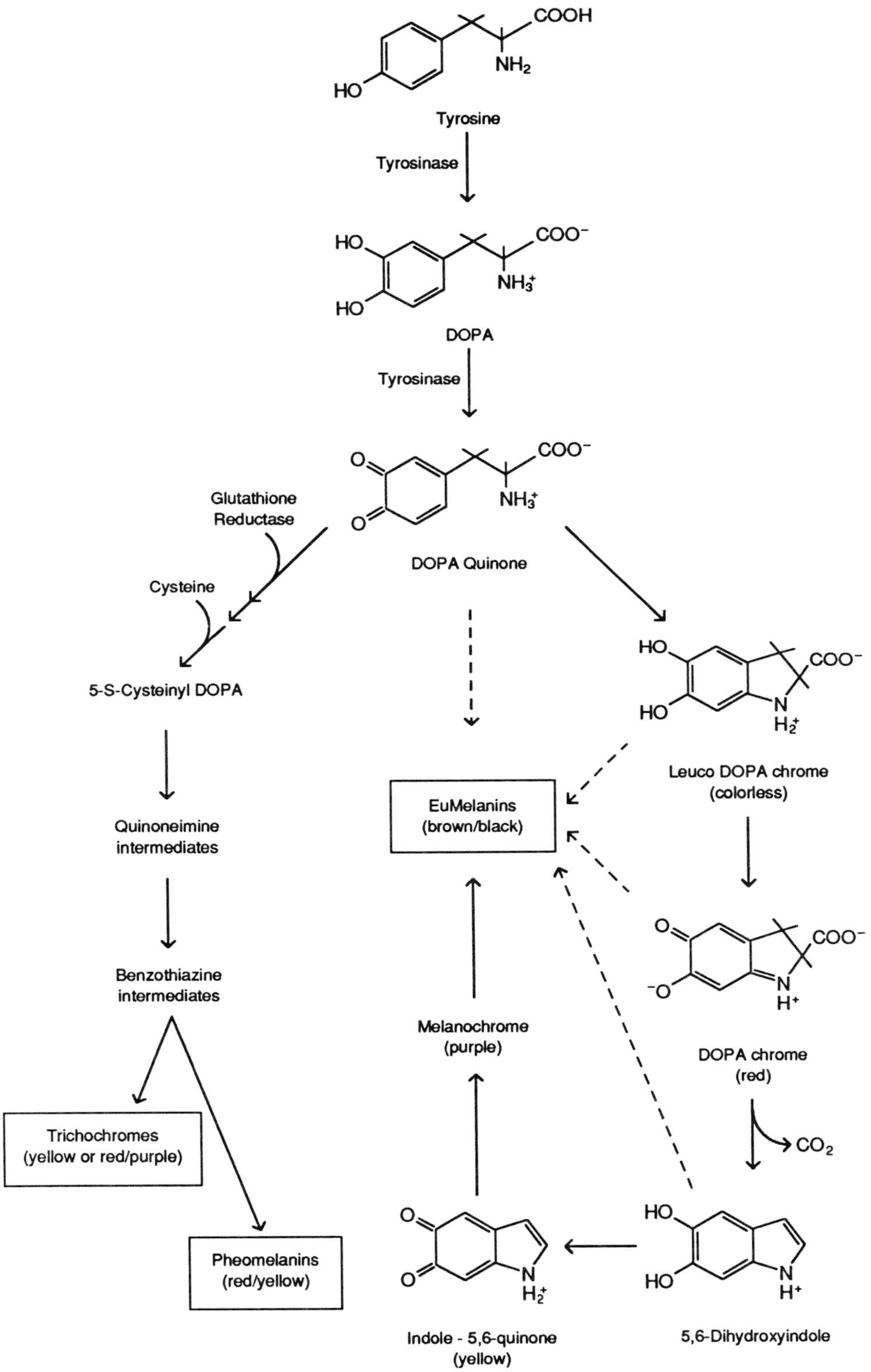

FIGURE 76–2. The role of tyrosine in pigmentation.

lems because of a decreased need to maintain high levels of polyunsaturated fatty acids in membranes relative to cold-water species (Cowey et al., 1985), but this has not been carefully studied.

In summary, the proper feeding and nutrition of marine tropical fishes remains an art form, and considerably more information is needed. Careful investigation of the natural history of the fish being managed, attention to provision of a variety of properly handled foods in forms acceptable to the fishes, and close observation for signs that might relate to

nutritional imbalances can go a long way in preventing nutritional problems in marine tropical fishes.

LITERATURE CITED

Cowey, C.B., Mackie, A.M., and Bell, J.G. (eds.) (1985) Nutrition and Feeding in Fish. Academic Press, London.
Halver, J.E. (ed.) (1972) Fish Nutrition. Academic Press, New York.
Lovell, T. (1989) Nutrition and Feeding of Fish. Van Nostrand Reinhold, New York.
Tytler, P., and Calow, P. (eds.) (1985) Fish Energetics, New Perspectives. The Johns Hopkins University Press, Baltimore, Maryland.

Chapter 77

REPRODUCTION OF MARINE TROPICAL FISHES

RUTH FRANCIS-FLOYD

Although marine tropical fishes account for only a small percentage of all ornamental fishes sold, they are the among most valuable animals in the pet fish trade. The anemonefishes are the only marine tropical group reared in large numbers for commercial sale. A few other species have been reared by hobbyists on a small scale, but the vast majority of marine tropical fishes sold are taken from the wild. Mortality of collected fish is substantial during capture and shipping. Life expectancy of those individuals that do reach their final destination is poor. Efforts to improve successful reproduction of these fishes in captivity are crucial. Although marine fish are not recommended for beginning aquarists because they are much less tolerant of suboptimal environmental conditions than most freshwater species, the popularity of these animals continues to grow because of their exceptional beauty and bright coloration.

This chapter has two main sections. The first deals with the natural ecology of coral reef reproductive strategies. The tropical marine environment contains two unique habitats that have no counterpart in the temperate zone, the coral reef and mangrove systems (Johannes, 1978). Reef fishes are most commonly encountered in home aquaria, and between 6000 and 8000 species of fishes inhabit the reefs of the world (Erlich, 1975). The second part of this chapter examines the various stages of controlled reproduction in marine tropical fishes.

THE CORAL REEF ECOSYSTEM

Environmental Factors

In temperate zones, temperature and daylight cycles are important variables that affect the reproductive stage of fish. In contrast, for marine tropical fishes, variations in currents and prevailing winds are of greater significance (Johannes, 1978). The two seasons found in the tropics involve changes in prevailing wind patterns, currents, and precipitation, not length of day or temperature. Change in precipitation appears to have minimal influence on the reproduction of tropical marine fishes, whereas spawning activity does correlate with seasonal variation in current and prevailing wind patterns (Johannes, 1978).

The greatest spawning activity occurs when prevailing winds or prevailing currents are weakest. This suggests reproductive strategies may have evolved to increase the chance that offshore larvae will be carried inshore rather than be swept out to sea. Some Hawaiian reef fishes spawn in locations where local gyrals keep developing larvae close to the appropriate habitat, increasing the opportunity to successfully colonize near shore areas (Erlich, 1975).

Reproductive Strategies

There are three fundamental reproductive strategies encountered in tropical marine fishes that are distinguished by the type of egg produced. Within these broad categories there is additional variation (Fig. 77–1).

Production of Pelagic Eggs

The most frequently encountered strategy in marine tropical fishes is the production of pelagic eggs (Table 77–1). Pelagic eggs have a specific gravity equal to or less than that of water (Thresher, 1984). They remain in the water column and frequently float in open water. Larvae hatched from pelagic eggs live in the planktonic soup for hours to months, depending on the species. This provides the advantage that larval fishes will be less susceptible to predation (Johannes, 1978). Protection from predation pressure is perhaps even more important than food abundance to the success of tropical marine fishes (Johannes, 1978).

Fishes that lay pelagic eggs can be further subdivided into pelagic spawners and benthic broadcasters (Thresher, 1984). Pelagic spawners are more common. Smaller fish species tend to swim up in the water column and release their gametes at the peak of a spawning ascent. The advantage of this strategy for smaller fish may be the ability to remain close to a home range, decreasing vulnerability to predation while releasing reproductive products high enough in the water column to be carried offshore by current and wind action (Johannes, 1978). Benthic broadcasters release pelagic eggs, but do not swim up in the water column to do so. The eels (Anguilliformes) are the only known reef inhabitants categorized as benthic broadcasters. Many species of eel participate in lengthy offshore migrations prior to spawning (Breder and Rosen, 1966; Thresher, 1984).

Production of Demersal Eggs

The second major reproductive strategy of marine tropical fishes is to lay demersal eggs that have a specific gravity greater than water and remain on the bottom (Thresher, 1984). Fishes that lay demersal eggs are further categorized as demersal spawners or as egg scatterers. Demersal spawners provide some type of parental care such as nest preparation or mouth-brooding. Egg scatterers do not provide parental care. These fish swim up in a spawning ascent, releasing eggs that settle to the bottom, where they are randomly scattered among the bottom sediment (Thresher, 1984). Examples of demersal spawners and egg scatterers are listed in Table 77–1.

Release of Free-Swimming Young

The third reproductive strategy practiced by tropical marine fishes is the release of free-swimming young into the water column. This is the least com-

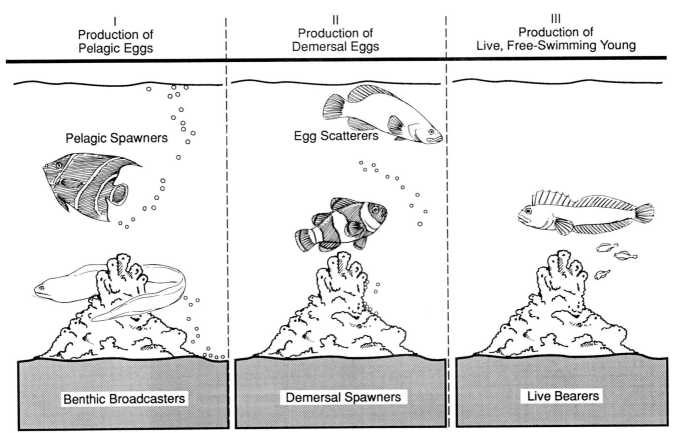

FIGURE 77–1. Schematic of reproductive strategies of tropical marine fishes.

TABLE 77–1. Reproductive Strategies in Marine Tropical Fishes

Common Name	Principal Reproductive Strategy	Reproductive Mode	Type of Eggs	Type of Larvae	Spawned in Captivity	Larvae Reared in Captivity
Surgeonfishes and Tangs	Pelagic spawners	Short spawning ascent Pair spawning/ group spawning	Pelagic	Planktonic	No	No
Eels	Benthic broadcaster	Migratory (Sargasso sea) Pelagic spawners	Pelagic	Planktonic	No	No
Cardinalfishes	Demersal spawner	Mouth-brooders Demersal spawners	Egg mass, large mucus-bound	Planktonic	Yes	No
Trumpetfishes	Unknown	Spawning ascent	Unknown	Unknown	No	No
Triggerfishes and Filefishes	Dermersal spawner	Harem-based Spawning occurs in female's territory	Demersal, adhesive; guarded by female	Planktonic	Yes	No
Combtooth Blennies	Demersal spawner	In crevice near bottom	Demersal, attached to roof of nest; guarded by male	No yolk sac; actively swim and feed immediately after hatching Planktonic	Yes	Yes
Brotulas	Variable (some livebearers)	Viviparous, ovoviviparous, and oviparous species	Variable	Planktonic	No	No
Dragonets	Pelagic spawner	Spawning ascent Male-dominated harem	Pelagic	Planktonic	Yes	No
Jacks, Pompano	Pelagic spawners	Offshore aggregates	Pelagic	Planktonic?	Yes?	No?
Pearlfishes	Unknown	Unknown	Pelagic stage	Planktonic	No	No
Butterflyfishes	Pelagic spawner	Permanent pair spawning; spawning ascent	Pelagic	Planktonic		
Pike Blennies	Demersal spawner	Spawn on bottom near shelter	Demersal; guarded by male	Unknown	Yes	No
Morwongs	Unknown	Unknown	Pelagic	Yolk sac Planktonic	No	No
Hawkfishes	Unknown	Spawning pairs; spawning ascent	Unknown	Planktonic	Yes	No
Blennies	Livebearers and demersal spawners	Viviparous and ovoviviparous; spawn in crevices near bottom	Gelatinous mass attached to roof of cave or algal mat; guarded by male	Variable (some species planktonic for 24 hours then actively seek bottom)	Yes	No
Porcupinefishes	Variable (pelagic and demersal spawners)	Variable, spawning ascent (female pushed to surface)	Variable (demersal or pelagic)		Yes	Yes
Spadefishes	Unknown	Offshore migration suspected Pelagic schooling fish	Unknown	Unknown	No	No
Cornetfishes	Unknown	Unknown	Pelagic	Unknown	No	No
Clingfishes	Demersal spawners	Spawn under rock or shell External and/or internal fertilization	Adhesive demersal Tended by male	Planktonic	Yes	Yes
Gobies	Demersal spawners	Protogynous hermaphroditism	Adhesive demersal Attached to roof or cavity	Planktonic	Yes	Yes
Soapfishes	Egg scatterers?	Spawning ascent Some species hermaphroditic	Demersal?	Planktonic	No	No
Grunts	Unknown	Unknown	Pelagic	Planktonic	No	Yes
Squirrelfishes	Unknown	Unknown	Pelagic?	Planktonic	No	No
Chub	Unknown	Unknown	Unknown	Unknown (note: juveniles collected in floating sargassum)	No	No

TABLE 77–1. Reproductive Strategies in Marine Tropical Fishes *Continued*

Common Name	Principal Reproductive Strategy	Reproductive Mode	Type of Eggs	Type of Larvae	Spawned in Captivity	Larvae Reared in Captivity
Wrasse	Pelagic spawner	Migrate to specific spawning site Spawning ascent Protogynous hermaphrodite (see text)	Pelagic	Planktonic	Yes	Yes
Snappers	Pelagic spawner	Spawning migration Group spawning Spawning ascent	Pelagic	Planktonic for 4 weeks	Yes	Yes
Other Lutyanoid Fishes	Variable (pelagic and demersal spawners)	Spawning ascent or nesting	Pelagic or demersal Demersal eggs are adhesive and tended by male	Planktonic until 25 mm	Yes	Yes
Tilefishes	Pelagic spawners	Spawning ascent	Pelagic	Planktonic until 16 mm	Yes	Yes
Mullets	Pelagic spawners	Offshore spawning migrations (variable) Spawning aggregation	Pelagic	Planktonic for 3 days	No	No
Sand Perch	Pelagic spawner	Protogynous hermaphrodite Spawning ascent	Pelagic	Planktonic (1–2 months)	No	No
Goatfishes	Pelagic spawner	Short migration (from inshore water to outer edge of reef) Pair and group spawning Spawning ascent	Pelagic	Planktonic until 40–60 mm	No	No
Trunkfishes	Pelagic spawner	Haremic Spawning ascent	Pelagic	Planktonic for 114 hours Juveniles in grassbeds	No	Yes
Marine Catfishes	Demersal spawner	Nest construction by male Spawn in nest	Demersal Tended by male	Free-swimming after 10 days	Yes	Yes
Marine Anglefishes	Pelagic spawner	Protogynous hermaphrodite Spawning ascent Pair spawning	Pelagic floating egg raft	Planktonic for 3–5 wks	Yes	Yes
Damselfishes	Demersal spawner	Sequential hermaphrodite	Demersal eggs Guarded until hatch (±3–7 days)	Planktonic (15–20 days)	Yes	Yes (but only confirmed report was to 30 days)
Anemonefishes	Demersal spawner	Protandrous hermaphrodite	Demersal eggs	Planktonic (short)	Yes	Yes
Bigeyes	Unknown	Unknown	Pelagic?	Planktonic	No	No
Basslets	Demersal spawner	Sequential hermaphrodites? Spawn in nest or sheltered area Mouth-brooders or tended by male	Demersal Egg balls formed	Planktonic up to 3 months Large larvae	Yes	No
Lionfishes	Pelagic spawner	Nocturnal Paired ascents	Gelatinous egg balls	Planktonic Feed 4 days after hatch settle 10–12 mm	Yes	No
Jawfishes	Demersal spawner	Pair spawn in burrow Mouth-brooders Eggs tended by male	Demersal Hatch in 7–19 days at 25–26°C	Planktonic settle 15–18 days	Yes	Yes
Sweepers	Unknown	Unknown (note: group spawning is suspected)	Unknown (note: pelagic eggs suspected)	Unknown	No	No

Table continued on following page

Common Name	Principal Reproductive Strategy	Reproductive Mode	Type of Eggs	Type of Larvae	Spawned in Captivity	Larvae Reared in Captivity
Parrotfishes	Pelagic spawner	Protogynous hermaphrodites Migrate to outer edge of reef Pair or group spawning Spawning ascent	Pelagic	Planktonic	One report Note: too large to spawn in home aquaria	No
Drums and Jackknifefish	Unknown	Unknown for reef-associated species	Pelagic	Benthic (some species)	Yes, induced spawning for food fish species	Yes Food fish species only
Scorpionfish	Variable	*Helicolenus* and *Sebastes* are livebearers *Scorpaena* produce egg mass	Ovoviviparous floating gelatinous egg mass	Planktonic	Yes (public aquaria)	No
Sea Perches	Unknown	Protogynous hermaphrodites; monandric (i.e., all males are derived from females Pair spawning	Pelagic?	Planktonic	Yes	No
Groupers	Pelagic spawner	Protogynous hermaphrodites; fish migrate to local "spawning grounds" Pair spawning Spawning ascent	Pelagic nonadhesive Spherical	Planktonic 30–40 days	Yes, hormone induced	Yes
Sea Basses	Pelagic spawner	Simultaneous hermaphrodites form spawning pairs (pair members successively alternate male and female roles) Streaker males compete with other males during spawning ascent; self-fertilization in belted sandfish	Pelagic Spherical nonadhesive	Planktonic	Yes	Yes (see Tucker, 1984)
Rabbitfishes	Egg scatterer?	Form spawning aggregates; spawning migration to specific sites; no parental care reported	Demersal Spherical, adhesive, colorless, small (0.42–0.66 mm) Scatter on bottom	Planktonic 25 days	Yes	Yes
Barracuda	Pelagic spawner	Migrate to specific spawning areas in spawning aggregates	Pelagic Spherical Transparent	Planktonic until 18 mm	No	Yes
Lizardfishes	Pelagic spawner	Pair spawning with spawning ascent	Pelagic Large spherical	Planktonic settle at 30–35 mm	No	No
Puffers	Unknown	Unknown for reef Some temperate species spawn on beach	Demersal Adhesive in temperate species; unknown in reef species Egg tending not reported	Planktonic, settle after 30 days in *Lagocephalus lunau*	Yes	Yes
Triplefin Blennies	Demersal spawner	Spawning pairs Satellite males may disrupt pairs Nest preparation	Sticky threads anchor eggs to nest site	Planktonic for 40 days	Yes	Yes
Moorish Idols	Unknown	Pair spawning?	Pelagic?	Long planktonic stage suspected	Yes	Yes

mon strategy encountered among tropical marine fishes. Livebearers may be less common in tropical marine environments than in freshwater environments because of the disadvantages of decreased fecundity and the increased vulnerability of gravid adults (Johannes, 1978).

Hermaphroditism

Hermaphroditism is common among reef fishes. Most hermaphroditic marine tropical fishes are sequential hermaphrodites. Except for a brief transitional period, they are either male or female depending on the stage of their life cycle. Protogynous hermaphrodites, such as the parrotfish, function first as females and later as males (Choat and Robertson, 1975). In some species, rapid acceleration in the growth rate is associated with sex changes from female to male, as in the saddleback wrasse (Ross, 1987). The evolutionary advantage of rapid growth associated with sex change may be to decrease the period of sexual dysfunction associated with transition.

Protoandric hermaphrodites function first as males and later as females. Anemonefishes are an example. Laboratory and field studies with orange-finned anemonefish and skunk-striped anemonefish show that change from male to female occurs when the dominant female is removed (Fricke and Fricke, 1977). This provides a mechanism for maintaining a monogamous pair in an environment of low population density caused by the random distribution of host anemones throughout reef systems.

A few species of porgies and several sea basses function as simultaneous hermaphrodites and can function as either male or female at any given time (Thresher, 1984). In certain sea basses, all fish initially function as simultaneous hermaphrodites, but as they mature, ovary tissue is resorbed and the fish function only as males (Hastings and Petersen, 1986; Petersen, 1987). These larger males establish territories inhabited by a small number (one to eight) of simultaneous hermaphrodites that serve as a harem. This is a rare gender allocation pattern that may benefit fish that live at the periphery of the reef, in rock or sand habitats, and do not migrate to the outer margins of the reef prior to spawning (Petersen, 1987).

CAPTIVE REPRODUCTION OF MARINE TROPICAL FISHES

There are many reasons why few tropical marine fishes have been successfully spawned and reared in captivity, not the least of which is the difficulty of providing an acceptable substitute for the reef environment. In addition, the life histories of many of these fishes are complex and not well understood. Even if fishes are successfully spawned, larval rearing remains a major challenge to completion of the life cycle in captivity.

Anemonefishes and neon gobies are cultured in Florida for commercial sale (Frakes and Hoff, 1983). Anemonefishes can be spawned in the home aquarium with a minimum of effort (Thresher, 1984). They are sequential hermaphrodites, and so breeding pairs can be formed by maintaining a number of individuals in the same tank. Their demersal eggs are more conducive to aquarium conditions than the pelagic eggs of other species, and hatching occurs after 7 or 8 days. Feeding the newly hatched larvae can be difficult, but a marine rotifer, *Brachionis plicatilis*, can be used successfully until fry are large enough to be fed brine shrimp (*Artemia* sp.) (Frakes and Hoff, 1983; Thresher, 1984).

Other marine tropical species have been naturally spawned in captivity. Aquarium spawning of six species of angelfishes has been achieved in the laboratory with no attempt to rear developing larvae beyond the period of yolk absorption (120 hours) (Bauer and Bauer, 1981). Perhaps these species could be successfully reared if an appropriate food item were found for the youngest larvae.

Broodstock Conditioning and Induced Spawning

A number of marine tropical fish species have been successfully spawned using hormone injections to induce ovulation. Used more extensively in the management of reproduction of freshwater tropical fishes, induced spawning has great potential for use in controlled reproduction of marine tropical fishes. A prerequisite to successful hormone spawning is broodstock conditioning. A breeding animal can only be induced to spawn if mature gametes are present to be released.

To condition broodstock, they must be well fed, and manipulation of environmental conditions may be required. When these techniques are used initially on new species, the art of good animal husbandry is probably more important than the sciences of endocrinology or theriogenology.

A number of regimens have successfully induced spawning in marine fishes (Hoff et al., 1972; Roberts et al., 1978; Tucker, 1984). All require egg sampling prior to hormone administration to ensure mature oocytes are present. The appearance of mature oocytes must be determined for each new fish species spawned. Oocyte staging data are available for the red drum (Roberts et al., 1978).

Once the presence of mature oocytes has been confirmed, the female fish is injected intramuscularly or intraperitoneally. Intraperitoneal injection is easier in small fish. Human chorionic gonadotropin (HCG) or carp pituitary hormone are most frequently used to induce ovulation. Human chorionic gonadotropin at a dosage of 0.7 to 1.7 IU/g body weight, followed in 24 hours by a second injection of 0.6 to 0.8 IU HCG/g body weight, induces ovulation in black sea bass (Tucker, 1984). The next day, ovarian biopsies of anesthetized females are used to identify ripe fish for stripping. The eggs are then fertilized by wet fertilization. Milt is collected from male fish with a tuberculin syringe without a needle and mixed with the ripe eggs in filtered seawater. Then the eggs are washed and placed in rearing tanks. Dry fertilization is described in Chapter 66. A few reef species have been spawned using similar techniques (Table 77–1).

Larval Rearing

Once fish have been successfully spawned, the major hurdle of larval feeding must still be overcome. Successful spawning in captivity is more frequently achieved than successful larval rearing. Most larvae of tropical marine fishes are planktonic, spending a few hours to many months floating in surface waters of the open ocean. The ocean environment is extremely stable, a condition difficult to reproduce under captive conditions. In addition, food items needed by various larvae may not be readily available in captivity. Candidate fish species for captive propagation must be selected carefully for large larval size at hatching and for relatively short planktonic periods. These fish hold the most promise for successful captive rearing in the near future.

Successful feeding of larval fish is critical for captive rearing. Food particles must be small enough to be ingested and must be sufficiently abundant for larvae to "bump into." Behavioral cues for ingestion of food items (i.e., olfactory or visual stimuli) may limit initial feeding in some species. As new culture technologies continue to develop for food fish production, there will be advances of immediate benefit to those attempting to rear ornamental fishes.

In the past, the principal food item for young fish has been brine shrimp or newly hatched brine shrimp nauplii, both of which are available from pet stores. These items are simply too large to be ingested by many larval fish, including many marine tropical species. Brine shrimp and newly hatched nauplii are acceptable foods for older fish and will likely be required in the culture of most tropical marine species. Brine shrimp can be reared in mass culture for feeding fish in commercial culture facilities (Sorgeloos, 1973; Persoone and Sorgeloos, 1975). Decapsulation is recommended prior to feeding brine shrimp newly hatched from commercially sold freeze-dried eggs. Decapsulation removes the hard outer layer (chorion) from the encapsulated embryo shrimp with a dilute hypochlorite solution (Campton and Busack, 1989). Decapsulated nauplii that do not hatch are still available as food, and decapsulation avoids fatal intestinal obstruction secondary to ingestion of shells by young fish.

Rearing rotifers as food for larval fishes is a more recent technology. Rotifer culture is much more complex than brine shrimp culture (Hirayama and Nakamura, 1976), but many larval fish can be fed rotifers until they are large enough to ingest brine shrimp.

LITERATURE CITED

Bauer, J.A., Jr., and Bauer, S.E. (1981) Reproductive biology of pigmy angelfishes of the genus *Centropyge* (Pomacanthidae). Bull. Marine Sci. 31:495–513.

Breder, C.M., and Rosen, D.E. (1966) Modes of Reproduction in Fishes. T.F.H. Publications, Neptune, New Jersey.

Campton, D.E., and Busack, C.A. (1989) Simple procedure for decapsulating and hatching cysts of brine shrimp (*Artemia* spp.). Progressive Fish Culturist 51:176–179.

Choat, J.H., and Robertson, D.R. (1975) Protogynous hermaphroditism in fishes in the family Scaridae. In: Intersexuality in The Animal Kingdom (Reinboth, R. ed.). Springer-Verlag, Berlin, pp. 263–283.

Erlich, P.R. (1975) The population biology of coral reef fishes. Annu. Rev. Ecol. Syst. 6:211–248.

Frakes, T.A., and Hoff, F.H. (1983) Mass propagation techniques currently being used in the spawning and rearing of marine fish species. Zoo Biol. 2:225–234.

Fricke, H., and Fricke, S. (1977) Monogamy and sex change by aggressive dominance in coral reef fish. Nature 266:830–832.

Hastings, P.A., and Petersen, C.W. (1986) A novel sexual reproductive pattern in serranid fishes: simultaneous hermaphrodites and secondary males in *Serranus fasciatus*. Environ. Biol. Fish. 15:59–68.

Hirayama, K., and Nakamura, K. (1976) Fundamental studies on the physiology of rotifers in mass culture—V. dry *Chlorella* powder as food for rotifers. Aquaculture 8:301–307.

Hoff, F., Rowell, C., and Pulver, T. (1972) Artificially induced spawning of the Florida pompano under controlled conditions. Proc. World Mariculture Soc. 3:53–64.

Johannes, R.E. (1978) Reproductive strategies of coastal marine fishes in the tropics. Environ. Biol. Fish 3(1):65–84.

Persoone, G., and Sorgeloos, P. (1975) Technological improvements for the cultivation of invertebrates as food for fishes and crustaceans. I. methods and devices. Aquaculture 6:275–289.

Petersen, C.W. (1987) Reproductive behavior and gender allocation in *Serranus fasciatus*, a hermaphroditic reef fish. Anim. Behav. 35:1601–1614.

Roberts, D.E., Harpster, B.V., and Henderson, G.E. (1978) Conditioning and induced spawning of the red drum, *Sciaenops ocellata*, under varied regimens of photoperiod and temperature. Proc. World Mariculture Soc. 9:311–332.

Ross, R.M. (1987) Sex-linked growth acceleration in a coral-reef fish, *Thalassoma duperrey*. J. Exp. Zool. 244:455–461.

Sorgeloos, P. (1973) High density culturing of brine shrimp. Aquaculture 1:385–391.

Thresher, R.E. (1984) Reproduction of Reef Fishes. T.F.H. Publications, Neptune, New Jersey.

Tucker, J.W. (1984) Hormone-induced ovulation in black sea bass. Progressive Fish Culturist 46(3):201–203.

Chapter 78

BACTERIAL DISEASES OF MARINE TROPICAL FISHES

MICHAEL K. STOSKOPF

The bacterial diseases of marine tropical fishes have been less extensively studied than those of the commercial food fishes. Bacterial isolates are commonly obtained from moribund or dead fish, but few studies have investigated the pathogenic potential of these organisms. Table 78–1 lists the bacterial diseases found in marine tropical fishes.

DAMSELFISH ULCER DISEASE

SYNONYMS. Ulcer disease, vibriosis, red sore disease.

Host and Geographic Distribution

The original isolation of *Vibrio damsela* was from the blacksmith, a Pacific damselfish found in southern California coastal waters (Love et al., 1981). Early efforts showed infections in wild populations to be relatively confined to the damselfishes. The opaleye and representatives of the silversides, blennies, sculpins, surfperches, and gobies were resistant to challenge (Love et al., 1981). However, this apparent host specificity may not be complete. The organism has been cultured from captive brown sharks originating from the Atlantic ocean and causes mortality in experimentally infected spiny dogfish (Grimes et al., 1984), but infections could not be reproduced in lemon sharks (Grimes et al., 1985). The organism has also been cultured from wounds of humans and bottlenose dolphins (Morris et al., 1982; Kreger, 1984; Fujioka et al., 1988).

Clinical Signs

This disease is characterized by deep skin ulcers that cause muscle destruction and may be as large as a centimeter in diameter. Ulcers usually are seen on the caudal peduncle and at the base of the pectoral fins. There are no serologic tests available.

Pathology and Diagnosis

The pathology associated with this infection is described primarily as deep granulomatous ulcerative dermatitis and myositis. The organism is highly cytotoxic. Diagnosis is based upon isolation and characterization of the causative organism.

Culture and Identification

Vibrio damsela can be cultured by swabbing material from an ulcer onto brain-heart infusion agar supplemented with 5% (v/v) sheep blood or onto thiosulfate citrate bile salt sucrose agar. At 25°C incubation requires 2 to 4 days for growth.

The organism is a weakly motile gram-negative pleomorphic rod. It produces acid from glucose, but not from arabinose, mannitol, or sucrose, in contrast to *V. anguillarum*. *Vibrio damsela* is β-galactosidase and lysine decarboxylase negative. It does not produce indole, degrade gelatin or lipids, and cannot utilize citrate or malonate.

TABLE 78–1. Bacterial Diseases of Marine Tropical Fishes*

Disease	Organism	Host
Damselfish ulcer disease	*Vibrio damsela*	Blacksmith, other damselfishes, sharks
Vibrio septicemia	*Vibrio alginolyticus*	Gilthead sea bream, marine angelfishes, striped mullet, grunts, pinfish, soldierfishes, squirrelfishes, other reef species
Streptococcosis	*Streptococcus* spp.	Pinfish, spot, striped mullet, bluefish, spotted sea trout, stingrays, rainbow trout, yellowtail, ayu, tilapia, Atlantic croaker, channel catfish, golden shiner, sea catfishes, menhaden, and other species
Red pest	*Vibrio anguillarum*	Salmonids, marine cold water species, marine tropical fishes, eels, striped bass

See also Chapters 24, 48, and 67.

Transmission and Epidemiology

A seasonal incidence of the disease is thought to coincide with warmer water temperatures. Ulcers have been recorded on between 10 and 70% of blacksmiths in a southern Californian yacht basin and at an island harbor site on Catalina Island, California, in the summer months. Experimental infections can be achieved in blacksmiths through scarification. Trials with several species of Pacific fishes suggests considerable host specificity.

Treatment and Control

Methods of treatment or control of this disease have not been published. The isolation of *Vibrio damsela* from infected human wounds indicates the potential for zoonotic transmission. The organism occurs normally in the marine environment.

VIBRIO SEPTICEMIA

SYNONYMS. Vibriosis, gas gut disease.

Host and Geographic Distribution

Vibrio alginolyticus has been isolated from marine waters routinely, including marine aquaria. An extensive mortality in cultured gilthead sea bream in Israel is the best documented occurrence of the disease (Colorni et al., 1981). The organism has been reported in striped mullet (Burke and Rodgers, 1981). It is commonly isolated from reef fishes dying with signs of generalized septicemia in large marine aquaria, including marine angelfishes, grunts, pinfish, soldierfishes, and squirrelfishes. There is no reason to believe that the organism is geographically restricted in marine waters. All marine fishes should be considered susceptible until otherwise demonstrated.

Clinical Signs

The clinical picture seen in fish from which this organism is cultured is one of a generalized bacterial septicemia. Lethargy, skin darkening, scale loss, and occasionally ulcers can be seen. Fish become anorectic and may develop abdominal distension due to gas and fluid accumulation in the intestines. Respiratory rate may be increased, and gills are sometimes pale if anemia is present.

Pathology and Diagnosis

At postmortem examination, the liver, intestines, swimbladder, and peritoneum are congested. The intestines are often distended with fluid. The gallbladder is distended. Anemia may be a feature, resulting in pale gills and making congestion of the other organs difficulty to appreciate. Granulomatous ulcerative dermatitis may be present.

A diagnosis is made by obtaining pure or relatively pure cultures of *V. alginolyticus* from affected organs. Serologic tests are not available.

Culture and Identification

Vibrio alginolyticus can be cultured on tryptone soya agar supplemented with seawater, incubating at 15 to 25°C for 2 to 7 days (Austin and Austin, 1987). The organism grows in swarming colonies. It produces hydrogen sulfide, degrades urea, and produces a positive methyl red test. It does not produce β-galactosidase or produce acid from arabinose. It does produce acid from salicin.

Transmission and Epidemiology

Vibrio alginolyticus is common in marine waters. Attempts to fulfill Koch's postulates have not been particularly successful when attempted. Mortalities are often recorded after extensive handling (Colorni et al., 1981) or when environmental conditions have deteriorated; however, disease also occurs when no environmental or handling pressures are apparent. The organism has been reported to be a secondary invader (Burke and Rodgers, 1981). Considerably more work must be done to clarify the role of this organism in fish disease.

Treatment and Control

The possible role of *V. alginolyticus* as a secondary invader makes control of environmental and other stressors an important potential means of control of the disease. Chloramphenicol, tetracyclines, nitrofurazone, and gentamicin have been reported to be successful in treating clinical diseases with signs compatible with a diagnosis of vibrio septicemia. The lack of clinical confirmation of diagnosis makes speculation about therapeutic efficacy somewhat moot.

STREPTOCOCCOSIS

SYNONYMS. Streptococcicosis, popeye, yellowtail disease.

Host and Geographic Distribution

This disease was originally described in rainbow trout in Japan (Hoshina et al., 1958). The disease is of economic importance in the Japanese eel, ayu, tilapia, and yellowtail industries, and much of the work on *Streptococcus* spp. has been done in Japan.

The disease is also important in rainbow trout farms in South Africa (Barham et al., 1979) and occurs sporadically in Great Britain, Norway, and the United States. It has been reported in a wide variety of marine fishes, including pinfish, spot, striped mullet, bluefish, Atlantic croaker, spotted sea trout, stingrays, sea catfishes, and gulf menhaden. It is known to cause a rapidly fatal disease in many tropical reef fishes, particularly butterflyfishes. Similar acute diseases, apparently due to infection with *Streptococcus* spp., occur in freshwater golden shiners and channel catfish.

Clinical Signs

The clinical signs of this disease vary tremendously among affected fish species and even different outbreaks in the same species. In marine tropical fishes, mortality is usually peracute. Often no premonitory signs are seen. Fish eat and behave normally up to within hours of death. Sometimes fish will exhibit erratic swimming and extreme disorientation followed rapidly by death.

In the salmonid, it is sometimes difficult to differentiate streptococcosis from bacterial kidney disease and enteric red mouth. Signs include exophthalmia, often with hemorrhage into the anterior chamber as is commonly seen in enteric red mouth disease. Abdominal distention is another common sign. Affected fish darken and swim erratically just under the water surface. The disease in salmonids can also be relatively devoid of signs. Fish may appear normal or just a bit sluggish before dying acutely.

In golden shiners, raised areas of inflammation can be seen on the sides and dorsal aspect of affected fish. In bluefish and spotted sea trout, the fish may not show any signs of illness, but large abscesses containing streptococcal organisms destroy the meat.

Pathology and Diagnosis

In tropical marine species, diagnosis may be complicated by the peracute nature of the disease. Gross examination of the fish may not reveal any visible abnormalities. In some cases, an enlarged and friable spleen and/or signs of vasculitis may be evident. Microscopic cocci in internal organ smears can be indicative. In salmonids, the liver, anus, and intestine are often congested. In some cases, the kidney is significantly swollen. Gram-positive cocci can be demonstrated in smears of spleen, liver, kidney, and heart. Necrosis of the kidney, heart, and liver can be demonstrated histologically. Severe destruction of the intestines, vascular system, and liver are seen. Renal tubules are frequently filled with degenerating tubular epithelial cells. Skin or external lesions are rare.

Finding of gram-positive cocci on tissue smears should be confirmed with culture and identification of the organism. No serologic diagnostic tests are routinely available.

Culture and Identification

It is apparent from reviewing the taxonomic characteristics of the *Streptococcus* spp. associated with disease in fish that several bacterial species and strains are involved. These are placed in the genus *Streptococcus* on the basis of serologic studies. However, serologic studies have not been adequate to remove the confusion about precise species and strain identification. Isolates from different outbreaks have been placed in Lancefield group B (Cook and Lofton, 1975) and Lancefield group D (Boomker et al., 1979). Some isolations have not corresponded with any of the established Lancefield groups. Even species classification has proven difficult. Organisms have been isolated from fish die-offs that approximate the identification criteria of *Streptococcus faecalis*, *S. equinus*, *S. lactis*, *S. casseliflavus*, the pediococci, and aerococci. Other isolates have not matched the descriptions of any of the 28 recognized species phenotypes.

Streptococci infecting fish can be grown on blood agar (bovine, ovine, or lapine). They grow in temperature ranges between 22 and 37°C, showing small gray 1- to 2-mm colonies in up to 48 hours. Strains pathogenic to fish have been α-hemolytic (Kusuda et al., 1976), β-hemolytic (Robinson and Meyer, 1966), or nonhemolytic (Plumb et al., 1974). They are gram-positive cocci, usually seen in short chains or pairs.

Transmission and Epidemiology

The source of the original outbreak in Japanese rainbow trout was thought to be from contaminated food. It is known that foodborne transmission can occur (Taniguchi, 1983). Streptococci are present in fresh and frozen fish used in diets and can survive 6 months or more in frozen meat (Minami, 1979). The organism can also be transmitted by contact with infected fish (Robinson and Meyer, 1966). Pathogenic streptococci can be found in the environment throughout the year, with higher numbers found in the sea in summer months and in mud samples in autumn and winter (Kitao et al., 1979).

That these organisms grow at high incubation temperatures implies a mammalian origin and may have importance when one is considering the zoonotic potential of the bacteria.

Treatment and Control

Control of disease due to *Streptococcus* spp. centers on good management, including prompt removal of diseased fish. Vaccination has been pursued, but results have been disappointing (Iida et al., 1982). Drug therapy has shown some success with salmonids, although the peracute nature of the disease in marine tropical fishes makes it unlikely that antibiotics will be delivered in time. In yellowtail, erythromycin has provided better results than oxytetracycline or ampicillin (Kitao, 1982), although oxytetracycline (Shiomitsu et al., 1980) and doxycycline (Nakamura, 1982) have been effective in other outbreaks. Success has been reported using sodium nifurstyrenate (50 mg/kg) in the face of an outbreak (Kashiwagi et al., 1977a,b).

RED PEST

SYNONYMS. Vibriosis, pestis rubra anguillarum, saltwater furunculosis, boil disease, ulcer disease, Hitra disease, erysipelosis anguillarum.

Host and Geographic Distribution

This disease should best be described in the chapters on bacterial diseases of marine coldwater fishes, salmonids, or eels. It was first described in the 1700's as a disease of European eels and has become an important disease in salmonids reared in saltwater as well as in cultured turbot and other mariculture species. Cultured striped bass and striped bass hybrids in culture are frequently affected with this disease. The causative organism, *Vibrio anguillarum*, also affects marine tropical species, including marine angelfishes and wrasses. Vibriosis due to *V. anguillarum* occurs worldwide in fresh water as well as marine water but is more common in saline water.

Clinical Signs

Fish affected with red pest frequently show erythema of the mouth, vent, and base of the fins, much like the appearance of enteric redmouth *(Yersinia ruckeri)*. In addition, necrotic skin lesions and red lesions in the abdominal muscles are usually present. Affected fish rarely feed and are lethargic and depressed.

Pathology and Diagnosis

Affected fish often have distended intestines filled with clear mucoid fluid. Bacteremia, with an enlarged spleen, is commonly seen at postmortem. Diagnosis is based on culture and identification of *Vibrio anguillarum* from blood, spleen, or kidney in combination with characteristic external lesions.

Culture and Identification

Culture of *V. anguillarum* is relatively simple. Salt-supplemented (0.5 to 3% W/V tryptone soya

agar, nutrient agar, or brain-heart infusion agars are suitable for isolation. Incubation at 15°C may require up to 7 days for sufficient growth to occur. The organism grows well at 25°C.

Colonies are round, raised, shiny, and usually off-white. Individual bacteria are gram-negative motile rods. The organism is positive for catalase, oxidase, indole, β-galactosidase, and arginine dihydrolase and does not produce hydrogen sulfide or urease. *Vibrio anguillarum* produces acid from arabinose, cellobiose, galactose, glycerol, maltose, mannitol, sorbitol, sucrose, and trehalose, but not from lactose, inositol, or xylose. More detailed descriptions of taxonomic features of *V. anguillarum* are given in specialized bacteriology texts (Austin and Austin, 1987).

Transmission and Epidemiology

Vibrio anguillarum is a nearly ubiquitous organism in marine environments, with higher levels being present in warmer water. Although controversial, it is still thought that initial colonization of fishes with the organism occurs through the anus, in the colon. There appears to be some degree of species specificity in that strains of *V. anguillarum* that cause disease in one host fish species will often not cause disease in other fish species.

Epidemics tend to occur in the summer or when tank water becomes warm and dissolved oxygen is decreased. Stress and overcrowding often are associated with an outbreak of disease, with high mortality. Other stressors, such as heavy metal exposure, particularly copper, can precipitate an outbreak. Debate continues over whether exotoxins and/or endotoxins are produced and play a part in the pathogenesis of the disease. It seems likely that debilitation of the host is a major factor in the initiation of the disease.

Treatment and Control

Commercial vaccines are available for this disease. Vaccinated fish appear to grow and survive better than their unvaccinated counterparts, but the exact nature of the immunity conferred is not well characterized. Most products are bivalent vaccines containing formalin-killed cells of both *V. anguillarum* and *V. ordalii*. They are usually administered by immersion, although injectable vaccines are available, as are oral vaccines. Success with oral vaccines has been less good than that with injectable or immersion vaccines. Sonicated, heat-killed vaccines are also available and effective. Chemotherapeutic management of the disease is limited because of the usual lack of appetite in affected fish. Many strains have developed resistance to chloramphenicol, streptomycin, sulfonamides, and tetracycline.

LITERATURE CITED

Austin, B., and Austin, D.A. (1987) Bacterial Fish Pathogens: Disease in Farmed and Wild Fish. John Wiley & Sons, New York.

Barham, W.T., Schoonbee, H., and Smit, G.L. (1979) The occurrence of *Aeromonas* and *Streptococcus* in rainbow trout *(Salmo gairdneri).* J. Fish Biol. 15:457–460.

Boomker, J., Imes, G.D., Cameron, C.M., Naude, T.W., and Schoonbee, H.J. (1979) Trout mortalities as a result of *Streptococcus* infection. Onderstepoort J. Vet. Res. 46:71–77.

Burke, J., and Rodgers, L. (1981) Identification of pathogenic bacteria associated with the occurrence of "red spot" in sea mullet, *Mugil cephalus* L., in south-eastern Queensland. J. Fish Dis. 3:153–159.

Colorni, A., Paperna, I., and Gordin, H. (1981) Bacterial infections in gilthead sea bream *Sparus aurata* cultured at Elat. Aquaculture 23:257–267.

Cook, D.W., and Lofton, S.R. (1975) Pathogenicity studies with a *Streptococcus* sp. isolated from fishes in an Alabama-Florida fish kill. Trans. Am. Fish. Soc. 104:286–288.

Fujioka, R.S., Greco, S.B., Cates, M.B., and Schroeder, J.P. (1988) *Vibrio damsela* from wounds in bottlenose dolphins *Tursiops truncatus.* Dis. Aquatic Organ. 4:1–8.

Grimes, D.J., Stemmler, J., Hada, H., May, E.B., Maneval, D., Hetrick, F.M., Jones, R.T., Stoskopf, M., and Colwell, R.R. (1984) *Vibrio* species associated with mortality of sharks held in captivity. Microbiol. Ecol. 10:271–282.

Grimes, D.J., Gruber, S.H., and May, E.B. (1985) Experimental infection of lemon sharks, *Negaprion brevirostris* (Poey), with *Vibrio* species. J. Fish Dis. 8:173–180.

Hoshina, T., Sano, T. and Morimoto, Y. (1958) A *Streptococcus* pathogenic to fish. J. Tokyo Univ. Fish. 44:57–58.

Iida, T., Wakabayashi, H., and Egusa, S. (1982) Vaccination for control of streptococcal disease in cultured yellowtail. Fish Pathol. 16:201–206.

Kashiwagi, S., Sugimoto, N., Watanabe, O., Ohta, S., and Kusuda, R. (1977a) Chemotherapeutical studies on sodium nifurstyrenate against *Streptococcus* infection in cultured yellowtail I. In vitro studies on sensitivity and bacteriocidal effects. Fish Pathol. 12:11–14.

Kashiwagi, S., Sugimoto, N., Ohta, S., and Kusuda, R. (1977b) Chemotherapeutical studies on sodium nifurstyrenate against *Streptococcus* infection in cultured yellowtail. II. Effect of sodium nifurstyrenate against experimental streptococcal infection. Fish Pathol. 12:157–162.

Kitao, H. (1982) Erythromycin—the application to streptococcal infection in yellowtails. Fish Pathol. 17:77–85.

Kitao, T., Aoki, T., and Iwata, K. (1979) Epidemiological study on streptococcosis of cultured yellowtail *(Seriola quinquiradiata).* 1. Distribution of *Streptococcus* sp. in sea water and muds around yellowtail farms. Bull. Jpn. Soc. Sci. Fish. 45:567–572.

Kreger, A.S. (1984) Cytolytic activity and virulence of *Vibrio damsela.* Infect. Immun. 44:326–331.

Kusuda, R., Kawai, T., Toyoshima, T., and Komatsu, I. (1976) A new pathogenic bacterium belonging to the genus *Streptococcus,* isolated from an epizootic of cultured yellowtail. Bull. Jpn. Soc. Sci. Fish. 42:1345–1352.

Love, M., Teebken-Fisher, D., Hose, J.E., Farmer, J.J. III, Hickman, F.W., and Fanning, G.R. (1981) *Vibrio damsela,* a marine bacterium, causes skin ulcers on the damselfish *Chromis punctipinnis.* Science 214:1139–1140.

Minami, T. (1979) *Streptococcus* sp. pathogenic to cultured yellowtail, isolated from fishes for diets. Fish Pathol. 14:15–19.

Morris, J.G., Wilson, R., Hollis, D.G., Weaver, R.E., Miller, H.G., Tacket, C.O., Hickman, F.W., and Blake, P.A. (1982) Illness caused by *Vibrio damsela* and *Vibrio hollisae.* Lancet 1:1294–1297.

Nakamura, Y. (1982) Doxycycline. Fish Pathol. 17:67–76.

Plumb, J.A., Schachte, J.H., Gaines, J.L., Peltier, W., and Carrol, B. (1974) *Streptococcus* sp from marine fishes along the Alabama and northwest Florida coast of the Gulf of Mexico. Trans. Am. Fish. Soc. 103:358–361.

Robinson, J.A., and Meyer, F.P. (1966) Streptococcal fish pathogen. J. Bacteriol. 92:512.

Shiomitsu, K., Kusuda, R., Osuga, H., and Munekiyo, M. (1980) Studies on chemotherapy of fish disease with erythromycin.—II. Its clinical studies against streptococcal infection in cultured yellowtails. Fish Pathol. 15:17–23.

Taniguchi, M. (1983) Progress of streptococcosis in peroral inoculation. Bull. Jpn. Soc. Sci. Fish. 49:1171–1174.

Chapter 79

FUNGAL DISEASES OF MARINE TROPICAL FISHES

RENATE REIMSCHUESSEL

Table 79–1 lists the fungal diseases covered in this chapter.

EXOPHIALIOSIS

SYNONYMS.   *Exophiala* spp., sea horse disease.

Host and Geographic Distribution

Exophiala species have been reported in fish held in both fresh and saltwater (Richards et al., 1978; Fijan, 1969; Carmichael, 1966). An *Exophiala* sp. resembling *E. jeanselmei* has been reported in northern sea horses, and sargassum triggerfish among the marine tropical fishes, and probably can affect other species (Blazer and Wolke, 1979). A similar fungus, *E. pisciphila,* has not been reported in free-ranging fish, only in captive specimens. It has been incriminated as the cause of an epizootic in channel catfish (Fijan, 1969) and may affect salmonids, although the organism *E. salmonis* is considered the pathogen of salmonids.

Clinical Signs

In affected sea horses, the primary clinical sign is lethargy, with the appearance of nonulcerative

TABLE 79–1. Fungal Diseases of Marine Tropical Fishes

Disease	Organism	Host
Exophialiosis	*Exophiala* spp.	Northern sea horse, sargassum triggerfish
Ichthyophoniasis	*Ichthyophonus hoferi*	Many species

*See Chapters 25, 37, and 68.

dermal masses externally. Disorientation and abnormal swimming may also be noted.

Diagnosis

Diagnosis is based on identification of typical fungal elements in histologic sections (Fig. 79–1) or by culture and identification of the organism. No serologic tests are available.

Pathology

Internal lesions due to *Exophiala* spp. in marine tropical fishes appear as raised, white to yellow areas that can be found on multiple organs, but most frequently the liver. They can be raised but more often are slightly depressed. Histologically the inflammatory reaction can be classified as either acute nonproliferative or chronic proliferative. The early acute response consists of necrosis with heterophil and macrophage invasion; in experimental infections little or no inflammatory response may occur, and only necrosis will be evident. Hyphae can be distinguished in the tissues. Chronic cases have lesions characterized by granuloma formation with central necrosis and mineralization. These lesions resemble mycobacteriosis.

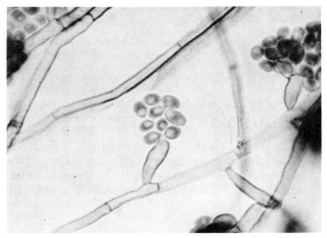

FIGURE 79–1. Wet mount of *Exophiala pisciphila* showing conidia (1900×). (Courtesy of L. Ajello. From Neish, F.A., and Hughes, G.A. [1980] Diseases of Fishes: Book 6: Fungal Diseases of Fishes. [Snieszko, S.F., and Axelrod, H.R., eds.]. T.F.H. Publications, Neptune, New Jersey, p. 107.)

Culture and Identification

Exophiala spp. are imperfect fungi (Deuteromycetes) in the Hyphomycetes class. These fungi produce yellow-brown, subglobose to ovoid conidia on an annellide. The ends of these annelloconidia are rounded and truncate at the proximal end. The hyphae are aseptate, 2 by 3 to 5 μm long. *Exophiala pisciphila* can be grown at 25°C on potato-dextrose, cereal, or V–8 juice agar. Black or gray colonies 25 to 28 mm in diameter appear in 14 days. They do not grow well on Sabouraud's agar.

Transmission, Epidemiology, Pathogenesis, Treatment, and Control

Little is known of the transmission, epidemiology, or pathogenesis of this disease. No effective treatment or control measures are reported for *Exophiala* infections.

ICHTHYOPHONIASIS

SYNONYMS.   *Ichthyophonus hoferi*, ichthyophonosis, Traummelkrankheit, reeling disease, sandpaper disease.

Host and Geographic Distribution

By far the most commonly reported marine fungal pathogen is *Ichthyophonus hoferi*. Other species have, however, been reported in marine and estuarine fishes. Oomycetes, *Saprolegnia*, and *Aphanomyces* were isolated from the Atlantic menhaden (Noga and Dykstra, 1986). Oomycetes are usually responsible for superficial dermal mycotic infections of freshwater fish. Lesions in the menhaden were also dermal but extended into the muscles, and sometimes into the peritoneal cavity. The microscopic host reaction was an intense chronic inflammatory response with the development of granulomas.

Clinical Signs

Clinical signs may include corkscrew swimming or other abnormal swimming patterns, but this is less common in marine tropical species than in salmonids. In fine-scaled species, a granular, rough appearance to the skin may be evident from multiple small subcutaneous granulomas. The appetite usually remains good until the terminal stages of the disease. Lethargy or listlessness may be noted. Some fish will develop a dark color on the lateral line, which progresses to complete darkening. The variability in clinical signs is undoubtedly related to the site of the fungal invasion.

Diagnosis

Ichthyophonus hoferi is a well known marine fungal pathogen of an uncertain class. The genus has a complicated taxonomic history that has been well described (Wolke, 1975; Neish and Hughes, 1980; Alderman, 1982; McVicar, 1982).

The organism has a prominent "resting spore" stage. It is a spherical, thick-walled multinucleated cell varying from 10 to 250 μm in diameter. The nuclei are 2 to 4 μm in diameter. The cytoplasm contains glycogen and is PAS-positive (periodic acid–Schiff stain). The spore wall, which contains polysaccharides, is also strongly PAS-positive and ranges in thickness from 2 to 11 μm. Its thickness may be a function of host response. No serologic diagnostic tests are available.

Pathology

Infected fish often have white nodules in affected organs and connective tissue (Gartner and Zwerner, 1988; Neish and Hughes, 1980; Wolke, 1975). A severe focal granulomatous response is common. Organs rich in blood supply appear to be most frequently affected, although any organ can harbor the organism. Microscopically, the spores are usually surrounded by mononuclear cells, macrophages, and fibroblasts (McVicar and McLay, 1985; McVicar, 1982; Neish and Hughes, 1980). Macrophages may contain phagocytosed endospores. Multinucleated giant cells, heterophils, eosinophilic granular cells, and melanin deposition occur in lesions in some fish species (McVicar and McLay, 1985).

Culture and Identification

Some of the variation in developmental stages found in the literature may be due to differing culture conditions and nutrients (McVicar, 1982). The fungus grows on Sabouraud's dextrose medium supplemented with 1% beef serum incubated at 10°C.

Most authors agree that *Ichthyophonus hoferi* has a simple life cycle, with no sexual reproduction. Multinucleated spores subdivide into smaller endospores either by formation of hyphae or by rupture (Fig. 79–2). The spores germinate, especially rapidly after death, producing hyphae of varying numbers. Cytoplasm from the spore moves into the hyphae,

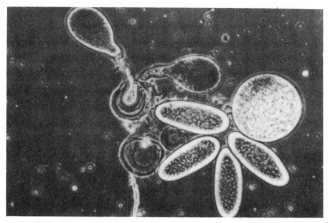

FIGURE 79–2. *Ichthyophonus* sp. germinating with the formation of hyphal bodies in culture (wet mount). (From McVicar, A.H. [1982] *Ichthyophonus* infections of fish. In: Microbial Diseases of Fish. [Roberts, R.J., ed.]. Academic Press, New York, p. 254.)

undergoes endogenous cleavage, and produces daughter spores that vary in size and the number of nuclei. Other methods of reproduction have been described. Formation of daughter spores that are released by rupture of the resting spore, without formation of hyphae, has been noted. Rupture of the resting spore, releasing nuclei and bits of cytoplasm that develop walls, is also known (Daniel, 1933; Fish, 1934). Division at the tips of cytoplasmic tubes can produce numerous small hyphal bodies (endospores), which have been noted both in infected tissues (Dorier and Degrange, 1961) and *in vitro* (McVicar, 1982). Several authors have observed ameboid movement of the endospores (McVicar, 1982). Conidia-like bodies in marine fish have also been reported (Reichenback-Klinke, 1956).

Transmission, Epidemiology, and Pathogenesis

The mode of transmission is most likely ingestion of food containing infective spores (Chien et al., 1979; Dorier and Degrange, 1961; Sindermann and Scattergood, 1954). Once the endospores are released they are disseminated throughout the body. These then develop into the larger multinucleated spores and resting spores. Spores are frequently found in heart, kidney, liver, muscle, and skin.

Treatment and Control

There are no chemotherapeutic measures documented for this disease. Good hygiene and pasteurization of potentially infected food is used as a preventive measure. Removal of dead or dying fish from aquaria prevents ingestion of infective spores.

LITERATURE CITED

Alderman, D.J. (1982) Fungal diseases of aquatic animals. In: Microbial Diseases of Fish. (Roberts, R.J., ed.). Academic Press, New York, pp. 189–242.

Blazer, V.S., and Wolke, R.E. (1979) An *Exophiala*-like fungus as the cause of a systemic mycosis of marine fish. J. Fish Dis. 2:145–152.

Carmichael, J.W. (1966) Cerebral mycetoma of trout due to a *Phialophora*-like fungus. Sabouraudia 5:120–123.

Chien, C., Miyazaki, T., and Kubota, S.S. (1979) Studies on *Ichthyophonus* disease of fishes. VI. Artificial infection. Bulletin of the Faculty of Fisheries, Mie University 6:153–159.

Daniel, G. (1933) Studies on *Ichthyophonus hoferi*, a parasitic fungus of the herring *(Clupea harengus)*. I. The parasite as it is found in the herring. Am. J. Hyg. 17:267–276.

Dorier, A., and Degrange, C. (1961) L'evolution de l'*Ichthyosporidium (Ichthyophonus) hoferi* (Plehn et Mulsow) chez les salmonides d'elevage (truite arc-en-ciel et saumon de fontaine). Trav. Lab Hydrobiol. Piscic. Univ. Grenoble 1960/1961:7–44.

Fijan, N. (1969) Systemic mycosis in channel catfish. Bull. Wildl. Dis. Assoc. 5:109–110.

Fish, F.F. (1934) A fungus disease in fishes of the Gulf of Maine. Parasitology 26:1–16.

Gartner, J.V., Jr., and Zwerner, D.E. (1988) An *Ichthyophonus*-type fungus in the deep-sea pelagic fish *Scopelogadus beanii* (Gunther) (Pisces:Melanmphaidae): pathology, geographic distribution and ecological implications. J. Fish Biol. 32:459–470.

McVicar, A.H. (1982) *Ichthyophonus* infections of fish. In: Microbial Diseases of Fish. (Roberts, R.J., ed.). Academic Press, New York, pp. 242–269.

McVicar, A.H., and McLay, H.A. (1985) Tissue response of plaice, haddock, and rainbow trout to the systemic fungus *Ichthyophonus*. In: Fish and Shellfish Pathology. (Ellis, A.E., ed.). Academic Press, New York, pp. 329–346.

Neish, B.A., and Hughes, G.C. (1980) Diseases of Fishes. Book 6: Fungal Diseases of Fishes. (Snieszko, S.F., and Axelrod, H.R., eds.). T.F.H. Publications, Neptune, New Jersey.

Noga, E.J., and Dykstra, M.J. (1986) Oomycete fungi associated with ulcerative mycosis in menhaden, *Brevoortia tyrannus* (Latrobe). J. Fish Dis. 9:47–53.

Reichenback-Klinke, H.H. (1956) Die vermehrungsformer des zoophagen pilzes *Ichthyosporidium hoferi* (Plehn and Mulsow) (Fungi, Phycomycetes) in wirt. Veroff. Inst. Meeresforsch, Bremerh 4:214–219.

Richards, R.H., Holliman, A., and Helgason, S. (1978) Naturally occurring *Exophiala salmonis* infection in Atlantic salmon *(Salmo salar* L.) J. Fish Dis. 1:357–369.

Sindermann, C.J., and Scattergood, L.W. (1954) Diseases of fishes of the western North Atlantic. II. *Ichthyosporidium* disease of the sea herring *(Clupea harengus)*. Res. Bull. Dept. Sea Shore Fish. Me. 19:1–40.

Wolke, R.E. (1975) Pathology of bacterial and fungal diseases affecting fish. In: The Pathology of Fishes. (Ribelin, W.E., and Migaki, G., eds.). University of Wisconsin Press, Madison, Wisconsin, pp. 33–116.

Chapter 80

MARINE TROPICAL FISH VIRUSES

PHILIP E. McALLISTER   MICHAEL K. STOSKOPF

Although several viral diseases are suspected in marine tropical fishes (Table 80–1), few efforts have been undertaken to characterize them. Undoubtedly more viral diseases of marine fishes will be discovered and characterized as more sophisticated efforts are brought to marine tropical fish medicine.

TIGER PUFFER VIRUS

SYNONYM. *Kuchihiro-sho.*

Host and Geographic Distribution

An ulcerative disease, known as *kuchihiro-sho*, occurs in young, cultured tiger puffers in Kagoshima and Nagasaki Prefectures (Japan) (Nakauchi et al., 1985; Wada et al., 1986). The disease has not been reported elsewhere.

Clinical Signs and Pathology

The disease is characterized by eroded ulcers that occur on the mouth and snout (Nakauchi et al., 1985; Wada et al., 1986). In addition to the ulcerative lesions, affected fish are dark and develop aggressive biting behavior. Internally, a linear superficial hemorrhage occurs in the liver. Pathologic changes include epithelial desquamation, hyperplasia of melanophores, and congestion of the dermis. Secondary bacterial invasion of the ulcers also occurs. Degenerative changes are seen in the nerve cells of the eighth to tenth cranial nerves and in the supramedullary neuron. Affected nerve cells show distortion of the nucleus, condensation of chromatin and nucleoli, karyolysis, and formation of intranuclear inclusion bodies. Degenerative changes in the medulla oblongata occur in conjunction with necrosis of affected nerve cells.

Diagnosis

The disease is presumptively diagnosed by correlating clinical signs and species. The diagnosis is confirmed by isolation of virus in cell culture and by visualizing appropriately sized viral particles in electron micrographs of nerve cells.

TABLE 80–1. Viral Diseases of Marine Fishes*

Disease	Virus	Host
Tiger puffer ulcer disease (*Kuchihiro-sho*)	Tiger puffer virus	Tiger puffer
Lymphocystis	Lymphocystis virus	Over 125 species
Viral erythrocytic necrosis	Erythrocytic necrosis virus	Wrasses, comb-toothed blennies
Infectious pancreatic necrosis	Infectious pancreatic necrosis virus	Over 20 species
Angelfish encephalitis	Uncharacterized rhabdovirus	Gray angelfish French angelfish
Tang fingerprint disease	Uncharacterized	Blue tang Ocean surgeon Doctorfish

See also Chapters 26, 38, and 99.

Virus Detection and Identification

Although virus has been isolated in cell culture, kuchihiro-sho was initially designated as a viral infection based on electron microscopic observations (Wada et al., 1985). Thin sections of affected nerve cells show viruslike particles 110 to 140 nm in diameter, arrayed in aggregates adjacent to an intranuclear inclusion and scattered along the nuclear membrane. The viruslike particles have not been assigned to a taxonomic grouping.

Virus can be isolated using PFG cells incubated at 20°C; cytopathic changes are seen in cells inoculated with homogenates of brain and kidney after about 20 days of incubation (Inoue et al., 1986). No serologic tests for virus identification have been described.

Transmission, Epizootiology, and Pathogenesis

Tiger puffers can be experimentally infected, using tissue extracts from infected fish or using medium from cell culture virus assays. Challenged fish develop the same clinical signs and histopathologic changes seen in naturally infected fish (Wada et al., 1986). The incubation time to mortality decreases with increasing titer of virus inoculum (Inoue et al., 1986). Under natural conditions, the disease is presumably transmitted horizontally by waterborne and contact exposure.

Treatment and Control

No methods for treatment or control have been described.

LYMPHOCYSTIS (see also Chap. 26)

SYNONYM. Lymphocystis disease.

Hosts and Geographic Distribution

Lymphocystis occurs in marine and freshwater fishes. In marine tropicals, it is by far more common in the angelfishes, although it is also seen in wrasses, grunts, pinfish, puffers, boxfish, porcupinefishes, snappers, porgies, drums, goatfishes, scats, butterflyfishes, blennies, and gobies. It appears to have a very wide host range. The geographic range is probably global.

Clinical Signs and Pathology

The virus induces hypertrophied cells that form unsightly nodular tumorlike growths, frequently described as pearl-like. These growths do not always have the classic white hyaline appearance of pearls, but they can be cream-colored, brown, or gray. If massive, they can show redness due to vascularity. Internal manifestations are very uncommon, although concomitant infection with other viruses is common. Affected fish may show no behavioral aberrations. Lesions on the mouth may cause difficulty in feeding.

Histologic diagnosis is based on finding large nonneoplastic-appearing hypertrophied dermal fibroblasts that may be up to 2 mm in diameter. The nuclei of these cells are enlarged proportionally, and the cells are surrounded by hyaline layers. Affected cells contain large basophilic cytoplasmic inclusion bodies, which are often horseshoe-shaped and contain viral particles. The size of the viral particles appears to vary considerably, depending on the species of fish involved.

Diagnosis

Lymphocystis lesions must be differentiated from chlamydial epitheliocystis in which the nucleus of affected cells is pushed peripherally; clusters of trematode cysts with moving trematodes; or dermal sarcoma virus lesions, which consist of solid masses of normal-sized cells with cytoplasmic inclusions. Often, occasional ciliates or other protozoa are found in squash smear preparations of lymphocystis lesions, but these are not thought to be involved in the pathogenesis of the disease. Instead, they are considered incidental findings. A mixed inflammatory response is common.

Virus Detection and Identification

Lymphocystis is caused by an iridovirus or family of morphologically similar iridoviruses.

Transmission, Epizootiology, and Pathogenesis

Carrier states are postulated, but nothing is known about transmission. Lymphocystis is commonly found on fish that are compromised by other problems, particularly stressful environmental or behavioral problems.

Treatment and Control

Although lymphocystis lesions are unsightly, they rarely endanger the fish directly. An exception would be proliferations around the mouth or eyes, which can become large enough to interfere with feeding. In these cases, the hypertrophied tumors can be surgically removed under anesthesia and the area carefully cauterized with povidone-iodine compounds. The ocular form of this disease affects the choroid coat of the eye and does not appear operable. Unless conditions stressing the fish are altered, surgical treatment will only be a temporary measure, and the masses frequently return.

If the lesions are not interfering with feeding, a conservative course is recommended because the disease is self-limiting if stressful conditions are alleviated. Examples of stressors include social conditions, water quality, and filtration problems. The remission of lymphocystis involves complete involution of the lesions with no residual scar. Recrudescence is probable if conditions are allowed to become stressful again.

VIRAL ERYTHROCYTIC NECROSIS

SYNONYMS. VEN, piscine erythrocytic necrosis (PEN), erythrocytic necrosis virus (ENV).

Hosts and Geographic Distribution

In tropical marine species, viral erythrocytic necrosis (VEN) has been confirmed in wrasses and the comb-toothed blennies. It may affect other reef fishes as well.

Clinical Signs and Pathology

This disease is characterized by pale gills and pale visceral organs. Blood from affected fish clots slowly, if at all, and low hematocrits are seen. Hematopoietic tissue is usually hyperactive when examined histologically. Circulating erythrocytes are affected, usually showing a small eosinophilic inclusion in the cytoplasm and a vacuolated or degenerating nucleus.

Diagnosis

The disease is diagnosed by staining blood films with Giemsa-based stain and finding the distinct eosinophilic cytoplasmic inclusions. Confirmation is based on electron microscopy of the inclusions revealing icosahedral virions. A method for electron microscopic diagnosis using lysed erythrocytes has been published (Smail and Egglestone, 1980).

Virus Detection and Identification

The virus is a cytoplasmic icosahedral DNA virus that is considered an iridovirus, although it has not been isolated in cell culture. In different hosts, the virus is dramatically different in size (150 to 500 nm). The largest virus is reported in the only report of the disease in a shark (see Chaps. 88 and 99).

Transmission, Epizootiology, and Pathogenesis

Transmission is thought to be waterborne, but other means have not been excluded. The incubation period ranges between 5 and 30 days. It is more common for young fish to be infected.

Treatment and Control

No treatment or control measures are reported.

INFECTIOUS PANCREATIC NECROSIS

Hosts and Geographic Distribution

An infectious pancreatic necrosis–like virus has been isolated from several species of tropical Caribbean reef fish maintained at 78°F. Infectious pancreatic necrosis (IPN) is an acute, highly contagious viral disease, which has been best characterized in salmonids maintained in intensive rearing facilities.

Clinical Signs and Pathology

Affected marine tropical fish die relatively acutely but do not show classic pancreatic necrosis. Signs in affected fishes include anorexia followed by acute onset of disorientation, swimming upside-down, and lethargy. Ascites is a component of the disease in many cases. Petechial hemorrhages at the bases of fins occur frequently. Although classic necrosis of the pancreas is not noted, epithelial slough-ing in the gut is present.

Diagnosis

Diagnosis is based upon isolation of the virus from gut tissue.

Virus Detection and Identification

The virus, indistinguishable from IPN virus on the basis of in vitro testing, will grow on a variety of cell lines and gives every indication of having an extremely wide range of host infectability. It has not been tested for virulence against salmonids.

Transmission, Epizootiology, and Pathogenesis

No work has been done on the viruses isolated from marine tropical species. (See Chapter 38 for information about the virus that infects salmonids.) The disease should be considered a potential differ-ential in diagnosing acute, high-mortality diseases associated with equilibrium loss in marine tropicals, particularly if salmonids are maintained in the same or nearby facilities.

Treatment and Control

No therapeutic or control measures are known.

ANGELFISH ENCEPHALITIS

SYNONYM. Angelfish rhabdovirus infection.

Hosts and Geographic Distribution

This disease was first described in 1983 in adult gray angelfish and French angelfish collected in the Florida Keys and placed in a large, closed-system, artificial reef. The disease was seen again in 1984 and 1985, but was not a factor in the collection in 1986 or 1987.

Clinical Signs and Pathology

Clinically affected animals become anorectic and lethargic and display the milky appearance of excess mucus secretion. Subsequently, they lose equilibrium and die.

Diagnosis

Diagnosis is based upon virus isolation from explanted brain or kidney tissue.

Virus Detection and Identification

A rhabdovirus has been cultured from kidney and brain. This virus is unusual for fish rhabdovi-ruses because in culture it is warm adapted, growing best above 72°C. No reinfectivity studies have been performed.

Transmission, Epizootiology, and Pathogenesis

No information on the pathogenesis or epizo-otiology is currently available.

Treatment and Control

No treatment or control method is known.

TANG FINGERPRINT DISEASE

Hosts and Geographic Distribution

Similar symptoms have been seen in the blue tang, ocean surgeon, and doctorfish collected from the Florida Keys.

Clinical Signs and Pathology

The lesions resemble fingerprints, and in early cases, first identified in recently caught and shipped fish, there was suspicion that they were skin lesions due to careless handling of the fish. Later, the disease was seen to occur spontaneously during stressful periods. Careful histologic examination of the skin in the areas showing discoloration have been unfruit-ful. Affected fish initially continue to feed and behave relatively normally.

Diagnosis

Diagnosis is currently based upon the character-istic clinical signs of skin lesions, which appear as large oval discolorations on the sides of the fish.

Virus Detection and Identification

This disease is only suspected to be of viral etiology on the basis of epidemiology and the failure to identify any other agent. The virus has NOT been isolated. It received its name because of the characteristic appearance of a mottled patch bilaterally on the dorsal body of affected fish.

Treatment and Control

If overcrowding or water-quality problems are corrected, spontaneous recovery is common. If the syndrome is ignored in a system, morbidity will approach 100% within a few days. Mortalities do occur, possibly due to secondary infections and other complications, although alternate causes of death are not always identifiable. Oral antibiotic therapy with chloramphenicol or tetracycline does not appreciably affect the course of the disease. To date, the only management of the disease is to correct environmental and social stresses, in which case, the disease

tends to be self-limiting with minimal loss and no permanent scarring.

LITERATURE CITED

Inoue, K., Yasumoto, S., Yasunaga, N., and Takami, I. (1986) Isolation of a virus from cultured tiger puffer, *Takifugu rubripes*, infected with "Kuchijiro-sho" and its pathogenicity. Fish Pathol. 21:129–130.
Nakauchi, R., Miyazaki, T., and Shiomitsu, T. (1985) A histopathological study on "Kuchijiro-sho" of tiger puffer. Fish Pathol. 20:475–479.
Smail, D. A., and Egglestone, S. I. (1980) Virus infections of marine fish erythrocytes: electron microscopical studies on the blenny virus. J. Fish Dis. 3:47–54
Wada, S., Fujimake, Y., Hatai, K., Kubota, S.S., and Isoda, M. (1985) Histopathological findings of cultured tiger puffer *Takifugu rubripes* naturally infected with "Kuchijiro-sho." Fish Pathol. 20:495–500.
Wada, S., Hatai, K., Kubota, S.S., Inoue, K., and Yasunaga, N. (1986) Histopathological findings of tiger puffer, *Takifugu rubripes*, artificially infected with "Kuchijiro-sho." Fish Pathol. 21:101–104.

Chapter 81

PARASITIC DISEASES OF MARINE TROPICAL FISHES

PAUL CHEUNG

Rapid breathing, panting, scratching, fraying of fins, gray dusty appearance of the skin, white spots, black spots, cloudy cornea, bloody eyes, extravasation, and ulcerations are all common observable external signs of ectoparasitic infestations in aquarium fishes. Some of the same distressing signs can be induced by adverse environmental factors, such as a change in pH, salinity, dissolved oxygen, carbon dioxide, ammonia, nitrite, nitrate, organic matter, or heavy metal levels. This chapter considers several of the most important protozoan and metazoan diseases of marine tropical fishes, including detail about the life cycle and morphologic characteristics of the parasites.

Ectoparasites on the skin and gills of fish are infectious and can often inflict severe damage and high mortality on fish maintained in tanks and aquaria, but the signs of different parasitic infections can be quite similar. Thus, correct identification of the parasite involved is important in prescribing suitable treatments to control parasitic diseases. Skin scrapings and gill biopsies of infected individual fish should be examined under the compound microscope to confirm a diagnosis. On the other hand, endoparasitic infections are difficult to diagnose ex-

cept by inference from pathologic examinations. At the present time, information on endoparasitism is scanty, especially for parasites that require intermediate hosts. Many endoparasitic diseases are often well tolerated by the fish host if the initial exposure to infective stages of the parasite is low enough to allow the fish to develop immunity.

DISEASES CAUSED BY AMEBA

Information on amebic parasites in tropical marine fishes is lacking, but there is no reason to suspect that this group of fishes would not on occasion harbor these protozoa. Certainly the parasites are known to occur in other marine fishes. Examples include *Entamoeba gadi* in pollock from the Atlantic (Bullock, 1966) and *E. molae* in ocean sunfish from the Pacific (Noble and Noble, 1966). These *Entamoeba* are endocommensals in the digestive tract causing no apparent damage. More recently, *Paramoeba pemaguidensis* was incriminated as the cause of severe gill damage and epithelial hyperplasia in seawater-reared coho salmon in Washington (Kent, 1988). This gill ameba is resistant to formalin, copper sulfate, and malachite green treatment but can be eradicated by reducing salinity to 10 ppt. Similar parasites may be found in marine tropical species.

DISEASES CAUSED BY FLAGELLATES

Amyloodinium

Ectoparasitic flagellates infesting marine tropical fishes belong to the family Blastodiniidae, in which two genera of dinoflagellates, *Amyloodinium* and *Crepidoodinium*, are serious pathogens. *Amyloodinium ocellatum (Oodinium ocellatum)* is a ubiquitous parasitic dinoflagellate, infecting gills and skin of tropical marine and estuarine fishes (Brown, 1951, 1963; Brown and Hovasse, 1946). Detailed morphology, cytology, life history, and the ultrastructure of the attachment rhizoids and surface structures of various stages of the parasite are known (Nigrelli, 1936; Brown and Hovasse, 1946; Lom and Lawler, 1973).

The fish skin infested with *A. ocellatum* appears dusty with characteristic gray patches often referred to as "velvet disease." Heavily infested fish show frequent flashing and hemorrhage of the skin. Fish with *A. ocellatum* infestation in their gills show feeble movement and rapid breathing characteristic of hypoxic fish. Pathologic features include depletion of mucous cells (Papperna, 1980), extensive cellular damage due to rhizoid penetration of infected cells (Lom and Lawler, 1973), and epithelial irritation.

The life cycle of *A. ocellatum* is shown in Figure 81–1. The parasitic trophonts (feeding stage) are nonmotile and attach to gills or skin with rhizoids that penetrate deep into the epithelium. Trophonts leave by undergoing encystment and division. Rhizoids and stomopodes are gradually retracted into the parasite and a cellular cap secreted to seal the cyst. When this process is completed, division is initiated. The encysted, or palmella, stage represents the reproductive phase of the life cycle of *Amyloodinium*. The first division forms a two-cell stage 10 to 15 hours after encystment. Subsequent divisions occur synchronously to produce 256 active, swimming, oval dinospores, measuring about 12×8 μm. These dinospores have the red pigment bar and two flagella (transverse and sulcal) characteristic of dinoflagellates. The dinospore lacks armored structures and appears smooth.

Under natural conditions a free-swimming dinospore invades the branchial chamber of the fish, becomes attached to a gill filament, and metamorphoses into the parasitic trophont. The rate of encystment, reproduction, and subsequent excystment is temperature- and salinity-dependent. *A. ocellatum* can withstand a wide range of temperatures (7 to 30°C) and salinities (7 to 31 ppt) (Cheung et al., 1978); however, the optimal conditions for dinospore development are 25 to 30°C at 14 to 31 ppt salinity.

The tomont of *A. ocellatum* has been reported in the fish intestine and may survive after intestinal passage (Lawler, 1967). *A. ocellatum* can occur in internal organs, such as the submucosa, muscle, and connective tissue of the pharynx, the hematopoietic tissue of the head kidney, the Stannius corpuscle, and the mesentery adjacent to the liver of the porkfish. The precystic trophonts, from 17×17 μm to 78×86 μm, are observed in deep tissues, indicating continuation of growth of the dinospores after making the entry in the host. However, no apparent cellular changes are associated with internal *A. ocellatum* infection.

Amyloodiniasis is very difficult to treat because the life cycle of *Amyloodinium ocellatum* involves an encapsulated tomont, or reproductive, stage that is resistant to most parasiticides. Ionic copper is still the treatment of choice for this disease. With recent success in culturing *A. ocellatum* in the laboratory (Noga, 1987) many therapeutic chemicals or antiprotozoan drugs can be tested in vitro for possible application for the eradication of this disease. Also, the immune response on the infective stage of fishes can be evaluated.

Trypanosomes

Thirteen established species of *Trypanosoma* from marine teleosts and elasmobranchs are reported (Becker, 1977). Trypanosomes have a single flagellum, a well-developed undulating membrane, a nucleus, and a kinetoplast. Some fish trypanosomes are monomorphic, consisting of one size only, whereas others are noticeably dimorphic or polymorphic. The stage observed in fish blood is the trypomastigote. The parasite is transmitted by aquatic leeches. Piscine trypanosomiasis is rare in aquarium fish because the leech vectors are usually excluded from the tanks. Furthermore, information pertaining to the pathogenesis and pathology of trypanosome infection, especially on tropical marine fishes, is lacking.

Trypanoplasma

Hemoflagellates of the genus *Trypanoplasma* superficially resemble trypanosomes but differ in having two flagella and kinetosomes. Only four species infecting marine fishes have been reported. *Trypanoplasma beckeri* and *T. bullocki* are two extensively studied species. Their life cycles require a vector, the leech. In the gut of the leech, they produce a series of morphologically and physiologically different stages. The infective stages migrate to the proboscis sheath for transmission (Burreson, 1979, 1982). *Trypanoplasma bullocki* is widely distributed and infects at least 10 species of marine fishes along the Atlantic coast of North America and in the Gulf of Mexico. Young fish are more susceptible. Heavily infected fish are anemic and may show abnormal swellings. Although trypanoplasmosis is often found in wild fish, it has not been reported in tropical coral reef fishes.

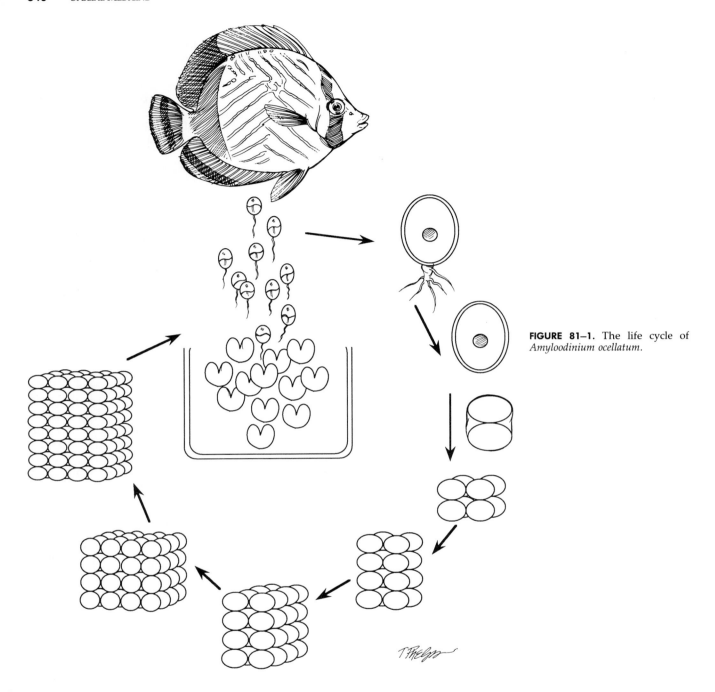

FIGURE 81–1. The life cycle of *Amyloodinium ocellatum.*

Cryptobia

Members of the genus *Cryptobia* are biflagellates that have been observed in the gills and skin of freshwater fishes but they also are found in the digestive tract and gallbladder of marine fishes. They lack an intermediate host and reproduce asexually by binary fission. Transmission of the parasite is by direct transfer. *Cryptobia* organisms are triangle-shaped, with the kinetoplast and kinetosome in anterior-lateral positions. One flagellum extends in front of the body and the other runs backward along the body, sometimes forming a narrow, undulating membrane.

Hexamita

Hexamita and the trichomonads of the genera *Monocercomonas* and *Protrichomonas* are intestinal flagellates of marine fishes (Lavier, 1936; Noble and Noble, 1966; Brugerolle, 1980). These flagellates are endocommensals with no apparent pathogenic effects on the hosts.

DISEASES CAUSED BY CILIATES

The phylum Ciliophora has more than 7600 established species (Corliss, 1979). Important ectoparasites, epibionts, ectocommensals, endocommensals, and facultative and obligatory parasites of marine fishes occur in six families. Important representative species of ciliate parasites are given in Table 81–1.

Cryptocaryon

The parasitic holotrichous ciliate *Cryptocaryon irritans* resembles *Ichthyophthirius multifiliis* the well-known "ich" of freshwater fishes. It was first reported as *Ichthyophthirius marinus* (Sikama, 1937). The disease reached enzootic proportions in the aquarium of the Zoological Society of London (Brown, 1951) and in the New York Aquarium (Nigrelli, 1958) in the 1950s and is believed to have been introduced from the Far East through marine fish importation.

The skin and gills of heavily infested fish show many white papules and petechiae. Since the trophonts (feeding stage) burrow vigorously into the epithelium causing extreme irritation, fish often flash and swallow sand in attempts to rid themselves of the parasites. Scanning electron microscopic studies show that the buccal apparatus of the trophont consists of a single ring of 65 to 75 cirri-like structures surrounding the mouth opening (Fig. 81–2). Each cirri-like structure is composed of a row of three cilia fused at the tip to form a pointed spike and arranged in a circular sawlike collar. The burrowing and rasping actions of the collar probably account for the irritating effects of the parasite that result in excessive production of mucus on the body and in the gills of affected fish. Fusion of gill lamellae, epithelial hyperplasia, sloughing of excess mucus, hemorrhages, and lesions of secondary bacterial infection are common clinical signs of cryptocaryoniasis in addition to the typical white spots.

The life history of *C. irritans* had been described (Brown, 1951, 1963; Sikama, 1937, 1961) and is in many respects similar to *Ichthyophthirius multifiliis* (Fig. 81–3). The living trophonts are oval and vary from 48 × 27 to 450 × 350 μm. Once the trophont leaves the host, it adheres to the substrate and in 24 hours becomes encysted, forming the reproductive tomont stage. Within the cyst the parasite multiplies, producing a number of similarly sized tomites. The

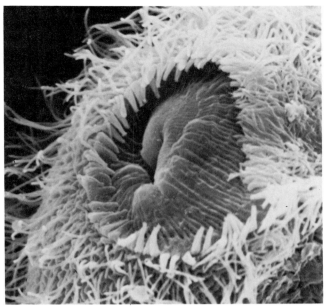

FIGURE 81–2. Scanning electron micrograph of the buccal apparatus of *Cryptocaryon irritans* showing a ring of 65 to 76 cirri surrounding the oral opening and cytopharynx.

complete development to emergence of infective stages takes 6 to 9 days at 22°C. The number of tomites produced depends on the size of the tomont. As many as 200 tomites may be formed from a large tomont. Fully developed tomites are motile within the cyst and emerge from a small opening. Newly emerged tomites are pear-shaped, measuring 56 × 35 μm, with a characteristic four-lobed nucleus. They are phototropic (Nigrelli and Ruggieri, 1966) and actively search for a host. The tomite stage is very sensitive to chemotherapeutic treatments. Formalin and copper, chelated copper, citrated copper, and copper sulfate all have been used successfully to treat cryptocaryoniasis at this stage.

Cytolysis of tomonts occurs at salinities of 16 ppt or lower, and hyposalinity is suggested as an alternative method of treating *C. irritans* infestation of euryhaline species of fishes (Cheung et al., 1979a; Colorni, 1985). The optimum conditions for tomont development are 30°C at a salinity of 31 ppt (Cheung et al., 1979a). At low temperature (7°C), trophonts remain inactive and fail to encyst or divide. Cryptocaryoniasis does not develop at temperatures below 19°C (Nigrelli and Ruggieri, 1966; Wilkie and Gordin, 1969). This may explain why *C. irritans* infestation is not commonly found in feral fish from northern waters.

Brooklynella

Brooklynella hostilis, a highly lethal *Chilodonella*-like parasite in the gills and skin of marine fishes, has been reported in sporadic outbreaks in 13 species of aquarium fishes (Lom and Nigrelli, 1970). The

TABLE 81–1. Important Representative Species of Ciliate Parasites Affecting Marine Fishes

Family Ichthyophthiriidae	Family Trichodinidae
Cryptocaryon	*Trichodina*
Cryptocaryon irritans	*Trichodina spheroidesi*
Family Hartmannulidae	*Trichodina halli*
Brooklynella	Family Scyphidiidae
Brooklynella hostilis	*Scyphidia arctice*
Family Uronematidae	*Ambiphyra miri*
Uronema	*Caliperia brevipes*
Uronema marinum	*Clausophyra*
Family Philasteridae	
Miamiensis	
Miamiensis avidus	

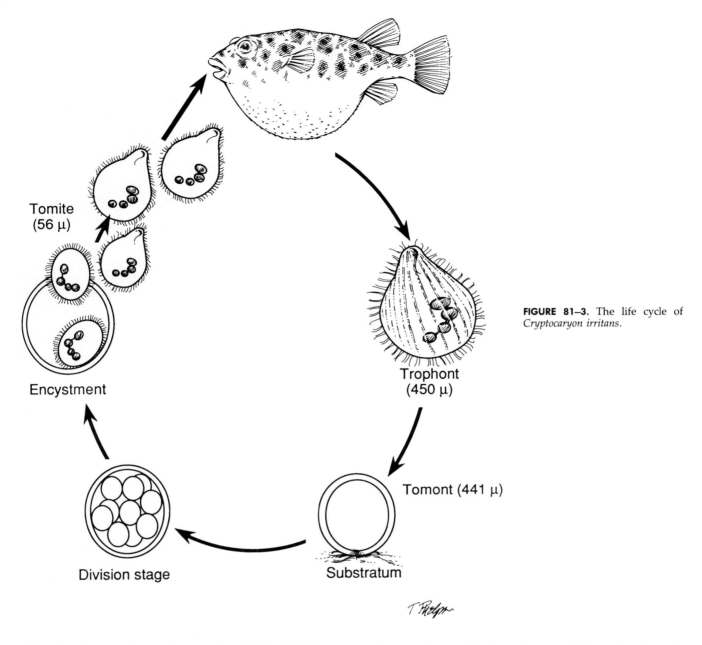

FIGURE 81–3. The life cycle of *Cryptocaryon irritans*.

Tomite
(56 μ)

Encystment

Division stage

Substratum

Tomont (441 μ)

Trophont
(450 μ)

T. Phelps

ultrastructure and morphogenesis of *B. hostilis* have been studied in detail (Lom and Corliss, 1971). These ciliates are bean- to kidney-shaped and glide on the surface of their ventral side. The organisms are 56 to 86 × 32 to 50 μm. The cytopharyngeal tube of *B. hostilis* is basketlike, characteristic of *Chilodonella*, and the parasite has a posterior adhesive organelle. This ciliate reproduces by binary fission and requires no secondary host.

In light infestations, fish infected with *Brook-lynella* appear healthy. Outbreaks of brooklynelliasis are probably due to changes in environmental conditions altering the host-parasite balance to favor the growth and multiplication of the parasites. In heavily infested fish, desquamation, massive hemorrhage, and respiratory difficulties are observed (Lom and Nigrelli, 1970). The disease can be controlled by restoring the optimal water conditions for the affected fish or by chemotherapeutic treatment with copper to reduce the number of the parasites.

Miamiensis and Uronema

Two opportunistic scuticociliatid ciliates, *Miamiensis avidus* and *Uronema marinum*, invade internal organs of marine fishes. *Miamiensis avidus* has been observed in the body of the sea horse (Moewus, 1962), *Uronema marinum* has been reported in nine species from four families of aquarium marine fishes (Cheung et al., 1980). These ciliates are closely related and are characterized by a shallow elongated buccal cavity with a tetrahymenal buccal apparatus. The undulating membrane is on the right border of the buccal cavity, and there are three small linearly arranged membranelles (Thompson, 1963). The ciliary meridians vary in number from 10 to 16 with a long, 34 μm, caudal cilium. The parasites are elongated and oval and measure 34 × 15 μm. *Uronema marinum* is free-living and can be cultured in fish broth (Cheung et al., 1980). The parasites reproduce by fission.

External ulceration is often associated with *Uronema* infestations (Fig. 81–4). In sea horses, muscle and skin become hemorrhagic and necrotic, and aneurysms of the gills and epithelial detachment of the epidermis are common. Infected fish are lethargic but not emaciated. The disease is believed to be related to the debilitating effects of adverse environmental conditions on the host immune system. It is still uncertain how the ciliate gains entrance into the host, but once it establishes itself, the tissue destruction is very rapid, with death occurring quickly. At the present time, no treatment is available for this disease.

Trichodina

There are about 70 marine species of *Trichodina* described to date. The mobiline peritrichs are turban-shaped with an adhesive disc and a characteristic denticulate ring (Fig. 81–5). These ciliates may irritate gills by gliding on the epithelium or by attaching themselves temporarily to the epithelial cells. Under normal conditions, the trichodinids are harmless, feeding on suspended particles in water. Binary fission and conjugation are described in *T. sphoeroidesi* and *T. halli* (Padnos and Nigrelli, 1942).

Trichodina species can be ectoparasitic and endoparasitic of the urinary, intestinal, and reproductive tracts. They occur in a wide range of tempera-

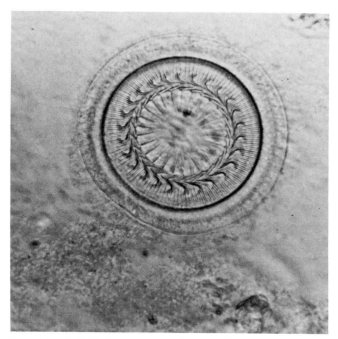

FIGURE 81–5. *Trichodina* sp. from the skin of a wolf eel showing the denticular ring.

tures, from 0 to 25°C, and apparently do not live well in high salinity or temperature. The first case of trichodiniasis in a marine fish was reported in a northern puffer from the New York and New Jersey coast at 16 to 20°C and 28 ppt salinity (Padnos and Nigrelli, 1942). Later, the disease was identified as a major problem in flatfish mariculture (McVicar, 1978). The parasites often contain host blood cells in vacuoles and are capable of considerable tissue destruction. Serious outbreaks of trichodiniasis are not common in aquarium fishes, and the intensity of infestation is varied in relation to ecologic conditions. Trichodinids are transmitted directly. The endozoic trichodinids are pathogens rather than endocommensals. A yellow mucoid exudate is associated with heavy infection (Khan, 1972).

DISEASES CAUSED BY APICOMPLEXA

These sporozoan parasites, phylum Apicocomplexa, are intracellular and are equipped with an apical complex consisting of polar rings, rhoptries, conoid, and micronemes (Levine, 1970). The life cycle requires two hosts, a vertebrate and an invertebrate. Infective stages are vermicular sporozoites formed within spores and oocysts.

Hemogregarines

The intraerythrocytic parasites of marine fishes are found in two subclasses, Coccidia and Piroplasmia. Hemogregarines (subclass Coccidia) were first observed in a sole and in two species of blennies

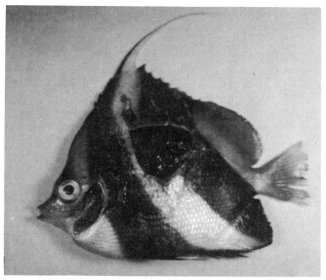

FIGURE 81–4. Heniochus butterflyfish infected with *Uronema marinum,* showing extensive dermal ulceration.

from the coast of France (Laveran and Mesnil, 1901). More than 80 species of the genus *Haemogregarina* have been described from red and white blood cells of marine fishes. The piscine hemogregarines are transmitted by leeches, isopods, or copepods.

Infected blood cells are hypertrophied and have a disfigured nucleus, which ultimately disintegrates. Blood of affected fish shows an increase in immature leukocytes (Ferguson and Roberts, 1975). There are no apparent external signs of disease.

Piroplasmas

Three genera with three described species of piroplasmas infect blood cells of marine fishes. *Haemohormidium beckeri* (Khan, 1980) has been reported in four species of marine fishes. *Haematractidium* infects mackerel (Henry, 1913), and *Babesiosoma rubrimarensis* infects at least six species of tropical marine fishes (Saunders, 1960). Reports on piroplasma in marine fishes are relatively uncommon. Erythrolysis and atypical leukocytes are pathologic signs of the infection (MacLean, 1980).

Coccidia

Three families of coccidia, Eimeriidae, Cryptosporiidae, and Calyptosporidae, are found in marine fishes, with more than 50 species described. The eimerid coccidia are predominant and are represented by four genera. *Eimeria* species are characterized by the presence of Stieda and sub–Stieda bodies in the sporocyst and a complete intracellular life cycle in the fish host. *Epieimeria* species have an *Eimeria*-like sporocyst with epicellular schizogony and gamogony. *Goussia* species have two valves forming the sporocyst wall and lack Stieda bodies (Lom and Dykova, 1982). *Crystallospora* species are characterized by a crystal-shaped sporocyst wall opening along an equatorial line.

Intestinal mucosa infected with eimerid coccidia shows different degrees of necrosis and sloughing of epithelium. Sporulated oocysts are discharged in the feces. Secondary bacterial infections and hemorrhages can be observed at the site of eimerid infection (Cheung et al., 1979b).

Cryptosporidium nasoris attaches on the surface of the intestinal epithelial cells of tropical naso tangs (Hoover et al., 1981). Infected fish are characterized by emaciation, intermittent anorexia, regurgitation of food, and feces with undigested food.

Extraintestinal coccidia commonly invade and sporulate in the liver, testicles, and connective tissues of the swimbladder. They also sporulate in the kidneys, blood stream, intestinal submucosa, and the muscular layers of the gallbladder and urinary bladder. Cellular degeneration and fibrocytic infiltration are common host reactions to extraintestinal coccidia. Gonadal infection may result in castration of the host. Spores can be released when the host is de-

voured by a predator or from body decomposition after the death of the host. Autoinfection has been assumed as a possible explanation for extremely heavy infections.

DISEASES CAUSED BY MICROSPORIDIANS

Microsporidiosis can be fatal and highly contagious. The life cycle of a microsporidian species consists of two distinct phases: a multiplicative stage, schizogony, and a spore-forming stage, sporogony. The infection is invasive with diffuse infiltration of tissues. The parasites are found in the intestines, pyloric ceca, bile ducts, liver, mesenteric lymph nodes, muscles, neural ganglia, subcutaneous tissues, testes, and ovaries. Autogamy appears to initiate spore formation at the end of schizogonic activity. Oral ingestion is the mode of transmission; however, intermediate hosts, such as rotifers and planktonic crustaceans, may be required in the life cycle of the parasites (Stunkard and Lux, 1965).

The microsporidian spore is ovoid and has a thick wall without any opening. The infective germ, the sporoplasm, is extruded to the exterior through a hollow, coiled polar tube that is everted after the spore has been ingested by a specific host. The sporoplasm is injected into the host cell and undergoes multiple binary fission, producing an enormous number of cells. The parasites do not cause host cell degeneration but stimulate hypertrophy and abnormal development into a xenoparasitic complex, or xenoma. In heavy infections, the gut wall can be largely supplanted by cysts. The intestine appears chalk-white and pebbled and has a rigid, thickened, hard wall. The epithelium of the intestine is denuded, and the lumen of the cecum may be almost occluded (Stunkard and Lux, 1965). Mechanical distention of the intestinal tissue and starvation are thought to be the cause of death (Scarborough and Weidner, 1979). No effective chemotherapeutics have been suggested for the control of the disease.

Sixty species from 11 genera of the order Microsporida are reported in marine fishes (Lom, 1984). The genera *Glugea*, *Pleistophora*, and *Spraguea* (*Nosema*) contain very pathogenic species. The following *Glugea* species have been studied extensively. *Glugea stephani* is an important parasite in flatfish mariculture (McVicar, 1975); *G. hertwigi* is an agent causing epizootic infection in European and American smelts (Nepszy et al., 1978); *G. anomala* infects the subcutaneous tissue and internal organs of sticklebacks and accounts for the high mortality of those fish (Weissenberg, 1968); and *G. heraldi* forms white cysts on the subcutaneous tissue of Atlantic sea horses (Blasiola, 1979).

Pleistophora macrozoarcidis is an important parasite of the ocean pout (Nigrelli, 1946). *Spraguea lophii* invades the ganglionic cells of anglerfishes and produces a xenoma with grapelike tumors in the nervous system (Loubes et al., 1979).

DISEASES CAUSED BY MYXOSPORIDIANS

Myxosporidians are parasites of fish, with the exception of a few species that infect amphibians or reptiles. They are characterized by polar capsules in the spore, and endogenous cell cleavage in trophozoite and sporogony stages. Spores contain one to seven or more polar capsules, sporoplasm, and a shell with valves. Classification of myxosporans is based on the number of shell valves and the position of the polar capsules in the spore (Shulman, 1959). Members of the order Bivalvulida have two spore wall valves, and those of Multivalvulida have three or more valves in the spore wall. There are more than 1100 species of myxosporidians reported in the literature, but only a few are described in marine aquarium fishes. Figure 81–6 summarizes the representative species of 24 genera of myxosporans found in marine fishes. These parasites either infect the gallbladder and urinary tract (celozoic) or are found as intercellular or intracellular parasites of muscle or connective tissue (histozoic). Trophozoites of celozoic species attach to the epithelium of the gallbladder and urinary bladder during their reproductive cycles with no apparent damage to the host and without initiating a host reaction. Nearly all marine tropical fishes collected from the wild harbor species of myxosporans from the genera *Ceratomyxa*, *Myxidium*, or *Leptotheca* in their gallbladders. In heavily infected fish, the bile appears cloudy and opaque often with an amorphous cheeselike substance. The function of the gallbladder can be impaired.

All species of Multivalvulida and a few Bivalvulida are important histozoic parasites inflicting serious injuries to the hosts. For example, species from genera *Kudoa* (many reported species), *Unicapsula* (three species), *Pentacapsula* (three species), and *Hexacapsula* (one species) are found in myocytes and have an intracellular reproductive cycle. The infected muscle fibers become enlarged and replaced by cysts filled with mature spores that may be encapsulated by the host's connective tissue. Muscular liquefaction is due to a proteolytic enzyme released by the parasites after the death of the host.

The following myxospores are described from tropical marine fishes. *Pentacapsula muscularis* was observed in the dorsal musculature of collare butterflyfish from the Indo-Pacific and Philippine Islands (Cheung et al., 1983). An unidentified *Pentacapsula* species has been found in the muscle of smooth anglerfish (Cheung and Nigrelli, 1988). *Septemcapsula plotosi* var. *yasunagai* was found infecting the nervous tissue of coral catfish, causing the fish to whirl before death (Cheung and Nigrelli, 1988). *Coccomyxa hoffmani*, a single encapsulated bivalvulid, infected the cartilage of the gill filament and arches of the coral catfish, causing damage to the gill lamellae (Cheung and Nigrelli, 1988).

The life cycle of the myxosporidians has not been fully elucidated and requires future investigation. However, evidence seems to indicate that an intermediate host is needed. It is also noted that many genera contain only one or two species, suggesting that more species and perhaps genera are waiting to be discovered in marine fishes.

DISEASES CAUSED BY CNIDARIANS

Cnidarians that parasitize fish are rare. There is one reported case in an aquarium-held sea horse. Various species of *Hydractinia*, *Hydrichthella*, *Stylactis*, *Stylactella*, and *Podocoryne* have been reported on marine fishes (Hand, 1957), especially on slow-moving and bottom-feeding fish.

Members of the genus *Hydrichthys* are truly parasitic, attacking mainly young hosts or small fish species. Hydroid colonies of *H. pietschi* (Martin, 1975) on the skin of lanternfishes from Hawaii cause intensive host tissue response.

DISEASES CAUSED BY TURBELLARIA

A turbellarian on the skin and fins of yellow tangs causes epithelial disruption and eventual mortality of the fish (Blasiola, 1976). Fishes other than the yellow tang are also affected, including surgeonfishes, marine angelfishes, marine butterflyfishes, parrotfishes, and wrasses. The turbellarian parasite has not been identified but probably belongs to the order Eulecithophora in the genus *Ichthyophaga* (Kent, 1981). Outbreaks of turbellarian infestation are apparently due to crowding and high levels of organic waste accumulated in the aquarium system. A variety of treatments, including formalin dip, masoten, and lowered salinity, are reported (Kent, 1981).

DISEASES CAUSED BY MONOGENETIC TREMATODES

Monogenetic tremataodes are commonly found on gills, skin, or fins, but a few invade the rectal cavity, ureters, body cavity, and even the blood vascular system. Since monogeneans require only one host, transmission is direct from host to host. The oncomiracidia are hatched in water and are free-swimming ciliated larvae.

Neobenedenia melleni (*Epibdella melleni*) (MacCallum, 1927) has been a major cause of death of marine fishes at the New York Aquarium (Nigrelli, 1940). This parasite belongs to the family Capsalidae and has an opisthohaptor armed with three pairs of dissimilar anchors. The parasite is found mainly on the skin. Many species of marine tropical fishes, especially from the West Indies, are susceptible to *N. melleni* infestation under aquarium conditions. However, *Neobenedenia* species are quite host-specific in nature (Tripathi, 1959). Heavily infested fish swim erratically, flashing and rubbing against the bottom

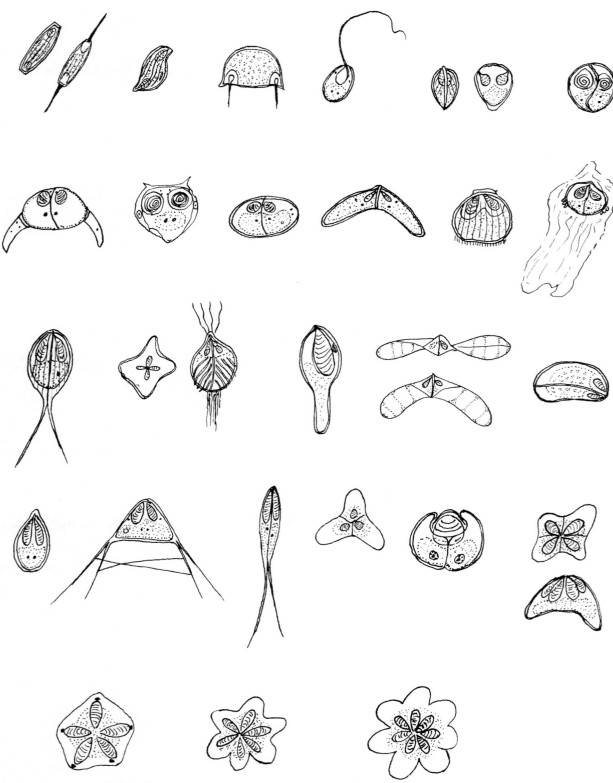

FIGURE 81–6. Representative myxospores of the 24 genera that infect marine tropical fishes.

of the tank. This results in dermal ulceration with secondary bacterial infection. *Neobenedenia* on the eyes often causes destruction of the cornea and eventually blindness. Freshwater dips effectively control *Neobenedenia* infestations; however, complete elimination of the worms from an aquarium system requires more aggressive treatment.

Microcotyle spp. are monogeneans with many paired clumps in their opisthohaptor. They are often observed in the gills of marine fishes. More than 100 species have been reported. The worms cause irritation, epithelial hyperplasia, and hemorrhage of the gills. Heavy infestations in gills of blackfish cause the gills to appear white owing to the severe blood loss inflicted by the worms.

Members of families Dactylogyridae and Gyrodactylidae are small monogeneans found on gills. Many species of the genera *Haliotrema, Ancyrocephalus, Pseudoancyrocephalus, Cleithrarticus, Neohaliotrema*, and *Pseudempleurosoma* are reported on tropical marine fishes (Yamaguti, 1968). Extensive damage to the gill tissues and hyperplastic epithelium are observed at the attachment sites of the armed haptors of the worms.

DISEASES CAUSED BY DIGENETIC TREMATODES

Digenetic trematodes have a rather complicated life cycle with at least two hosts. The fish may be the final or one of the intermediate hosts. Life cycles of several marine trematodes are known (Stunkard, 1930; Koie, 1976, 1978; Wolfgang, 1955). The digeneans parasitize primarily the digestive tract, but a few infect the gallbladder, blood, and peritoneal cavity. Yamaguti (1970) described 227 new species of the total of 314 digenetic trematodes studied from 144 species of marine fishes collected in Hawaiian waters. The digeneans belong to 160 genera of 72 subfamilies in 30 families.

The Didymozoidae are tissue parasites, living in pairs, encysted in the gills, skin, mouth, muscle, or connective tissue. The fluke *Paracardicola hawaiensis* causes liver damage in the balloonfish (Martin, 1960), whereas the adult trematodes in the digestive tract of the fish are usually not a cause of serious disease. The migrating larvae, cercariae, and metacercariae are of greatest significance to the fish host.

Cercariae of *Cryptocotyle lingua* (Creplin) invade and encyst in the fins and integument of herring, cunner, and a number of inshore western Atlantic species, causing the formation of "black spots" on the skin (Stunkard, 1930). Massive cercarial invasion will blind and kill immature herring (Sinderman and Rosenfield, 1954). Penetrated cercariae cause extensive muscle degeneration and invasion and proliferation of inflammatory cells (Sommerville, 1981). Exophthalmia, cataract, granuloma formation, and in extreme cases complete destruction of the eye are some of the effects of metacercariae invasion of the

fish eye. However, such massive invasion of metacercariae does not often occur in aquaria, where fish are isolated from mollusks and crustaceans, the intermediate hosts of the parasite.

DISEASES CAUSED BY CESTODES

The cestodes of fish have a life cycle requiring at least one other host. Fish may serve as final or intermediate hosts for cestodes. Only some species of the Tetraphylliade, Spathebothriidae, Trypanorhyncha, and Pseudophyllidea have been studied in detail with regard to effects on fish hosts (Rohde, 1984). Adult cestodes are occasionally harmful parasites in the digestive tract of fishes, but the larval stages, plerocercoids, are of greatest concern in marine fishes. The elongated trypanorhynch larvae of *Poecilancistrium robustum* are called "spaghetti worms" in the flesh of drum in the Gulf of Mexico (Chandler, 1954). "Wormy couta" is another example of heavy infestation of tapeworm larvae, *Gymnorhynchus thyrsites*, in Australian barracuda.

Adult cestodes may occur in significant numbers in the digestive tract of fish; however, their prevalence in marine teleost is low. Massive infestation of adult worms can have a severe effect on the growth of the host. It may obstruct the intestine, causing irritation and scaring. Cestodiasis is not a major problem in captive marine tropical fish because the intermediate hosts required in the life cycles of the cestodes are usually eliminated in an aquarium.

DISEASES CAUSED BY NEMATODES

Adult nematodes may live in various organs and tissues of marine fishes, but they occur primarily in the digestive tract. The larvae in fishes can be histozoic, causing mechanical and toxic damage to hosts. Nematode sexes are separate. Fertilized eggs develop first to a larva that molts four times to become a reproductive adult. The life cycle can require one or two intermediate hosts. Crustaceans often are the first intermediate host. Host specificity of marine nematodes varies greatly; most parasites are not strictly specific to one host fish species.

Nematodes that infect marine fishes are mainly represented by the following superfamilies and genera: Ascaridoidea (*Contracaecum, Anisakis, Terranova, Hysterothylacium*, and *Raphidascaris*), Spiruroidea (*Ascarophis* and *Metabronema*), Camallanoidea (*Cucullanus, Camallanus*, and *Spirocamallanus*), and Dracunculoidea (*Philometra* and *Philonema*).

Most members of Spiruroidea, Camallanoidea, and Dracunculoidea have two host life cycles in which fish are the final hosts. The worms are found living or encysted in various tissues. Species of *Spirocamallanus* (Camallanoidea) have been found in 363 specimens representing 16 species of 10 genera of marine tropical fishes from Hawaiian waters (Rychlinski and Deardorff, 1982). They also have been implicated as serious parasites of marine aquarium fishes.

Members of Dracunculoidea in marine fishes are histozoic, belonging to the family Philometridae, genus *Philometra*. Adults commonly occur in the gonads and other tissues, causing marked pathologic effects. Visceral adhesion, edema, and granuloma are common pathologic findings. Heavy infections have been reported in white spotted pufferfish from Hawaiian waters (Deardorff and Stanton, 1983). The intensity of nematode infections is usually low in aquarium fish owing to the captive conditions in which further exposure to infective stages of the worms is often limited. Only isolated cases of severe nematodiasis are observed in routine necropsies of long-term captive fishes.

DISEASES CAUSED BY ACANTHOCEPHALANS

Adult acanthocephalan worms usually live in the intestine of fish. They absorb the intestinal contents of the host through their surface. The life cycle requires one other host (amphipods). Species from the genera *Pomphorhynchus* and *Echinorhynchus* are found in marine fishes. However, acanthocephalan infections are rarely encountered in marine reef fishes.

DISEASES CAUSED BY LEECHES

Parasitic leeches are blood-sucking worms that are important vectors for hemogregarines or hemoflagellates (Burrenson, 1982). The life history involves copulation, cocoon deposition, embryonic development, and hatching. Temperature plays an important part in the distribution of the parasite. Attached leeches on the skin of fish cause inflammation, displacement, and erosion of the dermal layers. Hyperplasia of the epithelium, ulcerated patches, and extensive scars on the body are seen (Sanjeeva-Raj, 1974).

Leeches are rarely observed in aquarium fish. Occasionally a few are encountered from newly acquired wild-caught fishes. Exhibited tropical marine fishes are usually subjected to vigorous prophylactic treatments for external parasites, and leeches are usually eliminated by these procedures.

DISEASES CAUSED BY BRANCHIURANS

The majority of branchiurans that parasitize fishes belong to the genus *Argulus*. Only a few species are reported in marine fishes. *Argulus* organisms are dioecious and can move freely over the surface of the host, feeding on tissue fluid, blood, and predigested tissues of the fish. However, the effects of *Argulus* on marine fishes have not been proved harmful, and the parasites are not commonly reported in captive tropical marine fish.

Argulus funduli has been observed on the skin of spotfin butterfly fish from North Carolina waters (Pearse, 1947). *Argulus intectus* has been found on the gills of scup.

DISEASES CAUSED BY COPEPODS

The parasitic Copepoda are separated into three suborders, Siphonostomoida, Poecilostomatoida, and Cyclopoida (Kabata, 1979). The majority of the marine forms belong to the Siphonostomoida and the Poecilostomatoida. The Cyclopoida are mainly parasites of freshwater fishes. Virtually all copepods parasitizing the outer surfaces of fishes belong to the Siphonostomatoida. Some are freely mobile and some are burrowing. The rarely observed endoparasitic forms are found in the genera *Colobomatus*, *Lerneascus*, and *Sarcotaces* of the suborder Poecilostomatoida (Kabata, 1984).

Members of the Cecropidae, Caligidae, Hatschekiidae, Lernanthropidae, Ergasilidae, and Chondracanthidae are found on the gills or skin of fish. The parasites damage the gills by grasping and anchoring, causing tissue irritation, occlusion of blood vessels, destruction of filaments, and epithelial hyperplasia. The parasites damage skin, causing epithelial thickening, erythema, fibroblast proliferation, infiltration of macrophages and lymphocytes, and dermal hemorrhage.

The members of Pennellidae, Sphyriidae, Lernaeopodidae, and Chondracanthidae penetrate the skin and burrow deeply into tissues (Nigrelli and Firth, 1939). Capsulation, leukocytic infiltration, and formation of a black tumorlike structure at the point of attachment are noticeable tissue reactions of the host. The changes are characteristic of chronic inflammation.

The transmission of these parasites is direct, requiring no intermediate hosts, except in some members of Pennellidae. The nauplian and copepodids are free-swimming stages that undergo several molts before metamorphosing to adults. The larval stages are sensitive to chemicals, especially copper.

DISEASES CAUSED BY ISOPODS

Five families of isopods have species parasitic on fishes, the Cymothoidae, Aegidae, Anilocridae, Gnathiidae, and Corallanidae (Kabata, 1970; 1984). Members of Gnathiidae are parasitic during the young stage only, and the Cymothoidae are parasitic only as adults. Aegids are only facultative, temporary parasites that have no preference for a specific site on the host. Anilocrids are more specific in site selection and limited to the skin of their hosts. Their association with host fishes is obligatory, and their attachment is more permanent. Corallanids are closely related to the cymothoids, but their life cycles are more like those of gnathiids. The adult stage leaves the host and takes up a secluded, demersal mode of life.

Livoneca ovalis, a cymothoid, attached to the gills and the branchial chamber of several hosts, namely, striped bass, bluefish, scup, weakfish, ocean sunfish, menhaden, and kingfish, causes gill erosion and hemorrhage. Marked swellings produced on the surface of lionfish infested with *Ichthyotaces pteroisicola* have been reported (Shiino, 1932). Each swelling acts as a protective sac for a parasite.

LITERATURE CITED

Becker, C.D. (1977) Flagellate parasites of fish. In: Parasitic Protozoa. Vol. 1. (Kreier, J.P., ed.). Academic Press, New York, pp. 357–416.

Blasiola, G.C., Jr. (1976) Ectoparasitic turbellaria. Marine Aquarist 7(2):53–58.

Blasiola, G.C., Jr. (1979) *Glugea heraldi* n.sp. (Microsporida, Glugeidae) from the seahorse *Hippocampus erectus* Perry. J. Fish Dis. 2:493–500.

Brown, E.M. (1951) (A new parasitic protozoan the causal organism of a white spot disease in marine fish . . . *Cryptocaryon irritans* gen. & sp.n.). Agenda Science Meetings, Zoological Society of London, 1950, No. 11:1–2.

Brown, E.M. (1963) Studies on *Cryptocaryon irritans* Brown. Proceedings of the International Congress of Protozoology, Prague, Aug. 1961. Progress in Protozoology, Academia Publishing House, Prague, pp. 284–287.

Brown, E.M., and Hovasse, R. (1946) *Amyloodinium ocellatum* (Brown), a peridinian parasitic on marine fishes. A complementary study. Proc. Zool. Soc. Lond. 116:33–46.

Brugerolle, G. (1980) Ultrastructural study of the flagellate *Protrichomonas legeri* (Leger 1905) parasite of the stomach of the boops (Box boops). Protistologica 16:353–358.

Bullock, W.L. (1966) *Entamoeba gadi* sp.n. from the rectum of the pollock, *Pollachius virens* (L. 1758), with some observations on its cytochemistry. J. Parasitol. 52:679–684.

Burreson, E.M. (1979) Structure and life cycle of *Trypanoplasma beckeri* sp.n. (Kinetoplastida), a parasite of the cabezon, *Scorpaenichthys marmoratus*, in Oregon coastal waters. J. Protozool. 26(3):343–347.

Burreson, E.M. (1982) The life cycle of *Trypanoplasma bullocki* (Zoomastigophorea: Kinetoplastida). J. Protozool. 29:72–77.

Chandler, A.C. (1954) Cestoda. In Gulf of Mexico, its origin, waters, and marine life. Fish. Bull. U.S. Fish Wildlife Serv. 55:1–604.

Cheung, P.J., and Nigrelli, R.F. (1988) A histozoic myxosporean (Pentacapsulidae) in the muscle of smooth angler fish, *Histiophryne bougainvilli*. Fish Health Sect./Am. Fish. Soc. Newslett. 16(3):6.

Cheung, P.J., Nigrelli, R.F., and Ruggieri, G.D. (1979a) Effects of temperature, salinity and pH in endozootics of protozoan diseases in captive fishes (abstract). Wildlife Disease Association Conference, Stillwater, Oklahoma.

Cheung, P.J., Nigrelli, R.F., and Ruggieri, G.D. (1979b) Coccidian parasite of black fish, *Tautoga onitis* (L.): Life cycle and histopathology. Am. Zool. 19(3):abstract.

Cheung, P.J., Nigrelli, R.F., and Ruggieri, G.D. (1980) Studies on the morphology of *Uronema marinum* Dujardin (Ciliata: Uronematidae) with a description of the histopathology of the infection in marine fishes. J. Fish Dis. 3:295–303.

Cheung, P.J., Nigrelli, R.F., and Ruggieri, G.D. (1983) *Pentacapsula muscularis* sp. nov. (Myxosporea: Pentacapsulides); a histozoic parasite of butterfly fish, *Chaetodon collare* Bloch. J. Fish Dis. 6:393–395.

Cheung, P.J., Nigrelli, R.F., and Ruggieri, G.D. (1984) *Philometra saltatrix* infecting the heart of the 0+ class bluefish, *Pomatomus saltatrix* (L.) (abstract) The Annual Meeting of Midwest Fish Disease Workshop, Little Rock, Arkansas.

Cheung, P.J., Ruggieri, G.D., and Nigrelli, R.F. (1978) Effects of temperature and salinity on the developmental cycle of *Oodinium ocellatum* Brown (Mastigophore: Phytomastogophoresa: Dinoflagellida) (abstract). The Fourth International Congress of Parasitology in Poland.

Colorni, A. (1985) Aspects of the biology of *Cryptocaryon irritans*, and hyposalinity as a control measure in cultured gilt-head sea bream *Sparus aurata*. Dis. Aquatic Organ. 1:19–22.

Corliss, J.O. (1979) The Ciliated Protozoa Characterization, Classification and Guide to the Literature. 2nd ed. Pergamon Press, Elasford, NY, pp. 1–455.

Deardorff, T.L., and Stanton, F.G. (1983) Nematode-induced abdominal

distention in the Hawaiian pufferfish, *Canthigaster jactator* (Jenkins). Pacif. Sci. 37:45–47.

Ferguson, H.W., and Roberts, R.J. (1975) Myeloid leucosis associated with sporozoan infection in cultured turbot (*Scophthalmus meoticus* L.). J. Comp. Pathol. 85:317–326.

Fournie, J.W., and Overstreet, R.M. (1983) True intermediate hosts for *Eimeria funduli* (Apicomplexa) from estuarine fishes. J. Protozool. 30:672–675.

Hand, C. (1957) Table 1. Host relationships of some symbiotic hydroids. Interrelations of organisms. A. Commensalism. In: Treatise on Marine Ecology and Paleoecology. Vol. 1 (Hedgpeth, J.W., ed.). Geol. Soc. Amer. Mem. 67, pp. 392–394.

Henry, H. (1913) A new haemosporidian from *Scomber scomber*, the common mackerel. J. Pathol. Bacteriol. 18:228–231.

Hoover, D.M., Hoerr, F.J., Carlton, W.W., Hinsman, E.J., and Ferguson, H.W. (1981) Enteric cryptosporidiosis in a naso tang, *Naso lituratus* Bloch and Schneider. J. Fish Dis. 4:425–428.

Kabata, Z. (1970) Crustacea as enemies of fishes. In: Diseases of Fishes, Book 1 (Snieszko, S.F., and Axelrod, H.R., eds.). T.F.H. Publications, Neptune, New Jersey.

Kabata, Z. (1979) Parasitic Copepoda of British Fishes. Ray Society, London.

Kabata, Z. (1984) Diseases caused by metazoans: Crustaceans. In: Diseases of Marine Animals, Vol. IV, Part 1, Introduction, Pisces (Kinne, O., ed.). Biologische Anstalt Helgoland, Hamburg, FG, pp. 321–399.

Kent, M.L. (1981) The life cycle and treatment of a Turbellarian disease of marine fishes. Freshwater and Marine Aquarium 4:11–13.

Kent, M.L. (1988) *Paramoeba pemaquidensis* infestation of coho salmon gills (abstract). International Fish Health Conference, Vancouver, B.C., Canada, July 19–21, 1988.

Khan, R.A. (1972) Taxonomy, prevalence, and experimental transmission of a protozoan parasite, *Trichodina oviducti* Polyansky (Ciliata: Peritrichida), of the thorny skate, *Raja radiata* Donovan. J. Parasitol. 58:680–686.

Khan, R.A. (1980) The leech as a vector of a fish piroplasm. Can. J. Zool. 58:1631–1637.

Koie, M. (1976) On the morphology and life history of *Zooqonoides viviparus* (Olsson, 1868) Odhner, 1962 (Trematoda, Zoogonidae). Ophelia 15:1–14.

Koie, M. (1978) On the morphology and life history of *Derogenes varicus* (Muller, 1784) Looss 1901 (Trematoda, Hemiuridae). Z. Parasit. Kde 59:67–78.

Laveran, A., and Mesnil, F. (1901) Deux hemogregarines nouvelles des poissons. C.R. Acad. Sci. Paris 133:572–577.

Lavier, G. (1936) Sur quelques flagelles intestinaux de poissons marins. Ann. Parasitol. Hum. Comp. 14:278–289.

Lawler, A.R. (1967) *Oodinium cyprinodontum* n.sp., a parasitic dinoflagellate on the gills of Cyprinodontidae of Virginia. Chesapeake Sci. 8:67–68.

Levine, N.D. (1970) Taxonomy of the sporozoa. J. Parasitol. 56(4):208–209.

Lom, J. (1984) Diseases caused by Protistans. In: Diseases of Marine Animals, Vol. IV, Part 1, Introduction, Pisces (Kinn, O., ed.). Biologische Anstalt Helgoland, Hamburg, pp. 114–168.

Lom, J., and Corliss, J.O. (1971) Morphogenesis and cortical ultrastructure of *Brooklynella hostilis*, a dysteriid ciliate ectoparasitic on marine fishes. J. Protozool. 18(2):261–281.

Lom, J., and Dykova, I. (1982) Some marine fish coccidia of the genera *Eimeria* Schneider, *Epieimeria* Dykova and Lom and *Goussia* Labbe. J. Fish Dis. 5:309–321.

Lom, J., and Lawler, A.R. (1973) An ultrastructural study on the mode of attachment in dinoflagellates invading gills of cyprinodontidae. Protistologica 1(2):293–309.

Lom, J., and Nigrelli, R.F. (1970) *Brooklynella hostilis* n.g., n.sp., a pathogenic cyrtophorine ciliate in marine fishes. J. Protozool. 17(2):224–232.

Loubes, C., Maurand, J., and Ormieres, R. (1979) Etude ultrastructurale de *Spragues lophii* (Doflein, 1898), Microsporidie parasite de la Baudroie: essai d'interpretation du dimorphisme sporal. Protistologica 15:43–54.

MacLean, S.A. (1980) Study of *Haematractidium scombri* in Atlantic mackerel, *Scomber scombrus*. Can. J. Fish. Aquatic Sci. 37:812–816.

Martin, W.E. (1960) Hawaiian helminthes. IV. *Paracardicola hawaiensis* n.gen., n.sp. (Trematoda: Sanguinicolidae) from the balloon fish, *Tetraodon hispidus* L. J. Parasitol. 46:648–650.

Martin, W.E. (1975) *Hydrichthys pietschi*, new species (coelenterata), parasitic on the fish, *Ceratias holboelli* Bull. 5th Cal. Acad. Sci. 74:1–5.

McVicar, A.H. (1975) Infection of plaice *Pleuronectes platessa* L. with *Glugea* (*Nosema*) *stephani* (Hagenmuller 1899) (Protozoa: Microsporidia) in a fish farm and under experimental conditions. J. Fish Biol. 7:611–619.

McVicar, A.H. (1978) Flatfish at risk—trials pinpoint dangers from disease. Fish Farmer 2:32–33.

Moewus, L. (1962) Studies on marine parasitic *Tetrahymena* species. J. Protozool. 9(Suppl.):13.

Nepszy, S.J., Budd, J., and Dechtiar, A.O. (1976) Mortality of young-of-the-year rainbow smelt (*Osmerus mordax*) in Lake Erie associated with the occurrence of *Glugea hertwigi*. J. Wildlife Dis. 14:233–239.

Nigrelli, R.F. (1936) The morphology, cytology and life-history of *Oodinium ocellatum* Brown, a dinoflagellate parasite on marine fishes. Zool. N.Y. 21:129–164.

Nigrelli, R.F. (1940) Mortality statistics for specimens in the New York Aquarium, 1939. Zool. N.Y. 25:525–552.

Nigrelli, R.F. (1946) Studies on the marine resources of southern New England. V. Parasites and diseases of the ocean pout, *Macrozoarces americanus*. Bull. Bingham Oceanogr. Collect. 9:187–202.

Nigrelli, R.F. (1958) Causes of diseases and death of fishes. Transactions of the Northeast Wildlife Conference, 10th Annual Meeting, pp. 375–377.

Nigrelli, R.F., and Firth, F.E. (1939) On *Sphyrion lumpi* (Kroyer), a copepod parasite on the redfish *Sebastes marinus* (Linnaeus) with special reference to the host-parasite relationships. Zool. N.Y. 23:1–10.

Nigrelli, R.F., and Ruggieri, G.D. (1966) Enzootics in the New York Aquarium caused by *Cryptocaryon irritans* Brown, 1951 (= *Ichthyophthirius marinus* Sikama, 1961), a histophagous ciliate in the skin, eyes and gills of marine fishes. Zool. N.Y. 51(9):97–107.

Noble, G.A., and Noble, E.R. (1966) *Monocercomonas molae* n.sp., a flagellate from the sunfish *Mola mola*. J. Protozool. 13:257–259.

Noga, E. (1987) Propagation in cell culture of the dinoflagellate *Amyloodinium*, an ectoparasite of marine fishes. Science 236:1302–1305.

Padnos, M., and Nigrelli, R.F. (1942) *Trichodina spheroidesi* and *Trichodina halli* spp. nov. parasitic on the gills and skin of marine fishes, with special reference to the life-history of *T. spheroidesi*. Zool. N.Y. 27(2):65–72.

Papperna, I. (1980) *Amyloodinium ocellatum* (Brown, 1931) (Dinoflagellida) infestations in cultured marine fish at Eilat, Red Sea: epizootiology and pathology. J. Fish Dis. 3:363–372.

Pearse, A.S. (1947) Parasitic copepods from Beaufort, North Carolina. J. Elisha Mitchel Sci. 63(1):1–16.

Rohde, K. (1984) Disease caused by metazoans: Helminths. In: Diseases of Marine Animals. Vol. VI, Part I, Pisces (Kinne, O., ed.). Biologische Anstalt Helgoland, Hamburg, pp. 193–319.

Rychlinski, R.A., and Deardorff, T.L. (1982) Spirocamallanus: a potential fish health problem. Freshwater and Marine Aquarium, Febr. 22–23.

Sanjeeva-Raj, P.J. (1974) A review of the fish-leeches of the Indian Ocean. J. Marine Biol. Assoc. Ind. 16:381–397.

Saunders, D.C. (1960) A survey of the blood parasites in the fishes of the Red Sea. Trans. Am. Microscop. Soc. 79:239–252.

Scarborough, A., and Weidner, E. (1979) Field and laboratory studies of *Glugea hertwigi* (microsporida) in the rainbow smelt *Osmerus mordax*. Biol. Bull. 157:334–343.

Shiino, S.M. (1932) *Ichthyotaces pteroisicola* n.g., and n.sp., a copepod parasitic on the fish, *Pterois lunulata* Temminck and Schlegel. Ann. Zool. Jpn. 13:417–433.

Shulman, S.S. (1959) Osnovnye napravleniya evolyutsii V otryade Myxosporidia. (Basic trends of evolution in the order Myxosporidia (in Russian, English summary). Zool. Zh. 38:1481–1497.

Sikama, Y. (1937) "Preliminary report on the white spot disease in marine fish" (in Japanese). Suisan-Gakukai 7(3):149–160.

Sikama, Y. (1961) On a new species of *Ichthyophthirius* found in marine fishes. Sci. Rep. Yokosuka City Mus. 6:66–70.

Sindermann, C., and Rosenfield, A. (1954) Diseases of fishes of the western North Atlantic. I. Diseases of the sea herring. Dept. Sea Shore Fish. Res. Bull. 18:1–23.

Sommerville, C. (1981) A comparative study of the tissue response to invasion and encystment by *Stephanochasmus baccatus* (Nicoll, 1907) (Digenea: Acanthocolpidae) in four species of flatfish. J. Fish Dis. 4:53–68.

Stunkard, H.W. (1930) The life history of *Cryptocotyle linqua* (Creplin) with notes on the physiology of the metacercaria. J. Morphol. 50:143–191.

Stunkard, H., and Lux, F.E. (1965) A microsporidian infection of the digestive tract of the winter flounder, *Pseudopleuronectes americanus*. Biol. Bull. 129:371–385.

Thompson, J.C., Jr. (1963) A redescription of *Uronema marinum*, and a proposed new family, Uronematidae. Va. J. Sci. 15:80–87.

Thompson, J.C., Jr., and Moewus, L. (1964) *Miamiensis avidus* n.g., a marine facultative parasite in the ciliate order Hymenostomatida. J. Protozool. 11:378–381.

Tripathi, Y.R. (1959) Monogenetic trematodes from fishes of India. India J. Helminthol. 9:1–49.

Weissenberg, R. (1968) Intracellular development of the microsporidian *Glugea anamala* Moniez in hypertrophying migratory cells of the fish *Gasterosteus aculeatus* L., an example of the formation of 'Xenoma tumours.' J. Protozool. 15:44–57.

Wilkie, D.W., and Gordin, H. (1969) Outbreak of cryptocaryoniasis in marine aquaria at Scripps Institute of Oceanography. Cal. Fish Game 55(3):227–236.

Wolfgang, R.W. (1955) Studies of the trematode *Stephanostomum baccatum* (Nicoll, 1907). III. Its life cycle. Can. J. Zool. 3:113–128.

Yamaguti, S. (1968) Monogenetic Trematodes of Hawaiian Fishes. University of Hawaii Press, Honolulu.

Yamaguti, S. (1970) Digenetic trematodes of Hawaiian fishes. Keigaku Publishing, Tokyo.

Chapter 82

NEOPLASIAS OF MARINE TROPICAL FISHES

ERIC B. MAY

Fish grouped under this heading of marine tropical fishes are those tropical and migratory species that spend most, if not all, of their life cycle in tropical marine waters. This represents a difficult group to summarize, as reports are scattered and many are very old and unconfirmed. No clear picture of causation or of predisposing factors to neoplasias can be drawn. A list of tumors reported in this group of fishes is given in Table 82–1.

TABLE 82–1. Tumors Reported in Marine Tropical Fishes

Site/Neoplasia	Fish	References
Nervous System		
Neurilemmoma	Gray snapper	Lucke, 1942
	Dog snapper	Lucke, 1942
Neurofibroma	Gray snapper	Harshbarger, 1965–1981
	Sculpin	Harshbarger, 1965–1981
Schwannoma	Bicolor damselfish	Schmale et al., 1983
Xanthophoroma	Blenny	Lucke, 1942
Cardiovascular (Including Organs of Hematopoiesis)		
Mesothelioma	Jewfish	Shields and Popp, 1979
Gastrointestinal System		
None reported		
Urinary System		
None reported		
Endocrine System		
Thyroid adenoma	Serpentine goby	Homa and Ishiyama, 1982
	Unspecified sea bass	Marsh and Von Willer, 1916
Adenocarcinoma	Kelp bass	Blasiola et al., 1981

LITERATURE CITED

Blasiola, G.C., Turnier, J.C., and Hurst, E.E. (1981) Metastatic thyroid adenocarcinomas in a captive population of kelp bass, *Paralabrax clanthatus*. J. Natl. Cancer Inst. 66:51–59.

Harshbarger, J.C. (1965–1981) RTLA supplement. Registry of Tumors in Lower Animals. Smithonian Institution, Washington, D.C.

Homma, Y., and Ishiyama, M. (1982) A case of adenomatous goiter developed in the thyroid gland of a serpentine goby, *Pterobobius elapoides*, reared in aquarium. Ann. Rep. Sado Biol. Stat., Niigata Univ. 12:27–31.

Lucke, B. (1942) Tumors of the nerve sheaths in fish of the snapper family (Lutianidae). Arch. Pathol. 34:133–150.

Marsh, M.C., and Von Willer, P. (1916) Thyroid tumor in the sea bass (*Serranus*). J. Cancer Res. 1:183–196.

Schmale, M.C., Hensley, G., and Udey, L.R. (1983) Animal model of human disease. Neurofibromatosis, von Recklinghausen's disease, multiple schwannomas, malignant schwannomas: Multiple schwannomas in the bicolor damselfish, *Pomacentrus partitus* (Pisces, Pomacentridae). Am. J. Pathol. 112:238–241.

Shields, R.P., and Popp, J.A. (1979) Intracardial mesotheliomas and a gastric papilloma in a giant grouper, *Epinephelus itajara*. Vet. Pathol. 16:191–198.

Chapter 83

PHARMACOLOGY OF MARINE TROPICAL FISHES

MICHAEL K. STOSKOPF

The problems faced by clinicians selecting therapeutic drugs for marine tropical fishes are similar to those enumerated in Chapter 72. The choices of route of delivery are the same with similar precautions and recommendations. Unfortunately the basis for selecting drug doses is perhaps even less well documented. Extrapolation from anecdotal and incomplete information is the rule rather than the exception. Considerably more work needs to be done in this area of fish medicine.

The one major factor that distinguishes chemotherapeutic considerations in marine tropicals from those in freshwater tropicals is the nature of the environment. The interaction of drugs and chemicals with salt water can have a significant impact on the availability of drugs provided to be taken per os, or used as a dip or bath. This has been best studied for the common use of divalent copper ions to treat protozoan infections. In addition, the physiologic adaptations of fishes to marine environments may have significant effects on drug disposition and kinetics.

COPPER

A variety of copper compounds have been used as therapeutic and prophylactic agents for fishes in both fresh and salt water (Table 83–1). Copper may account for 50% of the disease treatment products available to saltwater hobbyists. Unfortunately, the efficacy of copper therapy is not well documented, even though treatment techniques have not changed appreciably in 2 decades. There is, however, strong anecdotal confidence in the efficacy of copper against protozoan and even some metazoan parasites.

It is critically important to understand the interaction of copper with various ions and water conditions to understand why a treatment that might be suitable for marine tropical fishes can be devastating in a freshwater system. Anything that affects the solubility or binding strength of copper complexes will affect bioavailability and bioactivity. The toxicity of copper depends on its speciation. Free cupric ion is most toxic, with complexed forms being less toxic. In natural seawater, copper is complexed with organic and inorganic ligands.

Dissolved copper can chelate with hydroxides, carbonates, amino acids, and polypeptides to form neutral, anionic, or cationic complexes in marine waters (Fig. 83–1). Ammonia or amines generally form positive complexes with copper. A less stable neutral complex is formed between copper and acetate. In marine water, chloride ions bind strongly to copper ions and form stable divalent negatively charged soluble complexes that are less available to biologic systems than the hydrated complexes of copper ions. These chloride-copper complexes will break down at the alkaline pH of most seawater, causing copper to precipitate out in the form of insoluble salts and copper carbonate.

Copper depletion occurs owing to equilibrium with any calcium or magnesium carbonate present in a tank, such as coral, oyster shell, or dolomite (Keith, 1981). Changes in system dynamics, such as increased salinity or decreased pH, can redissolve precipitated or adsorbed copper suddenly, resulting in toxic levels (Cardeilhac and Whitaker, 1988).

Toxicity

Copper causes toxic changes in the nervous system, gills, liver, kidneys, and the immune system of fishes (Cardeilhac et al., 1979; Gardner and La-Roche, 1973). Fish exposed to acute overdoses of copper become dark and lethargic. At this stage of copper toxicity, gill lesions consist of blunting of the gill filaments with the presence of thick, dilated mucous cells and congested capillaries (Cardeilhac et al., 1979). With further exposure, fish become indifferent to external stimuli and are easy to catch. If

TABLE 83–1. Copper Treatment Stock Solutions

Copper Citrate
  3 g copper sulfate pentahydrate
  2 g citric acid monohydrate
  Bring to 750 ml with distilled water in a volumetric flask
  Final concentration 1 mg/ml of copper

Copper Sulfate
  3 g copper sulfate pentahydrate
  Bring to volume in 750-ml flask with distilled water
  Final concentration 1 mg/ml copper

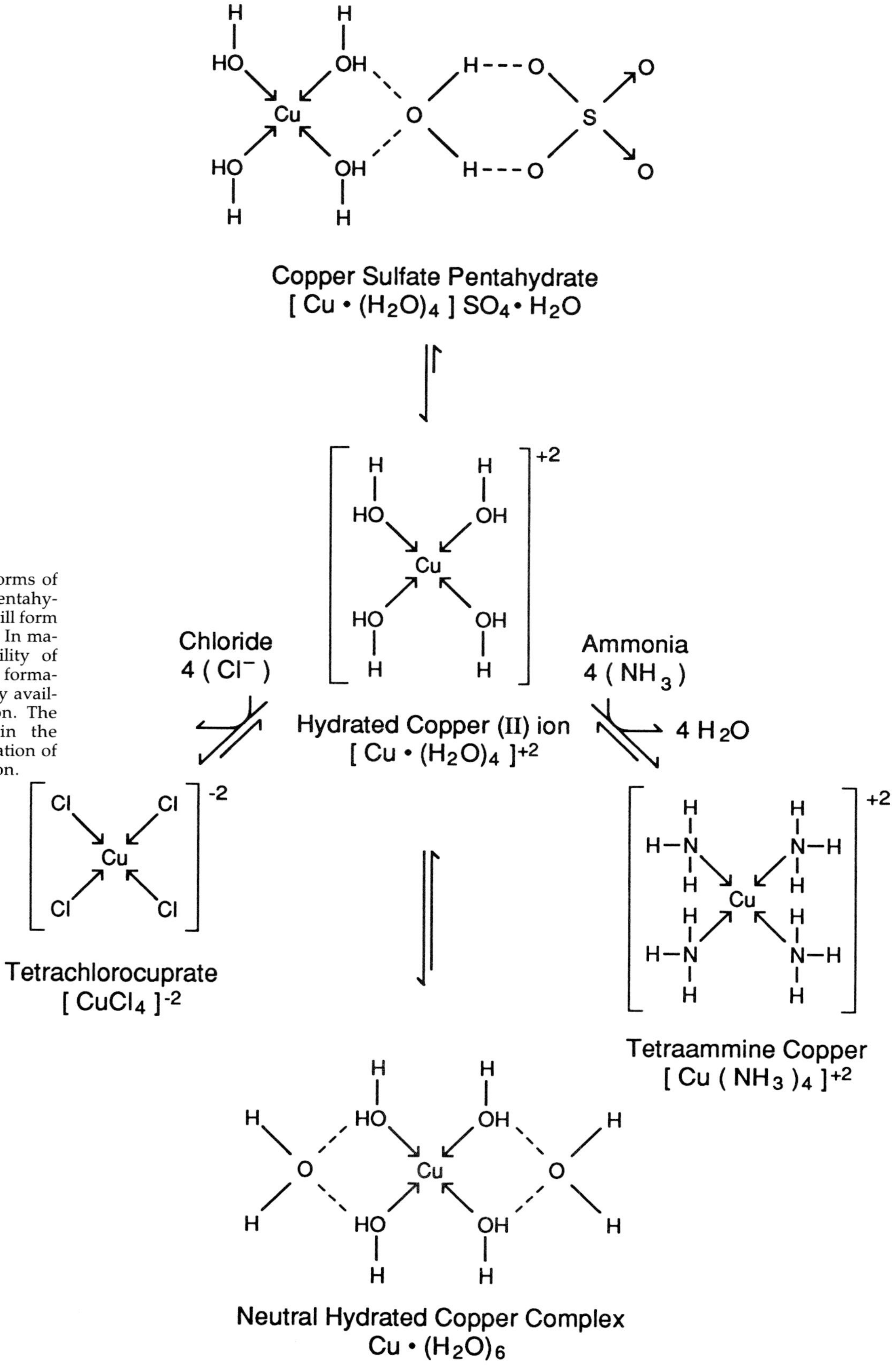

Copper Sulfate Pentahydrate
$[Cu \cdot (H_2O)_4] SO_4 \cdot H_2O$

Hydrated Copper (II) ion
$[Cu \cdot (H_2O)_4]^{+2}$

Chloride
$4 (Cl^-)$

Ammonia
$4 (NH_3)$

$4 H_2O$

FIGURE 83–1. Important forms of copper. Copper sulfate pentahydrate dissolved in water will form hydrated copper (II) ions. In marine waters, the availability of chloride ions will favor formation of the less biologically available tetrachlorocuprate ion. The presence of ammonia in the water will allow the formation of tetraammine copper (II) ion.

Tetrachlorocuprate
$[CuCl_4]^{-2}$

Tetraammine Copper
$[Cu (NH_3)_4]^{+2}$

Neutral Hydrated Copper Complex
$Cu \cdot (H_2O)_6$

exposure continues, fish become uncoordinated and disoriented, losing normal posture. Finally, they become moribund and die.

As the toxicity progresses, serum potassium increases, probably due to cellular damage. In addition, exposure to even low levels of copper causes an increase in hematocrit, serum glucose, and serum levels of hepatic enzymes, as well as decreased immunoglobulin production. Hepatic lesions frequently consist of vacuolar degeneration (Pearl and Cardeilhac, 1982). Direct effects of copper on lateral line mechanoreceptors are documented, possibly explaining some of the postural changes seen (Cardeilhac et al., 1979).

Fish exposed to slowly rising copper levels can adapt to the presence of the metal by inducing metallothionine production in the liver. This is the reason for the slow introduction of fish to therapeutic copper levels. Metallothionine binds copper and facilitates its internal storage without toxic effects.

Treating with Copper

When treating marine systems, be sure there are no water-quality problems before the treatment. Studies on the effects of copper on nitrification have been inconsistent, but negative effects have been documented at levels of 0.2 ppm copper (Bower and Turner, 1982). The negative impact of copper on the nitrification beds usually remains much longer than the actual copper treatment. This may be due to the difficulties involved in removing copper from a system. Before treating, always test water first to see how much copper is inadvertently in the tank. Remove any sensitive animals such as invertebrates and particularly sensitive fishes before treating.

Routine prophylactic copper treatment is probably not a wise course. However, in the case of marine tropicals coming in from the wild or undefined sources, the risk and prevalence of ciliate parasitism is usually high enough to warrant prophylactic copper therapy. A 3-week course of copper levels of 0.15 ppm will effectively reduce surface parasitism. It is not effective in eliminating internal parasites or parasites encysting in gut tissues. A 3-week course actually takes about 4 weeks to implement, since copper levels should be brought to 0.15 gradually over a period of 3 days and then stabilized. Keep in mind that colorimetric methods only determine total copper, and to judge therapeutic effectiveness, you need to know the free copper ion concentration. On the market are several chelated copper products. These are purported to be less toxic to fishes. Curiously, since the active ingredient of copper is the copper ion, a product that relies on chelation to reduce toxicity should be proportionally less effective against the parasites it is intended to treat.

Treating with copper in tanks containing calcium carbonate materials considerably slows the process of reaching therapeutic levels. Carbonate materials take about 55% of the copper in solution within the first 2 hours of initial treatment with copper sulfate. Another 20% of the copper ions are absorbed over the next 22 hours. Within 24 hours of the initial treatment, nearly 75% of the copper added for treatment is unavailable if carbonate materials are present (Cardeilhac and Whitaker, 1988).

Copper is not magic, and coppered tanks should not be considered sterilized, a common misconception. Many organisms survive copper therapy. Contagion between coppered tanks and other systems is a reasonable expectation if the opportunity for cross-contamination is allowed to arise. There are no studies documenting any germicidal effect at therapeutic levels against viral diseases and the direct effect of copper on bacteria and fungi may well be overshadowed by the impact of copper on the immune system of fishes.

The immunosuppressive nature of copper is a major practical drawback of copper therapy. Recently shipped fish are transiently immunosuppressed from the cortisol surges caused by the stress of packing and shipping. Unless there is an ongoing outbreak of protozoan disease upon or early after arrival, it is generally a good idea to wait at least a week after arrival for the fish to settle and acclimate before starting copper treatment. During copper therapy, the appearance of severe bacterial disease, which will not be affected by copper treatment, may require the suspension of the antiparasitic prophylaxis to allow the immune system to respond adequately to the bacterial or viral diseases. Similarly, fish showing signs of viral or bacterial disease on arrival should not be subjected to copper until the other problems are under control. This highlights the importance of diagnostics in a quarantine protocol.

It takes at least 3 or 4 days to remove the copper from a system at the end of treatment. Even then, only a portion of the copper is usually removed. Chelated copper compounds may take considerably longer to remove. Copper is generally removed with activated carbon filtration, which will bind copper ions. The removal of copper with activated carbon is not appreciably affected by temperature or pH. Water changes are also used to speed the removal process. The most effective way to speed the removal of copper from a treated tank is to remove any corals and carbonate structures from the system (Bower, 1982).

TETRACYCLINES

The tetracyclines are another chemotherapeutic group that has significantly different activity and kinetics in marine systems compared to freshwater systems (Fig. 83–2). The tetracyclines are antibiotics derived from the elaboration products of *Streptomyces* spp. They are very stable and have found uses for treating diseases in a wide variety of species, ranging from man to palm trees. Their mechanism of action

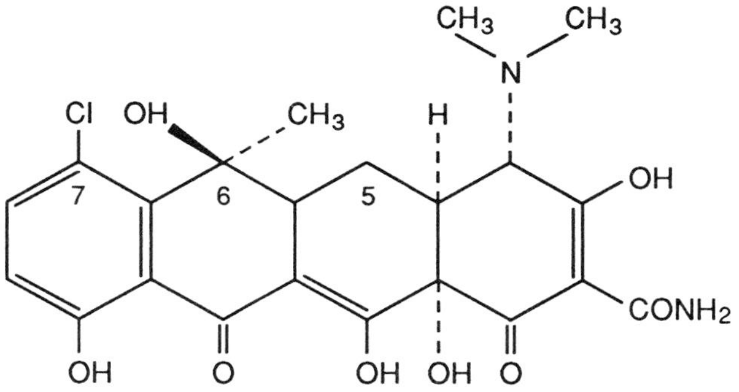

Chlortetracycline

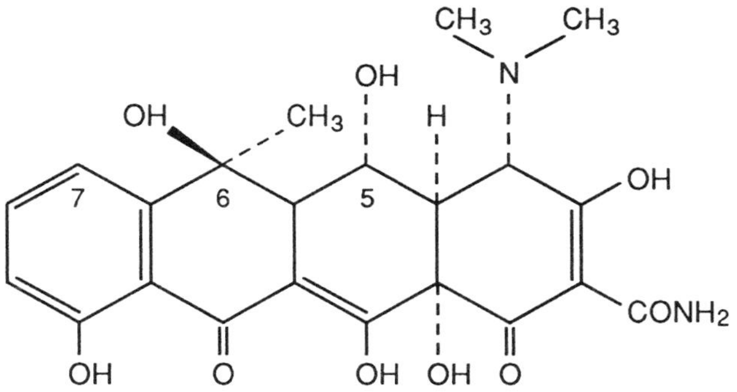

Oxytetracycline

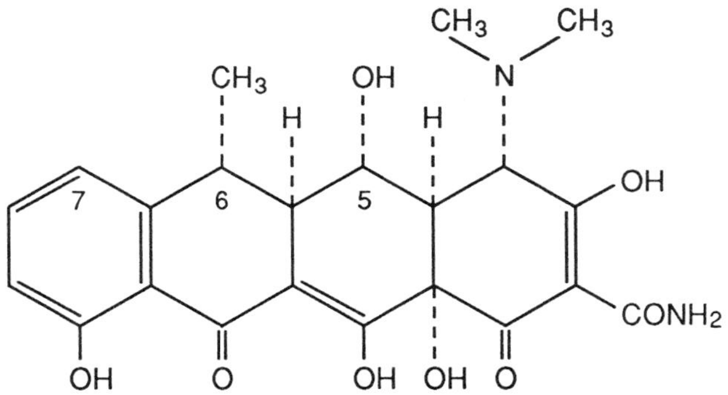

Doxycycline

FIGURE 83–2. The structure of selected tetracyclines.

is to inhibit protein synthesis. Much like the aminoglycosides, tetracyclines bind specifically to 30-S ribosomes, interfering with transcription.

They are generally supplied in the form of a hydrochloride salt and are soluble in water. Oxytet-

racycline, for example, is highly soluble, up to 1 kg/ L of water. However, on standing, it hydrolyses and precipitates out as a crystalline hydrochloride. The closely related chlortetracycline (Aureomycin) differs from oxytetracycline by the presence of a chlorine atom at the 7 position of the polycyclic aromatic skeleton and the absence of a hydroxyl group at the 5 position. It is considerably less soluble in water (0.5 to 0.6 g/L), and even more readily forms stable insoluble crystalline salts.

As a crystalline hydrochloride, oxytetracycline is so stable it retains potency when frozen, exposed to pH 1 environments, or even when heated for 4 days at 100°C. It loses less than 5% activity when heated to 56°C for 4 months, but it is less resistant to alkaline pH. The half-life of oxytetracycline at pH 8.5 (37°C) is 33 hours. In marine waters, this susceptibility to alkaline pH, combined with a strong affinity for calcium ions to form stable insoluble calcium complexes, significantly reduces the effectiveness of tetracyclines. Actually, tetracyclines can bind to a range of divalent and trivalent cations, including magnesium, to form complexes that can in turn bind to larger molecules, including proteins. Recent work has shown that at pH 8, in seawater, only about 5.3% of oxytetracycline remains as therapeutically active free drug after complexing with the polyvalent cations of seawater (Lunestad and Goksoyr, 1990). The same workers demonstrated significant effects on antibiotic sensitivity testing when marine salts are supplemented in the agar base of the media at levels simulating seawater (Lunestad and Goksoyr, 1990). This has important implications on the selection of tetracyclines as therapeutic agents in marine systems. There is undoubtedly a marked underestimation of organism resistance to tetracyclines when unsupplemented media are used for sensitivity testing (Lunestad and Goksoyr, 1990).

Tetracyclines are very broad spectrum. When they were first introduced, they were highly effective against rickettsiae, chlamydiae, and gram-positive and gram-negative bacteria. Unfortunately, organisms which are resistant to one tetracycline often are resistant to others, and frequently are also moderately insensitive to chloramphenicol. Resistance factors can be actively accumulated by certain bacteria, and plasmids containing resistance markers (called R factors) are readily transferred between even different species of bacteria. This, combined with evidence of considerable stability of tetracyclines in bottom sediments (Samuelsen et al., 1988), makes the use of these drugs in the marine environment a questionable practice. The main mechanism for oxytetracycline degradation in the environment appears to be photodecomposition (Oka et al., 1989), a relatively ineffective mechanism in bottom sediments, particularly in deeper waters.

Deleterious effects of tetracyclines have been recorded in a variety of species. These include allergic responses, angioedema, photophobia, anaphylaxis, glossitis, gastrointestinal irritation, leukocytosis, formation of atypical lymphocytes, thrombopenia, weight loss, negative nitrogen balance, renal dysfunction, and delayed blood coagulation due to calcium chelation. There is no reason not to believe that many of these effects may affect fishes treated with these drugs.

LITERATURE CITED

Bower, C.E. (1982) Copper treatment: The dark side of the story. Drum and Croaker 20(1):39–44.

Bower, C.E., and Turner, D.T. (1982) Effects of seven chemotherapeutic agents on nitrification in closed seawater culture systems. Aquaculture 29:331.

Cardeilhac, P.T., and Whitaker, B.R. (1988) Tropical fish medicine. Copper treatments, uses and precautions. Vet. Clin. North Am., Small Anim. Pract. 18(2):435–448.

Cardeilhac, P.T., Simpson, C.F., Lovelock, R.L., Yosha-Calderwood, H.W., and Gudat, J.C. (1979) Failure of osmoregulation with apparent potassium intoxication in marine teleosts: a primary toxic effect of copper. Aquaculture 17:231.

Gardner, G.R., and LaRoche, G. (1973) Copper-induced lesions in estuarine teleosts. J. Fish. Res. Bd. Can. 30:363.

Keith, R.E. (1981) Loss of therapeutic copper in closed marine systems. Aquaculture 24:355.

Lunestad, B.T., and Goksoyr, J. (1990) Reduction in the antibacterial effect of oxytetracycline in sea water by complex formation with magnesium and calcium. Dis. Aquatic Organ. 9:67–72.

Oka, H., Ikai, Y., Kawamura, N., Yamada, M., Harada, K., Ito, S., and Suzuki, M. (1989) Photodecomposition products of tetracycline in aqueous solution. J. Agric. Food Chem. 37:226–231.

Pearl, D.S., and Cardeilhac, P.T. (1982) Mechanism of copper toxicity to marine fish when different routes of administration are used. Proc. Int. Assoc. Aquatic Anim. Med. 13:2.

Samuelsen, O., Torsvik, V., Hansen, P.K., Pittman, K., and Ervik, A. (1988) Organic waste and antibiotics from aquaculture. Int. Coun. Explor. Sea Comm. Meet. (Mariculture Comm.) F:14:1–14.

Weinstein, L. (1975) Antimicrobial agents, tetracyclines and chloramphenicol. In: The Pharmacological Basis of Therapeutics (Goodman, L.S., and Gilman, A., eds.). Macmillan, New York, pp. 1183–1200.

Windholz, M., Budavari, S., Blumetti, R.F., and Otterbein, E.S. (eds.) (1983) The Merck Index. Merck & Co, Rahway, New Jersey.

SECTION VII

MARINE COLD-WATER

FISHES

GERALD JOHNSON, *Section Editor*

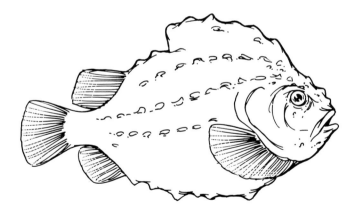

Chapter 84

MARINE COLD-WATER COMMERCIAL FISH TAXONOMY AND NATURAL HISTORY

RICHARD E. ZURBRIGG

Marine cold-water commercial food fishes are a heterogeneous group whose species should not be viewed as minor variations on a theme (i.e., the horse, the dog, the fish). For example, the Pacific cod and Pacific halibut are mutually less "related" than are the African elephant and Florida manatee. An awareness of such divergence through a knowledge of taxonomy (classification), systematics (relationships), and natural history (biology) brings valuable insight to any study of species-specific problems.

The "North American" marine cold-water fishes examined here are a select few whose artificial propagation and/or husbandry is feasible. As representatives of large taxonomic orders, they constitute only a partial list of saltwater species having such potential.

GADIDS ("CODS")

Cod, haddock, pollock, and hake all are members of the broadly defined Gadidae, much sought for their fine, firm flesh. (Note that the common names cod, hake, and pollock refer to a wide variety of forms.) This family includes some 70 marine species worldwide, the burbot or ling being the only freshwater exception. Some close relatives are the moras or flatnose cods, grenadiers or rattails, and cusk-eels. More distant are the bizarre anglers and batfishes.

Gadids belong to a side branch (Paracanthopterygii) in the evolution of the "higher" fishes (Acanthopterygii). They are distinguished by many esoteric osteologic characters but are usually identified as being elongate yet heavy-bodied, with large heads and mouths containing abundant well-developed teeth. A chin barbel is often present. The prominent soft-rayed fins include large pectorals and jugular/thoracic pelvics. The scales are small and smooth. As

in most advanced fishes, gadids lack a pneumatic duct to their swimbladder. Consequently, these fishes suffer gross swimbladder distention and oral eversion of the digestive tract when hauled from the depths to the surface.

COD

The Atlantic cod and Pacific cod (Fig. 84–1) share a similar morphology and biology. They exhibit three dorsal and two anal fins, an inferior mouth, and a chin barbel. Color is muted and variably gray, green, or brown, often with numerous spots. The lateral line is conspicuously pale, and the belly off-white. The infamous oily liver is best forgotten by those unfortunate generations raised on its extracts.

Cod occur as distinct populations, or "stocks," migrating locally over subarctic and temperate continental shelves and preferring waters under 10°C. Northern stocks initiate their mid-water spawning in winter with a progressively later start southward, ending as late as September. This correlates with the accelerated hatching of the myriad 1.0- to 1.5-mm pelagic eggs (as many as 12 million per female) in warmer southern waters where spawning duration is 6.0 versus 1.5 weeks. The eggs and larvae float in the less saline coastal waters. Larvae absorb their yolk sacs in 1 to 2 weeks. When they are about 5 cm

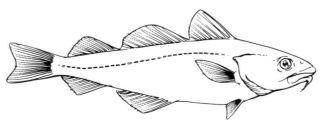

FIGURE 84–1. The Pacific cod.

long, the young cod sink to the bottom where growth depends largely on temperature and food availability. Ravenous feeders, juveniles and young adult cod favor benthic invertebrates, whereas older fish (4 to 5 years) frequently venture into the water column (0 to 55°M) seeking such prey as capelin, sand lance, rockfish, and herring. Cod mature at 5 to 8 years, with fork lengths of 40 to 60 cm and weights of 1 to 2 kg. An age of 27 years and a weight of 95 kg have been recorded; however, 4 to 8 year olds are the rule. Young cod are food for many predators, not the least of which are larger cod. Adults are devoured by aquatic mammals, particularly seals, and are the intermediate hosts for *Phocanema decipiens*, the sealworm.

Norway has artificially propagated cod since the nineteenth century. The controlled culture and release of fry bypasses the astronomical early losses in nature and is a valued adjunct to the local fishery. More recent attempts at actual cod farming have begun to deal effectively with cannibalism. North America is beginning to follow the lead and consider the similar potential of haddock and pollock, but progress may be impeded by recreational, navigational, industrial, and municipal constraints.

SABLEFISHES

The sablefish (Fig. 84–2) and skilfish are the sole representatives of the family Anoplopomatidae (collectively known as sablefishes), found only in the north Pacific Ocean. The sablefish, also called blackcod or coalfish, is particularly valued on the west coast as fresh and smoked products, whereas the skilfish is commercially important only in the Far East. The flesh of both species is fine-grained and tasty, but very oily. The phylogeny of sablefishes is poorly known. They possess a bony "strut" extending from the orbital base to the anterior operculum or mail cheek. They are currently considered allied to lumpfishes and rockfish, or ocean perch, greenlings, sculpins, and searobins.

The sablefishes are distinguished by their slender form, two well-spaced dorsal fins, thoracic single-spined pelvic fins, fine patchy teeth in a small but broad mouth, and a large slit posterior to the last gill arch. The adult coloration is a reticulate slate green/blue-to-black dorsally and a light gray ventrally. The jet-black inner operculum is very characteristic. As in cods, the liver is rich in oil; however, the swim-

bladder is entirely absent. Consequently, sablefishes often remain quite lively when first caught, even when taken from very deep waters.

Despite occasional extensive migrations, adult sablefishes are basically sedentary deep-water forms typically found below 200 m (exceptionally to 2000 m). They school on the continental shelf in progressively deeper water from Alaska to northern Mexico. More or less distinct stocks spawn below 300 m from January to March, producing millions of 2-mm bathypelagic eggs. These hatch by May or June, the postlarvae initially feeding on plankton. The lightly colored juveniles soon move into shore waters where they eat crustaceans, worms, and small fish. They are especially attracted by effluents from food-processing plants. Growth is optimal at 6 to 8°C and steady to age 3 to 4 years (40 to 45 cm, 0.5 kg), at which time the subadults move into deep water to forage principally on rockfish, herring, and squid. Maturity occurs at 5 years, commonly at lengths of 50 to 60 cm and weights near 1 kg. The legal catch limit is 55 cm. The fishery typically includes individuals from 4 to 35 years old, with lengths to about 1 m and weights up to 15 kg. An age of 55 years and a weight of 57 kg have been reported.

Sablefishes are placid and resistant to disease and are easily handled. They thrive in well-managed impoundments and are quite receptive to culture, but artificial hatching is difficult, necessitating collection of juveniles at sea. This dependence on the vagaries of year-class strength is most undesirable. Attempts at catching and fattening small legal-sized sablefishes have met with mixed success. Mortalities have been associated with high summer temperatures (>10°C), low salinities from run-off, density stress, and infected wounds. Another problem is food, for although sablefishes are indiscriminate feeders, raw fish and offal transmit diseases such as anasakid parasites and mycobacteria. An acceptable synthetic diet with controlled composition and sterility would seem most desirable.

Despite setbacks, the potential for sablefish culture is great. The current demand for smoked and fresh sablefish products far outstrips the fishery's maximum sustainable yield of 3500 metric tons per year.

LUMPFISHES

The homely lumpfishes are classified in the Cyclopteridae, a worldwide family of 177 temperate-/cold-water fishes. Nearly all genera exhibit small gill openings, a loss of the lateral line, and pelvic fins that are modified to form a thoracic disc capable of adhering to a substrate (Fig. 84–3). Some relatives have been listed with the sablefishes. The sculpins and the obscure, sculpinlike Psychrolutidae are the nearest affiliates.

The lumpfish is particularly prized for its quality roe, although some Europeans also enjoy the flesh. It is characterized by a short stout scaleless body, a

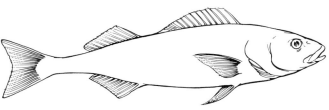

FIGURE 84–2. The sablefish.

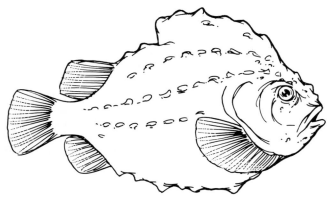

FIGURE 84–3. The lumpfish.

mixed cartilaginous-gelatinous back hump enveloping the dorsal fin, and a leathery skin covered in hard tubercles; the larger tubercles are arranged in seven rows. Color varies with surroundings, although dorsal blue-gray or green-brown with ventral yellow or white is common. Breeding males have red bellies that are brightest near the sucking disc. The adults lack a swimbladder.

Lumpfishes are found in the north Atlantic Ocean from Chesapeake Bay north to Hudson Bay and southeast from Greenland to northern Portugal. Adults are not highly migratory, and at age 5 years or older move shoreward in spring to spawn when the water temperature reaches 4°C. Lumpfishes home in on the previous years' sites over rocky bottoms and abundant kelp and seaweed. The smaller males precede the females to establish territories. The colorful spongy egg masses are attached to rocks by females laying several batches at 8- to 14-day intervals. These are guarded and aerated by the males until the 5-mm larvae hatch in 6 to 8 weeks. The young grow rapidly to 45 to 75 mm in their first year, continuing to feast on the plankton associated with surface seaweed.

Although weak swimmers, adult lumpfishes pursue a semipelagic lifestyle in the upper 50 to 60 m of the ocean, becoming gradually demersal in winter before spawning. A seaward fall migration initiates a period of heavy feeding on crustaceans, jellyfish, comb jellies, sand lance, and small herring. Lumpfishes may be precocious at 3 years and 11 cm in length, but females usually mature when 4 to 5 years old at lengths of 30 to 40 cm. Weight gains occur at a relatively faster rate than increases in length, with females far outstripping males. Females average 3.5 kg and 44 cm at age 5 to 9 years when caught in the fishery. Maximum sizes taken are 64 cm and 10 kg. Seals are significant predators, although lumpfishes have also been found as stomach contents in Greenland sharks and sperm whales.

Gill nets trap a narrow size range of large female lumpfishes in spring, bringing a lucrative return. The eggs are best excised when they are mature red to purple rather than when overripe and red-orange. Up to 1 kg of roe (140,000 eggs) may be harvested

from a 45-cm female, with rare counts to 400,000 eggs in very large specimens. The end product of a washing, sieving, salting, and curing process is a choice caviar regarded as a delicacy on both sides of the Atlantic. In Europe, a limited market exists for the smoked flesh of breeding males. Successful small-scale culturing of lumpfish indicates that these fishes have significant potential for commercial rearing, impoundment, and caviar production.

TUNA

The name *tuna* or *tunny* collectively represents 13 of the 48 species within the Scombridae, which also incorporates the mackerels and bonitos. Many of these warm-water speedsters are prized both for food and for sport. The swordfishes, louvar, and billfishes are relatives.

The tunas are exquisite, highly evolved, pelagic swimming and feeding machines. Their powerful, round fusiform bodies are streamlined with a tightly closed mouth, fared eyes, anterior paired fins, two separate dorsal fins in fitted slots, dorsal and ventral finlets on the slender double-keeled caudal peduncle, a lunate caudal fin, and smooth fine scales.

Bluefin Tuna

Bluefin tuna undergo vast migrations through the north Pacific and north Atlantic oceans. Although they are not strictly cold-water fishes, large individuals invade the productive northern climes each summer to gorge themselves on fishes and squid. This is facilitated by the bluefin tuna's internal thermoregulation that can maintain body temperatures up to 15°C warmer than the ambient temperature. This species may be the largest of all the bony fishes (to 4.3 m, 910 kg), and one of the swiftest (70 to 88 km/hour). As a tuna, the bluefin is characterized by its huge size, specific meristics, and color (Fig. 84–4). It is a deep metallic blue-black (without stripes) dorsally graduating to silver laterally and white ventrally, with yellowish finlets and no black spots below the pectoral fin. The swimbladder is present in this perpetually swimming species.

Pelagic schools of voracious bluefin tuna roam throughout the upper reaches of the oceans in pur-

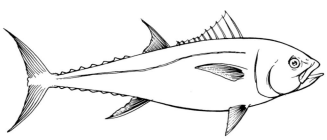

FIGURE 84–4. The bluefin tuna.

suit of prey. Large tuna, solitary or in small compact schools, best tolerate environmental extremes and dominate the cool fringes of the species' range. Adults aged 10 years and over are the principal spawners in the subtropical spring, with fecundities of 5 to 60 million eggs per female. The buoyant 1-mm eggs hatch in a few days at 25 to 30°C. The fraction of juveniles surviving early predation exhibit amazing growth to 4 kg by 1 year, doubling in weight each subsequent year to first maturity at age 4 or 5. Rapid increase in length continues to about 2.5 m or an age of 12 years. Thereafter, fattening occurs. Each summer between June and early November, the "giants" indiscriminately devour prey off Canada and the northern United States. These fish must eat frequently to compensate for a small stomach and high metabolic rate. While members of this species may reach an age of 38 years, the failing fishery comprises largely 15 to 30 year olds. Other than man, the few predators of mature bluefin tuna include killer whales and mako sharks.

Bluefin tuna are usually marketed fresh or frozen, but they are now scarce. For example, few "giants" remain to be trapped in St. Margaret's Bay, Nova Scotia, for seasonal impoundment. Their fattening, slaughter, and air transport to lucrative Japanese markets was a most successful enterprise. The familiar canned tuna includes mostly albacore as "white meat tuna" versus the "light meat tuna" of other species such as skipjack and yellowfin tuna. The latter should not be confused with the yellowtail, a member of the Carangidae extensively cultured in Japan.

FLATFISHES

The flatfishes constitute the specialized order Pleuronectiformes, many of whose 538 species are commercially prized as food. Their identification as halibut, flounder, plaice, turbot, sole, dab, brill, and so forth is extremely imprecise and confusing. For example, the plaice, or righteye flounders, Dover sole, true soles, and turbot, or the lefteye flounders, caught or cultured in European waters are totally different species from similarly named fishes living off North American shores.

A lively debate exists concerning the classification and evolutionary placement of the Pleuronectiformes. Many researchers classify the group as closely related to such "advanced" fishes as the dominant Perciformes. Others regard them as specialized offshoots derived from an earlier phylogenetic line. Whatever the case, flatfishes are very distinctive forms.

In general, adult flatfishes are demersal and carnivorous, possessing highly compressed, unsymmetric bodies with both eyes on the slightly rounded pigmented "top" side. Usually the "blind" side is flat and unpigmented, the median fins long, the body cavity small, and the swimbladder absent. Ontogeny involves a conventional bilaterally sym-

metric postlarva that metamorphoses via eye migration and complex osseous, nervous, and muscular modifications to the future adult form. Individual species and families are often exclusively left- or right-sided, referring to the eyed side.

The North American fauna includes a bewildering array of commercially important flatfishes. A short list of Atlantic cold-water forms might include American plaice, Atlantic halibut, witch flounder, or "sole," yellowtail flounder, winter flounder, and Greenland turbot (also called the Greenland halibut). Favored Pacific species are petrale sole, or "brill," Pacific halibut, rock sole, yellowfin sole, "Dover sole," and "English sole." This mixed assemblage defies general description, each member having a unique life history and environmental niche. A closer look at two savory righteye flounders from the family Pleuronectidae illustrates this point.

American Plaice

The American plaice is also known as Canadian plaice, plaice, dab, sand dab, rough dab, long rough dab (U.K.), flounder, and sole! Occurring from the Gulf of Maine to Greenland, it constitutes half of all Canadian flatfish landings, and is valued for the excellent quality and flavor of its flesh. The highly regarded rock sole fills a similar economic niche on the west coast. The American plaice has a small head but large jaws with modest conical teeth, and a long dorsal fin starting over the moderately sized eyes (Fig. 84–5). It has a prominent preanal spine, convex caudal fin, arched lateral line over the pectoral, and red to gray-brown color on the eyed side with white dorsal and anal fin tips. The blind side is white.

American plaice prefer temperatures of –0.5 to 1.5°C (range –1.5 to 13°C), depths of 90 to 250 m (range 0 to 700 m), and fine sandy or mud bottoms. They are relatively sedentary despite offshore winter and onshore spring movements. Bottom spawning takes place from April to June at temperatures of 0 to 2.5°C. Females produce up to 1.5 million eggs (1.5 to 2.8 mm). These float to the surface after fertilization and drift widely to provide virtually the only intermingling of the geographically distinct stocks. Hatching time varies with temperature (11 to 14 days at 5°C), to produce 4- to 6-mm larvae. Metamorphosis

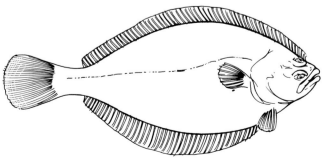

FIGURE 84–5. The American plaice.

occurs at 18 to 34 mm. Youngsters settle down to grow slowly on a diet of mysids, amphipods, brittle stars, and polychaete worms. Individuals over 30 cm add larger echinoderms, bivalve molluscs, and fishes such as capelin and sand lance to their diet. Females are larger, mature later, and live longer than males. Females become adults at lengths of 30 to 50 cm and ages 8 to 11 years. The largest plaice on record was a female 81 cm long, weighing 6.3 kg gutted. Maximum age for this species is approximately 25 years.

The American plaice biomass is particularly sensitive to overexploitation of the young adults and subadults that constitute most of the population. This species responds to stock depletion by a progressive earlier maturation of diminutive individuals. Any assessment of American plaice's potential for culture should account for its susceptibility to a cornucopia of parasites. Also, gonad development can deplete muscle protein, producing a temporarily flaccid, jellylike flesh undesirable for sale and consumption. A high incidence of lymphocystis infection has been reported in several stocks.

Pacific Halibut

The Pacific halibut and the probably conspecific Atlantic halibut are by far the largest and most valuable of the flatfishes. The halibut is more elongate than most flatfishes (Fig. 84–6). Its length is three times its width. It has a large head and well-

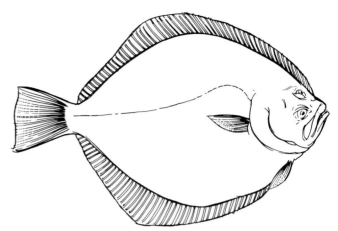

FIGURE 84–6. The Pacific halibut.

armed jaws, a long dorsal fin starting over the prominent projecting eyes, a lunate caudal fin, an arched lateral line over the pectoral, and olive, dark brown, or black color on the eyed side, frequently decorated with irregular lighter blotches. The blind side is usually white. The flesh is of premium quality.

Pacific halibut are demersal inhabitants of deep ocean waters in winter (to over 1200 m) and fringes of continental shelves or banks in summer (30 to 250 m), preferring temperatures of 3 to 8°C. They are distributed from Japan, across to Alaska, and south to California, sometimes moving tremendous dis-

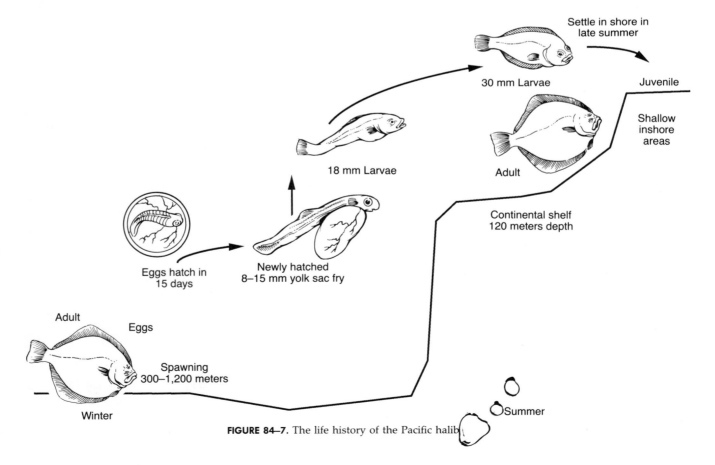

FIGURE 84–7. The life history of the Pacific halibut.

tances (up to 4000 km). Halibut stocks are thus extensively interrelated and not distinct. Spawning occurs in winter along the edge of the continental shelf at depths of 275 to 412 m (Fig. 84–7). Fecundity increases with size, from 0.5 to over 4.0 million eggs per female. The mid-water eggs (3.0 to 3.5 mm) hatch in about 15 days to symmetric, upright larvae (8 to 15 mm) with huge yolk sacs drifting below 200 m. At 18 mm in length, the postlarvae have lost the yolk sac and are feeding on plankton. By this time the left eye has already initiated its migration to the right side, and metamorphosis is completed as the postlarvae slowly rise to 100-m depths as 30-mm juveniles. When approximately 6 months old, the youngsters exhibit an adult form and settle to the bottom in shallow inshore areas for the next 2 to 3 years. Here they eat small crustaceans and tiny fish. They subsequently move into deeper waters, migrating most extensively in winter to the southeast. This counterbalances the passive northeasterly drift of eggs and larvae. Halibut are powerful swimmers and active predators that devour anything they can catch, including octopus, squid, crabs, clams, herring, sablefishes, gadids, rockfish, and flatfishes including young halibut. Females grow faster, mature later, and live longer than males. The average age to maturity is 8 years for males and 12 years for females. At 10 years, the average lengths for males and females are 97 cm (9 kg) and 120 cm (17 kg), respectively. Few males exceed 36 kg, and all halibut over 45 kg are females. Specimens approaching 3 meters in length and 320 kg have been taken, but the average landed size is about 16 kg. Maximum recorded ages are 27 years for males and 42 years for females.

The Pacific halibut fishery is comprehensively managed by the International Pacific Halibut Commission to sustain yields, markets, and prices. Studies by this agency indicate that halibut now grow and mature significantly faster than in the 1920s, presumably a positive response to fishing pressure and changing environmental factors. This contrasts sharply with the negative impact of heavy fishing on American plaice stocks.

The Commission has long battled the use of the name *Greenland halibut* for the fatty, inferior Greenland turbot, a related flatfish. This was sold competitively as halibut, misleading consumers and confounding dietitians. Consequently, the United States now requires that Greenland turbot not be marketed as halibut. True halibut flesh is sold principally as the fresh or frozen product. Most canning efforts have been stymied by organoleptic deterioration and short shelf life.

Research into the propagation and culture of halibut has brought promising results through the application of biologic knowledge. For example, the previous unacceptable mortality rates associated with controlled hatching, initial growth, and metamorphosis have been reduced by imitating such natural conditions as low ambient light. The halibut is regarded as a very clean fish, and its capacity for accelerated growth implies a great potential for aquaculture.

LITERATURE CITED

Anonymous (1987) Annual report 1986. International Pacific Halibut Commission, Seattle.

Anonymous (1987) The Pacific halibut: biology, fishery, and management. International Pacific Halibut Commission Tech. Rep. 22:59.

Anonymous (1988) Atlantic Groundfish Management Plan. Department of Fisheries and Oceans, Ottawa.

Bakken, E. (1987) Growth, biomass, and production of a small unexploited plaice stock in St. Margaret's Bay, Nova Scotia. Can. Tech. Rep. Fish. Aquatic Sci. 1555(7):51.

Bardach, J.F., Ryther, J.H., and McLarney, W.O. (1972) Aquaculture. The Farming and Husbandry of Freshwater and Marine Organisms. John Wiley & Sons, New York.

Beacham, T.D. (1982) Some aspects of growth and exploitation of American plaice (*Hippoglossoides platessoides*) in the Canadian Maritimes area of the Northwest Atlantic. Can. Tech. Rep. Fish. Aquat. Sci. 1080(3):43.

Bell, F.H. (1981) The Pacific Halibut, the Resource, and the Fishery. Alaska Northwest Publishing, Anchorage.

Bell, G.R., Slind, D., and Bagshaw, J.W. (1986) Pictorial atlas of histology of the sablefish (*Anoplopoma fimbria*). Can. Spec. Publ. Fish. Aquatic Sci. 94:93.

Benfey, T.J., and Methven, D.A. (1986) Pilot-scale rearing of larval and juvenile lumpfish (*Cyclopterus lumpus* L.), with some notes on early development. Aquaculture 56:301–306.

Bigelow, H.B., and Schroeder, W.C. (1953) Fishes of the Gulf of Maine. U.S. Fish Wildlife Serv. Fish. Bull. 74(53):577.

Bone, Q., and Marshall, N.B. (1982) Biology of Fishes. Blackie and Son, Glasgow.

Bowering, W.R. (1982) Witch Flounder. Underwater World. Department of Fisheries and Oceans, Ottawa.

Bowering, W.R. (1983) Turbot (Greenland halibut). Underwater world. Dep. Fish. Oceans, Ottawa.

Bowering, W.R. (1986) The distribution, age and growth and sexual maturity of the Atlantic halibut (*Hippoglossus hippoglossus*) in the Newfoundland and Labrador area of the Northwest Atlantic. Can. Tech. Rep. Fish. Aquat. Sci. 1432(4):34.

Breder, C.M., Jr., and Rosen, D.E. (1966) Modes of Reproduction in Fishes. T.F.H. Publications, Neptune, New Jersey.

Clay, D., and Hurlbut, T. (1988) Bluefin Tuna. Underwater World. Department of Fisheries and Oceans.

Cohen, D.M. (1989) Papers on the Systematics of Gadiform Fishes. Natural History Museum of Los Angeles County, Science Service 32(9):262.

Davenport, J., and Thorsteinsson, V. (1989) Observations on the colours of lumpsuckers, *Cyclopterus lumpus* L. J. Fish. Biol. 35(6):829–838.

Fisher, R. (1988) Assessments and observations of a cod farming operation in Newfoundland, Canada. Can. Ind. Rep. Fish. Aquatic Sci. 194(6):71.

Forrester, C.R., and Thomson, J.A. (1969) Population studies on the rock sole (*Lepidopsetta lineata*) of Northern Hecate Strait, British Columbia. Can. Tech. Rep. Fish. Res. Bd. Can. 108(2):104.

Funk, F., and Bracken, B.E. (1984) Status of the Gulf of Alaska sablefish (*Anoplopoma fimbria*) resource in 1983. Alaska Dept. Fish. Game, Informational Leaflet 235:55.

Gavaris, S. (1985) Lumpfish. Underwater World. Department of Fisheries and Oceans, Ottawa.

Gosline, W.A. (1971) Functional Morphology and Classification of Teleostean Fishes. University Press of Hawaii, Honolulu.

Greenwood, P.H., Miles, R.S., and Patterson, C. (eds.) (1973) Interrelationships of Fishes. Zool. J. Linnean Soc., Suppl. 1. Academic Press, London.

Hart, J.L. (1973) Pacific fishes of Canada. Bull. Fish. Res. Bd. Can. 180:740.

Haug, T., Huse, I., Kjorsvik E., and Rabben, H. (1989) Observations on the growth of juvenile Atlantic halibut (*Hippoglossus hippoglossus* L.) in captivity. Aquaculture 80:79–86.

Lagler, K.F., Bardach, J.E., Miller R.R., and Passino, D.R.M. (1977) Ichthyology. 2nd ed. John Wiley & Sons, New York.

Lear, W.H. (1989) Atlantic cod. Underwater World. Department of Fisheries amd Oceans, Ottawa.

Liewes, E.W. (1984) Culture, feeding and diseases of commercial flatfish species. A.A. Balkema, Rotterdam.

Love, M.S., and Cailliet, G.M. (eds.) (1979) Readings in Ichthyology. Goodyear Publishing, Santa Monica, California.

Mason, J.C., Beamish, R.J. and McFarlane, G.A. (1983) Sexual maturity, fecundity, spawning and early life history of sablefish (*Anoplopoma fimbria*) off the Pacific Coast of Canada. Can. J. Fish. Aquatic Sci. 40:2126–2134.

McClane, A.J. (ed.) (1974) McLane's New Standard Fishing Encyclopedia and International Angling Guide. Holt, Rinehart & Winston, New York.

McFarlane, G.A., and Nagata, W.D. (1988) Overview of sablefish mariculture and its potential for industry. In: Proceedings of the Fourth Alaska Aquaculture Conference, University of Alaska Sea Grant College Program (Keller, S., ed.). Fairbanks, Report 88–4:105–120.

Migdalski, E.C., and Fichter, G.S. (1976) The Fresh and Salt Water Fishes of the World. Alfred A. Knopf, New York.

Moyle, P.B., and Cech, J.J., Jr. (1988) Fishes: An Introduction to Ichthyology. 2nd ed. Prentice-Hall, Englewood Cliffs, New Jersey.

Naas, K. (1987) Current status of cod (Gadus morhua) culture in Norway—an overview of the pond method. In: Proceedings of the Third International Symposium on Reproductive Physiology of Fish (Idler, D.R, Crim, L.W., and Walsh, J.M., eds.). Memorial University, St. John's, Newfoundland, p. 82.

Nelson, J.S. (1984) Fishes of the World. John Wiley & Sons, New York.

Pitt, T.K. (1983) Yellowtail flounder. Underwater World. Department of Fisheries and Oceans, Ottawa.

Pitt, T.K. (1984a) American plaice. Underwater World. Department of Fisheries and Oceans, Ottawa.

Pitt, T.K. (1984b) Winter flounder. Underwater World. Department of Fisheries and Oceans, Ottawa.

Pritchard, G.I. (ed.) (1984) Proceedings of the National Aquaculture Conference—strategies for aquaculture development in Canada. Can. Spec. Publ. Fish. Aquatic Sci. 75:131.

Rivas, L.R. (1978) Preliminary models of annual life history cycles of the North Atlantic bluefin tuna. In: The Physiological Ecology of Tunas. Proceedings of the Tuna Physiology Workshop, Southwest Fisheries Center, La Jolla, California, 1977 (Sharp, G.D., and Dixon, A.E., eds.). Academic Press, New York, pp. 369–393.

Roache, J.F. (ed.) (1987) Atlantic Canada Aquaculture Workshop—Proceedings. General Education Series #5, Vol. I: p. 229; Vol. II: p. 191.

Scott, W.B., and Scott, M.G. (1988) Atlantic fishes of Canada. Can. Bull. Fish. Aquatic Sci. 219:731.

Shepherd, C.J., and Bromage, N.R. (eds.) (1988) Intensive Fish Farming. BSP Professional Books, Oxford, England.

Stevenson, S.C., and Baird, J.W. (1988) The fishery for lumpfish (Cyclopterus lumpus) in Newfoundland waters. Can. Tech. Rep. Fish. Aquatic Sci. 1595:26.

Wheeler, A. (1975) Fishes of the World. An Illustrated Dictionary. Macmillan, New York.

Chapter 85

COLD-WATER COMMERCIAL MARINE FISH ANATOMY AND PHYSIOLOGY

CAROL M. MORRISON   RICHARD E. ZURBRIGG

Marine fishes from cold waters show extensive variations in body shape and physiology as a result of adaptations to the wide spectrum of environments found in the sea. This chapter discusses a few selected topics of marine cold-water commercial food-fish anatomy and physiology that are related to special adaptations.

ANATOMY

Codfishes

The Atlantic cod is a fish most people know. It is of great commercial value and has been cultured in closed bays in Norway and in sea-cages in Newfoundland (Waiwood et al., 1988), although culture is not yet economically rewarding. The cod is relatively unspecialized, inhabiting North Atlantic inshore waters and continental shelves (Scott and Scott, 1988). Its anatomy has been well studied (Knorr et al., 1974; Morrison, 1987, 1988, 1990).

The head of the cod is large, and there are three dorsal fins, two anal fins, and large paired pectoral and jugular/thoracic pelvic fins (Fig. 85–1). Ribs from the vertebrae of the trunk surround the body cavity. When the body cavity is opened (Fig. 85–2), the large liver can be seen, which contains much lipid in the fall but is depleted by spring when the cod spawns. Unlike the salmonids, little fat is found in the mes-

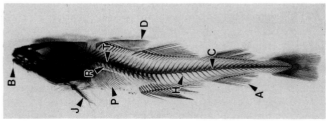

FIGURE 85–1. Juvenile cod treated with trypsin and stained with Alcian blue for cartilage and alizarin red for bone, and cleared in glycerine: (A) anal fin, (B) barbel, (C) caudal vertebrae, (D) dorsal fins, (H) hemal arches, (J) pelvic fins, (P) pectoral fins, (R) ribs, (T) thoracic vertebrae. (Specimen provided by C. Annand and D. Beanlands.) (Photo courtesy of C. Morrison.)

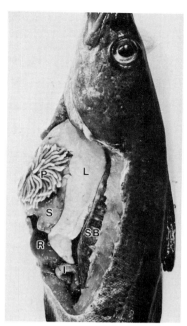

FIGURE 85–2. A cod with the body wall removed to show organs in situ: (I) intestine, (L) liver, (P) pyloric ceca, (R) rectum, (S) stomach, (SB) swimbladder. (Courtesy of C. Morrison.)

enteries between the organs. In Figure 85–3, the digestive tract has been removed from the body cavity to show the different parts of the stomach, the gallbladder, the spleen, and the sites at which the pyloric ceca and bile duct enter the digestive tract.

The internal surface of the esophagus is finely ridged, whereas the stomach has large folds, or rugae (Fig. 85–4). The pyloric ceca branch, unlike those of the salmonids (Grassé, 1958), so that while there are many pyloric ceca, there are few openings into the intestine. The pyloric ceca have a lining similar to that of the intestine and presumably aid digestion by increasing the surface area. A caudally directed internal valve separates the intestine from the rectum (Fig. 85–5). Intestinal flagellates (Poynton and Morrison, 1990) are common in the rectum but rarely found in the rest of the intestine. Apparently, the valve prevents their spread from the relatively wide, flaccid rectum, which can probably be invaded by foreign organisms through the anus.

Cod have abundant well-developed teeth (Figs. 85–6 and 85–7), which occur not only on tooth plates on the jaws and in the pharynx but also on projections on the gill arches. The projections fit into each other when the arches are closed, so that there is a complete circle of teeth around the pharynx. Cod often feed on smaller fish, so this arrangement stops prey from escaping through the gill arches and prevents damage to the delicate gill filaments. The teeth are conical and constantly replace each other, so teeth at all stages of development can be seen.

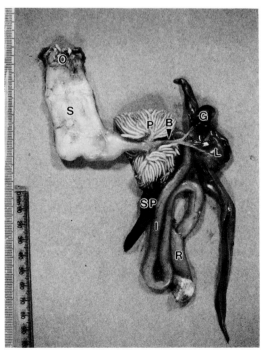

FIGURE 85–3. The digestive tract of a cod removed from the body: (B) bile duct, (G) gallbladder, (I) intestine, (L) liver, (O) esophagus, (P) pyloric ceca, (R) rectum, (S) stomach, (SP) spleen. (Courtesy of C. Morrison.)

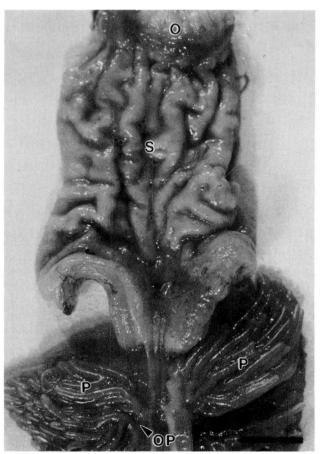

FIGURE 85–4. The anterior digestive tract of a cod opened to show the internal surfaces: (O) esophagus, (P) pyloric ceca, (S) stomach, (OP) opening of pyloric ceca into the intestine. (Courtesy of C. Morrison.)

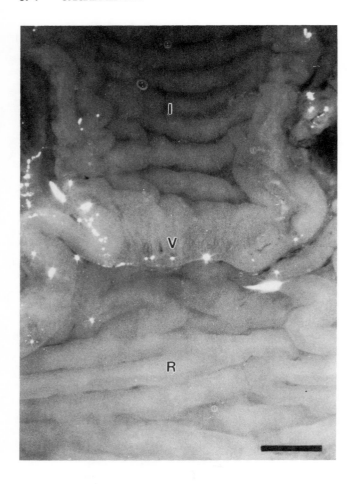

FIGURE 85–5. The posterior portion of the digestive tract of a cod opened to show the caudally directed valve (V) separating the narrow intestine (I) from the wider rectum (R). (Courtesy of C. Morrison.)

FIGURE 85–6. The roof of the mouth of a cod. Teeth (T) are located on the premaxilla, vomer, and pharyngeal tooth plate. (Courtesy of C. Morrison.)

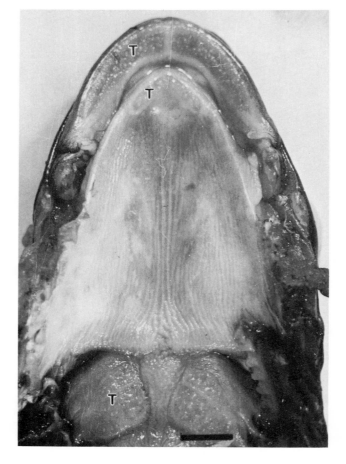

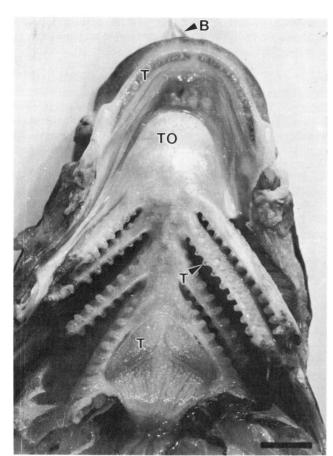

FIGURE 85–7. The floor of the mouth of a cod. The barbel (B) can be seen below the jaw. There are teeth (T) on the dentary, pharyngeal tooth plate, and projections on the gill arches. (TO) tongue. (Courtesy of C. Morrison.)

Cod have four pairs of gill arches (Fig. 85–8). Each arch has two rows of gill filaments. The first arch has a row of gill rakers and a row of tooth-bearing projections, and the second and third have no rakers but two rows of tooth-bearing projections. The fourth arch has only one row of projections, since its posterior border is attached to the floor of the pharynx, where there is a tooth plate.

The genital and urinary systems open caudal to the anus, at a urogenital papilla. The swimbladder lacks a pneumatic duct (physoclistous) and contains a gas gland and foramen ovale to regulate the gases in the swimbladder. The gonads are fused posteriorly and are supplied by genital vessels that run in mesenteries suspended from the swimbladder. When the cod is sexually mature, the gonad (which in the female can contain several million eggs) fills and distends the body cavity (Fig. 85–9). The mature testes are extensively folded and white, whereas the ovaries contain eggs, which become opaque and visible to the naked eye as they mature, then hydrate and become translucent just before spawning.

The Pacific cod is morphologically similar to the Atlantic cod and is also economically important. Another member of the family found in the Atlantic Ocean is the haddock. This is a prime food fish but is not as easy to keep in captivity as the cod and has not been seriously considered for aquaculture. Its anatomy (Knorr et al., 1975a) is generally similar to that of the cod, but male haddock, especially, have a well-developed sound muscle attached to the cranial part of the swimbladder. When this muscle contracts, it produces sounds that are probably important in mating behavior.

Sablefishes

Sablefishes appear similar to cod, although they are sleeker and belong to a different family. They are active fish, capable of very fast bursts of swimming to catch the fish and squid found in their diet. Sablefishes live in both shallow and deep waters of the North Pacific (benthopelagic), and the larvae are pelagic. The small, pointed teeth are arranged in patches on the tooth plates. The arrangement of the organs in the body cavity is similar to that in the cod, as is the histologic appearance of the major organs (Bell et al., 1986). The gonads are thin, lobed

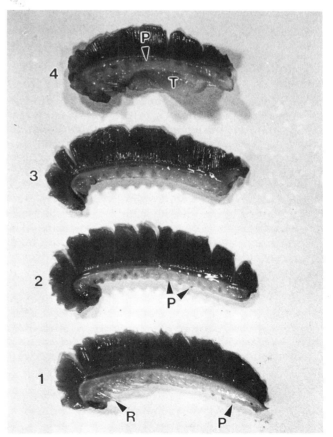

FIGURE 85–8. The gill arches (1, 2, 3 and 4) from the left side of a cod. Rakers (R) are present on the first gill arch. One row of projections (P) bears teeth on the first and fourth gill arch. Two rows of projections are present on the second and third gill arches. The inner surface of the fourth gill arch is attached to the pharyngeal tooth plate (T). (Courtesy of C. Morrison.)

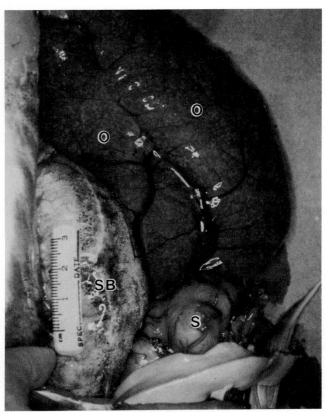

FIGURE 85–9. Ovaries of a mature cod (O) fill the body cavity. (S) stomach, (SB) swimbladder. (Courtesy of C. Morrison.)

threads in immature fish, then in the maturing male, the testis becomes white and develops folds. As the female matures, the eggs become white, opaque, and visible to the naked eye, and then translucent just before spawning. The liver is a good source of vitamins A and D (Hart, 1973), and fat is also stored in the muscle, making the flesh oily, but tasty when smoked. There is no swimbladder.

Juveniles grow quickly, but growth becomes much slower as they reach sexual maturity. The growth rings on scales and the otoliths of the inner ear are usually used for aging sablefishes. However, the rings are difficult to distinguish, especially in older specimens, because they become closer together as growth slows. A special technique for preparing the otoliths for aging (Beamish et al., 1983) has shown that many of these fishes are much older than was previously thought. A study of western Canada found that the majority of fish caught were 4 to 35 years old, but some fish reached an age of 55 years (McFarlane and Beamish, 1983).

Flatfishes

The flatfishes are a large group that have become specialized for bottom dwelling. They include many commercially important species. Some general anatomy of the flounder is discussed in Chapter 1. The

bilaterally symmetric larvae of flatfishes become asymmetric by a curious process of development, so that the flattened adult lies on one side. This is unlike the skates and rays, which are dorsoventrally flattened. The changes involved in metamorphosis include movement of one eye to the other side of the head, so that the underside is blind. Some flatfishes lie on the left side, with both eyes on the right (righteye flounders). Off the U.S. and Canadian coasts these belong mainly to the Pleuronectidae. These include the American plaice, found in the Atlantic, the Atlantic halibut, and the Pacific halibut (the two halibut species may be indistinguishable) (Scott and Scott, 1988). The rest of the flounders lie on their right (lefteye flounders). Reversal is occasionally encountered. Pigmentation is normally present only on the eyed side of the fish. Occasionally, specimens lack areas of pigmentation or have regions of coloration on the blind side.

Both the European plaice (Knorr et al., 1975b) and the American plaice (known as the "long rough dab" in Europe) have dorsal, anal, and caudal fins, which form an almost continuous ridge. The body cavity is small, and a flat liver and a digestive tract with a few short, blunt pyloric ceca are present. The gonads lie on either side of the pterygiophore, and the mature ovaries extend caudally into the tail musculature. A swimbladder is present in the larva but is lost when the fish starts living on the bottom.

As the eyes relocate during metamorphosis, the skull becomes twisted to varying degrees in different flatfishes (Bürgin, 1986). The skull is nearly symmetric in visual feeders such as the halibut and turbot, which take mainly free-swimming food. The halibut has a large mouth and bites into its prey with strong jaws that have well-developed teeth. The turbot can enlarge the mouth cavity to suck in its prey. Plaice usually feed on slowly moving prey such as worms, bivalves, and crustaceans and have a more asymmetric skull, so that the mouth points to the bottom when opened. They depend mainly on sight, but also on chemical sensors. Soles also have a very asymmetric mouth and are specialized for more sedentary living on muddy bottoms. The eyed side of the mouth is used mainly for respiration, and the teeth are reduced or lost. The blind side is used mainly for feeding on sessile organisms, which are found mainly by smell and touch (deGroot, 1971; Holmes and Gibson, 1983).

Herrings

The herrings, which include the alewife, shad, sardine, menhaden, and anchovy as well as the Atlantic herring, and the very similar Pacific herring, are anatomically specialized for a pelagic life. They are small, schooling fish with a laterally compressed, slender body and small head. They feed on plankton, so the teeth are minute or absent (Scott and Scott, 1988). Herring support extensive commercial fisheries but have little potential for aquaculture because they are available in large quantities in the wild, and their value per unit weight is low. Moreover, they are difficult to maintain in tanks, largely because the scales are easily lost during handling. Fat is stored in the flesh as well as the liver, as in sablefishes, and is highest before spawning. The swimbladder is connected to the intestine (physostomous) (Knorr et al., 1980). The gonads are not fused caudally, and the testis is straight, not convoluted as in the cod. Apart from their small size, herring are not generally accepted as fresh food fish because they are so bony. This is because the neural spines and ribs are long, and "fish" or "pin" bones are present between the muscles. The fish bones are ossifications of the connective tissue of the septa between the muscles, so they are not, strictly speaking, part of the skeletal system (Harder, 1975).

Mackerels

Like the herrings, the mackerels are pelagic. The tunas, such as the bluefin tuna, and the mackerels are both important food fishes off the Atlantic coast, although only the former has been cultured. Tunas have a high growth rate, so it is economically feasible to keep them in large net enclosures and feed them to increase their market size. Like flatfishes, the larvae of the mackerels have swimbladders, but these are lost in the adults, which must therefore swim continuously, making maintenance in tanks for aquaculture difficult. Externally, mackerels and tunas are very similar (Grassé, 1958). They are both strong, active swimmers, and their bodies have beautifully streamlined fusiform shapes, with a keeled, narrow caudal peduncle. They have distinctive deeply forked rigid caudal fins with longs lobes for stability. Some of the fins are retractable, and the scales are few in number and small, so friction is reduced. The gill surface area is high, and there is a large blood volume and high hemoglobin content (Waiwood et al., 1988), which helps active swimming. Tunas, especially, undergo extensive migrations (Scott and Scott, 1988).

Internally, the pyloric ceca of tunas and mackerels show the highest degree of organization found in fish (Grassé, 1958). They are embedded in connective tissue and surrounded by an epithelium, forming a pyloric organ. As in the herrings, fat is stored in the flesh as well as the liver and varies in quantity according to the time of year. The red muscle is highly vascularized and very distinct from the white muscle.

The main difference between mackerels and tunas is size. Mackerels are relatively small, but tunas used for aquaculture usually weigh over 136 kg and can weigh over 680 kg (Waiwood et al., 1988). Tunas have a unique system of cutaneous arteries and veins supplying blood to the muscle (Grassé, 1958). A rete of small arteries and veins forms a slab of vascular tissue on the dorsal and ventral surfaces of the red muscle (Carey and Teal, 1969), acting as a counter-current heat exchanger and preventing heat loss

through the gills. A similar system of parallel cutaneous arteries and veins also helps to prevent heat loss from the mainly white musculature of the tail (Harder, 1975). A rete of blood vessels is also found on the liver of bluefin tuna, which helps to conserve heat in the interior of the animal. These adaptations, together with the heat generated by continuous muscular activity, result in a body temperature higher than that of the surrounding water. The temperature is highest around the red muscle, which drives the tuna at its cruising speed. The body cavity is small, which helps to conserve heat and also leaves more room for muscular development.

Lumpfishes

Lumpfishes have a stout body with a short, blunt head and are covered with a thick leathery skin and hard tubercles instead of scales. There are seven rows of large tubercles, one along the midline of the back, two on each side, and one on each edge of the flattened ventral surface. The rest of the body is covered with small tubercles, so that it feels rough to the touch (Cox, 1920). There are numerous small, simple, conical teeth arranged in several rows on the jaws. In adult fish, the intestine is long, being more than twice the length of the body. There are numerous (36 to 79) pyloric ceca (Davenport, 1985). The histology of the digestive tract is similar to that of the cod (Timeyko, 1986).

Larval and juvenile lumpfishes are semipelagic. The adults spawn on inshore rocky or stony bottoms on both sides of the North Atlantic, but it has been found that they also live semipelagically, often far from land, feeding on large zooplankton such as small jellyfish and crustaceans. This seems odd for a fish that has no swimbladder and weak swimming ability. However, lumpfishes have an almost neutral buoyancy in seawater. This is partly because the skeleton is made of uncalcified cartilage, and also because there is a partly cartilaginous, partly gelatinous hump of low osmolality on the back (Davenport and Kjorsvik, 1986). This hump engulfs the first dorsal fin. The pelvic fins are modified and surrounded with a flap of skin to form a ventral suction disc, which is well developed at hatching and is probably important for attaching the buoyant fish to floating weeds or to the rocky bottom during spawning.

The mature female is usually larger than the male, and the main commercial value of lumpfishes is the roe, which is used as caviar. Up to 400,000 eggs can be produced by a ripe female, although 100,000 is closer to the average. The ovaries and oviducts are fused, forming a single pink roe that fills up to two-thirds of the body cavity in the ripe female (Davenport, 1985). The large dorsal muscles of the gravid female are watery, counteracting the negative buoyancy of the eggs and making the flesh inedible. This may be partly why lumpfish flesh has not received general acceptance, although the flesh has been described as being normally rich, tender, well flavored, and nourishing (Cox, 1920). Another reason is probably the homely appearance of the fish, and the fact that the thick skin and hump have to be removed before an acceptable fillet is found. Lumpfishes are easy to spawn and grow in captivity (Benfey and Methven, 1986) but have not yet been cultured commercially.

PHYSIOLOGY

A comprehensive review of marine cold-water commercial food fish physiology would constitute thousands of text pages. The literature is extensive (Breder and Rosen, 1966; Alexander, 1967; Lagler et al., 1977; Hoar and Randall, 1978; Love and Cailliet, 1979; Bone and Marshall, 1982; Smith, 1982; Rankin et al., 1983; Moyle and Cech, 1988; Rowley et al., 1988; Roberts, 1989). This chapter focuses on special adaptations related to intensive culture.

Digestion

Codfishes

In contrast to many other fishes, the cod stomach contains crypts and compound tubular glands in the mucosa and lamina propria. In addition to acid and pepsin, the stomach of cod produces chitinase and chitobiase, which disrupt the exoskeletons of ingested crustaceans. The efficacy of cod pancreatic triglyceride lipase appears dependent on the presence of bile salts, versus mammals, in which inhibition is the rule (Gjellesvik et al., 1989). Cod have a specialized ileorectal valve, which prevents both reflux and the entrance of pathogens from the flaccid rectum.

Tunas

The highly evolved tunas deserve special note. Their pyloric ceca are organized into a definite "cecal mass," which constitutes a very major component of the viscera. Presumably, this is an aid to efficient digestion. The pancreas is much more discrete than that of most teleosts (as are the compact kidneys). Bluefin extend thermoregulation to the viscera and tripartite liver, the latter being remarkable in its lobulation and dorsal retia mirabilia heat exchangers. The resultant high internal body temperature speeds digestion and absorption to stoke the metabolic furnaces of this active species (Carey et al., 1971; Collette, 1978).

Flatfishes

American plaice include many invertebrates in their diet, unlike the mainly piscivorous halibut. The former has a relatively longer intestine than the latter to deal with chitinous and shelled forms, although the softer protruding portions of prey are often ingested preferentially. When the stomach of flatfishes is distended, aboral neurogenic rings of contraction and myogenic nonpropagating contractions are initiated. Indigestible items such as pieces of skeleton and shell are collected and passed separately through the pyloric sphincter. Gastric emptying slows significantly with single meals. The pyloric appendices of plaice are tiny in comparison to those of halibut. In the latter species, these diverticula considerably increase the digestive area, expediting digestion of large prey.

Metabolism

Protein and Carbohydrate

Insulin in marine cold-water fishes enhances proteogenesis (and lipogenesis) but suppresses gluconeogenesis. Its major role in most teleosts is to regulate protein metabolism, unlike the case in mammals, in which glucose homeostasis is critical to the functional integrity of the brain and central nervous system. This is less important in fish because of their higher brain glycogen reserves. As insulin in fish seems geared to oxidative clearance of glucose rather than its disposition as glycogen, it may almost be viewed as a growth hormone. Similarly, elevated insulin levels are associated with gonad development and reproduction (Smith, 1982; Ince, 1983).

Lipids

Awareness of lipid intake, storage, and metabolism in cold-water marine fishes is crucial to our understanding of their form, function, and condition. These provide for acclimatization, buoyancy, and energy storage specifically tailored to these organisms' individual physiology. For example, cod and flatfishes principally use the liver for lipid storage, tunas mainly place reserves in the muscle, and sablefishes employ both sites (Lagler et al., 1977; Lie et al., 1986; Jobling, 1988).

Cold-water fishes easily assimilate unsaturated fats (natural diet), dealing poorly with saturated, solid fats (experimental diet). Although each species manufactures its own unique blend of body lipids, this complement can be significantly influenced by intake (Privol'nev and Brizinova, 1964). At the extreme, a surfeit of saturated fatty acids can result in excessive protein catabolism, nitrogen loss, and permanent deposition of unusable solid fat, giving the fish an appearance that belies its true condition. The low–melting point fatty acids in these fishes reflect enzyme systems operating in temperature regimens near (even below) the freezing point, whose activation brings an adaptive exothermic bonus. Such compounds as oleic, gadoleic, and clupanodonic acids combine with saturated compounds such as palmitic acid to produce the overall unsaturated, eutectic mixtures of oils found in the liver of cod and muscle of sablefishes. These diffuse energy stores can complicate accurate visual assessment of body condition.

Sablefishes undergo extensive migrations and can withstand pressure changes imposed by rapid vertical movements in the water column. They remain slightly negative in buoyancy, suiting their punctuation of active swimming with periodic passive sinking and resting on the bottom. Their ability to cope with radical temperature and pressure changes relates largely to the insulation and residual buoyancy provided by a high, low-density oil content, coupled with the absence of a swimbladder (Kulikov, 1964). However, unlike other tissues, the bones of this species average 50% lipid by dry weight, primarily as triglycerides lacking polyunsaturation. This energy source is probably synthesized internally from two-carbon units, in contrast to polyunsaturated phospholipids whose composition reflects the dietary intake of fatty acids (Lee et al., 1975). Cod are also replete with oils (liver), but their gradual vertical movements are tempered by the need to adjust swimbladder volume. If pressure is reduced quickly to about 70% of the adapted level, the weak wall of the cod swimbladder will burst. Affected fish may survive with internal scarring, with the rupture having acted as a safety valve.

Assessing Condition and Meat Quality

In cod, a large creamy liver indicates a good state of nutrition, whereas a small red/brown one, depletion. However, relative liver size can be misleading. Migratory codfishes lay down most lipid for fuel. Thus, even satiated fishes may not have large livers, and the level of liver lipid is no guide to the state of the muscle.

A pale straw-colored bile indicates continuous feeding, whereas a large, taut, green to deep-blue gallbladder indicates deprivation. A blue but "wrinkled" gallbladder implies resumption of feeding.

Until recently, it was assumed that because farmed cod that were fed rations with a protein energy–to–total energy ratio under 0.45 developed enlarged fatty livers, a high-protein/low-lipid diet was optimal. Paradoxically, this categorizes the natural food of cod (e.g., herring, sandeel, and capelin) as nutritionally poor! In fact, these enlarged livers indicate obesity. Formulated feeds are emptied overrapidly from the cod stomach, leading to intestinal overloading, reduction in absorption efficiency, changes in nutrient supply, and increased fat synthesis and deposition. Amino acids not required for protein synthesis are deaminated, and the carbon chains catabolized or used for lipid synthesis (liver triglycerides). It would be ideal to feed impounded cod with natural prey, but its long-term storage is compromised by lipid degeneration and loss of vitamin content due to thiaminase action. Suggested solutions include the incorporation of coarse-ground fish chunks into a moist pellet feeding regimen, or alternating formulated feed with whole fish to pro-

long the flow of nutrient-rich chyme from the stomach (Jobling, 1988).

At very low temperatures cod may feed well, have full gastrointestinal tracts, yet appear to be starving. One explanation is that food moves very slowly through the gut, and that absorption lags behind metabolic requirements.

In cod muscle there is only 1% lipid (wet weight), and the organoleptic degeneration of fillets in long-term storage results mainly from breakdown products of structural proteins rather than from oxidative degeneration of triglycerides. Nevertheless, meat from well-fed cod has a shorter shelf life than that from starved fishes, because oxidation of unsaturated fatty acids in even small amounts affects quality.

"Gaping" is seen in fillets of cod and other fishes that are frozen stale (with a low pH). This is more pronounced in smaller fish with lower glycogen reserves, although there is some overall seasonal variation associated with the resumption of feeding following starvation. The cause is a weakened collagen framework affected by lowered pH. Anaerobic accumulation of lactic acid reaches a maximum in cod fillets within 15 hours of death. Struggling does not exacerbate the condition, as the same amount of lactic acid forms regardless (Love, 1970, 1980).

Following the capture and storage of tuna, the flesh of some individuals may be very pale, soft, and unappealing, a condition termed "tuna burn." This is apparently a reflection of oxygen depletion in white muscle, resulting in a cellular calcium influx activating autocatalytic proteases that disassemble myofilaments. In brief, the phenomenon is stress related (Hochachka and Brill, 1987).

Respiration

Fish are amazingly efficient at extracting oxygen from water (Preston, 1960; Shelton, 1970; Satchell, 1971; Smith, 1977). Respiration is critical, and osmoregulatory losses incurred by increased ventilation rates are tolerated in the short term (Butler and Metcalfe, 1983).

For many fishes, a continuous flow of water over the gills is achieved by the balanced operation of the buccal pressure pump and opercular suction pump. Cod expand the buccal and opercular cavities slowly and contract them quickly, at a cost of 1 to 2% of the resting metabolic rate (Alexander, 1967). They asphyxiate at oxygen levels under 0.8 ppm, but 3.0 ppm is the critical level below which consumption depends on concentration. They are independent of ambient oxygen above this critical level, although respiratory volume is adjusted according to activity (Jobling, 1988). Cod display an adaptive response as oxygen demands increase in warm water while oxygen content diminishes (Becker et al., 1958). Blood parameters change such that from 16 to 8°C, MCHC (19/18.8 g/dl) is unaffected by temperature, MCH (47/41 pg) and MCV (249–219 fl) are lower, and RBC ($1.03/1.31 \times 10^6$/ml), Hct (25.3/27.9%), Hb (4.80/5.35

g/dl) are higher. Erythrocyte enzyme production (prostaglandins, leukotrienes, and so forth) and membrane structure also adapt as fatty acid content changes (Lie et al., 1989).

Tuna forego the pump mechanism altogether. These active fishes attain a critical size, such that their normal cruising speed exceeds that required to support passive gill ventilation. Mature tuna realize significant metabolic savings and streamlining from open-mouth swimming (ram gill ventilation) but have become obligated to move in order to respire. Their extensive array of gill filaments is strengthened by cross linkages and fusion along edges to withstand and effectively channel the high-velocity water flow. The result is the removal of proportionately more dissolved oxygen from the water than any other fish known. Restrictive impoundment of bluefin results in hypoxia, resulting in strong "coughing" and thrashing by affected fish (Roberts, 1975, 1978). The efficient respiration and high metabolic needs of the bluefin correlate with its erythrocyte count of 2.3×10^6/ml and hematocrit of 41.0%, which overlap mammalian values.

Flatfishes such as plaice have enlarged opercular cavities, accentuating the suction phase of the respiratory cycle while preventing damage from sand reflux via opercular valve action (Lagler et al., 1977). Their slow ventilation rate reflects high oxygen extraction (to 80%) but low oxygen consumption.

Excretion and Osmoregulation

Carnivorous fishes, such as the marine cold-water species considered here, excrete urea produced principally in the liver from uric acid and purine nucleotides (Smith, 1982). Ingested monovalent ions are excreted mainly across the gills, whereas most divalent ions remain in rectal fluids. Any divalent ions absorbed are excreted by the kidneys. The glomerular filtration rate is the major factor controlling urine volume and composition, with the exception of divalent ions, creatine, and some organic acids, which are actively secreted by the proximal tubules. This is vital to maintaining low internal Mg^{2+} levels, as demonstrated by the effects of scale loss where high Mg^{2+} influx blocks myoneural junctions and fish die with flaccid muscular paralysis. The bladder is key in the fish's net reabsorption of water and maintenance of high Mg^{2+} ion concentrations in the urine (Hickmann Jr., 1968a, b; Smith, 1982).

Cod can tolerate salinities to 2 to 3 ppt if temperatures are low (5 to 6°C) for a short time. At 10°C they are obviously distressed in 7 to 8 ppt salinity, suffering some mortality, and they become most agitated below 4 to 5 ppt (Jobling, 1988).

Autonomic Control

The effects of stress on fish, such as result from captivity, are mediated by catecholamines (short term) and cortisol (long term). For example, handling flatfishes (netting, placing them upside down, and so forth) gives immediate high blood plasma ionic levels followed by a persistent hyperglycemia (up to 24 hours). Chromaffin cells in the cranial kidney are the principal catecholamine producers in fishes, releasing their products into the circulation via the posterior cardinal vein. These cells do occur in other sites depending on species; for example, in several of the autonomic ganglia of cod (Eddy, 1981; Smith, 1982).

Cod synthesize epinephrine intraneuronally from norepinephrine, apparently being able to release both catecholamines and acetylcholine from the same neuron. The α-adrenoreceptors in cod include the iris sphincter, swimbladder, celiac arteries, spleen, kidney, and urinary bladder where smooth muscle constriction is mediated. The pyloric sphincter of flatfishes is also closed by α-receptor stimulation. Cod β-adrenoreceptors occur in the gills, swimbladder, and urinary bladder to inhibit (relax) smooth muscles. β-receptors also occur in the heart, where their vagosympathetic adrenergic stimulation produces variable responses according to circumstance. The postganglionic neuronal receptors in cod are nicotinic, whereas postganglionic cholinergic nerve endings act on the muscarinic receptors of the effector organs similar to other vertebrates. However, cod celiac artery and visceral vascular beds show little sensitivity to cholinergic drugs. In cod, the gills are innervated by the branchial nerves, the glossopharyngeal and the vagus (Nilsson et al., 1983).

The control of physoclist swimbladder volume, as exemplified by cod, is far more complex than that of physostomes such as salmonids (Steen, 1970). The secretory and resorbent portions of the organ are very richly endowed with the adrenergic nerve fibers of a vagosympathetic trunk. Stimulation of secretion is mediated by α-receptors, whereas β-receptors respond by causing the resorbent oval to enlarge. This exposes a capillary network for passive gas absorption by relaxing a thin mucosal impermeable membrane associated with the swimbladder inner epithelium. Administration of acetylcholine has no effect on secretion but has a contracting influence on a resorbent swimbladder. Bilateral vagotomy in cod totally abolishes swimbladder volume control (Alexander, 1967; Nilsson et al., 1983).

Swimming and Muscle Metabolism

Fishes exhibit two distinct muscle types, dark and white. Mitochondria-rich dark muscle aerobically metabolizes resident fatty acids to conserve its glycogen stores and maintain contraction. White muscle weakens as its extensive glycogen reserves rapidly deplete to lactic acid via anaerobic glycolysis. Recovery occurs as the lactate is oxidatively recycled to glycogen with only a small fraction released to the blood and lost by excretion (Lindsey, 1978; Smith, 1982).

Exercise of starved cod results in conservation of the dark muscle powering sustained swimming, despite marked watery degeneration of the "expendable" white muscle masses used for sudden acceleration and activity bursts. High levels of mRNA and myosin heavy chains are retained at the expense of other muscle proteins. This preserves contractibility and retains the potential for fast recovery when food supplies are reestablished (Von der Decken, 1989). Larval cod initially possess only white muscle, moving about by a series of quick darts. Adult cod maintain a muscle temperature slightly above their surroundings, which increases remarkably in "burst" activities, a bonus because vertebrate muscle gains threefold in power for each 10°C rise in temperature (Driedzic and Hochachka, 1978; Lindsey, 1978). In contrast to mammals, the number of muscle fibers of cod increases throughout life.

Sablefishes are streamlined and capable of high-speed bursts. However, these fishes are restricted to sustained swimming velocities of 2.0 to 2.5 body lengths per minute by limits in oxygen uptake and lack of muscle power (Smith, 1982). Lumpfishes are not speedy and have little red muscle.

Giant bluefin tuna are specialized, thermoregulated, swimming machines capable of bursts to over 22.6 m/second (81.4 km/hour). At sustained speeds of 2.4 to 3.8 m/second, individuals swim 86 to 260 km/day or 94,608 km/year, more than twice the equatorial circumference of the Earth (Wardle et al., 1989). They represent the ultimate in streamlining. The paired fins fit into custom grooves, the eyes are "faired in," the narrowly tapered caudal peduncle has bony keels—even the tongue has special ridges to add lift. Muscle activity is translated into propulsion via the powerfully oscillating tail, with the distance traveled for each full oscillation being termed the "stride."

Tuna red muscle is virtually indefatigable in the maintenance of sustained high-speed swimming. This is due in part to core retention of metabolic heat by the complex retia of countercurrent blood vessels stemming from a prominent subcutaneous blood supply. Elevation of internal temperatures is influenced by the degree of activity. In bluefin tuna, muscle temperatures can exceed an inner 31°C and a superficial 21°C, despite any cold external environment. As a result, these giants can modulate their intense metabolism over large changes in rate and are free to exploit the rich food supply of the cooler latitudes (Carey and Teal, 1966; Carey, 1973; Sharp and Pirages, 1978).

The high-quality white flesh of most flatfishes reflects their behavior in vivo. Plaice and halibut do not habitually indulge in sustained swimming and require little red muscle. Instead, absence of a swimbladder allows them to attain negative buoyancy and stability against bottom currents. They prefer to stalk and catch their prey by final spurts of activity, although they can swim in midwater by body undulation and synchronized wide amplitude flexures of dorsal and anal fins.

SENSORY SYSTEMS

Vision

The eyes of fishes incorporate a high-quality, spherical lens producing an image almost free of aberration. Fishes accommodate by varying the distance between the lens and retina, and as a group have more visual pigments than all other vertebrates combined. Individual teleosts have specialized eye structures and wavelength sensitivities, correlated with behavior and movement within the water column. Tuna and flatfishes deserve special mention here.

As evidenced by the disproportionately large optic tectum and cerebellum of their brains, the tunas place a premium on vision. Reaction times to visual stimuli in bluefin are very swift. The conduction of nerve impulses is expedited by the elevated eye and brain temperatures generated via cranial retia mirabilia. Tuna are basically surface feeders yet tend to actually hunt from below. Descending light is very blue with few yellow or green wavelengths. Tuna then are somewhat exceptional as epipelagic teleosts that lack multiple visual pigments and color vision. They possess only one basic rhodopsin (probably in both the rods and the cones) of an approximate absorbance wavelength of 483 nm, a spectral match to the background light. This aids the partial binocular vision of tuna in detecting surface prey silhouetted against a bright surface (McFarland and Munz, 1975).

The eyes of flatfishes are perched upon one side of the head as a consequence of complex bone, nerve, and muscle modifications occurring in metamorphosis. Unlike many teleosts, these forms have excellent accommodation and, in some cases, a pupillary operculum to control light intensity reaching the retina. The very active, independent movements of their protruding eyes cannot be fully appreciated unless viewed in nature. Adult halibut are particularly dependent on their vision to actively pursue fishes in front of or upward from the head. The more bottom-oriented plaice make good use of both upper eyes and the shielded anterior lateral line receptors on the underside to detect substrate disturbances made by benthic invertebrate prey.

Gustation and Olfaction

More than most other marine cold-water food fishes, benthic-feeding codfishes are strongly influenced by taste and odors (Kleerekoper, 1969; Jónsson, 1980). The chin barbel of the cod is equipped with taste buds and free nerve endings for chemoreception. Its function includes probing the bottom for invertebrate prey, with a sensitivity to even dilute concentrations of individual amino acids. The prominent olfactory tract forms a nervelike connection between the brain and olfactory organ, being divided into four bundles of massed fibers, each collectively controlling specific behaviors (Guthrie, 1983):

1. Outer lateral: head-down swimming, as in bottom feeding and foraging
2. Inner lateral: very active swimming and jaw snapping, as in feeding
3. Outer medial: head-up positioning with quivering flanks, as in reproductive behavior
4. Inner medial: substrate pressing and color changes to flank stripes and dorsal spots

Knowledge of the precise stimuli eliciting these activities could prove valuable in promoting desirable behaviors for intensive culture of cod.

Auditory and Lateral Line Sensors

Marine organisms are immersed in a world of currents, vibrations, sounds, pressures, and disturbances far beyond our limited abilities to experience. Water is an excellent medium for long-range sound transmission, with speeds almost five times faster than that in air. Fishes are finely attuned to their surroundings. The effects of many human activities unremarkable to us impact profoundly on fishes' behavior, physiology, and biology (Tavolga, 1971; Smith, 1982).

Most species of fishes make good use of their lateral line near-field receptors for detecting currents, barriers, bottoms, predators, and prey. Schooling cod and tuna use these pressure sensors to orient with nearby fish. Some of the burrowing flatfishes have extensive anterior receptors on their underside. These are covered by flaps to prevent fouling and are used to sense any nearby movement of prey (Alexander, 1967).

Cod hear low-frequency sounds under 200 Hz. These are detected by the inner ear with amplification via gas in the anterior vermiform horns of the swimbladder. This corresponds with their own production of sounds at frequency peaks of 50 Hz. Grunts produced by muscular action on the swimbladder are associated with aggression, flight, and the spawning preliminaries of males attracting females (Fish and Mowbray, 1970). The successful Norwegian pond culture of cod includes conditioning of fry to respond to sound signals at feeding sites, where they may easily be trapped for harvesting, transportation, and vibriosis vaccination (Naas, 1987).

Sablefishes, lumpfishes, tunas, and flatfishes are not known as noteworthy noise makers. Bluefin tuna hear well over a wide frequency range, being most attentive to sounds in the 200 to 800 Hz middle range (Fish and Mowbray, 1970; Tavolga, 1971).

The saccular otoliths employed for hearing are of singular value to managers in determining the age and growth of fish. Accurate readings are a product of knowledge, care, and experience. For example, the age of sablefishes has been severely underestimated until recent years, as rapid growth to maturity is succeeded by barely detectable annual increments.

A similar situation exists for flatfishes, whereas such aging of cod and tuna is unreliable. In the latter species, fin ray sections yield more accurate growth estimates (Chilton and Beamish, 1982).

REPRODUCTION AND GROWTH

Ovarian group synchrony with "leading clutches" is most common in marine cold-water commercial food fishes (de Ulaming, 1983). Hepatic glycogen and lipid are the energy sources that supply the metabolic needs of ovarian growth and spawning. In cod, estrogen mobilizes these stores to elevate lipid plasma levels during vitellogenesis. These species accumulate larger amounts of lipid in successive years, presumably to supply the gonads that grow disproportionately in relation to the body. Spawning in cod coincides with the maximal water content in white muscle, as gonad requirements are given priority (Lagler et al., 1977; Smith, 1982; Hemre et al., 1989).

Many extruded cod eggs fail to be fertilized and die. The gauntlet continues for the newly hatched cod, because unlike salmonids they require microscopic food immediately (Smith, 1982). Cannibalism is highest in cultured cod fry at lengths of 12 to 30 mm, especially when fed only dry food. The ultimate result is a very low survival rate. Metamorphosis occurs at 40 days, followed by vibriosis vaccination at 4 months in artificial rearing ponds (Hislop, 1984; Naas, 1987).

Young immature cod are more adapted to cold water than are adults, showing higher food conversions and growth at 6°C. This possibly relates to the added metabolic cost of living at higher temperatures (Brown et al., 1989). Young cod also have much higher blood levels of antifreeze glycoproteins than do older fish, initiating their production when the temperature sinks to 1°C. Colder temperatures dramatically elevate antifreeze glycoprotein levels. This trait allows young cod to exploit the food supplies of cold coastal areas in the winter (Fletcher et al., 1987a, b).

As adults, smaller cod grow optimally at 11 to 15°C, whereas larger individuals do best at 9 to 12°C. Adult cod cannot adapt well to temperatures above 15 to 16°C (Pedersen and Jobling, 1989). This may relate to their notoriously thermounstable collagen, myofibrillar proteins, and central nervous system lipids. Interestingly, cod collagen is annually renewed, retaining characteristics of "young collagen." Thus an annual cycle of depletion and thickening of connective tissue occurs, with cod collagen remaining quite soluble in acid buffer throughout life, unlike collagen of aging mammals (Love, 1970, 1980).

Successful sablefish spawning is highly dependent on a favorable environment plus a critical population size. Large year classes of this long-lived species (to 65+ years) may be spaced 10 years or more apart. Egg production remains high (average 500,000/female) in readiness for those relatively rare conditions conducive to larval survival. A single annual spawning is presumed, with juveniles growing well at temperatures below 10°C (Mason et al., 1983; Funk and Bracken, 1984).

In British Columbia, gonadotropin-releasing hormone (GnRH) and analogues have been used in sablefishes to induce gonadal hydration and ovulation within 5 to 20 days, resulting in fertilization success rates up to 76% (Solar et al., 1987). Dopamine inhibitor does not potentiate this induction. Some similar work in flatfishes indicates a parallel effect (Zohar, 1989). Weight changes and increased diameter of cannulated eggs are reliable indications of an ovulatory response. Mammalian hormones are effective, available commercially, and nonimmunogenic and require only low dosages (economical). The time of administration may be important for females (February, not September). However, a giant hurdle for sablefish culture from eggs has been larval to postlarval metamorphosis, for which the exact requirements are unknown (McFarlane and Nagata, 1988).

Lumpfish adults can be readily maintained in aquaria on frozen whole capelin and will readily spawn under such conditions. The larvae are easily reared on trout starter sprinkled from a salt shaker, which they take from the surface as it hits. Brine shrimp gives even better growth rates. Hatching and eye-up are synchronous, with newly hatched lumpfishes being well developed (Benfey and Methven, 1986).

Some flatfish species (for example, winter flounder) may build only limited lipid reserves in a bad season and produce no gametes, electing for growth and postponing reproduction until a better year (Smith, 1982). In plaice, phospholipids are the major lipid class in serum and gonads, although the exact type is influenced by food supply (White and Fletcher, 1987). A rise in hypothalamic gonadotropin-releasing hormone in this species is a solid indicator of increased gonadal activity. In Pacific halibut, the occurrence of a specific serum factor may be an indicator of sexual maturation (Utter and Ridgway, 1967).

In addition to extrinsic factors, adequate thyroxine and growth hormone levels are key to efficient food conversion, proper growth, metamorphosis, and gonadal development (Bell, 1981; Inui and Miwa, 1985; Billard, 1989). In halibut larvae, high temperature (9 to 11°C) and exposure to light (3 to 300 LUX) during the resorption of the yolk sac result in serious jaw and body deformities (Bolla and Holmefjord, 1988).

Cold-water marine flatfishes exhibit an endogenous rhythm of reproduction cued to photoperiod, rather than temperature, to ensure gamete production on a 12-month cycle. This helps ensure that larvae hatch when conditions most favor their survival. In artificial situations, manipulation of photoperiod can induce up to a 5-month advance in flatfish spawning, with a very compressed 6-month cycle being the limit. The influence of photoperiod is exerted via the central nervous system. In spring and during summer, growth hormone promotes feeding and anabolism while blocking the transcription of antifreeze glycoprotein genes in the liver. In fall, shorter day lengths inhibit the release of growth hormone, while antifreeze glycoproteins are produced. Artificial initiation of continuous long day lengths by September (October at the latest) greatly expedites growth for commercial marketing (Bye, 1987; Fletcher et al., 1989; Haug et al., 1989).

LITERATURE CITED

Alexander, R.McN. (1967) Functional design in fishes. Hutchinson and Son, London.

Beamish, R.J., McFarlane, G.A., and Chilton, D.E. (1983) Use of oxytetracycline and other methods to validate a method of age determination for sablefish. In: Proceedings of the International Sablefish Symposium. Alaska Sea Grant Report 83–8, pp. 95–118.

Becker, E.L., Bird, R., Kelly, J.W., Schilling, J., Solomon, S., and Young, N. (1958) Physiology of marine teleosts. 2. Hematologic observations. Physiol. Zool. 31:228–231.

Bell, F.H. (1981) The Pacific Halibut, the Resource, and the Fishery. Alaska Northwest Publishing, Anchorage.

Bell, G.R., Slind, D., and Bagshaw, J.W. (1986) Pictorial atlas of histology of the sablefish (Anoplopoma fimbria). Can. Spec. Publ. Fish Aquatic Sci. 94:1–93.

Benfey, T.J., and Methven, D.A. (1986) Pilot-scale rearing of larval and juvenile lumpfish (Cyclopterus lumpus L.), with some notes on early development. Aquaculture 56:301–306.

Billard, R. (1989) Endocrinology and fish culture. Fish Physiol. Biochem. 7(1–4):49–58.

Bolla, S., and Holmefjord, I. (1988) Effect of temperature and light on development of Atlantic halibut larvae. Aquaculture 74:355–358.

Bone, Q., and Marshall, N.B. (1982) Biology of Fishes. Blackie and Son, Glasgow.

Breder, C.M., Jr., and Rosen, D.E. (1966) Modes of Reproduction in Fishes. T.F.H. Publications, Jersey City, New Jersey.

Brown, J.A., Pepin, P., Methven, D.A., and Somerton, D.C. (1989) The feeding, growth, and behaviour of juvenile cod, Gadus morhua L., in cold environments. J. Fish Biol. 35:373–380.

Bürgin, T. (1986) The syncranial morphology of the bastard sole Macrochirus theophila (Risso, 1810) (Pleuronectiformes, Soleidae). Neth. J. Zool. 36:117–161.

Butler, P.J., and Metcalfe, J.F. (1983) Control of respiration and circulation. In: Control Processes in Fish Physiology (Rankin, J.C., Pitcher, T.J., and Duggan, R.T., eds.). Wiley-Interscience, New York, pp. 41–65.

Bye, V.J. (1987) Environmental management of marine fish reproduction in Europe. Proceedings of the Third International Symposium on Reproductive Physiology of Fish. (Idler, D.R., Crim, L.W., and Walsh, J.M., eds.). Memorial University, St. John's, Newfoundland, pp. 289–298.

Carey, F.G. (1973) Fishes with warm bodies. Sci. Am. 228(2):36–44.

Carey, F.G., and Teal, J.M. (1966) Heat conservation in tuna fish muscle. Proc. Natl. Acad. Sci. 56:1464–1469.

Carey, F.G., and Teal, J.M. (1969) Regulation of body temperature by the bluefin tuna. Comp. Biochem. Physiol. 28:205–213.

Carey, F.G., Teal, J.M., Kanwisher, J.W., Lawson, K.D., and Beckett, J.S. (1971) Warm-bodied fish. Am. Zool. 11:137–145.

Chilton, D.E., and Beamish, R.J. (1982) Age determination methods for fishes studied by the Groundfish Program at the Pacific Biological Station. Can. Spec. Publ. Fish. Aquatic Sci. 60:1–102.

Collette, B.B. (1978) Adaptations and systematics of the mackerels and tunas. In: The Physiological Ecology of Tunas (Sharp, G.D., ed.). Proceedings of the Tuna Physiology Workshop, Southwest Fisheries Center, La Jolla, California, 1977. Academic Press, New York, pp. 7–39.

Cox, P. (1920) Histories of new food fishes. 11. The lumpfish. Bull. Biol. Bd. Can. 2:28.

Davenport, J. (1985) Synopsis of biological data on the lumpsucker Cyclopterus lumpus (Linnaeus, 1758). FAO Fish. Synop. 147:1–31.

Davenport, J. and Kjørsvik, E. (1986) Buoyancy in the lumpsucker. J. Marine Biol. Assoc. U.K. 66:159–174.

Driedzic, W.R., and Hochachka, P.W. (1978) Metabolism in fish during exercise. In: Fish Physiology (Hoar, W.S., and Randall, D.J., eds.). Academic Press, New York, pp. 503–543.

Eddy, F.B. (1981) Effects of stress on osmotic and ionic regulation in fish. In: Stress and Fish (Pickering, A.D., ed.). Academic Press, London, pp. 77–102.

Fish, M.P., and Mowbray, W.H. (1970) Sounds of Western North Atlantic Fishes. Johns Hopkins Press, Baltimore.

Fletcher, G.L., Idler, D.R., Vaisius, A., and Hew, C.L. (1989) Hormonal regulation of antifreeze protein gene expression in winter flounder. Fish Physiol. Biochem. 7(1–4):387–393.

Fletcher, G.L., King, M.J., and Kao, M.H. (1987a) Low temperature regulation of antifreeze glycopeptide levels in Atlantic cod (Gadus morhua). Can. J. Zool. 65:227–233.

Fletcher, G.L., Shears, M.A., King, M.J., Kao, M.H., Hew, C.L., and Davies, P.L. (1987b) Antifreeze protein gene transfer: a potential solution to ocean pen culture of salmon in icy waters. In: Proceedings of the Third International Symposium on Reproductive Physiology of Fish (Idler, D.R., Crim, L.W., and Walsh, J.M., eds.). Memorial University, St. John's, Newfoundland, p. 306.

Funk, F., and Bracken, B.E. (1984) Status of the Gulf of Alaska sablefish (Anoploploma fimbria) resource in 1983. Alaska Dept. Fish. Game, Informational Leaflet 235:1–55.

Gjellesvik, D.R., Raae, A.J., and Walther, B.T. (1989) Partial purification and characterization of a triglyceride lipase from cod (Gadus morhua). Aquaculture 79:177–184.

Grassé, P.P. (1958) Traité de Zoologie. Anatomie, Systématique, Biologie. Vol. 13, Agnathes et Poissons. Paris, Masson.

deGroot, S.J. (1971) On the interrelationships between morphology of the alimentary tract, food and feeding behaviour in flatfishes (Pisces: Pleuronectiformes). Neth. J. Sea Res. 5:121–196.

Guthrie, D.M. (1983) Integration and control by the central nervous system. In: Control Processes in Fish Physiology (Rankin, J.C., Pitcher, T.J., and Duggan, R.T., eds.). Wiley-Interscience, New York, pp. 130–154.

Harder, W. (1975) Anatomy of Fishes (Part I: text; part II: figures and plates). E. Schweizerbart'sche Verlagsbuchhandlung (Nägele u. Obermiller), Stuttgart.

Hart, J.L. (1973) Pacific fishes of Canada. Bull. Fish. Res. Bd. Can. 180:740.

Haug, T., Huse, I., Kjorsvik, E., and Rabben, H. (1989) Observations on the growth of juvenile Atlantic halibut (Hippoglossus hippoglossus L.) in captivity. Aquaculture 80:79–86.

Hemre, G.-I., Lie, O., Lied, E., and Lambertsen, G. (1989) Starch as an energy source in feed for cod (Gadus morhua): digestibility and retention. Aquaculture 80:261–270.

Hickman, C.P., Jr., (1968a) Glomerular filtration and urine flow in the euryhaline southern flounder, Paralichthys lethostigma, in seawater. Can. J. Zool. 46:427–437.

Hickman, C.P., Jr. (1968b) Urine composition and kidney tubular function in the euryhaline southern flounder, Paralichthys lethostigma, in seawater. Can. J. Zool. 46:439–455.

Hislop, J.R.G. (1984) A comparison of the reproductive tactics and strategies of cod, haddock, whiting, and Norway pout in the North Sea. In: Fish Reproduction: Strategies and Tactics (Potts, G.W., and Wootton, R.J., eds.). Academic Press, London, pp. 311–329.

Hoar, W.S., and Randall, D.J. (1978) Fish Physiology (10 vols.). Academic Press, New York.

Hochachka, P.W., and Brill, R.W. (1987) Autocatalytic pathways to cell death: a new analysis of the tuna burn problem. Fish Physiol. Biochem. 4(2):81–87.

Holmes, R.A., and Gibson, R.N. (1983) A comparison of predatory behaviour in flatfish. Anim. Behav. 31:1244–1255.

Ince, B.W. (1983) Pancreatic control of metabolism. In: Control Processes in Fish Physiology (Rankin, J.C., Pitcher, T.J., and Duggan, R.T., eds.). Wiley-Interscience, New York, pp. 89–102.

Inui, Y., and Miwa, S. (1985) Thyroid hormone induces metamorphosis in flounder larvae. Gen. Comp. Endocrinol. 60:450–454.

Jobling, M. (1988) A review of physiological and nutritional energies of cod (Gadus morhua), with particular reference to growth under farmed conditions. Aquaculture 70:1–19.

Jónsson, L. (1980) Chemical stimuli: role in the behaviour of fishes. In: Environmental Physiology of Fishes (Ali, M.A., ed.). Plenum Press, New York, pp. 353–367.

Kleerekoper, H. (1969) Olfaction in Fishes. Indiana University Press, Bloomington, Indiana.

Knorr, G., Meyer, V., Kreff, G., and Lillelund, K. (1974) Atlas zur Anatomie und Morphologie der Nutzfische. 1. Gadus morhua. Verlag Paul Perey, Hamburg and Berlin.

Knorr, G., Meyer, V., Kreff, G., and Lillilund, K. (1975a) Atlas zur Anatomie und Morphologie der Nutzfische. 4. Melanogrammus aeglefinus. Verlag Paul Perey, Hamburg and Berlin.

Knorr, G., Meyer, V., Kreff, G., and Lillilund, K. (1975b) Atlas zur Anatomie und Morphologie der Nutzfische. 2. Pleuronectes platessa. Verlag Paul Perey, Hamburg and Berlin.

Knorr, G., Meyer, V., Kreff, G., and Lillilund, K. (1980) Atlas zur Anatomie und Morphologie der Nutzfische. 6. Clupea harengus. Verlag Paul Perey, Hamburg and Berlin.

Kulikov, M.Y. (1964) (On the adaptation of sablefish Anoplopoma fimbria [Pallas] to sudden changes in pressure.) Isv. Tikhookeans Nauchn.—Issled. Inst. Rybu. Khoz. i Okeanogr. 55:247–248; Biol. Abstr. 48, 552 (1967).

Lagler, K.F., Bardach, J.E., Miller, R.R., and Passino, D.R.M. (1977) Ichthyology. 2nd ed.. John Wiley and Sons, New York.

Lee, R.F., Phleger, C.F., and Horn, M.H. (1975) Composition of oil in fish bones: possible function in neutral buoyancy. Comp. Biochem. Physiol. 50B:13–16.

Lie, O., Lied, E., and Lambertsen, G. (1986) Liver retention of fat and of fatty acids in cod (Gadus morhua) fed different oils. Aquaculture 59:187–196.

Lie, O., Lied, E., and Lambertsen, G. (1989) Hematological values and fatty acid composition of erythrocyte phospholipids in cod (Gadus morhua) fed at different water temperatures. Aquaculture 79(1–4):137–144.

Lindsey, C.C. (1978) Form, function, and locomotory habits in fish. In: Fish Physiology. (Hoar, W.S., and Randall, D.J., eds.). Academic Press, New York, pp. 1–100.

Love, M.S., and Cailliet, G.M. (1979) Readings in Ichthyology. Goodyear Publishing, Santa Monica, California.

Love, R.M. (1970) The Chemical Biology of Fishes. Academic Press, London.

Love, R.M. (1980) The Chemical Biology of Fishes. Vol. 2: Advances 1968–1977. Academic Press, London.

Mason, J.C., Beamish, R.J., and McFarlane, G.A. (1983) Sexual maturity, fecundity, spawning, and early life history of sablefish (Anoplopoma fimbria) off the Pacific coast of Canada. Can. J. Fish. Aquatic Sci. 40:2126–2134.

McFarland, W.N., and Munz, F.W. (1975) The evolution of phototopic visual pigments in fishes. Vision Res. 15:1071–1080.

McFarlane, G.A., and Beamish, R.J. (1983) Biology of adult sablefish (Anoplopoma fimbria) in waters off western Canada. Proceedings of the International Sablefish Symposium, pp. 59–80, Alaska Sea Grant Report, pp. 83–88.

McFarlane, G.A., and Nagata, W.D. (1988) Overview of sablefish mariculture and its potential for industry. In: Proceedings of the Fourth Alaska Aquaculture Conference (Keller, S., ed.). University of Alaska Sea Grant College Program, Fairbanks, Report 88:161–120.

Morrison, C.M. (1987) Histology of the Atlantic cod, Gadus morhua: an atlas. Part One. Digestive tract and associated organs. Can. Spec. Publ. Fish. Aquatic Sci. 98:1–219.

Morrison, C.M. (1988) Histology of the Atlantic cod, Gadus morhua: an atlas. Part Two. Respiratory system and pseudobranch. Can. Spec. Publ. Fish. Aquatic Sci. 102:1–91.

Morrison, C.M. (1990) Histology of the atlantic cod, Gadus morhua: an atlas. Part Three. Reproductive Tract. Can. Spec. Publ. Fish. Aquatic Sci.

Moyle, P.B., and Cech, J.J., Jr. (1988) Fishes: An Introduction to Ichthyology. 2nd ed. Prentice-Hall, Englewood Cliffs, New Jersey.

Naas, K. (1987) Current status of cod (Gadus morhua) culture in Norway—an overview of the pond method. In: Proceedings of the Third International Symposium on Reproductive Physiology of Fish (Idler, D.R., Crim, L.W., and Walsh, J.M., eds.). Memorial University, St. John's, Newfoundland.

Nilsson, S., Holmgren, S., and Fange, R. (1983) Autonomic nerve functions in fish. In: Control Processes in Fish Physiology. (Rankin, J.C., Pitcher, T.J., and Duggan, R.T., eds.). Wiley-Interscience, New York, pp. 1–22.

Pedersen, T., and Jobling, M. (1989) Growth rates of large, sexually mature cod, Gadus morhua, in relation to condition and temperature during an annual cycle. Aquaculture 81:161–168.

Potts, G.W., and Wootton, R.J. (1984) Fish Reproduction: Strategies and Tactics. Academic Press, London.

Poynton, S.L., and Morrison, C.M. (1990) Morphology of diplomonad flagellates: Spironucleus torosa n. sp. from Atlantic cod Gadus morhua L., and haddock Melanogrammus aeglefinus (L.) and Hexamita salmonis Moore from brook trout Salvelinus fontinalis (Mitchill). J. Protozool. 37(5):369–383.

Preston, A. (1960) Red blood values in the plaice (Pleuronectes platessa L.). J. Marine Biol. Assoc. U.K. 39:681–687.

Privol'nev, T.I., and Brizinova, P.N. (1964) Melting point of fish fats. In: Fish Physiology in Acclimatization and Breeding (Privol'nev, T.I., ed.). Bull. State Scientific Res. Inst. of Lake and River Fisheries, Leningrad 58; Israel Program for Scientific Translations, Jerusalem, 1970, pp. 45–56.

Rankin, J.C., Pitcher, T.J., and Duggan, R.T. (1983) Control Processes in Fish Physiology. Wiley-Interscience, New York.

Roberts, J.L. (1975) Active branchial and ram gill ventilation in fishes. Biol. Bull. 148:85–105.

Roberts, J.L. (1978) Ram gill ventilation in fish. In: The Physiological Ecology of Tunas. Proceedings of the Tuna Physiology Workshop (Sharp, G.D., and Dixon, A.E., eds.). Southwest Fisheries Center, La Jolla, California, 1977. Academic Press, New York, pp. 83–88.

Roberts, R.J. (1989) Fish Pathology. 2nd ed. Baillière Tindall, London.

Rowley, A.F., Hunt, T.C., Page, M., and Mainwaring, G. (1988) Fish. In: Vertebrate Blood Cells (Rowley, A.F., and Ratcliffe, N.A., eds.). Cambridge University Press, Cambridge.

Satchell, G.H. (1971) Circulation in Fishes. Cambridge University Press, London.

Scott, W.B., and Scott, M.G. (1988) Atlantic fishes of Canada. Can. Bull. Fish. Aquatic Sci. 219:731.

Sharp, G.D., and Pirages, S.W. (1978) The distribution of red and white swimming muscles, their biochemistry, and the biochemical phylogeny of selected scombrid fishes. In: The Physiological Ecology of Tunas (Sharp, G.D. and Dixon, A.E., eds.). Proceedings of the Tuna Physiology Workshop, Southwest Fisheries Center, La Jolla, California, 1977. Academic Press, New York, pp. 41–78.

Shelton, G. (1970) The regulation of breathing. In: Fish Physiology. Vol. IV. The Nervous System, Circulation, and Respiration. (Hoar, W.S., and Randall, D.J., eds.). Academic Press, New York, pp. 293–359.

Smith, J.C. (1977) Body weight and the haematology of the American plaice, *Hippoglossoides platessoides*. J. Exp. Biol. 67:17–28.

Smith, L.S. (1982) Introduction to fish physiology. T.F.H. Publications, Neptune, New Jersey.

Solar, I.I., Baker, I.J., and Donaldson, E.M. (1987) Induced ovulation in sablefish *(Anoplopoma fimbria)* using gonadotropin-releasing hormone analogues. In: Proceedings of the Third International Symposium on Reproductive Physiology of Fish (Idler, D.R., Crim, L.W., and Walsh, J.M., eds.). Memorial University, St. John's, Newfoundland, p. 101.

Steen, J.B. (1970) The swim bladder as a hydrostatic organ. In: Fish Physiology. Vol. IV, The Nervous System, Circulation, and Respiration (Hoar, W.S., and Randall, D.J., eds.). Academic Press, New York, pp. 413–443.

Tavolga, W.N. (1971) Sound production and detection. In: Fish Physiology, Vol. V. Sensory Systems and Electric Organs (Hoar, W.S., and Randall, D.J., eds.). Academic Press, New York, pp. 135–205.

Timeyko, V.N. (1986) The digestive systems of white sea cod, *Gadus morhua*

marisalbi, and lumpfish, *Cyclopterus lumpus*, at different stages of ontogeny. J. Ichthyol. 26:72–82.

Ulaming, V., de (1983) Oocyte development patterns and hormonal involvements among teleosts. In: Control Processes in Fish Physiology (Rankin, J.C., Pitcher, T.J., and Duggan, R.T., eds.). Wiley-Interscience, New York, pp 176–199.

Utter, F.M., and Ridgway, G.J. (1967) A serologically detected serum factor associated with maturity in English sole, *Parophys vetulus*, and Pacific halibut, *Hippoglossus stenolepis*. U.S. Fish Wildlife Serv., Fishery Bull. 66:47–58.

Von der Decken, A. (1989) Ration size in the feeding of cod *(Gadus morhua)*: effect on skeletal muscle proteins, with special reference to myosin heavy chain. Aquaculture 79:47–52.

Waiwood, K., Goff, G., and Brown, J. (1988) Marine Finfish Culture in Atlantic Canada: Status and Potential. Aquaculture International Congress and Exposition. Congress Proceedings. Aquaculture International Congress, Vancouver.

Wardle, C.S., Videler, J.W., Arimoto, T., Franco, J.M., and He, P. (1989) The muscle twitch and the maximum swimming speed of giant bluefin tuna *(Thunnus thynnus* L.). J. Fish Biol. 35(1):129–138.

White, A., and Fletcher, T.C. (1987) Polar and neutral lipid composition of the gonads and serum in the plaice, *Pleuronectes platessa* L. Fish Physiol. Biochem. 4(1):37–43.

Zohar, Y. (1989) Endocrinology and fish farming: aspects in reproduction, growth, and smoltification. Fish Physiol. Biochem. 7(1–4):395–405.

Chapter 86

CLINICAL PATHOLOGY OF COLD-WATER MARINE FISHES

BARBARA HORNEY

HEMATOLOGY

Baseline hematologic values can be found in Tables 86–1 and 86–2.

CELLULAR MORPHOLOGY

Erythrocytes

Mature piscine erythrocytes are ellipsoidal with a central nucleus. Immature cells are smaller and more rounded (Blaxhall and Daisley, 1973). Supravital stained reticulocytes of albacore and skipjack tuna (3 to 9% of erythrocytes) contain a loose, dis-

connected reticulum around the nucleus (Alexander et al., 1980). Mature cells in these species have a mean size of 9.0×6.6 μm (Alexander et al., 1980).

Abnormal erythrocyte morphology has been associated with *Haemogregarina platessa* infection in tongue sole (Obiekezie, 1986) and in viral infections of cod and blenny (Reno et al., 1986; Smail and Egglestone, 1980). Erythrocyte counts are lower in bluefin tuna prior to spawning compared to post-spawning (Alexander et al., 1980).

Thrombocytes

Spiked and spindle-shaped thrombocytes are predominant in plaice when the blood is collected

TABLE 86–1. Baseline Hematologic Parameters of Marine Cold-Water Fishes: Leukocyte Indices

Species	Heterophils (%)	Band Cells (%)	Monocytes (%)	Lymphocytes (%)	Eosinophils (%)	Basophils (%)	Other (%)	References
Albacore tuna	24	0	6	51	13	0	6	Alexander et al., 1980
Skipjack tuna	33	0	6	46	11	0	4	Alexander et al., 1980

TABLE 86–2. Baseline Hematologic Parameters of Marine Cold-Water Fishes: Erythrocyte Indices

Species	N	RBCs (mil/ml)	Hct (%)	Hb (g/dl)	References
Albacore tuna	NA	2.3–3.0	42–57	11–17	Alexander et al., 1980
Skipjack tuna	NA	2.5–4.8	42–66	15.8–22.3	Alexander et al., 1980
Starry flounder	NA		11–20		Wood et al., 1977
Winter flounder	NA	2.7–2.9	30–32	6.8–7.6	Fletcher, 1975

with minimal stress to the fish and the sample is carefully and quickly processed (Ellis, 1976). Turbot thrombocytes are 11.3 × 5 μm (Burrows and Fletcher, 1987) and those of plaice 7.0 × 2.5 to 12.0 × 4.0 μm (Ellis, 1976).

Lymphocytes

A large, indented nucleus and a thin rim of basophilic cytoplasm (9 μm in diameter) characterize the lymphocytes of the turbot (Burrows and Fletcher, 1987). Larger lymphocytes with more abundant cytoplasm are rare in this species (Burrows and Fletcher, 1987). Occasional azurophilic granules are present in albacore lymphocytes (Alexander et al., 1980). Lymphocytes of plaice are usually 4 to 6 μm in diameter and appear to lack phagocytic activity (Ellis, 1977).

Monocytes

Turbot monocytes are large (11.5 μm), vacuolated cells with round or horseshoe-shaped nuclei (Burrows and Fletcher, 1987). They have also been described in plaice (Ellis, 1976), albacore, and skipjack (Alexander et al., 1980). Increased numbers of immature leukocytes identified as monocytes have been associated with a sporozoan infection in turbot (Ferguson and Roberts, 1975).

Granulocytes

Nuclei of heterophils from plaice or albacore tuna are monolobed or occasionally bilobed (Alexander et al., 1980; Ellis, 1976). Heterophils from turbot only occasionally have multilobed nuclei (Burrows and Fletcher, 1987), in contrast to salmonid heterophils that commonly are multilobed (Ellis, 1977). Eosinophils are present in albacore and skipjack (Alexander et al., 1980), but are usually not seen in plaice (Ellis, 1976; Ferguson, 1976). Basophils are not seen in skipjack, albacore tuna (Alexander et al., 1980), or plaice (Ellis, 1976; Ferguson, 1976), but are present in low numbers in some other cold-water marine fishes (Ellis, 1977).

Antifreeze Glycoprotein

Atlantic cod (Hew et al., 1981) and winter flounder (Fletcher and Smith, 1980) may have a plasma component, which depresses the freezing temperature of the plasma without altering the melting temperature. These glycoproteins are believed to be essential for the survival of many fish residing in ice-laden seawater (Hew et al., 1981). Timing of the cycle of production of this glycoprotein may differ between populations of winter flounder in a manner unrelated to environmental stimuli (Fletcher and Smith, 1980). These proteins may interfere with osmolality values measured by a freezing point depression method creating a false elevation of the measured value (Fletcher, 1975).

Serum Enzymes

Many methods applied to human sera are acceptable for the assay of enzyme activity in fish blood, although the optimal pH for the assay of alanine aminotransferase (ALT) and aspartate aminotransferase (AST) of English sole is lower than that for humans (Casillas et al., 1982). Normal ranges of serum activity vary between species and normal values must be produced from a representative population of each species (Sandnes et al., 1988; Mawdesley-Thomas and Barry, 1970). Large variations in documented enzyme activities in fish may be due in part to differences in methodology (Hille, 1982). Associations between alterations in serum enzyme activity and the pathophysiology of fish have been documented in several studies. Serum alkaline phosphatase activity is positively correlated to hepatic lesions in yellowtail tuna (Sandnes et al., 1988). High levels of AST and ALT activity are found in the liver and kidney of English sole. Elevations of these enzymes in serum correlate with histologic liver lesions in sole after acute exposure to carbon tetrachloride (Casillas et al., 1983).

Serum chemistry and electrolyte values for marine cold-water fishes are given in Table 86–3.

Minerals

Serum calcium is subject to changes in water characteristics (Wood et al., 1988) and kidney function (Casillas et al., 1983). Inorganic phosphorus was elevated in the serum of English sole with kidney lesions induced by intraperitoneal injection of carbon tetrachloride. Magnesium is reported to be altered by kidney damage in this species (Casillas et al., 1983).

TABLE 86–3. Serum Chemistry and Electrolyte Values of Marine Cold-Water Fishes

Species (Refs.)	Parameter	Values
English sole (Casillas et al., 1983)	Bilirubin (mg/dl)	0.0–0.14
	Serum urea nitrogen (mg/dl)	2.9–7.1
	AST (U/L)	<89
	ALT (U/L)	<29
Winter flounder (Fletcher, 1975)	Total protein (g/dl)	5.7–6.2
	Na (mM/L)	218–225
	Cl (mM/L)	190–194
	K (mM/L)	1.0–1.2
	Osmolality (mOsm/L)	704–722*

Most likely a false elevation due to the presence of antifreeze glycoproteins.

Other Serum Chemical Parameters

Serum creatinine alterations are associated with kidney damage in English sole (Casillas et al., 1983). Bilirubin is not elevated with experimentally induced toxic liver damage in English sole (Casillas et al., 1983). Blood urea nitrogen is not elevated in association with toxic liver and kidney damage in English sole (Casillas et al., 1983). Urea is not a major end product of protein metabolism in most fish (Casillas et al., 1983) and urea is diffusible over the gills (Audet et al., 1988).

Elevation of blood glucose was found associated with intraperitoneal carbon tetrachloride injection as well as acute liver and kidney damage in English sole (Casillas et al., 1983). There is marked variation of serum glucose within populations (Hille, 1982). Forced, exhausting activity results in acidosis and increased CO_2 and lactate levels (Wood et al., 1977).

LITERATURE CITED

Alexander, N., Laurst, R.M., McIntosh, A., and Russel, S.W. (1980) Haematological characteristics of albacore, *Thunnus alalunga* (Bonnaterre), and skipjack, *Katsuwonus pelamis* (Linnaeus). J. Fish Biol. 16:383–395.

Audet, C., Munger, R.S., and Wood, C.M. (1988) Long-term sublethal acid exposure in rainbow trout (*Salmo gairdneri*) in soft water: Effects on ion exchanges and blood chemistry. Can. J. Fish. Aquatic Sci. 45:1387–1398.

Blaxhall, P.C., and Daisley, K.W. (1973) Routine haematological methods for use with fish blood. J. Fish Biol. 5:771–781.

Burrows, A.S., and Fletcher, T.C. (1987) Blood leucocytes of the turbot *Scophthalus maximus* L. Aquaculture 67:214–215.

Casillas, E., Sundquist, J., and Ames, W.E. (1982) Optimization of assay conditions for, and the selected tissue distribution of, alanine aminotransferase and aspartate aminotransferase of English sole, *Parophrys vetulus* Girard. J. Fish Biol. 21:197–204.

Casillas, E., Myers, M., and Ames, W.E. (1983) Relationship of serum chemistry values to liver and kidney histopathology in English sole (*Parophrys vetulus*) after acute exposure to carbon tetrachloride. Aquatic Toxicol. 3:61–78.

Ellis, A.E. (1976) Leucocytes and related cells in the plaice *Pleuronectes platessa*. J. Fish Biol. 8:143–156.

Ellis, A.E. (1977) The leucocytes of fish: a review. J. Fish Biol. 11:453–491.

Ferguson, H.W. (1976) The ultrastructure of plaice (*Pleuronectes platessa*) leucocytes. J. Fish Biol. 8:139–142.

Ferguson, H.W., and Roberts, R.J. (1975) Myeloid leucosis associated with sporozoan infection in cultured turbot (*Scophthalmus maximaus* L.) J. Comp. Path. 85:317–326.

Fletcher, G.L. (1975) The effects of capture "stress" and storage of whole blood on the red blood cells, plasma proteins, glucose, and electrolytes of the winter flounder (*Pseudopleuronectes americanus*). Can. J. Zool. 53:197–206.

Fletcher, G.L., and Smith, J.C. (1980) Evidence for permanent population differences in the annual cycle of plasma "antifreeze" levels of winter flounder. Can. J. Zool. 58:507–512.

Hew, C.L., Slaughter, D., Fletcher, G., and Joshi, B. (1981) Antifreeze glycoproteins in the plasma of newfoundland Atlantic cod (*Gadus morhum*). Can. J. Zool. 59:2186–2192.

Hille, S. (1982) A literature review of the blood chemistry of rainbow trout, *Salmo gairdneri* Rich. J. Fish Biol. 20:535–569.

Mawdesley-Thomas, L.E., and Barry, D.H. (1970) Acid and alkaline phosphatase activity in the liver of brown and rainbow trout. Nature 227:738–739.

Obiekezie, A.I. (1986) Haematozoa of the tongue sole, *Cynoglossus senegalensis* (Kaup, 1958) (Teleostei, Cynoglossidae) from the West African coast. Rev. Zool. Afr. 99:255–261.

Reno, P.W., Kleftis, K., Sherburne, S.W., and Nicholson, B.L. (1986) Experimental infection and pathogenesis of viral erythrocytic necrosis (VEN) in Atlantic cod, *Gadus morhua*. Can. J. Fish Aquatic Sci. 43:945–951.

Sandnes, K., Lie, O. and Waagbo, R. (1988) Normal ranges of some blood chemistry parameters in adult farmed Atlantic salmon, *Salmo salar*. J. Fish Biol. 32:129–136.

Smail, D.A., and Egglestone, S.I. (1980) Virus infections of marine fish erythrocytes: prevalence of piscine erythrocytic necrosis in cod *Gadus morhua* L. and blenny *Blennius pholis* L. in coastal and offshore waters of the United Kingdom. J. Fish Dis. 3:41–46.

Wood, C.M., McMahon, B.R., and McDonald, D.G. (1977) An analysis of changes in blood pH following exhausting activity in the starry flounder, *Platichthys stellatus*. J. Exp. Biol. 69:173–185.

Wood, C.M., Playle, R.C., et al. (1988) Blood gases, acid-base status, ions, and hematology in adult brook trout (*Salvelinus fontinalis*) under acid/aluminum exposure. Can. J. Fish Aquatic Sci. 45:1575–1586.

Chapter 87

MARINE COLD-WATER FISH NUTRITION

SANTOSH P. LALL   OLE J. TORRISSEN

The culture of marine cold-water fishes is a comparatively recent development, and, unlike the case with salmonid culture, there is no established body of nutritional knowledge. The nutrient requirements and feeding practices of some cold-water species such as cod and halibut are just beginning to be understood. In a natural environment, these fishes sieve phytoplankton or graze algae to catch small fish or invertebrates. They are the top of the food chain.

In the early attempts to rear marine fishes in captivity, natural foods were used, such as small fish, shrimp, and other fishery by-products. Later, having studied the chemical composition of natural foods, nutritionists tried to formulate balanced diets by substituting other food materials of animal and plant origin and supplementing them with micronutrients. Commercial diets are now manufactured for cod and turbot cultures in Europe, and an attempt to produce a successful halibut diet continues. Whole or ground fish is still used to feed fish species for which the nutrient requirements are poorly understood and in situations where it has not been practical to use dry or semimoist feed.

PROTEIN AND AMINO ACIDS

In the natural diet of most marine fishes, protein constitutes the largest single nutrient essential for growth and maintenance. The requirement for protein is mainly for the constituent amino acids. The nutritional quality of proteins from various food sources may differ because of the differences in their amino acid composition and the bioavailability of constituent amino acids. Protein requirements, therefore, have two components. Essential amino acids are required because fish cannot synthesize them or are unable to synthesize them rapidly enough, and nonessential amino acids are required to provide a source of nonessential nitrogen. Most cold-water fishes do not utilize carbohydrates efficiently; therefore, some protein is metabolized for energy. In order to obtain maximum growth and protein utilization, the protein source should be selected to create an amino acid supply close to that required. It is also desirable to meet the requirement for each amino acid as closely as possible, avoiding excess. High-quality fishmeal supplies all essential amino acids at appropriate levels and is widely used as the major source of protein in fish diets.

Only the crude protein requirements of plaice have been estimated using dose-response growth curves. These are in the range of 50% of the diet (Cowey et al., 1972). The protein requirement may vary owing to differences in fish size, water temperature, daily feed allowance, amount of nonprotein energy in the feed, and quality of the dietary protein. The gross protein requirements are highest when fish just start feeding and may decrease during the later stages of development. In order to achieve a maximum growth rate, fry must receive a diet in which nearly half of the digestible ingredients consist of a balanced protein.

Utilization of protein depends on digestion and hydrolysis of the peptide bond. Ingested protein is hydrolyzed to free amino acids and di- and tripeptides by digestive enzymes secreted into the gastrointestinal tract. These products are absorbed by the mucosal cells where digestion of small peptides occurs. There are some distinct anatomic differences in the digestive systems of various cold-water marine species, which may affect protein digestion (Glass, 1989). The early larval stages of flatfishes have rudimentary digestive tracts with no distinguishable stomach or gastric glands. These larvae are incapable of hydrolyzing protein, and it takes several days before proteolytic activity begins. They rely on live foods such as unicellular algae, rotifers, and brine shrimp napulii, and it appears that direct absorption of small peptide molecules from these organisms may be the source of essential amino acids for early growth and development.

LIPIDS

Lipids are an important source of energy and essential fatty acids. They also act as a carrier for fat-soluble vitamins and pigments, give diets a suitable texture, affect gastric emptying time, and cushion visceral organs. The natural diets of cold-water marine fishes consist of aquatic organisms rich in lipids containing highly unsaturated fatty acids. Marine fish lipids are characterized by a relatively high concentration of long-chain (20 and 22 carbon) ω3 polyunsaturated fatty acids and the presence of lipid classes such as wax esters (esters of a fatty acid and a long-chain fatty alcohol), hydrocarbons, and alkyldiacylglycerols, which are either uncommon or occur in small concentrations in terrestrial animals. Unlike other animals, marine fishes utilize wax esters efficiently. The subject of lipid nutrition and metabolism is complex, and several comprehensive reviews have been published (Sargent et al., 1989; Watanabe, 1982; Cowey and Sargent, 1979).

Like all living organisms, marine fishes contain polar lipids, largely phospholipid present in biomembranes, and neutral lipids that are fundamentally metabolic energy reserves. Fatty acids occur in nature as esters in these lipids. The neutral lipids are among the most abundant fatty acid derivatives in fish. Triglycerides, the esters of the fatty acids with glycerol, constitute the major fraction of neutral lipid. Other neutral lipids found in marine organisms are alkyldiacylglycerols, sterol esters, wax esters, and pigments. Crustaceans and a few species of fishes contain high amounts of wax esters, where the long-chain fatty acid is esterified to a long-chain fatty alcohol such as hexadecanol. The principal phospholipids in fish are phosphatidylcholine and phosphatidylethanolamine. Other phospholipids in marine fishes include phosphatidylserine, phosphatidylinositol, plasmalogens, and sphingomyelin. Fish tissues also contain cerebrosides and gangliosides.

In most fishes, most lipids are found in flesh in the form of triglycerides, except for the codfishes, which have higher levels of lipid in their livers than their flesh. The liver lipid in cod and haddock may reach levels as high as 80% of the total liver weight, which ranges from 4 to 10% of the body weight. These stored lipids are largely triglycerols, although

some cholesterols, fat-soluble vitamins, and pigments also are stored. The phospholipids are generally considered to be associated with membrane structure, and while the level of neutral lipids (triglycerides) fluctuates with total lipid levels, the level of phospholipids tends to remain more consistent at 0.5 to 1.5% of the wet weight of most tissues and organs. In general, the fatty acids of storage lipids contain more saturated and monounsaturated fatty acids than structural lipids, which have a high content of polyunsaturated fatty acids.

The most commonly accepted shorthand designation used to identify fatty acids involves two numbers separated by a colon. The carbon chain length of the fatty acid is indicated by the first number, and the second number following the colon identifies the number of double bonds. Saturated fatty acids have 0 for the second number (e.g., palmitic acid 16:0). For unsaturated fatty acids, it is important to know the position and configuration of the double bonds. A third number following ω indicates the number of carbon atoms between the first double bond and the methyl terminal. Thus, 18:2ω6 indicates a fatty acid with 18 carbons and two double bonds with the first double bond located between the sixth and seventh carbon atoms counting from the methyl end of the chain. The term *polyunsaturated fatty acid* refers to fatty acids with two or more double bonds, such as, linoleic acid (18:2ω6), linolenic acid (18:3ω3), or eicosapentaenoic acid (20:5ω3). The principal families of the fatty acids are shown in Figure 87–1.

The nature and level of lipid intake by fish in captivity or in a natural environment significantly influence their fatty acid composition and total lipid content. Several other factors, including temperature, depth, pressure, salinity, and season, may also influence the fatty acid composition of fish oils (Sargent et al., 1989). Table 87–1 summarizes the fatty acid

TABLE 87–1. Fatty Acid Analyses of Total Lipid or Flesh from Certain Marine Fishes (% by Weight)

Fatty Acid	Atlantic Herring*	Atlantic Cod*	Mackerel†	Menhaden†
14:0	5.1	3.7	4.9	8.0
16:0	10.9	12.6	28.2	28.9
16:1	12.0	9.3	5.3	7.9
18:0	1.2	2.3	3.9	4.0
18:1ω9	12.6	22.7	19.3	13.4
18:2ω6	0.7	1.5	1.1	1.1
18:3ω3	0.3	0.6	1.3	0.9
18:4ω3	1.5	0.6	3.4	1.9
20:1ω9	16.1	7.5	3.1	0.9
20:4ω6	0.4	1.4	3.9	1.2
20:4ω3	0.4	0.6		
20:5ω3	7.4	12.9	7.1	10.2
22:1ω9	19.8	6.2	2.8	1.7
22:5ω6	0.4	0.3		0.7
22:5ω3	1.1	1.7	1.2	1.6
22:6ω3	3.9	12.7	10.8	12.8
Σ Saturated	17.8	19.7	37.0	40.9
Σ Monounsaturated	61.5	47.1	30.5	23.9
Σ ω6	1.9	3.7	5.0	3.0
Σ ω3	14.6	29.1	23.8	27.4
ω3/ω6	7.7	7.9	4.8	9.1

*Whole fish lipid (Ackman, 1967).
†Flesh lipid (Gruger et al, 1964).

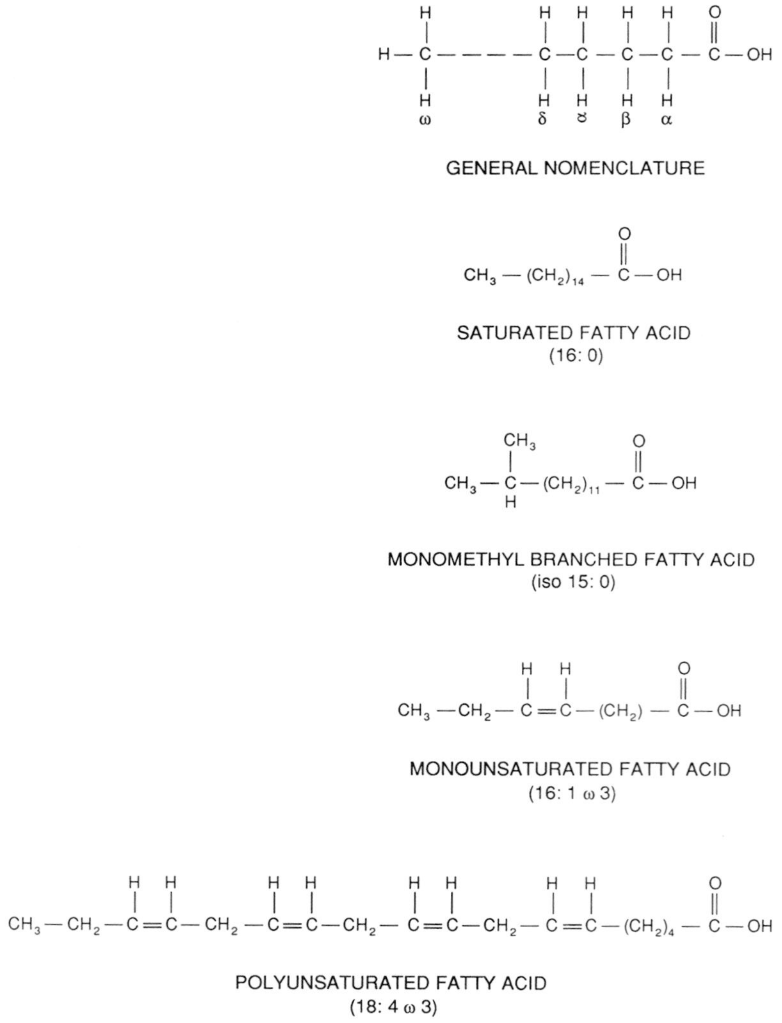

GENERAL NOMENCLATURE

SATURATED FATTY ACID
(16: 0)

MONOMETHYL BRANCHED FATTY ACID
(iso 15: 0)

MONOUNSATURATED FATTY ACID
(16: 1 ω 3)

POLYUNSATURATED FATTY ACID
(18: 4 ω 3)

FIGURE 87–1. Principal families of fatty acids.

composition of Atlantic herring, Atlantic cod, Atlantic mackerel, and Atlantic menhaden. A large intake of lipid correlates with higher lipid deposition in the fish, and the fatty acid composition of tissue neutral lipids generally reflects the lipid composition of the diet.

Essential Fatty Acids

Fish, like terrestrial animals, do not possess the desaturase enzymes needed to synthesize either 18:2ω6 or 18:3ω3 fatty acids. These must be supplied in the diet to maintain cellular function and normal growth (Fig. 87–2). The essential fatty acid requirements of fishes depend on the ability of the species to elongate and further desaturate parent fatty acids of the ω3 or ω6 series to longer-chain and more highly unsaturated fatty acids. The essential fatty acid requirements of most cold-water marine fishes have not been established. However, their body lipid compositions show higher concentrations of ω3 polyunsaturated fatty acid, which is generally derived from natural food sources.

Young turbot grow well on cod liver oil but cannot utilize 18:2ω6, 18:3ω3, or 20:4ω6 efficiently (Cowey et al., 1976). Also, most cold-water marine fishes appear to require 20:5ω3 and 22:6ω3 in their diet. The activity of the enzyme responsible for converting 20:5ω3 to 22:6ω3 is low in turbot, and both of these fatty acids are essential in their diet (Bell et al., 1985). It appears that diets for marine carnivorous fishes must be supplemented with lipids rich in C_{20} and C_{22} polyunsaturated fatty acids in addition to linolenic acid (Kanazawa, 1985).

Young turbot require 0.8% of their diet as long-chain ω3 polyunsaturated fatty acids (Gatesoupe et al., 1977). Turbot larvae have a higher requirement for ω3 fatty acids (1.3%) of chain length C_{20} or greater. Generally, the ω3 fatty acid contents of many marine fish eggs range from 5 to 10% of the total egg dry weight. This may reflect higher essential fatty acid requirements for larval and young fingerlings. Work conducted in Japan on marine larval fish shows that 22:6ω3 has a higher value than 20:5ω3, particularly for red sea bream (Watanabe, 1983a,b). Larval red sea bream feeding on rotifers containing 22:6ω3 show lower mortality and avoid essential fatty acid defi-

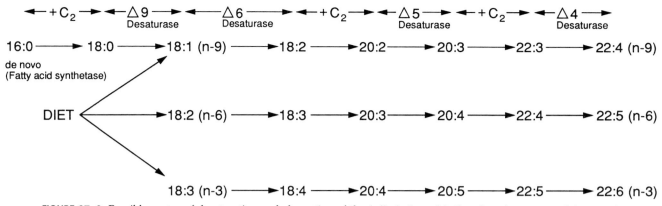

FIGURE 87–2. Possible routes of desaturation and elongation of the (ω9), (ω6), and (ω3) series of unsaturated fatty acids.

ciency. This suggests that diets of rotifers containing chlorella, which are cultured as larval feed for marine fishes, should be enriched with 22:6ω3. Both 20:5ω3 and 22:6ω3 are required for the optimum growth of the larvae; however, rotifers fed chlorella alone supply only high levels of 20:5ω3 (Watanabe, 1983a,b).

The signs of essential fatty acid deficiency in cold-water marine fishes have not been well characterized. In freshwater and other marine fishes, deficiency signs include poor growth and feed efficiency. Other signs include shock, fin erosion, low hatchability of eggs, and embryonic deformities (Sargent et al., 1989). Turbot fed diets devoid of polyunsaturated fatty acids show adipocyte membrane damage (Cowey et al., 1976) and damage to chloride cells in the gills (Bell et al., 1985).

CARBOHYDRATES

Most carnivorous fishes have a limited ability to use carbohydrate for energy. Although the basic pathways of carbohydrate metabolism in fish are similar to those of other animals, there are some basic differences. Starch derived from cereal grains is poorly digested by marine cold-water fishes, but heat processing improves the availability of carbohydrates in milled feeds. Excessive carbohydrates in juvenile marine fish diets produce abnormally high liver glycogen levels and mortality.

ENERGY

Nutritional and physiologic energetics of marine fishes have received limited attention with the exception of some studies on Atlantic cod (Jobling, 1988). Since fish are poikilothermic, their metabolic rate is commensurate with body temperature, and environmental temperatures may have a marked influence on energy requirements and feed intake. The metabolic rate of flat fishes appears to be low in comparison to round-bodied fishes measured under similar conditions (Jobling, 1982). The physiologic and nutritional energetics of fish have been reviewed in the literature (Brett and Groves, 1979; Cho and Kaushik, 1990).

VITAMINS

The discovery of vitamins as nutrients in the early nineteenth century led to the isolation of vitamins A and D in a wide variety of marine cold-water species. Fish liver oil was recognized as a natural source of these vitamins, and many marine fishes were exploited for their commercial production. A comprehensive review on the distribution of vitamins in fish has been published (Higashi, 1962). Later, the successful commercial synthesis of vitamins A and D resulted in a gradual decline in the use of fat-soluble vitamins from marine sources.

To date, information on the vitamin requirements of cold-water marine fishes is confined to a few species, even though distribution of most vitamins in tissues have been reported for Atlantic cod, haddock, turbot, halibut, and other food fishes. In natural diets, vitamins occur in sufficient amounts to supply the very limited quantities necessary for normal metabolic functions. However, when fish are raised on artificial diets, various factors, including the selection of food constituents and the rapid deterioration that may occur in some vitamins, may lead to specific deficiencies that impair body function. Unlike terrestrial animals, the gastrointestinal tracts of most cold-water marine fishes do not contain adequate microorganisms for a significant microbial synthesis of vitamins in the intestine. Deficiency signs of most vitamins in marine fishes have not been reported, with the exception of vitamin C deficiency observed in Atlantic halibut (Fig. 87–3).

MINERALS

The mineral requirements of most cold-water marine fishes have not been studied. The exchange of ions from the marine environment across gills and skin and their influx during the drinking of seawater complicates the determination of the quantitative

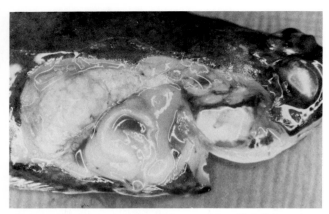

FIGURE 87–3. Tyrosinemia caused by ascorbic acid deficiency in an Atlantic halibut. (Courtesy of O.M. Rodseth.)

dietary requirements. Fish absorb calcium, magnesium, sodium, potassium, iron, zinc, and copper from the environment to partially satisfy their requirements; however, phosphates and sulfates are more effectively utilized from food sources. Despite the ability of fishes to absorb elements from the surrounding water, most commercial diets require some mineral supplementation to overcome problems of mineral bioavailability and various metabolic antagonisms and interactions (Lall, 1989).

The calcium requirements of marine cold-water fishes are met in large part directly from the environment. Calcium influx and efflux occurs across gills, fins, and buccal epithelia. The gills are the most important site of calcium regulation in these fishes. Marine fishes obtain magnesium by drinking and excrete the excess via the kidney. It appears that magnesium supplementation is not necessary unless there is an imbalance caused by an excessive amount of other minerals present in the diet. The main source of phosphorus in cold-water marine fishes is dietary, apparently because seawater phosphate concentrations are relatively low.

Some absorption of iron takes place across gill membranes; however, the intestinal mucosa is considered to be the major site of iron absorption, and food is considered the major source of metabolic iron. Supplementation of Atlantic halibut broodstock diets with zinc and manganese is considered essential to ensuring reproductive performance and production of good-quality eggs (Goff and Lall, 1989).

FEED FORMULATION AND PROCESSING

The main objective of ration formulation is to use knowledge of nutrient requirements and locally available feed ingredients to develop nutritionally balanced feeds that will be eaten in sufficient amounts to provide optimum production at the lowest possible cost. The basic information required for feed formulation includes nutrient requirements of

the species cultivated and their feeding habits; the local availability, cost, and nutrient composition of feed ingredients; the ability of fish to utilize nutrients from various sources; the type of ration desired (e.g., larval, starter, grower, and broodstock); the expected feed consumption; the feed additives required; and the feed processing desired.

Certain feed components are added for purely processing needs. Binders may be necessary to improve the firmness of pellets and reduce the loss of fine particles during feed manufacture. Widely used binders are sodium and calcium bentonites, lignosulfonates, hemicellulose, carboxymethylcellulose, alginates, and guar gum. Cereal grains provide starch, which gelatinizes to give a water-stable pellet. Other ingredients such as whey, wheat gluten, gelatinized starches, and molasses, alone or in combinations, permit the production of stable pellets. Antioxidants prevent rancidity during processing and storage. Common synthetic antioxidants added to fish feeds are BHT (3,5-di-tert-butyl–4-hydroxytoluene), BHA (2[3]-tert-butyl–4-hydroxyanisole), and ethoxyquin (1,2-dihydro–6-ethoxy–2,2,4-trimethylquinoline).

Other food items are known to be gustatory feeding stimulants and must be considered in feed formulation. Some of these organisms or their by-products, including nethrops, scallop wastes, shrimp, krill, crustacean by-products, squid, and other molluscs, have been successfully used to induce feeding (Carr, 1982). However, the chemosensitivity to these cues varies among fish species. Several chemical compounds, either alone or in combination, also involve feeding responses in carnivorous fishes, including glycine, proline, taurine, valine, betane, and inosine (Mackie, 1982). Since cold-water marine fishes detect food by olfaction or sight, the acceptability of feed can depend on appearance (size, shape, color), smell, feel, and taste (Carr, 1982; Mackie and Mitchell, 1985).

Often, the addition of humectants (propylene glycol and sodium chloride), which lower water activity and prevent bacterial growth, and fungistats (propionic and sorbic acid), which retard mold growth, is required in moist or semimoist diets. The high moisture content in these diets also enhances the oxidation of vitamin C. The composition of a typical halibut moist feed is shown in Table 87–2.

FEEDING PRACTICES

The amount of feed consumed by fishes varies among species and is generally affected by water temperature, salinity, body weight, energy content of the diet, feed palatability, and particle size. The feeding practices of most marine fishes, with the exception of cod, are based on ad libitum feeding. Feeding once a day is considered adequate for cod.

The feeding rate of fish is commonly expressed as a percentage of body weight fed per day. Gener-

TABLE 87–2. Composition of a Moist Diet for Atlantic Halibut

Ingredients	Percent by Weight
Whole herring, ground	45
Shrimp waste	10
Fishmeal	16
Extruded wheat	14
Vitamin mixture, mineral mixture, and binder meal	15
Chemical Composition (dry weight basis)	
Protein	55
Lipid	12
Nitrogen-free extract (including carbohydrate)	20
Ash	10
Other	3

From Ronnestad, I. (1988) For og foring. In: Oppdrett av Kveite (Hippoglossus hippoglossus) (Ronnestad, I., ed.). Institute of Marine Research, Bergen. Report Akva 8806 (in Norwegian), pp. 22–24.

ally, small fish require a higher percentage of their body weight fed per day as compared with larger fish. Fry and fingerlings require more frequent feeding than adult or growing fish. Fish fed too high an intake show poor feed conversion, partly because of feed wastage but also because of incomplete digestion and increased activity. On the other hand, underfeeding results in a lower growth rate.

The size, hardness, and texture of the pellet, the photoperiod, water quality, and stress may greatly influence feed intake. Since fish do not feed as actively at low temperatures, more time must be spent feeding. Changes in the particle size must be gradual and should be particularly avoided at low temperatures, or when fish are infected or stressed. Broodstock do not require frequent feeding, but the quality of feed is important. They generally stop feeding prior to spawning. After the spawning, broodstock fish should be gradually brought back to full feeding to replenish depleted nutrient reserves.

Larval Nutrition

Most pelagic fish larvae are visual feeders, and their digestive and sensory systems are not completely developed. Hatchery feeding strategies for propagation of marine fish larvae, postlarvae, and fry stage generally consist of live planktonic foods such as rotifer (*Branchionus plicatilis,* 100 to 400 μm) and brine shrimp (*Artemia salina,* 420 to 520 μm) napulii. Turbot, sole, and cod have been successfully weaned on complete formulated dry feeds. Although microencapsulated, microparticulate, or flaked larval diets have also been developed, they are more successful when used in conjunction with live foods. A variety of food types, including moist and dry crumbles, freeze-dried and powdered aquatic organisms and animal tissues, and pastes, have been fed along with supplemental vitamins, minerals, and feeding stimulants with varied success.

The mass production of live organisms for the rearing of larvae is relatively expensive. The nutritive value of the live organisms produced may be quite variable and depends on the strain, source, and culture method. Often, rotifers cultured on yeast are deficient in polyunsaturated fatty acids. The rotifer diet must be enriched to overcome essential fatty acid deficiencies in marine fish larvae reared on rotifers. Live food organisms may also harbor pathogens that can be transferred to fish larvae. On the other hand, artificial feeds can fail because of poor water stability, leaching of nutrients, improper feed presentation, or lack of knowledge of feeding behavior. A better understanding of the nutrient requirements, feeding behavior, digestion and absorption of food, feeding stimulants, feed manufacturing, and rearing techniques would revolutionize the use of artificial larval diets.

Cod

Two strategies are used for the production of juvenile cod, a semi-intensive system involving dammed estuarine ponds and intensive rearing in circular fiber glass tanks. The semi-intensive system has been more successful. In this system, 4- to 5-day-old larvae are transferred to estuarine ponds. These generally rely on natural food organisms for growth during the first 2 to 3 weeks, feeding mainly on napulii and rotifers, then gradually switching to copepodites, copepods, and decapod larvae. During the initial feeding period, chlorophyll and large numbers of dinoflagellates, diatomites, and silicates are found in the digestive tracts of cod larvae. The significance of algae in the initial feeding of cod larvae is not clear. Approximately 30 to 50% of these larvae survive through the metamorphosis period of about 35 days. Mortality is mainly attributed to shortages of food supplies that lead to cannibalism (Kvenseth and Oyestad, 1984; Oyestad et al., 1985).

In the intensive system, larval fish are wholly dependent on rotifers (*Brachionus plictalis*). The nutritional value of these rotifers is important, and their composition is often manipulated by supplementation with essential fatty acids and proteins. In both systems, juveniles are weaned to formulated diets when they weigh approximately 1 g.

Fingerling and adult cod are carnivorous and feed principally on crustaceans and small fish. In nature, they swallow prey whole. The exoskeltons of crustaceans contain a complex carbohydrate, chitin. Unlike salmonids, cod have chitinase and readily hydrolyze chitin. The natural prey of cod supply mainly protein and fat (Jobling, 1982). The cod uses its liver as a major energy storage organ, and it may contain as much as 45 to 75% fat. The cod liver accounts for 8.0 to 10.5% of the total body weight (Losnegard et al., 1986; Lie et al., 1988), and the size of the liver is linearly correlated to the amount of lipid in the diet.

Artificial moist and dry diets for cod have been

developed. The protein energy–to–total energy ratio in cod diets should be between 0.45 and 0.5. When this ratio falls below 0.45, enlarged fatty liver develops. Therefore, high-protein and low-fat diets for cod are desirable to avoid the fatty liver syndrome (Fig. 87–4). Fatty fishes, such as herring, capelin, mackerel, or sand eel, may cause fatty liver problems when incorporated into cod diets. Both herring and capelin have high lipid contents during the summer and are therefore considered unsuitable as a sole source of cod feed.

Cod have a limited capacity to digest complex carbohydrates. Incorporation of 10 to 40% precooked starch in cod diets causes reduced growth and significantly higher plasma glucose levels (Hemre et al., 1989). Incorporation of gustatory stimulants such as squid or prawn in cod diets increases feed consumption, feed conversion, and protein utilization (Lie et al., 1989a, b).

Like other cold-water fishes, the feeding, metabolism, and growth of cod are greatly influenced by water temperature and fish size. Generally, the appetite increases with the increasing temperature, reaches a peak, then declines as the temperature continues to increase (Jobling, 1988). Feeding once a day is considered adequate to maintain optimum growth rate. There is a slight reduction in growth rate when fish are fed alternate days. It takes several days for the food consumed in a single meal to be emptied from the stomach. Although feeding guides for most marine fishes have not been developed, Jobling (1988) has estimated food consumption for Atlantic cod in relation to fish size and water temperature (Table 87–3).

Halibut

The methods for juvenile halibut production are currently being researched. Halibut eggs normally hatch after 14 days at 6 to 7°C at a salinity of 34.0 to 34.5 ppt. Despite a relatively good hatching rate (75 to 80%), the survival of larvae is poor. During hatching and a relatively long yolk sac period (30 to 50 days), both eggs and larvae are extremely sensitive

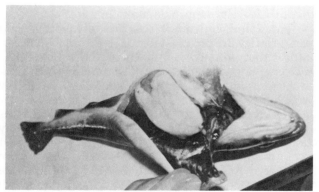

FIGURE 87–4. Enlarged fatty liver of an Atlantic cod. (Courtesy of O. Lie.)

TABLE 87–3. Food Consumption (Kilojoules per Day) for Atlantic Cod in Relation to Fish Size and Water Temperature

Fish Size (g)	Temperature (° C)			
	4	8	12	16
250	28.1	40.6	53.7	62.4
500	49.1	70.7	93.6	108.8
750	67.9	97.9	129.5	150.6
1000	85.5	123.3	163.1	189.7
1500	118.4	170.6	225.8	262.6
2000	149.1	215.0	284.4	330.7

From Jobling, M. (1988) A review of the physiological and nutritional energetics of cod, Gadus morhua L., with particular reference to growth under formed conditions. Aquaculture 70:1–19.

to environmental stress, including contact with tank walls, water currents, light, temperature, salinity, and contamination of the water with bacterial pathogens. Halibut larvae increase from 6 mm at hatching to 11 to 12 mm when the yolk sack has been reabsorbed. The activity of the larvae increases at the age of 25 to 30 days (Pittman et al., 1988), and trypsin activity in the gut is evident from day 35, indicating that the larvae are ready for feeding. These larvae accept feed particles as large as 2 to 3 mm.

Many unsuccessful attempts have been made to develop larval feeds for halibut. Diets based on cod roe have given the maximum survival; however, none of the larvae have completed metamorphosis. Larvae are usually fed natural zooplankton or nutrient-enriched rotifers or Artemia (Naas et al., 1988). After metamorphosis, the fry are weaned to dry crumble diets. Often the moistening of the crumbles with fresh water makes acclimation to the diet easier. Halibut fingerlings readily accept diets containing high-quality fishmeal without any supplementation with feed stimulants (Hjertnes, 1989).

Generally, wild halibut are difficult to feed initially. Feeding live sand eels, shrimp, or small fish and/or short periods of starvation interspersed with feeding are often necessary to evoke an early feeding response. Gradually, fresh whiting, herring, or capelin can successfully replace the live food. Vitamin and trace mineral supplements are necessary for broodstock (Goff and Lall, 1990). In Norway, commercial dry pellets are used to culture halibut weighing up to 2 kg. These fish are often switched to moist diets at that weight because the manufacture of the larger pellets (>11 mm) required by fish to ensure the proper prehension and consumption of food is not feasible (Ronnestad, 1988).

Halibut feed reasonably well at 4 to 5°C, but feed intake increases significantly above 6.5°C. The feeding rate may decrease when halibut are exposed to direct sunlight during long summer months. Approximately 58% protein is necessary to achieve maximum growth of juvenile halibut (Hjertnes and Opstvedt, 1990); however, this requirement may decrease with later stages of development. Halibut use somewhat higher levels of lipid than cod, although carbohydrate utilization is limited.

The natural food of flatfishes varies widely, but these fishes have been classified into three broad categories on the basis of shape, relative dimensions of the alimentary tract, and the type of food eaten (de Groot, 1971). These groups are fish, crustacean, and polkychaete-mollusc feeders. Flatfishes can also be classified by the visual and chemical stimuli they respond to. Visual feeders search for food by sight, mixed feeders search for food visually and by olfaction, and olfactory feeders search for food mainly by olfaction cues. The feeding behavior of commercially important flatfishes such as halibut has not been well studied.

Mackerel

In nature, Atlantic mackerel feed on a variety of food items, including euphausiids, copepods, chaetoganths, fish eggs and larvae, cladocerans, and larval invertebrates. Copepods form a large part of the typical mackerel diet. In late summer and autumn, mackerel also feed heavily on juvenile fish. During these intense feeding periods, mackerel increase their muscle volume and fat content. The fat content accumulates in the skin and red and white muscle fibers and may reach 30% of body weight. No systematic work has been done on feeding and nutrition of mackerel. Atlantic mackerel have been successfully reared in captivity on a diet consisting of finely chopped herring (D'Amours and Landry, 1989).

Tuna

The natural food of tuna captured in the Atlantic ocean consists mainly of juvenile pelagic fish, macrozooplankton, and cephalopods. Tuna may also consume fish larvae, crustaceans, and other molluscs. Although the type of food consumed by various tuna species does not vary much, some distinct dietary preference differences have been reported between juvenile and adult tuna. Juvenile tuna feed primarily on crustaceans, but adult tuna rely primarily on fish.

Adult bluefin tuna have been successfully reared in net impoundments in St. Margaret's Bay of Nova Scotia in Canada for a short durations of approximately 4 months using mackerel-based diets. These fish grow rapidly without signs of vitamin deficiencies.

NUTRITIONAL DISEASES

Nutritional deficiency diseases are uncommon in the wild marine environment, where fish obtain all of their nutrient need from natural food organisms. Fish reared in laboratory or intensive fish culture systems rely on the provision of nutritionally complete diets throughout their life cycle. Although

nutritional diseases of unknown etiology are often reported in these fish owing to an imbalance of several nutrients or feed rancidity, single nutrient deficiencies rarely are reported on marine fish farms. Some signs of ascorbic acid (see Fig. 87–3) and thiamine deficiency have been reported in flatfishes being fed purified diets under experimental conditions.

Most nutritional deficiencies develop slowly over an extended period of time. Often, early signs are difficult to characterize. Subclinical signs of certain vitamin deficiencies have been determined by measuring sensitive enzyme activities in tissues or erythrocytes. For example, erythrocyte transketolase, muscle aminotransferase, and liver acetyl-CoA carboxylase activities are reduced in deficiencies of thiamine, pyridoxine, and biotin, respectively. Marginal nutritional deficiencies predispose fish to infectious diseases, and so signs of nutritional deficiencies are often masked. Diagnosis of nutritional deficiencies requires gross examination of internal and external signs, clinical chemistry of blood and tissues, measurement of specific nutrient concentrations in tissues, and histopathologic examination.

Excess intake of either an essential or a nonessential nutrient over a prolonged period can cause toxicity. Furthermore, increased use of growth stimulants, preservatives, binders used to improve feed stability, nutrient supplements, or the presence of pesticide residues and contaminants may affect the health of fish. Nutrient toxicity problems in fish feeds are restricted primarily to fat-soluble vitamins, copper, selenium, and fluoride. Unlike salmonids and freshwater fishes, most cold-water marine fishes accumulate very high concentrations of vitamins A and D without showing signs of toxicity. Excessive intake of dietary fat causes fatty infiltration of the liver in cod.

Pathologic signs associated with eating rancid fish feed are frequently observed in cold-water marine fishes. Marine fish oil containing polyunsaturated fatty acids is incorporated in fish diets to meet the essential fatty acid requirements of the fish being fed. High levels of polyunsaturated fatty acids increase vitamin E requirements and make feed more susceptible to lipid oxidation during processing and storage. During lipid auto-oxidation, chemical degradation products are formed that react with vitamins, proteins, and other lipids, reducing their nutritional value. Rancid fats cause liver lipid degeneration, microcytic anemia, and steatitis in fish.

One of the common problems observed in fish culture is the refusal to accept food. Several factors may be responsible for this condition, including inadequate feeding, feed rancidity, nutrient deficiencies, improper particle size, overfeeding affecting water quality, mechanical obstruction of feed intake, physiologic stress, and behavioral problems. If food refusal continues for a prolonged period of time, there is a substantial loss of weight, fin erosion, skin ulceration, and darkening. Heavy mortality is common if the starvation continues for a long time.

LITERATURE CITED

Ackman, R.G. (1967) Characteristics of the fatty acid composition and biochemistry of some fresh-water fish oils and lipids in comparison with marine oils and lipids. Comp. Biochem. Physiol. 22:907–922.

Bell, J.G., Henderson, R.J., Pirie, B.J.S., and Sargent, J.R. (1985) Growth, gill structure and fatty acid composition of phospholipids in the turbot (Scophthalmus maximus) in relation to dietary polyunsaturated fatty acid deficiencies. In: Nutrition and Feeding in Fish (Cowey, C.B., Mackie, A.M., and Bell, J.G., eds.). Academic Press, London, pp. 365–369.

Brett, J.R., and Groves, T.D.D. (1979) Physiological energetics. In: Fish Physiology, Vol. VIII (Hoar, W.S., Randall, D.J., and Brett, J.R., eds.). Academic Press, Orlando, Florida, pp 280–352.

Carr, W.E.S. (1982) Chemical stimulation of feeding behavior. In: Chemoreception in Fishes (Hara, T.J., ed.). Elsevier, Amsterdam, pp. 259–373.

Cho, C.Y., and Kaushik, S.J. (1990) Nutrition energetics: Energy and protein utilization in rainbow trout (Salmo gairdneri). World Rev. Nutr. Diet. 61:132–172.

Cowey, C.B., and Sargent, J.R. (1979) Nutrition. In: Fish Physiology. Vol. VIII (Hoar, W.S., Randall, D.J., and Brett, J.R., eds.). Academic Press, Orlando, Florida, pp 1–69.

Cowey, C.B., Pope, J.A., Adron, J.W., and Blair, A. (1972) Studies on the nutrition of marine flatfish. The protein requirement of plaice (Pleuronectes platessa). Br. J. Nutr. 28:447–456.

Cowey, C.B., Adron, J.W., Owen, J.M., and Roberts, R.J. (1976) The effect of different dietary oils on tissue fatty acids and tissue pathology in turbot, Scophthalmus maximus. Comp. Biochem. Physiol. B 53:399–403.

D'Amours, D., and Landry, J. (1989) Capture and husbandry of juvenile (O-year) Atlantic mackerel (Scomber scombrus). Can. Tech. Rep. Fish Aquatic Sci. 1679:11.

Gatesoupe, F.J., and Luquet, P. (1981) Practical diet for mass culture of rotifers (Brachionus plicatilis): Application to larval rearing of sea bass (Dicentrarchus labrax). Aquaculture, 22:149–163.

Gatesoupe, F.J., Leger, C., Metailler, R., and Luquet, P. (1977) Turbot lipid requirements. Ann. Hydrobiol. 8:89–97.

Glass, H.J., MacDonald, N.L., Moran, R.M., and Stark, J.R. (1989) Digestion of protein in different marine species. Comp. Biochem. Physiol. 94B:607–611.

Goff, G., and Lall, S.P. (1989) An initial examination of the nutrition and growth of Atlantic halibut (Hippoglossus hippoglossus) fed whole herring with a vitamin supplement. Bull. Aquatic Assoc. Can., 89–3:56–58.

Groot, S.J. de (1971) On the interrelationships between morphology of the alimentary tract, food and feeding behavior in flatfishes (Pisces: Pleuronectiformes). Neth. J. of Sea Res. 5:121–196.

Gruger, E.H., Jr., Nelson, R.W., and Stansby, M.E. (1964) Fatty acid composition of oils from 21 species of marine fish, freshwater fish and shellfish. J. Am. Oil Chem. Soc. 41:662–667.

Hardy, R.W. (1989) Diet preparation. In: Fish Nutrition. 2nd ed. (Halver, J.E., ed.). Academic Press, New York, pp. 475–548.

Hemre, G.I., Lie, O., Lied, E., and Lambertsen, G. (1989) Starch as an energy source in feed for cod (Gadus morhua): Digestibility and retention. Aquaculture 80:261–270.

Higashi, H. (1962) Vitamins in fish with special reference to edible parts. In: Fish as Food. Vol. 1 (Borgstrom, G., ed.). Academic Press, New York, pp. 411–486.

Hjertnes, T. (1989) Yngelfor til marine oppdrettsarter. Sildolje og Sildemelindustriens Forskningsinstitutt, Bergen, SSF—Rapport C227:1–18.

Hjertnes, T., and Opstvedt, J. (1990) Effect of dietary protein levels on growth in juvenile halibut (Hippoglossus hippoglossus L.). In: Proceedings of the Third International Symposium Feeding and Nutrition in Fish (Takeda, M., and Watanabe, T., eds.), Tokyo University of Fisheries, Japan, pp. 189–193.

Jobling, M. (1982) Food and growth relationship for cod, Gadus morhua L. with special reference to Balsfjord, north Norway. J. Fish. Biol. 21:357–371.

Jobling, M. (1988) A review of the physiological and nutritional energetics of cod, Gadus morhua L., with particular reference to growth under farmed conditions. Aquaculture 70:1–19.

Kanazawa, A. (1985) Essential fatty acid and lipid requirement of fish aquaculture. In: Nutrition and Feeding in Fish (Cowey, C.B., Mackie, A.M., and Bell, J.G., eds.). Academic Press, London, pp. 281–298.

Kvenseth, P.G., and Oyestad, V. (1984) Large-scale rearing of cod fry on natural food production in an enclosed pond. In: The Propagation of Cod, Gadus morhua L. (Dahl, E., Danielsen, D.S., Moksness, E., and Solemdal, P., eds.). Flodevigen Rapportser, Norway, pp. 645–655.

Lall, S.P. (1989) The minerals. In: Fish Nutrition. 2nd ed. (Halver, J.E., ed.), Academic Press, New York, pp. 220–257.

Lie, O., and Lambertsen, G. (1985) Digestive lipolytic enzymes in cod (Gadus morhua). Comp. Biochem. Physiol. 80B(3):447–450.

Lie, O., Lied, E., and Lambertsen, G. (1988) Feed optimization in Atlantic cod (Gadus morhua): Fat versus protein content in the feed. Aquaculture 69:333–341.

Lie, O., Lied, E., and Lambertsen, G. (1989a) Feed attractants for cod (Gadus morhua). Fisk. Dir. Skr. Ser. Ernaering. 2:227–233.

Lie, O., Julshamn, K., Lied, E., and Lambertsen, G. (1989b) Growth and feed conversion in cod (Gadus morhua) on different feeds, retention of some trace elements in the liver. Fisk. Dir. Skr. Ser. Ernaering. 2(7):235–244.

Losnegard, N., Langmyhr, E., and Madsen, D. (1986) Oppdrettstorsk, kvalitet og anvendelse. I. Kjemisk sammensetning som funksjon av arstiden.Fiskeridir. Rapp. 11/86:1–17.

Mackie, A.M. (1982) Gustatory feeding stimulants. In: Chemoreception in Fishes (Hara, T.J., ed.), Elsevier, Amsterdam, pp. 275–291.

Mackie, A.M., and Mitchell, A.I. (1985) Identification of gustatory feeding stimulants for fish-applications in aquaculture. In: Nutrition and Feeding in Fish (Cowey, C.B., Mackie, A.M., and Bell, J.G., eds.), Academic Press, London, pp. 177–190.

Naas, K., Nyhammer, G., and Jensen, A.M. (1988) Startforingsfasen. In: Oppdrett av kveite (Hippoglossus hippoglossus L.) (Ronnerstad, I., ed.). Institute of Marine Research, Bergen, Report Akva 8806 (in Norwegian), pp. 83–90.

Oyestad, V., Kvenseth, P.G., and Folkvord, A. (1985) Mass production of Atlantic cod juveniles, Gadus morhua, in a Norwegian saltwater pond. Trans. Am. Fish. Soc. 114:590–595.

Pittman, K., Skiftesvik, A.B., and Harboe, T. (1988) Effect of temperature on growth rates and organogenesis in the yolk sac larvae of halibut (Hippoglossus hippoglossus L.). International Council for Exploration of the Sea, Report F:95.

Roberts, R.J., and Bullock, A.M. (1989) Nutritional pathology. In: Fish Nutrition., 2nd ed. (Halver, J.E., ed.). Academic Press, New York, pp. 424–473.

Ronnestad, I. (1988) For og foring. In: Oppdrett av kveite (Hippoglossus hippoglossus L.) (I. Ronnerstad, ed.), Institute of Marine Research, Bergen. Report Akva 8806 (in Norwegian), pp. 22–24.

Sargent, J.R., Henderson, R.J., and Tocher, D.R. (1989) In: Fish Nutrition. 2nd ed. (Halver, J.E., ed.). Academic Press, New York, pp. 154–218.

Smith, R.R. (1989) Nutritional energetics. In: Fish Nutrition. 2nd ed. (Halver, J.E., ed.). Academic Press, New York, pp. 1–29.

Tacon, A.G.J. (1985) Nutritional Fish Pathology. FAO Publ., ADCP/REP/85/22.

Watanabe, T. (1982) Lipid nutrition in fish. Comp. Biochem. Physiol. 73B:3–15.

Watanabe, T., Kitajima, C., and Fujita, S. (1983a) Nutritional value of live organisms used in Japan for mass propagation of fish: a review. Aquaculture 34:115–143.

Watanabe, T., Tamiya, T., Oka, A., Hirata, M., Kitajima, C., and Fujita, S. (1983b) Improvement of dietary value of live foods for fish larvae by feeding them on ω3 highly unsaturated fatty acids and fat-soluble vitamins. Bull. Jpn. Soc. Sci. Fish. 49(3):471–479.

Wilson, R.P. (1989) Amino acids and proteins. In: Fish Nutrition. 2nd ed. (Halver, J.E., ed.), Academic Press, New York, pp. 111–151.

Chapter 88

COLD-WATER MARINE FISH VIRUSES

PHILIP E. McALLISTER

Estuarine and marine fishes are susceptible to a variety of viral infections. Some infections cause epizootic mortality, while others debilitate the infected fish, predisposing it to secondary infections. Some viruses are associated with neoplastic conditions, and others have no readily detectable effect on the overall health of the host. Many of the viral agents have been detected only by electron microscopy. The viruses listed in Table 88–1 are found in estuarine and marine fishes.

ATLANTIC COD EPIDERMAL HYPERPLASIA

SYNONYM. Atlantic cod adenovirus.

Host and Geographic Distribution

Atlantic cod captured in the Baltic Sea were found to have hyperplastic skin lesions (Jensen and Bloch, 1980). This is the only report of the epidermal lesions in cod, but similar lesions are seen in dab taken in the eastern North Sea (Bloch et al., 1986).

Clinical Signs and Pathology

The skin lesions are slightly raised, transparent plaques, 3 to 20 mm in diameter, distributed over the whole body, particularly the caudal portion. Histologically, the plaque is an epidermal hyperplasia (Jensen and Bloch, 1980). The epithelium is smooth and normal in appearance, but is about four times normal thickness. The affected area contains few mucous cells, and cells in the germinal layer are shorter than normal. Vascularity is greatly increased below the basement membrane. Pigment cells no longer appear as a uniform layer, but are dispersed, granule-containing aggregates. Electron micrographs of affected skin show that the epidermis is increased in thickness, but epidermal cells generally appear normal.

Diagnosis

The presumptive diagnosis is based upon histologic examination and is confirmed by demonstrating adenoviruslike particles in lesion tissue by electron microscopy.

Virus Detection

The virus has not been isolated in cell culture but has been demonstrated by electron microscopy. Electron micrographs show hyperplastic cells that are generally normal in appearance, but some cells at the periphery of the epidermis contain intranuclear aggregates of viral particles. The particles are unenveloped icosahedra about 77 nm in diameter, with a centrally placed, electron-dense nucleoid. The nucleoid is surrounded by an outer capsid about 10 nm thick, and fibers 20 to 25 nm long radiate from the capsid vertices. Based on particle ultrastructure and intranuclear location, the virus is tentatively classified as an adenovirus (Jensen and Bloch, 1980).

Transmission, Epidemiology, and Pathogenesis

No attempts to experimentally transmit the disease have been reported, and the disease has been described only once. A similar skin lesion occurs in dab (Bloch et al., 1986).

Treatment and Control

No methods for treatment or control have been described.

DAB EPIDERMAL HYPERPLASIA

SYNONYM. Dab adenovirus.

Host and Geographic Distribution

Epidermal hyperplasias and papillomas were found on dab captured in the eastern North Sea (Bloch et al., 1986). Skin lesions of similar gross appearance are seen in Atlantic cod (Jensen and Bloch, 1980).

TABLE 88–1. Viral Diseases of Coldwater Marine Fishes*

Disease	Virus	Host
Atlantic cod epidermal hyperplasia	Atlantic cod adenovirus	Atlantic cod
Dab epidermal hyperplasia	Dab adenovirus	Dab
Turbot epithelial cell giantism	*Herpesvirus scophthalmi*	Turbot
Pacific cod ulcerative epidermal hypertrophy	Pacific cod herpesvirus	Pacific cod
Smelt papillomatosis	Smelt herpesvirus	Smelt
Atlantic cod ulcus syndrome	Iridovirus and rhabdovirus	Atlantic cod
Viral erythrocytic necrosis	Erythrocytic necrosis virus	At least 29 genera
Unknown (fish and marine mammals) Vesicular exanthem (swine)	Opaleye calicivirus (San Miguel sea lion virus)	Opaleye Various marine mammals Swine
Unknown	Eel rhabdovirus B12	European eel
Unknown	Eel rhabdovirus C30	European eel
Epizootic mortality	Eel virus—American	American eel Rainbow trout
Unknown (eel)	Eel virus—European X	European eel
Epizootic mortality	*Rhabdovirus olivaceus*	Japanese flounder, Ayu, chum salmon, coho salmon, Masou salmon, rainbow trout
Papilloma	Gilthead sea bream papilloma–associated virus	Gilthead sea bream
Epidermal papilloma	Pleuronectid epidermal papilloma–associated virus	Several species of pleuronectids
Epidermal papilloma	Winter papilloma–associated virus	Winter flounder
Epidermal papilloma	Stomatopapilloma-associated viruses: Eel virus (Berlin), EV-1, EV-2, unnamed syncytium-forming virus	European eel

See also sections on white sturgeon adenovirus, lymphocystis virus, 13p2 reovirus, Esox epidermal hyperplasia retrovirus, Esox lymphosarcoma retrovirus, and Esox sarcoma retrovirus in Chapter 26; Herpesvirus salmonis, steelhead herpesvirus, Oncorhynchus masou virus, Yamame tumor virus, infectious pancreatic necrosis virus, chum salmon virus, Atlantic salmon fibrosarcoma retrovirus, Atlantic salmon papilloma retrovirus, infectious hematopoietic necrosis virus, viral hemorrhagic septicemia virus, and ulcerative dermal necrosis–associated virus in Chapter 38; and Herpesvirus cyprini in Chapter 50.

Clinical Signs and Pathology

The hyperplasias are smooth, round, semitransparent, creamy white patches that are 2 to 10 mm in diameter. The papillomas have a highly vascularized rough texture and are 5 to 15 mm in diameter. Hyperplasia may be the initial developmental stage of the papilloma (Bloch et al., 1986).

Histologically, the epithelium appears normal but becomes up to 50 cell layers thick. The lesions are composed of several strata. A layer of vertically oriented, cuboidal basal cells is overlaid by a central zone of horizontally arrayed, polyhedral epidermal cells and by a superficial surface layer of horizontally oriented, elongated, and flattened cells. Few mucous cells are seen, and pigment cells are dispersed. The histologic profile of the lesions resembles that of the epidermal hyperplasia in Atlantic cod (Jensen and Bloch, 1980).

Diagnosis

Presumptive diagnosis is based on histologic examination of the skin lesion and confirmed by finding adenoviruslike particles in electron micrographs of lesion tissue.

Virus Detection

Virus has not been isolated in cell culture, but electron micrographs of hyperplastic tissue show intranuclear inclusions of adenoviruslike particles. Virus is seen in otherwise normal-appearing cells in the outer one-third of the epidermis (Bloch et al., 1986). The particles are unenveloped icosahedra about 80 nm in diameter and consist of an electron-dense, but not homogeneously staining, nucleoid surrounded by a capsid about 7 nm thick. The virus particles closely resemble those seen in the hyperplastic epidermis from Atlantic cod (Bloch et al., 1986; Jensen and Bloch, 1980).

Transmission, Epidemiology, and Pathogenesis

No attempts to transmit the tumor have been reported. Affected fish are captured in the wild, and lesions occur only in fish more than 3 years old.

Treatment and Control

No methods of treatment or control have been described.

TURBOT EPITHELIAL CELL GIANTISM

SYNONYMS. Turbot epithelial hypertrophy, turbot giant cells, turbot herpesvirus, *Herpesvirus scophthalmi.*

Host and Geographic Distribution

Young turbot develop epithelial cell giantism in the skin and gills that is of putative herpesvirus etiology (Buchanan et al., 1978; Richards and Buchanan, 1978). Epizootic losses from the disease occur in both feral and cultured turbot. A survey of preserved specimens suggests that the disease is endemic in feral turbot in Scotland.

Clinical Signs and Pathology

Clinical signs are few and hardly distinctive. Affected fish are lethargic and inappetent, but otherwise appear healthy up to death.

The hypertrophied epithelial cells are found primarily on the gills and on the dorsal skin surface, and appear to be derived from malpighian cells. In severe infections, adjacent gill lamellae fuse, and surrounding malpighian cells become hyperplastic. No pathologic changes are seen in other organs and tissues. The hypertrophied cells form by cell fusion, creating syncytia 45 to 130 μm in diameter. Although the giant cells are occasionally multinucleated, recruited nuclei generally fuse to form a single, enlarged nucleus occupying up to 90% of the cell volume. Coarse, Feulgen-positive inclusions develop in the cytoplasm and nucleus.

Diagnosis

The disease is diagnosed by correlating histopathologic examination with findings of herpesvirus particles in giant epithelial cells.

Virus Detection

Attempts to culture the virus have been unsuccessful, but large accumulations of virus can be detected in skin scrapings by electron microscopy (Buchanan and Madeley, 1978). Electron micrographs of giant cells show that osmophilic inclusions in the nucleus are arrays of unenveloped herpesviruslike capsids, and that the cytoplasm is filled with membrane-bound aggregates of enveloped viral particles.

Transmission, Epidemiology, and Pathogenesis

No experimental transmission trials have been reported (Buchanan and Madeley, 1978). However, the disease is considered endemic in feral turbot, and epizootic mortality occurs in intensively cultured fish, suggesting that the disease is at least horizontally transmissible (Buchanan et al., 1978; Richards and Buchanan, 1978). Horizontal transmission seemingly can occur under intensive culture conditions when fish are exposed to virus released from sloughed epidermal tissue (Richards and Buchanan, 1978).

Mortality can reach 30% during the 6 months after young-of-the-year fish are put into intensive culture. The mortality rate in intensively cultured fish fluctuates considerably, but deaths increase within 5 days of culture stress, such as transportation, temperature fluctuation, and change in water quality, indicating that the viral infection may remain latent until activated by stress (Buchanan et al., 1978; Richards and Buchanan, 1978).

Treatment and Control

No methods of treatment or control have been described. Seemingly, management practices that reduce culture stress might reduce losses or delay activation of latent infection in intensive culture (Richards and Buchanan, 1978).

PACIFIC COD ULCERATIVE EPIDERMAL HYPERTROPHY

SYNONYM. Pacific cod herpesvirus.

Host, Geographic Distribution, and Clinical Signs

Two types of skin lesions are seen in Pacific cod from the Bering Sea (McArn et al., 1978). One lesion is a round, hemorrhagic ulceration, 1 to 50 mm in diameter. The second is a raised, circular or ring-shaped lesion, 5 to 20 mm wide and 10 to 50 mm in diameter, that is a cream-colored, sometimes hemorrhagic band surrounding normal-appearing epidermis (McCain et al., 1979).

Pathology

Pathologic changes in the ringlike lesion or band are in the epidermis and underlying stratum spongiosum. The lesion contains cystlike structures or hypertrophied cells with a PAS-positive hyaline coat (McArn et al., 1978; McCain et al., 1979). Within the hypertrophied cells or cystlike structures, small eosinophilic bodies are seen at the periphery and throughout the basophilic center. Inflammatory cells migrate adjacent to hypertrophied cells.

Diagnosis

The skin lesions are presumptively diagnosed based on clinical signs and pathologic changes. Diagnosis is confirmed by finding herpesviruslike particles in the hypertrophied, cystlike cells (McArn et al., 1978).

Virus Detection

Virus has not been isolated in cell culture, but herpesviruslike particles are reportedly associated with the hypertrophied, cystlike cells (McArn et al., 1978). Viruslike particles, 80 to 110 nm in diameter, as well as developmental forms, are evident in the nucleus, and larger particles, 120 to 170 nm in diameter, are seen in the cytoplasm (Wolf, 1988).

Transmission, Epidemiology, and Pathogenesis

No attempts to experimentally transmit the disease have been reported, nor has the pathobiology of the disease been described. The skin lesions have been seen only in feral Pacific cod.

Treatment and Control

No methods of treatment or control have been described.

SMELT PAPILLOMATOSIS

SYNONYM. Smelt spawning papillomatosis (see also section on carp pox in Chapter 50).

Host and Geographic Distribution

An epidermal papilloma occurs in a significant proportion of adult smelt captured during spring spawning migrations in the Elbe, Eider, and Weser Rivers, Kiel Canal, and Schlei Fjord in northern Europe (Anders, 1984; Anders and Moller, 1985).

Clinical Signs and Pathology

The smooth, whitish, epidermal papillomas occur as single or multiple growths of variable shape on the skin surface, predominantly the head region and fins. The nuclei of papilloma cells are pleo-

morphic and contain Cowdry type A inclusion bodies. The papillomas appear to be quite similar to carp pox lesions (Anders and Moller, 1985).

Diagnosis

Diagnosis is based on correlating clinical signs, histopathology, and the species of concern. The smelt papilloma is described as being very similar and possibly identical to carp pox, but definitive comparisons have not been made.

Virus Detection and Identification

Electron micrographs of papilloma tissue show intracytoplasmic and intranuclear accumulations of herpesviruslike particles (Anders and Moller, 1985), but the virus has not been isolated in cell culture.

Transmission, Epidemiology, and Pathogenesis

No transmission trials have been reported. The papilloma occurs at a prevalence up to 5.5% and is seen only during the spring spawning season (February to May) in fish about 16 cm in length (Anders and Moller, 1985). The growths occur most frequently in brackish as opposed to freshwater or marine environments.

Treatment and Control

No methods of treatment or control have been described.

ATLANTIC COD ULCUS SYNDROME

SYNONYMS. Atlantic cod ulcer disease, cod ulcus-syndrome iridovirus, cod ulcus-syndrome rhabdovirus (see also section on viral hemorrhagic septicemia virus in Chapter 38).

Host and Geographic Distribution

Ulcus syndrome is an infectious disease that occurs primarily among 1- to 2-year-old cod in the Baltic coast region of Denmark.

Clinical Signs

Ulcus syndrome is characterized by papuloulcerative lesions found mainly on lateral body surfaces. The skin lesions develop progressively from multiple vesicular eruptions, 2 to 8 mm in diameter, to eroded ulcerations, 2 to 8 cm in diameter, and finally to small depigmented scarred areas of healing (Jensen and Larson, 1979).

Pathology

Pathologic changes appear initially as severe loose connective tissue edema in the epidermis and dermis. Edema, necrosis, and cellular infiltration progress to the underlying musculature before healing (Jensen and Larsen, 1979).

Diagnosis

Primary diagnosis is based on clinical signs. The etiologic significance of virus isolated from cod with ulcus syndrome has not been conclusively established.

Virus Isolation

Two viruses, an iridovirus and a rhabdovirus, have been isolated from cods with ulcus syndrome (Jensen et al., 1979). An iridovirus was isolated on the third blind passage of homogenized papule tissue inoculated onto EPC cells. Virus was not isolated from internal organs. The virus replicates well in EPC cells at 15°C, but poorly in PS cells. Electron micrographs of infected cell cultures show iridovirus particles arrayed in the cytoplasm and budding from cellular membranes, but no virus is seen in papule tissue.

A rhabdovirus was isolated on the second blind passage from homogenized papule tissue inoculated onto PS cells. Virus was not isolated from internal organs. The rhabdovirus replicates well in PS cells at 15°C, but poorly in EPC cells. Typical rhabdoviral particles are seen in electron micrographs of infected cell cultures, but not in papule tissue. Infectivity neutralization and immunofluorescence assays show that the cod ulcus syndrome rhabdovirus is indistinguishable from viral hemorrhagic septicemia virus (Vestergard Jorgensen and Olesen, 1987).

Transmission, Epidemiology, and Pathogenesis

Ulcus syndrome can be experimentally transmitted by cohabitation and by applying papule homogenate to scarified skin (Jensen and Larsen, 1982). Results are variable with intraperitoneal inoculation of papule homogenate, and no transmission occurs by intranasal inoculation.

Ulcus syndrome has been induced by intracardiac but not by intraperitoneal inoculation of cell culture–grown iridovirus. Unfortunately, the experimental challenges were flawed because wild-captured fish were used for the transmission trials, and no attempts were made to reisolate the iridovirus from experimentally infected fish. Thus, the iridovirus etiology of ulcus syndrome has not been definitively established.

Ulcus syndrome is not induced by intraperitoneal or intracardiac inoculation of cell culture–grown rhabdovirus, and the role, if any, of the rhabdovirus in ulcus syndrome is unknown (Jensen and Larsen, 1982).

The lesions of ulcus syndrome are most prevalent through the summer and early autumn. Healing is observed mainly in the late autumn when water temperatures are about 7°C. Environmental stress and pollution may be significant factors in provoking outbreaks of ulcus syndrome (Larsen and Jensen, 1982).

Treatment and Control

No methods of treatment or control have been reported.

VIRAL ERYTHROCYTIC NECROSIS

SYNONYMS. Viral erythrocytic necrosis (VEN), piscine erythrocytic necrosis (PEN).

An erythrocytic disease of putative viral etiology occurs in some marine, estuarine, and anadromous fishes of North America and Europe. The disease, originally called piscine erythrocytic necrosis, is now designated viral erythrocytic necrosis (VEN) (Evelyn and Traxler, 1978; Laird and Bullock, 1969). An iridovirus, designated erythrocytic necrosis virus (ENV), is associated with infected erythrocytes (MacMillan et al., 1980; Rohovec and Amandi, 1981). Although virus has not been isolated in cell culture, viral etiology is supported by experimental transmission of the disease.

Similar erythrodegenerative conditions are recognized in various poikilothermic vertebrates and are described as protozoan infections by species of *Pirhemocyton, Toddia, Immanoplasma,* and others (Johnston, 1975; Johnston and Davies, 1973). Inclusions and viruslike particles in fish erythrocytes have sometimes been described as *Pirhemocyton*-like in appearance (Appy et al., 1976; Johnston and Davies, 1973; Laird and Bullock, 1969; Walker, 1971).

Host and Geographic Distribution

Viral erythrocytic necrosis occurs in species from 23 genera (*Alosa, Anguilla, Brevoortia, Clupea, Gadus, Hemitripterus, Leiostomus, Limanda, Liparis, Macrozoarces, Melanogrammus, Merluccius, Microgadus, Myoxocephalus, Osmerus, Paralichthys, Pholis, Pollachius, Pseudopleuronectes, Raja, Scophthalmus, Tautoga,* and *Urophyscis*) found on the Atlantic coast of North America from the Carolinas in the United States through Greenland (Khan and Newman, 1982; Laird and Bullock, 1969; Philippon et al., 1977; Reno et al., 1985; Sherburne, 1977; Sherburne and Bean, 1979; Walker and Sherburne, 1977). The disease occurs in three genera (*Clupea, Oncorhynchus,* and *Salmo*) from the Pacific northwest of North America and in four genera (*Blennius, Gadus, Mugil,* and *Platichthys*) in the Atlantic waters of Europe (Eiras, 1984; Evelyn and Traxler, 1978; Johnston and Davies, 1973; Meyers et al., 1986; Rohovec and Amandi, 1981; Smail and Eggleston, 1980a,b). Viral erythrocytic necrosis can be experimentally transmitted to *Salvelinus* species (MacMillan and Mulcahy, 1979), and an erythrodegenerative disease in the Mediterranean dogfish could also be viral erythrocytic necrosis (Johnston, 1975; Johnston and Davies, 1973).

Clinical Signs

Few clinical signs are associated with mild viral erythrocytic necrosis infections, but severely affected fish appear darkly pigmented and show signs of severe anemia, including pale gills and internal organs and depressed hematocrit values (Evelyn and Traxler, 1978; MacMillan et al., 1980; Meyers et al., 1986; Philippon et al., 1977; Sherburne, 1973; Walker and Sherburne, 1977). Mortality directly attributable to viral erythrocytic necrosis is low, although two instances of epizootic mortality have been reported in Pacific herring (Meyers et al., 1986). Generally, infected fish succumb to secondary bacterial infections, usually vibriosis or bacterial kidney disease (Evelyn and Traxler, 1978).

Pathology

Histologic examination reveals mitotic hyperactivity in renal hematopoietic tissues compatible with erythroblastosis, but no significant anomalies in other tissues. Gross pathologic changes are confined to erythrocytes (Appy et al., 1976, Evelyn and Traxler, 1978; Johnston and Davies, 1973; MacMillan et al., 1980; Philippon et al., 1977; Reno and Nicholson, 1981; Reno et al., 1978; Rohovec and Amandi, 1981; Sherburne, 1973; Walker and Sherburne, 1977). Degenerative intracytoplasmic and intranuclear changes occur in both mature and immature erythrocytes. In some cases, virtually 100% of the erythrocytes are infected. Affected erythrocytes generally develop a rounded, irregular morphology and are more fragile. The cytoplasm contains a single (rarely multiple) amorphous inclusion, 0.3 to 4.0 µm in diameter (the largest inclusions occur in immature cells). Marked cytoplasmic vacuolation is sometimes seen. The nucleus develops an atypical, irregular morphology and is sometimes displaced. The nuclear membrane remains intact, but chromatin accumulates at the periphery, creating the appearance of an intranuclear pseudovacuole. An intranuclear inclusion has sometimes been seen (MacMillan et al., 1980; Reno and

Nicholson, 1981; Reno et al., 1978; Walker and Sherburne, 1977).

Diagnosis

Viral erythrocytic necrosis can be presumptively diagnosed by examining Giemsa-stained erythrocytes for cytoplasmic inclusions, and is confirmed by electron microscopy. Cytoplasmic accumulations of iridoviruslike particles are seen in electron micrographs of infected erythrocytes. In salmonid fishes, the viral particles are about 150 to 200 nm in diameter, whereas in other species, the viral particles are about 200 to 500 nm in diameter (Wolf, 1988).

Viral Detection and Identification

The erythrocytic necrosis virus has not been isolated in cell culture. Attempts to isolate the virus from filtrates of chum and pink salmon kidney and spleen have been unsuccessful (Evelyn and Traxler, 1978). The virus-containing, infectious filtrate was inoculated onto CHSE–214, FHM, RTG–2, and rainbow trout ovary cells and incubated at 8 and 15°C for 3 weeks, but no cytopathic changes were seen. Similarly, attempts to isolate virus from lysed blenny erythrocytes in primary cultures of dab ovary were unsuccessful (Smail, 1982). These attempted isolations were probably unsuccessful because inappropriate or refractory cell types were used to replicate an apparently erythrocyte-specific virus.

Infected erythrocytes can be maintained in vitro for up to 2 weeks (Reno and Nicholson, 1980). Some evidence of viral replication in peripheral blood can be obtained, but attempts to infect erythrocytes in vitro have been unsuccessful. Infection seemingly occurs at early stages in erythrogenesis.

Transmission and Epidemiology

Although virus has not been isolated, viral erythrocytic necrosis can be experimentally transmitted. Atlantic cod are infected by intraperitoneal injection of infected cod erythrocytes (Nicholson and Reno, 1981). The disease can be transmitted to chum and pink salmon by intraperitoneal injection of membrane (0.45 µm)–filtered homogenates of kidneys and spleen from infected chum salmon and Pacific herring. Injection of heated filtrates (60°C for 15 min) does not induce disease (Evelyn and Traxler, 1978). Ten species of salmonids are known to be susceptible to erythrocytic necrosis virus by intraperitoneal injection of membrane-filtered erythrocyte lysate, and two species have been infected via immersion challenge (MacMillan and Mulcahy, 1979). Empirical observations and some experimental results indicate that younger fish are more susceptible to infection than older fish. Although the virus can be experimentally transmitted in fresh water, few natural occurrences have been reported in freshwater fish.

The mechanisms for transmission in nature are unknown, but the disease is probably contracted in the marine environment (Evelyn and Traxler, 1978). Prevalence in the wild varies, but approaches 100% in some populations. Stress conditions might activate latent infections, exacerbate existing infections, or enhance waterborne transmission (Smail, 1982).

The disease occurs in pre- and postspawning anadromous alewives, but not in juveniles in fresh water (Sherburne, 1977). Viral erythrocytic necrosis occurs in spawning coho and chinook salmon and steelhead trout, and the virus might be vertically transmitted, as virus has been detected in yolk-sac fry and alevin chum salmon (Rohovec and Amandi, 1981). Further, blood-sucking ectoparasites such as the salmon louse (*Lepeophtheirus* sp.) or gill maggot (*Salmincola* sp.) have been indicted as possible mechanical vectors (Smail, 1982).

Pathogenesis

Fish with viral erythrocytic necrosis usually succumb to secondary bacterial infections rather than to the virus. Infected chum salmon have a threefold greater mortality from vibriosis, a decreased tolerance to oxygen depletion, and a decreased ability to osmoregulate (MacMillan et al., 1980). In contrast, no significant alteration is seen in the osmoregulatory capacity of erythrocytic necrosis virus–infected cod or alewives, but infected cod have more difficulty coping with stressful situations than uninfected fish (Reno et al., 1985). In infected Pacific herring, epizootic mortality is attributed to osmoregulatory stress (Meyers et al., 1986).

Hematopathologic parameters vary with each fish species (Evelyn and Traxler, 1978; MacMillan et al., 1980; Reno et al., 1985). In general, hematocrit values and erythrocyte counts are depressed, but compensatory erythroblastosis is also seen. Plasma electrolytes and hemoglobin concentration are sometimes depressed. In infected cod, herring, and alewives, species-related changes occur in erythrocyte ATP synthesis and in glucose–6-phosphatase, lactate dehydrogenase, and citrate synthetase enzyme activity, but no significant changes occur in plasma protein levels (Reno et al., 1985). These species-related physiologic changes may reflect adaptive responses to infection that could be influenced by varying environmental pressures (Reno et al., 1985).

Treatment and Control

No methods of treatment or control have been described.

OPALEYE CALICIVIRUS

SYNONYM. San Miguel sea lion virus.

Host and Geographic Distribution

Several caliciviruses are isolated from apparently healthy opaleye, an omnivorous marine perchlike fish common to shallow rocky waters and tide pools along the coast of southern California and Mexico. The opaleye isolates are now known to be pathogenic for marine and terrestrial mammals. The opaleye calicivirus is antigenically indistinguishable from the San Miguel sea lion virus (Smith et al., 1980). The San Miguel sea lion virus is isolated from California sea lions (*Zalophus californianus*), northern elephant seals (*Mirounga angustirostris*), northern fur seals (*Callorhinus ursinus*), walruses (*Odobenus rosmarus*), and from a liver fluke of the California sea lion (*Zalophatrema* sp.) (Smith et al., 1983). Neutralizing antibody to the virus has been detected in walrus and bowhead whales (*Balaena mysticetus*) (Smith et al., 1983).

The San Miguel sea lion virus is considered the causative agent of vesicular exanthema of swine, a viral disease that ravaged swine production in California beginning in 1932 and spread throughout the United States.

Clinical Signs and Pathology

Neither naturally or experimentally infected opaleye show clinical signs or histologic changes associated with disease.

Diagnosis

Calicivirus infection is diagnosed by isolation of the virus in cell culture and identification of the virus using specific immune serum. The opaleye calicivirus is antigenically indistinguishable from San Miguel sea lion virus.

Virus Detection and Identification

Calicivirus can be isolated from opaleye (10 to 15 cm long) collected from tide pools on the southern California coast. Whole viscera and individual samples of kidney, liver, spleen, gut, muscle, and gills are homogenized and inoculated onto Vero kidney cells. The cultures are incubated at 37°C, and cytopathic changes are seen after two to three passages. Higher virus titer and more rapid virus detection occur with sea lion and seal isolates (Smith et al., 1981). This could indicate that the cell culture and incubation conditions may not be optimal for recovery of the virus from a poikilothermic host; however, no alternative isolation protocols have been tested with fish. In infectivity neutralization assays, the opaleye calicivirus is antigenically indistinguishable from San Miguel sea lion virus (Smith et al., 1980).

Transmission, Epidemiology, Pathogenesis

The opaleye can be infected by intraperitoneal inoculation and oral exposure. The virus persists for 31 days in orally exposed fish. In injected fish, a generalized infection develops and the virus replicates, with the highest virus titers being found in the spleen (Smith et al., 1981).

Vesicular exanthema can be experimentally induced in swine by injection or contact exposure to San Miguel sea lion virus or virus from opaleyes (Smith et al., 1980, 1981). The historical epizootics of vesicular exanthema were probably caused by calicivirus in raw fish scraps fed to swine (Smith et al., 1980). The opaleye seems to be at least one natural reservoir for a marine calicivirus that infects a variety of homeothermic and poikilothermic species, and parasites are possible vectors in the marine environment (Smith et al., 1980).

Treatment and Control

No methods for treatment or control of viral infection in opaleyes have been described.

EEL RHABDOVIRUSES

SYNONYMS. Eel virus-American (EVA), eel virus-European X (EVEX), C30 virus, B12 virus.

Host and Geographic Distribution

Two rhabdoviruses (EVA and EVEX) were isolated from eels imported to Japan. The EVA was isolated from moribund American eels from Cuba, and EVEX from apparently healthy European eels from France (Sano, 1976; Sano et al., 1977). In addition, two rhabdoviruses (C30 and B12) were isolated from apparently healthy, feral European eels in France (Castric and Chastel, 1980; Castric et al., 1984). Viruses EVEX and B12 are endemic in the elver population of the Loire estuary (France) (Castric et al., 1984). Rainbow trout fry are susceptible to EVA and EVEX (Nishimura et al., 1981), whereas Japanese eels and elvers are refractory to EVEX (Sano, 1976).

Clinical Signs and Pathology

Clinical signs of disease in fish infected with EVA and EVEX are very similar and resemble the clinical signs and histopathologic changes of infectious hematopoietic necrosis and viral hemorrhagic septicemia (see Chap. 38) (Hill et al., 1980; Nishimura et al., 1981; Sano, 1976). Affected fish become dark and lethargic. Hemorrhaging occurs in the pectoral

and anal fins, over the abdominal skin, in the skeletal muscle, and in the kidneys. Histopathologic changes include hemorrhagic degeneration of the skeletal muscle, intensive necrosis and hemorrhage of kidney hematopoietic tissue, hemorrhaging into the kidney tubules and Bowman's space, and focal necrosis of the liver, spleen, and pancreas. No clinical signs of disease or pathology are reported for C30 and B12 eel rhabdoviruses.

Diagnosis

Diagnosis is based on isolation of virus in cell culture and identification by serologic reactivity with specific antiserum.

Virus Detection and Identification

The EVA and EVEX viruses are isolated in FHM and RTG–2 cells at 15° C and in EPC cells from 10 to 25°C. The B12 virus replicates in EPC cells at 10 and 14°C, but not at 20°C, and will not replicate in RTG–2 cells. Thus, EVA, EVEX, and B12 viruses can all be detected using EPC cells incubated at 14°C. Detection of various eel viral isolates was monitored in several eel and other fish cell lines (Sorimachi, 1982).

Among the rhabdoviruses isolated from eels, at least three are antigenically distinct. Viruses EVEX and C30 are most probably identical (Castric et al., 1984). Viruses EVA and EVEX are closely related, but antigenically distinct, and are most probably strains of the same virus (Hill et al., 1980). Structurally, EVA and EVEX are rhabdoviruses of the vesiculovirus subgroup, and B12 is a rhabdovirus of the lyssavirus subgroup.

The EVA and EVEX isolates are serologically distinct by infectivity neutralization assay from B12, infectious hematopoietic necrosis, viral hemorrhagic septicemia, and infectious pancreatic necrosis viruses (see Chap. 38). They are also distinct from the perch rhabdovirus and ulcerative disease rhabdovirus of the snakehead (see Chap. 26) (Frerichs et al., 1989; Hill et al., 1980). The B12 virus isolate is serologically distinct by infectivity neutralization (Castric and Chastel, 1980; Castric et al., 1984).

Transmission, Epidemiology, and Pathogenesis

Isolations of B12 and EVEX viruses from apparently healthy elvers from the Loire estuary suggest that the elvers are asymptomatic virus carriers (Castric et al., 1984). Experimental challenge of elvers, young eels, and rainbow trout fry at various temperatures by immersion and intraperitoneal injection of B12 and EVEX viruses did not produce mortality, although the rainbow trout may have been beyond the susceptible age (Castric and Chastel, 1980). Others find that rainbow trout fry are susceptible to EVA and EVEX by intraperitoneal injection and that mortality from EVA is greatest at 20°C and from EVEX at temperatures above 10°C (Nishimura et al., 1981). No mortality occurs in Japanese eels or elvers injected with EVEX. Naturally infected young American eels, reared at 20 to 27°C, sustain about 60% mortality (Sano, 1976).

Treatment and Control

No methods for treatment or control of the eel rhabdoviruses have been described.

JAPANESE FLOUNDER RHABDOVIRUS

SYNONYMS. Hirame rhabdovirus, *Rhabdovirus olivaceus*.

Host and Geographic Distribution

A virus, designated *Rhabdovirus olivaceus* or hirame rhabdovirus, was isolated from diseased pen and seawater tank–cultured hirame (Japanese flounder) and seawater tank–cultured ayu fry in Hyogo, Kagawa, and Hokkaido prefectures (Japan) (Gorie and Nakamoto, 1986; Kimura et al., 1986). Various species of salmonid fishes have been experimentally infected with the virus (Kimura et al., 1986). The viral disease is not known to occur in North America.

Clinical Signs and Pathology

Affected hirame show focal hemorrhage of the skeletal muscle and fins, accumulation of ascites, and congestion of the gonads. Necrotic changes are seen in the hematopoietic tissues of the kidneys and spleen. Hyperemia and hemorrhage occur in the interstitial tissue of the kidneys and gonads, in the splenic pulp, and in capillary vessels of skeletal muscle (Oseko et al., 1988a). No pathologic changes are seen in the liver. In affected ayu fry, the only clinical signs and pathologic changes described are exophthalmia and petechial hemorrhages on the opercula.

Diagnosis

The disease is presumptively diagnosed by correlating clinical signs and species, but confirmed diagnosis requires isolation and serologic identification of the virus.

Virus Detection and Identification

The hirame rhabdovirus was originally isolated in RTG–2 cells, but cytopathic effects are also seen in fathead minnow cells. The virus replicates in cell culture at temperatures from 5 to 20°C but not at or above 25°C. No cytopathic effects or virus yield occur in CHH–1, CHSE–214, or KO–6 cells. The virus is serologically distinct from other fish rhabdoviruses (IHNV, VHSV, SVCV, PFR, EVA, and EVEX) and from a fish herpesvirus (OMV).

Transmission, Epidemiology, and Pathogenesis

Hirame rhabdovirus is pathogenic for several fish species. Fingerling rainbow trout, but not fingerling masou salmon, can be lethally infected by intramuscular injection, and virus can be recovered (Kimura et al., 1986). Few or no mortalities occur when chum, coho, and masou salmon fry or ayu fry are exposed by immersion. Virus has been recovered from some dead and from some surviving fish exposed in this manner, but the immersion trial results are suspect because water temperatures may not have been optimal in these trials (Kimura et al., 1986).

When juvenile hirame are exposed to hirame rhabdovirus by intramuscular or intraperitoneal inoculation, mortality occurs in both test groups at 10°C but in neither at 15°C (Gorie and Nakamoto, 1986). Virus can be recovered from kidney tissues of fish that die. Juvenile hirame exposed to hirame rhabdovirus by intraperitoneal injection and held at 5, 10, 15, and 20°C show highest mortality at the lower temperatures (40% at 5°C and 60% at 10°C) (Oseko et al., 1988b). Pathologic changes are most severe and virus titers are greatest in fish exposed at 5°C. Virus-specific neutralizing antibody can be recovered from challenged fish, and antibody titers increase with increasing water temperature (Oseko et al., 1988b). Under natural conditions, deaths in juvenile hirame range from 3.3 to 25%. The highest levels of mortality occur in winter at water temperatures of 2 to 5°C.

Treatment and Control

No method of treatment or control has been described.

GILTHEAD SEA BREAM PAPILLOMA

Host and Geographic Distribution

Maxillary tumors containing viruslike particles were found on 7 of 39 gilthead sea bream collected in salt mine flats on the coast of Spain (Gutierrez et al., 1977). The tumors have not been described elsewhere.

Clinical Signs and Pathology

The maxillary tumor appears to be a benign fibroepithelial papilloma. The basal membrane of the tumor is intact, and no invasion or metastasis is observed. Marked disparity in the ratios of length to weight in tumor-bearing fish indicates that the tumor interferes with feeding.

Diagnosis

The tumor is presumptively diagnosed by correlating species, clinical signs, and pathology. Viruslike particles are seen in electron micrographs of tumor tissue.

Virus Detection

Electron micrographs of tumor tissue show viruslike particles occurring singly or in aggregates in cytoplasmic vacuoles and in association with or possibly budding from cellular membranes. The particles are 35 to 65 nm in diameter and appear to have an envelope arrayed with peplomers. Many particles are electron-lucent, but some have a centrally placed, somewhat electron-dense nucleoid (Gutierrez et al., 1977). No attempts to isolate virus have been reported.

Transmission, Epidemiology, and Pathogenesis

No data have been reported.

Treatment and Control

No methods for treatment or control have been described.

PLEURONECTID EPIDERMAL PAPILLOMA

Host and Geographic Distribution

Several species of European and North American flatfishes (Pleuronectiformes) are affected by a benign epidermal papilloma (Cooper and Keller, 1969; Nigrelli et al., 1965; Wellings et al., 1965, 1966, 1976). The tumor appears to be of significance only in flatfishes on the Pacific coast of North America.

Clinical Signs and Pathology

The single or multiple epidermal tumors occur on any body surface and show some invasiveness but no metastasis. Marked retardation in growth and extensive tumor involvement appear to decrease the probability of survival (Cooper and Keller, 1969; Miller and Wellings, 1971; Wellings et al., 1964).

Several types of lesions are observed during tumor development (Cooper and Keller, 1969; Miller and Wellings, 1971; Nigrelli et al., 1965; Wellings, 1970; Wellings et al., 1964, 1965, 1976). The earliest lesion is the angioepithelial nodule, which is 1 to 2 mm in diameter, smooth in texture, and pink to red. This occurs only in fish 6 to 12 months old and is composed of a highly vascularized connective tissue stroma with an overlying thin layer of hyperplastic epidermis. The transition from an angioepithelial nodule to a mature epidermal papilloma or to the less frequently observed angioepithelial polyp occurs in fish 8 to 12 months old. Both the mature papilloma and the polyp are 0.5 to 5 cm in diameter and 0.5 to 1.5 cm thick. They have a nodular undulating texture and are pink to gray brown. The papilloma is composed of thick layers of hyperplastic epidermis overlaying a meager stratum of vascularized connective tissue. In contrast, the polyp is composed primarily of vascularized connective tissue covered by a thin layer of epidermis. The epidermal and connective tissue components of all three lesion types contain unique, pathognomonic tumor cells, "X-cells" (Brooks et al., 1969). The X-cells show glycocalyxlike encapsulation and are considered by some to be transformed cells (Wellings et al., 1976).

Diagnosis

Presumptive diagnosis is based on observing clinical signs in the species of concern, and the diagnosis is confirmed by histologic examination.

Virus Detection and Identification

The epidermal papilloma is of suspected viral etiology, but as yet attempts to isolate virus from homogenates of tumor tissue have been unsuccessful. Attempts to detect tumor cell–specific nucleic acids by density gradient centrifugation have also failed. Inoculation of pleuronectid cell cultures with papilloma cells produces no evidence of cytopathic effect or cell transformation (Wellings et al., 1976).

Electron microscopic examination of tumor-specific X-cells reveals intracytoplasmic, viruslike particles and a possible virogenic structure (Brooks et al., 1969; Nigrelli et al., 1965; Wellings and Chuinard, 1964; Wellings et al., 1965, 1976). One particle type appears to be an enveloped spheroid about 45 nm in diameter that contains a centrally placed, electron-dense nucleoid 6 nm in diameter. This type of particle is often observed in association with amorphous, electron-dense structures approximately 150 nm in diameter. These structures may represent the site of 45-nm particle formation or a developmental stage of a second viruslike particle designated the granular body (Wellings et al., 1965, 1976). The membrane-bound granular body is about 160 to 200 nm in diameter and contains numerous electron-dense granules. A particle similar to the granular body has been observed in epidermal papilloma tissue from the goby (Ito et al., 1976).

Transmission, Epidemiology, and Pathogenesis

Attempts to transmit the tumor in young feral pleuronectids by injection of tumor cells or tumor homogenates yielded equivocal results (Wellings et al., 1976). In all cases, the epidermal papilloma occurred with equal frequency in control and experimental populations.

The tumor occurs at a frequency of 5 to 10%, but can approach 50% in some populations. Fish of both sexes are affected, and those 8 months to 3 years old show the most extensive tumor involvement (Miller and Wellings, 1971; Wellings, 1970; Wellings et al., 1964). Environmental factors can affect tumorigenesis, but apparently bear no direct causal relation to the tumor (Miller and Wellings, 1971; Wellings et al., 1976).

Treatment and Control

No methods of treatment or control have been described.

WINTER FLOUNDER PAPILLOMATOSIS

Host and Geographic Distribution

Papilloma-type lesions are seen on the dorsal surface of winter flounder captured in Conception Bay (Newfoundland), an estuary receiving relatively high-level discharges of mutagenic hydrocarbons (Emerson et al., 1985).

Clinical Signs and Pathology

The lesions are irregular, blisterlike swellings in which intercellular spaces are distended and cells are in contact only at desmosomes. In affected cells, the nucleus is lobate and the nuclear membrane swollen. The cytoplasm is vacuolated and filled with numerous enlarged and degenerative mitochondria. The cisternae of the endoplasmic reticulum are distended, and tonofilaments are reduced in number. The cytologic changes and virus-like particles seen with the lesions are very similar to those reported for X-cell tumors in Pacific flatfishes and ulcerative dermal necrosis in Atlantic salmon (Emerson et al., 1985).

Diagnosis

Presumptive diagnosis is based on correlating clinical signs and the species of concern. Confirmed diagnosis is based on histologic and electron microscopic examination.

Virus Detection and Identification

Although no virus has been isolated in cell culture, electron micrographs of lesion cells show unenveloped viruslike particles in the cytoplasm and nucleus. Particles in the cytoplasm are about 30 nm in diameter and are found free and in membrane-bound aggregates and vacuoles. Degenerated particles in vacuoles may be segregated and held in membrane-bound aggregates as part of a cell defense mechanism (Emerson et al., 1985). In the nucleus, accumulations of particlelike granules and, occasionally, crystalline arrays of 25-nm particles are seen in proximity to 30-nm particles in the adjacent cytoplasm. The intranuclear crystalline arrays may be "virus factories" (Emerson et al., 1985). Based on cytochemical staining, distribution in the cell, and effects of DNAse treatment, the particles are not glycogen granules or other cellular products, but are putative DNA viruses most closely resembling papovaviruses or parvoviruses (Emerson et al., 1985).

Transmission, Epidemiology, and Pathogenesis

No data have been reported.

Treatment and Control

No methods of treatment or control have been described.

STOMATOPAPILLOMA OF EEL

SYNONYMS. Stomatopapilloma, "cauliflower" disease, eel virus (Berlin), EV-1, EV-2, unnamed syncytium-forming virus, blumenkohlkrankheit.

Host and Geographic Distribution

Stomatopapilloma, or "cauliflower" disease, occurs in European eels but not in American or Japanese eels (Deys, 1976; Koops and Mann, 1966). The condition was first observed in the early 1900s in eels captured from the Baltic Sea but aroused little interest until the 1940s, when the prevalence and geographic distribution of the disease became economically significant (Christiansen and Jensen, 1950; Nagel, 1907; Wolff, 1912). Affected eels are now found in the Baltic, North, and Black Seas and their tributaries in north-central Europe (Christiansen and Jensen, 1950; Peters and Peters, 1979; Radulescu and Angelescu, 1973). Eels with stomatopapilloma were also captured in rivers in England and Scotland (Delves-Broughton et al., 1980; Hussein and Mills, 1982). The disease has not been described elsewhere.

Clinical Signs and Pathology

Eels with stomatopapilloma show single or multiple epidermal proliferations principally about the mouth and head. In some areas, up to 40% of the eels caught are affected by the disease (Koops and Mann, 1969; Peters et al., 1972b). Empirical evidence suggests that the tumor occurs with the greatest frequency in eels 15 to 35 cm long (Hussein and Mills, 1982; Peters and Peters, 1977). The growths are inconspicuous in the early stages of development but can increase to a volume of several hundred cubic millimeters in a matter of weeks (Peters, 1975). The round-to-oval proliferations have a nodular, undulating texture and a firm-to-soft or spongy consistency (Peters and Peters, 1977). Pigmentation appears light reddish gray to fleshy red or slate blue–gray, depending on the degree of vascularity (Christiansen and Jensen, 1950). The papilloma can obstruct feeding, and affected eels can become emaciated (Koops and Mann, 1966). If the growth detaches, severe scarring usually develops.

Pathologic changes associated with stomatopapilloma are confined to the epidermis. The tumor rarely invades the surrounding tissue or metastasizes (Koops et al., 1970; Deys, 1976). Normal epidermis is composed of well-differentiated basal, mucous, and club cells (Bremer and Ernst, 1972). The developing tumor replaces the normal structure with undifferentiated epidermal cells beginning at the basal layer (Fig. 88–1) (Schmid, 1969). Mucous and club cells are seldom found in the tumor. Extensive intercellular spaces develop, and cellular interdigitations are reduced. Tumor cells are stellate to oval and contain irregular, swollen mitochondria and nuclei. Degenerating or regressing tumors show marked lymphocyte infiltration (Peters and Peters, 1977).

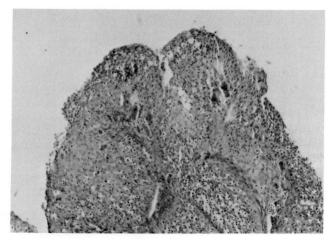

FIGURE 88–1. Papillomatosis virus lesion from the skin of European eel (100×) (courtesy M. Stoskopf).

Diagnosis

Stomatopapilloma is readily diagnosed by correlating clinical signs and affected species. Although several viruses have been isolated from eels with stomatopapilloma, their etiologic significance is uncertain.

Virus Detection and Identification

Several viruses have been isolated from and viruslike structures seen in eels with stomatopapilloma, but the viral etiology of the disease has yet to be proved. During attempts to isolate virus from homogenates of tumor tissue and whole eel, a virus was recovered from the blood of affected eels (Pfitzner and Schubert, 1969). The virus, designated eel virus (Berlin), caused lytic cytopathic effects in RTG–2 cells incubated at 16 to 18°C. Electron microscopy of infected RTG–2 cells revealed intracellular membrane-bound aggregates or "cysts" of polyhedral viral particles about 55 nm in diameter.

The sequential appearance of intranuclear viruslike structures and cytoplasmic aggregates of virus in RTG–2 cells suggested that virogenesis began in the nucleus (Pfitzner, 1969, 1973; Schubert, 1969). Although originally considered to be a papovavirus (Schwanz-Pfitzner, 1976), the eel virus (Berlin) is now considered to be a birnavirus (Schwanz-Pfitzner et al., 1984). No 55-nm particles were seen in electron micrographs of tumor tissue. Instead, in some instances, numerous intracellular icosahedral particles 30.0 nm in diameter and bundles of 2.5-nm needlelike structures, which reached 100.0 nm or more in length and diameter, were seen (Koops et al., 1970; Schubert, 1969) in the cytoplasm, or sometimes in a "cyst" in the nucleus of tumor cells (Deys, 1969; Pfitzner, 1973; Schubert, 1969). The significance of these structures has not been determined.

A second virus, designated EV–1, was isolated from tumor and internal organ homogenates (Wolf and Quimby, 1970). When homogenates were inoculated onto RTG–2 and FHM cells, pyknotic, necrotic foci in association with massive syncytia developed in both cell lines. These cytopathic effects were very different from those reported for the eel virus (Berlin). Electron micrographs of infected cells showed cytoplasmic accumulations of a small icosahedral virus. The virus has not been characterized, and no infectivity trials were performed.

When frozen stocks of EV–1 were reexamined some years later, a virus different from EV–1 was isolated (Nagabayashi and Wolf, 1979). The virus, designated EV–2, replicated in FHM cells but not in RTG–2, BB or BF–2 cells. The temperature range of viral replication was 10 to 25°C (optimum 15°C). At 15°C, pyknotic cell masses, syncytia, and cell lysis were seen, whereas only pyknosis and lysis occurred at 20 and 25°C. Electron micrographs of negatively stained, purified virus showed pleomorphic particles,

90 to 140 nm in diameter, having radially arranged peplomers, 10 nm in length. Based on biochemical, biologic, and physical characteristics, EV–2 was considered to be similar to an orthomyxovirus (Nagabayashi and Wolf, 1979).

Another syncytium-forming virus, as yet unnamed, was isolated from European eels with stomatopapilloma (Ahne and Thomsen, 1985). The virus was not neutralized by antiserum to EV–2. Few other characteristics and no pathogenicity trials were reported. The relationships among the various lytic and syncytium-forming virus isolates, their pathogenicity for eels, and their relevance to stomatopapilloma are unresolved issues.

Transmission, Epidemiology, and Pathogenesis

The results of infectivity trials using the various cell culture virus isolates are difficult to interpret. In some trials, virus could not be consistently recovered from eels that died. In others, the test eels were found to be carrying other perhaps different viruses. Nevertheless, no papillomatous lesions were induced in any of the attempts to transmit the tumor using cell culture–grown virus.

Attempts to initiate tumor production by implantation of tumor tissue and by scarification or injection of tumor homogenates or blood from affected eels have been unsuccessful (Deys, 1969; Koops et al., 1970; Schwanz-Pfitzner, 1976). Transmission by cohabitation or other techniques have been difficult to interpret because the health history of the experimental fish is unknown (Christiansen and Jensen, 1950; Deys, 1976; Koops and Mann, 1966).

Stomatopapillomas can be induced by exposure to various chemicals. Epidermal proliferations develop in glass eels and young eels exposed to sodium fluoride (15 mM) or sodium monoiodoacetate (1.5 to 1.75 mM) (Peters and Wilke, 1972; Peters and Peters, 1970). The proliferations do not develop if test fish are simultaneously exposed to inorganic diphosphate (1 mM), sodium pyruvate (5 to 20 mM), or oxygen at double the normal atmospheric partial pressure (320 mmHg).

Environmental factors markedly affect development of the stomatopapilloma. The tumor expands rapidly at temperatures of 15 to 22°C and regresses (though remnants persist) at 5 to 8°C and above 22°C (Peters, 1975, 1977; Peters and Peters, 1977; Pfitzner, 1973). This temperature dependency is reflected in annual fluctuations in the occurrence of the disease. Tumor prevalence and size are low in autumn, winter, and spring and high in summer (Hussein and Mills, 1982). Fluctuations in temperature, dissolved oxygen, salinity, and pollutants may increase physiologic stress, precipitating tumor development (Deys, 1976; Peters, 1975, 1977; Peters and Peters, 1977; Schwanz-Pfitzner, 1976). In addition, the demersal habits of the eel provide the opportunity for prolonged contact with the seemingly unfavorable environment of bottom sediments.

Treatment and Control

Because eels are captured as feral fish, control of stomatopapilloma in an aquaculture sense is not possible. However, several studies have reported successful treatment of tumors. Transitory tumor regression and cellular redifferentiation occur when eels are held in a saline environment (Peters and Peters, 1979). Quinine sulfate (15 to 60 mg/L) promotes cellular redifferentiation and reduction of tumor size, but the proliferation of undifferentiated cells resumes if treatment is discontinued (Peters et al., 1972a,b). Tumor regression purportedly involves an interaction between the quinine and the cell's energy-producing metabolic pathways (Peters et al., 1972a,b). Treatment with 2 mM inorganic diphosphate ($Na_2P_2O_7$•PPi) reportedly promotes cellular redifferentiation, as well as destruction and sloughing of the tumor (Peters, 1970; Peters and Peters, 1970). Increased numbers of lymphocytes and macrophages in adjacent tissues are interpreted as possible immunologic responses to tumor tissue.

LITERATURE CITED

Ahne, W., and Thomsen, I. (1985) The existence of three different viral agents in a tumour-bearing European eel (*Anguilla anguilla*). Zentralbl. Veterinaermed. Reihe B 32:228–235.
Anders, K. (1984) Preliminary results of histopathological and epidemiological studies on two "new" diseases of smelt (*Osmerus eperlanus* L.). Bull. Eur. Assoc. Fish. Pathol. 4:62–63.
Anders, K., and Moller, H. (1985) Spawning papillomatosis of smelt, *Osmerus eperlanus* L., from the Elbe estuary. J. Fish. Dis. 8:233–235.
Appy, R.G., Burt, M.D.B., and Morris, T.J. (1976) Viral nature of piscine erythrocytic necrosis (PEN) in the blood of Atlantic cod (*Gadus morhua*). J. Fish. Res. Bd. Can. 33:1380–1385.
Bloch, B., Mellergaard, S., and Neilsen, E. (1986) Adenovirus-like particles associated with epithelial hyperplasias in dab, *Limanda limanda* (L.). J. Fish Dis. 9:281–285.
Bremer, H., and Ernst, P. (1972) Ein beitrag zur onkologie der blumenkohlgeschwulste bei Anguilla anguilla. Z. Binnenfisch. DDR. 19:167–176.
Brooks, R.E., McArn, G.E., and Wellings, S.R. (1969) Ultrastructural observations on an unidentified cell type found in epidermal tumors of flounders. J. Natl. Cancer Inst. 43:97–110.
Buchanan, J.S., and Madeley, C.R. (1978) Studies on *Herpesvirus scophthalmi* infection of turbot *Scophthalmus maximus* (L.) ultrastructural observations. J. Fish Dis. 1:283–295.
Buchanan, J.S., Richards, R.H., Sommerville, C., and Madeley, C.R. (1978) A herpes-type virus from turbot (*Scophthalmus maximus* L). Vet. Rec. 102:527–528.
Castric, J., and Chastel, C. (1980) Isolation and characterization attempts of three viruses from European eel, *Anguilla anguilla*. Preliminary results. Ann. Virol. 131 E:435–448.
Castric, J., Rasschaert, D., and Bernard, J. (1984) Evidence of lyssaviruses among rhabdovirus isolates from the European eel, *Anguilla anguilla*. Ann. Virol. 135E:35–55.
Christiansen, M., and Jensen, A.J.C. (1950) On a recent and frequently occurring tumor disease of eel. Rep. Danish Biol. Sta. 50:29–44.
Cooper, R.C., and Keller, C.A. (1969) Epizootiology of papillomas in English sole, *Parophrys vetulus*. Natl. Cancer Inst. Monogr. 31:173–185.
Delves-Broughton, J., Fawell, J.K., and Woods, D. (1980) The first occurrence of "cauliflower disease" of eels *Anguilla anguilla* L. in the British Isles. J. Fish Dis. 3:255–256.
Deys, B.F. (1969) Papillomas in the Atlantic eel, *Anguilla vulgaris*. Natl. Cancer Inst. Monogr. 31:187–193.
Deys, B.F. (1976) Atlantic eels and cauliflower disease (orocutaneous papillomatosis). Prog. Exp. Tumor Res. 20:94–100.

Eiras, J.C. (1984). Virus infection of marine fish: prevalence of viral erythrocytic necrosis (VEN) in *Mugil cephalus* L., *Blennius pholis* L., and *Platichthys flesus* L. in coastal waters of Portugal. Bull. Eur. Assoc. Fish Pathol. 4:52–56.

Emerson, C.J., Payne, J.F., and Bal, A.K. (1985) Evidence for the presence of a viral non-lymphocystis type disease in winter flounder, *Pseudopleuronectes americanus* (Walbaum), from the north-west Atlantic. J. Fish Dis. 8:91–102.

Evelyn, T.P.T., and Traxler, G.S. (1978) Viral erythrocytic necrosis: natural occurrence in Pacific salmon and experimental transmission. J. Fish. Res. Bd. Can. 35:903–907.

Frerichs, G.N., Hill, B.J., and Way, K. (1989) Ulcerative disease rhabdovirus: cell-line susceptibility and serological comparison with other rhabdoviruses. J. Fish Dis. 12:51–56.

Gorie, S., and Nakamoto, K. (1986) Pathogenicity of a virus isolated from Hirame (Japanese flounder). Fish Pathol. 21:177–180.

Gutierrez, M., Crespo, J.P., and Arias, A. (1977) Particulas virus-like en un tumor en boca de dorado *Sparus aurata* L. (Virus-like particles in a mouth tumor of gilthead seabream, *Sparus aurata* L.) Invest. Pesq. 41:331–336.

Hill, B.J., Williams, R.F., Smale, C.J., Underwood, B.O., and Brown, F. (1980) Physicochemical and serological characterization of two rhabdoviruses isolated from eels. Intervirology 14:208–212.

Hussein, S.A., and Mills, D.H. (1982) The prevalence of "cauliflower disease" of the eel, *Anguilla anguilla* L., in tributaries of the River Tweed, Scotland. J. Fish Dis. 5:161–165.

Ito, Y., Kimura, I., and Miyake, T. (1976) Histopathological and virological investigations of papillomas in soles and gobies in coastal waters of Japan. Prog. Exp. Tumor Res. 20:86–93.

Jensen, N.J., and Bloch, B. (1980) Adenovirus-like particles associated with epidermal hyperplasia in cod *(Gadus morhua)* Nord. Veterinaermed. 32:173–175.

Jensen, N.J., and Larsen, J.L. (1979) The ulcus-syndrome in cod *(Gadus morhua)* I. A pathological and histopathological study. Nord. Veterinaermed. 31:222–228.

Jensen, N.J., and Larsen, J.L. (1982) The ulcus-syndrome in cod *(Gadus morhua)*. IV. Transmission experiments with two viruses isolated from cod and *Vibrio anguillarum*. Nord. Veterinaermed. 34:136–142.

Jensen, N.J., Bloch, B., and Larsen, J.L. (1979) The ulcus-syndrome in cod *(Gadus morhua)*. III. A preliminary virological report. Nord. Veterinaermed. 31:436–442.

Johnston, M.R.L. (1975) Distribution of *Pirhemocyton* Chatton and Blanc and other, possibly related, infections of poikilotherms. J. Protozool. 22:529–535.

Johnston, M.R.L., and Davies, A.J. (1973) A *Pirhemocyton*-like parasite of the blenny, *Blennius pholis* L. (Teleostei: Blenniidae) and its relationship to *Immanoplasma* Neumann, 1909. Intern. J. Parasitol. 3:235–241.

Khan, R.A., and Newman, M.W. (1982) Blood parasites from fish of the Gulf of Maine to Cape Hatteras, Northwest Atlantic Ocean, with notes on the distribution of fish hematozoa. Can. J. Zool. 60:396–402.

Kimura, T., Yoshimizu, M., and Gorie, S. (1986) A new rhabdovirus isolated in Japan from cultured hirame (Japanese flounder) *Paralichthys olivaceus* and ayu *Plecoglossus altivelis*. Dis. Aquatic. Organ. 1:209–217.

Koops, H., and Mann, H. (1966) The cauliflower disease of eels in Germany. Bull. Off. Int. Epizoot. 65:991–998.

Koops, H., and Mann, H. (1969) Die blumenkohldrankheit der aale vorkommen und verbreitung der krankheit. Arch Fischereiwiss. 20:5–15.

Koops, H., Mann, H., Pfitzner, I., Schmid, O.J., and Schubert, G. (1970) The cauliflower disease of eels. In: A Symposium on Diseases of Fishes and Shellfishes (Sniegko, S.F., ed.). Am. Fish. Soc. Spec. Publ. 5, pp. 291–295.

Laird, M., and Bullock, W.L. (1969) Marine fish haematozoa from New Brunswick and New England. J. Fish. Res. Bd. Can. 26:1075–1102.

Larsen, J.L., and Jensen, N.J. (1982) The ulcus-syndrome in cod *(Gadus morhua)* V. Prevalence in selected Danish marine recipients and a control site in the period 1976–1979. Nord. Veterinaermed. 34:303–312.

MacMillan, J.R., and Mulcahy, D. (1979) Artificial transmission to and susceptibility of Puget Sound fish to viral erythrocytic necrosis (VEN). J. Fish. Res. Bd. Can. 36:1097–1101.

MacMillan, J.R., Mulcahy, D., and Landolt, M. (1980) Viral erythrocytic necrosis: some physiological consequences of infection in chum salmon *(Oncorhynchus keta)*. J. Fish. Res. Bd. Can. 37:799–804.

McArn, G.E., McCain, B., and Wellings, S.R. (1978) Skin lesions and associated virus in Pacific cod *(Gadus macrocephalus)* in the Bering Sea. Fed. Proc. 37:937.

McCain, B.B., Gronlund, W.D., Myers, M.S., and Wellings, S.R. (1979) Tumours and microbial diseases of marine fishes in Alaskan waters. J. Fish. Dis. 2:111–130.

Meyers, T.R., Hauck, A.K., Blankenbeckler, W.D., and Minicucci, T. (1986) First report of viral erythrocytic necrosis in Alaska, USA, associated with epizootic mortality in Pacific herring, *Clupea harengus pallasi* (Valenciennes). J. Fish. Dis. 9:479–491.

Miller, B.S., and Wellings, S.R. (1971) Epizootiology of tumors on flathead sole *(Hippoglossoides elassodon)* in East Sound, Orcas Island, Washington. Trans. Am. Fish. Soc. 100:247–266.

Nagabayashi, T., and Wolf, K. (1979) Characterization of EV-2, a virus isolated from European eels *(Anguilla anguilla)* with stomatopapilloma. J. Virol. 30:358–364.

Nagel, X. (1907) Die blumenkohlkrakheit der aale auch in den deutschen bennengewassern beobachtet. Deut. Fisch. Zt. Stettin. 4:1960.

Nicholson, B.L., and Reno, P.W. (1981) Viral erythrocytic necrosis (VEN) in marine fishes. In: Proceedings of Republic of China–United States Cooperative Science on Fish Diseases at University of Washington, Seattle, 23–26 July 1979 (Kou, G.H., Fryer, J.L., and Landolt, M.L., eds.). NSC Symp. Ser. No. 3, pp. 59–65.

Nigrelli, R.F., Ketchen, K.S., and Ruggieri, G.D. (1965) Studies on virus diseases of fishes. Epizootiology of epithelial tumors in the skin of flatfishes of the Pacific coast, with special reference to the sand sole *(Psettichthys melanosticus)* from northern Hecate Strait, British Columbia, Canada. Zoologica 50:115–122.

Nishimura, T., Toba, M., Ban, F., Okamoto, N., and Sano, T. (1981) Eel rhabdovirus, EVA, EVEX and their infectivity to fishes. Fish Pathol. 15:173–184.

Oseko, N., Yoshimizu, M., Gorie, S., and Kimura, T. (1988a) Histopathological study on diseased hirame (Japanese flounder; *Paralichthys olivaceus*) infected with *Rhabdovirus olivaceus* (hirame rhabdovirus; HRV). Fish Pathol. 23:117–123.

Oseko, N., Yoshimizu, M., and Kimura, T. (1988b) Effect of water temperature on artificial infection of *Rhabdovirus olivaceus* (hirame rhabdovirus: HRV) to hirame (Japanese flounder, *Paralichthys olivaceus*). Fish Pathol. 23:125–132.

Peters, G. (1975) Seasonal fluctuations in the incidence of epidermal papillomas of the European eel *Anguilla anguilla* L. J. Fish Biol. 7:415–422.

Peters, G. (1977) The papillomatosis of the European eel *(Anguilla anguilla* L.): analysis of seasonal fluctuations in the tumor incidence. Arch. Fischereiwiss. 27:251–263.

Peters, G., and Peters, N. (1977) Temperature-dependent growth and regression of epidermal tumors in European eel *(Anguilla anguilla* L.). Ann. N.Y. Acad. Sci. 298:245–260.

Peters, G., and Peters, N. (1979) The influence of salinity on growth and structure of epidermal papillomas of the European eel *Anguilla anguilla* L. J. Fish Dis. 2:13–26.

Peters, N. (1970) Abstossung von tumoren unter einwirkung von anorganischem diphosphat. Experientia 26:1135.

Peters, N., and Peters, G. (1970) Tumorgenese, ein energieproblem der zelle? Untersuchungen an papillomen des europaischen aals, *Anguilla anguilla* (L). Arch. Fischereiwiss. 21:238–257.

Peters, N., and Wilke, H. (1972) Proliferation der fischepidermis nach der einwirkung von inhibitoren des glykolytischen energiestoffwechsels. Experientia 28:315–317.

Peters, N., Frohlich, K.H., and Bresching, G. (1972a) Experimentelle reversion von tumorzellen in vivo. Experientia 28:319–321.

Peters, N., Peters, G., and Bresching, G. (1972b) Redifferenzierung und wachstumshemmung von epidermalen tumoren des europaischen aals unter einwirkung von chininsulfat. Arch. Fischereiwiss. 23:47–63.

Pfitzner, I. (1969) Zur atiologie der blumenkohlkrankheit der aale. Arch. Fischereiwiss. 20:24–35.

Pfitzner, I. (1973) Untersuchungen zur klarung der atiologie der "blumenkohlkrankheit der aale" und zum einfludieses tumors auf ernahrung und wachstum. Verhandl. Inter. Verein. Limnol. 18:1666–1673.

Pfitzner, I., and Schubert, G. (1969) Ein virus aus dem blut mit blumenkohlkrankheit behaftetes aale. Z. Naturforsch. 24b:790a–790b.

Philippon, M., Nicholson, B.L., and Sherburne, S.W. (1977) Piscine erythrocytic necrosis (PEN) in the Atlantic herring *(Clupea harengus):* evidence for a viral infection. Fish Health News 6:6–10.

Radulescu, I., and Angelescu, N. (1973) Un caz de papilomatoza la *Anguilla anguilla* (L) capturata in marea neagra. Bull. Cercet. Piscic. 31:133–136.

Reno, P.W., and Nicholson, B.L. (1980) Viral erythrocytic necrosis (VEN) in Atlantic cod *(Gadus morhua)*: in vitro studies. Can. J. Fish. Aquatic. Sci. 37: 2276–2281.

Reno, P.W., and Nicholson, B.L. (1981) Ultrastructure and prevalence of viral erythroctyic necrosis (VEN) virus in Atlantic cod, *Gadus morhua* L., from the northern Atlantic Ocean. J. Fish Dis. 4:361–370.

Reno, P.W., Philippon-Fried, M., Nicholson, B.L., and Sherburne, S.W. (1978) Ultrastructural studies of piscine erythrocytic necrosis (PEN) in Atlantic herring *(Clupea harengus harengus)*. J. Fish. Res. Bd. Can. 35:148–154.

Reno, P.W., Serreze, D.V., Hellyer, S.K., and Nicholson, B.L. (1985) Hematological and physiological effects of viral erythrocytic necrosis (VEN) in Atlantic cod and herring. Fish Pathol. 20:353–360.

Richards, R.H., and Buchanan, J.S. (1978) Studies on *Herpesvirus scophthalmi* infection of turbot *Scophthalmus maximus* (L.): histopathological observations. J. Fish Dis. 1:251–258.

Rohovec, J.S., and Amandi, A. (1981) Incidence of viral erythrocytic necrosis among hatchery-reared salmonids of Oregon. Fish Pathol. 15:135–141.

Sano, T. (1976) Viral diseases of cultured fishes in Japan. Fish Pathol. 10:221–226.

Sano, T., Nishimura, T., Okamoto, N., and Fukuda, H. (1977) Studies on viral diseases of Japanese fishes—VII. A rhabdovirus isolated from European eel, *Anguilla anguilla*. Bull. Jpn. Soc. Sci. Fish. 43:491–495.

Schmid, O.J. (1969) Beitrag zur histologie und atiologie der blumenkohlkrankheit der aale. Arch. Fischereiwiss. 29:16–23.

Schubert, G. (1969) Electronenmikroskopische untersuchungen an der haut mit blumenkohlkrankheit behaftetes aale. Arch. Fischereiwiss. 20:36–49.

Schwanz-Pfitzner, I. (1976) Further studies of eel virus (Berlin) isolated from the blood of eels (Anguilla anguilla) with skin papilloma. Prog. Exp. Tumor Res. 20:101–107.

Schwanz-Pfitzner, I., Ozel, M., Darai, G., and Gelderblom, H. (1984) Morphogenesis and fine structure of eel virus (Berlin), a member of the proposed birnavirus group. Arch. Virol. 81:151–162.

Sherburne, S.W. (1973) Erythrocyte degeneration in the Atlantic herring, Clupea harengus L. U.S. Natl. Mar. Fish. Serv. Fish. Bull. 71:125–134.

Sherburne, S.W. (1977) Occurrence of piscine erythrocytic necrosis (PEN) in the blood of the anadromous alewife, Alosa pseudoharnegus, from Maine coastal streams. J. Fish. Res. Bd. Can. 34:281–286.

Sherburne, S.W., and Bean, L.L. (1979) Incidence and distribution of piscine erythrocytic necrosis and the microsporidian, Glugea hertwigi, in rainbow smelt, Osmerus mordax, from Massachusetts to the Canadian Maritimes. Fish. Bull. 77:503–509.

Smail, D.A. (1982) Viral erythrocytic necrosis in fish: a review. Proc. R. Soc. Edinb. Sect. B 81:169–176.

Smail, D.A., and Egglestone, S.I. (1980a) Virus infections of marine fish erythrocytes: prevalence of piscine erythrocytic necrosis in cod Gadus morhua L. and blenny Blennius pholis L. in coastal and offshore waters of the United Kingdom. J. Fish Dis. 3:41–46.

Smail, D.A., and Egglestone, S.I. (1980b) Virus infections of marine fish erythrocytes: electron microscopical studies on the blenny virus. J. Fish Dis. 3:47–54.

Smith, A.W., Skilling, D.E., Dardiri, A.H., and Latham, A.B. (1980) Calicivirus pathogenic for swine: a new serotype isolated from opaleye Girella nigricans, an ocean fish. Science 209:940–941.

Smith, A.W., Skilling, D.E., Prato, C.M., and Bray, H.L. (1981) Calicivirus (SMSV–5) infection in experimentally inoculated opaleye fish (Girella nigricans). Arch. Virol. 67:165–168.

Smith, A.W., Ritter, D.G., Ray, G.C., Skilling, D.E., and Wartzok, D. (1983) New calicivirus isolates from feces of walrus (Odobenus rosmarus). J. Wildl. Dis. 19:86–89.

Sorimachi, M. (1982) Susceptibility of fish cell lines to eel viruses. Fish Pathol. 17:119–123.

Vestergard Jorgensen, P.E., and Olesen, N.J. (1987) Cod ulcus syndrome rhabdovirus is indistinguishable from the Egtved (VHS) virus. Bull. Eur. Assoc. Fish Pathol. 7:73–74.

Walker, R. (1971) PEN, a viral lesion of fish erythrocytes. Am. Zool. 11:707.

Walker, R., and Sherburne, S.W. (1977). Piscine erythrocytic necrosis virus in Atlantic cod, Gadus morhua, and other fish: and distribution. J. Fish. Res. Bd. Can. 34:1188–1195.

Wellings, S.R. (1970) Biology of some virus diseases of marine fish. In: A Symposium on Diseases of Fishes and Shellfishes (Snieszko, S.F., ed.). Am. Fish. Soc. Spec. Publ. 5, pp. 296–306.

Wellings, S.R., and Chuinard, R.G. (1964) Epidermal papillomas with virus-like particles in flathead sole, Hippoglossoides elassodon. Science 146:932–934.

Wellings, S.R., Chuinard, R.G., Gourley, R.T., and Cooper, R.A. (1964) Epidermal papillomas in the flathead sole, Hippoglossoides elassodon, with notes on the occurrence of similar neoplasms in other pleuronectids. J. Natl. Cancer Inst. 33:991–1004.

Wellings, S.R., Chuinard, R.G., and Bens, M. (1965) A comparative study of skin neoplasms in four species of pleuronectid fishes. Ann. N.Y. Acad. Sci. 126:479–501.

Wellings, S.R., Cooper, R.A., and Chuinard, R.G. (1966) Skin tumors of pleuronectid fishes in Puget Sound, Washington. Bull. Wildlife Dis. Assoc. 2:66.

Wellings, S.R., McCain, B.B., and Miller, B.S. (1976) Epidermal papillomas in Pleuronectidae of Puget Sound, Washington. Prog. Exp. Tumor Res. 20:55–74.

Wolf, K. (1988) The viruses and viral diseases of fish. Cornell University Press, Ithaca, New York.

Wolf, K., and Quimby, M.C. (1970) Virology of eel stomatopapilloma. In: Progress in Sport Fishery Research 1970 (Resource Publ. 106), U.S. Fish and Wildlife Service, Washington, D.C., pp. 94–95.

Wolff, B. (1912) Uber ein blastom bei einem aal (Anguilla vulgaris) nebst bemerkungen zur vergleichenden pathologie der geschwulste. Arch Pathol. Anat. Physiol. 210:365–385.

Chapter 89

PARASITES OF COLD-WATER MARINE FISHES

SARAH L. POYNTON

Parasites can adversely affect their fish hosts by weakening them, rendering them more conspicuous, or less commonly by causing epizootics and mass mortalities (Sindermann, 1990). Chronic stock loss is usually associated with parasitic infections, and this may be more detrimental than acute stock loss (Sindermann, 1966). Parasitized marine fish can transmit infections to man. Conversely, they may be useful as biologic tags for stock identification (Lom, 1984) or as indicators of environmental changes (Sindermann 1966, 1985).

Therefore, today precise knowledge of the identity of marine fish parasites is crucial (Margolis and Kabata, 1984). Unfortunately, the extensive literature is highly dispersed, and much is published in Rus-

sian. Few compendia exist (Hargis, 1985; Margolis and Kabata, 1984) except for the recent Canadian works (Arai 1989a,b; Beverley-Burton, 1984; Bousfield and Kabata, 1988; Kabata, 1988; Margolis and Arthur, 1979; Rafi, 1988). Little is known about some groups of parasites such as the protozoans, leeches, amphipods, and isopods affecting cold-water marine fishes (Bousfield, 1987; Lom, 1986; Meyer and Khan, 1979; Rafi, 1988).

Protozoan diseases, often associated with crowding and poor water quality, are important in marine aquaculture. Helminths are not generally a significant problem, in part because of the difficulty in completing complex life cycles in culture systems (McVicar, 1978). However, disease organisms that are benign or unknown in wild host populations may cause serious problems in mariculture (Sindermann and Lightner, 1988). Information on the treatment of marine fish diseases is limited when compared with that on freshwater fishes (Liewes, 1984).

The following eight parasites causing disease of wild or cultured fishes of economic importance are considered in detail:

- Sarcomastigophora: *Cryptobia bullocki*
- Apicomplexa: *Eimeria* spp.
            Haemogregarina sachai
- Microspora: *Glugea stephani*
- Digenea: *Cryptocotyle lingua*
- Nematoda: *Anisakis* spp.
            Pseudoterranova decipiens
- Crustacea: *Lernaeocera branchialis*

See Table 89–1 for an extensive list of parasites of cold-water marine fishes.

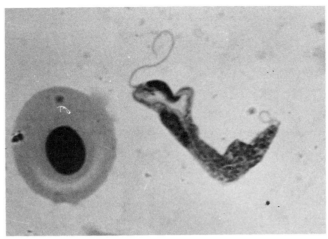

FIGURE 89–1. *Cryptobia (Trypanoplasma) bullocki* from a blood smear of a winter flounder. (Courtesy of P. Cheung.)

CRYPTOBIA *BULLOCKI*

SYNONYMS. *Trypanoplasma bullocki*, cryptobiasis, trypanosomiasis.

Hosts and Geographic Distribution

The flagellate *Cryptobia bullocki* has been recorded from many hosts but is most prevalent in flatfishes (Burreson and Zwerner, 1982). Hosts include American plaice, bay whiff, hogchoker, smooth flounder, summer flounder, windowpane, winter flounder, mummichog, Northern searobin, oyster toadfish, spot, spotted hake, striped bass, striped killifish, tautog, weakfish (Burreson, 1982; Burreson and Zwerner, 1982; Margolis and Arthur, 1979; Sindermann, 1985). *Cryptobia bullocki* is widely distributed along the Atlantic coast of North America, and in the Gulf of Mexico, it is usually most prevalent in young fish from brackish waters (Burreson, 1982).

Clinical Appearance and Diagnosis

Fish with cryptobiasis usually exhibit anemia, splenomegaly, and a grossly distended abdominal cavity caused by ascites (Burreson and Zwerner, 1984; Lom, 1984). *Cryptobia* sp. infection of laboratory-held summer flounder is characterized by ulceration and hemorrhagic lesions (Newman, 1978).

Hemoflagellates are readily observed in fresh plasma by their rapid, wriggling movements (Strout, 1965). In fixed and stained preparations, look for a slender, sinuous body (10.9 to 23.1 μm long, 1.2 to 6.0 μm wide) with a nucleus and kinetoplast, undulating membrane, and anterior and posterior flagella (Fig. 89–1) (5.8 to 19.1 and 4.4 to 18.2 μm long, respectively) (Strout, 1965).

Pathologic Effects and Pathogenesis

Crytobia bullocki has been implicated in extensive mortalities of juvenile flatfishes (Sindermann, 1985). In experimental infections, rapidly increasing parasitemias of *C. bullocki* are lethal to hogchoker and summer flounder (Burreson, 1982; Burreson and Zwerner, 1984). Low temperatures facilitate increased parasitemia (Burreson and Zwerner, 1982, 1984). In laboratory-held summer flounder, *Cryptobia* sp. infection is associated with edema, hemorrhage, and necrosis of the gastrointestinal tract. Large numbers of parasites are usually present in the gut and liver (Newman, 1978).

Life Cycle, Transmission, and Epidemiology

Cryptobia bullocki is transmitted by the estuarine leech *Calliobdella vivida* (Burreson, 1982; Sawyer, 1986). The flagellates divide in the crop and postceca of this vector, and the infective stages are found in the proboscis. These are injected into a new host at feeding (Lom, 1984). Infected leeches retain flagellates through three successive feedings (Burreson, 1982). In the fish, the flagellates divide in the peripheral blood and internal organs (Lom, 1984).

Treatment and Control

Calcium cyanamide and calcium oxide have been reported to be effective against *Cryptobia* spp., and pyrimethamine (Daraprim) antimalarial treatment may be effective (Herwig, 1979). None of these drugs are approved for use in food fishes. No public health concerns are known for this disease.

Text continued on page 727

TABLE 89–1. Parasites of Cold-Water Marine Fishes*

Parasite (Phyla and Genera)	Hosts	Location on/in Hosts	Method of Infection	Prevalence	References
SARCOMASTIGOPHORA					
Amyloodinium	Nonspecific	External surfaces, gills, skin	Direct	Common in aquaria	Moller and Anders, 1986
Cryptobia	Killifishes Lefteye flounders Lumpfishes Righteye flounders	Blood, stomach, urinary bladder	Vector, leech; host, fish	Common	Daily, 1978 Lom, 1984 Margolis and Arthur, 1979
Entamoeba	Codfishes	Rectum	Direct	Uncommon	Moller and Anders, 1986
Hexamita	Codfishes	Intestine	Direct	Common	Lom, 1984
Ichthyobodo	Codfishes Righteye flounders	External surfaces, gills	Direct	Unknown	Lom, 1984 Morrison et al., 1986
Monocercomonas	Molas	Gastrointestinal tract	Direct	Unknown	Moller and Anders, 1986
Spironucleus	Codfishes	Rectum	Direct	Common	Poynton and Morrison, 1990
Trypanosoma	Combtooth blennies Codfishes Eelpouts Righteye flounders Sculpins Snailfishes Soles Wolffishes	Blood	Vector, leech; host, fish		Margolis and Arthur, 1979 Sindermann, 1970
APICOMPLEXA					
Cyrilia	Eelpouts	Blood	Vector, leech; host, fish;	Common	Lom, 1984
Eimeria	Codfishes Grenadiers Herrings Sculpins	Intestine Kidney Liver Pyloric ceca Rectum Swimbladder Testes	Probably direct, invertebrate paratenic host may be needed	Common	Dykova and Lom, 1983 Lom, 1984 Margolis and Arthur, 1979 Sindermann, 1970
Goussia	Codfishes Grenadiers Herrings	Gallbladder Heart Hepatic vein, intestine, kidney, liver, swimbladder	Probably direct, invertebrate paratenic host may be needed	Common	Dykova and Lom, 1983 Lom, 1984 Moller and Anders, 1986 Morrison et al., 1986 Morrison and Poynton, 1989 Odense and Logan, 1976
Haematractidium	Mackerels	Blood	Vector, unknown; host, fish;	Common	Lom, 1984
Haemogregarina	Blennies Codfishes Eelpouts Gunnels Herrings Lefteye flounders Righteye flounders Sculpins Snailfishes Soles Wolffishes	Blood	Vector, leech or crustacean; host, fish	Common	Liewes, 1984 Lom, 1984 Margolis and Arthur, 1979 Morrison et al. 1986 Sindermann, 1970
Haemohormidium	Codfishes Righteye flounders Sand lances Sculpins	Blood	Vector, leech; host, fish	Unknown	Lom, 1984 Margolis and Arthur, 1979
Sarcocystis	Eelpouts	Musculature	Definitive host, fish; intermediate host, unknown	Unknown	Margolis and Arthur, 1979
MICROSPORA					
Glugea	Codfishes Grenadiers Herrings Lanternfishes Pipefishes Righteye flounders Smelts Sticklebacks	Branchial cavity Body cavity Connective tissue Eye Heart Gills Intestine Mesentery Ovary Pyloric ceca Skeletal muscle Viscera	Direct	Common	Canning and Lom, 1986 Margolis and Arthur, 1979 Sindermann, 1970
Ichthyosporidium	Wrasses	Body cavity	Direct	Unknown	Canning and Lom, 1986
Loma	Codfishes	Gills Kidney Spleen Viscera	Direct	Uncommon	Canning and Lom, 1986 Morrison et al., 1986
Microgemma	Mullets	Liver	Direct	Unknown	Canning and Lom, 1986
Microsporidium	Codfishes Gunnels Sculpins Smelts	Body cavity Liver Skeletal muscle Testes	Direct	Common	Lom, 1986 Canning and Lom, 1986

Table continued on following page

TABLE 89–1. Parasites of Cold-Water Marine Fishes* *Continued*

Parasite (Phyla and Genera)	Hosts	Location on/in Hosts	Method of Infection	Prevalence	References
Mrazekia	Codfishes	Pyloric ceca	Direct	Unknown	Moller and Anders, 1986
Nosema	Toadfishes Wrasses	Gallbladder and urinary bladder—hyperparasites of myxosporidia	Direct	Unknown	Canning and Lom, 1986
Pleistophora	Blennies Butterfishes Codfishes Eelpouts Goosefishes Herrings Mullets Righteye flounders Sculpins Soles Wolffishes	Liver Skeletal muscle	Direct	Common	Canning and Lom, 1986 Lom, 1984
Spraguea	Goosefishes	Ganglia of CNS	Direct	Common	Canning and Lom, 1986
Tetramicra	Lefteye flounders	Musculature	Direct	Common	Lom, 1986
Theragra	Lefteye flounders	Skeletal muscles	Direct	Common	Canning and Lom, 1986
CILIATA					
Brooklynella	Many species in aquaria	Gills	Direct	Common in aquaria	Lom, 1984
Cryptocaryon	Many species	Gills Skin	Direct	Uncommon in wild; common in aquaria	Lom, 1984 Sindermann, 1970
Euplotes	Eelpouts Righteye flounders Soles	Skin	Direct	Unknown	Lom, 1984, 1986
Helicostoma	Eelpouts Righteye flounders Soles	Skin	Direct	Unknown	Lom, 1984, 1986
Paratrichodina	Cusk-eels	Gills	Direct	Unknown	Lom, 1984
Scyphidia	Righteye flounders Sculpins Snailfishes Sticklebacks	Gills	Direct	Uncommon	Lom, 1984, 1986 Margolis and Arthur, 1979 Sindermann, 1970
Trichodina	Codfishes Eelpouts Herrings Lefteye flounders Lumpfishes Mullets Pricklebacks Righteye flounders Sculpins Sticklebacks	Fins Gills Skin	Direct	Common	Liewes, 1984 Lom, 1984 MacKenzie, 1987 Margolis and Arthur, 1979 Poynton and Lom, 1989
Uronema	Eelpouts Righteye flounders Soles	Gills, musculature, viscera	Direct	Unknown	Lom, 1984, 1986 Moller and Anders, 1986
MYXOZOA					
Alatosporum	Jacks Righteye flounders Searobins	Gall bladder	Life cycle of myxosporea poorly known, some need an intermediate host (Lom, 1986)	Unknown	Moller and Anders, 1986
Auerbachia	Grenadiers	Gallbladder	Life cycle at myxosporea poorly known, some need an intermediate host (Long, 1986)	Common	Margolis and Arthur, 1979 Zubchenko, 1985
Ceratomyxa	Codfishes Cusk-eels Cutlassfishes Eelpouts Grenadiers Herrings Righteye flounders Sculpins Sticklebacks Wrymouths	Bile ducts Gallbladder Kidney Intestine Musculature Viscera	Life cycle of myxosporea poorly known, some need an intermediate host (Long, 1986)	Common	Lom, 1984 Margolis and Arthur, 1979 Moller and Anders, 1986 Sindermann, 1970
Chloromyxum	Herrings Sculpins	Gallbladder	Life cycle of myxosporea poorly known, some need an intermediate host (Long, 1986)	Common	MacKenzie, 1987 Margolis and Arthur, 1979 Sindermann, 1970
Conispora	Codfishes	Kidney tubules	Life cycle of myxosporea poorly known, some need an intermediate host (Long, 1986)	Unknown	Margolis and Arthur, 1979
Davisia	Grenadiers	Kidney, urinary bladder	Life cycle of myxosporea poorly known, some need an intermediate host (Long, 1986)	Unknown	Margolis and Arthur, 1979

TABLE 89–1. Parasites of Cold-Water Marine Fishes* *Continued*

Parasite (Phyla and Genera)	Hosts	Location on/in Hosts	Method of Infection	Prevalence	References
Kudoa	Codfishes Eelpouts Gunnels Herrings Mackerels Righteye flounders Sculpins	Blood Intestine Kidney Musculature	Life cycle of myxosporea poorly known, some need an intermediate host (Long, 1986)	Common	Lom, 1986 Margolis and Arthur, 1979 Moller and Anders, 1986
Leptotheca	Codfishes Grenadiers Herrings Mackerels Molas Scorpionfishes	Gallbladder Kidney tubules	Life cycle of myxosporea poorly known, some need an intermediate host (Long, 1986)	Common	Lom, 1984 MacKenzie, 1987 Margolis and Arthur, 1979 Moller and Anders, 1986 Sindermann, 1970
Myxidium	Argentines Codfishes Grenadiers Lumpfishes Righteye flounders Sculpins Soles	Gallbladder Gills Intestine Kidney Urinary bladder	Life cycle of myxosporea poorly known, some need an intermediate host (Long, 1986)	Common	Lom, 1984 Margolis and Arthur, 1979 Moller and Anders, 1986 Morrison et al., 1986 Sindermann, 1970
Myxobilatus	Righteye flounders Sticklebacks	Kidney tubules Urinary bladder	Life cycle of myxosporea poorly known, some need an intermediate host (Long, 1986)	Unknown	Margolis and Arthur, 1979 Moller and Anders, 1986
Myxobolus	Codfishes Lumpfishes Mullets Righteye flounders	Gills Intestine Kidney Skeleton (head) Cranial cartilage	Life cycle of myxosporea poorly known, some need an intermediate host (Long, 1986)	Unknown	Lom, 1984 Moller and Anders, 1986 Sindermann, 1970
Myxoproteus	Codfishes Goosefishes Grenadiers Righteye flounders Sculpins	Gallbladder Urinary bladder	Life cycle of myxosporea poorly known, some need an intermediate host (Long, 1986)	Unknown	Margolis and Arthur, 1979 Moller and Anders, 1986
Ortholinea	Combtooth Blennies Herrings Righteye flounders	Kidney tubules	Life cycle of myxosporea poorly known, some need an intermediate host (Long, 1986)	Unknown	Lee et al., 1985 MacKenzie, 1987
Parvicapsula	Dragonets Righteye flounders	Urinary bladder	Life cycle of myxosporea poorly known, some need an intermediate host (Long, 1986)	Unknown	Moller and Anders, 1986
Sinuolinea	Dories Grenadiers	Urinary bladder	Life cycle of myxosporea poorly known, some need an intermediate host (Long, 1986)	Unknown	Margolis and Arthur, 1979 Moller and Anders, 1986
Sphaeromyxa	Herrings Pipefishes Righteye flounders Sculpins	Gallbladder	Life cycle of myxosporea poorly known, some need an intermediate host (Long, 1986)	Common	Lom, 1984, 1986 Moller and Anders, 1986
Sphaerospora	Mullets Righteye flounders Sticklebacks	Kidney Urinary bladder	Life cycle of myxosporea poorly known, some need an intermediate host (Long, 1986)	Common	Lom, 1984 Moller and Anders, 1986
Unicapsula	Righteye flounders	Musculature	Life cycle of myxosporea poorly known, some need an intermediate host (Long, 1986)	Unknown	Margolis and Arthur, 1979
Zschokkella	Codfishes Grenadiers	Gallbladder Kidney Urinary bladder	Life cycle of myxosporea poorly known, some need an intermediate host (Long, 1986)	Common	Lee et al., 1985 Margolis and Arthur, 1979 Moller and Anders, 1986 Zubchenko, 1985
CNIDARIA *Hydrichthys*	Jacks Lanternfishes Scorpionfishes	Body surface or hyperparasitic on copepods on body surface	Direct	Uncommon	Arai, 1989b Lauckner, 1984
Ichthyocodium	Scorpionfishes	Hyperparasitic on copepods on body surface	Direct	Uncommon	Lauckner, 1984
Perigonimus	Poachers	Body surface	Direct	Uncommon	Slauckner, 1984
TURBELLARIA *Udonella*	Codfishes Righteye flounders	On copepods on body surface	Direct	Uncommon	Beverley-Burton, 1984
MONOGENEA *Anthocotyle*	Codfishes	Gills	Direct	Common	Beverley-Burton, 1984 Moller and Anders, 1986
Axine	Needlefishes	Gills	Direct	Common	Llewellyn, 1956

Table continued on following page

TABLE 89–1. Parasites of Cold-Water Marine Fishes* *Continued*

Parasite (Phyla and Genera)	Hosts	Location on/in Hosts	Method of Infection	Prevalence	References
Benedenia	Scorpionfishes	Gills	Direct	Unknown	Beverley-Burton, 1984 Egorova, 1985
Capsala	Mackerels Molas	Body surface	Direct	Common	Moller and Anders, 1986 Rohde, 1984
Cyclocotyloides	Grenadiers	Gills	Direct	Common	Beverley-Burton, 1984
Diclidophora	Codfishes Grenadiers	Gills	Direct	Common	Beverley-Burton, 1984 Llewellyn, 1956 Moller and Anders, 1986 Rodjuk, 1985
Diclidophoroides	Codfishes	Gills	Direct	Common	Gaevskaya and Umnova, 1977
Diplectanum	Temperate basses	Gills	Direct	Unknown	Rohde, 1984 Silan and Maillard, 1986
Entobdella	Righteye flounders Scorpionfishes Soles	Body surface	Direct	Common	Beverley-Burton, 1984 Moller and Anders, 1986
Gastrocotyle	Jacks	Gills	Direct	Common	Llewellyn, 1956
Gyrodactyloides	Herrings Smelts	Gills Nasal cavities	Direct	Unknown	Beverley-Burton, 1984 MacKenzie, 1987
Gyrodactylus	Codfishes Herrings Killifishes Righteye flounders Sculpins Sticklebacks Surfperches	Body surface Fins Gills Pharynx	Direct	Common	Appy and Burt, 1982 Beverley-Burton, 1984 Moller and Anders, 1986
Kuhnia	Mackerels	Gills	Direct	Common	Beverley-Burton, 1984 Llewellyn, 1956
Laminiscus	Herrings Smelts	Gills	Direct	Unknown	Beverley-Burton, 1984 MacKenzie, 1987
Linguadactyla	Codfishes	Gills	Direct	Common	Moller and Anders, 1986
Macruricotyle	Grenadiers	Gills	Direct	Unknown	Beverley-Burton, 1984
Mazocraeoides	Herrings	Gills	Direct	Unknown	MacKenzie, 1987
Microcotyle	Butterfishes Greenlings Scorpionfishes Sea basses Temperate basses Wrasses	Gills	Direct	Common	Beverley-Burton, 1984 Llewellyn, 1956 Moller and Anders, 1986 Silan and Maillard, 1986
Octosoma	Mackerels	Gills	Direct	Common	Llewellyn, 1956
Plectanocotyle	Searobins	Gills	Direct	Common	Llewellyn, 1956
Pseudacanthocotyla	Porgies	Skin	Direct	Common	Gaevskaya and Umnova, 1977
Pseudaxine	Jacks	Gills	Direct	Common	Llewellyn, 1956
Tristoma	Swordfishes	Gills, branchial cavity	Direct	Common	Beverley-Burton, 1984
Trochopus	Scorpionfishes Searobins Sebastes	Gills	Direct	Common	Beverley-Burton, 1984 Egorova, 1985 Moller and Anders, 1986
DIGENEA *Accacladium*	Molas	Intestine	Definitive host, fish; 1st intermediate host, mollusc; 2nd intermediate host, worms and coelenterates	Unknown	Margolis and Arthur, 1979 Schell, 1985
Accacladocoelium	Molas	Intestine	Definitive host, fish; 1st intermediate host, mollusc; 2nd intermediate host, worms and coelenterates	Unknown	Margolis and Arthur, 1979 Schell, 1985
Anisorchis	Greenlings Sculpins	Intestine Pyloric ceca Stomach	Definitive host, fish; 1st intermediate host, mollusc; 2nd intermediate host, crustacean or mollusc	Common	Margolis and Arthur, 1979 Schell, 1985
Aporocotyle	Codfishes Grenadiers Mackerels Righteye flounders Scorpionfishes	Gills Heart Mesenteries Muscles	Definitive host, fish; 1st intermediate host, mollusc or polychete; 2nd intermediate host, invertebrate	Common	Margolis and Arthur, 1979 Moller and Anders, 1986 Morrison et al., 1986 Schell, 1985 Zubchenko, 1985
Brachyphallus	Codfishes Herrings Righteye flounders Sand lances Scorpionfishes Sticklebacks	Intestine Stomach	Definitive host, fish; 1st intermediate host, mollusc; 2nd intermediate host, unknown	Uncommon	Appy and Burt, 1982 Gaevskaya and Umnova, 1977 Margolis and Arthur, 1979 Schell, 1985
Bucephaloides	Codfishes	Intestine Nervous system	Definitive host, fish; 1st intermediate host, bivalve; 2nd intermediate host, fish	Common	Matthews, 1974 Smyth, 1976
Bucephalus	Gobies Righteye flounders Temperate basses	Digestive tract Liver	Definitive host, fish; 1st intermediate host, bivalve; 2nd intermediate host, fish	Common	Matthews, 1973 Smyth, 1976

TABLE 89–1. Parasites of Cold-Water Marine Fishes* *Continued*

Parasite (Phyla and Genera)	Hosts	Location on/in Hosts	Method of Infection	Prevalence	References
Cainocreadium	Righteye flounders Temperate basses	Muscles Pyloric ceca	Definitive host, fish; 1st intermediate host, mollusc; 2nd intermediate host, fish	Uncommon	Margolis and Arthur, 1979 Schell, 1985
Cryptocotyle	Codfishes Herrings Lefteye flounders Mackerels Righteye flounders Sculpins Wrasses	Fins Gills Liver Muscles Skin	Definitive host, bird; 1st intermediate host, snail; 2nd intermediate host, fish	Common	Margolis and Arthur, 1979 Morris et al., 1986 Smyth, 1976
Deretrema	Scorpionfishes	Gallbladder	Definitive host, fish; 1st intermediate host, mollusc; 2nd intermediate host, invertebrate	Common	Margolis and Arthur, 1979
Derogenes	Argentines Codfishes Goosefishes Grenadiers Herrings Mackerels Righteye flounders Sand lances Scorpionfishes Sculpins Smelts Sticklebacks Wolffishes Wrasses	Esophagus Intestine Stomach	Definitive host, fish; 1st intermediate host, mollusc; 2nd intermediate host, crustacean or worm	Common	Schell, 1985 Appy and Burt, 1982 Gaevskaya and Umnova, 1977 Margolis and Arthur, 1979 Schell, 1985 Zubchenko, 1985
Deropristis	Sturgeons	Intestine	Definitive host, fish; 1st intermediate host, mollusc; 2nd intermediate host, polychete	Common	Margolis and Arthur, 1979 Schell, 1985
Dihemistephanus	Codfishes Molas	Intestine Pyloric ceca	Definitive host, fish; 1st intermediate host, mollusc; 2nd intermediate host, invertebrate	Unknown	Margolis and Arthur, 1979 Schell, 1985
Diplostomum	Herrings	Eye	Definitive host, birds; 1st intermediate host, mollusc; 2nd intermediate host, fish	Unknown	MacKenzie, 1987
Fellodistomum	Codfishes Righteye flounders Scorpionfishes Wolffishes Wrymouths	Gallbladder Intestine Pyloric ceca Stomach	Definitive host, fish; 1st intermediate host, bivalve; 2nd intermediate host, brittle stars	Common	Appy and Burt, 1982 Margolis and Arthur, 1979 Moller and Anders, 1986 Schell, 1985
Galactosomum	Greenlings Herrings Sandlances Surfperches	Gill arches	Definitive host, bird; 1st intermediate host, mollusc; 2nd intermediate host, fish	Uncommon	MacKenzie, 1987 Margolis and Arthur, 1979 Schell, 1985
Genolinea	Greenlings Righteye flounders Sculpins	Ovary Stomach	Definitive host, fish; 1st intermediate host, mollusc; 2nd intermediate host, crustacean	Common	Margolis and Arthur, 1979 Schell, 1985
Gonocerca	Codfishes Grenadiers Righteye flounders	Stomach	Definitive host, fish; 1st intermediate host, mollusc; 2nd intermediate host, crustacean	Uncommon/common	Appy and Burt, 1982 Margolis and Arthur, 1979 Schell, 1985 Zubchenko, 1985
Helicometra	Scorpionfishes	Intestine	Definitive host, fish; 1st intermediate host, mollusc; 2nd intermediate host, arthropod or fish	Uncommon	Gaevskaya and Umnova, 1977 Margolis and Arthur, 1979 Schell, 1985
Hemiurus	Argentines Codfishes Grenadiers Herrings Righteye flounders Scorpionfishes Sculpins Smelts Sticklebacks Wrasses Wrymouths	Intestine Musculature Pyloric ceca Stomach	Definitive host, fish; 1st intermediate host, mollusc; 2nd intermediate host, crustacean	Common	Appy and Burt, 1982 Gaevskaya and Umnova, 1977 MacKenzie, 1987 Margolis and Arthur, 1979 Schell, 1985 Zubchenko, 1985
Lampritrema	Argentines Pomfrets	Gills Stomach	Definitive host, fish; 1st intermediate host, mollusc; 2nd intermediate host, crustacean	Common	Margolis and Arthur, 1979 Schell, 1985

Table continued on following page

TABLE 89–1. Parasites of Cold-Water Marine Fishes* *Continued*

Parasite (Phyla and Genera)	Hosts	Location on/in Hosts	Method of Infection	Prevalence	References
Lecithaster	Codfishes Cusk-eels Eelpouts Gobies Greenlings Herrings Pipefishes Pricklebacks Righteye flounders Sand lances Scorpionfishes Sculpins Smelts Snailfishes Sticklebacks Surfperches Wrasses Wrymouths	Intestine Pyloric ceca Rectum Stomach	Definitive host, fish; 1st intermediate host, mollusc; 2nd intermediate host, crustacean	Common	Appy and Burt, 1982 MacKenzie, 1987 Margolis and Arthur, 1979 Schell, 1985
Lecithochirium	Cusk eels Scorpionfishes	Stomach	Definitive host, fish; 1st intermediate host, mollusc; 2nd intermediate host, crustacean	Unknown	Margolis and Arthur, 1979 Schell, 1985
Lecithocladium	Mackerels	Stomach	Definitive host, fish; 1st intermediate host, mollusc; 2nd intermediate host, crustacean	Unknown	Moller and Anders, 1986
Lecithophyllum	Argentines Codfishes Greenlings Scorpionfishes Sculpins	Intestine Stomach	Definitive host, fish; 1st intermediate host, mollusc; 2nd intermediate host, crustacean	Common	Margolis and Arthur, 1979 Schell, 1985 Zubchenko, 1985
Lepidapedon	Butterfishes Codfishes Lefteye flounders Wrasses	Intestine Pyloric ceca	Definitive host, fish; 1st intermediate host, mollusc; 2nd intermediate host, invertebrate	Common	Appy and Burt, 1982 Gaevskaya and Umnova, 1977 Margolis and Arthur, 1979 Rodjuk, 1985 Schell, 1985
Lepidophyllum	Scorpionfishes Sculpins Wolffishes	Urinary bladder	Definitive host, fish; 1st intermediate host, mollusc; 2nd intermediate host, invertebrate	Common	Margolis and Arthur, 1979 Schell, 1985
Microphallus	Wrasses	Intestine Stomach	Definitive host, fish; 1st intermediate host, mollusc; 2nd intermediate host, arthropod	Uncommon	Margolis and Arthur, 1979 Schell, 1985
Neolepidapedon	Scorpionfishes	Intestine Pyloric ceca	Definitive host, fish; 1st intermediate host, mollusc; 2nd intermediate host, invertebrate	Unknown	Margolis and Arthur, 1979 Schell, 1985
Neophasis	Codfishes Righteye flounders Sculpins Wolffishes	Intestine Mesentery Stomach Urinary bladder	Definitive host, fish; 1st intermediate host, mollusc; 2nd intermediate host, invertebrate	Common	Appy & Burt, 1982 Margolis and Arthur, 1982 Schell, 1985
Neozoogonus	Surfperches	Intestine	Definitive host, fish; 1st intermediate host, mollusc; 2nd intermediate host, invertebrate	Common	Schell, 1985 Margolis and Arthur, 1979 Schell, 1985
Odhnerium	Molas	Intestine	Definitive host, fish; 1st intermediate host, mollusc; 2nd intermediate host, invertebrate	Unknown	Margolis and Arthur, 1979 Schell, 1985
Opechona	Herrings Scorpionfishes	Intestine Pyloric ceca	Definitive host, fish; 1st intermediate host, mollusc; 2nd intermediate host, invertebrate	Common	MacKenzie, 1987 Margolis and Arthur, 1979 Schell, 1985
Opecoeloides	Porgies	Intestine	Definitive host, fish; 1st intermediate host, mollusc; 2nd intermediate host, amphipod	Unknown	Gaevskaya and Umnova, 1977 Schell, 1985
Otodistomum	Codfishes Tonguefishes	Body cavity Liver	Definitive host, fish; 1st intermediate host, mollusc	Common	Appy and Burt, 1982 Schell, 1985
Parahemiurus	Codfishes Cusk-eels Eelpouts Greenlings Herrings Pipefishes	Intestine Pyloric ceca Stomach	Definitive host, fish; 1st intermediate host, mollusc	Uncommon	Margolis and Arthur, 1979 Schell, 1985

TABLE 89–1. Parasites of Cold-Water Marine Fishes* *Continued*

Parasite (Phyla and Genera)	Hosts	Location on/in Hosts	Method of Infection	Prevalence	References
Phyllodistomum	Scorpionfishes	Ureters Urinary bladder	Definitive host, fish; 1st intermediate host, mollusc; 2nd intermediate host, arthropod	Unknown	Margolis and Arthur, 1979 Schell, 1985
Plagioporus	Righteye flounders	Intestine Pyloric ceca	Definitive host, fish; 1st intermediate host, mollusc; 2nd intermediate host, arthropod	Unknown	Margolis and Arthur, 1979 Schell, 1985
Podocotyle	Codfishes Eelpouts Greenlings Gunnels Herrings Mackerels Poachers Pipefishes Righteye flounders Scorpionfishes Sculpins Sticklebacks	Intestine Pyloric ceca Stomach	Definitive host, fish; 1st intermediate host, mollusc; 2nd intermediate host, arthropod	Common	Appy and Burt, 1982 Margolis and Arthur, 1979 Schell, 1985
Prosorhynchus	Codfishes Cusk eels Righteye flounders Scorpionfishes Sculpins	Intestine, Muscle, and under Pyloric ceca Skin Stomach	Definitive host, fish; 1st intermediate host, mollusc; 2nd intermediate host, fish	Common	Appy and Burt, 1982 Korotaeva, 1985 Margolis and Arthur, 1979 Schell, 1985
Psettarium	Scorpionfishes	Heart	Definitive host, fish; 1st intermediate host, mollusc or annelid; 2nd intermediate host, unknown	Uncommon	Margolis and Arthur, 1979 Schell, 1985
Pseudopentagramma	Gobies Herrings Smelts	Intestine Pyloric ceca	Definitive host, fish; 1st intermediate host, mollusc; 2nd intermediate host, invertebrate	Uncommon	Margolis and Arthur, 1979 Schell, 1985
Ptychogonimus	Wrasses	Intestine	Definitive host, fish; 1st intermediate host, mollusc; 2nd intermediate host, crustacean	Uncommon	Margolis and Arthur, 1979 Schell, 1985
Rhipidocotyle	Cusk eels Herrings Sculpins	Fins Intestine Mouth Nasal cavities	Definitive host, fish; 1st intermediate host, mollusc; 2nd intermediate host, fish	Uncommon	MacKenzie, 1987 Margolis and Arthur, 1979 Schell, 1985
Steganoderma	Codfishes Grenadiers Righteye flounders Scorpionfishes Sculpins	Intestine Pyloric ceca	Definitive host, fish; 1st intermediate host, mollusc; 2nd intermediate host, invertebrate	Common	Appy and Burt, 1982 Margolis and Arthur, 1979 Schell, 1985 Zubchenko, 1985
Stenakron	Codfishes Righteye flounders Sculpins	Intestine Stomach	Definitive host, fish; 1st intermediate host, mollusc; 2nd intermediate host, invertebrate	Common	Appy and Burt, 1982 Margolis and Arthur, 1979
Stephanostomum	Codfishes Cusk eels Eelpouts Goosefishes Lefteye flounders Righteye flounders Scorpionfishes Sculpins Wrymouths	Fins Gills Intestine Musculature Pyloric ceca Rectum Skin	Definitive host, fish; 1st intermediate host, mollusc; 2nd intermediate host, fish	Common	Appy and Burt, 1982 Margolis and Arthur, 1979 Korotaeva, 1985
Steringotrema	Righteye flounders	Digestive tract Intestine Stomach	Definitive host, fish; 1st intermediate host, mollusc	Uncommon	Margolis and Arthur, 1979 Schell, 1985
Syncoelium	Pomfrets Scorpionfishes	Gills	Definitive host, fish; 1st intermediate host, mollusc; 2nd intermediate host, crustacean	Common	Margolis and Arthur, 1979 Schell, 1985
Telolechithus	Surfperches	Intestine	Definitive host, fish; 1st intermediate host, mollusc; 2nd intermediate host, mollusc	Uncommon	Margolis and Arthur, 1979 Schell, 1985
Tubulovesicula	Cusk-eels Lefteye flounders Pipefishes Righteye flounders Scorpionfishes Sculpins Surfperches Toadfishes	Intestine Stomach	Definitive host, fish; 1st intermediate host, mollusc; 2nd intermediate host, crustacean	Uncommon	Margolis and Arthur, 1979 Schell, 1985

Table continued on following page

TABLE 89–1. Parasites of Cold-Water Marine Fishes* *Continued*

Parasite (Phyla and Genera)	Hosts	Location on/in Hosts	Method of Infection	Prevalence	References
Zoogonoides	Righteye flounders	Digestive tract	Definitive host, fish; 1st intermediate host, mollusc; 2nd intermediate host, polychete	Common	Margolis and Arthur, 1979 Schell, 1979
CESTODA *Abothrium*	Codfishes Herrings Wrasses	Intestine Pyloric ceca	Definitive host, elasmobranch or fish; 1st intermediate host, crustacean; 2nd intermediate host, fish	Common	Appy and Burt, 1982 Margolis and Arthur, 1979 Rohde, 1984 Sindermann, 1970
Amphilina	Sturgeons	Body cavity	Definitive host, fish; 1st intermediate host, amphipod	Unknown	Rohde, 1984
Bothrimonus	Codfishes Eelpouts Righteye flounders Sculpins Sticklebacks	Intestine	Definitive host, fish; 1st intermediate host, amphipod	Unknown	Margolis and Arthur, 1979 Rohde, 1984
Bothriocephalus	Codfishes Eelpouts Gobies Greenlings Grenadiers Gunnels Herrings Jacks Lefteye flounders Righteye flounders Sand lances Scorpionfishes Sculpins Sticklebacks Smelts Wrasses	Intestine Pyloric ceca Stomach	Definitive host, fish; 1st intermediate host, copepod; 2nd intermediate host, fish	Unknown	MacKenzie, 1987 Margolis and Arthur, 1979 Rohde, 1984 Sindermann, 1970 Solonchenko, 1985 Zubchenko, 1985
Eubothrium	Smelts Wrasses	Intestine	Definitive host, fish; 1st intermediate host, crustacean; 2nd intermediate host, fish	Common	Margolis and Arthur, 1979 Moller and Anders, 1986 Sindermann, 1970
Gilquinia	Codfishes	Eye	Definitive host, elasmobranch; 1st intermediate host, copepod; 2nd intermediate host, fish and invertebrate	Common	Moller and Anders, 1986 Rohde, 1984
Grillotia	Codfishes Goosefishes Herrings Searobins	Body wall Mesentery Musculature Peritoneum Stomach wall Viscera	Definitive host, skate and ray; 1st intermediate host, copepod; 2nd intermediate host, fish and invertebrate	Common	Appy and Burt, 1982 Gaevskaya and Umnova, 1977 MacKenzie, 1987 Margolis and Arthur, 1979 Rohde, 1984 Zubchenko, 1985
Heptoxylon	Codfishes	Body cavity Viscera	Definitive host, elasmobranch; 1st intermediate host, copepod; 2nd intermediate host, fish and invertebrate	Common	Margolis and Arthur, 1979 Moller and Anders, 1986 Rohde, 1984
Lacistorhynchus	Herrings	Body cavity Intestine Musculature	Definitive host, elasmobranch; 1st intermediate host, crustacean; 2nd intermediate host-decapod and fish	Unknown	MacKenzie, 1987 Moller and Anders, 1986
Nybelinia	Codfishes Cusk-eels Eelpouts Herrings Scorpionfishes	Intestine Liver Mesenteries Musculature Stomach	Definitive host, elasmobranch; 1st intermediate host, copepod; 2nd intermediate host, fish	Common	Appy and Burt, 1982 Gaevskaya and Umnova, 1977 MacKenzie, 1987 Margolis and Arthur, 1979 Rohde, 1984
Phyllobothrium	Codfishes Cusk-eels Eelpouts Gobies Pipefishes Poachers Righteye flounders Sand lances Scorpionfishes Sculpins Smelts Sticklebacks	Gallbladder Intestine Stomach Pyloric ceca	Definitive host, elasmobranch and fish; 1st intermediate host, copepod; 2nd intermediate host, fish	Uncommon	Appy and Burt, 1982 Margolis and Arthur, 1979 Rohde, 1984

TABLE 89-1. Parasites of Cold-Water Marine Fishes* *Continued*

Parasite (Phyla and Genera)	Hosts	Location on/in Hosts	Method of Infection	Prevalence	References
Platybothrium	Sculpins	Intestine	Definitive host, elasmobranch or fish; 1st intermediate host, crustacean; 2nd intermediate host, fish	Uncommon	Margolis and Arthur, 1979 Rohde, 1984
Pyramicocephalus	Codfishes Lumpfishes Sculpins	Intestine Liver	Definitive host, pinniped; 1st intermediate host, crustacean; 2nd intermediate host, fish	Common	Margolis and Arthur, 1979 Rohde, 1984 Sindermann, 1970
Scolex	Numerous marine fishes	Alimentary canal Gallbladder Pyloric ceca	Definitive host, elasmobranch or teleost; 1st intermediate host, crustacean; 2nd intermediate host, fish and mollusc	Common	Gaevskaya and Umnova, 1977 MacKenzie, 1987 Rohde, 1984
Spatheobothrium	Codfishes Snailfishes	Stomach	Definitive host, fish; 1st intermediate host, amphipod	Uncommon	Appy and Burt, 1982 Rohde, 1984
Tentacularia	Codfishes	Mesentery	Definitive host, elasmobranch; 1st intermediate host, crustacean; 2nd intermediate host, fish or invertebrate	Uncommon	Appy and Burt, 1982 Rhode, 1984
NEMATODA *Anisakis*	All species are susceptible	Body cavity Intestine Mesenteries Muscle Stomach Viscera	Definitive host, cetacean; 1st intermediate host, crustacean; 2nd intermediate host, fish or squid; transport host, fish	Common	McClelland et al., 1983, 1985, 1987; pers. comm., 1989 Moller and Anders, 1986 Rohde, 1984
Ascarophis	Codfishes Greenlings Herrings Pricklebacks Scorpionfishes Sculpins Sticklebacks	Intestine Stomach Rectum	Definitive host, fish; 1st intermediate host, crustacean	Common	Appy and Burt, 1982 MacKenzie, 1987 Margolis and Arthur, 1979 Rohde, 1984 Sindermann, 1970
Camallanus	Mackerels	Intestine	Definitive host, fish; 1st intermediate host, crustacean	Unknown	Moller and Anders, 1986
Capillaria	Codfishes Eelpouts Greenlings Gunnels Righteye flounders Scorpionfishes Sculpins	Intestine Rectum Stomach	Definitive host, fish; 1st intermediate host, crustacean	Common	Appy and Burt, 1982 Gaevskaya and Umnova, 1977 Margolis and Arthur, 1979 Moller and Anders, 1986
Contracaecum	Anchovies Codfishes Cusk eels Eelpouts Gobies Greenlings Grenadiers Gunnels Herrings Lefteye flounders Mackerels Pipefishes Poachers Pricklebacks Sand lances Scorpionfishes Sculpins Smelts Sticklebacks Wrasses	Body cavity Intestine Liver Mesenteries Musculature Stomach Viscera	Definitive host, birds and mammals; 1st intermediate host, copepod; 2nd intermediate host, fish	Common	Appy and Burt, 1982 Gaevskaya and Umnova, 1977 Margolis and Arthur, 1979 Noble and Collard, 1970 Rohde, 1984 Zubchenko, 1985
Cucullanellus	Surfperches Wrasses	Intestine	Definitive host, fish; 1st intermediate host, planktonic invertebrate; 2nd intermediate host, fish	Common	Margolis and Arthur, 1979 Moller and Anders, 1986 Rohde, 1984
Cucullanus	Codfishes Cusk-eels Righteye flounders Scorpionfishes	Intestine Stomach Rectum	Definitive host, fish; 1st intermediate host, crustacean; 2nd intermediate host, fish	Common	Appy and Burt, 1982 Margolis and Arthur, 1979 Moller and Anders, 1986
Cystidicola	Herrings	Swimbladder	Definitive host, fish; 1st intermediate host, crustacean	Unknown	MacKenzie, 1987

Table continued on following page

TABLE 89–1. Parasites of Cold-Water Marine Fishes* *Continued*

Parasite (Phyla and Genera)	Hosts	Location on/in Hosts	Method of Infection	Prevalence	References
Hysterothylacium	Codfishes Eelpouts Herrings Mackerels	Body cavity Intestinal wall Mesentery Stomach	Definitive host, fish; 1st intermediate host, invertebrate; 2nd intermediate host, fish	Common	Appy and Burt, 1982 MacKenzie, 1987 Moller and Anders, 1986 Morrison et al., 1986 Rohde, 1984
Philometra	Codfishes Gunnels Righteye flounders Sticklebacks Swordfishes Wrasses	Body cavity Fins Gonad Head Intestine Subcutaneous tissue	Definitive host, fish; 1st intermediate host, copepod; 2nd intermediate host, fish	Common	Margolis and Arthur, 1979 Rohde, 1984
Phocascaris	Codfishes Wrasses	Intestinal wall Liver Viscera	Definitive host, mammal; 1st intermediate host, crustacean; 2nd intermediate host, fish	Unknown	Margolis and Arthur, 1979 McClelland et al., 1983 Moller and Anders, 1986
Pseudoterranova	All species are susceptible	Body cavity Mesenteries Musculature Viscera	Definitive host, seal; 1st intermediate host, invertebrate; 2nd intermediate host, fish	Common	McClelland et al., 1983, 1985, 1987; pers. comm., 1989
Thynascaris	Codfishes Cusk-eels Gunnels Herrings Mackerels Poachers Righteye flounders Sand lances Scorpionfishes Sculpins Sticklebacks	Body cavity Intestine Musculature Stomach Viscera	Unknown	Unknown	Margolis and Arthur, 1979
ACANTHOCEPHALA					
Bolbosoma	Codfishes	Intestine	Definitive host, cetacean; 1st intermediate host, crustacean; 2nd intermediate host, fish	Unknown	Arai, 1989a Dierauf, 1990
Cornyosoma	Codfishes Herrings Lefteye flounders Righteye flounders Sablefishes Scorpionfishes Sculpins Sturgeons Surfperches	Body cavity Intestinal wall Liver Mesenteries	Definitive host, pinniped, bird, or sea otter; 1st intermediate host, amphipod; transport host, fish	Common	Appy and Burt, 1982 Arai, 1989a Dierauf, 1990 Margolis and Arthur, 1979 Morrison et al., 1986 Rohde, 1984 Sindermann, 1970
Echinorhynchus	Codfishes Eelpouts Grenadiers Herrings Lefteye flounders Poachers Righteye flounders Sand lances Scorpionfishes Sculpins Smelts Sturgeons Surfperches Wolffishes Wrasses	Intestine Mesenteries Stomach	Definitive host, fish; 1st intermediate host, crustacean; transport host, fish	Common	Appy and Burt, 1982 Arai, 1989a Margolis and Arthur, 1979 Sindermann, 1970
Pomphorhynchus	Codfishes Eelpouts Herrings Righteye flounders Temperate basses	Gut wall Intestine Viscera	Definitive host, fish; 1st intermediate host, amphipod; transport host, fish	Common	MacKenzie, 1987 Moller and Anders, 1986 Rohde, 1984 Sindermann, 1970
Rhadinorhynchus	Herrings Sauries Swordfishes	Intestine	Definitive host, fish; 1st intermediate host, crustacean	Unknown	Arai, 1989a Margolis and Arthur, 1979
HIRUDINEA					
Abranchus	Sculpins	Body surface	Direct	Uncommon	Moller and Anders, 1986
Arctobdella	Righteye flounders	Body surface	Direct	Uncommon	Moller and Anders, 1986
Austrobdella	Lefteye flounders	Body surface	Direct	Common	Sawyer et al., 1975
Beringbdella	Codfishes	Buccal wall	Direct	Common	Madill, 1988
Branchellion	Lefteye flounders Wrasses	Body surface	Direct	Uncommon	Knight-Jones, 1962 Moller and Anders, 1986

TABLE 89–1. Parasites of Cold-Water Marine Fishes* *Continued*

Parasite (Phyla and Genera)	Hosts	Location on/in Hosts	Method of Infection	Prevalence	References
Calliobdella	Blennies Codfishes Eelpouts Goosefishes Herrings Lefteye flounders Righteye flounders Scorpionfishes Sculpins Searobins Toadfishes Wolffishes Wrasses	Body surface Fins	Direct	Uncommon	Appy and Dadswell, 1981 Knight-Jones, 1962 Madill, 1988 Meyer and Khan, 1979 Moller and Anders, 1986 Rohde, 1984 Sawyer, 1986 Sawyer et al., 1975
Ganymedebdella	Dragonets	Cloaca	Direct	Unknown	Knight-Jones, 1962
Hemibdella	Lefteye flounders Soles	Body surface	Direct	Uncommon	Moller and Anders, 1986 Anders, 1986 Sawyer, 1986
Johanssonia	Codfishes Eelpouts Righteye flounders Sculpins	Body surface Fins	Direct	Unknown	Margolis and Arthur, 1979 Sawyer, 1986
Janusion	Sculpins	Body surface	Direct	Uncommon	Moller and Anders, 1986
Malmiana	Codfishes Cusk-eels Righteye flounders Scorpionfishes Sculpins	Body surface Branchial cavity Eye Fins Gills	Direct	Common	Madill, 1988 Margolis and Arthur, 1979 Moller and Anders, 1986
Oceanobdella	Blennies Codfishes Eelpouts Lumpfishes Righteye flounders Sculpins	Body surface Branchial cavity Gills Fins Mouth	Direct	Common	Appy and Dadswell, 1981 Madill, 1988 Margolis and Arthur, 1979 Moller and Anders, 1986 Sawyer, 1986
Ostreobdella	Scorpionfishes	Body Head	Direct	Unknown	Madill, 1988
Ottoniobdella	Sculpins	Body surface	Direct	Uncommon	Moller and Anders, 1986
Piscicola	Scorpionfishes	Body surface	Direct	Unknown	Margolis and Arthur, 1979
Platybdella	Eelpouts Righteye flounders Sculpins Snailfishes Wolffishes Wrasses	Body surface Branchial cavity Gills Mouth	Direct	Uncommon	Knight-Jones, 1962 Madill, 1988 Meyer and Khan, 1979 Moller and Anders, 1986 Sawyer, 1986
Sanguinothus	Sculpins	Body surface Fins	Direct	Uncommon	Knight-Jones, 1962 Moller and Anders, 1986
COPEPODA *Acanthochondria*	Lefteye flounders Righteye flounders Sculpins Soles	Branchial cavity Buccal cavity	Direct	Common	Kabata, 1979, 1988
Alella	Porgies	Gills	Direct	Unknown	Kabata, 1979
Anchistrotos	Codfishes Lefteye flounders Sea basses	Gills Fins	Direct	Uncommon	Appy and Burt, 1982 Kabata, 1979
Anthosoma	Molas	Musculature/external	Direct	Uncommon	Kabata, 1979
Advena	Mackerels	Not noted	Direct	Uncommon	Kabata, 1979
Bomolochus	Codfishes Greenlings Herrings Pipefishes Sculpins Soles Sticklebacks Surfperches	Branchial cavity Nasal capsules	Direct	Common	Gaevskaya and Umnova, 1977 Kabata, 1979, 1988
Brachiella	Drums Mackerels Scorpionfishes	Fins	Direct	Common	Kabata, 1979

Table continued on following page

TABLE 89–1. Parasites of Cold-Water Marine Fishes* *Continued*

Parasite (Phyla and Genera)	Hosts	Location on/in Hosts	Method of Infection	Prevalence	References
Caligus	Chimaeras Codfishes Conger eels Dories Eelpouts Gobies Goosefishes Greenlings Herrings Jacks Lefteye flounders Lumpfishes Mackerels Molas Mullets Pomfrets Porgies Righteye flounders Sauries Scorpionfishes Searobins Soles Sticklebacks Temperate basses Wrasses	Buccal cavity Fins Skin	Direct	Common	Appy and Burt, 1982 Kabata, 1979, 1988 MacKenzie, 1987
Cecrops	Molas	Gills	Direct	Common	Kabata, 1979, 1988
Chondracanthodes	Grenadiers	Branchial cavity	Direct	Unknown	Kabata, 1988
Chondracanthus	Codfishes Cusk-eels Dories Dragonets Goosefishes Grenadiers Gunnels Righteye flounders Scorpionfishes Sculpins Swordfishes	Branchial cavity Gills Nasal capsules	Direct	Common	Katata, 1979, 1988
Claavella	Codfishes Dragonets Eelpouts Greenlings Grenadiers Scorpionfishes Sculpins Surfperches	Anal region Branchial cavity Fins Gills Mouth	Direct	Common	Appy and Burt, 1982 Kabata, 1979, 1988
Clavellisa	Herrings Mackerels	Gills	Direct	Uncommon	Kabata, 1979, 1988
Clavellistes	Opas	Eye Gills	Direct	Uncommon	Kabata, 1979
Clavellodes	Wolffishes	Gills	Direct	Common	Kabata, 1979, 1988
Clavellomimus	Grenadiers	Fins	Direct	Unknown	Kabata, 1988
Colobomatus	Scorpionfishes	Cephalic sensory canal	Direct	Common	Kabata, 1988
Congericola	Conger eels	Gills	Direct	Common	Kabata, 1979
Dichelesthium	Sturgeons	Branchial cavity	Direct	Common	Kabata, 1979, 1988
Diocus	Eelpouts Sculpins	Fins Branchial cavity	Direct	Uncommon	Kabata, 1988
Ergasilus	Herrings Mullets Silversides Smelts Sticklebacks Surfperches	Fins Gills Skin	Direct	Common	Kabata, 1979, 1988
Euryphorus	Mackerels Puffers	Body surface	Direct	Common	Kabata, 1979
Hemobaphes	Codfishes Dragonets Eelpouts Greenlings Gunnels Pipefishes Poachers Pricklebacks Righteye flounders Sand lances Scorpionfishes Sculpins Smelts Snailfishes Sticklebacks Surfperches	Branchial cavity	Definitive host, fish; 1st intermediate host, invertebrate or fish	Common	Kabata, 1979, 1988

TABLE 89–1. Parasites of Cold-Water Marine Fishes* *Continued*

Parasite (Phyla and Genera)	Hosts	Location on/in Hosts	Method of Infection	Prevalence	References
Hatschekia	Goatfishes Pomfrets Porgies Righteye flounders Wrasses	Gills	Direct	Common	Kabata, 1979, 1988
Holobomolochus	Codfishes Greenlings Lumpfishes Righteye flounders Scorpionfishes Sculpins; Sticklebacks Surfperches Wrasses	Branchial cavity	Direct	Common	Appy and Burt, 1982 Kabata, 1979, 1988
Lateracanthus	Grenadiers	Branchial cavity	Direct	Common	Zubchenko, 1985 Kabata, 1988
Lepeophtheirus	Codfishes Cusk-eels Greenlings Herrings Lefteye flounders Molas Righteye flounders Sablefishes Sand lances Scorpionfishes Sculpins Soles Sticklebacks Sturgeons Swordfishes	Branchial cavity Buccal cavity Gills Skin	Direct	Common	Kabata, 1979, 1988 Liewes, 1984
Lernanthropus	Drums Sea Basses	Gills	Direct	Common	Kabata, 1979
Lernaeocera	Codfishes Conger eels Dragonets Gobies Gunnels Herrings Lefteye flounders Lumpfishes Poachers Righteye flounders Sand lances Sculpins Sea basses Snailfishes Soles Wrasses	Blood vessels Body surface Gills Heart	Definitive host, usually gadids; intermediate host, usually righteye flounders; direct life cycle on dragonets and soles	Common	Appy and Burt, 1982 Kabata, 1979, 1988 Liewes, 1984 MacKenzie, 1987
Lernentoma	Searobins	Branchial cavity	Direct	Uncommon	Kabata, 1979
Luetkenia	Louvars	Gills Skin	Direct	Uncommon	Kabata, 1979
Lophoura	Cutthroat eels Grenadiers	Musculature	Direct	Uncommon	Kabata, 1979, 1988
Naobranchia	Lefteye flounders Righteye flounders Sablefishes Scorpionfishes Sculpins	Gill filaments	Direct	Unknown	Kabata, 1988
Nectobrachia	Codfishes Righteye flounders Scorpionfishes	Gills	Direct		Kabata, 1988
Neobrachiella	Codfishes Drums Righteye flounders Scorpionfishes Searobins	Gills Gill rakers	Direct	Common	Kabata, 1979, 1988
Orthagoriscicola	Molas	Body surface	Direct	Common	Kabata, 1979, 1988
Paeonocanthus	Deep-sea smelts	Musculature	Direct	Uncommon	Kabata, 1988
Peniculus	Scorpionfishes Sculpins	Fins	Definitive host, fish; intermediate host, invertebrate	Common	Kabata, 1988
Pennella	Frogfishes Goosefishes Mackerels Molas Porcupinefishes Swordfishes	Blood vessels Internal organs Musculature	Definitive host, fish; intermediate host, invertebrate or fish	Uncommon	Hogans, 1988 Kabata, 1979, 1984, 1988

Table continued on following page

TABLE 89–1. Parasites of Cold-Water Marine Fishes* *Continued*

Parasite (Phyla and Genera)	Hosts	Location on/in Hosts	Method of Infection	Prevalence	References
Philichthys	Swordfishes	Ducts and sinuses of frontal bones	Direct	Uncommon	Kabata, 1979
Philorthagoriscus	Sturgeons Molas	Body surface Eye	Direct	Common	Kabata, 1979, 1988
Phrixocephalus	Lefteye flounders Righteye flounders	Eye	Definitive host, fish; intermediate host, invertebrate or fish	Common	Kabata, 1988
Pseudocaligus	Codfishes Gobies	Body surface	Direct	Common	Kabata, 1979
Sarcotaces	Codfishes Scorpionfishes	Body wall Muscle Rectum	Direct	Unknown	Kabata, 1988
Sarcotretes	Lanternfishes	Musculature	Definitive host, fish; intermediate host, invertebrate or fish	Unknown	Kabata, 1988
Scianophilus	Drums	Body surface	Direct	Uncommon	Kabata, 1979
Sphyrion	Codfishes Grenadiers Lumpfishes Moras Righteye flounders Scorpionfishes Wolffishes	Musculature/external	Direct Direct	Common	Kabata, 1979, 1988
Tanypleurus	Eelpouts	Gills	Direct	Unknown	Kabata, 1988
Thersitina	Sticklebacks	Branchial cavity	Direct	Common	Kabata, 1979
Vanbenedenia	Chimaeras	Dorsal spine	Direct	Uncommon	Kabata, 1979
BRANCHIURA					
Argulus	Codfishes Greenlings Herrings Killifishes Righteye flounders Silversides Scorpionfishes Surfperches	Body surface Fins Skin	Direct	Common	Kabata, 1988 MacKenzie, 1987
ISOPODA					
Aega	Codfishes Righteye flounders Sculpins	Skin	Direct	Uncommon	Appy and Burt, 1982 Rafi, 1988 Richardson, 1905
Cirolana	Codfishes	Ovaries	Direct	Unknown	Moller and Anders, 1986 Schultz, 1982
Lironeca	Cusk-eels Herrings Jacks Lefteye flounders Scorpionfishes Surfperches Temperate basses	Branchial cavity Buccal cavity	Direct—juveniles may temporarily attach to fish species other than that on which they mature	Unknown	Brusca, 1981 Rafi, 1988 Schultz, 1982 Sindermann, 1970
Rocinela	Codfishes Righteye flounders Scorpionfishes	Skin	Direct	Common	Rafi, 1988 Richardson, 1905 Schultz, 1982
AMPHIPODA					
Lafystius	Codfishes Eelpouts Goosefishes Righteye flounders Sculpins Sturgeons	Body surface Fins Mouth Operculum Skin	Direct	Common	Bousfield, 1987, Bousfield and Kabata, 1988
Normanion	Codfishes Goosefishes	Skin	Direct	Common	Bousfield, 1987 Sars, 1895
Opisa	Codfishes Greenlings Righteye flounders Scorpionfishes	Body surface Fins Gills	Direct	Unknown	Bousfield, 1987
Paralafystius	Scorpionfishes	Skin	Probably Direct	Unknown	Bousfield, 1987
Protolafystius	Righteye flounders	Gills	Probably Direct	Unknown	Bousfield, 1987
MOLLUSCA					
Mytilus	Codfishes	External—parasitic on copepods	Direct	Uncommon	Moller and Anders, 1986

*The table lists parasites, their hosts, life cycle, prevalence, and references. Names of fishes and their geographical distribution are in accordance with Eschmeyer et al. (1983), Robins et al (1980), Scott and Scott (1988), and Wheeler (1987). The terminology of parts of the life cycles follows Post (1987).

EIMERIA SPP.

SYNONYMS. Coccidiosis, eimeriasis.

Hosts and Geographic Distribution

Eimeria is a member of the phylum Apicomplexa, subclass Coccidiasina (Lee et al., 1985). Eimeriid coccidia are common parasites in marine fishes and may infect most coastal species, particularly members of the herring family (Lom, 1984).

Clinical Appearance and Diagnosis

Fish infected with *Eimeria* usually show few or no obvious clinical signs. *Eimeria* spp. may infect the intestine or other sites, such as the kidney, liver, swimbladder, and testes. The thin-walled, spherical oocysts of *Eimeria* found in fish range from 20 to 40 μm in diameter. Each contains four sporocysts that contain two curved, elongated sporozoites. The egg-shaped sporocyst has a steida body plugging the polar aperture for sporozoite release (Dykova and Lom, 1981; Lom, 1984; Moller and Anders, 1986). In most species, little more than the oocysts and the site of infection in their hosts has been described (Dykova and Lom, 1981).

Pathologic Effects and Pathogenesis

The pathogenicity of coccidia infecting fish is poorly known (Dykova and Lom, 1981). The pathology caused by species, such as *Eimeria variabilis,* that infect the digestive tract is generally low (Lom, 1984). The extent of damage and the nature of the tissue reaction is dependent upon the intensity of the infection and the depth in the intestinal wall reached by the developmental stages of the parasite (Dykova and Lom, 1981). Certain extra-intestinal infections may be fatal (Lom, 1984). In *Eimeria funduli* infections in killfishes, organ changes are characterized by a decrease or elimination of functional parenchyma. Other *Eimeria* sp. infections in the liver may be accompanied by inflammation, granulomas, and destruction of host tissue (Dykova and Lom, 1981).

Life Cycle, Transmission, and Epidemiology

The life cycle of coccidia is completely intracellular (Lom, 1984) and usually involves only the fish host. The cycle comprises (1) reproduction (merogony), (2) formation and copulation of gametes (gametogony), and (3) development of the zygote into sporozoite infective stages (sporogony). Infection is by oral ingestion. An invertebrate paratenic host may be necessary for the life cycle of some species of *Eimeria* (Dykova and Lom, 1981; Lom, 1984).

Treatment and Control

Acetarsone, calcium chloride, and furoxone have been used to treat *Eimeria* infection (Herwig, 1979). None of these drugs is approved for use in food fishes, and efficacy is questionable. There are no known public health concerns with this parasite.

HAEMOGREGARINA SACHAI

SYNONYM. Parasitic myeloid leukosis.

Hosts and Geographic Distribution

Hemogregarines are the most common blood parasites of marine fishes. They belong to the suborder Adeleorina of the subclass Coccidiasina (Lee et al., 1985). *Haemogregarina* spp. infect cod, lefteyed flounders, righteyed flounders, sculpins, eelpout, and gunnel. In North American waters, they have more frequently been recorded from the Atlantic than the Pacific (Margolis and Arthur, 1979).

Clinical Appearance and Diagnosis

Cultured turbot infected with *Haemogregarina sachai* show subcutaneous or ulcerated nodules, prolapsed rectums, pigmentary nervous control failure, and exophthalmos (Ferguson and Roberts, 1975). All of these signs can be ascribed to space occupying granulomas. Ascites and tumorlike lesions with necrotic centers occur in lymphoreticular tissue, musculature, and viscera (Ferguson, 1989; Ferguson and Roberts, 1975; Kirmse, 1980; Kirmse and Ferguson, 1976; Lom, 1984). The granulomatous lesions are creamy white–yellow, up to 4 cm in diameter, with a thick, fibrous capsule that contains the parasites (Ferguson and Roberts, 1975; Kirmse, 1980; Kirmse and Ferguson, 1976). Approximately one-third of blood cells may be parasitized. Parasites in the white blood cells are 5.2 to 8.1 μm long and ovoid to slender (Fig. 89–2). Those in the red blood cells are 6.2 μm long. More than one parasite may be present per cell (Kirmse, 1978, 1980). Other stages are free in the plasma. Invaded blood cells are hypertrophied (Kirmse, 1978).

Pathologic Effects and Pathogenesis

Lethal myeloid leukosis in cultured turbot has been attributed to *Haemogregarina sachai* (Ferguson and Roberts, 1975). There is a leukocytosis and anemia as well as a marked parasitemia (Ferguson and Roberts, 1975; Ferguson, 1989). For many years these parasites have been considered benign, but recently their pathogenic potential in aquaculture has been demonstrated (Sindermann, 1985).

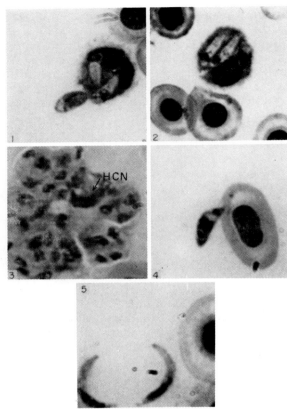

FIGURE 89–2. *Hemogregarina sachai. A.* Merozoite entering or leaving a monocyte, which already contains two merozoites (1600×). *B.* Monocyte with two merozoites (1250×). *C.* Large schizont with 36 nuclei, some of which are undergoing further division. The host cell nucleus (HCN) is laterally compressed (2500×). *D.* Merozoite penetrating an erythrocyte (E) (2750×). *E.* A pair of free microgametocytes among erythrocytes (2000×). (From Kirmse, P. D. [1978] *Haemogregarina sachai* n.sp. from cultured turbot *Scophthalmus mahimus* in Scotland. J. Fish Dis. 1:337–342.)

Life Cycle, Transmission, and Epidemiology

The life cycle of *Haemogregarina* spp. involves a fish and an invertebrate. Proliferative stages occur in the white and then red blood cells of a vertebrate host (Kirmse, 1978). Gamete and spore production occur in blood-sucking invertebrate vectors such as the leech, *Hemibdella solea,* and the crustaceans, *Gnathia* (isopods), and *Lernaeocera* sp. (copepods) (Lom, 1984; Moller and Anders, 1986). Fish probably become infected by the feeding activities of blood-sucking parasites, or by eating isopods that have mature sporozoites in their intestine. There have been some reports of apparently spontaneous infections (Lom, 1984).

Treatment and Control

No effective treatment or control measures are reported. There are no known public health considerations with this disease.

GLUGEA STEPHANI

SYNONYM. *Nosema stephani* (Canning and Lom, 1986).

Host and Geographic Distribution

Glugea stephani (phylum Microspora) is a small, unicellular parasite that commonly infects righteye flounders, such as plaice, flounders, and sole along both coasts of North America, the North Sea, the Baltic Sea, the Black Sea, and seas around England.

Clinical Appearance and Diagnosis

Abdominal enlargement may be evident in fishes infected with with *Glugea.* Whitish xenomas (hypertrophic host cells) 1 mm in diameter are present in the gut wall and may replace its structure. The gut becomes rigid and thickened, with a chalk-white, pebbled appearance. The mucosal epithelium may be lost. In heavy infections, xenomas may also be in the mesentery, liver, bile duct, pancreas, mesenteric lymph nodes, and ovary.

Cylindrical, dividing meronts have three to eight nuclei (Fig. 89–3). Sporoblast mother cells are in groups of eight or more per sporophorous vesicle. Fresh, oval spores are 4.2 to 5.2 × 2.3 to 2.8 μm. The posterior vacuole, with a straight anterior limit, reaches the middle of the spore. The polar filament has 12 to 14 coils (Canning and Lom, 1986).

Pathologic Effects and Pathogenesis

The infected host cell absorbs nutrients from surrounding tissue and enlarges to accommodate proliferating parasites. The nucleus enlarges, with multiple nucleoli. Such hypertrophic cells are termed xenomas. In heavy infections, the intestine is nonfunctional, and fish lose weight rapidly. Mortalities associated with *Glugea stephani* have occurred in

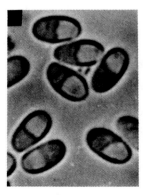

FIGURE 89–3. Fresh spores of *Glugea stephani.* (From Canning, E. U., and Lom, J. [1986] The Microsporidia of Vertebrates. Academic Press, London.)

aquaria and a farm (Canning and Lom, 1986; Liewes, 1984).

Life Cycle, Transmission, and Epidemiology

Glugea stephani is an obligate, intracellular parasite with a direct life cycle needing only a fish. Crustacean prey may act as reservoirs of infection (Canning and Lom, 1986). Ingested spores hatch in the gut and enter epithelial cells for development or transport to the developmental site. A minute tube, the polar filament, then everts through the spore wall and penetrates a host cell. The infective agent, or sporoplasm, passes via the filament to the host cytoplasm, where multiplication or merogony occurs. The second developmental stage, sporogony, produces spores packed in vesicles or membranes. *Glugea* spores may be released from the skin, in feces, in urine, or on death of the host (Canning and Lom, 1986). For establishment and development of infections, 16°C or higher is necessary (Lom, 1986). Juvenile fish are particularly susceptible to infection (Canning and Lom, 1986).

Treatment and Control

Calcium cyanamide is reported to be effective in destroying *Glugea* spores (Herwig, 1979). This compound is not approved for use in food fishes. No public health considerations are known for this parasite.

CRYPTOCOTYLE LINGUA

SYNONYMS. Black spot, black spot disease, melanosis, pigment spot disease.

Hosts and Geographic Distribution

Many species of coastal fishes often exhibit pinhead-sized black spots in their skin, fins, and eyes caused by larval digenean trematodes. In the north Atlantic, the condition is usually caused by the metacercaria of *Cryptocotyle lingua*. *Cryptocotyle lingua* infects many fishes, particularly herring and cod, from shallow waters where the first intermediate hosts, the snails *Littorina* spp., are found (Moller and Anders, 1986; Sindermann et al., 1978). Fishes with very thick or slimy skins do not become infected (Moller and Anders, 1986). *Cryptocotyle lingua* is very common in northern Europe and North America.

Clinical Appearance and Diagnosis

Black spots about 1 mm in diameter are seen in the skin, fins, and eyes. The disease is most obvious in fishes with white or silver skins, such as herring or smelt.

The cyst, containing a metacercaria, usually lies just beneath the epidermis. Less frequently it is found in the fillet or on internal organs. Melanin is deposited in the cyst membrane and in the surrounding host tissue capsule. The metacercaria resembles the adult digenean, having an oral and ventral sucker and a bifurcate gut.

Pathologic Effects and Pathogenesis

The thin, flexible cyst secreted by the cercaria becomes surrounded by host tissue (Rohde, 1984; Smyth, 1976). Development to the metacercaria elicits the gradual accumulation of melanophores around the cysts, resulting in a black spot. The size and intensity of the spot is dependent upon length of time after invasion (Sindermann et al., 1978).

Fish larvae and juveniles may be killed by a few cercariae if they penetrate the brain or heart. The effect on adult fish is minimal unless vital organs are infected. Metacercariae in the eye cause exophthalmos and blindness (Mawdesley-Thomas and Young, 1967; Sindermann and Rosenfield, 1954). Heavy infestations are fatal (Rohde, 1984; Sindermann and Rosenfield, 1954).

Life Cycle, Transmission, and Epidemiology

Cryptocotyle lingua has an indirect life cycle requiring three hosts. The definitive host, usually a sea gull, harbors adult flukes in its digestive tract. Eggs, in which miracidia develop, are shed in the feces. When miracidia infect shore snails (*Littorina* spp.), they develop into sporocysts, rediae, and cercariae. Subsequently, free-swimming ceracariae, with two distinct dark eye spots, emerge and penetrate the surface of a fish. There they encyst and transform into metacercariae. The cycle is completed when a bird eats an infected fish (Sindermann et al., 1978; Smyth, 1976).

Treatment, Control, and Public Health Considerations

Di-*N*-butyl tin oxide, among other compounds, has been used to treat for digenetic trematodes (Herwig, 1979; Stoskopf, 1988); however, this compound is not approved for use in food fishes and has severe detrimental environmental effects. Copper sulfate can be used against snails, the intermediate host (Schnick, 1988), but is also environmentally damaging.

Although *C. lingua* may be transferred to man via ingestion of infected raw fish, the pathologic effect is usually not serious (Moller and Anders,

1986). Heavy infections may hinder fish marketing due to esthetic and health concerns.

ANISAKIS SPP.

SYNONYMS. Anisakiasis, herring worm disease.

Hosts and Geographic Distribution

Nematodes of the genus *Anisakis* cause disease in fish and in man and reduce the commercial value of affected fish (Rohde, 1984); larvae of *A. simplex,* the most common species, occur worldwide and all species of fishes are susceptible.

Clinical Appearance and Diagnosis

Fishes with anisakiasis, or herring worm disease, show no external signs. In live fish, larvae may be free or coiled in capsules of host connective tissue. They can be found on or in the viscera, body cavity, skeletal muscles, and mesenteries (Fig. 89–4). The distribution varies with fish host age and length (Smith and Wootten, 1978). After the host fish dies, larvae leave the capsules and can enter skeletal muscles, especially the hypaxial parts around the body cavity. Larvae in fish flesh can be viewed by candling (examining fillets on a glass screen, light from below). The colorless larvae, 10 to 25 mm long, lie in spirals in the muscle and may be moving.

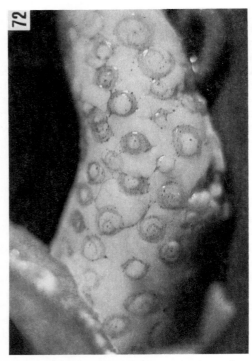

FIGURE 89–4. Larvae of *Anisakis simplex* in the liver of a codfish. (From Möller, H., and Anders, K. [1986] Diseases and Parasites of Marine Fishes. Verlag Möller, Kiel.)

Pathologic Effects and Pathogenesis

Anisakis larvae are not serious pathogens of marine fishes (Moller and Anders, 1986; Rohde, 1984; Smith and Wootten, 1978). However, larvae attached to or embedded in the liver may cause compression and mechanical damage. They may also rupture blood vessels, causing hemorrhage and thrombus formation (Hauck and May,1977; Mikhailova et al., 1964; Prusevich, 1964; Rohde, 1984).

Life Cycle, Transmission, and Epidemiology

Anisakis has an indirect life cycle requiring at least krill (Euphausiidae) and baleen whales. Adult nematodes commonly occur in whales, dolphins, and porpoises. Eggs shed with the host feces hatch in seawater. Emerged larvae swim and are eaten by planktonic crustaceans, particularly euphausiids (McClellend et al., 1983), and molt to the third stage. When these crustaceans are eaten by a fish or squid, larvae penetrate the host's digestive tract. Larvae may pass through a series of nektonic hosts without further molts. Gradually, larvae are concentrated in several large predatory fish species. The life cycle is completed when these fish are eaten by marine mammals.

Treatment, Control, and Public Health Considerations

The spread of *Anisakis* to freshwater fishes is minimized by avoiding marine trash fishes as aquacultural feeds (Smith and Wootten, 1978). No effective methods of treatment are known. Live third-stage larvae consumed in raw or inadequately pickled or cooked fish do not complete maturation in man. They do cause serious gastrointestinal damage, manifested by acute pain, vomiting, diarrhea, fever, and blood in stools. Chronic lesions may also be present (Moller and Anders, 1986). Larvae can penetrate the digestive tract and enter the body cavity (Ishikura et al., 1967). The treatment of the infection in humans involves endoscopic removal of the parasite. No effective drug therapy is known.

Anisakiasis can be avoided by rapid evisceration of caught fish, trimming of hypaxial parts of the body muscle when preparing fillets, deep freezing to $-30°C$, and sufficient marination or thorough cooking.

PSEUDOTERRANOVA DECIPIENS

SYNONYMS. *Phocanema, Porrocaecum decipiens, Terranova decipiens,* Codworm, Sealworm.

Hosts and Geographic Distribution

Pseudoterranova decipiens, an anisakid nematode, is one of the most common nematodes of marine fishes. The larvae are pathogenic to fish, can infect man, and are a serious problem for the fishing industry (McClellend et al., 1983). All marine fishes are susceptible to infection, particularly bottom fishes belonging to the cod, flatfish, and sculpin families (McClellend et al., 1983). Larvae are most common in fish from coastal areas or near islands. Increasing infection in certain Canadian cod stocks has precluded their exploitation.

Clinical Appearance and Diagnosis

The infection is most conspicuous in smelts, sculpin, and flatfishes in which the parasite can be seen through the skin. Heavily infected fishes are emaciated and in poor condition.

Larval distribution in infected fish and the proportion of worms that are encapsulated or free varies between host species (Kahl, 1938). In cod, worms are most common in muscle and in the body cavity. Only some parasites are encapsulated (McClelland et al, 1983). In smelt, larvae are most common in the head and tail and are found in large cavities in the muscle.

The infective L3 stage of *P. decipiens* is the largest larval nematode in fish. It reaches up to 60 mm long (McClelland et al., 1983). When the loose connective tissue capsules and worms degenerate, the worms turn from red to brown.

Pathologic Effects and Pathogenesis

The impact of *P. decipiens* varies according to host species. *P. decipiens* commonly infects West German smelt, causing extensive tissue damage, emaciation, and a decrease in condition factor (Klatt, 1985; Rohde, 1984). In Icelandic cod, the number of larvae and the condition of the host fish are positively correlated. Both parameters increase with the amount of food eaten (Palsson et al.,1985).

Life Cycle, Transmission, and Epidemiology

Pseudoterranova decipiens has an indirect life cycle (Fig. 89–5). It needs benthic macrofauna and a seal to complete the cycle. However, in the usual cycle, adult worms in the seal final host produce eggs that are shed with the seal feces and sink. Emerging larvae attach to the bottom substrate and are eaten by benthic meiofauna, mainly copepods. Then benthic macrofauna, such as amphipods and polychetes, eat the meiofauna or are infected directly. Demersal fishes are infected by eating benthic

macrofauna. Piscivorous demersal fishes acquire *P. decipiens* from their prey. The cycle is completed when seals eat infected fishes (McClelland et al., 1983).

Pseudoterranova decipiens abundance in fishes varies with geographic area and increases with the growth of seal populations. The prevalence and abundance in fishes increases with fish host length (McClellend et al., 1985; 1987).

Treatment, Control, and Public Health Considerations

Biologic and technical solutions to the sealworm problem are discussed by McClelland et al. (1983). No effective drug therapy is available. Consumed live larvae cause epigastric pain when they enter the gastric mucosa, but the disease is self-limiting, as larvae die. Most human infections occur in Japan (Margolis, 1977). Larval detection and removal from fish for cosmetic and health reasons increases processing costs.

LERNAEOCERA SPP.

SYNONYMS. Three species of *Lernaeocera* are valid (Kabata, 1979). Their synonyms are (1) *Lernaeocera branchialis—Lernaea branchialis, Lernaea gobina, Lernaeocera caparti, Lernaeocera megacephala, Lernaeocera obtusa, Lernaeocera wilsoni, Lernoela branchialis;* (2) *Lernaeocera lusci—Lernaea lusci, Lernaeocera brevicollis, Lernaeocera mulli, Lernaeocera phycidis;* (3) *Lernaeocera minuta—Lernaea minuta* (Kabata,1979).

Hosts and Geographic Distribution

Lernaeocera spp. are parasitic crustaceans (subclass Copepoda, family Pennellidae) with large pathogenic hematophagous adult females (Kabata, 1979). *Lernaea branchialis,* the most common species, occurs in the North Atlantic and adjacent seas. *Lernaea lusci* occurs in the European Atlantic Ocean and *L. minuta* throughout the North Sea. Hosts include blennies, bullrout, codfishes, dragonets, eelpout, left-eyed flatfishes, righteyed flatfishes, goby, hakes, hooknose, lumpsuckers, and sea snails, sandeels, snailfishes, soles, weevers, and wrasse (Kabata 1979, 1988; Khan, 1988).

Clinical Appearance and Diagnosis

Numerous juvenile parasites may infect the gill tips of intermediate hosts. Adult females, the most common stage seen, attach in low numbers at the bases of the gill arch of the definitive host fish. The female parasite's dark red body, readily seen under the operculum, grows from a sticklike shape to a thick S shape with egg strings attached. Its head

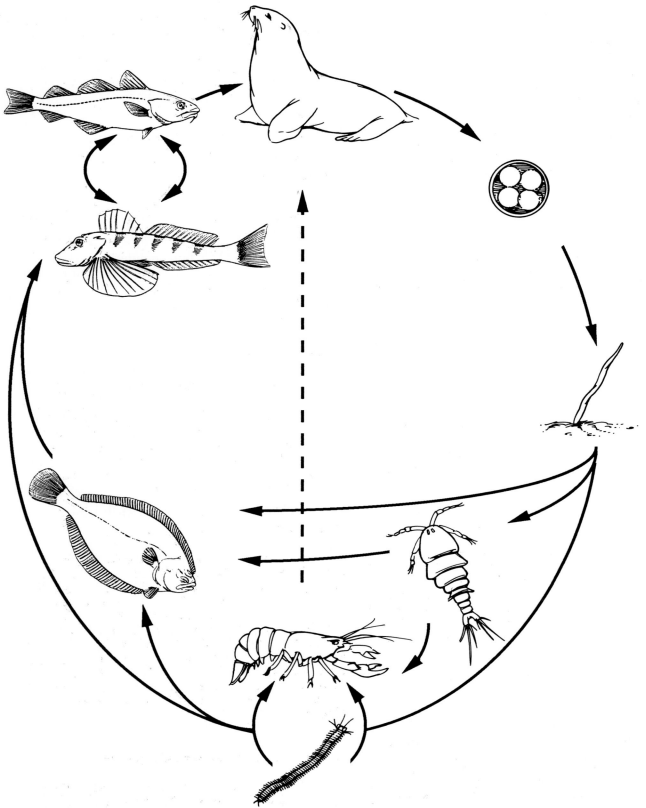

FIGURE 89–5. The life cycle of *Pseudoterranova decipiens,* the seal worm. Harbor, ringed, gray, and other seals pass developing ova in the feces. On hatching the larva adhere to substrates. Benthic copepods and macroinvertebrates carry larvae in their hemocoeles. Fish become infected by ingesting crustacean hosts or other infected fish. Seals are reinfected through ingestion of infected fishes or crustaceans.

embeds in a major blood vessel, often in the heart. *Lernaea branchialis* may reach 60 mm in length (Kabata, 1988). After the parasite has died, a granuloma remains. *Lernaea lusci* may attach near the pectoral fins. Affected fish may be thinner than uninfected fish.

The holdfast, or attachment structure, of the parasite has one dorsal and two lateral branching antlers. The neck expands abruptly into the trunk, which, jointly with the abdomen, is sigmoid. Egg sacs loop irregularly around a stalk (Kabata, 1988).

Pathologic Effects and Pathogenesis

Juvenile parasites can be benign or may induce swollen gills and poor condition (Kabata, 1979; Moller and Anders, 1986). The adult female parasite causes pressure atrophy of the gills, impaired opercular function, and increased hydrodynamic resistance (Smith, 1975). Attachment into the circulatory system causes connective tissue hypertrophy, blood-filled spaces, thickening of the heart walls (reducing its volume), and probable occlusion of major blood vessels (Khan, 1988; Sindermann, 1966). *Lernaeocera branchialis* induces blood loss, emaciation, open lesions, and reductions in fat content and reproductive capacity. Up to 30% of fish hosts die (Khan, 1988). This parasite causes serious economic problems (Kabata, 1979) and may transmit the protozoan *Hemogregarina simondi* (Moller and Anders, 1986).

Life Cycle, Transmission, and Epidemiology

Lernaeocera branchialis needs two hosts. The youngest nauplius stages are free-living. On the intermediate host, usually a flatfish, the copepodid stage attaches and develops through four attached chalimus larval stages. At the preadult stage, mating occurs. After copulation males die, and females swim to the final host, usually a gadoid (Moller and Anders, 1986). *Lernaeocera lusci* needs only the sole for completion of its life cycle. *Lernaeocaera branchialis* is more prevalent on young than old fish (Khan, 1988).

Treatment and Control

Although a variety of anticrustacean treatments exist, none are particularly effective. Manual removal may be appropriate (Stoskopf, 1988). There is no known public health significance.

LITERATURE CITED

Appy, R.G., and Burt, M.D.B. (1982) Metazoan parasites of Cod, *Gadus morhua* L., in Canadian Atlantic Waters. Can. J. Zool. 60:1573–1579.

Appy, R.G., and Dadswell, M.J. (1981) Marine and estuarine piscicolid leeches (Hirudinea) of the Bay of Fundy and adjacent waters with a key to species. Can. J. Zool. 59:183–192.

Arai, H.P. (1989a) Acanthocephala. In: Guide to the Parasites of Fishes of Canada. Part III (Margolis, L., and Kabata, Z., eds.). Canadian Special Publication of Fisheries and Aquatic Sciences, 107:95, pp. 1–90.

Arai, M.N. (1989b) Cnidaria. In: Guide to the Parasites of Fishes of Canada. Part III (Margolis, L., and Kabata, Z., eds.). Canadian Special Publication of Fisheries and Aquatic Sciences, 107:95, pp. 91–95.

Beverley-Burton, M. (1984) Monogenea and turbellaria. In: Guide to the Parasites of Fishes of Canada. Part I (Margolis, L., and Kabata, Z., eds.). Canadian Special Publication of Fisheries and Aquatic Sciences, 74:209, pp. 5–209.

Bousfield, E.L. (1987) Amphipod parasites of fishes of Canada. Can. Bull. Fish. Aquatic Sci. 217:37.

Bousfield, E.L., and Kabata, Z. (1988) Amphipoda. In: Guide to the Parasites of Fishes of Canada. Part II—Crustacea (Margolis, L., and Kabata, Z., eds.). Canadian Special Publication of Fisheries and Aquatic Sciences, 101:184, pp. 149–163.

Brusca, R.C. (1981) A monograph on the Isopoda Cymothoidae (Crustacea) of the eastern Pacific. Zool. J. Linnean Soc. 73:117–199.

Burreson, E.M. (1982) The life cycle of *Trypanoplasma bullocki* (Zoomastigophorea: Kinetoplastida). J. Protozool. 29:72–77.

Burreson, E.M., and Zwerner, D.E. (1982) The role of host biology, vector biology, and temperature in the distributions of *Trypanoplasma bullocki* infections in the lower Chesapeake Bay. J. Parasitol. 6:306–313.

Burreson, E.M., and Zwerner, D.E. (1984) Juvenile summer flounder, *Paralichthys dentatus*, mortalities in the western Atlantic Ocean caused by the hemoflagellate *Trypanoplasma bullocki*: evidence from field and experimental studies. Helgolander Meeresuntersuchungen 37:343–352.

Canning, E.U., and Lom, J. (1986). The Microsporidia of Vertebrates. Academic Press, London. p. 289.

Conservation and Utilization Division, North East Fisheries Center (1988). Status of the Fishery Resources off the Northeastern United States for 1988. National Oceanic and Atmospheric Administration (NOAA), Technical Memorandum NMFS–F/NEC–63, U.S. Department of Commerce, Washington, D.C.

Daily, D.D. (1978) Marine fish hematozoa from Maine. J. Parasitol. 64(2):361–362.

Dierauf, L.A. (1990) CRC Handbook of Marine Mammal Medicine. CRC Press, Boca Raton, Florida.

Dykova, I., and Lom, J. (1981) Fish coccidia: critical notes on life cycles, classification and pathogenicity. J. Fish Dis. 4:487–505.

Dykova, I., and Lom, J. (1983) Fish coccidia: an annotated list of described species. Folia Paraiitol. (Praha) 30:193–208.

Egorova, T.P. (1985) New data on the capsalid fauna of the World Ocean and questions of its specificity. In: Parasitology and Pathology of Marine Organisms of the World Ocean (Hargis, W.J., ed.). NOAA Technical Report NMFS 25. U.S. Department of Commerce, National Oceanic and Atmospheric Administration, National Marine Fisheries Service, Washington, D.C. pp. 75–76.

Eschmeyer, W.N., Herald, E.S., and Hammann, H. (1983) A Field Guide to Pacific Coast Fishes. Houghton Mifflin, Boston.

Ferguson, H.W. (1989) Systemic Pathology of Fish. Iowa State University Press, Ames, pp. 263.

Ferguson, H.W., and Roberts, R.J. (1975) Myeloid leucosis associated with sporozoan infection in cultured turbot (*Scophthalmus maximus*). J. Comp. Pathol. 85:317–326.

Gaevskaya, A.V., and Umnova, B.A. (1977) Parasitic fauna of the principal commercial fishes of the Northwest Atlantic. Sov. J. Marine Biol. 3:274–280.

Hargis, W.J. (ed.). (1985) Parasitology and pathology of marine organisms of the world ocean. NOAA Technical Report NMFS 25. U.S. Department of Commerce, National Oceanic and Atmospheric Administration, National Marine Fisheries Service, Washington, D.C., pp. 135.

Hauck, A.K., and May, E.B. (1977) Histopathologic alterations associated with *Anisakis* larvae in Pacific herring from Oregon. J. Wildlife Dis. 13:290–293.

Herwig, N. (1979) Handbook of Drugs and Chemicals Used in the Treatment of Fish Diseases. Charles C Thomas, Springfield, Illinois, p. 272.

Hogans, W.E. (1988) Redescription of *Penella sagitta* (Copepoda: Pennellidae) from *Histrio histrio* (Pisces) in the North-West Atlantic Ocean with a provisional revision of the genus *Pennella*. J. Zool. 216:379–390.

Ishikura, H., Hayasaka, H., and Kikuchi, Y. (1967) Acute regional ileitis at Iwanai in Hokkaido—with special reference to intestinal anisakiasis. Sapporo Med. J. 32:183–196.

Kabata, Z. (1979) Parasitic Copepoda of British Fishes. The Ray Society, London.

Kabata, Z. (1984) Diseases caused by metazoans: Crustaceans. In: Diseases of Marine Animals. Vol. IV. Part 1, Introduction and Pisces (Kinne, O., ed.). Biologische Anstalt Helgoland, Hamburg, pp. 321–399.

Kabata, Z. (1988) Copepoda and Branchiura. In: Guide to the Parasites of Fishes of Canada. Part II—Crustacea (Margolis, L., and Kabata, Z., eds.). Canadian Special Publication of Fisheries and Aquatic Sciences, 101:184, pp. 3–127.

Kahl, W. (1938) Nematoden in Seefischen. I. Erhebungen uber die durch larven von *Porrocaecum decipiens* Krabbe in fischwirten hervorgerufenen geweglichen veranderungen und kapselbildungen. Z. Parasitenkunde 10:415–431.

Khan, R.A. (1988) Experimental transmission, development, and effects of a parasitic copepod, *Lernaeocera branchialis*, on Atlantic Cod, *Gadus morhua*. J. Parasitol. 74:586–599.

Kirmse, P.D. (1978) *Haemogregarina sachai* n.sp. from cultured turbot *Scophthalmus maximus* in Scotland. J Fish Dis. 1:337–342.

Kirmse, P.D. (1980) Observations on the pathogenicity of *Haemogregarina sachai*. Kirmse, 1978 in farmed turbot *Scopthalmus maximus* L. J. Fish Dis. 3:101–114.

Kirmse, P.D., and Ferguson, H. (1976) *Toxoplasma*-like organisms as the possible causative agents of a proliferative condition in farmed turbot (*Scopthalmus maximus*). In: Wildlife Diseases (Page, L.A., ed.). Plenum Press, New York, pp. 561–564.

Klatt, G. (1985) Populationdynamik des Parasitischen Nematoden *Phocanema decipiens* im Stint. Thesis, University of Kiel, Germany, p. 53.

Knight-Jones, E.W. (1962) The systematics of marine leeches. In: Leeches (Hirudinea)—Their Structure, Physiology, Ecology, and Embryology (Mann, K.H., ed.). Pergamon Press, New York, pp. 169–186.

Korotaeva, V.D. (1985) Trematodes (digeneids) of commercial fish of the Pacific of practical importance. In: Parasitology and Pathology of Marine Organisms of the World Ocean (Hargis, W.J., ed.). NOAA Technical Report NMFS 25. U.S. Department of Commerce, National Oceanic and Atmospheric Administration, National Marine Fisheries Service, Washington, D.C., pp. 63–64.

Lauckner, G. (1984) Diseases caused by metazoans: Cnidarians. In: Diseases of Marine Animals. Vol. IV. Part 1. Introduction and Pisces (Kinne, O., ed.). Biologische Anstalt, Helgoland, Hamburg, pp. 180–192.

Lee, J.J., Hutner, S.H., and Bovee, E.C. (1985) An Illustrated Guide to the Protozoa. Society of Protozoologists, Lawrence, Kansas.

Liewes, E.W. (1984) Culture, Feeding and Diseases of Commercial Flat Fish Species. A.A. Balkema, Rotterdam.

Llewellyn, J. (1956) The host specificity, micro-ecology, adhesive attitudes and comparative morphology of trematode gill parasites. J. Marine Biol. 35:113–127.

Lom, J. (1984) Diseases caused by protistand. In: Diseases of Marine Animals. Vol. IV. Part 1. Introduction and Pisces (Kinne, O., ed.). Biologische Anstalt, Helgoland, Hamburg, pp. 114–168.

Lom, J. (1986) Protozoan infections in fish. In: Pathology in Marine Aquaculture (Vivares, C.P., Bonami, J.R., and Jaspers, E., eds.). European Aquaculture Society, Special Publication No. 9, Bredene, Belgium, pp. 95–104.

MacKenzie, K. (1987) Relationships between the Herring, *Clupea harengus* L., and its parasites. Adv. Marine Biol. 24:263–319.

Madill, J. (1988) New Canadian records of leeches (Annelida: Hirudinea) parasitic on fish. Can. Field Natural. 102:685–688.

Margolis, L. (1977) Public Health aspects of "codworm" infection: a review. J. Fisher. Res. Bd. Can. 34:887–898.

Margolis, L., and Arthur, J.R. (1979) Synopsis of the parasites of fishes of Canada. Bull. Fisher. Res. Bd. Can. 199: pp. 269.

Margolis, L., and Kabata, Z. (1984) General Introduction. In: Guide to the Parasites of Fishes of Canada. Part I (Margolis, L., and Kabata, Z., eds.). Canadian Special Publication of Fisheries and Aquatic Sciences, 74:209, pp. 1–4.

Matthews, R.A. (1973) Life cycle of *Bucephalus haimeanus* Lacaze-Duthiers, 1854 from *Cardium edule* L. Parasitology 67:341–350.

Matthews, R.A. (1974) Life cycle of *Bucephaloides gracilescens* (Rudolphi, 1819) Hopkins, 1954 (Digenea: Gasterostomata). Parasitology 68:1–12.

Mawdesley-Thomas, L.E., and Young, P.C. (1967) Cutaneous melanosis in a flounder (*Platichthys flesus* L.). Vet. Rec. 81:384–385.

McClelland, G., Misra, R.K., and Marcogliese, D.J. (1983) Variations in Abundance of Larval Anisakines, Sealworm (*Phocanema decipiens*) and Related Species in Cod and Flatfish from the Southern Gulf of St. Lawrence (4T) and the Breton Shelf (4Vn). Canadian Technical Report of Fisheries and Aquatic Sciences, No. 1201.

McClellend, G., Misra, R.K., and Martell, D.J. (1985) Variations in Abundance of Larval Anisakines, Sealworm (*Pseudoterranova decipiens*) and Related Species, in Eastern Canadian Cod and Flatfish. Canadian Technical Report of Fisheries and Aquatic Sciences, No. 1392.

McClellend, G., Misra, R.K., and Martell, J.D. (1987) Temporal and Geographical Variations in Abundance of Larval Sealworm *Pseudoterranova* (*Phocanema*) *decipiens* in the Fillets of American Plaice (*Hippoglossoides platessoides*) in Eastern Canada: 1985–86 Surveys. Canadian Technical Report of Fisheries and Aquatic Sciences No. 1513.

McVicar, A. (1978) Flatfish at risk—trials pinpoint dangers from disease. Fish Farmer 2:32–33.

Meyer, M.C., and Khan, R.A. (1979) Taxonomy, biology and occurrence of some marine leeches in Newfoundland waters. Proceed. Helminthol. Soc. Wash 46:254–264.

Mikhailova, J.G., Prazdenkov, E.V., and Prusevich, T.O. (1964) Morphological changes in fish tissue around the larvae of some parasitic worms (in Russian). Trans. Murmansk Sea Biol. Inst., 5:251–264. (English translation, Fisheries Research Board of Canada, translation no. 580.)

Moller, H., and Anders, K. (1983) Diseases and Parasites of Marine Fishes. Verlag Moller, Kiel, Germany, pp. 365.

Morrison, C.M., and Poynton, S.L. (1989) A new species of *Goussia* (Apicomplexa, Coccidia) in the kidney tubules of the cod, *Gadus morhua* L. J. Fish Dis. 12:533–560.

Morrison, C.M., McClelland, G., Cornick, J., and Marcogliese, D. (1986) Parasites and Diseases of Some Marine Finfish Off Nova Scotia. Canadian Technical Report of Fisheries and Aquatic Sciences, 1424.

Nelson, J.S. (1976) Fishes of the World. John Wiley & Sons, New York, p. 416.

Newman, M.W. (1978) Pathology associated with *Cryptobia infection* in a summer flounder (*Paralichthys dentatus*). J. Wildlife Dis. 14:299–304.

Noble, E.R., and Collard, S.B. (1970) The parasites of midwater fishes. In: A Symposium of Diseases of Fish and Shellfish (Snieszko, S.F., ed.). American Fisheries Society, Special Publication, 5:57–68.

Odense, P.H., and Logan, V.H. (1976) Prevalence and morphology of *Eimeria gadi* (Fiebiger, 1913) in the haddock. J. Protozool. 23:564–571.

Palsson, J., Sveinbjornsson, S., Steinarsson, B.A., and Stefansson, G. (1985) A Preliminary Report on the Possible Relationship Between Larval Anisakidae (Nematoda) Abundance in Cod and the Condition Factor of the Host. International Council for the Exploration of the Sea, C.M./ N:16.

Post, G. (1987) Textbook of Fish Health. T.F.H. Publications, Neptune, New Jersey, p. 288.

Poynton, S.L., and Lom, J. (1989) Some ectoparasitic trichodinids from Atlantic Cod, *Gadus morhua* L., with a description of *Trichodina cooperi* n.sp.. Can. J. Zool. 67:1793–1800.

Poynton, S.L., and Morrison, C.M. (1990) Morphology of diplomonad flagellates: *Spironucleus torosa* N. Sp. from Atlantic Cod *Gadus morhua* L. and Haddock *Melanogrammus aeglefinus* L., and *Hexamita salmonis* Moore from brook trout *Salvelinus fontinalis* (Mitchill). J. Protozool 37:369–383.

Prushevich, T.O. (1964) On the study of the formation of capsules around *Anisakis* sp. larvae in the tissues of the shorthorn sculpin *Myoxocephalus scorpius* (Russ.). Trudy Murmansk. Morsk. Biol. Inst. Akad. Nauk USSR, 5, 265–273. (English translation, Fisheries Research Board of Canada, translation no. 581.)

Rafi, F. (1988) Isopoda. In: Guide to the Parasites of Fishes of Canada. Part II. Crustacea (Margolis, L., and Kabata, Z., Eds.). Canadian Special Publication of Fisheries and Aquatic Sciences, 101:184, pp. 129–148.

Richardson, H. (1905) A monograph of the Isopods of North America. Bull. U.S.N.M. 54:1–727.

Robins, C.R., Bailey, R.M., Bond, C.E., Brooker, J.R., Laschner, E.A., Lea, R.N., and Scott, W.B. (1980) A List of Common and Scientific Names of Fishes from the United States and Canada. 4th ed. American Fisheries Society, Special Publication No. 12, Bethesda, Maryland, pp. 174.

Rodjuk, G.N. (1985) Parasitic fauna of the Atlantic part of the Antarctic (South Georgia Island and South Shetland Isles). In: Parasitology and Pathology of Marine Organisms of The World Ocean (Hargis, W.J., ed.). NOAA Technical Report NMFS 25. U.S. Department of Commerce, National Oceanic and Atmospheric Administration, National Marine Fisheries Service, Washington, D.C. pp. 31–32.

Rohde, K. (1984) Diseases caused by metazoans: helminths. In: Diseases of Marine Animals. Vol. IV, Part 1. Introduction and Pisces (Kinne, O., ed.). Biologische Anstalt Helgoland, Hamburg, pp. 193–320.

Sars, G.O. (1895) An Account of the Crustacea of Norway. Vol. I. Amphipoda (Text). Alb. Cammermeyers Forlag, Christiana and Copenhagen.

Sawyer, R.T. (1986) Leech Biology and Behavior. Vol. II. Feeding Biology, Ecology and Systematics. Oxford University Press, New York, pp. 419–793.

Sawyer, R.T., Lawler, A.R., and Overstreet, R.M. (1975) Marine leeches of the eastern United States and Gulf of Mexico, with a key to species. J. Natural Hist. 9:633–667.

Schell, S.C. (1985) Handbook of Trematodes of North America North of Mexico. University Press of Idaho, Moscow, Idaho.

Schnick, R.A. (1988) Chemotherapeutants for marine aquaculture. In: Disease diagnosis and control in North American marine aquaculture. 2nd rev. ed. (Sinderman, C.J., and Lightner, D.V., eds.). Developments in Aquaculture and Fisheries Science. Vol. 17. Elsevier, New York, pp. 402–412.

Schultz, G.A. (1982) Isopoda. In: Synopsis and Classification of Living Organisms. Vol. 2 (Parker, S.P., ed.). McGraw-Hill, New York, pp. 249–254.

Scott, W.B., and Scott, M.G. (1988) Atlantic fishes of Canada. Can. Bull. Fish. Aquatic Sci. 219:731.

Silan, P., and Maillard, C. (1986) Modalites de l'infestation par *Diplectanum auquans* monogene ectoparasite de *Dicentrarchus labrax* en aquiculture. Elements d'epidemiologie et de prophylaxie. In: Pathology in Marine Aquaculture (Vivares, C.P., Bonami, J.P., and Jaspers, E., eds.). European Aquaculture Society, Special Publication No. 9, Bredene, Belgium, pp. 139–152.

Sindermann, C.J. (1966) Diseases of Marine Fishes. T.F.H. Publications, Jersey City, New Jersey

Sindermann, C.J. (1970) Principal Diseases of Marine Fish and Shellfish. Academic Press, New York, pp. 369.

Sindermann, C.J. (1985) Recent studies on marine fish parasites and diseases. In: Parasitology and Pathology of Marine Organisms of the World Ocean (Hargis, W.J., ed.). NOAA Technical Report NMFS 25. U.S. Department of Commerce, National Oceanic and Atmospheric Administration, National Marine Fisheries Service, Washington, D.C. pp. 7–14.

Sindermann, C.J. (1990) Principal Diseases of Marine Fish and Shellfish. 2nd ed. Vol. 1. Diseases of Marine Fish. Academic Press, San Diego, pp. 521.

Sindermann, C.J., and Lightner, D.V. (Eds.). (1988) Disease Diagnosis and Control in North American Marine Aquaculture. 2nd rev. ed. Developments in Aquaculture and Fisheries Science. Vol. 17. Elsevier, New York.

Sindermann, C.J., and Rosenfield, A. (1954) Diseases of fishes of the western North Atlantic. III. Mortalities of sea herring (Clupea harengus) caused by larval trematode invasion. Maine Dept. Sea Shore Fish. Res. Bull. 21:1–16.

Sindermann, C.J., Ziskowski, J.J., and Anderson, V.T. (1978) A Guide to the Recognition of Some Disease Conditions and Abnormalities in Marine Fish. U.S. National Marine Fisheries Service, Technical Series Report No. 14, Washington, D.C. p. 60.

Smith, F.G. (1975) Crustacean parasites of Marine Fishes. In: The Pathology of Fishes (Ribelin, W.E., and Migaki, G., eds.). University of Wisconsin Press, Madison, pp. 189–203.

Smith, J.W., and Wootten, R. (1978) Anisakis and anisakiasis. Adv. Parasitol. 16:93–163.

Smyth, J.D. (1976) Introduction to Animal Parasitology. 2nd ed. Hodder & Stroughton, London, pp. 466.

Solonchenko, A. (1985) Development of larval stages of Bothriocephalus scorpii. In: Parasitology and Pathology of Marine Organisms of the World Ocean (Hargis, W.J., ed.). NOAA Technical Report NMFS 25. U.S. Department of Commerce, National Oceanic and Atmospheric Administration, National Marine Fisheries Service, Washington, D.C., pp. 83–84.

Stoskopf, M.K. (1988) Fish chemotherapeutics. Vet. Clin North Am. Small Anim. Pract. 18:(2)331–348.

Strout, R.G. (1965) A new haemoflagellate (genus Cryptobia) from marine fish of northern New England. J. Parasitol. 51:654–659.

Wheeler, A. (1978) Key to the Fishes of Northern Europe. Frederick Warne, London.

Zubchenko, A.V. (1985) Use of parasitological data in studies of local groupings of rock grenadier, Coryphaenoides rupestris Gunner. In: Parasitology and Pathology of Marine Organisms of the World Ocean. (Hargis, W.J., ed.). NOAA Technical Report NMFS 25. U.S. Department of Commerce, National Oceanic and Atmospheric Administration, National Marine Fisheries Service, Washington, D.C., pp. 19–24.

Chapter 90

NEOPLASIA IN COLD-WATER MARINE FISHES

ERIC B. MAY

Cold-water marine fishes are migratory species that spend most, if not all, of their life cycle in marine water. The bulk of the literature on neoplasias in these fishes was published prior to 1950 and represented the results of surveys in which the discovery of a tumor or neoplasm was incidental. In two cases (American sole and Winter flounder), clear environmental correlations could be made (Malins et al., 1985; Murchelano and Wolke, 1985). Aside from these observations, no clear picture of causation or predisposing factors can be drawn. A list of tumors reported in cold-water marine fishes is given in Table 90–1.

LITERATURE CITED

Charlton, M.M. (1929) A tumor of the pineal organ with cartilage formation in the mackerel, Scomber scombrus. Anat. Rec. 43:51–59.

Haddow, A., and Blake, I. (1933) Neoplasms in fish: a report of six cases with a summary of the literature. J. Pathol. Bacteriol. 36:41.

Harshbarger, J.C. (1965–1981) RTLA supplement. Registry of Tumors in Lower Animals. Smithsonian Institution, Washington D.C.

Huizinga, H.W., and Budd, J. (1983) Mephroblastoma in the smelt, Osmerus mordax (Mitchill). J. Fish Dis. 6:389–391.

Ingleby, H. (1929) Melanotic tumor in Lophius piscatorius (abstract). Arch. Pathol. 8:1016–1017.

Johnstone, J. (1915) Diseased and abnormal conditions of marine fishes. Proc. Trans. Liverpool Biol. Soc. 29:80–118.

TABLE 90–1. Tumors Reported in Cold-Water Marine Fishes

Site/Neoplasia	Fish	References
Nervous System		
Ganglioneuroma	Flatfishes	Takahashi, 1929
	La morue	Thomas, 1927
	Megrim	Haddow and Blake, 1933
Neurilemmoma	Anchovy	Harshbarger, 1965–1981
	Dover sole	Harshbarger, 1965–1981
	Lingcod	Harshbarger, 1965–1981
Neurofibroma	Pacific cod	Wellings, 1969
Melanoma	Haddock	Prince, 1982
	Atlantic cod	Prince, 1982
	Atlantic halibut	Johnstone, 1915
	Plaice	Johnstone, 1923–1925
	Goosefish	Ingleby, 1929
Cardiovascular System (Including organs of hematopoesis)		
Hemangioma	Atlantic cod	Harshbarger, 1965–1981
	Pollock	Harshbarger, 1965–1981
	Mackerel	Harshbarger, 1965–1981
	Plaice	Harshbarger, 1965–1981
Gastrointestinal System		
Hepatomas	English sole	Malins et al., 1985
	Winter flounder	Murchelano and Wolke, 1985
	Atlantic tomcod	Smith et al., 1979
Cholangiomas	English sole	Malins et al., 1985
	Winter flounder	Murchelano and Wolke, 1985
Urinary System		
Nephroblastoma	Smelt	Huizinga and Budd, 1983
Endocrine System		
Pineal chondroma	Mackerel	Charlton, 1929

Johnstone, J. (1923–1925) Malignant tumors in fishes. J. Marine Biol. Assoc. U.K. 13:447–471.

Malins, D.C., Krahn, M.M., Brown, D.W., Rhodes, L.D., Myers, M.S., Mcain, B.B., and Chan, S.L. Toxic chemicals in marine sediment and biota from Mukilteo, Washington: relationships with hepatic neoplasms and other hepatic lesions in English sole (Parophrys vetulus). J. Natl. Cancer Inst. 74:487–494.

Murchelano, R.A., and Wolke, R.E. (1985) Epizootic carcinoma in the winter flounder, Pseudopleuronectes Americanus. Science 228:587–589.

Prince, E.E., and Steven, J.L. (1982) On two large tumors in a haddock and a cod. Rep. Fish. Bd. Scotl. 10:323–325.

Smith, C.E., Peak, T.H., Klauda, R.J., and McLaren, J.B. (1979) Hepatomas in Atlantic tomcod, Microgadus tomcod (Walbaum), collected in the Hudson River Estuary in New York. J. Fish Dis. 2:313–319.

Takahashi, K. (1929) Studie uber die fishgeschwulste. Z. Krebsforsch. 29:1–73.

Thomas, L. (1927) Sur un cas de ganglioneurome abdominal ches la morue. Bull. Assoc. Franc. Etude Cancer 16:282–286.

Wellings, S.R. (1969) Neoplasia and primitive vertebrate phylogeny: echonoderms, prevertebrates, and fishes—a review. Natl. Cancer Inst. Monogr. 31:59–128.

SECTION VIII

SHARKS, SKATES, AND

RAYS

MICHAEL K. STOSKOPF, *Section Editor*

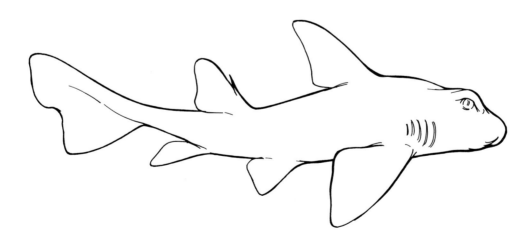

Chapter 91

TAXONOMY AND NATURAL HISTORY OF SHARKS, SKATES, AND RAYS

MICHAEL. K. STOSKOPF

SHARKS

There are approximately 350 living species of sharks (Compagno, 1984). Of these, only about half are of any use to fisheries, and less than 7% represent major fisheries species. Even fewer species are important display animals. The eight orders of sharks are relatively easily differentiated by external characteristics.

Angel Sharks

Three of the eight orders of sharks have no anal fin. Of these, the Squatiniformes, or angel sharks, are raylike but have a terminal mouth (Fig. 91–1). This order has a single family with one genus that includes about 12 species. Angel sharks are often found buried in the mud or sand in the daytime. They are nocturnal sharks that feed on small fish, crustaceans, cephalopods, gastropods, and bivalves. Their jaws are highly protrusable. Angel sharks are usually moderate in size, with only one species reaching 2 m.

Saw Sharks

The Pristiophoriformes, or saw sharks, also have no anal fin. They have a ventral mouth and an elongated, sawlike snout (Fig. 91–2). There are two genera and five species in this order. Saw sharks are little-known benthic inhabitants of temperate and tropical continental and insular shelves. Only one species is a deep-water inhabitant. These are small, slender sharks and should not be confused with the batoid sawfishes. Saw sharks are abundant where they occur. They are ovoviviparous, with litters of 7 to 17. Their large lateral rostral teeth erupt before birth but lay flat against the rostrum until after parturition. The smaller rostral teeth erupt postpartum. Saw sharks probably prey on small fish, crustaceans, and squid.

Dogfish Sharks

The Squaliformes, or bramble, rough, and dogfish sharks, have no anal fin but are not dorsoventrally flattened (Fig. 91–3). They do have a short

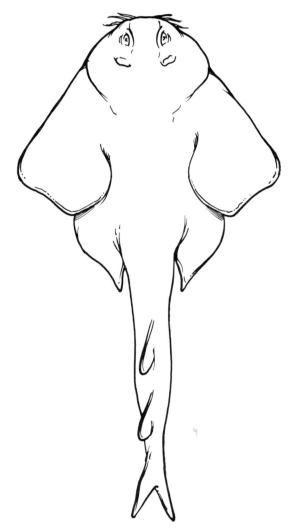

FIGURE 91–1. Angel shark.

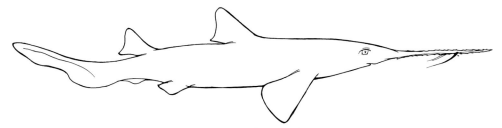

FIGURE 91–2. Saw shark.

rostrum and ventral mouth. There are three families in the order, with 20 genera. The majority of these genera are in the family Squalidae, or dogfish sharks. Most people are familiar with the small dogfish species in this family, found along continental and insular shelves, ranging close inshore in cool water. However, there are two species in the family that grow to longer than 6 m. The majority of the diversity in the family is found in the deep water species. Some species are solitary, and others form large nomadic schools with regular yearly migrations. All species studied in this family are ovoviviparous without placental attachment. Litter sizes vary from 1 to over 20 young. They feed on a wide variety of prey. Several species may feed communally and may attack cooperatively.

Frill and Cow Sharks

The members of the order Hexanchiformes, or frill and cow sharks, have only one dorsal fin and six or seven gill slits. The frill sharks have an elongated body and an eel-like, terminal mouth. They are represented by only one genus and two species. Frill sharks are benthic, deep-water species living on outer continental and insular shelves of all continents. They grow to nearly 2.0 m and mature at 1.0 m for males and 1.3 m for females. Frill sharks are ovoviviparous, with a long gestation period, producing 8 to 12 young per litter. They probably feed on cephalopods and bottom fish and are not considered dangerous.

The cow sharks make up the second family of

this order with four species, the broadnose and bigeye sixgill sharks (Fig. 91–4) and the sharpnose and bluntnose sevengill sharks. These sharks are distributed worldwide and are primarily deep-water species, but they can be found in shallow bays. Cow sharks range in size from very large to very small. They feed on other sharks, rays, bony fishes, crustaceans, and carrion. They are ovoviviparous and lack a yolk-sac placenta.

Requiem Sharks

Four of the eight shark orders have two dorsal fins and five gill slits. The Carcharhiniformes, or requiem sharks, have no fin spines, a mouth located behind the cranial margin of the eyes, nictitating eyelids, and a spiral or scroll-type intestinal valve. The majority of shark species are in this order. There are eight families in the order, the catsharks, finback cat sharks, false cat shark, barbel hound shark, hound sharks, weasel and snaggletoothed sharks, hammerhead sharks, and requiem sharks.

Carcharhiniformes sharks are found primarily in tropical and warm water, usually over continental shelves and along their edges. This is also the only group with members that swim far up freshwater rivers. The bull shark, a large dangerous species, has been found in tropical rivers and lakes. The Ganges shark, Pondicherry shark, reef blacktip shark, and spadenose shark all have been recorded in rivers.

The majority of unprovoked shark attacks on people are by requiem sharks (Fig. 91–5). About 21 species of sharks are considered dangerous or very

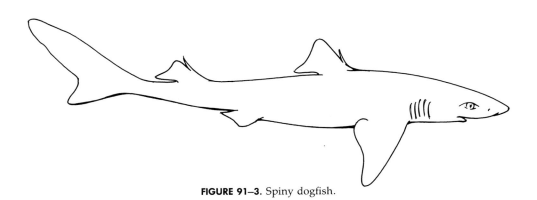

FIGURE 91–3. Spiny dogfish.

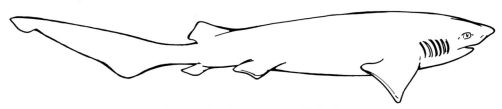

FIGURE 91–4. Broadnose sixgill shark.

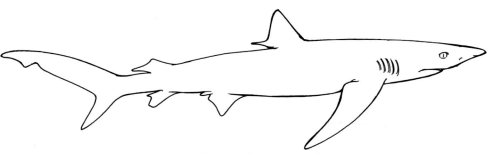

FIGURE 91–5. Blue shark (a requiem shark).

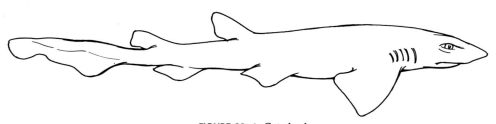

FIGURE 91–6. Cat shark.

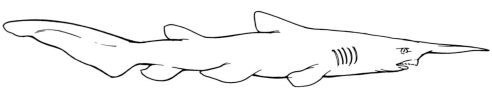

FIGURE 91–7. Goblin shark.

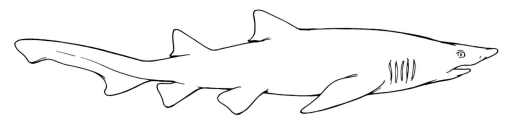

FIGURE 91–8. Sand tiger shark.

dangerous, and 14 of these are requiem sharks. Of the 12 species suspected of attacking people, 8 are requiem and hammerhead species. This does not imply that requiem sharks pose a major danger to humans. Worldwide, shark attacks are infrequent relative to other accidents causing human deaths at sea. It is estimated that 30 to 50 shark attacks are reported each year (Gilbert, 1981), and the combined reported and unreported attack rate is probably less than 100 per year (Compagno, 1988). In contrast, the human attack rate on sharks through fishing is estimated to be 150,000 times higher, with approximately 4.5 million shark fatalities due to humans occurring each year (Compagno, 1988). An exception would be the occurrence of disasters at sea. At these times, sharks can encounter large numbers of humans in the water and surplus killing may occur. The olfactory stimulus of blood in the water can spur on a feeding and killing frenzy. Ocean whitetip, silky, and blue sharks can be responsible for dozens of human fatalities in a very short time (Compagno, 1988).

The feeding patterns and habitats of this group of sharks are as varied as their morphology. Smaller cat sharks tend to feed on invertebrates and smaller fishes (Fig. 91–6). Requiem sharks feed primarily on fish. The reproductive modes of 159 species of this order are known. Thirty-three percent, including almost all of the cat sharks, are oviparous. Nearly half of the Carcharhiniformes species are viviparous. Half of the hound sharks are ovoviviparous, without any yolk-sac placentation.

Mackerel Sharks

The Lamniformes, or mackerel sharks, have physical features similar to those of the requiem sharks but have a ring-type intestinal valve and no nictitating eyelid. This order includes seven families, the goblin sharks (Fig. 91–7), megamouth shark, thresher sharks, sand tiger sharks, crocodile sharks, mackerel sharks, and basking sharks. The shark most commonly displayed in captivity from this group is the sand tiger shark. This shark is a relatively unaggressive, slow-swimming animal common in temperate and tropical water. It is often found near or on the bottom but also swims in midwater or on the surface. It is most active at night and is found in small to large schools. In some parts of the sand tiger shark's range, the species is migratory. It is known to swallow air at the surface, presumably to achieve neutral buoyancy. The sand tiger shark is capable of hovering motionless in the water like a bony fish, again presumably because of its ability to hold air in its stomach.

The numerous protruding teeth give the sand tiger shark a more dangerous appearance than is warranted by its behavior (Fig. 91–8). While the sand tiger shark is known as the gray nurse shark in Australia and is considered a maneater, this is apparently due to confusion with other species. The sand tigers are unaggressive when not provoked, although their large size demands respect. They feed on a variety of fishes, other sharks, rays, squids, and benthic crustaceans. They have been observed feeding cooperatively, surrounding and bunching prey fish. They are ovoviviparous, without a yolk-sac placenta. Intrauterine cannibalism is a fetal nutrition strategy.

Another well-known member of the Lamniformes is the megamouth shark (Fig. 91–9), a filter-feeding species that was originally discovered when the type specimen became entrapped on the sea anchor of a naval research vessel in open ocean. This

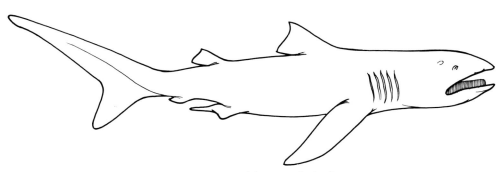

FIGURE 91–9. Megamouth shark.

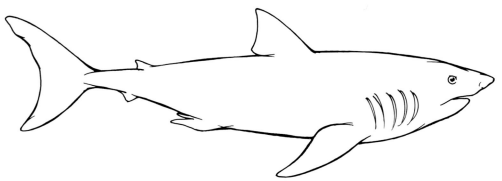

FIGURE 91–10. Great white shark.

shark is a giant plankton and euphasid filter feeder. The holotype was 4.46 m long.

The great white shark, a member of the mackerel shark family, is perhaps even better known (Fig 91–10). This immense, predatory shark inhabits coastal and offshore waters, most commonly in cold and temperate water, but it can be found in tropical water. The great white shark is a powerful swimmer, capable of an average cruising speed in excess of 3 km/hour. It is capable of sudden high-speed dashes. Little is known about its biology. The great white shark is usually found as a single animal or in a pair. It will feed on a wide variety of prey, which includes sea turtles, gannets, gulls, penguins, marine mammals, fishes, and invertebrates. It is presumably an ovoviviparous shark with intrauterine cannibalism, but this has not been confirmed, since gravid females are rarely caught.

Also well known are the thresher sharks, which have characteristic long dorsal lobes on their caudal fins (Fig. 91–11). It is thought that the common thresher shark strikes and stuns prey fish with its tail. These sharks are thought to be harmless to humans but deserve respect because of their size and the power of their tails. Their reproductive pattern is similar to that of the sand tiger shark.

Carpet Sharks

The Orectolobiformes, or carpet sharks, have their mouth well in front of their eyes and have no fin spines, differentiating them from the Heterodontiformes, the bullhead and horn sharks, which do have fin spines. This order comprises seven families, including the whale shark, zebra sharks, wobbegongs (Fig. 91–12), nurse sharks, carpet sharks, blind sharks, and longtail carpet sharks.

The most familiar species of this order are the nurse sharks, which are common display sharks (Fig. 91–13). There are two species of nurse sharks, the shorttailed nurse shark, found in the Western Indian Ocean off the coast of Tanzania and Kenya, and the common nurse shark, found in American waters. The common nurse shark has longer barbels and a first dorsal fin that is much larger than the second dorsal fin. This shark is an inshore bottom-dwelling animal found off both the east and west coasts of North and South America as well as the west coast of Africa. They are nocturnal sharks that often aggregate into schools of 3 to 36 animals. Nurse sharks grow to over 4.3 m, but are usually less than 3 m when adult. Males mature at 2.25 m, and females mature at about 2.3 to 2.4 m. They feed on bottom invertebrates and a variety of fishes, and may also feed on marine algae. These sharks have been kept very successfully in captivity for up to 25 years and have been bred in captivity. Nurse sharks are ovoviviparous, without yolk-sac placentation. Litters of 21 to 28 pups are born in the late spring.

Another member of the order of carpet sharks is the whale shark, an immense filter-feeding species with worldwide tropical and warm-temperate water distribution (Fig. 91–14). They are often found asso-

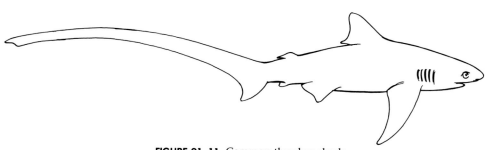

FIGURE 91–11. Common thresher shark.

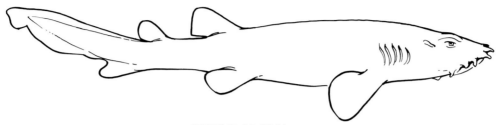

FIGURE 91–12. Wobbegong.

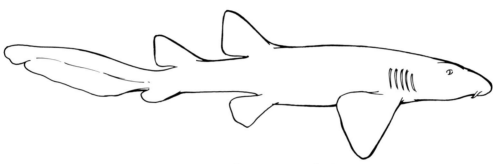

FIGURE 91–13. Common nurse shark.

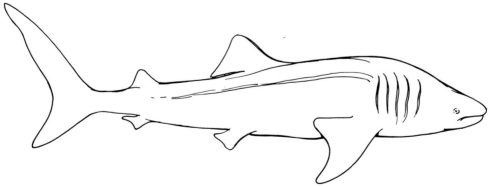

FIGURE 91–14. Whale shark.

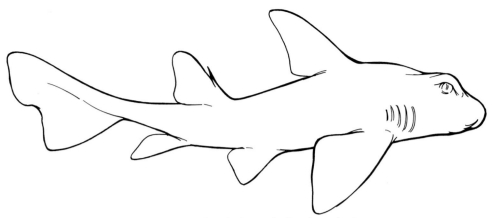

FIGURE 91–15. Port Jackson shark, a hornshark.

ciated with schools of pelagic fishes. Whale sharks can reach a length of 18 m but are rarely more than 12 m long. They are considered the largest fish in the world. Whale sharks are suction feeders, ingesting plankton, small crustaceans, and small fishes. Their suction feeding mechanism is more versatile than that of the basking shark, which has little or no capability to develop suction. This feature is important in the adaptation of whale sharks to captivity, a feat that has been accomplished in Japan. The whale shark does not require forward motion to feed, making captive management possible.

The carpet shark order also includes some of the smallest species of sharks. The bamboo sharks are small species that are usually oviparous and feed mainly on invertebrates. The blind sharks are not so named because they cannot see, but because of how they close their eyes when taken from the water.

Bullhead and Horn Sharks

The Heterodontiformes, or bullhead and horn sharks, are classified in a single family and genus (Fig. 91–15). These sharks are easily recognized by the dorsal fin, spine, and anal fin. They have a short, rounded snout and large, molariform teeth in the back of the mouth. They are sluggish tropical bottom sharks most often found in water less than 100 m deep. They are nocturnal and favor rocky crevices and caves in the daytime. At least one species is migratory. They are oviparous, producing large, spiral-flanged egg cases, which take over 5 months to hatch. They feed on benthic invertebrates and prefer sea urchins. They also feed on other invertebrates and, rarely, small fish.

BATOIDS

The batoids, or skates and rays, are closely related to the sharks. They are dorsoventrally flattened and often sport venomous spines. Taxonomi-

cally they are divided into a variable number of families. The batoids are not commercially exploited to the extent that the sharks are, but smaller forms are popular display species.

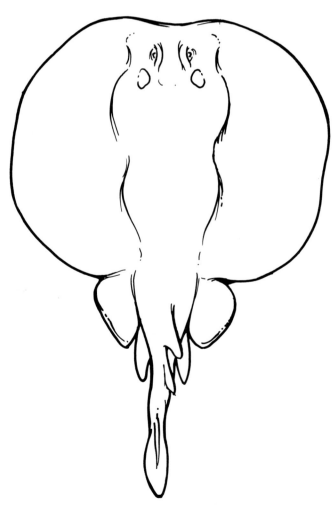

FIGURE 91–16. Torpedo.

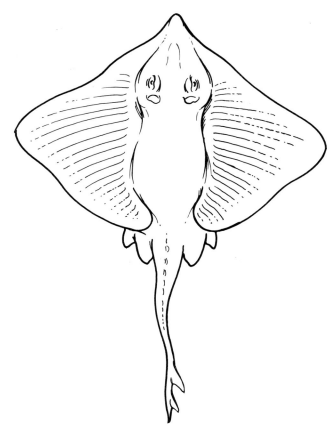

FIGURE 91–17. Clear-nosed skate.

Electric Rays

The electric rays include 30 species worldwide. They have a disc-shaped body that is thicker and softer than that of the other rays. They have a sharply demarcated tail, which is thicker at the base than most rays. Each electric ray has two electric organs, one on each side of the anterior disc. These fish are not strong swimmers. They live buried in sand or mud and use their electric organs to stun prey upon contact. Electric rays eat crustaceans, molluscs, worms, and fish. They are ovoviviparous. The most studied species of this group is the torpedo, which is found on both sides of the Atlantic (Fig. 91–16). These grow up to 2 m in length and may weigh up to 90 kg. Torpedoes can produce about 220 volts.

Skates

Skates are usually found in shallow water, but some species are known to live at great depth. There are about 120 species in 9 genera of skates. Skates have slender tails that are less than twice as long as the body. They normally have two dorsal fins. They lack a venomous caudal spine. Skates live on the bottom, burying themselves in the sand or gravel with their wings. They will pursue prey to the surface.

A common skate caught inshore and sometimes displayed in aquaria is the clear-nosed skate that is seen in the Chesapeake and Delaware Bays in April (Fig. 91–17). It grows to about 1 m long. The winter skate is about the same size as the clear-nosed skate and is also found in the continental waters of the western north Atlantic. This skate has a single spot on the dorsal surface of each wing. It prefers sand or gravel bottoms and cool water. It disappears when water temperatures rise in the summer, and it reappears in the winter. All skates are oviparous.

River Rays

The stingrays found in fresh water are classified in their own family. Only a few species are known, but they are abundant in the waters of South America and Thailand. These rays have a long, slender process directed forward from the pelvis. Their venomous spine is similar to that of the round stingrays. They spend much of their time buried in the mud in turbid river waters. River rays feed primarily on small invertebrates and fishes and are usually small themselves, being less than 1 m long. They are ovoviviparous. One species of South American fresh water ray, the motoro ray, which also frequents brackish water, is considered extremely dangerous. The venom is heat labile and is destroyed by acid and alcohol.

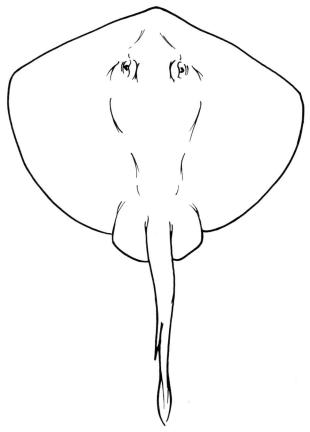

FIGURE 91–18. Stingray.

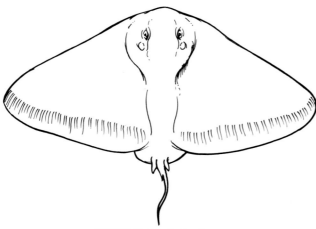

FIGURE 91–19. Butterfly ray.

Stingrays

The stingrays are divided into at least 30 species in at least three genera on the basis of their shape (Fig. 91–18). They are round, diamond-shaped, or kite-shaped. Stingrays all are characterized by a lack of caudal, dorsal, and separate cephalic fins. They are often found lying on the bottom of shoals and river mouths or on patches of sand where they are partially buried. This increases their hazard to swim-

mers and waders. Their tail is long and whiplike. The sting is large and located in the distal portion of the basal or middle third of the tail. Most species have only one sting, but many have two, and a few have three or more. The point, or sting, may be 15 to 30 cm long and is fringed with small barbs to hold it in a wound. It is covered by a thin sheath. The sheath is thought to contribute venom to the sting. Older rays have often lost their sheath and then inflict only mechanical injury. The stingrays feed on worms, molluscs, and crustaceans as well as small fishes. They are frequently preyed upon by sharks. They are ovoviviparous.

Butterfly Rays

The butterfly rays are divided into two genera, those with dorsal fins and those without (Fig. 91–19). These rays are closely related to the stingrays. They differ primarily in having wings that are much broader than the length of their tail. Some species of these rays have stings, and some do not. Butterfly rays have unusual color patterns for rays and are capable of changing colors to match backgrounds. These are slow-swimming, bottom-dwelling rays that feed on molluscs and crustaceans. They are ovoviviparous.

Round Stingrays

The round stingrays are smaller and have shorter, stouter muscular tails than the stingrays.

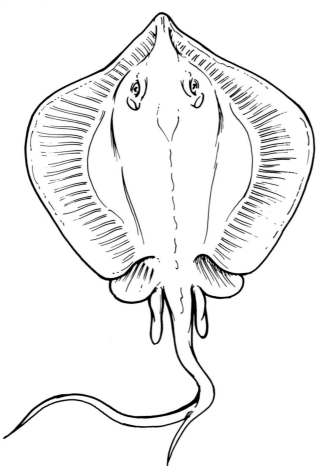

FIGURE 91–20. Atlantic stingray.

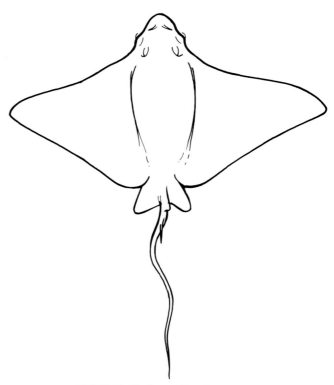

FIGURE 91–21. Spotted eagle ray.

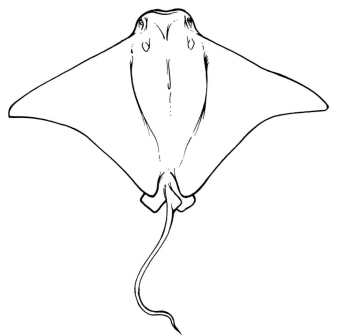

FIGURE 91–22. Atlantic cow-nose ray.

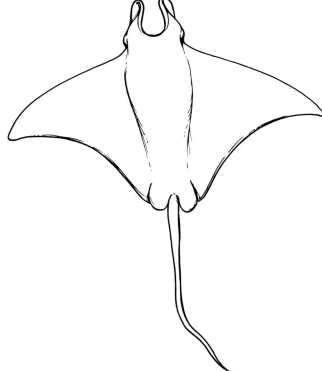

FIGURE 91–23. Giant devil ray (manta).

Some taxonomists would group the two families into one. Like the other stingrays, these spend much of their time buried in the mud. They feed principally on worms and crustaceans. Atlantic stingrays (Fig. 91–20) are generally found in shallow water and present a major hazard to fishermen and swimmers. The venom is heat labile. Another common species in the Atlantic, the yellow stingray, is found in large numbers in Jamaican waters and from the Florida Keys to the coast of North Carolina. It can grow to about 25 by 50 cm. The round stingrays are ovoviviparous.

Eagle Rays

Eagle rays are found in tropical and temperate seas worldwide (Fig. 91–21). They swim with a flying motion near the bottom or at the surface and are usually found in relatively shallow water. They have pavementlike teeth for crushing molluscs, which they dig from the bottom by flapping their wings when they detect currents from the siphons of buried clams and other molluscs.

The spotted eagle ray is sometimes also referred to as the spotted duck-billed ray. Schools of several thousand have been reported, although they are not generally considered common. This eagle ray is found on both sides of the Atlantic, in the Pacific and Indian Oceans, and in the Red Sea. The spotted eagle ray grows to 250 kg in weight and 2 m in width. It can have up to five venomous spines on the base of its long tail. Eagle rays are ovoviviparous.

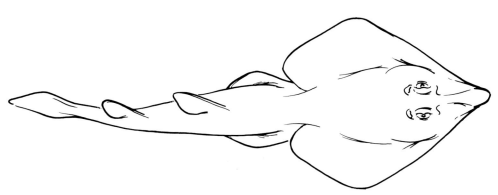

FIGURE 91–24. Guitarfish.

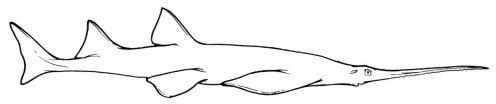

FIGURE 91–25. Common sawfish.

Cow-Nose Rays

These rays are set apart from the other rays by their distinctive square nose. Some taxonomists group them with the eagle rays. There is only one genus, and the principal species is the Atlantic cow-nose ray, which can grow to 45 kg in weight and 2 m in width (Fig. 91–22). These rays are usually seen in large schools. They feed primarily on molluscs and crustaceans. They are ovoviviparous. Their sting has been reported to be fatal for humans, but these reports involve wounds into the abdomen.

Devil Rays

This family of rays, named for the hornlike appearance of their rolled cephalic fins, is divided into three genera on the basis of the placement of the teeth. The lesser devil rays have teeth in both jaws. There are four species, divided on the presence or absence of a venomous spine and their geographic range. The most common species found in western Atlantic coastal waters grows to 1.3 m wide. The lesser devil rays are often seen in schools. They tend to use their cephalic horns to grasp anything that touches their head and can trap themselves on posts or anchor lines this way.

The giant devil ray has teeth only in its lower jaw (Fig. 91–23). This ray, also called the manta ray, can grow up to 6 m wide and can weigh over 1300 kg. Like all of the devil rays, these rays live at or near the surface. They are found in tropical and subtropical water of all oceans. They often leap up to 1.5 m out of the water, a behavior that has been postulated to be for removing ectoparasites. Giant devil rays are reported to copulate ventral to ventral, with the male on top. Usually only a single young is born, but it can weigh over 12 kg and can be 1.3 m wide. The third genus of this family has teeth only in the upper jaw. Less is known about this genus.

Guitarfishes

The guitarfishes look like a cross between a ray and a shark (Fig. 91–24). They are sometimes also called fiddler rays or banjo sharks. There are over 30 species in this family, found in tropical and warm temperate coastal water of all oceans. They may even occur in freshwater in Australia. In contrast to the rays, these fish propel themselves with their tail. Most species grow to a maximum of 2 m. They are ovoviviparous.

Sawfishes

The sawfishes are sometimes confused with sharks (Fig. 91–25). They have a more elongated body than most of the batoids. They are classified as rays because of the placement of their gill slits on their ventral surface. Their long, flat snout looks like a saw and has 16 to 32 large, widely spaced teeth on each side. The tooth count is used to differentiate species. Sawfishes use their unusual snouts to impale and capture prey by striking laterally. They can be a hazard to unwary humans. The green sawfish of Australian waters can grow to nearly 8 m long. The common sawfish grows up to 6 m long and can weigh over 300 kg. Sawfishes are ovoviviparous, giving birth to up to 24 young, which are born with their teeth encased in a protective membrane that is sloughed after birth.

LITERATURE CITED

Compagno, L.J.V. (1988) Sharks of the Order Carcharhiniformes. Princeton University Press, Princeton, New Jersey.

Compagno, L.J.V. (ed.) (1984) FAO Species Catalogue, Vol. 4, Sharks of the World. United Nations Development Programme, Rome.

Gilbert, P.W. (1981) Introduction to Sharks. Oceanus 24(4):3–4.

Halstead, B.W. (1988) Poisonous and Venomous Marine Animals of the World, 2nd rev. ed. Darwin Press, Princeton, New Jersey.

McCormick, H.W., Allen, T., and Young, W. (1963) Shadows in the Sea, the Sharks, Skates and Rays. Weathervane Books, New York.

Chapter 92

ANATOMY AND PHYSIOLOGY OF SHARKS

MICHAEL K. STOSKOPF

An introduction to the general anatomy and physiology of sharks is given in the section on general medicine. Actually the sharks, skates, and rays constitute one of the more homogeneous groups of fishes. That is a relative statement of course, but there are perhaps more similarities among the members of the group than differences (Fig. 92–1). Nevertheless, there are many more adaptations and specializations within the elasmobranchs than can be accommodated in this chapter, which will have to focus on a few major issues.

CARTILAGINOUS SKELETON

All of the elasmobranchs have cartilaginous skeletons, and although mineralization of cartilage occurs, particularly in the vertebral column, there is no true bone in these fishes. In some species, the mineralization of the cartilage matrix, primarily with calcium phosphates and carbonates, which form an apatite, can closely resemble bone. However, there are no canaliculi or any evidence of a haversian canal system similar to that found in true bone. Nor are the cell types of true bone found.

Phylogenetically, this lack of true bone has routinely been interpreted as a primitive feature of the elasmobranchs, but this is probably a misrepresentation. Examination of fossilized evidence in early sharks has demonstrated the presence of osteocytes in denticles. This finding supports the more current theory that the cartilaginous fishes derive from ancestors that lost the ability to form bone rather than from primitive forms that never developed the capability (Zangerl, 1966).

The adaptation of a cartilaginous skeleton has some unique features. Increased flexibility and decreased density of the skeletal system would be numbered among advantages for animals that do not require structural rigidity to combat gravity. Interestingly, the cartilaginous skeleton gives excellent protection to the central nervous system of elasmobranchs. The cranium of sharks, skates, and rays is not made up of separate pieces of cartilage in a manner analogous to the many bones of the teleost or mammalian skull. Instead the skull is one cartilaginous block with a chamber for the brain and foramina for the cranial nerves.

One of the more dramatic structural modifications of the skull of sharks is the dorsoventrally compressed and laterally expanded head of the hammerhead sharks. The benefits of this adaptation to survival are unknown, but it is not a unique modification. Some larval teleosts have a similarly shaped

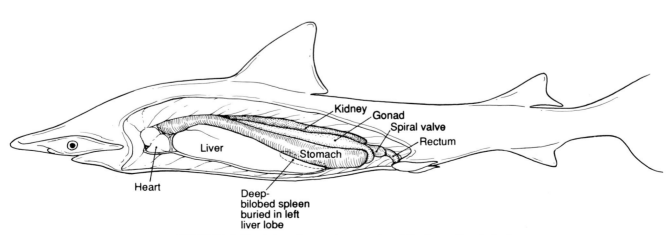

FIGURE 92–1. The internal organ topography of the bonnethead shark.

head that has resulted in their erroneous classification as distinct species from their adult forms. In these teleosts, the lateral wings of the skull are reabsorbed as they become adults. One postulate of the function of these cranial extensions is to serve as a hydroplane for facilitating rapid ascent and descent as well as assisting the pectoral hydroplanes in making quick lateral turns. This may or may not be true. The agility of the hammerheads has not been compared rigorously to other sharks to see if the head structure actually offers an advantage.

An alternative postulate is that the wide displacement of sensory organs may facilitate orientation. This is particularly interesting with the displacement of the nostrils that may provide what is in effect stereo smell. Again, there is no rigorous evidence to support this hypothesis (Murphy and Nichols, 1916).

The jaws of sharks are only loosely attached to the cranium. In the cow sharks, they make contact with the cranium in only two places, and the hyomandibular apparatus has no supporting role. In other sharks, a single muscular ligament connects the upper jaw to the skull and a cartilaginous hyomandibular apparatus supports the base of the upper jaw (Budker, 1971).

TEETH

The teeth of sharks are structurally enlarged placoid scales, which themselves have many of the structural components of a mammalian tooth. They consist of a mass of dentinelike material surrounding a central pulp cavity. They are covered with a varying thickness of an enameloid, hard, smooth substance.

Any classification of the teeth of sharks is probably an oversimplification, since variations in tooth

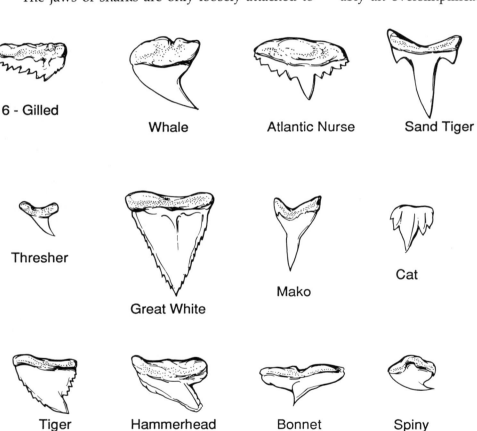

6 - Gilled   Whale   Atlantic Nurse   Sand Tiger

Thresher   Great White   Mako   Cat

FIGURE 92–2. Shark teeth are characteristic of genus and often species. This figure shows typical configurations of teeth from a variety of well-known sharks.

Tiger   Hammerhead   Bonnet   Spiny Dogfish

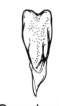

Greenland   Angel

morphology are often adequate for the identification of sharks down to species (Fig. 92–2). There are, however, two main types of teeth in the sharks and another more commonly found in the rays. The classic shark tooth is the triangular, sharp, cutting tooth found in the great white shark and other members of the Carcharhinidae. These flat teeth are exceptionally well adapted for cutting and tearing pieces of larger prey. The other major type of tooth found in sharks is the awl-shaped tooth found in the sand tiger shark. These teeth have a bifurcate root and a large cusp that is round in cross section. They are not functional for cutting prey but serve well for holding prey to be swallowed whole. Sharks with this type of teeth are best adapted for feeding on smaller fishes and squids. Of course, the skates and rays, which feed on crustaceans and molluscs, would be poorly served with these tooth forms. They have a molariform grinding tooth system that enables them to crush the shells of their sedentary prey.

The teeth of sharks are not embedded in sockets in the manner of mammalian teeth. They are merely attached at the base by a dense connective tissue. Sharks routinely shed their teeth, which are replaced, usually by auxiliary rows of teeth that migrate into active position. In the lemon shark, tooth replacement takes between 7 and 8 days if the animal is receiving good nutrition but can take several days longer in starved sharks (Moss, 1967).

There are some major adaptive structural changes in the teeth of some shark species. An example is the basking shark, which has long thin denticular modifications that serve as gill rakers for straining the plankton that it feeds upon. These are essentially modified teeth and apparently are shed periodically, leaving the animal unable to feed until they are replaced (Matthews, 1962). Another plankton-feeding shark, the whale shark, uses an entirely different strategy. This shark does not have modified denticles but instead uses many long thin cartilaginous rods tipped with a fine mesh of spongiform tissue and filling the spaces between the gill arches to form a straining net for plankton (Budker, 1971).

GILLS

Early physiologists believed that sharks did not have a vascular countercurrent mechanism in their gills similar to that found in teleosts. This was used to explain an apparent intolerance of sharks to low-oxygen water. Recent studies have shown that sharks do indeed have both a respiratory and a nonrespiratory blood supply to the gills and a countercurrent mechanism is functioning. There are, of course, differences between the generalized structure of shark gills and those of teleosts. These differences are less compelling, however, than the similarities. One distinction is the occurrence of a corpus cavernosum between the afferent filament arteries and the afferent lamellar arterioles, which has been best demonstrated in dogfish (Metcalfe and Butler, 1986). The

function of this structure is not resolved. It has been postulated to serve as a pulse-smoothing, capacitance system, but if this is the case, it is not very effective because postbranchial blood pressure remains pulsatile in the dogfish. A more likely function is that of a hydraulic skeleton. The corpus cavernosum of the dogfish occupies the same position in the gill filament as skeletal cartilage in teleost gills (Metcalfe and Butler, 1986).

CARDIOVASCULAR FUNCTION

A number of assumptions about the cardiovascular system of sharks need further investigation. It has been long accepted, for example, that the use of intramuscular drugs in these animals would be ineffective because of "poor vascular supply" to the muscles. Of course, physiologically there is no evidence that this postulated poor perfusion has any real impact on drug absorption, and clinical and pharmacologic evidence argues against it. The basis for the poor perfusion theory is the apparent requirement for muscular activity to assist venous return to the heart of sharks. Studies of shark cardiac output have often shown that venous return to the heart is weak and have supported postulations of very low blood flow.

An assumption that has contributed to this view has been the generalization that sharks must maintain negative pericardial pressure to optimize cardiac function. Again the interest is focused on the relatively poor cardiac output performance seen in experimental sharks. This question has recently been studied in horn sharks through the use of indwelling pericardial catheters (Abel et al., 1986).

The sharks have a rigid pericardium that maintains a negative pericardial pressure that becomes more negative with the ejection phase of the ventricle (Fig. 92–3). When the pericardium is punctured, interrupting the negative pressure in the chamber, venous return and cardiac output decrease dramatically. However, the pericardial space is not a closed space. It is connected to the peritoneal space through a valved duct, the pericardioperitoneal canal. This duct may function as a pressure-regulating device. It

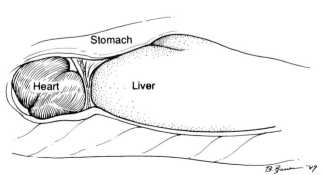

FIGURE 92–3. A substantial rigid pericardium separates the pericardial cavity of the shark from the abdominal cavity.

is normally closed, and pericardial fluid is allowed to flow only into the peritoneum, lowering pericardial pressure.

Studies using indwelling pericardial catheters have shown that venous return in a resting or moderately active shark is more dependent upon a pulsatile pericardial pressure than the maintenance of a constant mean negative pressure (Abel et al., 1986). Of further interest is that merely handling a shark can cause ejection of between 10 and 26% of the pericardial fluid through the canal and consequently a lowering of pressure in the pericardial cavity (Abel et al., 1986). This is somewhat analogous to what is found in a rapidly swimming shark, which increases the pulsatile venous return through active muscle contractions.

VISION

The design of elasmobranch eyes is similar to terrestrial eyes with only a few notable exceptions. One difference is the lens of a shark eye is abnormally large and spherical rather than flattened. The need for a more powerful lens is most likely the result of the inability of the cornea to contribute to focusing the image. The density differences between water and the cornea do not allow for significant refraction. The large spherical lens makes accommodation very difficult for sharks. Changing the shape of the lens, as occurs in mammals, is not practical for a spherical lens. Movement of the lens in relation to the retina, as has been demonstrated in the octopus and teleosts, may occur in the sharks, but it has not been proved (Cohen, 1981).

Nevertheless, shark vision is generally rather acute. Young lemon sharks are hypermetropic or farsighted by 2.76 diopters (Cohen, 1981). This finding indicates that while they may require glasses for reading, lemon sharks would not be at any disadvantage in focusing on remote objects, and their vision would be predicted to be adaptive to their predatory lifestyle.

Many skates and rays also have a ramp retina as a focusing mechanism. A ramp retina is actually only a variation in the distance between the lens of the eye and the retina, which allows the animal to move its eyes or bend its head to bring the image into focus on an appropriately distanced portion of the retina.

The question of color and night vision in sharks has intrigued physiologists for many years. It was once accepted that sharks had a rod-only or certainly a rod-dominated retina. However, ultrastructural studies have demonstrated that sharks, and with a few exceptions skates and rays, do have both rods and cones. This bireceptor retina is compatible with both nocturnal and daylight activity and some degree of color vision. There are certain differences in the spectral sensitivity of that color vision, however (Gruber et al., 1975).

The rod of most sharks absorbs in the green

range at 500 nm, the maximum transmittance wavelength in surface ocean waters (Cohen et al., 1977). Deep-water sharks have a golden visual pigment, chrysopsin, which has a maximum absorbency nearer blue in the 470 to 480 nm range. It is thought that this is more adaptive for vision in the deep sea, where much of the 500 nm light has been filtered by the water.

In addition to special visual pigments, sharks have a tapetum lucidum to maximize the use of all available light. Species that spend appreciable time near the surface also have a pigment layer that can project over the tapetum to protect the eye from bright light.

ELECTRORECEPTION

Scientists have been intrigued with the ampullae of Lorenzini, the special tubule sensory organs found distributed on the heads of sharks, skates, and rays. They have postulated a variety of functions for the mucus-filled canals that open to the outside environ-

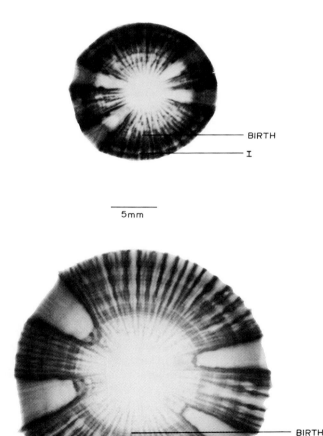

FIGURE 92–4. Transilluminated sections of vertebral bodies from thresher sharks showing the rings used in studies of age determination. (Courtesy of G.M. Cailliet.)

ment and contain a bundle of sensory cells innervated by multiple neurons. These functions have included the registration of depth and the detection of tactile stimuli. The sensors do react to many stimuli, including temperature shifts, salinity changes, pressure differences, and, of particular interest, electric potentials. The ampullae of Lorenzini are the sensory receptors elasmobranchs use to detect very weak electric fields.

The smooth dogfish and blue shark are able to detect electric fields as weak as 0.005 μV or 5 nV/cm at a distance of one-third of a meter (Ryan, 1981). This is considerably more sensitive than would be required to detect the electric fields generated by gill movements of plaice, which are in excess of 1000 μV/cm (Kalmijn, 1966). It is thought that this may be a major method of prey detection for those species that feed on flatfishes and molluscs, which lay sessile under the bottom mud and sand. It may also be a factor in pelagic species such as the blue shark, which prey on swimming foods. The blue shark executes feeding behavior in response to electric fields and will attack an electrically charged target in preference to an olfactory/taste target (Ryan, 1981).

The ampullae of Lorenzini may also function as a compass for sharks. When sharks, skates, and rays swim actively, they induce local electric fields with voltage gradients that have strength variations dependent upon the compass heading of the fishes' progress. These fields are strong enough for elasmobranchs to detect even when swimming at very low speeds. It remains to be demonstrated whether these fields are used to help elasmobranchs orient to the earth's magnetic field and navigate migrational paths.

AGE DETERMINATION AND GROWTH RATES

The determination of age and growth rate in free-living sharks is a complex and sometimes perplexing problem. Several methods are generally required to arrive at a reasonable estimate of the growth rate or to confirm age analysis. Age is often determined from examination of mineralized rings that appear in the centrum of the cartilaginous vertebrae of sharks (Fig. 92–4). In some species, these rings can be read with simple transillumination of a thin transverse microtomed slice of the vertebrae. Staining with 2% silver nitrate prior to transillumination facilitates visualization of the rings (Stevens, 1975). Unfortunately, it appears it may be necessary to determine the relationship between these rings and age for each species of shark and perhaps for different environmental situations.

Most studies indicate that two rings are laid down per year, but ring deposition may not occur every year. The vertebral rings of the shortfin mako shark are thought to be migration marks. Studies in lemon sharks have shown that probably three mineralized bands are laid down per year in this species.

Temporal analysis combined with tagging data and length frequency are used to correlate ring counts on the vertebrae of sharks. Tetracycline injections (10 to 20 mg/kg) can also be used to label cartilage in shark vertebrae. About a month after injection, deposition of a faint fluorescent band of tetracycline incorporated into the cartilage can be detected.

Growth rates of sharks vary considerably. The bull shark grows only 16 to 18 cm/year for its first 2 years and then slows to a fairly constant rate of only 11 to 12 cm/year (Thorson and Lacy, 1982). The lemon shark and brown shark are slower-growing and later-maturing species. Young lemon sharks grow between 10 and 20 cm/year. Captive specimens grow up to nine times faster than wild animals. Lemon sharks become sexually active when they are about 2.5 m in length, at about 12 years old.

The blue shark reaches an asymptotic growth rate of 21 cm/year at about 20 years of age (Stevens, 1975). The shortfin mako shark does not reach its asymptotic rate for about 45 years, and the common thresher shark at 50 years. The shortfin mako shark apparently has one of the most rapid growth rates of the sharks. It grows nearly twice as fast as the porbeagle and faster than the carcharhinids. The growth rate of the mako shark is commensurate with the growth rates of the large pelagic teleost fishes such as the dolphin, tunas, bluefish, and billfishes (Pratt and Casey, 1983). There is no difference in the growth rate of male and female shortfin mako sharks despite the size frequency differences that are normally seen. In the first year of life a mako shark will grow about 49 cm/year. This rate slows to 32 cm/year in the second year and stabilizes at an overall mean of approximately 25 cm/year (Pratt and Casey, 1983).

LITERATURE CITED

Abel, D.C., Graham, J.B., Lowell, W.R., and Shabetai, R. (1986) Elasmobranch pericardial function. 1. Pericardial pressures are not always negative. Fish Physiol. and Biochem. 1:75–83.

Budker, P. (1971) The Life of Sharks. Columbia University Press, New York.

Cohen, J.L. (1981) Vision in Sharks. Oceanus 24:17–22.

Cohen, J.L., Gruber, S.H., and Hamasaki, D.I. (1977) Spectral sensitivity and Purkinje shift in the retina of the lemon shark, *Negaprion brevirostris* (Poey). Vision Res. 17:787–792.

Gruber, S.H., Gulley, R.L., and Brandon, J. (1975) Duplex retina in seven elasmobranch species. Bull. Marine Sci. 25:353–358.

Kalmijn, A.J. (1966) Electro-perception in sharks and rays. Nature 212:1232–1233.

Matthews, L.H. (1962) The shark that hibernates. New Sci. 13:756–759.

Metcalfe, J.D., and Butler, P.J. (1986) The functional anatomy of the gills of the dogfish (*Scyliorhinus canicula*). J. Zool. Lond. 208:519–530.

Moss, S.A. (1967) Tooth replacement in the lemon shark, *Negaprion brevirostris*. In: Sharks, Skates and Rays (Gilbert, P.W., Mathewson, R.F., and Rall, D.P., eds.) Johns Hopkins Press, Baltimore, Maryland.

Murphy, R.C., and Nichols, J.T. (1916) The shark situation in the waters about New York. Brooklyn Mus. Qt. 3(4):145–160.

Pratt, H.L., and Casey, J.G. (1983) Age and growth of the shortfin mako, *Isurus oxyrinchus*, using four methods. Can. J. Fish. Aquatic. Sci. 40:1944–1957.

Ryan, P.R. (1981) Electroreception in blue sharks. Oceanus 24:42–44.

Stevens, J.D. (1975) Vertebral rings as a means of age determination in the blue shark (*Prionace glauca* L.) J. Marine Biol. Assoc. U.K. 55:657–665.

Thorson, T.B., and Lacy, E.J. (1982) Age, growth rate and longevity of *Carcharhinus leucas* estimated from tagging and vertebral rings. Copeia 1982:110–116.

Zangerl, R. (1966) A new shark of the family Edestidae, *Ornithoprion hertwigi*, from the Pennsylvanian Mecca and Logar Quarry shales of Indiana. Fieldiana Geol. 16:1–43.

Chapter 93

CLINICAL PATHOLOGY OF SHARKS, SKATES, AND RAYS

MICHAEL K. STOSKOPF

Although there has been a lot of detailed electron microscopy and cytochemistry done on the leukocytes of sharks, not much of practical clinical use is available (Fange, 1968; Fange and Mattisson, 1981; Hine and Wain, 1987a–d; Morrow and Pulsford, 1980).

METHODS

All principal mammalian leukocyte types are found in shark blood (Parish et al., 1986) (Table 93–1). However, a controversy remains about the nature of the heterophil in sharks. Workers have tried to establish the pink-staining polymorphonuclear cells in sharks as eosinophils, but all evidence is that they are true heterophils. They function much like the neutrophil of mammals (Mainwaring and Rowley, 1986). The problem is complicated because both eosinophils and heterophils of sharks are acid phosphatase and periodic acid–shift (PAS) positive (Hine and Wain, 1987a). Nevertheless, shark blood morphology can be readily accomplished using routine methodologies, and classification of cells into heterophils and eosinophils is relatively clear on the basis of cytoplasmic granule morphology and staining intensity in modified Wright-Giemsa stained smears.

One important methodologic problem is the determination of serum total protein in elasmobranchs (Table 93–2). Total protein determined with a refractometer is always artificially high because of the high serum urea nitrogen levels sharks maintain for osmotic balance. Refractometer values routinely read between two and three times higher than automated colorimetric assays.

RESPONSE TO INFECTIOUS DISEASE

Shark hematologic and serologic parameters (Tables 93–1 to 93–6) respond to infectious disease in much the same manner as would be expected from experience with mammalian systems. Bacterial infections routinely cause a marked leukocytosis that is most commonly a heterophilia. A distinct shift to the

left may be difficult to demonstrate in many cases because the nuclear morphology of the granulocytic series in sharks is less distinctly lobed in mature cells. This makes detection of young cells less certain (Fig. 93–1).

There has been little or no experience in the hematologic changes seen with viral or protozoal diseases in sharks. Overwhelming trematode infection can be accompanied by a leukocytosis, but it is difficult to say whether this is a response to the trematodes themselves or merely a generalized stress response. Serum chemistry shifts have been even less well studied in infectious diseases of sharks.

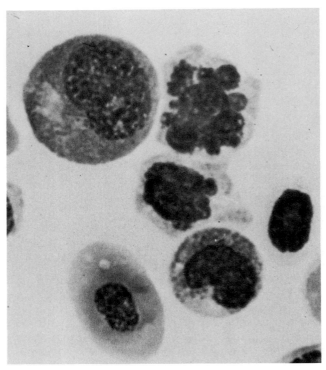

FIGURE 93–1. Occasionally bizarre blood cells are seen in shark blood. This figure shows two multinucleate cells, a binucleate cell, a blast cell, two erythrocytes, and an extruded erythrocyte nucleus circulating in the peripheral blood of a spiny dogfish. No medical history is available (Giemsa, 1000×).

TABLE 93–1. Baseline Hematologic Parameters of Elasmobranchs–Leukocyte Indices

Species	N	Total WBC × 10³/ml	Heterophils (%)	Band Cells (%)	Mono-cytes (%)	Lympho-cytes (%)	Eosinophils (%)	Basophils (%)	References
Brown shark (captive)	20	28.1	58	0	1	40	1	0	Stoskopf, unpublished
Lemon shark (captive)	3	25.9							
Nurse shark (wild)	5	27.8							
Nurse shark (captive)	7	27.2	56	0	1.4	30	0	0	Stoskopf, unpublished

TABLE 93–2. Baseline Hematologic Parameters of Elasmobranchs—Erythrocyte Indices

Species	N	Total RBC × 10⁶/ml	Hematocrit (%)	Hemoglobin (g/dl)	References
Blue shark	14	—	22.3	5.7	Johansson-Sjobeck, 1976
Brown shark (captive)	20	0.532	19.8	<4	Stoskopf, unpublished
Lemon shark (captive)	3	0.665	20.0	5.3	Stoskopf, unpublished
Nurse shark (wild)	5	0.366	10.3	4.0	Stoskopf, unpublished
Nurse shark (captive)	7	0.35	11.0	<4	Stoskopf, unpublished
Portuguese shark	1	—	13.0	—	Sherburne, 1973
Spiny dogfish	21	—	18.7	4.8	Torres et al., 1986

TABLE 93–3. Baseline Serologic Parameters of Elasmobranchs

Species	N	Urea Nitrogen (mg/dl)	Uric Acid (mg/dl)	Creatinine (mg/dl)	Total Protein (g/dl)	Albumin (g/dl)	Globulin (g/dl)	References
Brown shark (wild)	v*	848 (34)	0.45 (33)	0.45 (33)	2.2 (33)	0.5 (33)	1.7 (33)	Stoskopf, unpublished
Dusky shark (wild)	5	912	0.8	0.5	1.7	0.6	1.1	Stoskopf, unpublished
Scalloped hammerhead shark (wild)	4	880	1.0	0.4	2.5	0.4	2.1	Stoskopf, unpublished
Lemon shark (captive)	2	1,023	1.0	0.9	3.5	0.6	2.9	Stoskopf, unpublished
Nurse shark (wild)	9	1,147	0.2	0.4	2.6	0.6	2.2	Stoskopf, unpublished
Nurse shark (captive)	12	1,087	0.3	0.45	2.0	0.4	1.5	Stoskopf, unpublished
Sharpnose shark (wild)	10	847	1.1	0.5	2.1	0.4	1.7	Stoskopf, unpublished
Tiger shark (captive, compromised)	2	1,134	0.8	1.0	4.6	0.5	4.2	Stoskopf, unpublished

*v refers to a variable N indicated in parentheses after each value.

TABLE 93–4. Additional Baseline Serologic Parameters of Elasmobranchs

Species	N	Glucose (mg/dl)	Cholesterol (mg/dl)	Triglycerides (mg/dl)	AST (U/L)	ALT (U/L)	LDH (U/L)	References
Brown shark (wild)	v*	63 (33)	54 (32)	36 (9)	22 (35)	19 (37)	100 (28)	Stoskopf, unpublished
Dusky shark (wild)	5	115	29		24	4		Stoskopf, unpublished
Scalloped hammerhead shark (wild)	4	140	93		34	9	27	Stoskopf, unpublished
Lemon shark (captive)	2	77	75	126	4	15	238	Stoskopf, unpublished
Nurse shark (wild)	9	15.7	55	21.3	29.7	7.8	72.5	Stoskopf, unpublished
Nurse shark (captive)	12	25.1	53		18.5	4.4	74	Stoskopf, unpublished
Sharpnose shark (wild)	10	145	79		42.2	7.8	88	Stoskopf, unpublished
Tiger shark (captive, compromised)	2	164	69	52	131	22	463	Stoskopf, unpublished

*v refers to a variable N indicated in parentheses after each value.

TABLE 93–5. Baseline Serum Electrolyte Parameters of Elasmobranchs

Species	N	Sodium (mM/L)	Chloride (mM/L)	Potassium (mM/L)	Inorganic Phosphorus (mMl/L)	Calcium (mg/dl)	Magnesium (mg/dl)	References
Brown shark (wild)	v*	284 (27)	236 (25)	3.1 (32)	5.4 (30)	13.6 (33)		Stoskopf, unpublished
Dusky shark (wild)	5	287	239	4.0	7.0	17.0	4.2	Stoskopf, unpublished
Scalloped hammerhead shark (wild)	4	278	227	3.2	6.7	17.2	4.6	Stoskopf, unpublished
Lemon shark (captive)	2	285	235		5.2	15.4		Stoskopf, unpublished
Nurse shark (wild)	v	262 (6)	226 (6)	4.3 (9)	4.3 (9)	15.7 (8)		Stoskopf, unpublished
Nurse shark (captive)	11	263	228	3.9	4.1	14.7		Stoskopf, unpublished
Sharpnose shark (wild)	10	270	218	3.6	7.8	16.2		Stoskopf, unpublished
Tiger shark (captive, compromised)	2	284	257	3.2	7.4	13.1		Stoskopf, unpublished

*v refers to a variable N indicated in parentheses after each value.

TABLE 93–6. Baseline Serum Thyroid Parameters of Elasmobranchs

Species	N	Total T$_4$ (μg/dl)	T-Uptake Units	T$_3$ Uptake (%)	Free T$_4$ Index	References
Dusky shark (wild)	5	4.5	0.12	68.4	3.1	Stoskopf, unpublished
Scalloped hammerhead shark (wild)	4	2.9	0.2	65.2	1.8	Stoskopf, unpublished
Sharpnose shark (wild)	10	2.9	0.12	68.3	2.0	Stoskopf, unpublished

RESPONSE TO NONINFECTIOUS DISEASE

Certainly stress is a common factor in interpretation of shark hemograms and serum chemistry panels. Controlled studies in the spiny dogfish have confirmed that confinement stress in that species results in decreased erythrocyte counts, hematocrit, and hemoglobin levels (see Table 93–2). In addition to the anemia, the total leukocyte count increases dramatically, as does serum glucose (Torres et al., 1986). The stress leukogram of sharks can be difficult to differentiate from a response to bacterial septicemia. The leukocytosis is primarily due to a heterophilia. An eosinopenia may or may not be appreciated.

Heavy metal toxicity is the other major cause of hematologic changes due to noninfectious causes in sharks, skates, and rays. Copper exposure is a common problem, as sharks are much more sensitive to this metal than marine teleost fishes. In the spiny dogfish, exposure to physiologically compromising, but acutely sublethal concentrations of copper (2 ppm for 48 hours) results in a normochromic, normocytic anemia with decreased total erythrocyte count and hematocrit and a stable hemoglobin value. A leukopenia and decreased serum glucose are also seen (Tort et al., 1987). Exposure to higher levels (4, 6, 8, and 16 ppm) is fatal to spiny dogfish within 56 hours and gives a similar hematologic profile, although at higher concentrations hemoglobin begins to fall (Tort et al., 1987).

Zinc exposure in spiny dogfish also causes a hypochromic microcytic anemia characterized by a decreased hemoglobin but a normal hematocrit and an increased total erythrocyte count. A leukocytosis is present in contrast to copper exposure. Serum glucose is also depressed (Torres et al., 1986).

LITERATURE CITED

Fange, R. (1968) The formation of eosinophilic granulocytes in the oesophageal lymphomyeloid tissue of the Elasmobranchs. Acta Zool. 49:155–161.

Fange, R., and Mattisson, A. (1981) The lymphomyeloid (hemopoietic) system of the Atlantic nurse shark, Ginglymostoma cirratum. Biol. Bull. 160:240–249.

Hine, P.M., and Wain, J.M. (1987a) The enzyme cytochemistry and composition of elasmobranch granulocytes. J. Fish Biol. 30:465–475.

Hine, P.M., and Wain, J.M. (1987b) Composition and ultrastructure of elasmobranch granulocytes. I. Dogfishes (Squaliformes). J. Fish Biol. 30:547–556.

Hine, P.M., and Wain, J.M. (1987c) Composition and ultrastructure of elasmobranch granulocytes. II. Rays (Rajiformes). J. Fish Biol. 30:557–565.

Hine, P.M., and Wain, J.M. (1987d) Composition and ultrastructure of elasmobranch granulocytes. III. Sharks (Lamniformes). J. Fish Biol. 30:567–576.

Johansson-Sjobeck, M., and Stevens, J.D. (1976) Haematological studies on the blue shark, Prionace glauca L. J. Marine Biol. Assn. U.K. 56:237–240.

Mainwaring, G., and Rowley, A.F. (1986) Studies on granulocyte heterogeneity in elasmobranchs. In: Fish Immunology (Manning, M.J., and Tatner, H.F., eds.). Academic Press, London, pp.57–70.

Morrow, W.J.W., and Pulsford, A. (1980) Identification of peripheral blood leucocytes of the dogfish (Scyliorhinus canicula L.) by electron microscopy. J. Fish Biol. 17:461–475.

Parish, N., Wrathmell, A., Hart, S., and Harris, J.E. (1986) The leucocytes of the elasmobranch Scyliorhinus canicula L., a morphological study. J. Fish Biol. 28:545–561.

Sherburne, S.W. (1973) Cell types, differential cell counts and blood cell measurements of a Portuguese shark (Centrocymnus coelolepis) captured at 700 fathoms. Fish. Bull. 71(2):435–439.

Stoskopf, M.K. Unpublished data from Records of the National Aquarium in Baltimore.

Torres, P., Tort, L., Planas, J., and Flos, R. (1986) Effects of confinement stress and additional zinc treatment on some blood parameters in the dogfish Scyliorhinus canicula. Comp. Biochem. Physiol. 83C:89–92.

Tort, L., Torres, P., and Flos, R. (1987) Effects on dogfish haematology and liver composition after acute copper exposure. Comp. Biochem. Physiol. 87C:349–353.

Chapter 94

ENVIRONMENTAL REQUIREMENTS AND DISEASES OF SHARKS

MICHAEL K. STOSKOPF

Sharks, skates, and rays are found in most marine environments and even in fresh water. Obviously the requirements of each species vary considerably. There are few data on the species that inhabit the oceans. The focus of this chapter must then be primarily on the requirements of captive specimens. Traditionally sharks have not done particularly well in captivity. The number of species kept successfully for long periods is relatively limited, although successes in aquarium design and maintenance have expanded this list in recent years.

SELECTING SPECIES FOR CAPTIVITY

Several factors are important in selecting elasmobranchs for captive maintenance. Perhaps most important are the natural behaviors of the species. The majority of successes in long-term maintenance have been with animals that tend to be bottom dwellers or slower swimmers. Nonpelagic sharks that have done well in captivity include nurse sharks, cat sharks, and the lemon shark (Gruber and Keyes, 1981). Fast-swimming pelagic sharks have proved difficult to provide for.

Also important is the ultimate size of the specimen or specimens to be held. This has significant impact on the required size of the enclosure and the design of handling facilities. For example, although a 3 m long lemon shark will survive in a 2 m deep tank with dimensions of 13 by 7 m, a 2 m blacktip reef shark would not survive 24 hours in the same tank (Klay, 1977). On the other hand, a 1 m blacktip reef shark would do well in that much space. Several of the species that can be kept very successfully in captivity grow from relatively small animals to large specimens that require hoists and booms for effective manipulation out of the water. These animals seem to tolerate tighter spaces better than equal-sized wild specimens, but they still require a minimum rest-glide distance (Table 94–1).

Special dietary requirements can pose a significant obstacle to captive management of some species. Recent successes in managing the whale shark in captivity have shown that these factors can be overcome if careful attention is paid to the requirements of the shark. Another factor is the ease with which the species adapts to captive feeding on dead food. Rays are often very slow to adapt to food in captivity but do very well once they have begun to feed.

CAPTURE AND TRANSPORT

Capture

An important aspect of maintaining elasmobranchs in captivity is obtaining healthy, undamaged specimens. Capture methods for sharks, skates, and rays should minimize the time the animal is restrained. Trawling should be avoided. Trapping is only useful if the traps are checked very frequently. Cast netting is a popular method for capturing smaller sharks in clear shallow water but is not useful in deep or murky water. In such water, set lines are frequently used.

The type of set line can greatly influence survivability of caught sharks. One estimate suggests that set long lines (Fig. 94–1) can be expected to deliver only about 30% survivability compared to 90% survivability with set single lines (Fig. 94–2) (Klay, 1976). Much of this is certainly due to the time the animals spend on the hook. Frequent checking of long lines can provide much better survivability, but this is extremely labor intensive.

The handling of the animal during, and immediately after, capture is important to the quality of animal that will be obtained. Sharks should never be held vertically, whether with head up or down. They should always be held as close to horizontal as possible to avoid trauma to the ligaments of the internal organs. Sharks should be kept in a circulating live well on the trip to shore. There is always a necessary compromise between trying to reduce the transport time to shore and at the same time minimizing trauma to the animal through bouncing on the floor of the live well as the boat hits swells. The degree of trauma a shark can sustain from this trauma

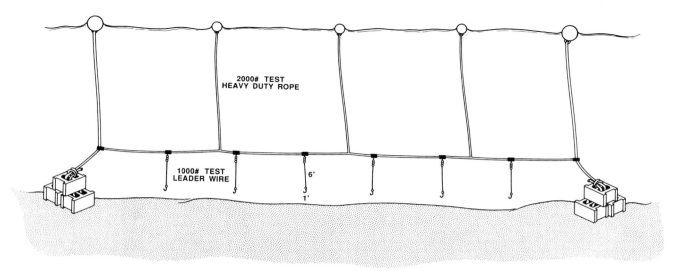

FIGURE 94–1. Typical long-line set-up for catching sharks in deeper water. Hook lines on long lines are spaced to prevent hooks from tangling. Anchors or weights are used to hold the ends of the line to the bottom. Large float buoys mark the anchors and, along with smaller buoys, suspend the catch line above the bottom. Hook lines on swivels are usually set a foot or so off the bottom.

is routinely underestimated, even by experienced collectors. Bruising of internal organs can severely compromise even bottom-dwelling sharks, which are usually relatively tolerant of captivity. A slower transport with less trauma is nearly always the best compromise.

Transport of Large Sharks

Transporting a captive shark requires careful consideration of the shark's needs. Large specimens should be accompanied by an attendant. These animals are routinely transported in boxes equipped with filtration and oxygen supplementation. Sharks for transport should have been held off feed for at least 1 day and preferably 2. This will reduce the risk of regurgitation and will keep nitrogenous waste production to a minimum.

Filtration should remove all particulate matter and maintain clear transport water. Ion exchange filtration can be used to remove nitrogenous waste products from the water. The transportation package should also include an oxygen cylinder capable of delivering 50 lb/hour for 40 hours and a battery that will supply 64 amp to drive the filtration pumps (Klay, 1976).

During the transport, do not tamper with the shark or container excessively, but there are some reasons to interfere. If foam builds up from regurgitation or defecation, remove the wastes immediately. If the pH of the water begins to fall, increase the aeration. Also, check the filter and possibly replace the calcareous gravel. If the water turns brown, either too little oxygen is being delivered or the pump to the filters is clogged and requires cleaning. Always carry a spare pump in the transport equipment.

If the shark begins to stiffen, massage the animal

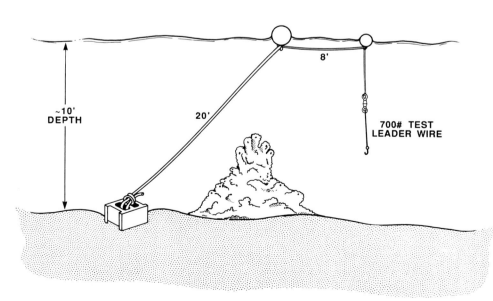

FIGURE 94–2. Setting a blockline for catching reef sharks. A typical set-up for catching lemon sharks in about 10 feet of water uses a 20-foot heavy line attached to cement blocks and a float. A second float suspends the hook line on a swivel above the bottom.

by slowly flexing the caudal peduncle. This will usually evoke swimming motions and help alleviate the build-up of lactate. Massage should be done every few minutes for a shark showing signs of stiffness. A system using a Neoprene sling supported with elastic bunge cords has proved very useful for preventing this problem in the transport of large brown sharks.

Temperature control is important to the safe transport of large sharks. If temperatures are too high, the animal will be hyperactive and difficult to manage in the transport box. Too low a temperature will result in very low respiratory rates.

Oxygen levels must be carefully monitored during transport of large specimens. Eight parts per million is usually considered optimal. Oxygen levels should not be allowed to exceed 15 ppm. Prolonged periods at up to 15 ppm do not seem to compromise the shark. Excessive oxygen levels above this level will cause neurologic damage and result in the death of the shark. Short-duration extreme hyperoxygenation episodes can burn gills. Sharks affected this way usually die 3 to 4 weeks after the episode. Sharks that are not getting enough oxygen begin to turn blotchy and increase their respiratory rate. Sharks receiving too much oxygen become pale and may cease to gill.

Shipping Small Sharks

Smaller shark specimens can be shipped with modifications of the methods used for marine tropical teleosts. Sharks that are not prone to biting can be shipped in closed plastic bags. Enough water is usually provided to cover the back of the shark. The water should be overlaid with pure oxygen at 0.35 kg/cm^2 over ambient air pressure (Fig. 94–3). This not only provides additional oxygen for exchange with the water and shark but also may have a slight anesthetic effect on the animal (Klay, 1976). This system will support a shark for between 10 and 15 hours during transport as long as the shark does not rupture the plastic bag with its teeth.

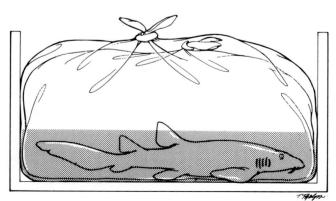

FIGURE 94–3. When shipping small sharks, enough water is provided to cover the back of the shark. The water is overlaid with pure oxygen at 0.35 kg/cm^2 over ambient air pressure.

Species that tend to be active biters should be transported in resin-coated or waterproof shipping tanks with smooth interior surfaces. These containers should not allow the shark to turn easily, or in the other extreme, should allow free swimming. This will reduce the likelihood of the shark's getting jammed in a compromising position.

Air Shipment

The shipment of sharks by air requires careful planning and anticipation of all possible problems (Klay, 1976). When shipping sharks by air it is important to have good relations with airline personnel. Shipments should be made on flights during nonpeak hours. Arrange all flight changes in advance, making personal contact with the people who will be responsible for moving the transport box from one flight to another. Always plan the shortest route with the minimum number of plane changes. The ground time between flights should be minimized, but it is also important to allow at least 2 hours for a plane change to avoid missing a connection.

Adhere to delivery times. Arrive at the airline 1 to 2 hours before flight time. The package must be labeled properly. Always ask for one of the first three positions on the plane that will be unloaded first (Klay, 1976). This will minimize the chance of missing a connection, a situation that could be fatal to the shark being shipped. Always notify the person responsible at the receiving institution of all plans and details of the shipment.

INTRODUCTIONS

Introduction of new sharks into a display or holding tank requires some thought. Newly caught sharks will represent a free meal to acclimated animals in the same tank if they are not about the same size as the established occupants. After capture and transport, new sharks are disoriented and at a serious disadvantage.

A tradition in shark introductions has been the "walking" of new animals. Although this tradition persists, it is rarely successful. If a shark is so compromised as to require additional oxygen, it is usually more effective to place an oxygenated water source in front of the mouth of the shark and allow the shark to rest on the bottom. If a shark is highly stressed, lactate accumulates and the oxygen-carrying capacity of the hemoglobin is decreased. Walking a shark contributes to this problem and defeats the delivery of more oxygen to tissues where it is needed. An acidotic shark becomes immobile, stiffens, and will die (Gruber and Keyes, 1981).

TANK CONFIGURATION

The configuration of tanks for sharks has long been a controversial subject, and that controversy

TABLE 94–1. Shark Rest-Glide Dimensions

Shark	Size (ft)	Turn (ft)	Cruise (ft)	Rest-Glide (ft)	Recovery (ft)	Cruise (ft)	Turn (ft)	Total (ft)
Blacktip	4	4	10–20	20	15	10–20	4	72+
Lemon	8	4–8	10–20	5	5	10–20	4–8	56
Bull	6	4–8	10–20	10	10	10–20	4–8	60
Brown	4	2–4	10	6	6	10	2–4	54
Porbeagle	5	2–4	20	20	20	10–20	4–6	84
Tiger	6	4–6	10–20	20	20	10–20	4–6	80

From Klay, G. (1977) Shark Dynamics and Exhibit Design. Drum and Croaker April:29–32.

will not be laid to rest in this chapter. Many shark managers feel that tank configuration is critical to the long-term health of captive sharks. Certainly it is important that any shark maintained in captivity be free to move unimpeded in any direction. Although contrary to popular belief, it is not necessary for sharks to ram ventilate, they do need to swim to facilitate cardiovascular return. Also, energetic concerns can become very limiting.

One aspect of tank configuration that is not intuitive is that the length of straightaways must allow swimming sharks to participate in a glide-rest phase of swimming (see Table 94–1). The faster a shark swims, the longer the straightaway needed for the glide-rest period. Normally a glide-rest is followed by an active swimming period. During the rest period, metabolic wastes are removed. During swimming they are accumulated. The metabolic implications for a shark not able to glide-rest are obvious.

Sharks will usually swim at the most energetically economical speed, or the speed that requires the least calories. During rest-glide, the shark moves without the aid of muscle strokes, which is even more energetically favorable. During the glide the shark will lose vertical position in the water column. The ratio of loss of position in the water column to gliding distance varies with each shark species. Pelagic blue or whitetip sharks have a sink:glide ratio of about 1:10. Inshore sharks have a much more favorable ratio, sinking much less per unit distance. This loss of water column position must be corrected with active swimming, and the cost of that swimming must be less than the energetic gain of the glide itself for the glide to function.

Pelagic sharks have much longer rest-glide requirements than inshore species. A 1.3 m blacktip reef shark requires between 24 and 25 m for a proper glide. Sharks that live inshore have shorter rest-glide periods, but they are more frequent. A 2.5 m bull shark requires only 20 to 21 m glide distance. Pelagic rays, like the eagle rays and manta rays, also have longer glide paths than near-shore rays and skates. Unfortunately, the rest-glide distance requirements do not increase linearly with increased length of a given species of shark. Happily, it is a decreasing function, with longer sharks of the same species requiring glide-rest distances proportionately shorter for their body length.

Also, experience with the tank can affect the required rest-glide distance of a shark. When first introduced, sharks require longer rest-glide periods than when they are acclimated. With the exception of lemon, nurse, bull, and sand tiger sharks, any shark over 2 m should have an introduction tank that is at least 35 m by 15 m to maintain normal swimming patterns.

Forced turns during cruising also cause loss of elevation in the water column, and in sharp turns there is a risk of stalling that stresses a shark. One theory proposes that to turn, swimming sharks must drop a significant portion of their lift surface on one side (Fig. 94–4). This initiates a turn much in the manner of an airplane. During the turn, the shark

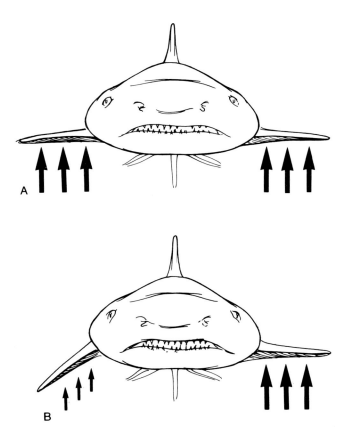

FIGURE 94–4. The primary lift surfaces for a shark are the pectoral fins. When a shark swims in a straight line, both pectoral fins provide approximately equal lift *(A)*. When a shark turns *(B)*, it lowers the pectoral to the center of the radius of the turn, effectively reducing lift on that side.

loses lift surface and would fall in the water column if it did not apply more forward momentum using its body and tail. This requires additional expenditure of energy and depletion of energy reserves. The theory proposes that if sharks are subjected to tanks with inadequate linear dimensions to allow straight glide paths, they can be put in an energy-deficit situation in which the amount of extra effort and energy used to constantly turn and yet maintain lift exceeds the energy intake of the animals. Support for this theory is fairly convincing. For example, lemon sharks significantly decrease their ad lib food consumption when they are moved to a larger pool and all other factors are controlled (Gruber and Keyes, 1981).

Also obvious from this theory would be the limitations of a round tank. The diameter of the tank would have to provide more than the minimum total glide-rest distance, including a turning radius at each end of the glide-rest. It has been observed that a totally round tank also usually results in a shark swimming continually in one direction.

Round tanks were once quite popular for sharks. The concept of the design was to avoid corners that might trap a swimming shark. However, sharks can turn in a very short radius and corners are usually not a problem for a healthy animal. In fact, sharks may have difficulty in perceiving a slightly curved wall. They seem to perceive straight walls better.

Light cycling into day and night patterns is also an important design consideration for sharks. Continuous illumination has been shown to damage the eyes of lemon sharks, eventually resulting in loss of pupillary responses (Gruber and Keyes, 1981).

A special consideration in maintaining sharks in captivity is their sensitivity to electrical fields. Elasmobranchs have special sensory organs that allow them to detect fields due to very low voltages on the order of the electrical currents generated by neuronal firing. This adaptation is apparently used in prey detection, but a positive adaptation in the wild can become extremely maladaptive in captivity if shark tanks are not shielded from electrical currents. Small short circuits and areas of increased resistance can generate disturbances that will cause a shark to become completely disoriented. Sharks will often attempt to attack walls or substrate in the area of a short circuit. Electrical problems should be placed in the differential diagnosis whenever behavioral changes are seen in captive sharks.

WATER QUALITY

Many shark facilities have the advantage of open water systems with flow-through exchange of the water. Closed systems require some special considerations for sharks. Biological filters are generally utilized for nitrate fixation, and particulate filtration is required. In addition, it is important to change at least 10 to 20% of the water volume in each month of operation (Gruber and Keyes, 1981). Old water can cause sharks to lose color or blanch. It can also result in pruritus, with sharks actively scratching on substrates and walls without any build-up of ectoparasites. Blatantly poor water quality, and the build-up of nitrogenous wastes, can cause overt neurologic signs in sharks, including what appear to be periodic seizures.

There are, of course, many different schedules for achieving water changes, but examining them suggests that a minimum of a 100% change annually is required to reduce the risk of goiter formation, scratching, blanching, or neurologic problems.

Water turnover through both the nitrate fixation and the particulate filtration systems should allow complete filtration of the tank volume every 2 hours in smaller-volume systems. Meeting these requirements, for example, would allow the management of a lemon shark in as little as 100 L/kg body weight; however, a ratio of 500 L/kg would be preferable.

Water temperature is most important in shark species that live at the extremes. Tropical sharks are much more susceptible to cold water, and sharks that live at depth or in cold water have severe problems with warm water. The bulk of species kept in captivity are relatively tolerant of temperature fluctuations.

Oxygen deficiency can be a severe problem in sharks in transport. Affected sharks develop white blotches on their pectoral fins. If not ameliorated, the condition can result in irreversible brain damage. On the other hand, supersaturation of water with oxygen, which causes "gas bubble disease," a recognized problem in teleost fishes, is also a problem in sharks, skates, and rays. The signs of this disease are similar to those seen in teleosts.

Salinity is a major problem in many shark species; however, some species that are frequently found in rivers, such as the lemon and bull sharks, can tolerate salinity changes much more readily than other sharks. Sharks subjected to sudden abnormally low salinity tend to have difficulty in swimming and spend most of their time on the bottom. A sudden change to an abnormally high salinity will cause a shark to swim with difficulty, often with the head partially out of the water.

Elasmobranchs are sensitive to water-quality issues related to pH shifts. A sudden drop of even 0.2 pH point can cause problems. Although most sharks tolerate short periods of pH flux well, and many aquaria maintain sharks in water with a pH as low as 7.4, care should be taken to maintain pH stability. Low pH can cause loss of appetite. Maintenance of sharks in low pH water is sometimes rationalized as an attempt to reduce the risk of ammonia toxicity. As little as 0.01 ppm un-ionized ammonia is toxic to sharks.

Sharks, skates, and rays are particularly susceptible to copper toxicity. They are severely compromised at levels that are considered therapeutic for marine teleost fishes. The olfactory bulbs of sharks are very sensitive to copper ions, and exposure causes the ampullae to become clogged with mucus and impairs their function (Gruber and Keyes, 1981). This problem relates to pH since very small decreases in pH can result in the dissolution of significant amounts of copper that may have plated out on substrates and tank walls if sharks are held in tanks that have been used for teleosts. Routine copper treatments of marine teleosts will plate out more than enough copper to cause severe problems in sharks if the pH shifts even 0.2 point toward acid.

LITERATURE CITED

Klay, G. (1976) Manual for Ocean Park, Ltd., Criteria for Collecting and Maintenance of Sharks and Other Large Fishes, Vols. I–III. S.Q. Oceanographic Inc., Marathon, Florida.

Klay, G. (1977) Shark Dynamics and Exhibit Design. Drum and Croaker April:29–32.

Gruber, S.H., and Keyes, R.S. (1981) Keeping sharks for research. In: Aquarium Systems (Hawkins, A.D., ed.). Academic Press, London, pp. 373–402.

Chapter 95

NUTRITION AND NUTRITIONAL DISEASES IN SHARKS

CHARLES S. PIKE, III   CHARLES A. MANIRE
SAMUEL H. GRUBER

Historically, the difficulties in developing a comprehensive nutritional plan for elasmobranchs have been compounded by the lack of directed studies (Gruber and Keyes, 1981). At the present time, nutritional requirements of sharks must still be extrapolated largely from studies of bony fishes (Halver, 1972) and studies on the bioenergetics of the lemon shark (Cortes, 1987; Schurdak and Gruber, 1989; Gruber, 1984; Cortes and Gruber, 1990; Wetherbee et al., 1990). Thus, the majority of information on nutritional requirements and deficiencies in sharks presented here is based on empirical studies carried out over the past 2 decades in a limited range of species.

IMPORTANCE OF DIET

In conjunction with the proper aquarium environment, diet is the most important aspect of maintaining sharks in captivity. Proper nutrition in the form of adequate food and vitamin and mineral supplementation is necessary to ensure that captive sharks grow at rates similar to those in the wild. Normal growth rates are usually indicative of healthy animals. Clinical disease may ensue when nutritional needs are not met (Cho, 1983). Only with healthy sharks, growing at normal rates, can data be collected from captive animals that can be compared and extrapolated to data collected from wild species.

The ultimate aim of nutrition research is to provide a quantitatively and qualitatively balanced diet, which will meet the requirements of the animal with respect to any one of a number of physiologic functions ranging from growth to reproduction. This aim cannot be attained without an understanding of the chemical role of each food component and a broad comprehension of the interplay between different food components (Cowey and Sargent, 1979). Once these relationships are understood, it is possible to provide for optimal performance of those functions with respect to any particular diet which might be designed or balanced. Formulas for balanced fish diets must include an energy source plus adequate essential amino acids, essential fatty acids, and vitamins and minerals to promote normal growth and ensure healthy animals (Halver, 1976).

NUTRITIONAL CONTENT

Protein

Energy becomes available to sharks in the form of protein, lipid, and, to a much lesser extent, carbohydrates when food is ingested. Ingested nutrients are useful only if they can be digested and absorbed. Enzymatic digestion is an important requirement for the utilization of metabolites for energy and other purposes. Proteins are the major organic materials in most animal tissues, making up about 67 to 75% of the total on a dry weight basis. Sharks must consume protein to furnish a continual supply of amino acids. After consumption, protein is digested or hydrolyzed to release free amino acids that are absorbed from the intestinal tract and distributed by the blood to various organs and tissues. These amino acids are then used to synthesize new protein. A regular intake of protein is required, since proteins are continually being used either to build new tissues or to repair worn or damaged tissues. If adequate protein is not provided in the diet, a rapid reduction or cessation of growth or a loss of weight will result, since protein is withdrawn from some tissues to maintain the functions of more vital ones. Conversely, too much protein results in proportionally less being used to make new protein, with the excess protein being metabolized to produce energy.

Proteins in the body tissues are built using approximately 23 amino acids. Ten are essential amino acids (arginine, histidine, isoleucine, leucine, lysine, methionine, phenylalanine, threonine, tryptophan, and valine), and all have been shown to be required by many species of bony fishes. The same is assumed to be true for sharks. The utilization of dietary protein is affected mainly by its amino acid pattern, by the level of protein intake, by the caloric content of the diet, and by the physiologic state of the animal. As an essential energy source for some critical body organs and tissues, certain amino acids are readily converted to glucose. Fish are more dependent upon amino acids as precursors to glucose than most other animals owing to the fact that carbohydrate is not prevalent in their natural diet and they have a limited ability (especially true in sharks) to metabolize it. Thus a portion of dietary protein is always used as an energy source (Cho, 1983).

Fish, as a group, are fundamentally different from other vertebrate animals in that they require more dietary protein (Tacon and Cowey, 1985; Wilson and Halver, 1986). Mammals and birds typically achieve maximum growth rates on diets comprising 12 to 25% protein, whereas fish require diets with 35 to 55% protein to reach maximum growth rates (Bowen, 1987). The level of protein intake necessary for maximal growth has been investigated in several fish species (De Long et al., 1958; Ogino and Saito, 1970; Jauncey, 1982). Optimum growth of chinook salmon occurs with a diet composed of 40% protein at 8.3°C and 55% at 19.5°C (De Long et al., 1958). Plaice require a diet of up to 70% protein for optimal growth at 15°C (Cowey et al., 1972). Carp and tilapia require similar high levels of dietary protein (Ogino and Saito, 1970). Juvenile tilapia have an estimated protein requirement of 40% of the diet (Jauncey, 1982). These and many other studies support an earlier prediction that the protein requirements of fishes should be markedly higher than those of birds and mammals (Gerking, 1955).

Lipids

Lipids fulfill two broad general functions. They play a major role in providing energy, and they are involved in maintaining the structural integrity of biologic membranes. Lipids are hydrolyzed by lipase and bile salts into diglycerides, monoglycerides, glycerol, and free fatty acids (Smith, 1980; Robinson and Mead, 1973). Absorption of lipids depends on the degree of saturation (Leger, 1985), decreasing as the melting point of the lipid increases (Nose, 1967). Triglycerides provide the bulk of fatty acids for oxidation in fishes. However, a major difference between fishes and terrestrial vertebrates is how lipids, and especially triglycerides, are stored as an energy reserve. Most fishes store very large quantities of lipid in their livers and muscles. This is especially true for sharks, since they store large quantities of lipids in their livers. Both proteins and lipids are highly digestible, and mechanisms of digestion and absorption are similar in elasmobranchs, teleosts, and other vertebrates (Braaten, 1979; Fange and Grove, 1979).

Carbohydrates

Dietary carbohydrates serve largely as a source of energy. The natural diet of most sharks contains relatively few carbohydrates. The small amounts of carbohydrates ingested are derived from muscle glycogen. Digestion of carbohydrates is related to structural complexity; simple saccharides are easily digested, whereas starches are poorly digested by fishes (Smith, 1971; Shimeno et al., 1977).

Vitamins and Minerals

Vitamins are organic compounds required in trace amounts by most forms of life for normal growth, reproduction, and health. Individual vitamin requirements are dependent on the intake of other nutrients, the size of the fish, and environmental stresses. Four fat-soluble and 11 water-soluble vitamins are known to be required by fishes, and the roles and functions of individual vitamins have been described (Halver, 1972, 1985; Anonymous, 1981, 1983). However, the exact vitamin requirements of sharks are unknown.

In fishes, minerals perform important roles in osmoregulation, intermediary metabolism, and formation of the teeth, skeleton, and scales (Lall, 1981). Mineral requirements are difficult to study because many minerals are required in only trace amounts, and others are absorbed from the water through the gills in significant quantities. Minerals required by fishes include calcium, cobalt, fluorine, iodine, iron,

TABLE 95–1. Dietary Supplements for Captive Sharks

Dietary Addition	Dosage (per kg Animal Weight per Week)
A	3570 IU
B$_1$	210.0 mg
B$_2$	0.39 mg
B$_6$	0.23 mg
B$_{12}$	0.9 mg
C	37.5 mg
Calcium pantothenate	0.6 mg
Choline	Trace
D	150 IU
E	37.5 IU
Ferrous gluconate	11.25 mg
Folic acid	Trace
Inositol	Trace
Kelp (iodine)	18 μg
Niacin	0.6 mg

Vitamins and minerals are furnished in a single multivitamin tablet. These supplements have been used successfully for 15 years on lemon sharks.

manganese, magnesium, phosphorus, selenium, and zinc (Anonymous, 1981, 1983).

Dietary levels for vitamins and minerals given in Table 95–1 are based on requirements of marine fishes and are modified for sharks. Using the formulation in Table 1, lemon sharks, nurse sharks, and bull sharks are successfully maintained for long periods (Gruber and Keyes, 1981). We have found that a single multivitamin tablet included in the food once per week is a simple, inexpensive way of providing such supplementation. Vitamin and mineral supplements are especially important when feeding sharks frozen fish, since vitamins are lost during prolonged storage. Water-soluble vitamins are labile and therefore subject to degradation (Cowey, 1981).

CAPTIVE HUSBANDRY

Types of Food

The types and nutritional content of foods given to sharks in captivity should be related to the diet that each species consumes in the wild. Since the diet of many sharks is composed primarily of bony fishes, diets in captivity often consist of either fresh or frozen fish. Depending on the size of the shark and the volume of the aquarium that it inhabits, either whole fish or filets of fish can be used. The feeding of whole fish leaves residues from uneaten portions. Scales and bones tend to clog the filtration system in small systems, and promote bacterial growth. If uneaten portions remain in the tank, the tank becomes badly contaminated with both particulate and soluble organic matter. This can be prevented for the most part in small systems by feeding boneless filets and properly cleaning immediately after feeding. Filets lack many nutrients, and this necessitates constant supplementation with vitamins and minerals.

Larger sharks have the ability to consume whole fish in one movement. Smaller sharks should be fed bite-size pieces of fish. The entire piece of food is ingested in one movement. If given a relatively large piece of food, a lemon shark will often remove bite-size pieces with lateral oscillation and twisting of its head. As it does so, small scraps torn from the food will enter the water and foul the tank. Lemon sharks will consume the flesh of many fish species but definitely prefer certain types (Cortes and Gruber, 1990). The local availability of food fish influences selection, but fresh food similar to the shark's natural diet is probably best.

Feeding Schedules

The feeding regimen adopted in the aquarium should meet the objectives for which the sharks are being held. For most physiologic, biochemical, or behavioral studies, the sharks must have a complete and nutritionally balanced diet. The same is true for any shark maintained in captivity unless special requirements are dictated for studies of metabolism or nutrition.

Absorption of nutrients across the wall of the gastrointestinal tract is one of the first steps in incorporating energy into the body. The nutritive value of food is dependent not only on the nutrient content but also on the ability of the animal to digest and absorb the nutrients (Smith, 1979).

Over the past 10 years we have been feeding our captive lemon sharks blue runner filets two or three times weekly at 2.0 to 2.5% of body weight per day with vitamin and mineral supplementation similar to that listed in Table 95–1. The growth rates obtained in captivity (9 to 12 cm/year) are only slightly slower than those of lemon sharks tagged internally in the wild (14 to 18 cm/year).

The frequency of feeding sharks in captivity should be related to how frequently the shark feeds in the wild. This frequency is ideally based on the nutritional content of the food and the shark's physiologic processes of gastric evacuation rates, total gut passage time, assimilation, and absorption efficiency. All of these dictate the amount of energy that can be extracted over time and used for growth. The food intake of captive lemon sharks is subject to substantial periodic variation, with a tendency toward 4-day cycles in peak consumption ad lib (Longval et al., 1982). Captive sharks fed to satiation refuse more food until some time passes. Hunger and satiation play a role in the shark's feeding behavior (Longval et al., 1982). In contrast, feeding by wild lemon sharks is asynchronous and intermittent (Cortes and Gruber, 1990). A pattern of periodicity can be discerned with peak consumption followed by a period of 36 hours of digestion (Cortes and Gruber, 1990).

Ration Levels and Growth Rates

Although an individual shark may not consume the same amount of food each day, or may not even feed daily, consumption expressed on a daily basis (daily ration) provides a useful means to compare ingestion rates for different organisms (Wetherbee et al., 1990). The daily ration of the lemon shark is about 1.6 to 2.2% of body weight per day (Cortes and Gruber, 1990). For brown sharks, this value is 1.1% of body weight (Medved et al., 1988). The daily ration of the spiny dogfish has been calculated at 1.3% of body weight (Brett and Blackburn, 1978), with some difference attributable to water temperature. The daily ration of the mako shark is 3.1% of body weight (Stillwell and Kohler, 1982). The higher level of consumption relative to other species is expected, since mako sharks are fast-swimming, highly active sharks, capable of maintaining a body temperature several degrees above that of ambient water (Carey and Teal, 1969). Digestion rate, rate of food passage, and consequent ingestion rate all may be increased at higher ambient temperatures (Kaushik, 1986).

It is apparent that sharks consume less on a percentage of body weight basis than most teleosts, which is reflected in slow growth. Many carnivorous teleosts consume 20 to 30% of their body weight per day (Brett and Groves, 1979), whereas the maximum ration voluntarily consumed by lemon sharks is less than 3% of body weight per day (Gruber, 1984).

DIGESTIVE PHYSIOLOGY

Gastric Evacuation and Total Gut Passage Time

Gastric evacuation rates (the time from ingestion to complete gastric emptying) and total gut passage times (the time from ingestion to complete gastrointestinal tract emptying) directly influence the amount of food consumed and the nutrients obtained from food. The longer a meal is in the digestive tract, the longer it is subject to the processes of enzymatic digestion and absorption and the greater the amount of nutrients absorbed (Windell, 1978). Captive lemon sharks require 24 hours and 41 hours to completely empty their stomach of fish filets and whole fish, respectively (Schurdak and Gruber, 1989). There is a time-dependent difference in the removal of carbohydrates and protein. In contrast, the time required for complete gastric evacuation in the brown shark is 71 to 92 hours (Medved, 1985). This difference in

time is greater than might be expected in these similar sharks with similar distribution, life history, and a close phylogenetic relationship. However, it is likely that methodologic differences, including food type, temperature, field conditions, and so forth, exaggerate actual differences in gastric evacuation rates. Other estimates of gastric evacuation rates for sharks are less (Table 95–2). The time for complete gastric emptying in the spiny dogfish was estimated by fitting a straight line to the data and extrapolating to zero food (Jones and Green, 1977). The time for complete gastric emptying for the mako shark is based on examination of stomach contents and information from other species of sharks (Stillwell and Kohler, 1982). Unfortunately, gastric evacuation rates have not been measured in either of these species. Brown sharks have food in their stomachs 48 hours after consumption of a meal, but time for complete gastric evacuation is not known (Wass, 1973). The average time for complete gastric evacuation of a meal measured for teleosts is about 12 hours (Fange and Grove, 1979). Based on the few actual measurements and partial measurements of gastric evacuation, it is apparent that a substantially longer period of time is required for food to be completely eliminated from the stomach of sharks than for teleosts.

Only limited data are available concerning the effect of increasing ration on gastric emptying for sharks (Cortes, 1987; Cortes and Gruber, 1990; Wetherbee et al., 1990; Wetherbee, 1988). There may be a positive correlation between ration level and total gut passage time. The total gut passage time of 70 to 100 hours for the lemon shark is slow in comparison with most teleosts, particularly for tropical species. Total gut passage time averages approximately 50 hours for 48 species of teleosts (Fange and Grove, 1979).

Absorption Efficiency

Absorption efficiency is a measure of the ability of an organism to digest and absorb nutrients from food (Buddington, 1979). The amount of nutrient absorbed represents energy extracted from food and reflects the quality of food and the adequacy with which an animal's digestive physiology is extracting energy (Brafield and Llewellyn, 1982). Absorption efficiency is fundamental to understanding growth of an individual or population (Talbort, 1985). Char-

TABLE 95–2. Estimates of Time Required for a Meal to be Completely Evacuated from the Stomachs of Sharks

Species	Hours for Complete Gastric Evacuation	Temperature (° C)	References
Spiny dogfish	124	10	Jones and Green, 1977
Brown shark	71–92	25	Medved, 1985
	48 +	—	Wass, 1973
Shortfin mako	36–48	—	Stillwell and Kohler, 1982
Lemon shark	28–41	20—29	Cortes and Gruber, 1990
	24	25	Schurdak and Gruber, 1989
Blue shark	24 +	—	Tricas, 1979

acteristics of the digestive physiology of an organism, as well as energy and nutrient requirements may be revealed by absorption efficiency (Cho et al., 1985). Absorption efficiency is one of the main indicators of the nutrient value in fish foods and has been used extensively in the evaluation of different foodstuffs and for the formulation and improvement of diets for cultured fishes (Cho et al., 1985). The efficiency with which the lemon shark is able to absorb energy, organic matter, and dry matter has been measured at five levels of energy intake (Wetherbee, 1988). Absorption efficiencies range from 62 to 83% for energy, 76 to 88% for organic matter, and 76 to 87% for dry matter. Absorption efficiencies increase as energy intake increases and decline at the highest level of intake, indicating that lemon sharks are capable of absorbing nutrients from food as efficiently as most teleosts.

Nutrient Utilization

Since food supply is the major factor controlling production of most animals, understanding the relationship between food supply and growth is important. A series of experiments established the relationship between feeding level and production in the juvenile lemon sharks (Cortes and Gruber, 1990). Increasing intake and the growth rate correlate directly until the growth rate levels off at high rations (Cortes and Gruber, 1990). The food-conversion efficiency of lemon sharks also continues to increase with increased ration, eventually leveling off at high rations (Wetherbee et al., 1990). Food is not converted to growth as efficiently at high-ration levels owing to decreased absorption efficiency or increased metabolic costs of processing the additional food (Warren and Davis, 1967). Growth does not appear to be limited by the ability of the lemon shark to absorb energy or to convert consumed energy to growth. The lemon shark has a metabolic rate comparable to active teleost predators, indicating that metabolic costs are not unusually high (Bushnell et al., 1989). The major factor responsible for slow rates of growth observed in lemon sharks is a relatively low level of consumption, which may, in turn, be limited by a slow rate of digestion (Wetherbee et al., 1990).

Nutritional Deficiencies

Even as there is little definitive information concerning nutrition in elasmobranchs, there is even less concerning nutritional deficiencies or nutritional diseases. On a broad basis, data must be extrapolated from that of other fishes, most of which is covered elsewhere in this book. Because of this and because it is rare for a single deficiency to manifest itself (Cowey and Roberts, 1978), our discussion is limited to deficiencies of major nutritional groups and possible differences between teleosts and elasmobranchs.

Protein Deficiency

In elasmobranchs, protein is the single most important nutritional group and may be the most common deficiency. Extreme lack of protein ingestion, whether induced by the animal or the caretaker, leads to starvation and mortality. Although the tiger shark (Clark, 1963), sand tiger shark, and horn shark are reputed to fast for months, the usual effects of starvation are catastrophic. Histologic and biochemical deterioration is documented in many tissues, including kidney, spleen, and muscle (Martini, 1978). Young lemon sharks lose about 1% of their in air body weight per day when experimentally fasted (Gruber and Keyes, 1981). As the shark falls below about 80% of its ad lib weight, physiologic changes become irreversible (Gruber and Keyes, 1981).

Less extreme protein deficiency leads to varying degrees of inhibited growth and reduced fecundity in mature teleosts (Springate et al., 1985; Watanabe, 1985). Possible causes of protein deficiencies in elasmobranchs include inadequate amounts being fed, inadequate amounts being eaten, competition for food, improper digestion caused by digestive dysfunction or parasites, or poor-quality protein. The only clinical feature recorded in virtually all amino acid deficiencies is retarded growth (Roberts, 1978), which in sharks frequently leads to a cachexic, emaciated body with a disproportionately large head, wrinkled and blotchy skin, and ragged fins.

Carbohydrate Deficiency

Since elasmobranchs have a very limited capacity for metabolism of carbohydrates, such deficiencies may be of no concern.

Lipid Deficiencies

Linolenic acid and to a lesser extent linoleic acid seem to be the only essential fatty acids in elasmobranchs (Kabata, 1985). Deficiencies of these lead to fatty infiltration of the liver. Excessive amounts of fat in the diet may lead to excessive accumulation in the liver, especially where rancidity may be involved. This may or may not be similar to the lipoid liver disease reported in other fishes (Smith, 1979; Gruber and Keyes, 1981). This condition may be prevented by supplementation with vitamin E (Smith, 1979).

Mineral Deficiencies

Since elasmobranchs absorb some minerals from their aqueous environment via skin and gills (Anonymous, 1983) as well as via intestinal absorption, most mineral deficiencies are probably caused by poor water quality, especially in artificial seawater. In general, symptoms of mineral deficiency would very rarely be encountered, as poor water quality would cause more acute problems long before mineral deficiency became a problem. Inadequate consumption may also contribute to mineral deficiencies when sharks are fed filets rather than whole fish. Supplementation of minerals in small amounts is encouraged, especially when artificial seawater is used, although its utility is not proven. Iodine deficiency has been implicated in thyroid hyperplasia in sharks, but other factors are probably also involved (Hoover, 1984).

Vitamin Deficiencies

Vitamin requirements have not been established for elasmobranchs. In general, vitamin deficiency leads to poor growth and an unhealthy appearance (including exophthalmia, ascites, and anemia). Oral multivitamin supplementation has prevented all vitamin deficiencies in our aquaria, but excessive supplementation of fat-soluble vitamins should be avoided (see Table 95–1). Addition of vitamin E is essential if a high-fat diet is being fed, to prevent problems related to rancid fat. Vitamin K, normally produced by the intestinal flora, may be depleted by the use of antibiotics, which suppress bacterial growth. This can lead to anemia and inhibited coagulation. Captive lemon sharks have exhibited symptoms of hypovitaminosis B_1 (lateral curvature of the body) when fed a diet containing large amounts of naturally occurring thiaminase (Gruber and Keyes, 1981). Again, supplementation prevents as well as reverses this condition.

LITERATURE CITED

Anonymous (1981) Nutrient Requirements of Coldwater Fishes. National Research Council (NRC). National Academy Press, Washington, D.C.

Anonymous (1983) Nutrient Requirements of Warmwater Fishes and shellfish. National Research Council (NRC). National Academy Press, Washington, D.C.

Bowen, S.H. (1987) Dietary protein requirements of fishes—a reassessment. Can. J. Fish. Aquatic Sci. 44:1995–2001.

Braaten, B.R. (1979) Bioenergetics—a review on methodology. In: Finfish Nutrition and Fishfeed Technology (Halver, J.E., and Tiews, K., eds.) Heenemann Gmblt., Berlin, pp. 461–504.

Brafield, A.E., and Llewellyn, M.J. (1982) Animal Energetics. Blackie and Sons, Glasgow.

Brett, J.R., and Blackburn, J.M. (1978) Metabolic rate and energy expenditure of the spiny dogfish, *Squalus acanthias*. J. Fish. Res. B. Can. 35:816–821.

Brett, J.R. and Groves, T.D.D. (1979) Physiological energetics. In: Fish Physiology. Vol. 8. (Hoar, W. S., Randall, D. J., and Brett, J. R., eds.). Academic Press, New York, pp. 279–352.

Buddington, R.K. (1979) Digestion of an aquatic macrophyte by *Tilapia zillii* (Gervais). J. Fish Biol. 15:449–455.

Bushnell, P.G., Lutz, P.L., and Gruber, S.H. (1989) The metabolic rate of an active, tropical elasmobranch, the lemon shark (*Negarprion brevirostris*). Exp. Biol. 48:279–283.

Carey, F.G., and Teal, J.M. (1969) Mako and porbeagle: warm-bodied sharks. Comp. Biochem. Physiol. 28:199–204.

Cho, C.Y. (1983) Nutrition and fish health. In: A Guide to Integrated Fish Health Management in the Great Lakes Basin. (Meyer, J. P., Warren, J. W., and Carey, T. G., eds.). Great Lakes Fishery Commission Special Publication 83–2, Ann Arbor, Michigan, pp. 63–73.

Cho, C. Y., Cowey, C.B., and Wantanabe, T. (1985) Methodological approaches to research and development. In: Finfish Nutrition in Asia. (Cho, C.Y., Cowey, C.B. and and Watanabe, T., eds.). IRAC, Ottawa, pp. 9–80.

Clark, E. (1963) The maintenance of sharks in captivity with a report on their instrumental conditioning. In: Sharks and Survival (Gilbert, P.W., ed.). D.G. Heath, Boston, pp. 115–150.

Cortes, E. (1987) Diet, Feeding Habits and Daily Ration of Young Lemon Sharks, *Negaprion brevirostris*, and the Effect of Ration Size on Their Growth and Conversion Efficiency. Master's Thesis, University of Miami, Miami, Florida.

Cortes, E., and Gruber, S.H. (1990) Food, feeding habits and first estimate of daily ration of young lemon sharks, *Negaprion brevirostris* (Poey). Copeia 1:204–208.

Cowey, C.B. (1981) The food and feeding of captive fish. In: Aquarium Systems. (Hawkins, A.D., ed.). Academic Press, New York, pp. 223–246.

Cowey, C.B., Pope, J.A., Aaron, J.W., and Blair, A. (1972) Studies on the nutrition of marine flatfish—the protein requirement of plaice (*Plueronectes platessa*). Br. J. Nutr. 28:447–456.

Cowey, C.B., and Roberts, R.J. (1978) Nutritional pathology of teleosts. In: Fish Pathology. (Roberts, R.J., ed.). Baillière Tindall, London, pp. 249–261.

Cowey, C.B., and Sargent, J.R. (1979) Nutrition. In: Fish Physiology. Vol. 8. (Hoar, W.S., Randall, D.J., and Brett, J.R., eds.). Academic Press, New York, pp. 1–70.

De Long, D. C., Halver, J.E., and Mertz, E.T. (1958) Nutrition of salmonid fishes VI. Protein requirements of Chinook salmon at two water temperatures. J. Nutr. 65:589–599.

Fange, R., and Grove, D. (1979) Digestion. In: Fish Physiology. Vol. 7. (Hoar, W.S., Randall, D.J., and Brett, J.R., eds.). Academic Press, New York, pp. 161–260.

Gerking, S.D. (1955) Influence of rate of feeding on body composition and protein metabolism of bluegill sunfish. Physiol. Zool. 28:267–282.

Gruber, S.H. (1984) Bioenergetics of the captive and free-ranging lemon shark. Proc. Amer. Assoc. Zool. Parks and Aquariums 60:340–373.

Gruber, S.H. and Keyes, R.S. (1981) Keeping sharks for research. In: Aquarium Systems. (Hawkins, A.D., ed.). Academic Press, New York, pp. 373–402.

Halver, J.E. (1972) The vitamins. In: Fish Nutrition. (Halver, J.E., ed.). Academic Press, New York, pp. 29–103.

Halver, J.E. (1976) Formulating practical diets for fish. J. Fish Res. Bd. Can. 33:1032–1039.

Halver, J.E. (1985) Recent advances in vitamin nutrition and metabolism in fish. In: Nutrition and Feeding in Fish. (Cowey, C.B., Mackie, A.M., and Bell, J.G., eds.). Academic Press, London, pp. 415–429.

Hoover, K.L. (1984) Hyperplastic thyroid lesions in fish. In: Use of Small Fish Species in Carcinogenicity Testing. Monograph Series National Cancer Institute 65, pp. 275–289.

Jauncey, K. (1982) The effects of varying dietary protein level on the growth, food conversion, protein utilization and body composition of juvenile tilapias (*Sarotherodon mossambicas*). Aquaculture 27:43–54.

Jones, B.C., and Geen, G.H. (1977) Food and feeding of spiny dogfish (*Squalus acanthias*) in British Columbia waters. J. Fish Res. Bd. Can. 34:2067-2078.

Kabata, Z. (1985) Parasites and Diseases of Fish Cultured in the Tropics. Taylor & Francis, Philadelphia, pp. 281–201.

Kaushik, S.J. (1986) Environmental effects on feed utilization. Fish Physiol. Biochem. 2:131–140.

Lall, S.P. (1981) Minerals—a review. In: Biological Aspects of Aquaculture Nutrition. Proceedings of the World Conference on Aquaculture International Trade Show September 20–23, Venice, Italy.

Leger, C. (1985) Digestion, absorption and transport of lipids. In: Feeding in Fish. (Cowey, C.B., Mackie, A.M., and Bell, J.G., eds.). Nutrition and Academic Press, New York, pp. 299–331.

Longval, M.J., Warner, R.M., and Gruber, S.H. (1982) Cyclical patterns of food intake in the lemon shark, *Negaprion brevirostris*, under controlled conditions. Fl. Sci. 45(1):25–33.

Martini, F.H. (1978) The effects of fasting confinement on *Squalus acanthias*. In: Sensory Biology of Sharks, Skates and Rays (Hodgson, E., and Mathewson, R., eds.). ONR, Arlington, Virginia, pp. 609–646.

Medved, R.J. (1985) Gastric evacuation in the sandbar shark *Carcharhinus plumbeus*. J. Fish. Biol. 26:239–253.

Medved, R.J., Stillwell, C.E., and Casey, J.G. (1988) The rate of food consumption of young sandbar sharks (*Carcharhinus plumbeus*) in Chincoteague Bay, Virginia. Copeia 1988:956–963.

Nose, T. (1967) Recent advances in the study of fish digestion. In: Symposium on Feeding in Trout and Salmon Culture (Gaudet, J.L., ed.). European Inland Fisheries Advisory Commission, Rome, pp. 83–94.

Ogino, C., and Saito, K. (1970) Protein nutrition in fish. The utilization of dietary protein by young carp. Bull. Jpn. Soc. Sci. Fish 36:250–254.

Roberts, R.J. (1978) Nutritional pathology of teleosts. In: Fish Pathology. (Roberts, R.J. ed.). Baillière Tindall, London, pp. 216–226.

Robinson, E.H., and Mead, J.F. (1973) Lipid absorption and deposition in rainbow trout (*Salmo gairdneri*). Can. J. Biochem. 51:1050–1058.

Schurdak, M.E., and Gruber, S.H. (1989) Gastric evacuation of the lemon shark *Negaprion brevirostris* (Poey) under controlled conditions. Exp. Biol. 48:77–82.

Shimeno, S., Hosokawa, S.H., Hirata, H., and Takeda, M. (1977) Comparative studies on carbohydrate metabolism of yellowtail and carp. Bull. Jpn. Soc. Sci. Fish. 43:213–217.

Smith, L.S. (1980) Digestion in teleost fishes. In: Fish Feed Technology. United Nations Development Program, FAO, Rome, pp. 3–18.

Smith, R.R. (1971) A method for measuring digestibility and metabolizable energy of fish feeds. Progressive Fish Culturist 33:132–134.

Smith, R.R. (1979) Methods for determination of digestibility and metabolizable energy of food stuffs for finfish. In: Finfish Nutrition and Fishfeed Technology. (Halver, J.E., and Tiews, K., eds.). Heenemann Gmblt., Berlin, pp. 453–459.

Springate, J.R.C., Bromage, N.R., and Cumaranatunga, P.R.T. (1985) The effects of different ration on fecundity and egg quality in the rainbow trout (Salmo gairdneri). In: Nutrition and Feeding in Fish. (Cowey, C.B., Mackie, A.M., and Bell, J.G., eds.). Academic Press, London, pp. 371–393.

Stillwell, C.E., and Kohler, N.E. (1982) Food, feeding habits and estimates of daily ration of the shortfin mako (Isurus oxyrinchus) in the northwest Atlantic. Can. J. Fish. Aquatic Sci. 39:407–414.

Tacon, A.G.T., and Cowey, C.B. (1985) Protein and amino acid requirements. In: Fish Energetics—New Perspectives (Tyler, P., and Calow, P., eds.). Johns Hopkins University Press, Baltimore, pp. 155–184.

Talbort, C. (1985) Laboratory methods in fish feeding and nutritional studies. In: Fish Energetics—New Perspectives (Tyler, P., and Calow, P., eds.). Johns Hopkins Univ. Press, Baltimore, pp. 125–154.

Warren, C.E., and Davis, G.E. (1967) Laboratory studies on the feeding, bioenergetics and growth of fish. In: The Biological Basis of Freshwater Fish Production (Gerking, S.D., ed.). Blackwell Scientific Publications, Oxford, England, pp. 175–214.

Wass, R.C. (1973) Size, growth and reproduction of the sandbar shark, Carcharhinus milberti in Hawaii. Pacif. Sci. 27:305–318.

Watanabe, T. (1985) Importance of the study of broodstock nutrition for further development of aquaculture. In: Nutrition and Feeding in Fish (Cowey, C.B., Mackie, A.M., and Bell, J.G., eds.). Academic Press, London, pp. 395–414.

Wetherbee, B.M. (1988) Absorption Efficiency of Juvenile Lemon Sharks, Negaprion brevirostris, at Varying Rates of Energy Intake. Master's Thesis, University of Miami, Miami, Florida.

Wetherbee, B.M., Gruber, S.H., and Cortes, E. (1990) Diet, feeding habits, digestion and consumption in sharks, with special reference to the lemon shark, Negaprion brevirostris. Environ. Biol. Fishes 29(1):59–66.

Wilson, R.P., and Halver, J.E. (1986) Protein and amino acid requirements of fishes. Annu. Rev. Nutr. 6:225–244.

Windell, J.T. (1978) Digestion and the daily ration of fishes. In: Ecology of Freshwater Fish Production (Gerking, S.D., ed.). John Wiley & Sons, New York, pp. 159–183.

Chapter 96

REPRODUCTION OF SHARKS, SKATES, AND RAYS

MICHAEL K. STOSKOPF

Reproduction of these species in captivity has been extremely limited, and we know very little about the cues, requirements, and medical problems associated with reproduction in sharks, skates, or rays. Certainly, several species have been born in captivity, including the bonnethead shark, several dogfish species, cat sharks, some skates, and rays. In many cases, fertilization has occurred prior to capture, but in others, the entire reproductive cycle has been completed in aquaria. Rarely have active measures been taken to facilitate reproduction. Besides a desire to provide a ready source for acclimated display specimens, there is considerable need to examine the reproductive requirements and problems in sharks to facilitate management of wild populations. The long gestation period and tendency toward production of few young have made shark populations extremely vulnerable to commercial fisheries. This vulnerability has had significant economic impact but, more critically, can threaten local shark populations.

COURTSHIP

Biting of the female's pectoral fins or back, between the two dorsal fins, is a common courtship display exhibited by male sharks of many species. It is possible that this allows the male to anchor itself in position with the swimming female prior to insertion of a clasper into the female's cloaca. In some species such as the cat sharks, the teeth of males are modified for this behavior, and the sex of an individual shark can be determined from examining only the teeth (Gilbert, 1981). Males of smaller shark species such as the cat sharks and dogfish wrap their bodies around the female in prelude to and during copulation. Copulation itself consists of insertion of the male clasper into the cloaca of the female shark. Usually only one clasper is inserted at a time.

In the gray bamboo shark, which has been bred in captivity (Dral, 1981), the male rubs his body against the female and then seizes the female's closest pectoral fin in his mouth, suddenly. The female will swim, but the male limits her forward motion by shaking her until she is nearly immobile. After further shaking by the male, the female will spread her pelvic fins wide, and open and close her cloaca in a distinct rhythm. The male will then bend the copulatory claspers craniad and use one of them to grip a pelvic fin of the female.

Attempts to induce courtship and mating behavior in sharks through injection of pituitary extracts similar to those frequently used in teleost fish have not been particularly successful in sharks and rays. However, use of aqueous solutions of dried pituitary may have induced mild courtship behavior in stingrays (Gilbert, 1981).

COPULATION

All sharks use internal fertilization schemes. Semen is introduced into the cloaca of the female, and eggs are fertilized in the anterior end of the female reproductive tract (Fig. 96–1). Male sharks can be recognized by distinctive claspers that are finger-like modifications of the medial aspects of their pelvic fins (Fig. 96–2). Claspers have a cartilaginous support that is often calcified. Grooves in the clasper are thought to carry semen to the female's cloaca.

In the gray cat shark, copulation lasts 5 to 15 minutes, with the couple either staying on the bottom or swimming slowly. After copulation, the male stays on the bottom, breathing rapidly and deeply. The male may touch the tips of its claspers together at this time. The female swims away nervously after copulation, swimming on her side (Dral, 1981).

EMBRYONIC DEVELOPMENT

Shark embryos are provided significant protection either within tough egg cases or by being re-

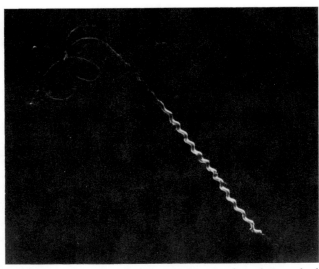

FIGURE 96–1. Scanning electron micrograph of sand tiger shark sperm (1950×). (From Gilmore, R.G., et al. [1983] Reproduction and embryonic development of the sand tiger shark, *Odontaspis taurus* [Rafinesque]. Fishery Bull. 18:201–225.)

tained within the female's body during development. All sharks, skates, and rays are born precocious and ready to survive on their own in a complex environment. All the embryonic development strategies in these animals are designed to produce such precocious offspring (Table 96–1).

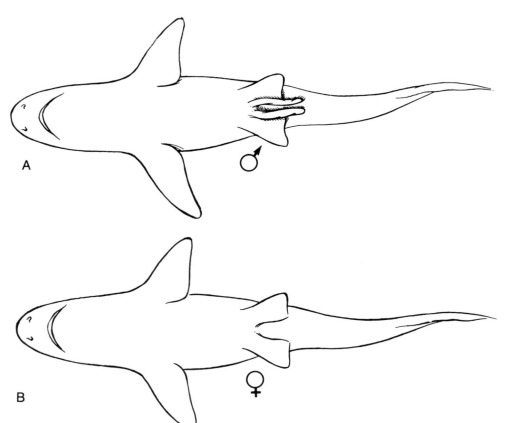

FIGURE 96–2. Sexual dimorphism in sharks. *A.* Male. *B.* Female.

TABLE 96–1. Shark Reproductive Data

Shark	Mode	Clutch Size
ANGEL SHARKS		
Pacific angel shark	Ovoviviparous	10
Sand devil	Ovoviviparous	—
COW SHARKS		
Sharpnose sevengill shark	Ovoviviparous	9–20
Bluntnose sixgill shark	Ovoviviparous	22–108
CARPET SHARKS		
Blind shark	Ovoviviparous	7–8
Common nurse shark	Ovoviviparous	21–28
Gray bamboo shark	Oviparous	40–80
CAT SHARKS		
Lesser spotted dogfish	Single oviparous	2
Skaamoong shark	Single oviparous	2
FINBACK CAT SHARKS		
Graceful cat shark	Single oviparous	2
Harlequin cat shark	Ovoviviparous?	2
FALSE CAT SHARK		
False cat shark	Ovoviviparous	2–4
BARBELED HOUNDSHARK		
Barbeled houndshark	Viviparous	
	Globular placenta	7
HAMMERHEAD SHARKS		
Scalloped hammerhead	Viviparous	15–31
Smooth hammerhead	Viviparous	29–37
Bonnethead	Viviparous	4–16
HORN SHARKS		
Horn shark	Oviparous	—
Mexican horn shark	Oviparous	—
Port Jackson shark	Oviparous	—
HOUNDSHARKS		
Gray smoothhound	Viviparous	2–5
Leopard shark	Ovoviviparous	4–33
Smooth dogfish	Viviparous	4–20
MACKEREL SHARKS		
Common thresher shark	Ovoviviparous	2–4
	Uterine cannibal	
Porbeagle	Ovoviviparous	1–5
	Uterine cannibal	
Sand tiger shark	Ovoviviparous	2
	Uterine cannibal	
Shortfin mako	Ovoviviparous	4–16
	Uterine cannibal	
REQUIEM SHARKS		
Brown shark	Viviparous	1–14
Bull shark	Viviparous	1–13
Dusky shark	Viviparous	3–14
Ocean whitetip	Viviparous	1–15
	Discoidal placenta	
Reef blacktip	Viviparous	2–4
	Discoidal placenta	
Silky	Viviparous	2–14
	Discoidal placenta	
Spinner shark	Viviparous	3–15
SAWSHARKS		
Shortnose sawshark	Ovoviviparous	7–17
WEASEL SHARKS		
Snaggletoothed shark	Viviparous	6–8
	Entire placenta	
Whitetipped weasel shark	Viviparous	2
	Entire placenta	

Data from Compagno, L.J.V. (1988) Sharks of the Order Carcharhiniformes. Princeton University Press, Princeton, NJ; and Compagno, L.J.V. (ed.) (1984) FAO Species Catalogue, Vol. 4, Sharks of the World. United Nations Development Programme, Rome, Italy.

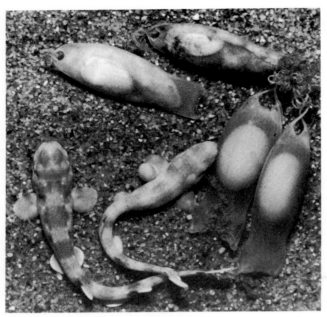

FIGURE 96—3. Newly hatched cat sharks and eggs in different stages of development. Each egg contains a single embryo. (From Studer, P. [1986] Fortpflanzung im Wasser. In: Nasse Welt. Zoologischer Garten, Basel, Switzerland, p. 189.)

Oviparous Strategies

A number of sharks, skates, and rays are oviparous, laying eggs that protect embryos as they develop outside of the mother's body (Fig. 96–3). These eggs have thick protective cases and usually only a single embryo in each. Eggs are laid, usually attached to substrate, and then are abandoned. Parental care is not a feature in shark reproduction.

The eggs of the gray bamboo shark are attached to branches of coral by tufts of filaments from the side edges of the egg capsule. The female bamboo shark swims nervously, rubbing her abdomen against a coral branch or protruding object. She circles around the object, and suddenly filaments are expressed from her cloaca and attach to the object the female is circling. The female continues to swim in circles, wrapping the filaments. With a final strong thrust, the egg is expelled, and the female repeats the process. In the gray bamboo shark the average clutch size is 4 eggs, each with a single embryo. It takes from 20 minutes to 2 days for a clutch to be laid. After laying each egg, the female sinks to the bottom, breathing hard in exhaustion. Clutches are laid about 9 days apart for about 6 months. After 6 months' rest, the female will usually resume laying.

After the egg is laid, the movements of the embryo circulate water freely through two holes in each end of the egg case. Initially, embryos develop external gills that disappear as gill slits develop. At hatching, the young shark exits the egg at the convex end. In captive breedings, sharks have been helped out of the egg when they are weak, but these animals rarely survive longer than a few days to weeks.

Other oviparous sharks include the Port Jackson shark, which produces a cone-shaped egg case about 6 inches long that contains a single embryo. Some workers think that this shark may carry its egg in its mouth and place it purposefully in a crevice (Gilbert, 1981). The question of oviparity is not as easy to establish as it might appear. For example, some workers consider the whale shark oviparous on the basis of an egg case 27 by 16 inches, found with a live embryo inside. However, since only one case has been found and on the basis of the thin wall of the case, much more similar to the egg cases of ovoviviparous sharks, many feel this large shark may be truly ovoviviparous.

Skates are oviparous and produce oblong egg capsules similar to those produced by oviparous sharks, but with stiff, pointed horns on all four corners of the rectangular case (Fig. 96–4). Skate eggs are usually coated on one side with a sticky substance to assist in holding the case to bottom substrate. Most skates prefer muddy or sandy bottoms for egg laying. Newly laid eggs are sealed with internal albumin coatings that cover the respiratory slits of the capsule. As albumin is absorbed by the embryonic skate, the slits are opened, and the egg case is bathed in a current of sea water. This makes it very easy to open skate eggs and observe the development of the embryo without harming it. Skate eggs take 4.5 to 15 months to hatch. At hatching, the young skate slips out of a thin slit in the case.

Viviparous and Ovoviviparous Strategies

The majority of sharks are viviparous or ovoviviparous and retain fertilized eggs in the uterus (McCormick et al., 1963). The difference between these two strategies might seem strange to scientists not familiar with the sharks; however, they do rep-

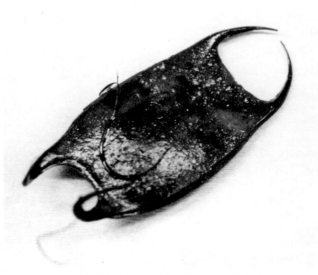

FIGURE 96—4. Egg of the clear-nosed skate.

resent two distinct strategies. In ovoviviparous sharks, no connection ever develops between the yolk sac and the womb. In contrast, viviparous sharks develop placenta and umbilical cord analogues during gestation.

Early in gestation in viviparous sharks, the embryo feeds on its yolk sac contents. As these are depleted, the yolk sac forms a close attachment to the womb of the female, and nourishment passes from the maternal blood to the embryo (McCormick et al., 1963). The requiem sharks and hammerhead sharks utilize a yolk-sac–placentation strategy. Hammerheads and the Pacific blackfin reef sharks have placentation so intimate that the yolk sac is interdigitated with the uterine wall with finger-like processes. Basking sharks and Greenland sharks are also apparently viviparous with a gestation period of 2 years or more.

Ovoviviparous sharks hatch within the uterus of the dam and are apparently supplied with oxygen and nutrients from the uterus, which becomes heavily vascularized. In the spiny dogfish, phosphates and sulfates are passed from maternal circulation to the uterine fluid, but pups do not seem to absorb these nutrients. In the spiny dogfish, the yolk-sac scar disappears within a few weeks of hatching, and the pup remains in the uterus for a gestation period that totals nearly 2 years. The average litter size is four to six.

Another strategy for nutrient provision in some of the ovoviviparous sharks is intrauterine cannibalism. This strategy is used by sand tiger sharks, mackerel sharks, and thresher sharks. The gestational strategy of the sand tiger shark has been particularly well studied (Gilmore et al., 1983). The breeding season runs from January to April, extending into September in the waters of the western mid-Atlantic states. In the reproductively active female sand tiger shark, only the right ovary is functional and enlarged. Both left and right oviducts bifurcate from a single osteum around the right ovary. As eggs are ovulated they pass through the oviduct and heart-shaped oviducal glands, which produce mucus, ovalbumin, and collagen. Sperm storage apparently occurs, but the site is unknown. However, it is reasonable to postulate that fertilization occurs proximal to the oviducal glands.

After the deposition of the protective capsule by the oviducal gland, egg capsules are deposited in each uterine horn. In sand tiger sharks as well as spiny dogfish, several fertilized eggs are enclosed in a single envelope, called a candle. Multiple candles of the same type and size are found in both uterine horns. Many of the candles may not be fertile and will not contain embryos.

Sand tiger shark embryos hatch within the uterus at 3 to 4 months of gestation, when they are about 49 to 63 mm in length. The young sharks have

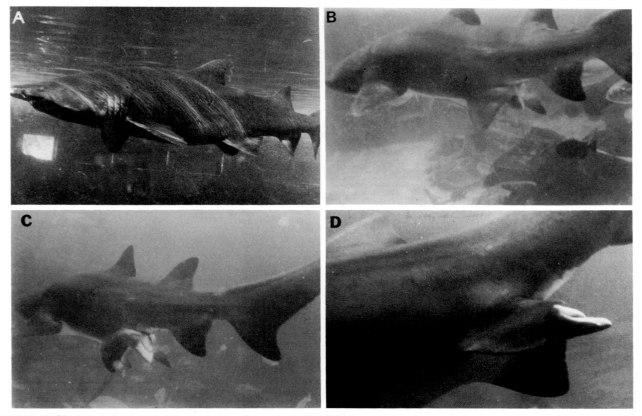

FIGURE 96–5. Sand tiger shark giving birth. *A.* Gravid female. *B.* Head-first presentation. *C.* Gill slits begin to emerge. *D.* Closer view of pup being born. (From Gilmore, R.G., et al. [1983] Reproduction and embryonic development of the sand tiger shark, *Odontaspis taurus* [Rafinesque]. Fishery Bull. 18:201–225.)

functional teeth even at this early stage. When they are about 100 mm in length and the yolk sac is depleted, the largest embryo proceeds to eat smaller embryos as they hatch or while they remain encapsulated. This is an active process consisting of intrauterine hunting and attacks. Scarred and wounded embryos are frequently found in the uterus. At this stage there are multiple embryos in each uterine horn, but soon only infertile eggs are available to nourish the successful embryo in each horn. After fertilization of ova has ceased and all other developing embryos have been consumed, the dam continues to ovulate, and unfertilized ova become the primary source of nutrition for the surviving embryos.

Late in the 9- to 12-month gestation, the stomachs of the two surviving pups become distended with the large amounts of yolk they are ingesting from the infertile eggs. This condition is referred to as the yolk stomach. Just prior to parturition the distention of the stomach reduces to nearly normal, and the liver size of the embryo increases dramatically. At the same time, the liver of the dam reaches a minimum weight as maternal ova production decreases.

Sand tiger shark pups can reach 1.2 m in length before parturition. Parturition may be preceded by a cloacal discharge. Birth is head first, as opposed to the carcharhinoids, which are normally born tail first (Wass, 1973; Mooney, 1975) (Fig. 96–5). The birth of the first pup can take over 30 minutes from the time the head is first visible. The second pup is usually born within a few minutes of the first. Pups are quite capable of turning within the uterus and may appear tail first initially, return to the uterus, and emerge head first. Pups may not feed for up to 25 days after birth, but once they begin to feed they gain considerable weight in first few months of life.

LITERATURE CITED

Compagno, L.J.V. (Ed.). (1984) FAO Species Catalogue, Volume 4, Sharks of the World. United Nations Development Programme, Rome, Italy.

Compagno, L.J.V. (1988) Sharks of the Order Carcharhiniformes. Princeton University Press, Princeton, New Jersey.

Dral, A.J. (1981) Reproduction en aquarium du Requin de fond tropical *Chiloscyllium griseum* Mull. et Henle (Orectolobides). Rev. fr. Aquariol. 7:99–104.

Gilbert, P.W. (1981) Patterns of shark reproduction. Oceanus 24:30–39.

Gilmore, R.G., Dodrill, J.W., and Linley, P.A. (1983) Reproduction and embryonic development of the sand tiger shark, *Odontaspis taurus* (Rafinesque). Fishery Bull. 81(2):201–225.

McCormick, H.W., Allen, T., and Young, W. (1963) Shadows in the Sea, the Sharks, Skates and Rays. Weathervane Books, New York.

Mooney, M.J. (1975) Hammerheads born in captivity. Sea Front. 21:359–361.

Wass, R.C. (1973) Size, growth, and reproduction of the sandbar shark, *Carcharhinus milberti*, in Hawaii. Pac. Sci. 27:305–318.

Chapter 97

BACTERIAL DISEASES OF SHARKS

MICHAEL K. STOSKOPF

There has been perhaps more interest in the bacterial flora of the shark mouth and its relation to sepsis in shark victims than there has in bacteria pathogenic for sharks. For example, the mouth of a great white shark yielded a variety of *Vibrio* species, including *V. alginolyticus, V. fluvialis,* and *V. parahaemolyticus* (Buck et al., 1984). Unfortunately, little is known about the bacterial diseases of sharks themselves compared to other groups of fishes. Few reports are found in the literature in which enough specific information is provided to be of clinical value. There is no reason to believe that this reflects reality. Sharks and the related skates and rays should be considered vulnerable to a variety of pathogenic bacteria until proved otherwise. Several species of *Vibrio*, including *V. alginolyticus, V. parahaemolyticus,*

V. damsela, and *V. harveyi* have been reported from Port Jackson sharks, epaulette sharks, and fiddler rays that developed septicemia and rapid death after heavy rains reduced the salinity of the water in which they dwelled. The disease was characterized by hemorrhage, congestion, and rapid mortality (Callinan, 1988). Boils have been noted on sand tiger sharks that have yielded bacteria identified as *Pseudomonas* spp., *Proteus* spp., and *Citrobacter freundi.* These lesions are usually raised and pigmented, containing variable amounts of purulent material. They respond well to broad-spectrum antibiotic therapy, but the syndrome has not been well studied.

There is also evidence that normal, healthy sharks may be colonized with bacteria in tissues other than the mouth and gastrointestinal tract (Knight et

TABLE 97–1. A Single Fairly Well-Documented Bacterial Disease of Sharks*

Disease	Organism	Host
Shark meningitis	*Vibrio carchariae*	Sand tiger shark Brown shark Lemon shark Spiny dogfish

See also sections on Aeromonas hydrophila *in Chapter 48;* Vibrio alginolyticus *in Chapter 78. Sharks are also susceptible to* Vibrio anguillarum *and* Vibrio parahaemolyticus.

al., 1987). Shark blood is usually sterile, but muscle, kidney, liver, and spleen from asymptomatic sharks can contain from 100 to 10,000 bacteria per gram of tissue (Grimes et al., 1985; Knight, 1987). The majority of bacteria isolated from sharks can hydrolyze urea and are capable of using urea as their only source of carbon and nitrogen (Grimes et al., 1984a). It is thought that these ureolytic bacteria may be functioning in the urea flux sharks use to adjust the osmolarity of their blood. In any event, the presence of these bacteria in internal organs is unusual. It has been postulated that during capture and maintenance in aquaria, the immune system of sharks may be compromised enough to allow a rapid systemic invasion by these resident bacteria. Since sharks do maintain high serum urea levels, it is also possible that these ureolytic bacteria could cause alkalinization of the blood through excessive urea hydrolysis (Grimes et al., 1984a).

There has been only one fairly well-documented bacterial disease of the shark group (Table 97–1). However, the astute clinician should be aware of the potential for bacterial disease in sharks and should not be lulled into a false sense of security because of the lack of work with these species in this discipline.

SHARK MENINGITIS

SYNONYM. Vibriosis.

Host and Geographic Distribution

Vibrio carchariae was originally isolated from brown sharks showing signs of clinical disease (Grimes et al., 1984a). A natural infection has occurred in a sand tiger shark. Experimental infections have been produced in lemon sharks and spiny dogfish (Grimes et al., 1985; Grimes et al., 1984a). Spiny dogfish died within 18 hours of intraperitoneal injection. Lemon sharks are more resistant to infection, and although histologic damage occurs in various internal organs, the experimental infections were not fatal. Other sharks are suspected to be susceptible. To date, all isolations have been from captive animals originally caught off the mouth of the Delaware Bay. The geographic distribution of the organism is not known.

Clinical Signs

Sharks with naturally occurring disease initially demonstrate lethargy and disinterest in their environment. This can be noted by alert aquarists days

before significant anorexia develops. Affected sharks fail to make eye contact with observers outside of the tank. Later they fail to make eye contact with other sharks in the tank. Anorexia is accompanied by progressive disorientation. Untreated, the disease progresses to convulsions, coma, and death. In some cases, large raised skin lesions filled with brown purulent exudate are present. Trematodes may or may not be present.

Pathology and Diagnosis

In brown sharks, meningitis is a prominent feature of the disease. *Vibrio carcarhiae* can be isolated from cerebrospinal fluid. The disease also affects the spleen, liver, and kidney. Kidney necrosis can be extremely severe. Intestinal and rectal gland lesions may also be seen. When present, dermal lesions in brown sharks yield pure cultures of the causative bacterium. In lemon sharks, subdermal cysts with necrosis have been observed and gram-negative rods are frequently found in these lesions.

Culture and Identification

Vibrio carchariae can be grown in thioglycolate broths. It is a gram-negative bacillus that is usually seen in pairs, chains, or clusters. It is a motile organism, with a polar flagellum. When *V. carchariae* is grown on solid media, a lateral flagellum is also present. The organism exhibits anaerobic growth and grows between 11 and 40°C. This vibrio of sharks is oxidase positive, decarboxylates lysine and ornithine, and reduces nitrate without producing gas. It produces indole and hydrolyzes urea, gelatin, and chitin. The organism grows well in media supplemented with up to 8% sodium chloride but is inhibited in 10% sodium chloride (Grimes et al., 1984b). It does not contain detectable plasmids (Grimes et al., 1984a).

Transmission and Epidemiology

The susceptibility of different shark species to the *V. carchariae* seems to vary considerably. The spiny dogfish is very susceptible, whereas the lemon shark appears more resistant. Experimental inoculations in well-maintained, healthy lemon sharks failed to produce clinical disease (Grimes et al., 1985). On the other hand, physiologically compromised lemon sharks developed lethal infections, implying that stress and physiologic compromise may play a role in the pathogenesis of the disease (Grimes et al., 1985). *Vibrio carchariae* has been isolated from *Dermophthirius* trematodes infesting the skin of lemon sharks (Grimes et al., 1984b), and it is thought that the flukes may play a role in transmission of the bacteria. *Vibrio* organisms are found in skin lesions on sharks associated with the feeding of these flukes. All reported isolations from naturally occurring cases have been from captive animals.

Treatment and Control

Control of shark meningitis is dependent upon the provision of proper environments for captive sharks. There are no bacterins or serological tests available to facilitate quarantine screening. This disease responds well to appropriate doses of tetracyclines, aminoglycosides, or chloramphenicol administered with the observation of early signs of the disease. Prophylactic administration of antibiotics is not recommended.

LITERATURE CITED

Buck, J.D., Spotte, S., and Gadbaw, J.J. (1984) Bacteriology of the teeth from a great white shark: Potential medical implications for shark bite victims. J. Clin. Microbiol. 20(5):849–851.
Callinan, R.B. (1988) Diseases of Australian native fishes. In: Fish Diseases: Refresher Course for Veterinarians, Proceedings 106, Post Graduate Committee of Veterinary Science, University of Sydney, Australia, p. 460.
Grimes, D.J., Colwell, R.R., Stemmler, J., Hada, H., Maneval, D., Hetrick, F.M., May, E.B., Jones, R.T., and Stoskopf, M.K. (1984a) *Vibrio* species as agents of elasmobranch disease. Helgolander Meeresuntersuchungen 37:309–315.
Grimes, D.J., Stemmler, J., Hada, H., May, E.B., Maneval, D., Hetrick, F.M., Jones, R.T., Stoskopf, M., and Colwell, R.R. (1984b) *Vibrio* species associated with mortality of sharks held in captivity. Microb. Ecol. 10:271–282.
Grimes, D.J., Gruber, S.H., and May, E.B. (1985) Experimental infection of lemon sharks, *Negaprion brevirostris* (Poey), with *Vibrio* species. J. Fish Dis. 8:173–180.
Knight, I.T., Grimes, D.J., and Colwell, R.R. (1987) Bacterial Hydrolysis of Urea in the tissues of carcharhinid sharks. Can. J. Fish. Aquatic Sci. 45:357–360.
May, E.B., Stoskopf, M.K., Jones, R.T., Andrews, J.C., and Jenkins, R.L. (1983) A Vibrio infection in brown sharks (*Carcharhinus plumbeus*): clinical gross pathology and histopathology. Proc. Int. Assoc. Aquatic Anim. Med. 14:26.

Chapter 98

FUNGAL AND ALGAL DISEASES OF SHARKS

MICHAEL K. STOSKOPF

Fungal and algal infections have been reported in sharks (Table 98–1). The impact of these diseases on wild populations is unknown. Most reports have been in captive specimens.

HYPHALOMYCOSIS

SYNONYMS. Fusarium mycosis, bonnethead disease.

Host and Geographic Distribution

This disease has been reported in two captive-born juvenile bonnethead sharks (Muhvich et al., 1989) and subsequently in four juvenile female bonnethead sharks in another facility 3 months after capture (Violetta et al., 1989). *Fusarium* infections are also reported in sea turtles, Atlantic salmon, red drum, and shrimp. Experimental infections have been produced in channel catfish.

TABLE 98–1. Fungal and Algal Diseases of Sharks

Disease	Organism	Host
Hyphalomycosis	*Fusarium solani*	Bonnethead shark Channel catfish (experimental)
Aureobasidiomycosis	*Aureobasidium* spp.	Pelagic stingray Carp (experimental)
Coccolithophorid algal dermatitis	Unidentified *Chrysophycophyta* spp.	Spiny dogfish

Clinical Signs

The initial two cases in sharks first presented with lethargy, mild progressive disorientation, and weight loss. Eventually, small skin ulcers and erosions were evident on the head. The second outbreak was described as beginning with the formation of papules on the dorsal and ventral surfaces of the head and along the lateral line (Violetta et al., 1989). These papules were easily ruptured, releasing white purulent exudate with traces of blood.

Diagnosis, Pathology, Culture, and Identification

Hyphalomycosis is characterized by chronic myositis and muscle necrosis with hyphal penetration into the cartilage (Fig. 98–1). Septate branching hyphae similar to those found in *Aspergillus, Penicillium, Pseudallescheria,* and *Acremonium* are seen in sections. *Fusarium solani* can be cultured on Sabouraud's (preferably without Actidione) and blood agar. Colonies are usually cottony and white. Microconidiophores of *F. solani* are elongate, and the macroconidia are thick-walled (Fig. 98–2) and asymmetrically septate

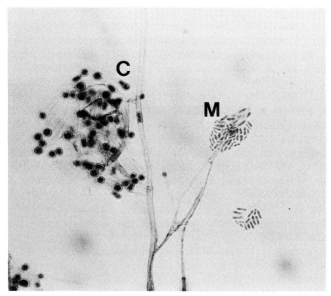

FIGURE 98–2. *Fusarium solani* segmented hyphae with chlamydospores (C) and banana-shaped macroconidia (M) (wet mount, Lactophenol cotton blue, 430×). (Courtesy of R. Reimschuessel.)

with a larger distal part. Hyphae have hyaline colorless walls.

Transmission, Epidemiology, and Pathogenesis

Fusarium solani is thought to be an opportunistic pathogen infecting severely debilitated hosts. Experimental infections have been achieved by injecting pure cultures isolated from sharks intramuscularly into channel catfish. The catfish developed lesions, and *Fusarium solani* was recultured.

Treatment, Control, and Public Health Significance

No treatment or control measures are reported. In humans, the organism is thought to infect primarily debilitated hosts (Rippon, 1988). Careful attention to environmental characteristics is warranted when this infection appears. *Fusarium* species are usually sensitive to amphotericin B and resistant to 5-fluorocytosine. Human cases have been cured with surgical excision, iodated alcohol treatments, and spontaneous cures also occur. *Fusarium solani* is the most common cause of mycotic keratitis in humans.

AUREOBASIDIOMYCOSIS

SYNONYMS. Phaeohyphomycosis, black yeast disease, pullulariosis.

Host and Geographic Distribution

The disease has been described once in a captive pelagic stingray, which died of unknown causes (Otte, 1964).

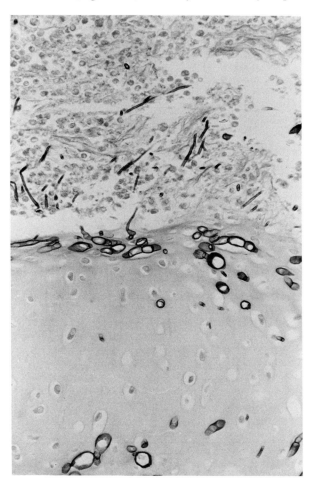

FIGURE 98–1. Section of the tail of a newborn bonnethead shark. Note the fungal hyphae in the necrotic muscle and the cartilage. Numerous mononuclear cells are present in the muscle (Grocott, 250×). (Courtesy of R. Reimschuessel.)

Clinical Signs

The affected stingray was ascitic with a swollen liver and splenomegaly. No other clinical signs were reported in the only description of this disease.

Diagnosis, Pathology, Culture, and Identification

In the one reported case, the infection was confined to the liver. The liver showed necrotic foci that contained cellular debris, lipid deposits, and numerous septate hyphae. There was an acute nonproliferative and chronic granulomatous response to the organism. Splenomegaly was apparent. *Aureobasidium* spp. are easily cultured on Sabouraud's agar, blood agar, or glucose blood agar (Fig. 98–3). Colonies usually begin as white and turn black with time. Hyphae are multiseptate with thick pigmented walls. Several conidia can often be seen aggregating around the conidiogenic cell of a hyphae. Conidia may bud from nonpigmented yeast forms that resemble *Candida*.

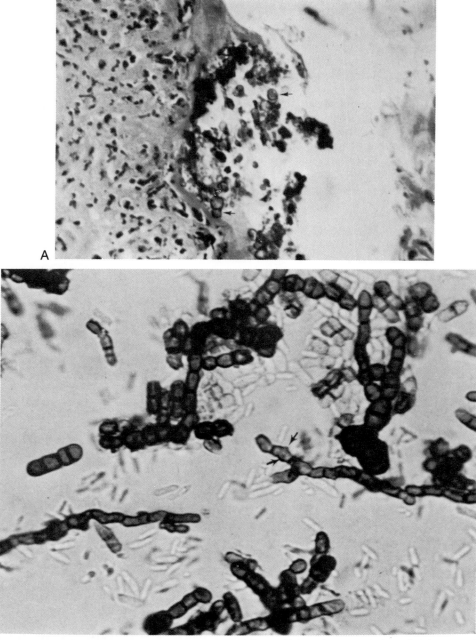

FIGURE 98–3. *A.* Cutaneous colonization of human skin with *Aureobasidium pullulans* showing thick-walled brown cells of the fungus. *B.* Wet mount of *Aureobasidium* sp. with a very septate mycelium giving rise to many hyaline ameroconidia, which bud. Peglike dentricles (arrows) on conidiogenous cells give rise to conidia (wet mount 800×). (From Rippon, J.W. [1988] Medical Mycology, 3rd ed. W.B. Saunders, Philadelphia.)

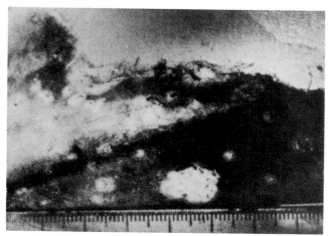

FIGURE 98–4. Dorsal fin and dorsum of a spiny dogfish severely affected with coccolithophorid algal dermatitis, showing composite and individual skin lesions (scale in cm). (From Leibovitz, L., and Leibovitz, S.S. [1985] A coccolithophorid algal dermatitis of the spiny dogfish, *Squalus acanthias* [L.]. J. Fish Dis. 8:351–358.)

Pure culture injected intraperitoneally into carp resulted in the carp developing lethal infections with histologic lesions similar to those observed in the stingray. The fungus was reisolated from lesions of the carp. Unfortunately, further taxonomic identification of the organism was not pursued.

Transmission, Epidemiology, Pathogenesis, Treatment, and Control

Nothing is known about the natural history of this disease. No methods of treatment or control are reported.

COCCOLITHOPHORID ALGAL DERMATITIS

SYNONYMS. Summer dermatitis, algal dermatitis.

Host and Geographic Distribution

This disease has been reported only in the spiny dogfish but may affect other sharks. Five cases are reported, one of which involved a wild-caught specimen (Leibovitz and Leibovitz, 1985). The other four sharks affected were in captivity at the time the disease was noted. Other species of sharks may be susceptible.

Clinical Signs

Lesions begin as petechial and ecchymotic skin hemorrhages that enlarge into raised vesicles 1 to 3 mm in diameter (Fig. 98–4). These focal lesions can occur on any part of the skin but most often are seen over the tail, fins, and dorsal surface of the body. The vesicles are easily desquamated, leaving an ulcer. Lesions frequently coalesce into larger lesions up to a centimeter in diameter, which often have a target appearance consisting of three rings. Over the course of the disease, lesions become progressively more generalized. Ulcers heal with granulation that may or may not be reepithelialized. Early cases continue to feed and swim relatively normally.

Diagnosis and Pathology

Hemorrhages from dermal capillaries beneath the basement membrane of the epidermis are the earliest histologic signs of the disease. Epidermal spongiosis followed by vesicular formation and excoriation of the necrotic surface results in characteristic target lesions with three distinct zones visible grossly. The central zone is an ulcer surrounded by epidermal ballooning degeneration. Cells in the middle zone contain intracellular, round organisms that have a nucleus and disk-shaped peripheral inclusions. These organisms can displace the host cell architecture into an outer capsule. Pseudomembranous collections of algal organisms may also be present. The outer zone of a typical lesion exhibits subepithelial hemorrhage and early epidermal degeneration. Melanocyte proliferation and dermal denticle lysis and fragmentation are seen. A mild degree of infiltration by inflammatory cells is seen in late stages of lesion formation.

Culture and Identification

The organism responsible for this disease has not been grown in culture, and specific identification of species has not been done. The distinct cell walls and polarized light-refringent rhombohedral crystalline cellular inclusions (7.1 by 5.85 μm), which form interlocking coccoliths, are considered characteristic of the division *Chrysophycophyta*, the golden and yellow-green algae (Fig. 98–5).

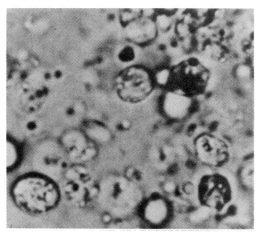

FIGURE 98–5. Direct fresh smear impression of coccolithophorid algal skin lesion examined by polarized light microscopy showing refractile rhomboidal crystals within algal organisms (wet mount 1500×). (From Leibovitz, L., and Leibovitz, S.S. [1985] A coccolithophorid algal dermatitis of the spiny dogfish, *Squalus acanthias* [L.]. J. Fish Dis. 8:351–358.)

Transmission, Epidemiology, and Pathogenesis

The life cycle of the organism responsible for the disease is not known. It has been postulated that the disease may represent the conversion of a symbiotic relationship to a pathogenic one (Leibovitz and Leibovitz, 1985). Coccolithophorid algae have complex life cycles that usually include motile flagellated stages in addition to the nonmotile stages seen in the skin lesions. The stage in the skin lesions probably represents the autospore stage of the algae characteristic of other algal symbionts found in animal tissues (McLaughlin and Zahl, 1966). The autospore stage appears to reproduce independently by binary fission. All cases of the disease reported have occurred between July and October. Four of the five cases were held in captivity at the time of discovery of the disease. The disease is progressive.

Treatment and Control

The lesions can be but are not necessarily self-limiting. No treatment or control measures are known.

LITERATURE CITED

Leibovitz, L., and Leibovitz, S.S. (1985) A coccolithophorid algal dermatitis of the spiny dogfish, *Squalus acanthias* L. J. Fish Dis. 8:351–358.
McLaughlin, J.A., and Zahl, O. (1966) Endozoic algae. In: Symbiosis. Vol. 1. Association of Microorganisms, Plants and Marine Organisms (Henry, S.M., ed.). Academic Press, London.
Muhvich, A.G., Reimschuessel, R., Lipsky, M.M., and Bennett, R.O. (1989) *Fusarium solani* isolated from newborn bonnethead sharks, *Sphyrna tiburo* (L.). J. Fish Dis. 12(1):57–62.
Otte, E. (1964) Eine Mykose bei einem Stachelrochen (*Trygon pastinaca* L). Wiener Tierarztl. Mschr. 51:171–175.
Rippon, J.W. (1988) Medical Mycology. 3rd ed. W.B. Saunders, Philadelphia.
Violetta, G.C., Dalton, L.M., and Crawley, R. (1989) A case history of *Fusarium* sp. in a captive population of bonnethead sharks, *Syhyrna tiburo* (sic). IAAAM Conf. Proceed. 20:64.

Chapter 99

SHARK VIRUSES

PHILIP E. McALLISTER   MICHAEL K. STOSKOPF

Reports of viral diseases in sharks are scarce, and few viral diseases of sharks have been studied. Undoubtedly, future investigations will reveal more viral diseases in sharks. Table 99–1 lists the reported viral diseases of sharks.

SMOOTH DOGFISH VIRAL DERMATITIS

SYNONYMS. Shark dermatitis, smooth dogfish herpesvirus, shark herpesvirus.

Host and Geographic Distribution

Wild-captured and laboratory-maintained populations of smooth dogfish from the Woods Hole area of Massachusetts (U.S.A.) developed a dermatitis of putative herpesvirus etiology (Leibovitz and Leibovitz, 1985).

Clinical Signs

Discrete, progressively developing skin lesions in addition to various traumatic wounds were found on 1 to 8% of newly captured and laboratory-maintained smooth dogfish. The skin eruptions are rounded, elevated, whitish-gray depigmented areas of skin 1 to 10 mm in diameter. The lesions contain three distinct zones: a small dark depressed central zone, a whitish-gray middle zone, and a granular, reddened, elevated outer zone (Leibovitz and Leibovitz, 1985). The lesions develop over the body

TABLE 99–1. Viral Diseases of Sharks

Disease	Virus	Host
Dermatitis	Shark herpesvirus	Smooth dogfish
Erythrocytic necrosis	Erythrocytic necrosis virus*	Smooth dogfish

See also Chapters 80 and 88.

surface, fins, and tail. Focal pigment deposition occurs as lesions heal.

Pathology

Normal epidermal structure is disrupted as the lesions develop. Lesions initially appear as foci of degenerating basal epidermal cells showing intracellular edema and intranuclear and intracytoplasmic DNA-positive inclusion bodies. Lesions enlarge by lysis and sloughing of necrotic epidermal cells, separation of epidermal layers, and vesicle formation within the epidermis. Subepithelial capillaries of the dermis become dilated and congested, further separating the epithelial and dermal layers. Hemorrhages occur over the surfaces of lesions from ruptured capillaries. Zones of pathologic change are seen in the lesions: a central focal zone with necrosis, sloughing epithelium, and melanin deposition; a middle zone with cellular degeneration and vesicle formation; and an outer zone with ballooning degeneration and hemorrhage. Electron micrographs of the lesions show progressive intracytoplasmic and intranuclear pathology.

Diagnosis

The diagnosis of smooth dogfish viral dermatitis is based on clinical signs, pathology, and electron micrographs showing herpesvirus-like particles in the skin lesions.

Virus Detection

The herpesvirus has not been isolated in cell culture. Electron micrographs of lesion tissue show particles with herpesvirus morphology budding from nuclear and cytoplasmic membranes and accumulations of particles forming cytoplasmic inclusions (Leibovitz and Leibovitz, 1985).

Transmission, Epidemiology, and Pathogenesis

No defined experimental transmission trials have been reported; however, disease lesions are more prevalent in long-term captive fish compared to newly caught ones. This could indicate that the virus is transmitted with cohabitation or that a latent infection is activated following capture and culture in an artificial environment.

Treatment and Control

No methods of treatment or control have been reported.

VIRAL ERYTHROCYTIC NECROSIS

SYNONYMS. VEN; Pirhemocyton; Toddia; Cytamoeba; Immanuoplasma; piscine erythrocytic necrosis; erythrocytic necrosis virus (ENV).

Hosts and Geographic Distribution

This virus was long thought to be a protozoan parasite. It has been reported in a wide range of species, including amphibians and reptiles. It has been reported in the smooth dogfish (Johnston, 1975) and other elasmobranchs (Kahn and Newman, 1982). Virus isolates from different hosts vary widely in size, which may indicate that several closely related iridoviruses, rather than a single virus, are responsible for the disease.

Clinical Signs and Pathology

Sharks with this disease have pale gills and pale visceral organs. Blood from affected sharks clots slowly, if at all, and low hematocrits are a sign of the disease. Hematopoietic tissue is usually hyperactive when examined histologically. Circulating erythrocytes usually show a small eosinophilic inclusion in the cytoplasm and a vacuolated or degenerating nucleus.

Diagnosis

Diagnosis is based on stained blood films showing the distinct eosinophilic cytoplasmic inclusions in erythrocytes. Confirmation is obtained from electron microscopy of the inclusions, revealing icosahedral virions (Smail and Egglestone, 1980).

Virus Detection and Identification

The virus is a cytoplasmic icosahedral DNA virus that is usually considered an iridovirus, although it has not been isolated in cell culture. In different hosts, the virus is dramatically different in size (150 to 500 nm). The largest virus is reported in the smooth dogfish (viral particles 450 to 500 nm).

Transmission, Epidemiology, and Pathogenesis

Transmission is thought to be waterborne, but other means have not been excluded. The incubation period ranges between 5 and 30 days. It is more common for young fish to be infected.

Treatment and Control

No treatment or control measures are reported.

LITERATURE CITED

Johnston, M.R.L. (1975) Distribution of *Pirhemocyton* Chatton and Blanc and other, possibly related, infections of poikilotherms. J. Protozool. 22:529–535.

Kahn, R.A., and Newman, M.W. (1982) Blood parasites from fish of the Gulf of Maine to Cape Hatteras, Northwest Atlantic Ocean, with notes on the distribution of fish hematozoa. Can. J. Zool. 60:396–402.

Leibovitz, L., and Leibovitz, S.S. (1985) A viral dermatitis of the smooth dogfish, *Mustelus canis* (Mitchill). J. Fish Dis. 8:273–279.

Smail, D.A., and Egglestone, S.I. (1980) Virus infections of marine fish erythrocytes: Prevalence of piscine erythrocytic necrosis in cod *Gadus mormua* L. and blenny *Blennias phocis* L. in coastal and offshore waters of the United Kingdom. J. Fish Dis. 3:41–46.

Chapter 100

PARASITIC DISEASES OF ELASMOBRANCHS

PAUL CHEUNG

The development of saltwater treatment technologies in recent years increases the capabilities of major aquaria to exhibit a large variety of sharks, skates, and rays. Wild-caught animals are usually infested with parasites, but if introduced untreated to a recirculating water system, the same fish can succumb to parasitic diseases. This is due partly to the rapid build-up of parasite populations in tanks and partly to the lowering of disease resistance of the hosts. The belief that elasmobranchs, especially the sharks, are not subject to sickness and diseases is far from correct (Cheung et al., 1982; May et al., 1983; Leibovitz and Leibovitz, 1985; Campbell, 1985; Benz, 1985). This chapter presents selected parasitic diseases of elasmobranchs and their pathologic features. Table 100–1 lists protozoan, helminth, and crustacean parasites of elasmobranchs.

PROTOZOA

Ameba have not been reported as parasites in sharks, skates, or rays. *Amyloodinium ocellatum* is a common parasite in marine tropical fishes but is rarely observed in elasmobranchs. However, Lawler (1980) experimentally induced amyloodiniasis in an Atlantic stingray under laboratory conditions. Five species of *Trypanosoma* are described in nurse hounds (Laveran and Mesnil, 1901) and skates (Laird, 1951; Laird and Bullock, 1969). Other flagellates, such as *Cryptobia*, *Trypanoplasma*, *Hexamita*, and *Trichomona*, have not been observed in elasmobranchs.

Trichodina oviducti and *T. rajae* are mobiline peritrichs that infect the urogenital tract of the thorny skate and cause a yellow, mucoid discharge from the fish (Khan, 1972; Eudokimova, 1969). No other tri-chodinids are found in sharks or rays. *Caliperia brevipes*, a symphoriontic sessile peritrich of the family Scyphiidae, was found attached to the gills of a little skate from the Bay of Fundy (Laird, 1959). However, the infestation was not considered to be harmful to the host.

Parasitic and opportunistic ciliates of marine fishes, such as *Cryptocaryon irritans*, *Brooklynella hostilis*, *Uronema marinum*, and *Miamiensis avidens*, have not been observed in elasmobranchs; however, smooth dogfish were susceptible to *Cryptocaryon* infection under laboratory conditions (Leibovitz and Leibovitz, 1985). An unidentified ciliate (probably *Uronema marinum*) invaded the gill tissues of a captive-born juvenile southern stingray at the New York Aquarium.

The intraerythrocytic hemogregarine *Haemogregarina delagei* was reported in three species of Californian skates (Love and Moser, 1976) and a spiny dogfish from New Brunswick (Laird and Bullock, 1969). The infected blood cells are hypertrophied, have a distorted shape, have a displaced and disfigured nucleus, and may ultimately disintegrate (Khan, 1972).

Coccidiosis in elasmobranchs is rare, only nine species of *Eimeria* are reported (see Table 100–1). Most of the species are found in the spiral valves of fish. *Eimeria quentini* can be found in peritoneal epithelial cells of the spotted eagle ray (Boulard, 1977), and oocysts of an as yet unidentified species of *Eimeria* have been seen embedded in the epithelial cells of the serosa of a cownose ray collected from New York Bight waters (Cheung et al., 1987). The infected area appeared hyperemic and caseated. Erosion of the outer reticulum and ruptures of the serosa were noted in heavily infected areas. Epithelial

Text continued on page 804

TABLE 100–1. Parasites Found in Elasmobranchs

Parasite	Host	Site of Infection	Location
PROTOZOA			
Phylum Sarcomastigophora			
Family Blastodiniidae			
Amyloodinium ocellatum	Atlantic stingray	Gills	Laboratory induced
Family Trypanosomatidae			
Trypanosoma spp.	Skates	Blood	N. Atlantic
Trypanosoma scyllii	Lesser spotted dogfish, cat shark	Blood	N.E. Atlantic
Family Trichodinidae			
Trichodina oviducti	Winter skate, thornback skate, thorny skate, winter skate, other skates	Urogenital tract	Barents Sea, Argentina, and world wide
Trichodina rajae	Scabina skate	Urogenital tract	Argentina
Family Scyphiidae			
Caliperia brevipes	Little skate	Gills	Bay of Fundy
Phylum Apicomplexa			
Family Haemogregarinidae			
Haemogregarina delagei	Little skate, thorny skate, smooth skate, spiny dogfish	Blood cells	California, New Brunswick
Eimeria lucida	Spiny dogfish, cat shark, smooth dogfish	Spiral valve	Not reported
Eimeria squali	Spiny dogfish	Spiral valve	Puget Sound
Eimeria southwelli	Spotted eagle ray	Spiral valve of intrauterine embryos	Sri Lanka
Eimeria rajarum	Gray skate	Intestine	France
Eimeria quentini	Spotted eagle ray	Peritoneum	Not reported
Eimeria zygaenae	Smooth hammerhead shark	Spiral valve	Not reported
Eimeria sp.	Cownose ray	Serosal membrane, uterine lining	New York
Eimeria gigantea	Porbeagle	Spiral valve	Not reported
Elmeria scylii	Unidentified cat shark	Intestine	Mediterranean
Class Microsporea	None		
Class Myxosporea			
Family Ceratomyxidae			
Ceratomyxa jamesoni	Leopard shark	Bile	California
Ceratomyxa lunata	Tiger shark	Bile	California
Ceratomyxa mesospora	Bonnethead shark, smooth hammerhead shark	Bile	N. Carolina
Ceratomyxa recurvata	Smooth hammerhead shark	Bile	N. Carolina
Ceratomyxa sp.	Gummy shark	Bile	Australia
Leptotheca agilis	Little skate	Bile	N. Carolina
Leptotheca fusiformes	Smooth hammerhead shark	Bile	N. Carolina
Leptotheca fisheri	Spotted ratfish	Bile	California
Family Chloromyxidae			
Chloromyxum leydigi	Winter skate, bonnethead shark, smooth hammerhead shark, spiny dogfish, Pacific torpedo ray	Bile	N. Carolina, England, California
Chloromyxum ovatum	Soupfin shark, gray smoothhound, brown smoothhound, spiny dogfish, Pacific electric ray, round stingray	Bile	California
Chloromyxum levigatum	Pacific angel shark	Bile	California
Chloromyxum sphyrnae	Bonnethead shark	Bile	Brazil
Chloromyxum obliquum	Gummy shark	Bile	Not reported
Chloromyxum scyliorhinum	Sand shark	Bile	Korea
Family Tetracapsulidae			
Kudoa sp.	Lesser electric ray	Muscle	Florida
Class Turbellaria			
Micropharynx parasitica	Barndoor skate, thorny skate	Back (no effect)	N. Atlantic

Table continued on following page

TABLE 100–1. Parasites Found in Elasmobranchs *Continued*

Parasite	Host	Site of Infection	Location
Monogenea (Monogenetic Trematodes)			
Family Acanthocotylidae			
Acanthocotyle lobianchi	Thornback skate	Skin, gills	Mediterranean
Acanthocotyle elegans	Thornback skate, miraletus skate	Skin	Naples, Italy
Acanthocotyle oligoterus	Thornback skate	Skin	Naples
Acanthocotyle grenni	Unidentified skate	Skin	England
Acanthocotyle pugetensis	Big skate, unidentified shark	Nostril, gills, filaments	Puget Sound, California
Pseudacanthocotyle williamsi	Unidentified skates	Skin	Aleutian Islands
Pseudocanthocotyle pacifica	Big skate, long-nose skate, starry skate	Skin	Puget Sound, California
Pseudocanthocotyle verrilli	Unidentified skate	Skin	Cape Cod
Family Capsalidae			
Benedeniella macrocolpa	Cownose ray	Skin	Sri Lanka
Benedeniella posterocolpa	Cownose ray	Skin	Florida
Entobdella bumpusii	Roughtail stingray	Skin, gills	Woods Hole, Massachusetts
Entobdella corona	Southern stingray, Atlantic stingray, bluntnose stingray	Gills	Florida
Entobdella diadema	Pelagic stinray, bluntnose stingray	Gills	Mediterranean
Entobdella guberleti	Round stingray	Gills	Mexico
Entobdella australis	Queensland stingray	Skin	Australia
Pseudoentobdella pacifica	Bat ray	Gills	California
Macrophyllida antarctica	Gummy shark	Gills	Australia
Sporstonia squatinae	Angel shark	Gills	Atlantic
Family Loimoidae			
Loimopapillosum dasyatis	Southern stingray, bluntnose stingray	Gills	Florida
Loimos salpinggoides	Dusky shark	Gills	Woods Hole, Massachusetts
Loimos scoliodoni	Sharpnose shark	Gills	Florida, Texas
Loimos secundus	Indian sharpnose shark	Gills	India
Loimosina wilsoni	Smooth hammerhead shark	Gills	Florida
Family Microbothriidae			
Asthenocotyle kaikourensis	Plunket's shark	Skin	New Zealand
Asthenocotyle tarankiensis	Prickly dogfish	Skin	New Zealand
Dermophthirius carcharhini	Dusky shark, Galapagos shark, blacktip shark	Skin	Woods Hole, Massachusetts, Bermuda, New Jersey
Dermophthirius maccallumi	Bull shark	Skin	Nicaraguan Lake
Dermophthirius nigrellii	Lemon shark	Skin	Florida
Dermophthirius penneri	Spinner shark, blacktip shark	Skin	New Jersey
Dermophthirius melanopteri	Blacktip reef shark	Skin	Hawaii
Dermophthiroides pristidis	Smalltooth sawfish	Skin	Florida
Leptobothrium pristiuri	Blackmouth dogfish	Skin	Ireland
Leptocotyle minor	European cat shark	Skin	Naples, Italy, England
Microbothrium apiculatum	Spiny dogfish, dusky shark	Skin	Chesapeake Bay, Woods Hole, Massachusetts
Microbothrium tolloi	Unidentified dogfish	Skin	Seno, Reloncavi
Leptomicrobothrium longiphallus	Carpet shark	Gills	New Zealand
Pseudocotyle squatinae	Angel shark	Skin	Mediterranean
Pseudocotyle lepidorhini	Unidentified dogfish	Skin	Atlantic
Family Monocotylidae			
Calicotyle kroyeri	Skates, ratfish, thorny skate, gray skate, cuckoo skate	Cloaca, rectal gland	Atlantic
Calicotyle affinis	Ratfish	Gills	North Sea
Calicotyle australis	Fiddler ray	Not given	S. Australia
Calicotyle macrocotyle	Skate	Spiral valve	Uruguay
Calicotyle ramsayi	Spiny dogfish, unidentified dogfish	Cloaca, spiral valve	New Zealand
Calicotyle stossichi	Smooth dogfish	Rectal gland	Mediterranean
Dictyocotyle coeliaca	Pale skate, thorny skate, cuckoo skate	Not given	North Sea
Gymnocalicotyle inermis	Saw shark	Oviduct	Australia
Dendromonocotyle octodiscus	Bluntnose stingray, yellow stingray	Skin, gills	Florida
Dendromonocotyle kuhlii	Blue spot stingray	Skin	Australia
Dendromonocotyle californica	Bat ray	Skin	California
Dendromonocotyle akajeii	Akaei stingray	Skin	Japan
Potamotrygonocotyle tsalickisi	Freshwater stingray	Gills	Brazil
Squalotrema llewellyni	Spiny dogfish	Nasal fossae	Plymouth, England

TABLE 100–1. Parasites Found in Elasmobranchs *Continued*

Parasite	Host	Site of Infection	Location
Cathariotrema selachii	Dusky shark, smooth hammerhead shark, thresher shark	Olfactory organ	Woods Hole, Massachusetts
Empruthotrema raiae	Little skate, winter skate, clear-nosed skate, rough skate	Olfactory organ, gills	Woods Hole, Massachusetts, Florida, New Zealand
Merizocotyle diaphana	Gray skate	Gills	Belgium
Merizocotyle minor	Long-nosed skate	Gills	Roscoff, France
Merizocotyle pugetensis	Big skate	Nostril	Puget Sound
Merizocotyle sinensis	Guitarfish	Gills	China
Thaumatocotyle concinna	Bluntnose stingray, little skate	Gills	Woods Hole, Massachusetts
Thaumatocotyle longicirrus	Bluntnose stingray	Gills	Florida
Thaumatocotyle pseudodasybatis	Spotted eagle ray	Gills	Florida
Thaumatocotyle retorta	Southern stingray	Gills	Woods Hole, Massachusetts
Dasybatotrema dasybatis	Bluntnose stingray	Gills	Woods Hole, Massachusetts
Dasybatotrema rajae	Porosa skate	Gills	China
Dasybatotrema spinosum	Black-spined skate	Gills	China
Heterocotyle pastinacae	Bluntnose stingray	Gills	Mediterranean
Heterocotyle aetobatis	Spotted eagle ray, bullnose ray	Gills	Florida, N. Carolina
Heterocotyle americana	Southern stingray	Gills	Florida
Heterocotyle minima	Bluntnose stingray, spiny dogfish, roughtail stingray	Gills	Woods Hole, Massachusetts
Heterocotyle papillata	Shovelnose guitarfish	Gills	California
Heterocotyle pseudomonima	Stingrays	Gills	Florida
Heterocotyle robusta	Common stingray	Gills	Sydney
Heterocotyle chinensis	Akaei stingray	Gills	China
Heterocotyle armata	Warnak's stingray	Gills	China
Heterocotyloides prici	Southern stingray	Gills	Florida
Heterocotyloides diademalis	Atlantic stingray	Gills	Florida
Horricauda rhynchobatis	White spotted ray, shovelnose guitarfish	Gills	India, Australia, China
Horricauda forficata	White spotted ray	Gills	China
Monocotyle myliobatis	Whip ray	Gills	Naples, Italy
Monocotyle undosocirrus	Unidentified skate	Gills	China
Monocotyle ancylostomae	Angel shark	Gills	China
Neoheterocotyle inpristi	Unidentified sawfish	Gills	Florida
Neoheterocotyle ruggieri	Smalltooth sawfish	Gills	Florida
Troglocephalus rhinobatidis	Shovelnose guitarfish	Gills	Australia
Spiruris lophosoma	Shovelnose guitarfish	Gills	California
Tritestis ijime	Bluntnose stingray	Mouth	Japan
Tympanocirrus spirophallus	Estuary stingray	Gills	Bay of Bengal
Family Dactylogyridae			
Amphibdella torpedinis	Marbled torpedo ray	Gills	Mediterranean
Amphibdella flavolineata	Torpedo ray	Gills	Woods Hole, Massachusetts
Amphibdella paronaperugiae	Various torpedo rays, Narce skate	Gills	Mediterranean
Amphibdella cuticulovagina	Fairchild's torpedo ray	Gills	New Zealand
Amphibdelloides maccalumi	Spiny dogfish, Pacific torpedo ray, marbled torpedo ray, Atlantic torpedo ray	Gills	California
Amphibdelloides cameroni	Torpedo ray	Gills	India
Amphibdalloides narcine	Lesser electric ray	Gills	Florida
Amphibdelloides vallei	Marbled torpedo ray	Gills	Mediterranean
Order Polyopisthocotylea			
Family Chimaericolidae			
Chimaericola leptogaster	Spotted ratfish, ratfish	Gills	Washington, Atlantic, N.E. Atlantic
Callorhynchiocola multitesticulatus	Elephant shark	Gills	
Callorhynchocotyle marplatensis	Elephant shark	Gills	Argentina
Family Hexabothriidae			
Dasyoncocotyle spiniphallus	Atlantic stingray	Gills	Florida
Hexabothrium appendiculatus	Spiny dogfish, European cat shark, unidentified cat shark	Gills	Plymouth, England, Naples, Italy
Hexabothrium akaroensis	School shark	Gills	New Zealand
Hexabothrium musteli	Smooth dogfish	Gills	Woods Hole, Massachusetts
Heterocotyle hypoprioni	Lemon shark	Gills	Florida
Heterocotyle leucas	Bull shark	Gills	Louisiana
Pseudohexabothrium rajae	Fylla's skate, brown smoothhound	Gills	Norway, California
Erpocotyle laevis	Smooth dogfish	Gills	Mediterranean
Erpocotyle abbreviata	Piked dogfish, spiny dogfish	Gills	Ireland, Pacific

Table continued on following page

TABLE 100–1. Parasites Found in Elasmobranchs *Continued*

Parasite	Host	Site of Infection	Location
Erpocotyle antarctica	Gummy shark	Gills	Australia
Erpocotyle borealis	Greenland shark, unidentified dogfish	Gills	Belgium, Norway, Iceland
Erpocotyle callorhynchi	Elephant sharks	Gills	S. Africa, New Zealand
Erpocotyle canis	Unidentified dogfish	Gills	Roscoff, France
Erpocotyle catenulata	Smoothhound, smooth dogfish, marbled torpedo ray	Gills	Naples, Italy
Erpocotyle francai	Sevengill shark	Gills	Angola
Erpocotyle ginglymostomae	Nurse shark	Gills	Florida
Erpocotyle grisea	Sixgill shark, smooth hammerhead shark	Gills	Naples, France
Erpocotyle laymani	Unidentified hound	Gills	Japan
Erpocotyle licha	European cat shark	Gills	Iceland
Erpocotyle maccallumi	Blacktip shark	Gills	Woods Hole, Massachusetts
Erpocotyle carcharhini	Bull shark	Gills	Rio San Juan, Nicaragua
Erpocotyle macrohystera	Sandbar shark	Gills	Woods Hole, Massachusetts
Erpocotyle mavori	Smooth hammerhead shark	Gills	Woods Hole, Massachusetts
Erpocotyle microstoma	Smooth hammerhead shark, smalleye hammerhead	Gills	N. Carolina
Erpocotyle somniosi	Sleeper shark	Gills	Alaska
Erpocotyle sphyrnae	Smooth hammerhead shark, scalloped hammerhead shark	Gills	Woods Hole, Massachusetts, Hawaii
Erpocotyle spinacis	Unidentified dogfish	Gills	Norway
Erpocotyle squali	Soupfin shark, spiny dogfish, brown smoothhound	Gills	California, Woods Hole, Massachusetts
Erpocotyle striata	Dogfish, spiny dogfish	Gills	Washington
Erpocotyle tiburonis	Bonnethead shark	Gills	Florida
Erpocotyle torpedinis	Marbled torpedo ray	Gills	Morocco
Erpocotyle tropai	Spiked dogfish	Gills	E. Africa
Erpocotyle taschenbergi	Sixgill shark	Gills	France
Erpocotyle tudes	Smalleye hammerhead shark	Gills	Paloma
Erpocotyle septistima	Smalleye hammerhead shark	Gills	Red Sea
Erpocotyle triakis	Leopard shark	Gills	California
Rajoncotyle battis	Skates	Gills	Washington
Rajoncotyle alba	Burton skate	Gills	Roscoff, France
Rajoncotyle kenojei	Unidentified skate	Gills	Japan
Rajoncotyle laevis	Barndoor skate	Gills	Woods Hole, Massachusetts
Rajoncotyle miraletus	Cuckoo skate	Gills	Ireland
Rajoncotyle prenanti	Long-nosed skate	Gills	Roscoff, France
Rajoncotyle clavata	Thornback skate	Gills	Ireland
Rajoncotyle emarginata	Skates	Gills	Roscoff, France Naples, Italy
Rajoncotyle wehri	Starry skate	Gills	Washington
Rajoncotyle blandae	Skates	Gills	Roscoff, France
Neoerpocotyle platensis	Smooth hammerhead shark	Gills	Uruguay
Rhinobatoncotyle cyclovaginata	Shovelnose guitarfish	Gills	California
Paraheteronchocotyle amazonensis	Freshwater stingray	Gills	Brazil
Family Multicalycidae			
Multicalyx cristata	Cownose ray, bullnose ray, sand tiger shark, scalloped hammerhead shark	Bile	Gulf of Mexico, N. Carolina, S. Africa
Multicalyx elegans	Spotted ratfish	Bile	Argentina
Multicalyx multicristatus	Scalloped hammerhead shark	Bile	S. Atlantic
DIGENEA (Digenetic Trematodes)			
Family Bucephalidae			
Bucephalopsis arcuatum	Dusky shark	Spiral valve	Woods Hole, Massachusetts
Prosorhynchus squamatus	Spiny dogfish	Spiral valve	Gulf of St. Lawrence
Prosorhynchus clavatum	Bluespot stingray	Spiral valve	China
Family Zoogonidae			
Steganoderma formosum	Spiny dogfish	Spiral valve	Newfoundland
Family Gorgoderidae			
Anaporrhutum albidum	Spotted eagle ray	Body cavity, pericardium	Pacific
Neoanaporrhutum sp.	Unidentified stingray	Not given	India
Nagmia Yorkei	Unidentified stingray	Rectum	Sri Lanka
Nagmia floridensis	Southern stingray, Atlantic stingray	Not given	Florida
Nagmia larga	Cownose ray, spotted eagle ray, nurse shark, unidentified cat shark, stingrays	Body cavity	Sri Lanka

TABLE 100–1. Parasites Found in Elasmobranchs *Continued*

Parasite	Host	Site of Infection	Location
Petalodistomum pacificum	Soupfin shark	Body cavity	Mexico
Petalodistomum polycladum	Bluespot stingray	Body cavity	Queensland
Staphylorchis cymatodes	Bluespot stingray	Body cavity	Queensland
Probolitrema richiardii	Spiny dogfish	Body cavity	Mediterranean
Probolitrema antarcticum	Gummy shark	Body cavity	Victoria
Probolitrema californiense	Bat ray, shovelnose guitarfish, thornback guitarfish	Body cavity	California
Probolitrema clelandi	Spotted smoothhound, spiny dogfish	Body cavity	Encounter Bay, Australia, New Zealand
Probolitrema mexicanum	Sicklefin smoothhound, unidentified stingray	Body cavity	Mexico
Probolitrema philippi	Bullhead shark, spiny dogfish	Body cavity	Australia, New Zealand
Probolitrema simile	Gummy shark	Body cavity	Encounter Bay, Australia
Probolitrema rotundatum	Carpet shark	Not given	New Zealand
Family Allocreadiidae			
Pedunculacetabulum ghardaguensis	Fantail ray	Not given	Red Sea
Pedunculacetabulum pedicellatum	Slender bamboo shark	Not given	India
Family Aphanhysteridae			
Aphanhystera monacensis	Portuguese shark	Stomach	Mediterranean
Family Azygiidae			
Otodistomum veliporum	Pacific angel shark, spiny dogfish, black shark, big skate, sixgill shark, long-nosed skate, barndoor skate,	Stomach, digestive tract	California, Canada, New Zealand, Oregon
Otodistomum cestoides	Gray skate, barndoor skate, shagreen skate, pale skate, thornback skate, thorny skate	Digestive tract	Belgium, Chile
Otodistomum plicatum	Sixgill shark	Digestive tract	Friday Harbor, Washington
Otodistomum hydrolagi	Ratfish	Body cavity	Washington
Otodistomum plunketi	Plunket's shark	Digestive tract	New Zealand
Otodistomum pristiophori	Nurse shark	Digestive tract	Australia
Otodistomum Scymni	Bramble shark, Portugese shark, marble electric ray, bramble shark, sixgill shark	Digestive tract	Golfe de Gascogne, French W. Africa, Roscoff, France
Otodistomum veliporum pachytheca	Torpedo rays	Digestive tract	Cote Atlantique du Maroc, New Zealand
Otodistomum veliporum valiporum	Sixgill shark, carpet shark	Stomach	Arcachon, British Columbia, Washington, New Zealand
Family Ptychogonimidae			
Ptychogonimus megastomus	Spotted smoothhound, smooth dogfish, rough skate, blue shark	Stomach, buccal cavity	Atlantic, Japan, New Zealand
Family Synoceliidae			
Syncoelium ragassii	Unidentified dogfish, mackerel shark	Branchial chamber	Not given
Otiotrema totosum	Unidentified dogfish, mackerel shark	Branchial chamber	Not given
Paronatrema vaginicola	Unidentified dogfish	Oviduct	New Guinea
Paronatrema mantae	Atlantic manta	Skin	Panama
Family Didymozoidae			
Tricharchen okenii	Brama ray	Gill chamber	Naples, Italy
Family Cephaloporidae			
Plectognathotrema hydrolagi	Ratfish	Stomach	Oregon
Family Heterophyidae			
Stictodora sawakinesis	Gray smoothhound	Metacercaria	USSR
Family Apocreadiidae			
Opecoeloides vitellosis	Knifenose chimaera	Not given	N.W. Atlantic
Family Hemiuridae			
Genarchopsis muelleri	Spiny dogfish	Stomach	Japan
Paravitellotrema overstreeti	Freshwater stingray	Not given	Colombia
Derogenes varicus	Spiny dogfish	Not given	Newfoundland
Hemiurus levinseni	Spiny dogfish	Not given	Gulf of St. Lawrence
Leicithocladium gulosum	Knifenose chimera	Not given	N.W. Atlantic
Family Rugogastridae			
Rugogaster hydrolagi	Ratfish	Rectal gland	Washington
Family Sanguinicolidae			
Salachohemecus olsoni	Sharpnose shark	Circulatory system	Florida

Table continued on following page

TABLE 100–1. Parasites Found in Elasmobranchs *Continued*

Parasite	Host	Site of Infection	Location
Chimaerohemecus trondheimensis	Ratfish	Circulatory system	Norway
Hyperandrotrema cetorhinin	Basking shark	Circulatory system	Tunisia
CESTODES			
Order Grocotylidea			
Family Gyrocotylidae			
Gyrocotyloides nybelini	Ratfish	Not given	Not given
Gyrocotyle spp.	Deep-water chimera, knifenose chimera, deep-water ratfish, spotted ratfish, elephant shark	Spiral valve	Canada, N.W. Atlantic, Washington, New Zealand
Family Bothriocephalidae			
Bothriocephalus squali-glanci	Blue shark	Spiral valve	Accidental host
Bothriocephalus squalii	Dogfish	Spiral valve	Accidental host
Family Echinobothriidae			
Echinobothrium typus	Skates, bluntnose stingray	Spiral valve	Mediterranean, Black Sea
Echinobothrium affine	Thornback skate, requiem sharks, guitarfish	Spiral valve	France
Echinobothrium benedeni	Skates	Spiral valve, stomach	Mediterranean
Echinobothrium boisii	Spotted eagle ray	Spiral valve	Sri Lanka
Echinobothrium brachysoma	Gray skate, thornback skate	Spiral valve	France
Echinobothrium longicolle	Bluespot stingray	Spiral valve	Sri Lankà
Echinobothrium mathiasi	Whip ray	Spiral valve	France
Echinobothrium musteli	Smoothhounds	Spiral valve	France
Echinobothrium raji	Thorny skate	Spiral valve	Canada
Echinobothrium rhinoptera	Cownose ray	Spiral valve	Sri Lanka
Echinobothrium coronatum	Spotted smoothhound	Spiral valve	New Zealand
Echinobothrium bonasum	Cownose ray	Spiral valve	Chesapeake Bay
Echinobothrium harfordi	Cuckoo skate	Spiral valve	English Channel
Echinobothrium euzeti	Lima skate	Spiral valve	Chile
Order Tetraphyllidea			
Family Phyllobothriidae			
Phyllobothrium lactuca	White shark, lemon shark, smooth dogfish, spiny dogfish, gummy shark, smoothhound, tiger shark, angel shark, leopard shark, mackerel shark, sixgill shark, stingrays, skates	Spiral valve	New Zealand, Belgium
Phyllobothrium brassica	Spiny dogfish	Spiral valve	Belgium
Phyllobothrium centrurum	Sixgill shark, Atlantic stingray	Spiral valve	Woods Hole, Massachusetts, Dry Torugas
Phyllobothrium dagnallium	Guitarfish, cat shark, tiger shark, blue shark, porbeagle, barndoor skate	Spiral valve	Sri Lanka, Canada
Phyllobothrium dasybati	Akaei stingray, lemon shark	Spiral valve	Japan, Florida
Phyllobothrium dentatum	Unidentified shark	Rectum	Antarctica
Phyllobothrium dohrnii	Sevengill shark, smooth dogfish, granular dogfish, European cat shark, sand tiger shark, sixgill shark, hounds, broadsnouted sevengill shark	Spiral valve	Naples, Italy, Woods Hole, Massachusetts, Porcupine Bank, Tirreno, Japan, New Zealand
Phyllobothrium fallax	Spiny dogfish	Spiral valve	Belgium
Phyllobothrium filiforme	Thresher shark, dusky shark	Spiral valve	Pacific Coast, Japan
Phyllobothrium foliatum	Roughtail stingray, dusky shark, Atlantic stingray	Spiral valve	Woods Hole, Massachusetts, Dry Tortugas
Phyllobothrium gracile	Marbled torpedo ray, angel shark, sevengill shark, guitarfish, spiny dogfish	Spiral valve	Europe, Catania, Japan
Phyllobothrium laciniatum	Sand tiger shark, dogfish, ratfish	Spiral valve	Woods Hole, Massachusetts, E. China Sea, Tirreno, Japan
Phyllobothrium loculatum	Bullhead shark	Spiral valve	E. China Sea
Phyllobothrium magnum	Pacific sleeper shark	Spiral valve	Puget Sound
Phyllobothrium marginatum	Angel shark	Spiral valve	Japan
Phyllobothrium microsomum	Nurse shark	Spiral valve	India
Phyllobothrium minutum	Blacktip shark	Spiral valve	Sri Lanka
Phyllobothrium musteli	Smooth dogfish	Spiral valve	Belgium
Phyllobothrium pammicrum	Blacktip shark, thorny ray	Spiral valve	India
Phyllobothrium prionacis	Blue shark	Spiral valve	Japan

TABLE 100–1. Parasites Found in Elasmobranchs *Continued*

Parasite	Host	Site of Infection	Location
Phyllobothrium radioductum	Big skate, long-nosed skate, California skate, leopard shark, brown smoothhound	Spiral valve, body cavity	Friday Harbor, California
Phyllobothrium riggii	Torpedo ray, marbled torpedo ray, European cat shark, thorny skate	Spiral valve	Woods Hole, Massachusetts, Mediterranean
Phyllobothrium rotundum	Sixgill shark	Spiral valve	Trieste
Phyllobothrium serratum	Cat shark	Spiral valve	Japan
Phyllobothrium squali	Spiny dogfish	Spiral valve	Japan
Phyllobothrium thridax	Angel shark, stingray, Greenland shark, hammerhead sharks, skates, spiny dogfish	Spiral valve	Belgium, Mediterranean, Japan
Phyllobothrium triacis	Cat shark, dogfish, sixgill shark	Spiral valve	Pacific Coast, Japan, Atlantic
Phyllobothrium tumidum	White shark, bonito shark, cat shark, sharpnose shark	Spiral valve	Woods Hole, Massachusetts, California, Florida
Phyllobothrium typicum	Lesser blue shark, milk shark, hound	Spiral valve	Madras, India
Phyllobothrium chiloscyllii	Cat shark, white spotted guitarfish, granular guitarfish, shovelnose shark	Spiral valve	Madras, India
Phyllobothrium minimum	White spotted guitarfish	Spiral valve	Madras, India
Phyllobothrium (Calyptrobothrium) chalarosomum	Carpet shark	Spiral valve	New Zealand
Phyllobothrium occidentale	Fairchild's electric ray	Spiral valve	New Zealand
Phyllobothrium sinuosiceps	Sixgill shark	Spiral valve	Chile
Phyllobothrium orectolobi	Wobbegong	Spiral valve	Australia
Phyllobothrium myliobatidis	Bull ray	Spiral valve	Rio de la Plata, Uruguay
Phyllobothrium piriei	Cuckoo skate	Spiral valve	
Phyllobothrium unilaterale	Angel shark	Spiral valve	Naples, Italy, France, British Isles
Anthobothrium cornucopia	Spiny dogfish, smooth dogfish, stingrays, thorny skate, winter skate, hammerhead sharks, sevengill shark, mackerel shark, blue shark	Spiral valve	Black Sea, Woods Hole, Massachusetts, Canada, France, California
Anthobothrium auriculatum	Dogfishes, skates, angel shark, marbled torpedo ray, cat shark, smooth dogfish, blue shark, sixgill shark, mackerel sharks, requiem sharks	Spiral valve	Atlantic, Mediterranean, France
Anthobothrium bifidum	Akaei stingray	Spiral valve	E. China Sea
Anthobothrium exiguum	Common thresher shark	Spiral valve	Japan
Anthobothrium hickmani	Tasmanian numbfish	Spiral valve	Tasmania
Anthobothrium laciniatum	Dusky shark, bull shark, requiem sharks, mackerel shark, dogfishes, smooth hammerhead shark, sharpnose shark, skates, milkshark, round stingray, blue shark, school shark	Spiral valve	Woods Hole, Massachusetts, Atlantic, California, New Zealand
Anthobothrium lintoni	Spotted guitarfish	Spiral valve	Sri Lanka
Anthobothrium minutum	Blue shark	Spiral valve	Iles du Cap Vent
Anthobothrium oligorchidum	Round stingray	Spiral valve	California
Anthobothrium panjadi	Eagle ray, spotted eagle ray	Spiral valve	Sri Lanka
Anthobothrium parvum	Hammerhead, brown smoothhound, hound, leopard shark	Spiral valve	Rovigno, Sea of Japan, California
Anthobothrium pristis	Largetooth sawfish	Spiral valve	Amazon
Anthobothrium quadribothria	Bluntnose stingray	Spiral valve	Woods Hole, Massachusetts
Anthobothrium rajae	Skate	Spiral valve	Japan
Anthobothrium variabile	Roughtail stingray, bluespot stingray, basking shark, winter skate, thorny skate	Spiral valve	Woods Hole, Massachusetts Sri Lanka, Adriatic, Canada
Anthobothrium septatum	Spotted guitarfish	Spiral valve	Madras, India
Anthobothrium crenulatum	Guitarfish	Spiral valve	Madras, India
Anthobothrium spinosum	Lesser blue shark, milk shark, blacktip shark	Spiral valve	Madras, India
Anthobothrium amuletum	Common shovelnosed ray	Spiral valve	Australia
Anthobothrium sasoonense	Granular shovelnose ray	Spiral valve	Sasson Dock, Bombay
Glyphobothrium zwerneri	Cownose ray	Spiral valve	Chesapeake Bay

Table continued on following page

TABLE 100–1. Parasites Found in Elasmobranchs *Continued*

Parasite	Host	Site of Infection	Location
Carpobothrium chiloscyllii	Slender bamboo shark, spotted guitarfish	Spiral valve	Sri Lanka
Carpobothrium megapallum	Gray bamboo shark	Spiral valve	Madras, India
Cyatocotyle marchesettii	Mackerel shark	Spiral valve	India
Dinobothrium septaria	Porbeagle, white shark	Spiral valve	Belgium, Woods Hole, Massachusetts
Dinobothrium plicitum	Basking shark, blue shark	Spiral valve	France
Dinobothrium keilini	Blue shark	Spiral valve	English Channel
Echeneibothrium minimum	Round stingray, cownose ray, skates, bluntnose stingray, requiem sharks	Spiral valve	California, Sri Lanka Atlantic
Echeneibothrium affine	Gray skate	Spiral valve	Scandinavia
Echeneibothrium austrinum	Unidentified skate	Spiral valve	Mossell Bay
Echeneibothrium bilobatum	Round stingray	Spiral valve	California
Echeneibothrium burgeri	Roughtail stingray	Spiral valve	Woods Hole, Massachusetts
Echeneibothrium cancellatum	Cownose ray	Spiral valve	Woods Hole, Massachusetts
Echeneibothrium ceylonicum	Unidentified stingray	Spiral valve	Sri Lanka
Echeneibothrium dolichophorum	Long-nosed skate	Spiral valve	California
Echeneibothrium dollfusi	European stingray	Spiral valve	France
Echeneibothrium flexile	Bat rays, stingrays, eagle rays	Spiral valve	California, Woods Hole, Massachusetts, Sri Lanka, Vankali Parr, Japan
Echeneibothrium gracile	Gray skate, bluntnose stingray	Spiral valve	Not given
Echeneibothrium hui	Akaei stingray	Spiral valve	China
Echeneibothrium javanicum	Cownose rray	Spiral valve	Java
Echeneibothrium julievansium	Skates	Spiral valve	Irish Sea, France
Echeneibothrium longicolle	Bullnose ray, roughtail stingray	Spiral valve	Woods Hole, Massachusetts
Echeneibothrium maccallumi	Roughtail stingray	Spiral valve	Woods Hole, Massachusetts
Echeneibothrium macrascum	California skate	Spiral valve	California
Echeneibothrium maculatum	Unidentified skate	Spiral valve	Plymouth, England
Echeneibothrium myzorhynchum	Big skate, bat ray	Spiral valve	Puget Sound, California
Echeneibothrium octorchis	Big skate, California skate	Spiral valve	California
Echeneibothrium opisthorchis	Bat ray	Spiral valve	California
Echeneibothrium oligotesticularae	Granular guitarfish	Spiral valve	India
Echeneibothrium verticillatum	Spotted guitarfish	Spiral valve	Madras, India
Echeneibothrium filamentosum	Granular guitarfish, shovelnose guitarfish	Spiral valve	Madras, India
Echeneibothrium palombi	Roughtail stingray, pelagic stingray	Spiral valve	Woods Hole, Massachusetts, France
Echeneibothrium rankini	Roughtail stingray	Spiral valve	Woods Hole, Massachusetts
Echeneibothrium shipleyi	Bluespot stingray, stingray	Spiral valve	Sri Lanka, Japan
Echeneibothrium tetrascaphium	Bat ray	Spiral valve	California
Echeneibothrium tobijei	Eagle ray	Spiral valve	Japan
Echeneibothrium trifidum	Stingray	Spiral valve	Sri Lanka
Echeneibothrium trygonis	Unidentified stingray	Spiral valve	Sri Lanka
Echeneibothrium tumidulum	Gray·skate, thornback skate, roundtail skate, torpedo ray, round stingray	Spiral valve	Ireland, California, France
Echeneibothrium urobatidium	Round stingray, winter skate, little skate, thorny skate	Spiral valve	California, Canada, Woods Hole, Massachusetts
Rhinebothrium rhinobati	Skates	Spiral valve	Chile, Tunis
Rhinebothrium flexile	Bluntnose stingray	Spiral valve	Tunis
Rhinebothrium chilensis	Chilean skate	Spiral valve	Chile
Rhinebothrium freitasi	Unidentified ray	Spiral valve	S. America
Rhinebothrium leiblei	Chilean skate	Spiral valve	Chile
Rhinebothrium scobinae	Chilean skate	Spiral valve	Chile
Rhinebothrium pearsoni	Bank's shovelnosed ray	Spiral valve	Australia
Rhinebothrium moralarai	Freshwater stingray	Spiral valve	Colombia
Rhinebothrium scorzai	Freshwater stingray	Spiral valve	Venezuela
Rhinebothrium ditesticulum	Round stingray	Spiral valve	S. California
Rhinebothrium tumidulum	Skates	Spiral valve	Not given
Acanthobothroides thorsoni	Stingray	Spiral valve	Colombia
Caulobothrium uruguayense	Eagle ray	Spiral valve	Rio de la Plata, Uruguay
Caulobothrium ostrowskiae	Eagle ray	Spiral valve	Rio de la Plata, Uruguay
Caulobothrium myliobatidis	Eagle ray	Spiral valve	Rio de la Plata, Uruguay
Caulobothrium opisthorchis	Bat rat	Spiral valve	California
Rhabdotobothrium dollfusi	Bluntnose stingray	Spiral valve	France
Rhinebothroides amazonensis	Freshwater stingray	Spiral valve	Brazil
Gastrolecithus planus	Basking shark, brown smooth-hound	Spiral valve	Woods Hole, Massachusetts, California
Marsupiobothrium alopias	Thresher shark	Spiral valve	Japan
Marsupiobothrium forte	Smooth hammerhead shark	Spiral valve	Woods Hole, Massachusetts

TABLE 100–1. Parasites Found in Elasmobranchs *Continued*

Parasite	Host	Site of Infection	Location
Monorygma perfectum	Greater spotted dogfish, Pacific sleeper shark, Greenland shark	Spiral valve	Naples, Italy, Alaska, Greenland
Monorygma galeocerdonis	Tiger shark	Spiral valve	Woods Hole, Massachusetts
Monorygma megacotyle	Swell shark	Spiral valve	Japan
Monorygma hyperapolytica	Black shark	Spiral valve	New Zealand
Myzophyllobothrium rubrum	Spotted eagle ray	Spiral valve	Sri Lanka
Orygamatobothrium versatile	Spiny dogfish, smooth dogfish, European cat shark, hound, spotted smoothhound	Spiral valve	Trieste, Japan, New Zealand
Orygamatobothrium musteli	Smoothhound, smooth dogfish, brown smoothhound, spiny dogfish, soupfin shark, European cat shark, leopard shark, hound	Spiral valve	European Atlantic, California, Japan
Orygamatobothrium plicatum	Skates	Spiral valve	Japan
Orygamatobothrium zschokkei	Smoothhound, smooth dogfish	Spiral valve	Atlantic
Pelichnibothrium speciosum	Smalltooth sand tiger shark, blue shark	Spiral valve	Medeira, Japan
Pithophorus tetraglobus	Spotted guitarfish	Spiral valve	Sri Lanka
Pithophorus muscutosus	Lesser blue shark, blacktip shark, milk shark, white spotted ray	Spiral valve	Madras, India
Pseudanthobothrium hanseni	Thorny skate	Spiral valve	Disko Bugt
Pseudanthobothrium vulpeculae	Thresher shark	Spiral valve	Japan
Reesium paciferum	Basking shark	Spiral valve	English Channel, Japan
Rhodobothrium pulvinatum	Roughtail stingray, spiny dogfish, bluespot stingray	Spiral valve	Woods Hole, Massachusetts, Sri Lanka, France
Rhodobothrium brachyascum	Bat ray	Spiral valve	California
Zyxibothrium kamienae	Smooth skate	Spiral valve	Gulf of Maine
Scyphophyllidium giganteum	Spiny dogfish, gray skate, thorny skate, soupfin shark	Spiral valve	Europe, Canada, California
Family Oncobothriidae			
Oncobothrium pseudo-uncinatum	Skates, stingrays, torpedo rays, dogfishes	Spiral valve	Atlantic, Canada
Oncobothrium convolutum	Hound	Spiral valve	Japan
Oncobothrium farmeri	Bluespot stingray	Spiral valve	Sri Lanka
Oncobothrium ganfini	European cat shark	Spiral valve	Naples, Italy
Acanthobothrium coronatum	Smoothhounds, skates, rays, torpedo rays, sharks, dogfishes	Spiral valve	Mediterranean, Atlantic, Indian and Pacific Oceans
Acanthobothrium aetobatis	Spotted eagle ray	Spiral valve	Lifu
Acanthobothrium benedeni	Thornback skate, pelagic stingray	Spiral valve	Naples, Italy
Acanthobothrium brachyacanthum	Big skate, California skate	Spiral valve	California
Acanthobothrium cestracii	Hammerhead	Spiral valve	Japan
Acanthobothrium crassicolle	Pelagic stingray, bluntnose stingray	Spiral valve	Black Sea, Europe
Acanthobothrium ponticum	Skates, round stingray	Spiral valve	Naples, Italy, New Zealand, California
Acanthobothrium dasybati	Akaei stingray, skates, round stingray	Spiral valve	Japan
Acanthobothrium dujardinii	Skates, stingrays, shovelnose guitarfish, Philippine guitarfish	Spiral valve	Belgium, Black Sea, Manche, Florida, Puget Sound, California, Woods Hole, Massachusetts, Tsing Tao
Acanthobothrium folicolle	Marbled skate, pelagic stingray, sixgill shark	Spiral valve	Roscoff, France, Naples, Italy, Trieste
Acanthobothrium gracile	Torpedo ray	Spiral valve	Japan
Acanthobothrium grandiceps	Akaei stingray	Spiral valve	East China Sea
Acanthobothrium harpago	Lemon shark	Spiral valve	Senegal
Acanthobothrium herdmani	Bluespot stingray	Spiral valve	Sri Lanka
Acanthobothrium heterodonti	Philippine horn shark	Spiral valve	Australia
Acanthobothrium hispidum	Pacific torpedo ray	Spiral valve	California
Acanthobothrium holorhini	Bat ray	Spiral valve	California
Acanthobothrium ijimai	Akaei stingray, electric ray, cat sharks	Spiral valve	Japan, Sri Lanka
Acanthobothrium latum	Akaei stingray	Spiral valve	Japan
Acanthobothrium macranthum	Thorny ray	Spiral valve	Sri Lanka
Acanthobothrium maculatum	Bat ray	Spiral valve	California
Acanthobothrium micracantha	Akaei stingray, lesser butterfly ray	Spiral valve	Japan

Table continued on following page

TABLE 100–1. Parasites Found in Elasmobranchs *Continued*

Parasite	Host	Site of Infection	Location
Acanthobothrium microcephalum	Bat ray	Spiral ray	California
Acanthobothrium musculosum	Pelagic stingray	Spiral valve	Naples, Italy
Acanthobothrium parviuncinatum	Pelagic stingray, California butterfly ray	Spiral valve	California
Acanthobothrium paulum	Stingrays, skates, bluntnose stingray, lesser butterfly ray	Spiral valve	Woods Hole, Massachusetts, Beaufort, North Carolina
Acanthobothrium indicum	Electric rays	Spiral valve	Madras, India
Acanthobothrium rhinobati	Shovelnose guitarfish	Spiral valve	California
Acanthobothrium robustum	Shovelnose guitarfish	Spiral valve	California
Acanthobothrium semivesiculum	Sephen stingray	Spiral valve	India
Acanthobothrium triacis	Smooth dogfish	Spiral valve	Japan
Acanthobothrium tsingtavense	Akaei stingray	Spiral valve	China
Acanthobothrium uncinatum	Dogfishes, stingrays, skates, torpedo ray	Spiral valve	France, Irish Sea, Sri Lanka
Acanthobothrium unilaterale	Bat ray	Spiral valve	California
Acanthobothrium woodsholei	Roughtail stingray	Spiral valve	Woods Hole, Massachusetts
Acanthobothrium zschokkei	Ocellate electric ray	Spiral valve	Naples, Italy
Acanthobothrium southwelli	Guitarfish	Spiral valve	Madras, India
Acanthobothrium rhynchobatidis	Spotted guitarfish	Spiral valve	Madras, India
Acanthobothrium wedli	Skates	Spiral valve	New Zealand
Acanthobothrium electricolum	Lesser electric ray	Spiral valve	Colombia
Acanthobothrium lintoni	Lesser electric ray	Spiral valve	Gulf of Mexico, Colombia
Acanthobothrium quinonesi	Freshwater stingray	Spiral valve	Magdalena River, Colombia
Acanthobothrium amazonensis	Freshwater stingray	Spiral valve	Brazil
Acanthobothrium terezae	Neotropical freshwater stingray	Spiral valve	Brazil
Acanthobothrium olseni	Round stingray, shovelnose guitarfish	Spiral valve	California
Acanthobothrium psammobati	Skate	Spiral valve	Chile
Acanthobothrium annapinkiensis	Chilean skate	Spiral valve	Chile
Acanthobothrium goldsteini	Thornback skate	Spiral valve	California
Acanthobothrium americanum	Southern stingray	Spiral valve	Chesapeake
Acanthobothrium lineatum	Southern stingray	Spiral valve	Chesapeake
Acanthobothrium brevissime	Round stingrays, clear-nosed skate	Spiral valve	Gulf of Mexico, Chesapeake Bay
Acanthobothrium floridensis	Clear-nosed skate	Spiral valve	Gulf of Mexico, Chesapeake Bay
Acanthobothrium quadripartitum	Cuckoo skate, thorny skate	Spiral valve	North Sea
Acanthobothrium colombianum	Spotted eagle ray, stingrays	Spiral valve	Colombia
Acanthobothrium electricolum	Lesser electric ray	Spiral valve	Colombia
Acanthobothroides thorsoni	Whip ray	Spiral valve	South America
Potamotrygonocestus magdalenensis	Freshwater stingray	Spiral valve	Magdalena River, Colombia
Potamotrygonocestus amazonensis	Freshwater stingray	Spiral valve	Brazil
Potamotrygonocestus travassosi	Freshwater stingray	Spiral valve	South America
Family Dioecotaenidae			
Dioecotaenia cancellata	Cownose ray	Spiral valve	Chesapeake Bay
Dioecotaenia campbelli	Cownose ray	Spiral valve	Colombia
Calliobothrium verticillatum	Dogfishes, angel shark, smooth dogfish, hounds, sixgill shark, blue shark, gummy shark	Spiral valve	Belgium, Mediterranean, Woods Hole, Massachusetts, Japan, France, England, Chile, New Zealand
Calliobothrium eschrichtii	Dogfishes, hounds, estuary stingray, gummy shark	Spiral valve	Europe, Woods Hole, Massachusetts, India, Japan, New Zealand
Calliobothrium leuckartii	Dogfishes, hounds	Spiral valve	Belgium, France, Tunis
Calliobothrium nodosum	Smooth dogfish	Spiral valve	Japan
Calliobothrium pellucidum	Gray smoothhound	Spiral valve	S. California
Calliobothrium tylotocephalum	Gummy shark	Spiral valve	New Zealand
Calliobothrium creeveyae	School shark	Spiral valve	Australia
Ceratobothrium xanthocephalum	Porbeagle shark, bonito shark, shortfin mako	Spiral valve	Italy, Woods Hole, Massachusetts, Japan, New Zealand
Cylindrophorus typicus	White shark	Spiral valve	Not reported
Cylindrophorus posteroporus	Blue shark	Spiral valve	California
Pedibothrium globicephalum	Nurse shark, sawfish	Spiral valve	Florida
Pedibothrium brevispine	Nurse shark	Spiral valve	Florida
Pedibothrium hutsoni	Nurse shark, tiger shark, guitarfish	Spiral valve	Sri Lanka
Pedibothrium longispine	Nurse shark, slender bamboo shark, guitarfish, tiger shark, angel shark	Spiral valve	Florida, India, Sri Lanka
Pedibothrium ottleyi	Zebra Shark	Spiral valve	Australia

TABLE 100–1. Parasites Found in Elasmobranchs Continued

Parasite	Host	Site of Infection	Location
Phoreiobothrium lasium	Smooth hammerhead shark, dusky shark, bull shark, blacktip shark, sandbar shark, tiger shark, sharpnose shark, thresher shark	Spiral valve	Woods Hole, Massachusetts
Phoreiobothrium exceptum	Smooth hammerhead shark, bull shark	Spiral valve	Woods Hole, Massachusetts
Phoreiobothrium pectinatum	Smooth hammerhead	Spiral valve	Woods Hole, Massachusetts
Phoreiobothrium triloculatum	Dusky shark, sharpnose shark, brown shark, sand tiger shark	Spiral valve	Woods Hole, Massachusetts
Phoreiobothrium tiburonis	Bonnethead shark	Spiral valve	Florida
Platybothrium cervinum	Blue shark, dusky shark	Spiral valve	Woods Hole, Massachusetts
Platybothrium auriculatum	Blue shark	Spiral valve	Japan
Platybothrium baeri	Blue shark	Spiral valve	Naples, Italy
Platybothrium hypoprioni	Lemon shark	Spiral valve	Florida
Platybothrium musteli	Unidentified dogfish	Spiral valve	Japan
Platybothrium parvum	Brown shark, bonito shark, smooth hammerhead shark, blue shark	Spiral valve	Woods Hole, Massachusetts, Canada
Pinguicollum pinguicollum	Skates	Spiral valve	California, Puget Sound
Spiniloculus mavensis	Smooth dogfish	Spiral valve	Australia
Thysanocephalum crispum	Spotted eagle ray, tiger shark, smooth hammerhead shark	Spiral valve	Woods Hole, Massachusetts
Thysanocephalum rugosum	Tiger shark	Spiral valve	Florida
Uncibilocularis trygonis	Stingrays	Spiral valve	Sri Lanka
Uncibilocularis mandleyi	Snaggletoothed shark	Spiral valve	Sri Lanka
Uncibilocularis indica	Gray bamboo shark	Spiral valve	Madras, India
Yorkeria parva	Slender bamboo shark	Spiral valve	Sri Lanka
Family Triloculariidae			
Trilocularia gracilis	Spiny dogfish, thorny skate	Spiral valve	Scandinavia
Trilocularia acanthiaevulgaris	Spotted spiny dogfish	Spiral valve	Canada, New Zealand
Order Lecanicephalidea			
Family Lecanicephalidae			
Lecanicephalum pellatum	Roughtail stingray, smalltooth sawfish, bluespotted stingray, lesser butterfly ray, Southern stingray	Spiral valve	Woods Hole, Massachusetts, Sri Lanka, Colombia
Discobothrium myliobatidis	Bat ray	Spiral valve	California
Discobothrium fallax	Thornback skate	Spiral valve	Belgium
Discobothrium japonicum	Japanese electric ray	Spiral valve	Japan
Discobothrium quadrisurculi	Estuary stingray, whitespotted shovelnose ray	Spiral valve	Bombay
Discobothrium redactum	Estuary stingray, whitespot shovelnose ray	Spiral valve	Bombay
Discobothrium arrhynchum	Eagle ray	Spiral valve	Rio de la Plata, Uruguay
Calycobothrium typicum	Spotted eagle ray	Spiral valve	Sri Lanka
Cephalobothrium aetobatidis	Spotted eagle ray, lesser butterfly ray, bluespot stingray	Spiral valve	Egypt, Sri Lanka
Cephalobothrium rhinobatidis	Guitarfish	Spiral valve	Madras, India
Cephalobothrium taeniurai	Fantail ray	Spiral valve	Egypt
Hexacanalis abruptus	Lesser butterfly ray	Spiral valve	Sri Lanka
Polypocephalus radiatus	Guitarfish, coach whip ray, bluespot stingray, estuary stingray, spotted guitarfish	Spiral valve	Sri Lanka, Madras, India
Polypocephalus affinis	Guitarfish	Spiral valve	Madras, India
Polypocephalus coronatus	Spotted guitarfish	Spiral valve	Madras, India
Polypocephalus lintoni	Spotted guitarfish	Spiral valve	Madras, India
Polypocephalus medusia	Roughtail stingray, bluntnose stingray, guitarfish, spotted guitarfish	Spiral valve	Woods Hole, Massachusetts, Beaufort, North Carolina, Madras, India
Polypocephalus pulcher	Estuary stingray	Spiral valve	Sri Lanka
Polypocephalus rhynchobatidis	Spotted guitarfish	Spiral valve	Madras, India
Polypocephalus rhinobatidis	Guitarfish	Spiral valve	Madras, India
Polypocephalus vitellaris	Spotted guitarfish	Spiral valve	Madras, India
Polypocephalus moretonensis	Estuary stingray	Spiral valve	Australia
Tylocephalum pingue	Cownose ray	Spiral valve	Woods Hole, Massachusetts
Tylocephalum campanulatum	Shark ray	Spiral valve	Australia
Tylocephalum aetobatidis	Spotted eagle ray, stingray	Spiral valve	Sri Lanka
Tylocephalum dierama	Eagle ray	Spiral valve	Sri Lanka

Table continued on following page

TABLE 100–1. Parasites Found in Elasmobranchs *Continued*

Parasite	Host	Site of Infection	Location
Tylocephalum marsupium	Spotted eagle ray	Spiral valve	Tortugas
Tylocephalum simile	Stingray	Spiral valve	Not given
Tylocephalum squatinae	Angel shark	Spiral valve	Japan
Tylocephalum translucens	Spotted eagle ray	Spiral valve	Sri Lanka
Tylocephalum yorkei	Spotted eagle ray	Spiral valve	India
Tylocephalum elongatum	White spotted ray	Spiral valve	Madras, India
Tylocephalum minimum	White spotted ray	Spiral valve	Madras, India
Family Adelobothriidae			
Adelobothrium aetobatidis	Spotted eagle ray, white spotted ray	Spiral valve	Loyalty Island, Torgugas, Sri Lanka
Family Balanobothriidae			
Balanobothrium tenax	Stingray	Spiral valve	Sri Lanka
Balanobothrium parvum	Stingrays, tiger shark	Spiral valve	Sri Lanka
Balanobothrium sp.	Zebra shark	Spiral valve	Australia
Family Disculicipitidae			
Disculiceps pileatus	Blacktip shark, dusky shark, mackerel shark, sharpnose shark, bull shark	Spiral valve	Australia, Woods Hole, Massachusetts, Bermuda, Bengal, France, Gulf of Mexico
Family Tetragonocephalidae			
Tetragonocephalum trygonis	Pelagic stingray, stingrays, bluespot stingray	Spiral valve	France, Sri Lanka, India
Order Trypanorhyncha			
Family Hepatoxylidae			
Hepatoxylon squali	Thresher shark, dogfishes, mackerel sharks, blue shark	Serous membrane of stomach and liver, exterior of liver	Atlantic, Pacific, Japan, California
Hepatoxylon megacephalum	Thresher shark, black shark, school shark, broadsnouted sevengill shark	Spiral valve, body cavity	New Zealand
Hepatoxylon trichuri	Shovelnosed spiny dogfish, mako shark, blue shark, spotted spiny dogfish, Fairchild's electric ray, white shark	Body cavity, spiral valve	New Zealand, Atlantic
Family Sphyriocephalidae			
Sphyriocephalus viridis	Cat sharks, granular dogfish, bigeye thresher shark, bonito shark	Spiral valve	Mediterranean, Japan, California
Sphyriocephalus pelorosoma	Bigeye thresher shark, bonito shark	Spiral valve	Japan
Sphyriocephalus tergestinus	Thresher shark	Spiral valve	France
Sphyriocephalus sp.	Pygmy shark	Stomach	Indian Ocean, Pacific
Sphyriocephalus alberti	Portuguese shark, false cat shark	Spiral valve	Mediterranean
Family Tentacularidae			
Tentacularia coryphaenae	White shark, dusky shark, ocean whitetip shark, smooth hammerhead shark, blue shark, tiger shark, sharpnose shark	Spiral valve, pyloric ceca	Woods Hole, Massachusetts, N. Mexico, Japan
Tentacularia megalobothrida	Bluntnose sixgill shark	Spiral valve	Puget Sound
Nybelina lingualis	Blue shark, smooth dogfish, thornback skate, spiny dogfish, angel shark, cat shark, bonito shark, smooth hammerhead shark	Spiral valve	Not given
Nybelina bisulcata	Dusky shark, brown shark, tiger shark, spiny dogfish	Spiral valve	Woods Hole, Massachusetts
Nybelina equidentata	Celanese stingray	Spiral valve	Sri Lanka
Nybelina herdmani	Celanese stingray	Spiral valve	Sri Lanka
Nybelina manazo	Hounds	Spiral valve	Japan
Nybelina narinari	Spotted eagle ray	Spiral valve	Woods Hole, Massachusetts
Nybelina perideraea	Ganges shark, tawny nurse shark	Spiral valve	Sri Lanka
Nybelina pintneri	Shortfin mako shark, blue shark	Spiral valve	Japan
Nybelina robusta	Dusky shark, roughtail stingray, shortfin mako shark, porbeagle	Spiral valve	Woods Hole, Massachusetts, France
Nybelinia tenuis	Roughtail stingray	Spiral valve	Woods Hole, Massachusetts
Nybelinia palliata	Smooth hammerhead shark	Spiral valve	Woods Hole, Massachusetts
Nybelinia sphyrnae	Smooth hammerhead shark	Spiral valve	Japan

TABLE 100–1. Parasites Found in Elasmobranchs *Continued*

Parasite	Host	Site of Infection	Location
Nybelinia syngenes	Smooth hammerhead shark	Spiral valve	Florida
Nybelinia anthicosum	Leopard shark	Stomach, spiral valve	California
Nybelinia lingualis	Shortfin mako shark	Spiral valve	Mediterranean
Nybelinia sp.	Broadnose sevengill shark	Spiral valve	California
Family Cathelocephalidae			
Cathelocephalus thatcheri	Bull shark	Spiral valve	Florida
Cathelocephalus sp.	Blacktip shark	Spiral valve	Australia
Family Dasyrhynchidae			
Dasyrhynchus varioucinatum	Brown shark, lemon shark	Not given	Woods Hole, Massachusetts, Gulf of Mexico
Dasyrhynchus ingens	Dusky shark, blue shark	Not given	Atlantic, Pacific
Dasyrhynchus talismani	Ocean whitetip shark, blue shark	Not given	N. Mexico, W. Africa
Dasyrhynchus giganteus	Bull shark	Not given	Florida
Callotetrarhynchus gracile	Lemon shark, dusky shark	Spiral valve	Florida
Callotetrarhynchus speciosum	Blue shark	Spiral valve	California
Callotetrarhynchus perilica	Lemon shark	Spiral valve	Florida
Callotetrarhynchus tumidulum	Smooth dogfish, smoothhound	Spiral valve	Woods Hole, Massachusetts
Floriceps lichiae	European cat shark	Encysted in liver	Naples, Italy
Floriceps saccatus	Dusky shark, broadnose sevengill shark, blue shark	Spiral valve	Atlantic
Family Eutetrarhynchidae			
Eutetrarhynchus ruficollis	Smooth dogfish, spiny dogfish, skates	Spiral valve	Atlantic, Mediterranean, France
Eutetrarhynchus schmidti	Round stingray, shovelnose guitarfish	Spiral valve	California
Eutetrarhynchus araya	Stingray, shovelnose guitarfish	Spiral valve	Amazon
Eutetrarhynchus leucomelanum	White spotted ray, bluespot stingray	Spiral valve	Sri Lanka
Eutetrarhynchus lineatum	Common nurse shark	Spiral valve	Florida
Eutetrarhynchus macrotrachelus	Gray smoothhound	Spiral valve	California
Eutetrarhynchus litocephalus	Gray smoothhound, leopard shark	Spiral valve	California
Christianella minuta	Angel shark, requiem shark	Spiral valve	Belgium, India
Christianella trygon-brucco	Stingray, round stingray	Spiral valve	Mediterranean, California
Parachristianella trygonis	Bluntnose stingray, round stingray	Spiral valve	Concarneau, California, Seal Beach, California
Parachristianella monomegacantha	Southern stingray	Spiral valve	Chesapeake Bay
Prochristianella trygonicola	Bluntnose stingray	Spiral valve	Concarneau
Prochristianella minima	Round stingray	Spiral valve	California
Prochristianella tennispinis	Roughtail stingray	Spiral valve	Woods Hole, Massachusetts
Prochristianella aetobatis	Unidentified eagle ray	Spiral valve	New Zealand
Prochristianella heteracantha	Guitarfish	Spiral valve	Chile
Prochristianella fragilis	Shovelnose guitarfish	Spiral valve	California
Prochristianella monomegacantha	Shovelnose guitarfish	Spiral valve	California
Mecistobothrium myliobati	Round stingray, bat ray	Spiral valve	California
Family Gilquiniidae			
Gilquinia squali	Spiny dogfish, dogfishes	Spiral valve	Atlantic, Mediterranean, Pacific
Gilquinia anteroporus	Piked dogfish	Spiral valve	Puget Sound
Gilquinia nannocephala	Blainville's dogfish	Spiral valve	Japan
Aporhynchus norvegicum	Velvetbelly shark	Spiral valve	Scandinavia
Family Gymnorrhynchidae			
Gymnorrhynchus gigas	Shortfin mako shark	Spiral valve	California
Gymnorrhynchus isuri	Shortfin mako shark	Spiral valve	New Zealand
Molicola horridus	Longfin mako shark	Spiral valve	Pacific, California
Molicola uncinatus	Common thresher shark	Spiral valve	Woods Hole, Massachusetts, Pacific
Family Lacistorhynchidae			
Lacistorhynchus tenuis	Spiny dogfish, gray smoothhound, smooth dogfish, common thresher shark, shovelnose guitarfish, leopard shark, school shark, brown smoothhound	Spiral valve	Atlantic, California, New Zealand California, New Zealand
Lacistorhynchus dollfusi	Gummy shark, saw shark, school shark, brown smoothhound, leopard shark	Spiral valve	Australia, California
Diesingium lomentaceum	Unidentified dogfish, smooth dogfish	Spiral valve	Panormi, Woods Hole, Massachusetts

Table continued on following page

TABLE 100–1. Parasites Found in Elasmobranchs *Continued*

Parasite	Host	Site of Infection	Location
Grillotia erinaceus	Skates, bluntnose sixgill shark, dusky shark, spiny dogfish	Spiral valve	Atlantic, Canada
Grillotia erinaceus	Skates, bluntnose sixgill shark, dusky shark, spiny dogfish	Spiral valve	Atlantic, Canada
Grillotia acanthoscolex	Bluntnose sixgill shark	Spiral valve	Porcupine Bank, Atlantic
Grillotia dolichocephala	Portuguese shark, false cat shark	Spiral valve	Azores, Iles du Cap Vent
Grillotia dollfusi	Chilean skate	Spiral valve	Chile
Grillotia institata	Sevengill shark, bluntnose sixgill shark, European catshark	Spiral valve	Naples, Italy, France
Grillotia megabothridia	Bluntnose sixgill shark	Spiral valve	Puget Sound
Grillotia minor	Unidentified dogfish	Spiral valve	Golfe de Gascogne
Grillotia pastinacae	Bluntnose stingray	Spiral valve	Finistere
Grillotia scolecina	Sevengill shark, bluntnose sixgill shark	Spiral valve	Naples, Chile
Grillotia heptanchii	Ocellated torpedo ray, European cat shark, broadsnouted sevengill shark	Spiral valve	Puget Sound, New Zealand
Grillotia smarisgora	European angel shark, Pacific angel shark	Spiral valve	Atlantic
Grillotia musculara	Bluntnose sixgill shark	Spiral valve	Puget Sound
Family Otobothriidae			
Otobothrium crenacolle	Smooth hammerhead shark, dusky shark, bull shark, sharpnose shark, spiny dogfish	Stomach	Chile, Woods Hole, Massachusetts, Beaufort, North Carolina, Gulf of Mexico
Otobothrium curtum	Tiger shark	Spiral valve	Dry Tortugas
Otobothrium penetrans	Smooth hammerhead shark, requiem sharks	Spiral valve	Florida
Otobothrium pronosomum	Bluntnose stingray	Spiral valve	Trieste
Otobothrium minutum	Requiem sharks	Spiral valve	Madras, India
Otobothrium dipsacum	Dusky shark	Spiral valve	Atlantic, Pacific
Otobothrium linstowi	Thailand sawfish, white spotted ray, unidentified sevengill shark	Spiral valve	Sri Lanka, Tsing Tao
Otobothrium propecysticum	Smooth hammerhead shark	Spiral valve	Mediterranean
Otobothrium pephrikos	Smooth hammerhead shark	Spiral valve	Mediterranean
Diplootobothrium springeri	Smalleye hammerhead shark	Spiral valve	Japan
Poecilancistrum caryophyllum	Bull shark, sharpnose shark	Spiral valve	Brazil
Poecilancistrum gangeticum	Ganges shark	Spiral valve	India
Poecilancistrum ilisha	Ganges shark	Spiral valve	India
Family Pterobothriidae			
Pterobothrium dasybati	Akaei stingray	Spiral valve	Japan
Pterobothrium filicolle	Roughtail stingray, tiger shark, smooth dogfish, smoothhound, brown shark, dusky shark, sharpnose shark, bluntnose stingray	Spiral valve	Woods Hole, Massachusetts, Beaufort, North Carolina
Pterobothrium fragile	Largetooth sawfish, deepwater shark	Spiral valve	Brazil
Pterobothrium lintoni	Bluntnose stingray	Spiral valve	Atlantic
Pterobothrium malleum	Roughtail stingray	Spiral valve	Woods Hole, Massachusetts
Pterobothrium platycephalum	Celanes stingray	Spiral valve	Sri Lanka
Pterobothrium heteracanthum	Tiger shark	Stomach	Woods Hole, Massachusetts
Halysiorhynchus macrocephalus	Celanes stingray, guitar ray	Spiral valve	Sri Lanka
Family Proteocephalidae			
Prosobothrium armigesum	Spotted spiny dogfish, unidentified hammerhead shark, requiem sharks, blue shark	Spiral valve	Atlantic, Mediterranean, Japan
Prosobothrium adhaerens	Smooth hammerhead, blue shark	Spiral valve	Woods Hole, Massachusetts
Family Mixodigmatiae			
Mixodigma leptaleum	Megamouth	Spiral valve	Hawaii
Family Rhinoptericolidae			
Rhinoptericola megacantha	Cownose ray	Spiral valve	Chesapeake Bay
Family Hornelliellidae			
Hornelliella macropora	Zebra shark, brownbanded bamboo shark	Spiral valve	Queensland, Australia
Hornelliella cobraformis	Spotted eagle ray	Spiral valve	Australia

TABLE 100–1. Parasites Found in Elasmobranchs *Continued*

Parasite	Host	Site of Infection	Location
Order Litobothridea			
Family Litobothridae			
Litobothrium gracile	Smalltooth sand tiger shark	Spiral valve	California
Litobothrium alopias	Bigeye thresher shark	Spiral valve	California
Litobothrium coniformis	Bigeye thresher shark	Spiral valve	California
NEMATODES			
Order Trichuridea			
Family Trichuridae			
Capillaria carcharini	Dusky shark	Not given	Woods Hole, Massachusetts
Capillaria hathawayi	Spiny dogfish	Not given	Gulf of Mexico
Capillaria spinosa	Brown shark	Not given	Woods Hole, Massachusetts
Order Ichthyostrongylidea			
Family Ichthyostrongylidae			
Ichthyostrongylus clelandi	Unidentified dogfish	Spiral valve	S. Australia
Order Oxyuridea			
Family Kathlaniidae			
Kathlania chiloscyllii	Slender bamboo shark	Not given	Sri Lanka
Order Ascarididea			
Family Heterocheiliidae			
Acanthocheilus quadridentatus	Dogfishes, gummy shark	Encysted in stomach wall	S. Africa, Australia, Japan, California
Acanthocheilus bicuspis	Cat sharks, dogfishes, saw shark	Coelomic cavity, encysted in stomach wall, digestive tract	California, North Sea, New Zealand, Mediterranean
Acanthocheilus intermedius	Smoothhound	Stomach	Not given
Acanthocheilus nudifex	Tiger shark, smooth hammerhead shark	Stomach	Woods Hole, Massachusetts
Brevimulticaecum sp.	Unidentified stingray	Stomach	Brazil
Contracaecum plagiostomorum	Basking shark, thorny skate	Gills	Sri Lanka
Contracaecum aduncum	Carpet shark, knifenose chimera	Intestine	New Zealand, N.W. Atlantic
Contracaecum clavatum	Spiny dogfish	Intestine	Newfoundland
Metanisakis rajae	Unidentified skate	Intestine	Japan
Paranisakis squatinae	European angel shark	Intestine	Egypt
Paranisakis pastinacae	Bluntnose stingray, marbled stingray, Queensland stingray	Intestine	Sri Lanka
Paranisakis taeniure	Queensland stingray	Intestine	Sri Lanka
Porrocaecum laymani	Akaei stingray	Intestine	Not given
Pseudanisakis australis	Gummy shark	Intestine	Europe
Pseudanisakis rotundata	Thorny skate	Spiral valve	North Sea
Raphidascaroides blochii	Unidentified hammerhead shark	Spiral valve	Pakistan
Terranova antarctica	Gummy shark	Stomach	Antarctic, New Zealand
Terranova brevicapitata	Tiger shark, dusky shark	Olfactory organ	Woods Hole, Massachusetts
Terranova cephaloscyllii	Unidentified cat shark	Intestine	Japan
Terranova chiloscyllii	Brownbanded bamboo shark, gummy shark	Intestine	Queensland
Terranova circularis	Unidentified sawfish	Intestine	Cameroon
Terranova galeocerdonis	Tiger shark, wobbegong, nurse shark, hammerhead sharks	Intestine	Sri Lanka, Australia
Terranova ginglymostomae	Common nurse shark	Intestine	Florida
Terranova petrovi	Skate	Intestine	Russia
Terranova pristis	Largetooth sawfish	Intestine	Australia
Terranova rochalimai	Dogfish, smalltooth sawfish	Intestine	Brazil, W. Africa
Terranova scoliodontis	Blue dog shark	Intestine	Australia
Terranova brooksi	Scalloped hammerhead	Intestine	Kaneohe Bay, Hawaii
Order Spiruridea			
Family Cucullanidae			
Cucullanus squali	Dogfishes	Intestine	Not given
Family Gnathostomatidae			
Echinocephalus uncinatus	Stingrays	Spiral valve	Trieste
Echinocephalus aebobati	Eagle ray	Spiral valve	Trieste
Echinocephalus spinossimus	Stingrays, bullhead shark	Spiral valve	Gulf of Manaar, Adriatic, Sri Lanka, Australia, W. Africa
Echinocephalus pseudouncinatus	Bat ray	Spiral valve	California
Echinocephalus daileyi	Freshwater stingray	Intestine	Rio Orinoco, S. America
Echinocephalus diazi	Whip ray	Intestine	Lake Marcaibo, Venezuela

Table continued on following page

TABLE 100–1. Parasites Found in Elasmobranchs *Continued*

Parasite	Host	Site of Infection	Location
Echinocephalus sinensis	Unidentified ray	Spiral valve	Deep Bay, Hong Kong
Echinocephalus mobulae	Ox ray	Spiral valve	India
Echinocephalus overstreeti	Port Jackson shark, wobbegong, rays, skates, elephant fish	Spiral valve	Australia
Paraleptus scyllii	Slender bamboo shark	Spiral valve	S. China
Paraleptus australis	Bullhead shark, gummy shark	Spiral valve	Australia
Proleptus acutus	Smoothhounds, spiny dogfish, thornback skate, cat shark, thornback guitarfish	Stomach, intestine	California, Mediterranean, Iceland
Proleptus australis	Tiger shark	Intestine	Queensland
Proleptus coronatus	Thorny skate, European catshark	Intestine	Not given
Proleptus elegans	Bluntnose sixgill shark	Intestine	Not given
Proleptus obtusus	European cat shark, spiny dogfish, brown smoothhound, thorny skate, leopard shark, spotted eagle ray	Intestine, stomach lining	Atlantic, California
Proleptus problematicus	Spiny dogfish	Spiral valve	Roscoff, France
Proleptus rajae	Gray skate	Not given	Ireland
Proleptus sordidus	Shovelnose guitarfish	Spiral valve	Uruguay
Proleptus trygonorrhinae	Fiddler ray	Spiral valve	S. Australia
Proleptus urolophi	Common stingray	Spiral valve	New South Wales
Family Spiruridae			
Ascarophis helix	Roughtail stingray	Spiral valve	Woods Hole, Massachusetts
Parascarophis sphyrnae	Scalloped hammerhead	Spiral valve	Senegal
Parascarophis galeata	Bonnethead shark	Esophagus	Beaufort, N.C.
Family Rhabdochonidae			
Cystidicola galeatus	Bonnethead shark	Spiral valve	N. Carolina
Pancreatonema torriensis	Cuckoo skate	Pancreatic duct	Scotland, North Sea
Order Philometridea			
Family Philometridae			
Phylctainophora squali	Spiny dogfish	Subcutaneous	California
Phylctainophora lamnae	Porbeagle, smooth dogfish	Hyomandibular arch and skull, tumor base of ventral and pectoral fins	Mediterranean
ACANTHOCEPHALANS Order Acanthocephala			
Family Echinorhynchidae			
Echinorhynchus gadi	Spiny dogfish	Spiral valve	Not given
LEECHES Order Hirudinea Suborder Rhynchobdella			
Family Piscicolidae			
Branchellion borealis	Thornback skate	Back	English Channel
Branchellion ravenelii	Leopard shark, bullnose ray, southern stingray	Gills, skin, ventral surface	California, Florida, S. Carolina
Branchellion torpedinis	Shovelnose guitarfish, thornback skate, torpedo ray, marbled electric ray, bluntnose stingray	Body	Mediterranean, North Sea, Iceland, Senegal
Branchellion lobata	Soupfin shark, Pacific angel shark, big skate, broadnose sevengill shark, leopard shark, spiny dogfish, leopard shark, brown smoothhound	Clasper, buccal cavity, fins, ventral surface of embryo, cloaca, body, fins	California
Branchellion parkeri	Rough skate, elephantfish, saw shark, stingrays, gummy shark	Body	Australia
Branchellion australis	Skates	Body	Australia
Calliobdella carolinensis	Elasmobranchs	Body	Atlantic
Calliobdella nodulifera	Gray skate, spiny dogfish	Body	Newfoundland
Notostomobdella laeve	Greenland shark	Body	Greenland
Oxytonostoma typica	Thorny skate	Body	Iceland, Greenland, Alaska
Pontobdella muricata	Gray skate, thornback skate, electric rays	Body	Mediterranean
Pontobdella benhami	Skates	Body	Australia
Pterobdella Kaburaki	Unidentified stingray	Body	Chilka Lake
Pterobdellina jenseni	Gray skate	Body	Faeroe Islands

TABLE 100–1. Parasites Found in Elasmobranchs *Continued*

Parasite	Host	Site of Infection	Location
COPEPODS			
Order Copepoda			
Suborder Siphonostomatoida			
Family Caligidae			
Caligus curtus	Ratfishes, skates, dogfishes	Body	Atlantic, Mediterranean, Scandanavia
Caligus coryphaenae	Spiny dogfish, shortfin mako shark	Body, fins	Indian Ocean, S. Africa, Japan
Caligus dasyaticus	Coach whip ray, akaei stingray	Body	Bombay, Japan
Caligus furcisetifer	Hammerhead shark	Body	Bombay
Caligus latigentitalis	Dogfishes, guitarfish	Body	Japan
Caligus mutabilis	Lesser electric ray	Body	Florida
Caligus elongatus	Barndoor skate, spiny dogfish	Body surface	Canada, Woods Hole, Massachusetts, Greenland
Caligus petersii	Mackerel shark	Branchial arch	Mediterranean
Caligus quadratus	Unidentified guitarfish	Body	Pacific Coast
Caligus rabidus	Tiger shark	Cloaca	Brighton, England
Caligus rapax	Dogfishes, ratfishes	Skin	Texas
Caligus torpedinis	Electric rays	Skin	Indian Ocean
Caligus clemensi	Ratfishes	Skin	Canada
Caligus praetextus	Bonnethead shark	Skin	Gulf of Mexico
Caligus gurnardi	Spiny dogfish	Skin	Scandanavia
Lepeophtheirus edwardsi	Little skate	Not given	Woods Hole, Massachusetts
Lepeophtheirus eurus	Blacktip shark	Not given	Barents Sea
Lepeophtheirus hippoglossi	Skates	Not given	Barents Sea
Lepeophtheirus longispinosus	Smooth hammerhead shark	Gills	North America
Lepeophtheirus parviventris	Big skate, longnosed skate	Gills	British Columbia
Lepeophtheirus robustus	Round stingray, skates	Gills	California, Greenland
Lepeophtheirus thompsoni	Roughtail stingray, bluntnose stingray	Gill cavity	Mediterranean
Lepeophtheirus pravipes	Big skate	Not given	British Columbia
Lepeophtheirus cuneifer	Big skate, spiny dogfish	Gills	Alaska
Calistes trigonis	Stingrays	Not given	Rio de Janeiro
Pupulina suhmi	Manta ray, Atlantic lesser devil ray	Not given	Galapagos Island, Gulf of Mexico
Pupulina minor	Atlantic lesser devil ray	Not given	Gulf of Mexico
Family Cecropidae			
Cecrops achantii-vulgaris	Piked dogfish	Not given	France
Cecrops exiguus	Requiem sharks	Not given	Florida
Enterpherus laminipes	Atlantic lesser devil ray	Gill rakers	Gulf of Mexico
Luetkenia astrodermi	Smooth dogfish	Not given	Mediterranean
Philorthagoriscus serratus	Spiny dogfish	Not given	Newfoundland
Family Dissonidae			
Dissonus furcatus	Wobbegongs	Not given	Sri Lanka
Dissonus intermedins	Leopard shark	Not given	China
Family Euryphoridae			
Albeion carchariae	Requiem sharks, scalloped hammerhead, shark, smalleye hammerhead shark	Body surface	Atlantic, Indian Ocean Australia
Alebion alatus	Requiem sharks	Body surface	S. India
Alebion crassus	Smooth hammerhead shark	Body surface	Woods Hole, Massachusetts, Japan
Alebion echinatus	Scalloped hammerhead shark, smooth hammerhead shark	Body surface	Hawaii, Senegal, Japan
Alebion elegans	Smalleye hammerhead shark, large blacktip shark, lemon shark	Body surface	Dakar, Senegal
Alebion fuscus	Dusky shark	Body surface	Woods Hole, Massachusetts
Alebion glaber	Dogfishes, sand tiger shark	Body surface	Woods Hole, Massachusetts, Long Island, New York
Alebion gracilis	Requiem sharks, dogfishes, sand tiger shark	Body surface	Woods Hole, Massachusetts, W. Florida, Indian Ocean, E. Pacific
Alebion maculatus	Requiem sharks	Not given	Not given
Alebion megacephalus	Requiem sharks	Body surface	Sri Lanka
Dysgamus atlanticus	Whale shark	Not given	Cuba
Dysgamus limbatus	Blacktip shark	Not given	Texas
Elytrophora hemiptera	Blue shark	Gill operculum	Japan
Paralebion elongatus	Requiem sharks	Mouth, fins	Chesapeake Bay, Dry Tortugas, Florida, Beaufort, N.C.

Table continued on following page

TABLE 100–1. Parasites Found in Elasmobranchs *Continued*

Parasite	Host	Site of Infection	Location
Family Pandaridae			
Pandarus bicolor	Dogfishes, blue shark	Body, fins	Atlantic, Mediterranean
Pandarus fissiform	Dogfishes, school shark, seven-gill sharks, soupfin shark, brown smoothhound, guitar-fishes, leopard shark, shortfin mako shark	Body, fins	Pacific, New Zealand, California
Pandarus affinis	Dogfishes, dusky shark	Body surface	Dakar, Senegal, North Africa
Pandarus longus	Requiem shark	Body surface	India
Pandarus cranchii	Blue shark, white shark	Body surface	Atlantic coast of France, Florida
Pandarus pallidus	Ocean whitetip shark	Body surface	Indian Ocean
Pandarus vulgaris	Dusky shark	Skin	Woods Hole, Massachusetts
Pandarus dentatus	Bull shark	Skin	Florida
Pandarus concinnus	Porbeagle, requiem sharks, soupfin sharks, thresher sharks, hammerhead sharks, leopard shark	Dorsal fin, Body surface, Dorsal fin, Body surface	W. Africa, Japan, California, Indian Ocean, Hawaii, Taiwan
Pandarus marcusi	Blacktip shark	Not given	Brazil
Pandarus niger	Requiem shark, soupfin shark	Not given	Sri Lanka, India
Pandarus satyrus	Blue shark, smooth hammerhead shark, thresher sharks, school shark, dusky shark, shortfin mako shark	Body surface, Buccal cavity, Skin	Atlantic, W. Pacific, Indian Ocean, Japan, New Zealand, Gulf of Mexico
Pandarus sinuatus	Spiny dogfish, requiem sharks, sand tiger, dusky shark, bull shark, porbeagle, sharpnose shark, bonnethead shark, thresher sharks	Fins, Body surface, Skin	Woods Hole, Massachusetts, Canada, Gulf of Mexico, Florida, Atlantic, Brazil, Indian Ocean
Pandarus smithii	Requiem sharks, sand tiger, white shark, porbeagle, shortfin mako shark, smooth hammerhead shark, blue shark	Body surface, Mouth	Atlantic, Florida, Brazil, Indian Ocean, Japan
Pandarus floridanus	White shark	Body surface	W. Florida
Pandarus katoi	Shortfin mako shark	Mouth, gills	S. America
Achtheinus oblongus	Leopard shark	Not given	California
Achtheinus chinensis	Dogfish	Not given	China
Achtheinus dentatus	Leopard shark, soupfin shark, thresher shark, smooth-hounds, sevengill shark, big skate, smooth hammerhead shark, dogfishes	Not given	California, Peru, Argentina, Angola
Achtheinus galeorhini	Leopard shark	Not given	Japan, China
Achtheinus intermedius	Leopard shark	Not given	China
Achtheinus japonicus	Spiny dogfish	Not given	Japan
Achtheinus parvidens	Piked dogfish	Not given	S. Africa
Demoleus hepatus	Bluntnose sixgill shark, spiny dogfish	Skin, Body surface	Nice, California, Britain
Demoleus latus	Dogfishes	Not given	New Zealand, Japan
Dinemoura affinis	Salmon shark	Not given	Japan
Dinemoura ferox	Greenland shark	Not given	New Zealand
Dinemoura producta	Basking shark, white shark, blue shark, thresher shark, shortfin mako shark	Body, Fins	Africa, New Zealand, Maine, California
Dinemoura latifolia	White shark, mako sharks, thresher sharks, porbeagle, mackerel shark, blue shark, school shark,	Gills, body, buccal cavity	Adriatic, Atlantic, Pacific
Dinemoura discrepans	Bigeye thresher shark	Body	Madagascar
Echthrogaleus coleoptratus	Porbeagle, requiem sharks, mako sharks, blue shark, European cat shark, salmon shark, leopard shark	Buccal cavity, Body surface	Woods Hole, Massachusetts, Canada, New Zealand, Pacific, Indian Ocean, Australia, Japan, Newfoundland, California
Echthrogaleus denticulatus	White shark, shortfin mako shark, blue shark, smooth hammerhead shark, thresher sharks	Body surface, Buccal cavity	Woods Hole, Massachusetts, California, Japan, Indian Ocean
Echthrogaleus disciarai	Manta ray	Body surface	Sea of Cortez
Echthrogaleus luetkeni	Skates	Not given	Shetlands
Echthrogaleus neozealanicus	Requiem sharks	Not given	New Zealand
Echthrogaleus torpedinis	Electric rays	Not given	Woods Hole, Massachusetts

TABLE 100–1. Parasites Found in Elasmobranchs *Continued*

Parasite	Host	Site of Infection	Location
Gangliopus pyriformis	Shortfin mako shark, common thresher shark, blue shark	Gills	Concarneau, S. America, Indian Ocean, N. Pacific
Gangliopus japonicus	Smooth hammerhead shark	Body	Japan
Laminifera cornuta	Blue shark, shortfin mako shark	Gill chamber	Friendly Island, New Zealand, S. America, Indian Ocean, Hawaii
Lepimacrus jourdaini	Porbeagle	Not given	France
Nesippus orientalis	White shark, blue shark, tiger shark, dusky shark, smooth hammerhead shark, bull shark, spiny dogfish, gummy shark, broadnose sevengill shark	Mouth, gills, body surface	Indian Ocean, Java, Florida, S. Africa, Angola, New Zealand
Nesippus alatus	Dusky shark, white shark, sharpnose shark, bonnethead shark, common thresher shark, smooth hammerhead shark	Mouth cavity, skin, throat	Woods Hole, Massachusetts, S. Africa, N. Carolina, Texas
Nesippus borealis	Shortfin mako shark	Mouth cavity	North Sea
Nesippus crypturus	Bull shark, ocean whitetip shark, white shark, tiger shark, smooth hammerhead shark	Mouth	Madagascar, W. Florida, Puerto Rico
Nesippus tigris	Tiger shark	Mouth	W. Florida
Nesippus gracilis	Dusky shark, blacktip shark	Mouth, skin	Puerto Rico, Florida
Parapandarus nodulosus	Smooth hammerhead shark, blue shark	Gills	Woods Hole, Massachusetts
Parapandarus doello-juradoi	Porbeagle	Not given	Argentina
Pagina tunica	Bigeye thresher shark	Not given	Madagascar
Perissopus dentatus	Dusky shark, bull shark, bonnethead shark, smooth hammerhead shark	Body surface	Atlantic, Indian Ocean, Florida, New Zealand
Perissopus communis	Requiem sharks, sharpnose sharks, bonnethead shark, smooth dogfish, dusky shark	Body surface	Mediterranean, N. America, Gulf of Mexico, Texas, Woods Hole, Massachusetts, Dry Tortugas, Brazil, Rio de Oro, N.W. Africa
Perissopus crenatus	Requiem sharks	Not given	Java
Perissopus oblongatus	Common thresher shark, smoothhounds, sevengill sharks, spiny dogfish, big skate, smooth hammerhead shark, leopard shark	Body surface	California, Angola
Pseudopandarus scyllii	Leopard shark	Pectoral fin	Japan
Prosaetes rhincodontis	Whale shark	Gills	Indian Ocean
Family Trebiidae			
Trebius spinifrons	Skates, dogfishes, butterfly ray, bat ray	Skin	N. Atlantic, Iceland, Mediterranean, Florida, Monterey Bay, Angola
Trebius akajeii	Akaei stingray	Not given	Japan
Trebius exilis	Cownose ray	Not given	Sri Lanka
Trebius longicaudatus	Clouded angel shark	Not given	Japan
Trebius latifurcatus	Round stingray, bat ray	Body surface	California
Trebius tenuifurcatus	Stingrays	Skin	Atlantic, Woods Hole, Massachusetts, California
Family Anthosomatidae			
Anthosoma crassum	Porbeagle, white shark, mackerel sharks, blue shark, dogfishes, school shark, shortfin mako shark, dusky shark, basking shark	Buccal cavity, gills	Atlantic, New Zealand, Africa, N. America, S. America, Mediterranean, Japan
Family Eudactylinidae			
Eudactylina acuta	European angel shark, spiny dogfish	Gills	Europe, Great Britain
Eudactylina acanthii	Spiny dogfish	Gills	Irish Sea, Canada
Eudactylina aspera	Sharpnose shark	Not given	Java, Mexico
Eudactylina breviabdomina	Blacktip shark	Not given	Texas
Eudactylina carchariae-glauci	Blue shark	Gills	France
Eudactylina complexa	European angel shark, thorny skate	Not given	Mauritania, Canada
Eudactylina corrugata	Little skate	Not given	Canada
Eudactylina longispina	Bonnethead shark	Gills	Gulf of Mexico

Table continued on following page

TABLE 100–1. Parasites Found in Elasmobranchs *Continued*

Parasite	Host	Site of Infection	Location
Eudactylina minuta	Bluntnose stingray	Not given	Scottish Sea
Eudactylina rachelae	Torpedo ray	Gills	Plymouth, England
Eudactylina similis	Thorny skate	Gills	Shetlands
Eudactylina spinifera	Brown shark, dusky shark	Gills	Woods Hole, Massachusetts, Gulf of Mexico
Eudactylina spinula	Atlantic angel shark	Gills	N. Carolina
Eudactylina squamosa	Cownose ray	Gills	Gulf of Mexico
Eudactylina valei	Spiny dogfish, smooth dogfish	Gills	Angola
Eudactylina versicolor	Smooth hammerhead shark	Not given	Jamaica
Eudactylina pusilla	Tiger shark	Gills	W. Florida, Indian Ocean
Eudactylina tuberifera	Pacific angel shark	Gills	Chile
Eudactylina chilensis	Black shark	Gills	Chile
Eudactylina rhinobati	Shovelnose ray	Gills	Tunis
Eudactylinella alba	Stingrays	Gills	Woods Hole, Massachusetts
Beriaka alopiae	Bigeye thresher shark	Gill filament	Indian Ocean
Eudactylinodes uncinata	Soupfin shark, sand tiger shark	Gills	La Jolla, California, Woods Hole, Massachusetts
Eudactylinodes keratiphagus	Horn shark, Mexican horn shark	Gills	California
Eudactylinodes nigra	Sand tiger shark, bonnethead shark	Gills	Buzzard Bay, Beaufort, North Carolina, Woods Hole, Massachusetts
Protodactylina sp.	Broadnose sixgill shark	Branchial rays	France
Family Kroyeriidae			
Kroyeria lineata	Mackerel sharks, dog sharks, dogfishes, smooth hammerhead shark, requiem sharks	Gills	Atlantic, Europe, N. America
Kroyeria acanthias-vulgaris	Spiny dogfish	Not given	Not given
Kroyeria deborahae	Shovelnose guitarfish	Gills	Mexico
Kroyeria aculeata	Blue shark	Gills	Mediterranean
Kroyeria benzorum	Common thresher shark, shortfin mako shark	Not given	Mexico
Kroyeria carchariae-glauca	Blue shark	Gills	Mediterranean
Kroyeria cortezensis	Silky shark	Gills	Mexico
Kroyeria dispar	Tiger shark	Not given	W. Florida
Kroyeria echinata	Smooth hammerhead shark	Body surface	Bombay
Kroyeria gracilis	Brown shark, blue shark, blacktip shark, smooth hammerhead shark, bull shark, ocean whitetipped shark, sharpnose shark, dusky shark	Nostrils, gills	Woods Hole, Massachusetts, Gulf of Mexico, Indian Ocean, Florida
Kroyeria papillipes	Smooth hammerhead shark, tiger shark, gray shark	Gills	Woods Hole, Massachusetts, Panama
Kroyeria spatulata	Sharpnose shark, sand tiger shark, blacktip shark	Not given	Beaufort, North Carolina, Bahamas, Texas
Kroyeria mobulae	Manta ray	Gills	Mexico
Kroyeria sphyrnae	Smooth hammerhead shark	Gills	Bombay
Kroyeria trecai	Scalloped hammerhead shark	Not given	Senegal
Kroyeria praelongacicula	Scalloped hammerhead shark	Gill cavity	Hawaii
Kroyeria caseyi	Night shark	Gills	Western North Atlantic
Kroyerina elongata	Blue shark, tiger shark	Gills	Woods Hole, Massachusetts
Nemesis lamna	Porbeagle, blue shark	Gills	Nice, Great Britain
Nemesis mediterranea	Requiem sharks, smalltooth sand tiger shark, thresher sharks, basking shark, mackerel sharks	Gills	Mediterranean, Woods Hole, Massachusetts, New Zealand, Florida, Africa, Japan, California
Nemesis atlantica	Sharpnose shark, common thresher shark, requiem sharks	Gills	Beaufort, N.C., Woods Hole, Massachusetts, Florida, Dry Tortugas
Nemesis carchariae-glauci	Blue shark, leopard shark	Gills	France, California
Nemesis macrocephalus	Blacktip reef shark	Not given	Japan
Nemesis pilosa	Sand tiger shark	Not given	Bahamas
Nemesis pallida	Thresher sharks, requiem sharks, sharpnose shark, bonnethead shark, smooth hammerhead shark	Gills	Woods Hole, Massachusetts, Gulf of Mexico, Florida, S. Africa
Nemesis robusta	Bluntnose stingray, dogfishes, blue shark, stingrays, long nosed skate, bluntnose sixgill shark, common thresher shark, smooth hammerhead shark, hammerhead, bull shark	Gills	Belgium, Mediterranean, Adriatic, Naples, Italy, New Zealand, Angola, Mauritania, Madagascar, Canada

TABLE 100–1. Parasites Found in Elasmobranchs *Continued*

Parasite	Host	Site of Infection	Location
Nemesis vermi	Sand tiger shark, basking shark	Gills	British water, New Zealand
Nemesis versicolor	Smooth hammerhead shark	Gills	Jamaica
Nemesis aggregatus	Common thresher shark	Gills	Indian Ocean
Nemesis spinulosus	Dusky shark	Gills	W. Florida
Nemesis sphyrnae	Smooth hammerhead shark	Gills	India
Family Lernaeidae			
Lernaenicus procerus	Sand tiger shark	Not given	New Jersey
Family Lerneopodidae			
Lerneopoda bidiscalis	Smoothhound, smooth dogfish, gray smoothhound	Claspers	Ireland, California
Lerneopoda etmopteri	Blackbelly lantern shark	Not given	Japan
Lerneopoda galei	Dogfishes, smoothhounds, whip ray, sharpnose shark	Gill, cloaca	Mediterranean, Adriatic, New Zealand, Barents Sea, Mauritania,
Lerneopoda longicaudata	Dogfishes	Not given	South Island, Japan
Lerneopoda musteli	Gummy shark	Cloaca	New Zealand
Lerneopoda mustelicola	Dogfishes	Cloaca	Plymouth, England, Argentina
Lerneopoda tenuis	Leopard shark	Not given	Chile
Lerneopoda scylicola	European cat shark, big skate, leopard shark	Pelvic fins, cloaca, head	Plymouth, England, California
Lerneopoda selachiorum	Smoothhound, whip ray	Male genital pore	Trieste
Lernaeopodina longimana	Skates	Not given	Canada
Lernaeopodina longibrachia	Deep-water chimera	Not given	Canada
Lernaeopodina relata	Barndoor skate	Not given	Maine
Lernaeopodina pacifica	Long-nosed skate	Gills	Canada
Ommatokoita elongata	Greenland shark	Cornea	Greenland, Canada, Iceland
Ommatokoita superba	Porbeagle, smooth dogfish, rough sagre shark	Cornea, skin	Belgium, St. Pierre Bank, Scotian Bank, N.W. Atlantic
Dendrata cameroni longi-clavata	California skate	Skin	British Columbia, Canada
Pseudolernaeopoda caudocapta	Leopard shark	Skin	Chile
Vanbendenia kroyeri	Ratfish	Not given	Kattegat, North Sea
Brianella corniger	Rays	Not given	Chile
Thomsonella parkeri	Skates, stingrays	Not given	New Zealand
Clavella uncinata	Greenland shark	Not given	Arctic Sea
Acepadia pomposa	Whale shark	Not given	E. China Sea
Brachiella concava	Stingrays	Not given	Jamaica, Woods Hole, Massachusetts, Texas
Pseudocharopinoides myliobatidos	Eagle rays	Gills	Chile
Pseudocharopinus bicaudatus	Gray smoothhound, spiny dogfish, big skate	Spiracles, body surface	California, Woods Hole, Massachusetts, Oregon, Canada
Pseudocharopinus dentatus	Long-nosed skate	Buccal cavity, gills, skin, clasper	British Columbia, Canada
Pseudocharopinus narcinae	Electric ray	Gills	India
Pseudocharopinus pteromylaei	Tunisian butterfly ray	Gills	Tunisa
Charopinus dalmanni	Gray skates, stingrays	Not given	Atlantic, Mediterranean, Barents Sea
Charopinus bicaudatus	Spiny dogfish, stingrays, angel shark, whip ray, bluntnose skate, dogfishes	Not given	Mediterranean, Castiglione, North Sea, Gulf of Mexico
Charopinus parkeri	Skates, stingrays	Gills	New Zealand
Charopinus chimaerae	Ratfish	Not given	Japan
Charopinus dentatus	Big skate	Not given	British Columbia, Canada
Charopinus dubius	Skates	Gills	Irish Sea, North Sea, Barents Sea
Charopinus malleus	Torpedo ray	Mouth cavity	Rimini
Charopinus markewitschi	Skates, stingrays	Not given	Khanton Bay, Japan
Charopinus pastinacae	Bluntnose stingray, spiny dogfish, whip ray	Nasal fossa	Atlantic
Charopinus ramosus	Skates	Not given	Europe, Irish Sea, Quebec
Clavellopsis dasyaticus	Coach whip ray	Not given	Bombay
Schistobrachia tertia	Big skate, long-nosed skate	Gills, buccal cavity	British Columbia, Canada
Family Sphyriidae			
Opimia exilis	Soupfin shark, dusky shark	Mouth, gills	La Jolla, California, Gulf of Mexico
Paeon ferox	Sharpnose shark, bonnethead shark	Gill cavity	Beaufort, N.C. Atlantic, Texas

Table continued on following page

TABLE 100–1. Parasites Found in Elasmobranchs *Continued*

Parasite	Host	Site of Infection	Location
Paeon elongatus	Brown shark, dusky shark, leopard shark	Gills	Woods Hole, Massachusetts, California
Paeon vaissieri	Hammerhead sharks	Gills	Senegal, Hawaii
Paeon versicolor	Spiny dogfish	Mouth	Beaufort, N.C.
Tripaphylus musteli	Smooth dogfish	Gills	Belgium, Irish Sea, Adriatic Sea
Suborder Poecilostomatoida			
Family Bomobochidae			
Taeniacanthus albidus	Bonnethead shark	Not given	Beaufort, N.C.
Taeniacanthus flagellans	Smooth hammerhead	Gill cavity	Jamaica
Anchistrotos onosi	Dogfishes	Not given	Scottish Sea
Irodes gracilis	Smooth hammerhead	Not given	Java
Family Ergasilidae			
Ergasilus myctarothes	Smooth hammerhead	Nasal tube	Jamaica
Order Philichthyidea			
Family Chondracanthidae			
Acanthochondrites spp.	Gray skates, smooth dogfish	Cloaca, gills, nasal fossa	North Sea, Canada, Japan
Acanthochondria spp.	Ratfish	Claspers, branchial cavity	Canada, California
Pharodes tortugensis	Sharpnose shark	Claspers, branchial cavity	Gulf of Mexico
ISOPODS			
Order Isopoda			
Family Cirolanidae			
Cirolana borealis	Spiny dogfish, brown shark, tiger shark, hammerhead sharks	Uterus, heart, gills	Norway, Florida
Family Gnathiidae			
Gnathia piscivora	Stingrays, shortfin mako sharks	Skin, gills, pharyngeal cavity	Red Sea
Family Cymothoidae			
Nerocila californica	Leopard shark, eagle rays	Fins	California
Livoneca ovalis	Common sawfish	Gills	California
Family Aegiidae			
Rocinela belliceps	Spotted ratfish	Not given	California
CIRRIPEDS			
Order Thoracica			
Family Lepadidae			
Anelasma squalicola	Velvetbelly shark	Dorsal muscle	North Sea
Conchoderma auritum	Basking shark	Gills	North Sea

detachment and leakage of blood and fluid occurred. The endometrium was also heavily infected.

Eimeria southwelli is described from the spiral valves of an embryonic spotted eagle ray from Ceylon (Halawani, 1930). The intrauterine ray feeding on the mucus and oocyst-infected uterine tissues of the mother may account for the coccidian infection of this unborn ray.

Microsporidian parasites are not found in elasmobranchs, whereas myxosporidians (15 coelozoic species) are reported in their gallbladders (see Table 100–1). One unidentified histozoic species of *Kudoa* has been observed in the electric organs of the lesser electric ray from Florida. The effects of such infection have not been evaluated.

MONOGENETIC TREMATODES

Monogenea are ectoparasites found on the gills and skin of sharks, skates, and rays with the exception of the members from the order Aspidocotylea, which are found in the gallbladder. The monogenea that infest skin and gills belong to two orders, Monopisthocotylea and Polyopisthocotylea (Yamaguti, 1963a). The order Monopisthocotylea contains six families with 81 species in 35 genera, and the order Polyopisthocotylea with two families, Hexabothriidae and Chimaericolidae, consists of 50 species from nine genera. Chimaericolidae is a family with a single genus and species that infests only ratfish.

The members of Microbothriidae are exclusively parasites of sharks, mainly on the skin, causing extreme irritation to the hosts. Captive lemon sharks heavily infested with *Dermophthirius nigrellii* show early manifestations of erratic swimming, flashing, and rubbing on the bottom of the tank. Later, grayish patches and open wounds appear on the skin with the placoid scales detached at the site of monogenean attachment (Fig. 100–1). The ulcerated skin lesions become secondarily infected with bacteria, which cause the eventual death of the shark.

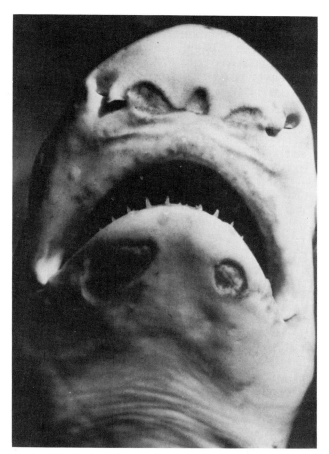

FIGURE 100–1. Lemon shark infested with *Dermophthirius nigrellii.* Many transparent trematodes barely visible on the live shark caused the lesions around the oral cavity shown here.

Dermophthirioides pristidis is another monogenean parasite causing skin ulceration in captive smalltooth sawfish (Cheung and Nigrelli, 1983). The disease is similar to that described for the lemon shark. The reproduction of the monogene is quite rapid, and the larvae hatched from eggs can reinfest the host directly. A mature worm can release more than 100 triangular eggs into the water in 20 minutes, and the development of the disease in a recirculating seawater system can occur within 3 months.

Monogenea infesting the gills of sharks, skates, and rays are difficult to detect. However, mortality occurs owing to massive infestations of *Entobdella bumpusii* in the gills of southern stingrays, *Dendromonocotyle octodiscus* in yellow stingrays, *Erprocotyle triakis* in leopard sharks, and *Heterocotyle triakis* in spotted eagle rays. The infested gills are hemorrhaged with epithelial proliferation. Sand grains are usually found in gill filaments of affected animals because they suck in sand in attempts to rub off the parasites.

The direct transmission of the parasites and the rapid increase of the parasite population in a recirculating system facilitate outbreaks of monogenean infestations. Thus, all wild-caught elasmobranchs should be subjected to vigorous prophylactic treatment for ectoparasites, especially the monogenea.

DIGENETIC TREMATODES

Digenetic trematodes are not commonly observed in elasmobranchs. About 53 described species of digenea are found in sharks, skates, and rays (see Table 100–1), representing 15 families and 27 genera. Nearly all of the families reported have only one genus and one species that parasitize elasmobranchs. The outbreak of trematodiasis and the mortality of sharks due to digenean infections rarely occur in nature or in captivity. The life cycles of digeneans require at least one intermediate host, usually a mollusc, and fish may serve as a second intermediate host.

CESTODES

Adult cestodes are commonly observed in the spiral valves of elasmobranchs. There are about 400 described species of cestodes from sharks, skates, and rays worldwide. Elasmobranchs harbor a large number of cestodes in their digestive tracts. It is quite common for several species of cestodes to be found in a single host, or members of a single cestode species to infect several different hosts.

The life cycle of a cestode requires at least one intermediate host, which can be a fish or an invertebrate such as a pelecypod, gastropod, cephalopod, or crustacean. Sharks, skates, and rays are usually the final hosts for cestode parasites. Although no significant rate of mortality of elasmobranchs is due to cestode infection, various pathologic signs are observed at the sites of attachment. Cavitation and localized hemorrhage of the epithelial lining, or merely compression of the intestinal microvilli with no marked harmful effects, may be observed (Williams, 1968; Rees and Williams, 1965).

NEMATODES

The number of nematodes found in elasmobranchs is relatively small. Only 68 species from 21 genera of 9 families in 5 orders are reported. Most of the worms belong to two families, the Heterocheiliidae (29 of the species) of the order Ascarididea and the Cucullanidae (32 species) of the order Spiruridea.

Nematodes are found primarily in the digestive tract but are also found in the coelomic cavity, gills, olfactory organ, esophagus, pancreatic duct, subcutaneous tissue, hyomandibular arch, skull, and fins and encysted in the stomach wall. Visible nodules form on the exterior of the intestine where the worms localize.

Nematodes of sharks require at least one intermediate host, usually a crustacean. For example, *Proletus acutus* (Gnathostomatidae), which infects the thornback skate, requires a decapod, *Carcinus maenas* or *Pagurus* spp., as an intermediate host (Wulker, 1929). However, *Eustoma rotundata,* found in the thorny skate and other elasmobranchs, requires a decapod, *Lithodes* sp., and a fish (Pleuronectidae or Gadidae), as a second intermediate host (Uspenskaya, 1955).

ACANTHOCEPHALANS

Acanthocephalan worms have harmful effects on bony fish hosts and are responsible for mass mortalities (Schultz, 1911). Acanthocephalan infection in elasmobranchs is extremely rare, only one species has been reported in the spiral valve of a spiny dogfish (Golvan, 1964).

LEECHES

About 15 species of leeches in 7 genera are reported in elasmobranchs of temperate waters. Leeches are found on the gills, skin, clasper, buccal cavity, and cloaca and in the spiral valve. No harmful effect or mortality of an elasmobranch host due to leech infestation is documented. However, eroded scars at the site of attachments are visible in heavily infested sharks. The blood-sucking species *Pontobdella muricata* is the vector for hematozoans, *Trypanosoma rajae* and *T. giganteum*, which are found in the blood of several species of skates. *Branchellion lobata* is capable of invading the embryos and the spiral valve of Pacific angel sharks (Moser and Anderson, 1977).

COPEPODS

About 280 species of parasitic copepods belonging to two suborders, Siphonostomatoida and Poecilostomatoida, infect elasmobranchs. The copepods are found attached to the gills, skin, head, nasal tube, branchial arch, oral cavity, mouth, fins, cornea, throat, claspers, and cloaca, in the male genital pore, or between teeth. The attachments can be superficial grasping, mobile, anchoring, or burrowing and cause localized irritation and hemorrhage.

Berland (1961) examined over 1000 specimens of the Greenland shark and found that the corneas of nearly all of the sharks were infested with the lernaeopodid copepod *Ommatokoita elongata*. The blinding effect on the hosts may severely affect the survival of the species in nature. *Anthosoma crassum*, a dichelesthiid parasite normally found in the flesh of host sharks, can be observed in clusters embedded in the eye (Kabata, 1984) and causing injury to the cornea and retinal distortion.

The damage due to copepod attachment is considered to be more severe than the feeding effect of copepods. The presence of the copepod can exert pressure and irritate gills, causing crypting (Friend, 1941) and destruction of the filament (Rokicki, 1982). Copepod bites on fins can cause severe erosion of the epidermis, fibroblast proliferation, and macrophage and lymphocyte infiltration. Fibroplasia and

the formation of dense granulation tissue occurs around the penetrating head of the copepod (Boxshall, 1977). Externally visible swelling occurs under each parasite. Heavy infections are accompanied by dermal hemorrhage.

ISOPODS

Isopods parasitizing elasmobranchs are rare; only a few species are reported. They are found on the skin and gills or in the heart, buccal cavity, or branchial cavity of the host. Some of the association is facultative and temporary, with no preference for a specific attachment site. The pranizae stage of *Gnathia piscivora* attacks the skin, gills, and pharyngeal cavity of stingrays and shortfin mako sharks impounded in marine cages. The parasites feed on blood and tissue fluid, causing extreme anemia and eventual death of the hosts.

Cirolana borealis attacks the heart tissues of sharks and sawfish by chewing through the musculature from the right pectoral fin (Bird, 1981). Ventricle abrasion and areas of necrosis are due to feeding activity of the isopods on heart tissues. Free isopods can be seen in the pericardial chamber, but none have been found in the interior of the heart or circulatory system. The same species of isopods also attaches to the cloacal opening and clasper, causing only minor injury to the hosts. Histopathologic examination of affected hearts shows myocardial necrosis, basophilic degeneration of myocardial fibers, inflammation, and endothelial degeneration. The high incidence of *Criolana borealis* infestation (60%) in sharks in Florida coincided with a sharp decline in the 1978 shark catch (Bird, 1981), suggesting a potential threat posed by the isopods to shark fishery.

BARNACLES

An obligate parasitic cirriped (barnacle) on the dorsum of a deep-sea shark is the only reported parasitic barnacle of sharks (Hickling, 1963). The stalk of the parasite embeds in the muscle, causing cavitation and emaciation of the host. Gonad maturation is suppressed in both sexes of infested sharks (Hickling, 1963). *Conchoderma auritum*, found on gills of the basking shark, is not a true parasite (Delamare Debouteville, 1948); however, tissue damage occurs at the site of attachment.

LITERATURE CITED

Averinzev, S. (1925) Neue Art von parasitaren Tricladen (micropharynx). Zool. Anz. 64.

Benz, G.W. (1980) Tissue proliferations associated with *Nemesis lamna* Risso, 1826 (Copepoda, Eudactylinidae) infestations on the gill filaments of shortfin makos *(Isurus oxyrinchus* Rafinesque). J. Fish Dis. 3:443–446.

Benz, G.W. (1985) Copepods as parasites of sharks. In: A Symposium on the Captive Maintenance of Elasmobranchs. An International Meeting, Baltimore (abstract).

Berland, B. (1961) Copepod *Ommatokoita elongata* (Grant) in the eyes of the Greenland shark—a possible case of mutual dependence. Nature, 191:829–830.

Bird, P. (1981) The occurrence of *Cirolana borealis* (isopoda) in the hearts of sharks from Atlantic coastal waters of Florida. Fish. Bull. 79:376–383.

Boulard, Y. (1977) Description d'*Eimeria quentini* n. sp., parasite intranucleaire du peritoine de la raie: *Aetobatis narinari* (Chondrichthyens, Myliobatidae) en malaisie. Protistologica T. XIII, fasc. 4:529–533.

Boxshall, G.A. (1977) The histopathology of infection by *Lepeophtheirus pectoralis* (Muller) (Copepoda: Caligidae). J. Fish Biol. 10:411–415.

Campbell, R.A. (1985) Helminth pathology in sharks. In: A Symposium on the Captive Maintenance of Elasmobranchs. An International Meeting, Baltimore (abstract).

Cheung, P.J., and Nigrelli, R.F. (1983) *Dermophthiriordes pristidis* n. gen., n. sp. (Microbothriidae) from the skin and *Neoheterocotyle ruggierii* n. sp. (Monocotylidae) from the gills of the smalltooth sawfish, *Pristis pectinata*. Trans. Am. Microsc. Soc. 102(4):366–370.

Cheung, P.J., Nigrelli, R.F., Ruggieri, G.D., and Cilia, A. (1982) Treatment of skin lesions in captive lemon sharks, *Negaprion brevirostris* (Poey), caused by monogeneans *(Dermophthirius sp.)*. J. Fish Dis. 5:167–170.

Cheung, P.J., Nigrelli, R.F., and Ruggieri, G.D. (1987) Coccidian Infection as the Cause of Death of the Cownose Ray, *Rhinoptera bonasus* (Mitchill). Northeast Fish and Wildlife Conference (abstract).

Cressey, R.F. (1967) Caligoid copepods parasitic on sharks of the Indian Ocean. Proc. U.S. Natl. Mus. 121 (No. 3572):1–21.

Delamare Debouteville, C. (1948) Sur un *Conchoderma auritum* (Crust. Cirripede) parasite branchial du squale pelerin (*Cetorhinus maximus* (Gunner)) a Banyuls. Bull. Mus. Natl. Hist. Nat., ser. 2, 20(5):448–449.

Eudokimova, E.B., Kuznecova, I.G., and Shtein, G.A. (1969) Parasitic ciliates of the family Urceolariidae (Peritricha, Mobilia) of some fishes of southwest Atlantic (in Russian). Zool. Zh. 48:1451–1455.

Friend, G.F. (1941) The life history and ecology of the salmon gill-maggot, *Salmincola salmonea* (L.). Trans. R. Soc. Edinb. 60:503–541.

Ginetsinskaya, T.A. (1956) Biological adaptations of the larval stages and parthenitae of trematodes in the search for and in the infection of animal hosts. Vestn. LGU 3:71–84.

Golvan, Y.J. (1964) An Illustrated Key to the Genera of Acanthocephala (Transl. by I. Pratt). Oregon State University, Corvallis, Oregon.

Halawani, A. (1930) On a new species *Eimeria (E. southwelli)* from *Aetobatis narinari*. Ann. Trop. Med. Parasitol. 24:1–3.

Hickling, C.F. (1963) On the small deep-sea shark *Etmopterus spinax* L. and its cirripede parasite, *Anelasma squalicola* (Loven.) J. Linn Soc. Lond. (Zool.) 45:17–24.

Jagerskiold, L.A. (1896) *Micropharynx parasitica*. Ofversigt Vetensk. Akad. Forhandl. Stockholm 53.

Kabata, Z. (1984) Diseases caused by metazoans: Crustaceans. In: Diseases of Marine Animals Vol. IV, Part 1, O. Kinne editor, Biologische Anstalt Helgoland, Hamburg. Pp. 321–399.

Khan, R.A. (1972) Taxonomy, prevalence, and experimental transmission of a protozoan parasite, *Trichodina oviducti* Polyansky (ciliata: Peritrichida) of the thorny skate, *Raja radiata* Donovan. J. Parasitol. 58:680–685.

Ko, R.C., Morton, B., and Wong, P.S. (1975) Prevalence and histopathology of *Echinocephalus sinensis* (Nematoda: Gnathostomatidae) in natural and experimental hosts. Can. J. Zool. 53:550–559.

Laird, M. (1951) Studies on the trypanosomes of New Zealand fish. Proc. Zool. Soc. Lond. 121:285–309.

Laird, M. (1959) *Caliperia brevipes* n. sp. (Ciliata: epizoic in *Raja erinacea* Mitchell at Saint Andrews, New Brunswick. Can. J. Zool. 37:283–288.

Laird, M., and Bullock, W.L. (1969) Marine fish haematozoa from New Brunswick and New England. J. Fish. Res. Bd. Can. 26:1075–1102.

Laveran, A., and Mesnil, F. (1901) Deux hemogregarines nouvelles des poissons. C.R. Acad. Sci. Paris 133:572–577.

Lawler, A.R. (1980) Studies on *Amyloodinium ocellatum* (Dinoflagellata) in Mississippi Sound: Natural and experimental hosts. Gulf Res. Rep. 6:403–413.

Leibovitz, L., and Leibovitz, S.S. (1985) Skin diseases of sharks. In: A Symposium on the Captive Maintenance of Elasmobranchs. An International Meeting, Baltimore (abstract).

Love, M.S., and Moser, M. (1976) Parasites of California Marine and Esturaine Fish. Marine Science Institute University of California, Santa Barbara, pp. 1–517.

May, E.G., Grimes, D.J., Jones, R.T., Stemmler, J., Hetrick, F.M., and Colwell, R.R. (1983) A *Vibrio* infection of brown sharks (*Carcharhinus plumbeus*): biochemical characterization of two unique *Vibrio* species— 14th Annual Symposium of the International Association for Aquarium Animal Medicine, Long Beach, California.

McVicar, A.H. (1972) The ultrastructure of the parasite-host interface of three tetraphyllidean tapeworms of the elasmobranch *Raja naevus*. Parasitology 65:77–88.

McVicar, A.H., and Fletcher, T.C. (1970) Serum factors in *Raja radiata* toxic to *Acanthobothrium quadripartitum* (Cestode: Tetraphyllidea), a parasite specific to *R. naevus*. Parasitology 61:55–63.

McVicar, A.H., and Gibson, D.I. (1975) *Pancreatonema torriensis* gen. nov., sp. nov. (Nematoda: Rhabdochonidae) from the pancreatic duct of *Raja naevus*. Int. J. Parasitol. 5:529–535.

Moser, M., and Anderson, S. (1977) An intrauterine leech infection: *Branchellion lobata* Moore, 1952 (Piscicolidae) in the Pacific angel shark, *(Squatina californica)* from California. Can. J. Zool. 55:759–760.

Nakajima, K. (1972) Studies on a new trypanorhynchan larva, *Callotetrarhynchus* sp., parasitic on cultured yellowtail–XI. Growth of the adult in the valvular intestine of *Triakis scyllia* (Japan). Bull. Jpn. Soc. Sci. Fish. 38:945–954.

Rees, G., and Williams, H.H. (1965) The functional morphology of the scolex and the genitalia of *Acanthobothrium coronatum* (Rud.) (Cestoda: Tetraphyllidea). Parasitology 55:617–651.

Rokicki, J. (1982) *Lironeca indica* Edwards, 1840 (Crustacea, Isopoda) from *Salar crumenophthalmus* (Bloch). Wiad. Parazytol. 28:205–206.

Ruyck, R., and Chabaud, A.G. (1960) Un cas de parasitisme attribuale a les larves de *Phlyctainophora lamnae* Steiner chez un selacien, et cycle evolutif probable de nematode. Vie Milieu 11:386–389.

Sakanari, J., and Moser, M. (1985) Infectivity of, and laboratory infection with, an elasmobranch cestode, *Lacistorhynchus tenuis* (Van Beneden, 1858). J. Parasitol. 7(16):788–791.

Schultz, B. (1911) Untersuchungen uber Nahrung und Parasiten von Ostseefischen. Wiss. Meeresunters. N.S. Abt. Kiel 13:285–312.

Schuurman Stekhoven, J.H., Jr., and Botman, T.P.J. (1932) Zur Ernahrungsbiologie von *Proleptus obtusus* Duj und die von diesem Parasiten hervorgerufenen reaktiven Anderungen des Wirtsgewebes. Z. Parasitkde. 4:220–239.

Thulin, J. (1982) The morphology of the miracidium of *Chimaerohemecus trondheimensis* van der Land, 1967 (Digenea: Sanguinicolidae). J. Parasitol. 85:9–10.

Uspenskaya, A.V. (1955) The parasite fauna of the benthic crustaceans of the Barents Sea (Russ.). Beneden (Nematodes, Spirurata) (Russ.). Zool. Zh. 32:828–832.

Williams, A.D., and Campbell, R.A. (1977) A new tetraphyllidean cestode, *Glyphobothrium zwerneri* gen. et. sp. n., from the cownose ray, *Rhinoptera bonasus* (Mitchill 1815). J. Parasitol. 63:775–779.

Willliams, H.H. (1968) *Acanthobothrium quadripartitum* sp. nov. (Cestoda: Tetraphyllidea) from *Raja naevus* in the North Sea and English Channel. J. Parasitol. 58:105–110.

Williams, H.H., and Richards, D.H.H. (1968) Observations on *Pseudanisakis rotundata* (Rudolphi, 1819) Mozgovoi, 1950, a common but little known nematode parasite of *Raia radiata* Donovan in the northern North Sea. J. Helminth. 42:199–220.

Wulker, G. (1929) Der Wirtswechsel der parasitischen Nematoden von meeresfischen. Verh. Deutsch. Zool. Ges. J. 33:147–157.

Yamaguti, S. (1958) Systema Helminthum. I. The Digenetic Trematodes of Vertebrates. Interscience Publishers, New York and London.

Yamaguti, S. (1959) Systema Helminthum. II. The Cestodes of Vertebrates. Interscience Publishers, New York and London.

Yamaguti, S. (1961) Systema Helminthum. III. The Nematodes of Vertebrates. Interscience Publishers, New York and London.

Yamaguti, S. (1963a) Systema Helminthum. IV. Monogenea and Aspidocotylea. Interscience Publishers, New York and London.

Yamaguti, S. (1963b) Systema Helminthum. V. Acanthocephala. Interscience Publishers, New York and London.

Yamaguti, S. (1963c) Parasitic Copepoda and Branchiura of Fishes. Interscience Publishers, New York and London.

Chapter 101

NEOPLASIA IN SHARKS

MICHAEL K. STOSKOPF

The popular press occasionally reports a scientific "gee whiz" article stating that sharks do not develop cancer. The origin of this belief is difficult to discern. An angiogenesis inhibitor extracted from the cartilage of the basking shark was discovered several years ago when researchers examined shark cartilage as a substitute for cartilage from growing calves (Lee and Langer, 1983). It should be noted that calf cartilage also contains a less potent angiogenesis inhibitor (Lee and Langer, 1983). These workers commented on the rarity of neoplasms in elasmobranchs relative to those reported in mammals, teleost fishes, and amphibians. Considerable research seeking to identify the reason for an apparent "resistance to cancer" in sharks has been conducted since then.

A number of neoplastic lesions in sharks and particularly skates and rays were identified in the early 1900s, and until relatively recently, little effort has gone into identification of spontaneous tumors in this group of fishes. The vast majority of sharks caught and killed each year are not subjected to careful examination, and subtle, and frankly not so subtle, neoplastic changes would be readily missed unless they caused a major external deformity. With the successful maintenance of sharks in captivity for longer periods, and the advent of careful necropsy procedures in large aquaria, neoplasias in sharks are being identified. The undifferentiated hemoblastic response in a Pacific angel shark listed in Table 101–1 occurred in an animal held in captivity and subjected to treatment with chloramphenicol (Stoskopf et al., 1987).

TABLE 101–1. Neoplasia in Sharks

Neoplasm/Location	Fish	References
Nervous System		
Choroid plexus papilloma	Spiny dogfish (taxonomy uncertain)	Prieur, 1976
Neurilemmoma	Spiny dogfish (taxonomy uncertain)	Harshbarger, 1974
Cardiovascular System		
Hemangioma	Starry skate (taxonomy uncertain)	Drew, 1912
Hemoblastic response	Pacific angel shark	Stoskopf et al., 1987
Gastrointestinal System		
Hepatic adenoma	Blue shark	Schroeders, 1908
Urinary System		
None reported		
Endocrine System		
Thyroid tumor	Spiked dogfish	Cameron and Vincent, 1915
Reproductive System		
Seminoma	Thornback skate	Harshbarger, 1990
Musculoskeletal System and Connective Tissue		
Chondroma	Mediterranean dogfish	Thomas, 1933
	Spiked dogfish	Takahashi, 1929
Fibroepithelial polyps	Spiny dogfish	Wellings, 1969
Fibrosarcoma	Bull shark	Harshbarger, 1968–1990
	Long-nosed skate (taxonomy uncertain)	Drew, 1912
Odontoma	Mediterranean dogfish	Ladreyt, 1929
Osteoma	Mediterranean dogfish	Thomas, 1933
Reticulum cell sarcoma	Brown shark	Harshbarger, 1968–1990
Integumentary System		
Epidermoid carcinoma	Mediterranean dogfish	Stolk, 1956
Malignant melanoma	Thornback skate	Johnstone, 1910–1911
		Haddow and Blake, 1933
	Common skate	Johnstone, 1911–1912, 1913

LITERATURE CITED

Cameron, A.T., and Vincent, S. (1915) Notes on an enlarged thyroid occurring in an elasmobranch fish (Squalus suckleyi). J. Med. Res. 27:251–256.

Drew, G.H. (1912) Some cases of new growths in fish. J. Marine Biol. Assoc. U.K. 9:281–287.

Haddow, A., and Blake, I. (1933) Neoplasms in fish: A report of six cases with a summary of the literature. J. Pathol. Bacteriol. 36:41–47.

Harshbarger, J.C. (1968–1990) Registry of Tumors in Lower Animals. Smithsonian Institution, Washington, D.C.

Johnstone, J. (1910–1911) Internal parasites and diseased conditions of fishes. Proc. Trans. Liverpool Biol. Soc. 25:88–122.

Johnstone, J. (1911–1912) Internal parasites and diseased conditions of fishes. Proc. Trans. Liverpool Biol. Soc. 26:103–144.

Johnstone, J. (1913) Diseased conditions of fishes. Proc. Trans. Liverpool Biol. Soc. 27:196–218.

Ladreyt, F. (1929) Sur un odontome cutane chez un Scyllium catulus. Bull. Inst. Oceanogr. Monaco No. 539:1–4.

Lee, A., and Langer, R. (1983) Shark cartilage contains inhibitors of tumor angiogenesis. Science 221:1185–1187.

Prieur, D.J., Fenstermacher, J.D., and Guarino, A.M. (1976) A choroid plexus papilloma in an elasmobranch (Squalus acanthias). J. Natl. Cancer Inst. 56:1207–1209.

Schroeders, V.D. (1908) Tumors of Fishes. Dissertation in Russian. Translation in Army Medical Library, Washington, D.C. St. Petersburg.

Stolk, A. (1956) Tumours of fishes. IXA and IXB. Epithelioma of the oral mucosa in the scylliid Scylliorhinus catulus (L.). Proc. K. Ned. Akad. Wet. 59:196–210.

Stoskopf, M.K., May, E.B., Bennett, R.O., Sigler, R., and Lipsky, M.M. (1987) An undifferentiated hemoblastic response in an angel shark (Squatina dumerili). Proc. Int. Assoc. Aquatic Anim. Med. 18:11.

Takahashi, K. (1929) Studie uber die Fischgeschqulste. Z. Krebsforsch. 29:1–73.

Thomas, L. (1933) Sur deux cas de tumeurs tegumentaires chez la rousette. Bull. Assoc. Fr. Etude Cancer 22:306–315.

Wellings, S.R. (1969) Neoplasia and primitive vertebrate phylogeny: Echinoderms, prevertebrates, and fishes—a review. Natl. Cancer Inst. Monogr. 31:59–128.

Chapter 102

SHARK PHARMACOLOGY AND TOXICOLOGY

MICHAEL K. STOSKOPF

Captive sharks are susceptible to many infectious and noninfectious diseases that require medical treatment. Unfortunately, the current pharmaceutical knowledge pertaining to sharks is relatively primitive. Shark medicine has only recently become a routine component of aquarium management and certainly is not routinely considered in the wild.

The wide variety of shark species and their different habitats, along with the problem that most sharks are difficult to handle and examine closely, complicates the problem. There is little in the way of established baseline diagnostic parameters for shark species, and we are handicapped by our lack of knowledge of the metabolism and effects of therapeutic drugs on sharks. Nevertheless, a few clinicians are actively involved in correcting the situation (Stoskopf, 1990). In addition, sharks are quite susceptible to heavy metals and agricultural chemicals. Again, more work is needed to provide a practical picture of shark toxicology, but the little knowledge available suggests that this would be a worthwhile endeavor.

ANESTHESIA AND IMMOBILIZATION

Chemical immobilization is required to accomplish a thorough hands-on examination of most sharks of any size. Several drugs can be used. In the late 1950s, tricaine methane sulfonate (MS–222) supplanted many less satisfactory immersion anesthetics such as urethane, and immersion anesthesia became the method of choice for anesthetizing sharks (Gilbert and Wood, 1957). Unfortunately, immersion is not appropriate for larger animals because of the quantities of drugs required to reach effective concentrations in large water systems. Methods using sprayers to apply drugs to the gills (tricaine methane sulfonate to effect) (Gilbert and Kritzler, 1960) require prior restraint and are usually not suitable for closed systems where the water would be heavily contaminated. Recently, azaperone, a butyrophenone tranquilizer that blocks dopaminergic receptors of the mesolimbic and nigrostriatal pathways, has been reported to be effective for immobilizing spiny dogfish when applied to the gills at 4 mg/kg (Latas, 1987).

Considerable efforts are being directed toward identification of intramuscular agents for immobilizing, tranquilizing, or sedating free-swimming sharks (Stoskopf, 1986b). Intramuscular agents drastically reduce contamination of closed systems and can be delivered easily from the surface. Success has been achieved in several shark species with ketamine HCl, an analgesic and cataleptic cyclohexamine commonly employed in terrestrial carnivore anesthesia. Ketamine provides good peripheral analgesia in mammals through suppression of dorsal horn cell activity in the spinal cord but provides little visceral analgesia (White et al., 1982). In addition, seizurelike muscle spasms due to spinal reflex firing are occasionally noted. In carcharhinid sharks, doses between 12 and 20 mg/kg provide reasonable immobilization in captive specimens.

Xylazine, a thiazine derivative distantly related to the phenothiazine tranquilizers, is a convulsant in teleosts and causes major changes in the electrocardiogram (ECG) (Oswald, 1978). It has been used successfully in combination with ketamine HCl in several shark species to ameliorate the muscle spasms that can occur with ketamine alone, but some shark clinicians eschew its use out of concern about the cardiovascular effects of the drug. The effects of xylazine on the cardiovascular system of sharks have not been well studied. Xylazine is generally administered to sharks at a dose of 6 mg/kg when given in combination with ketamine at 12 mg/kg. These doses are based on empirical observations, and some individual animals will not respond as expected. There are undoubtedly species differences in response to these drugs, and occasional individuals within a species will tolerate these doses and show few, if any, signs of drug effect.

Tiletamine and zolazepam mixtures have been tested unsuccessfully in Atlantic carcharhinids (Stoskopf, 1986b). Although tiletamine is chemically closely related to ketamine and generally more potent in mammalian species given in combination with the diazepam analogue zolazepam, it did not produce immobilization or tranquilization in a sand tiger shark or a lemon shark in individual trials. Instead, increased irritability, rapid swimming, and unrestrained biting were observed. Similarly, carfentanil, a potent narcotic analogue of fentanyl, failed to achieve any effect in a lemon shark even when administered at massive doses (Stoskopf, 1986b).

Reversal agents for immobilization drugs promise to be useful in sharks. Doxapram HCl given intravenously in the caudal vein produces dramatic arousal in brown sharks immobilized with ketamine and xylazine combinations. A single trial with yohimbine in a nurse shark immobilized with ketamine and xylazine also generated arousal nearly immediately after intravenous administration. Further work remains to be done in the use of α blockers and other drug antagonists in sharks.

CHEMOTHERAPEUTICS

Routes of Administration

Topical Administration

The routes available for administration of chemotherapeutic agents to a shark or ray are limited. Direct, localized topical administration is possible only if the shark is relatively easily handled. In small skates and rays and occasionally small sharks, the use of topical preparations designed for terrestrial mammals to treat open wounds has been successful. Apply these daily by taking the animal to the surface in appropriate restraint and putting the ointment on the affected area. Hold the treated area out of the water for a minimum of 1 minute to allow drug absorption and release the patient to swim free. Most ointments are washed off by the water, but there is a reasonable rationale for treating lesions with locally active lipophilic drugs rapidly absorbed by tissues. These ointments are often in an oil base and foul the water surface unless there is adequate skimming action by the filters.

Another form of topical treatment used for smaller elasmobranchs is the bath or dip. These are best performed by removing the animal from the main system and exposing it to drug in a smaller volume of water. This avoids the expense of reaching effective drug levels in a large volume of water and minimizes the chance of a deleterious impact on biological filtration systems. The major disadvantage is the necessity of handling the animal. Although very large animals can be treated in this manner if necessary, it can be a difficult procedure. When holding a shark in a small treatment tank, monitor dissolved oxygen levels carefully throughout the treatment and add oxygen by bubbling air or pure oxygen if the level of dissolved oxygen falls below 6 ppm.

The addition of drugs to entire large systems for the treatment of external parasites has been recommended in the past, but this approach to topical treatment is dangerous and inappropriate. The intricacies of the kinetics of drugs in large systems containing multiple species are complex, making it hard to ensure an effective treatment that is at the same time safe for all of the inhabitants of the system, including the microflora and fauna of the nitrogen-fixing biota.

Oral Route

The route of choice for administering medications to sharks, skates, and rays is per os in the food. This route is relatively precise. Most captive sharks can be pole-fed individually and are not particularly sensitive to capsules or tablets hidden in their food. It is much easier to administer medication in the feed when large numbers of animals must be medicated on a routine basis than to provide individual injections. Many liquid drugs can be injected into the body of the fish to be fed the shark. Tablets and capsules can be slipped into the body cavity of the feed-fish, and the shark enticed to take the proffered meal whole.

A major disadvantage of the oral route is that it can be used only when a shark is actively feeding, a condition often lacking when sharks require delivery of antibiotics. Another disadvantage is that the bioavailability is not known for any of the drugs rou-

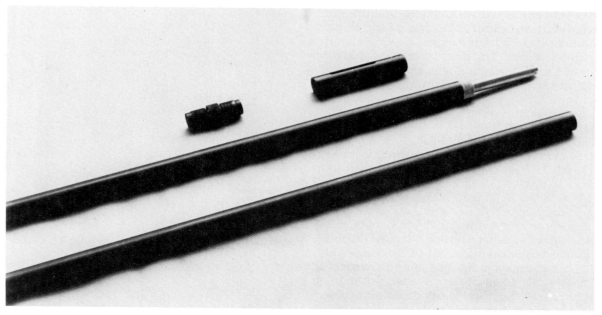

FIGURE 102–1. Pole syringe useful for making intramuscular injections in free-swimming sharks.

tinely delivered by this route. Drugs taken orally must retain activity and be readily absorbed from the gastrointestinal tract to be clinically useful.

Intramuscular Route

The advent of the pole syringe to shark medicine has made the intramuscular route of drug delivery very popular (Fig. 102–1). This route of medication is also relatively precise and is appropriate for a wider range of drugs than the oral route. It is more time-consuming, particularly when sharks become habituated to an injection at the appearance of the pole syringe. Aversion to feeding poles has been observed by some workers using this route of administration, but this is not usually a problem. The use of distinctly different-sized feeding poles and pole syringes helps avoid the problem.

The preferred type of pole syringe uses the pole as an extended plunger to the syringe, allowing injection with the thrust of the pole. This allows the operator to use both hands to target the injection. A cover on the syringe prevents breaking the tip of the syringe on impact. A cover also provides protection from bending the needle. Most pole syringe covers are friction fit over the disposable syringe used to deliver the drug. This should be modified by tying the cover to the pole with a short line or with a

length of adhesive tape to prevent the cover containing the syringe falling to the bottom of the tank if the needle catches momentarily in the skin of the shark.

Shark skin is very tough and resistant to puncture. Use a large-gauge needle for pole syringe injections. A 16-gauge needle is preferred in larger sharks, whereas 18-gauge needles are suitable for smaller animals. In some species, a 14-gauge needle is a major advantage. Too small a needle often results in the need to repeat injections and uncertainty about the total dose delivery when the needle bends during injection.

Most intramuscular injections to sharks should be delivered above the lateral line in a saddle region extending from behind the gill slits to the anterior aspect of the second dorsal (Fig. 102–2). This area consists of dorsal muscles and is free of vital structures which would be damaged by the injection.

Intraperitoneal Route

Intraperitoneal injections are useful for the delivery of drugs when rapid absorption is required and when intravenous injection is not feasible. The technique is generally restricted to restrained animals, although it is occasionally used inadvertently through inaccurate aim of the pole syringe. Drugs

FIGURE 102–2. The "saddle region" used for safe intramuscular injections of drugs in sharks.

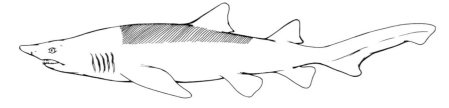

delivered intraperitoneally should be nonirritating. This includes dextrose and electrolyte solutions, most intramuscular steroid preparations, and the majority of intravenous drugs. The drug insert should always be examined for information about pH and possibly irritating preservatives before a drug is administered by this route.

Intravenous Route

Intravenous administration is limited to restrained sharks. The vein described for blood sampling (Fig. 102–3) is suitable for delivery of a variety of drugs including ketamine HCl, steroids, and intravenous antibiotics. Other sites for intravenous injection include veins running laterally behind the head just above the lateral line. These veins are accessible on larger animals. All of the same rules apply to intravenous administration of drugs to sharks that apply to intravenous administration to mammals. Sharks can develop infections at the injection site from injudicious use of contaminated needles, although this is rare. Basic attention to avoiding contamination of the needle in the water essentially eliminates this problem. Prepping shark skin with alcohol is very irritating and results in local erythema and induration. It is unnecessary and ineffective.

Antibacterial Treatments

Bacteria can cause primary disease in sharks or become secondary complications to other problems. Antibacterial drug treatment of sharks, skates, and rays is common and frequently contributes to the positive outcome of a case (Table 102–1). Evaluation of the need for antibacterial chemotherapy in elasmobranchs is based on several factors, and the selection of appropriate drugs is complex. The need for

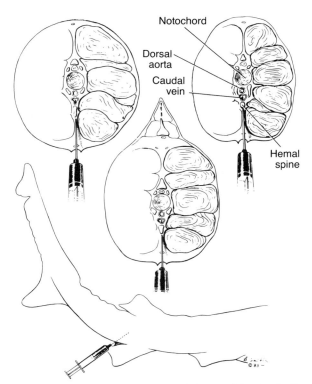

FIGURE 102–3. Venipuncture of the caudal vein of the shark. (From Smith, B., Stoskopf, M.K., and Klay, G. [1984] Clinical note: Blood sampling from captive sharks. J. Zoo Wild Anim. Med. 15[3]:116–117.)

culture, identification, and sensitivity testing is well established (Stoskopf, 1984; Nusbaum and Shotts, 1981; Wilford, 1967). The kinetics for a specific route of delivery, interactions with other drugs or environmental molecules, and any deleterious side effects must also be considered. Unfortunately, none of these data are complete for sharks. Kinetics studies of antibacterial antibiotics in sharks have been done,

TABLE 102–1. Antibacterial Treatments for Elasmobranchs

Antibiotic	Dose (mg/kg body wt)	Schedule and Route	Comments
Aminoglycosides			
Gentamicin	6	Every 6 days IM	Kinetics in brown sharks (Stoskopf et al., 1986)
Kanamycin	20	Daily IP or oral	500 mg/100 g of food
Neomycin	20	Daily oral	Use for enteritis
Tobramycin	6	Every 6 days IM	
Penicillins			
Ampicillin	10	Daily oral or IM	
Carbenicillin	200	Daily oral	Poor acceptance, odor to water
Quinolones			
Enrofloxin	5	Daily oral or IM	Broad spectrum
Nitrofurans			
Nitrofurazone	50	Daily oral	
Tetracyclines			
Chlortetracycline	10–20	Daily oral	
Oxytetracycline	10	Daily IM	
	50–75	Daily oral	
Miscellaneous			
Dihydrostreptomycin	10	Daily oral or IM	
Chloramphenicol succinate	40	Daily oral or IM	

but most of these studies examine the aminoglycosides (Fig. 102–4) (Stoskopf et al., 1986; Walsh, 1984). The majority of drugs remain unstudied. Information does exist for teleosts, humans, and other mammals and these should be considered in lieu of specific shark data (Kuhns, 1981; Herwig, 1979; Trust and Chapman, 1974; Wolf and Snieszko, 1964).

Experience suggests that underdosing or delivery failure is a more common cause of therapeutic failure with antibacterial drugs than overdosing or drug toxicity. The potential for developing resistant strains of organisms is high and it is important to rely heavily on culture and sensitivity results (Watanabe et al., 1971). If antibiotic sensitivity reports show resistance to the initial drug employed, switch to an effective drug.

Species-specific differences are not well documented for any antibiotics in sharks. This is not surprising considering the wide variety of sharks treated, but species variations undoubtedly exist. Therefore, when administering antibiotics, the patient should be monitored carefully for signs of toxicity or improvement of the condition, and doses adjusted. Successful dosing is usually rewarded with noticeable clinical improvement within 2 or 3 days, although the entire therapeutic course should be completed.

Antibiotic resistance and incomplete therapy are very real problems in fish medicine. Even though improvement is noted early in treatment, continue the treatment. A useful rule of thumb is to extend antibiotic therapy 1 week beyond the cessation of obvious signs of the disease being treated. This helps avoid relapses and decreases the number of resistant organisms created. The current state of the art in dosage timing is basically no different than judging mammalian treatments.

Antifungal Treatments

Fungal diseases affect sharks and are being diagnosed more frequently. Kinetic studies of antifungal drugs in sharks are not available. The doses provided here are purely empirical and should be used with caution. Miconazole and ketaconazole have been administered without untoward effects at doses of 5 and 10 mg/kg body weight in cases in which fungal disease has been suspected from the necropsy results of tank mates. Their efficacy and safety are not established.

Antiprotozoal Treatments

Protozoal diseases in captive sharks have not been as devastating as those in captive teleost medicine. As a result, experience and knowledge of chemotherapeutic remedies for protozoal disease in sharks is nearly nonexistent. The issue of sensitivity of sharks to copper remains controversial, although accidental exposures have resulted in signs of neural

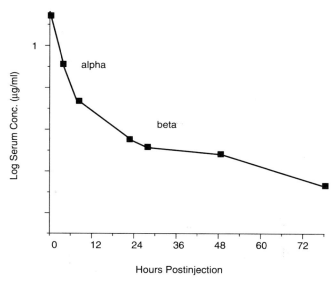

FIGURE 102–4. Kinetics of gentamicin in the brown shark.

dysfunction. Systemic antiprotozoal drugs such as metronidazole and emtryl hold promise, but their safety and efficacy in elasmobranchs remain to be demonstrated.

Antitrematode Treatments

Sharks are subject to parasitism by trematodes. The best-known trematode problem in captive sharks is the monogenean skin fluke *Dermopitherius* spp. that parasitizes the lemon shark (Gruber and Keyes, 1981). This trematode infestation can devastate host sharks and active treatment is required. Unfortunately, the therapeutic armamentarium for treating shark trematodes is quite limited. Many trematodes are not susceptible to copper at levels suitable for sharks. Praziquantel HCl has shown promise in teleost medicine but has not been studied in sharks (Fig. 102–5). It is a reasonable alternative to water treatments with organic pesticides. A dose of 400 mg/100 g of food, fed daily for 5 to 7 days, is a reasonable starting point for oral administration (Schmahl and Mehlhorn, 1985).

Trichlorfon (dimethyl-2,2,2-trichloro-l-hydroxyethylphosphonate), also marketed as Masoten, Dylox, or Neguvon as an agricultural pesticide, has

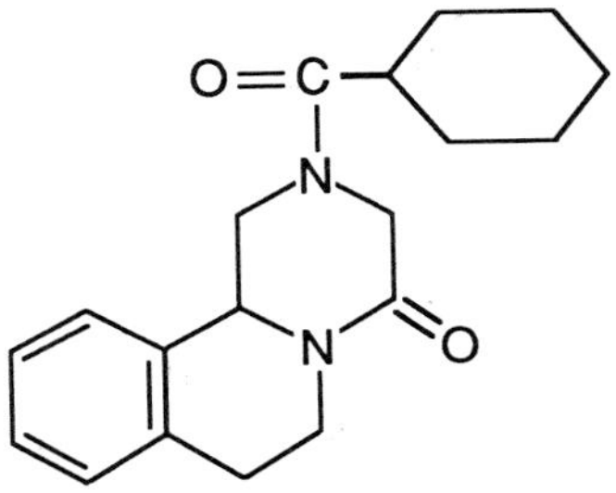

FIGURE 102–5. Structure of praziquantel.

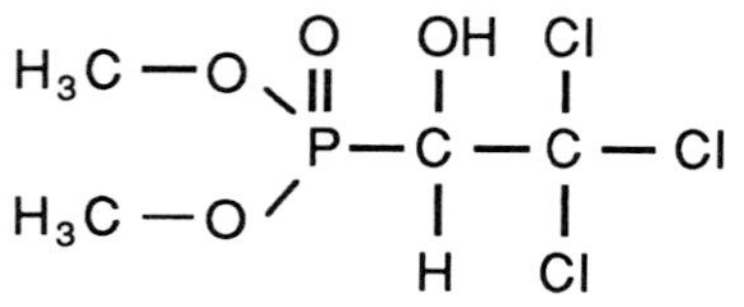

FIGURE 102–6. Structure of trichlorfon.

been used effectively to clear trematodes from captive sharks in both closed and open systems (Fig. 102–6). The compound is toxic and can be lethal to treated sharks. This pesticide should be handled and measured in a fume hood, wearing gloves. The dose of 0.25 mg/L is given for active ingredient, since preparations vary in the amount of binder used. The compound has also been used at 0.5 mg/L at 5-day intervals in a semiopen system and as a single exposure at 2.0 mg/L in a closed system (Gruber and Keyes, 1981). Trichlorfon is unstable in alkaline conditions and should be broken down relatively quickly in marine systems, but it is still preferable to perform treatments in tanks with minimal substrates rather than major system tanks. This chemical should not be used in water where divers will be exposed. After the treatments, water to be discarded should be brought to a pH of 11 with sodium hydroxide to ensure destruction of any residual drug.

Antinematode and Anticestode Treatments

Oral cambendazole (20 mg/kg), mebendazole (20 mg/kg), or levamisole (10 mg/kg) are effective nematode treatments (Fig. 102–7). Cestode infections can be treated with praziquantel or niclosamide. Suspected niclosamide toxicity has been observed in carcharhinid sharks in a closed system. Although no signs were seen upon oral administration of the drug, 2 days later animals became toxic and died. It was postulated that the excreted drug or a metabolite was toxic when absorbed by the gills (Beusse, 1988).

Anticrustacean Therapy

Early experiences with copepod infections in lemon sharks led to the use of intramuscular ivermectin in an experimental liposome formulation. Unfortunately, lemon sharks show signs of nervous system impairment, including disorientation and loss of equilibrium before the load of copepods is significantly reduced. Copepods are not usually susceptible to copper therapy at levels safe for the host sharks. Trichlorfon, discussed in the treatment of trematodes, is an effective copepod treatment, although the same precautions must be applied. Manual removal of copepods has been employed, but the mobile parasites will often hide in the mouth of the host shark, defying removal unless the animal is completely immobilized. Sprays of 2% buffered for-

malin are effective but cannot be used safely to remove parasites from the mouth and gills. Seventy percent isopropyl alcohol sprays are also effective but irritate the skin of the shark, causing hyperemia and excess mucus production.

Steroids and Anti-inflammatory Drugs

Steroids and nonsteroidal anti-inflammatory drugs are clinically useful in sharks with transport tetany, adrenal exhaustion after capture or transport, or chronic meningitis. Dexamethasone administered intravenously or intramuscularly, depending on the nature of the condition, has been most commonly employed. Prednisolone and long-acting steroids, including methylprednisolone acetate and fludrocortisone, have also been used effectively in appropriate cases. The longer-acting steroids are usually given subconjunctivally in conjunction with antibiotics to

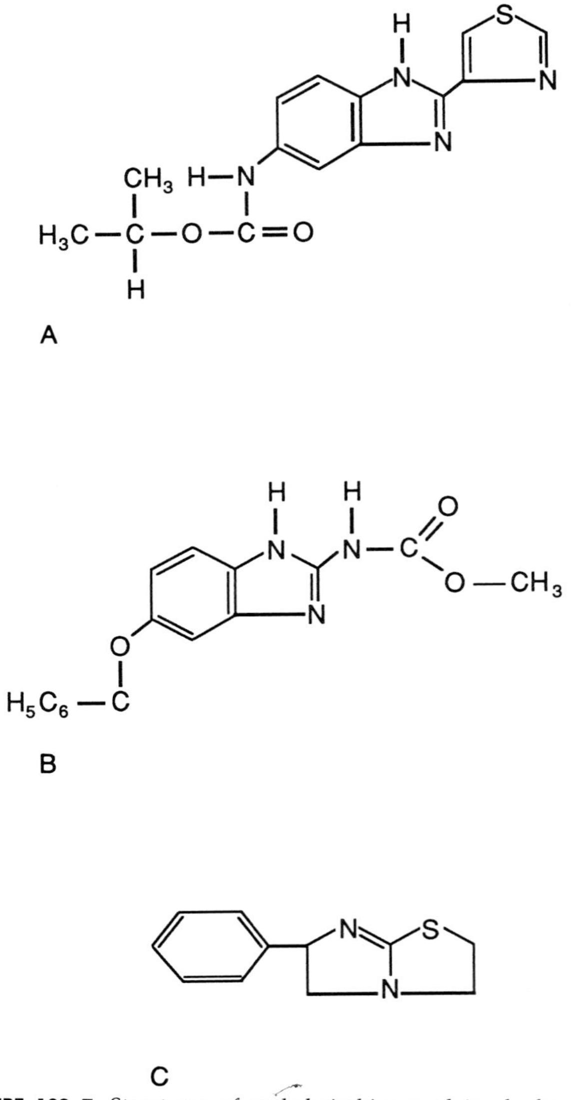

FIGURE 102–7. Structures of anthelminthics used in sharks. *A.* Cambendazole. *B.* Mebendazole. *C.* Levamisole.

treat corneal inflammation. Nonsteroidal anti-inflammatory drugs such as flunixin meglumine have also been employed in carcharhinid sharks using mammalian carnivore doses.

Fluid and Electrolyte Replacement

Sharks are subject to many of the same physiologic drains experienced by mammals during illness. A significant outcome of disease is dehydration. Living in a hyperosmolar environment, the shark is subject to dehydration through several mechanisms. Large wounds breaching the integument result in direct loss of water. Hepatic dysfunction impairing generation of blood urea nitrogen, critical for shark osmoregulation, also results in dehydration. Renal and particularly gill diseases also cause electrolyte imbalance and/or dehydration. Fluid replacement is a critical component to the care of an ill or injured shark.

Dehydrated sharks have elevated hematocrits and/or serum urea nitrogen levels. They can be successfully maintained by intravenous administration of 5% dextrose solution. Replacement rates should be balanced to the degree of dehydration but 20 ml/kg/day is a safe starting point. If intravenous administration is not possible, intraperitoneal fluids are effective in reducing the hematocrit. Administering fluids once in the face of severe metabolic or infectious disease is rarely adequate. Daily administration for several days until the shark begins feeding appears beneficial.

A more complex solution of shark ringers consisting of Eagle's medium for cell culture without the indicator dye and supplemented with physiologic concentrations of urea is useful for electrolyte replacement in sharks (Jones, 1987). This solution has the advantage of being isosmotic. It is used in situations in which electrolyte replacement is considered important.

Hormones

Hormone therapy in shark medicine has been limited. The extensive problem of goiter formation is related to a hypothyroid state with low levels of circulating thyroxine (T_4). Early detection of these hyperplastic noncolloid goiters and supplementation with oral or injected Synthroid (synthetic T_4 sodium levothyroxine) prevents the development of disfiguring goiter. The dose regimen required appears to be highly individual to the patient. Species differences may exist, but the data to establish these with certainty do not exist. Skates and rays seem to respond to treatment with much lower doses than the carcharhinid sharks. Oral administration is preferred. Both daily and every-other-day administration have proved clinically effective in maintaining reasonable circulating serum T_4 levels of 3 to 4 μg/ml.

A syndrome of ovarian degeneration has been observed in several species of long-term captive sharks maintained in indoor closed systems. The relationship between this condition and the more studied thyroid dysplasias has not been worked out. Some attempts have been made to supplement sharks suspected of this condition with estrogens. The clinical outcome of this effort is unclear.

Steroid supplementation in certain cases could be considered a form of hormone replacement. This is particularly true of the use of steroids for postcapture or posttransport adrenal exhaustion. Carcharhinid sharks in simulated transports have shown relatively rapid depletion of circulating cortisol. Administration of dexamethasone or prednisolone after capture or during long transports improves survivability.

Vitamins/Minerals

Vitamins and minerals are more completely covered in Chapter 95, but a major component of preventive therapeutics in captive sharks involves supplementation with specific vitamins and minerals in the food. The boundary between nutritional supplementation and therapeutics is always gray and indistinct.

Vitamin supplementation for sharks is generally focused on the water-soluble vitamins and the antioxidants. Water-soluble vitamins are leached out of fish when they are thawed and when they are placed in water. Of the water-soluble vitamins, thiamine or vitamin B_1 is usually given the most attention. The problems of thiaminase inactivation of thiamine are intrinsic in the feed-fish and not the predator species. Frozen fish feeds are usually supplemented at a level of 25 mg/kg fish fed (Geraci, 1986).

The fat-soluble vitamins, particularly vitamin E, are of concern for sharks being fed frozen fish. During storage, even at very cold temperatures, free radical attack and oxidation of double bonds degrade the fatty acid content of feed-fish and deplete antioxidant vitamins such as vitamin E and the water-soluble vitamin C. It is therefore reasonable to supplement with vitamin E to avoid steatitis. More likely of concern in sharks, however, is the possible role of vitamin E in preventing exertional myopathies. Levels for supplementation are not based on experimental data. Where frozen fish are used as feed, vitamin E should be supplemented at the levels commonly recommended for marine mammals, 100 IU/kg of fish fed (Geraci, 1986).

Mineral supplementation in sharks is even less well explored. Whole food is generally provided, and very little concern is given to calcium and phosphorus ratios or other traditional mineral imbalances. The major issue in mineral supplementation in sharks is related to goiter formation. Heavy supplementation of susceptible sharks with massive dietary iodine levels, 10 mg/kg body weight supplementation of potassium iodine (Sea World, 1985) in the feed once

TABLE 102–2. Emergency and Other Drugs Used in Sharks

Drug	Dose (per kg body wt)	Timing and Route	Indication
Atropine	0.1 mg/kg	IM, IP, or IV	Organophosphorus or chlorinated hydrocarbon toxicity
Flunixin meglumine	0.3 mg/kg	IM	Hyponatremia, adrenal exhaustion
Dexamethasone	1–2 mg/kg	IM, IP, or IV	Shock, adrenal exhaustion
Dextrose (5%)	20–30 ml/kg	IP or IV	Dehydration
Doxapram	5 mg/kg	IP or IV	Respiratory depression
Furosemide	2–3 mg/kg	IP or IM BID	Ascites or generalized edema
Prednisolone	1 mg/kg	IP, IV, or IM	Shock
Thyroxine	20 µg/kg	Orally daily IM every other day	Hypothyroidism
Vitamin A	500 U/kg	Orally daily for 2 weeks	Suspected deficiency

a week, is effective in avoiding the appearance of goiter in brown sharks. However, this level of iodine is not a simple supplementation to balance an iodine-deficient diet. In closed systems, the iodine content of the seawater will rise dramatically from the iodine excreted from sharks on this supplementation plan.

A list of emergency and other drugs used in sharks is given in Table 102–2.

LITERATURE CITED

Beusse, D.O. (1988) Personal communication.

Geraci, J.R. (1986) Nutrition and Nutritional Disorders in Zoo and Wild Animal Medicine (Fowler, M., ed.). W.B. Saunders, Philadelphia, pp. 760–764.

Gilbert, P.W., and Kritzler, H. (1960) Experimental shark pens at the Lerner Marine Laboratory. Science 132:424.

Gilbert, P.W., and Wood, F.G. (1957) Method of anesthetizing large sharks and rays safely and rapidly. Science 126:212–213.

Gruber, S.H., and Keyes, R.S. (1981) Keeping sharks for research. In: Aquarium Systems (Hawkins, A.D., ed.). Academic Press, New York, pp. 373–402.

Herwig, N. (1979) Handbook of Drugs and Chemicals Used in the Treatment of Fish Diseases. Charles C Thomas, Springfield, Illinois.

Jones, R. (1987) Personal communication.

Kuhns, J. (1981) FISHDRUG/TXT: a computer generated bibliographic index of the drugs and chemicals used in treating fish diseases. Aquariculture 2(1):4–18; 2(2):29–43; 2(3):45–58.

Latas, P.J. (1987) The use of azaperone in the spiny dogfish (Squalus acanthias). Ann. Proc. Int. Assoc. Aquatic Anim. Med. 18:157–165.

Nusbaum, K.E., and Shotts, E.B. (1981) Action of selected antibiotics on four common bacteria associated with disease of fish. J. Fish Dis. 4:397–484.

Oswald, R.L. (1978) Injection anesthesia for experimental studies in fish. Comp. Biochem. Physiol. 60C:19–26.

Schmahl, G., and Mehlhorn, H. (1985) Treatment of fish parasites 1. Praziquantel effective against Monogenea (Dactylogyrus vastator, Dactylogyrus extensus, Diplozoon paradoxum). Z. Parasitende. 71:727–737.

Sea World, Inc., Orlando, Florida (1985) Personal communication.

Stoskopf, M.K. (1984) Antibiotic therapy for fish. Proc. Am. Assoc. Zoo Vet. 29–30.

Stoskopf, M.K., Smith, B., and Klay, G. (1984) Clinical note: Blood sampling of captive sharks. J. Zoo Anim. Med. 15:116–117.

Stoskopf, M.K. (1986a) Feeding picivorous birds, a review. Ann. Proc. Am. Assoc. Zoo Vet. pp. 68–87.

Stoskopf, M.K. (1986b) Preliminary notes on the immobilization and anesthesia of captive sharks. Erkrankungen Der Zootiere. Akademie-Verlag, Berlin 28:145–151.

Stoskopf, M.K. (1990) Shark diagnostics and therapeutics: A short review. J. Aquariculture Aquatic Sci. 5(3):33–43.

Stoskopf, M.K., Kennedy-Stoskopf, S., Arnold, J., Andrews, J., and Perlstein, M.T. (1986) Therapeutic aminoglycoside antibiotic levels in brown sharks (Carcharhinus plumbeus). J. Fish Dis. 9(3):301–311.

Trust, T.J., and Chapman, D.C. (1971) Evaluation of aquarium antibiotic formulations. Antimicrob. Agents Chemother. 5(4):379–395.

Walsh, M. (1984) Abstracts of the Annual Meeting of the International Association for Aquatic Animal Medicine, Tampa, Florida, p. 21.

Watanabe, T., Aoki, T., Ogata, Y., and Egusa, S. (1971) R factors related to fish culturing. Ann. N.Y. Acad. Sci. 182:383–410.

White, P.F., Way, W.L., and Trevor, A.J. (1982) Ketamine—Its pharmacology and therapeutic uses. Anesthesiology 56:119–136.

Wilford, W.A. (1967) Toxicity of 22 Therapeutic Compounds to Six Fishes. Investigations in Fish Control, BSFW, FWS, U.S. Department of the Interior, Washington, D.C., No. 18, pp. 1–10.

Williams, T. (1988) Personal communication.

Wolf, K., and Snieszko, S.F. (1964) The use of antibiotics and other antimicrobials in therapy of diseases of fishes. Antimicrob. Agents Chemother. 1963:597–603.

Appendices

Appendix I

CONVERSION TABLES AND 37% FORMALDEHYDE ADDITIONS TABLE

Weight per Volume Conversions

ppm	mg/L	mg/gal	oz/1000 gal	g/cu ft	lb/acre-ft
0.1	0.1	.38	0.013	0.0028	0.27
1	1	3.8	0.134	0.0283	2.7
2	2	7.6	0.268	0.0567	5.4
3	3	11.4	0.402	0.0851	8.1
4	4	15.2	0.536	0.1134	10.8
5	5	19.0	0.670	0.1418	13.5
6	6	22.8	0.804	0.1701	16.2
7	7	26.6	0.938	0.1985	18.9
8	8	30.4	1.072	0.2268	21.6
9	9	34.1	1.206	0.2552	24.3
10	10	38	1.34	0.2835	27
20	20	76	2.68	0.562	54
100	100	380	13.4	2.835	270
1000	1000	3800	134	28.35	2700

37% Formaldehyde Additions

ppm	ml/L	ml/gal	qt/acre-ft
1	0.001	0.0038	1.304
2	0.002	0.0076	2.608
3	0.003	0.0114	3.912
4	0.004	0.0152	5.216
5	0.005	0.0190	6.520
6	0.006	0.0228	7.824
7	0.007	0.0266	9.128
8	0.008	0.0304	10.432
9	0.009	0.0343	11.736
10	0.010	0.0380	13.04
15	0.015	0.057	19.56
20	0.020	0.076	26.08
25	0.025	0.095	32.60
100	0.10	0.38	130.4
250	0.25	0.95	323
1000	1.0	3.8	1304

Conversions of Miscellaneous Units

To Convert	To	Multiply By	To Convert	To	Multiply By
Acre	Hectare	0.4057	Fluid ounces	Gallon	0.0078
	Square feet	43,560	*Continued*	Grams	29.57
Acre-foot	Cubic feet	43,560		Liter	0.0296
	Gallons	325,850		Milliliters	29.57
	Liters	1,233,342		Ounces	1.04
	Pounds of water	2,718,144		Pint	0.062
Centimeter	Inch	0.3937		Pound	0.065
Centiweight	Kilograms	45.3		Quart	0.031
	Pounds	100		Tablespoons	2
Centner (Zentner)	Kilograms	50		Teaspoons	6
Cubic centimeter	Cubic inch	0.0610	Foot	Centimeters	30.48
	Fluid ounce	0.034		Inches	12
	Gram water at 4°C	1		Meters	0.305
	Milliliter	1		Mile	0.000189
	Pint	0.002	Gallon (US)	Cubic foot	0.1337
	Quart	0.001		Cups	16
Cubic foot	Cubic centimeters	28,316		Drops	61,440
	Cubic inch	1728		Fluid ounces	128
	Fluid ounces	957.51		Grams of fresh water	3785.4
	Gallons	7.481		Liters	3.785
	Grams of water	28,355		Milliliters	3785.3
	Liters	28.311		Ounces	135.52
	Pints	59.844		Pints	8
	Pounds of fresh water	62.426		Pounds of water	8.345
	Ounces	998.816		Quarts (US)	4
	Pints	59.844	Gallon (Imp)	Cubic foot	0.1605
	Quarts	29.922		Cubic inches	277.42
Cubic foot per second	Gallons per 24 hours	646,300		Gallons (US)	1.2
	Gallons per minute	694		Liters	4.5459
Cubic inch	Cubic centimeters	16.387		Quarts (US)	4.845
	Cubic feet	0.00058	Grain	Dram	0.0166
	Fluid ounce	0.554		Drop	1
	Gallon	0.0043		Gram	0.065
	Grams	16.39		Milligrams	64.8
	Liter	0.0164		Minim	1
	Ounce	0.576		Ounce	0.35
	Pint	0.035		Scruple	0.05
	Pound	0.036	Grain per gallon (US)	Parts per million	19.12
	Quart	0.017		Pounds per million gallons	142.9
Cubic meter	Cubic feet	35.314	Gram	Fluid ounce	0.034
	Cubic inches	61,024		Grains	15.432
	Liters	1000		Kilogram	0.001
Cup	Fluid ounces	8		Milligrams	1000
	Large jigger	4		Ounce	0.03527
	Liter	0.236		Pint	0.002
	Milliliters	237		Pound	0.0022
	Pint	0.5	Hectare	Acres	2.47
	Quart	0.25		Square meters	10,000
	Tablespoons	16	Inches	Centimeters	2.54
	Teaspoons	48		Millimeters	25.4
Doppel zentner (Double centner)	Kilograms	100	Jigger	Fluid ounces	1.5
				Tablespoons	3
Dram	Drops	60	Jigger (large)	Cup	0.25
	Grains	60		Fluid ounces	2
	Grams	1.772	Kilogram	Grams	1000
	Ounce	0.125		Pounds	2.205
	Scruples	3	Kiloliter	Cubic feet	35.315
Drop	Grain	1		Gallons	264.18
	Milliliter	0.05		Liters	1000
	Minim	1	Kilometer	Mile	0.62
	Scruple	0.05	Liquid ounce	Milliliters	29.57
Fathom	Feet	6	Liter	Cubic inches of water	61.025
	Meters	1.8288		Cubic foot of water	0.0353
	Mile	0.0011		Cups	4.23
	Yards	2		Fluid ounces	33.8
Fluid ounces	Cubic centimeters	29.57		Kilogram of water	1
	Cubic inches	1.8			

Table continued on following page

Conversions of Miscellaneous Units *Continued*

To Convert	To	Multiply By	To Convert	To	Multiply By
Liter *Continued*	Milliliters	1000	Percent in food	Grams per pound feed	4.5
	Ounces	35.28		Ounce per pound	0.2
	Pints	2.1134		Grains per pound	83
	Pounds of water	2.205		Parts per million	10,000
	Quarts (US)	1.057	Percent solution (1%)	Gram per gallon (US)	38
	Tablespoons	67.6		Grams per liter	10
	Teaspoons	203		Milliliters per gallon	38
Meter	Centimeters	100		Milliliters per liter	10
	Feet	3.28		Ounces per gallon (US)	1.3
	Inches	39.37		Ounces per cubic foot	9.9
Microgram	Milligram	0.001		Pound per cubic foot	0.624
Mile	Feet	5284		Pound per gallon (US)	0.083
	Kilometers	1.61	Pint	Cups	2
	Yards	1760		Fluid ounces	16
Milligram	Grain	0.0154		Liter	0.473
	Gram	0.001		Quart (US)	0.5
	Micrograms	1000	Pound	Cubic foot of water	0.016
Milliliter	Drops	20		Gallon (US) water	0.12
	Cubic inch	0.061		Grams	453.6
	Gallon (US)	0.0003		Grains	7000
	Gram of water	1		Kilogram	0.4536
	Liter	0.001		Ounces	16
	Pound of water	0.002	Pounds per acre	Kilograms per hectare	1.121
	Teaspoon	0.20	Pounds per million gallons	Part per million	0.1199
Millimeter	Inch	0.03937	Quart (US)	Cubic foot	0.0334
Nautical mile (international)	Fathoms	1013.33		Cubic inches	57.75
	Feet	6076.12		Cups	4
	Kilometers	1.852		Fluid ounces	32
	Miles	1.1507		Gallon	0.25
Number per hundred cubic centimeters	Number per cubic foot	9.29		Grams of water	946.36
				Liter	0.95
Ounce	Cup	0.125		Milliliters	946.36
	Fluid ounce	0.96		Ounces	33.36
	Gallon	0.0075		Pints	2
	Grains	480		Pounds of water	2.086
	Grams	28.35	Scruple	Dram	0.33
	Liter	0.029		Drops	20
	Milliliters	29.5		Grains	20
	Pint	0.06	Square foot	Square centimeters	930
	Pound	0.0625		Square meter	0.093
	Quart	0.03	Square meter	Square centimeters	10,000
	Tablespoons	2		Square feet	10.764
	Teaspoons	6		Square inches	1550
Oxygen in milliliters per liter	Oxygen in parts per million	1.429	Stone	Pounds	14
Oxygen in parts per million	Oxygen in milliliters per liter	0.7	Tablespoon	Cup	0.0624
				Jigger	0.333
				Milliliters	15
Parts per million	Grain per acre foot	1233		Ounce	0.5
	Grain per gallon (US)	0.0586		Teaspoons	3
	Gram per cubic foot	0.0283	Teaspoon	Drops	60
	Gram per cubic meter	1		Ounce	0.166
	Gram per gallon (US)	0.0038		Milliliters	5
	Milligram per gallon (US)	3.8		Tablespoon	0.333
	Milligram per liter	1	Ton (metric)	Kilograms	1000
	Ounce per cubic foot	0.001		Pounds	2204.6
	Ounce per 1000 cubic feet	1	Ton (US)	Kilograms	906
	Ounce per 1000 gallons	0.134		Pounds	2000
	Pound per acre foot	0.37	Yard	Centimeters	91.44
	Pound per cubic foot	0.0000623		Feet	3
	Pound per million gallons water	8.34		Inches	36
				Meter	0.914
Parts per thousand (1:1000)	Grams per gallon	3.8	Zentner (Centner)	Kilograms	50
	Gram per 100 milliliters	0.1			
	Ounce per gallon	0.13			

Temperature Conversions

To °C	°F or °C	To °F	To °C	°F or °C	To °F	To °C	°F or °C	To °F	To °C	°F or °C	To °F
−40	−40	−40	−12.22	10	50.0	5.56	42	107.6	22.78	73	163.4
−34.44	−30	−22	−11.67	11	51.8	6.11	43	109.4	23.33	74	165.2
			−11.11	12	53.6	6.67	44	111.2			
−28.89	−20	−4	−10.56	13	55.4				23.89	75	167.0
−28.33	−19	−2.2	−10	14	57.2	7.22	45	113.0	24.44	76	168.8
−27.78	−18	−0.4				7.78	46	114.8	25	77	170.6
−27.22	−17	1.4	−9.44	15	59.0	8.33	47	116.6	25.56	78	172.4
−26.67	−16	3.2	−8.89	16	60.8	8.89	48	118.4	26.11	79	174.2
			−8.33	17	62.6	9.44	49	120.2			
−26.11	−15	5.0	−7.78	18	64.4				26.67	80	176.0
−25.56	−14	6.8	−7.22	19	66.2	10.0	50	122.0	27.22	81	177.8
−25	−13	8.6				10.56	51	123.8	27.78	82	179.6
−24.44	−12	10.4	−6.67	20	68.0	11.11	52	125.6	28.33	83	181.4
−23.89	−11	12.2	−6.11	21	69.8	11.67	53	127.4	28.89	84	183.2
			−5.56	22	71.6	12.22	54	129.2			
−23.33	−10	14.0	−5.0	23	73.4				29.44	85	185.0
−22.78	−9	15.8	−4.44	24	75.2	12.78	55	131.0	30.0	86	186.8
−22.22	−8	17.6				13.33	56	132.8	30.56	87	188.6
−21.67	−7	19.4	−3.89	25	77.0	13.89	57	134.6	31.11	88	190.4
−21.11	−6	21.2	−3.33	26	78.8	14.44	58	136.4	31.67	89	192.2
			−2.78	27	80.6	15	59	138.2			
−20.56	−5	23.0	−2.22	28	82.4				32.22	90	194.0
−20	−4	24.8	−1.67	29	84.2	15.56	60	140.0	32.78	91	195.8
−19.44	−3	26.6				16.11	61	141.8	33.33	92	197.6
−18.89	−2	28.4	−1.11	30	86.0	16.67	62	143.6	33.89	93	199.4
−18.33	−1	30.2	−0.56	31	87.8	17.22	63	145.4	34.44	94	201.2
			0	32	89.6	17.78	64	147.2			
−17.78	0	32.0	0.56	33	91.4				35.0	95	203.0
−17.22	1	33.8	1.11	34	93.2	18.33	65	149.0	35.56	96	204.8
−16.67	2	35.6				18.89	66	150.8	36.11	97	206.6
−16.11	3	37.4	1.67	35	95.0	19.44	67	152.6	36.67	98	208.4
−15.56	4	39.2	2.22	36	96.8	20	68	154.4	37.22	99	210.2
			2.78	37	98.6	20.56	69	156.2			
−15	5	41.0	3.33	38	100.4				37.78	100	212.0
−14.44	6	42.8	3.89	39	102.2	21.11	70	158.0	38.33	101	213.8
−13.89	7	44.6				21.67	71	159.8	38.89	102	215.6
−13.33	8	46.4	4.44	40	104.0	22.22	72	161.6	39.44	103	217.4
−12.78	9	48.2	5.0	41	105.8				40.0	104	219.2

This table permits conversion from degrees Celsius to degrees Fahrenheit or vice versa. Locate the number to be converted in the center (bold) columns. To convert the number to Celsius read to the left. To convert the number to Fahrenheit, read to the right.

CELL LINE ABBREVIATIONS

Abbreviation	Origin	American Type Culture Collection Designation	Abbreviation	Origin	American Type Culture Collection Designation
A6	South African clawed toad	CCL 102	KF-1	Kokanee	
AS	Atlantic salmon		KO-6	Kokanee ovary	
ASH	Atlantic salmon heart				
			LBF-1	Largemouth bass	
BB	Brown bullhead	CCl 59	LBF-2	Largemouth bass	
BF-W	Bluegill sunfish				
BF-2	Bluegill fry	CCL 91	McCoy	Mouse	
BGL	Bluegill		MDCK	Canine	CCL 34
Bhk-21	Syrian hamster	CCl 10	MHR	Milkfish heart	
CaPi	Common carp pituitary		PG	Northern pike gonad	
CAR	Goldfish		PH	Perch heart	
CCO	Channel catfish ovary		PL	Perch liver	
CE-1	Asagi carp embryo		PS	Pike sarcoma	
CE-2	Kohaku carp embryo				
CHH-1	Chum salmon heart		RTF-1	Rainbow trout fry	
CHSE-214	Chinook salmon embryo	CRL 1681	RTG-2	Rainbow trout gonad	CCL 55
CrF	Atlantic croaker		RTH-149	Rainbow trout hepatoma	
CSE	Coho salmon embryo		RTM	Rainbow trout mesothelioma	
CCS-119	Coho salmon embryo		RTS	Rainbow trout spleen	
CyA-1	Sand seatrout muscle		SH01	White sturgeon heart	
CyA-2	Sand seatrout muscle		SK	Porcine	
CyN-1	Spotted seatrout muscle		SP-1	Silver perch	
EPC	Common carp hyperplasia		SSE-5	Sockeye salmon embryo	
			SS-2	White sturgeon spleen	
FHM	Fathead minnow	CCL 42	STE-137	Steelhead trout embryo	
FT	Bullfrog	CCL 41	SWT	Red swordtail	
G1B	Walking catfish gill		TH-1	Box turtle	CCL 50
GD1I	Walking catfish gonad		TO-2	Tilapia ovary	
GE-4	Guppy embryo				
GF	Bluestriped grunt	CCL 58	Vero	African green monkey	CCL 81
GK	Grouper kidney		VH2	Russell's viper	CCL 140
GL1	*Gekko gecko*	CCL 111	VSW	Russell's viper	CCL 129
HeLa	Human	CCL 2	WC-1	Walleye dermal sarcoma	
HEp-2	Human	CCL 23	We-2	Walleye embryo	
			WF-2	Walleye fry	
IgH-2	Iguana	CCL 108	WI-38	Human	CCL 75
			WISH	Human	CCL 25
K1K	Walking catfish kidney		WO	Walleye ovary	
KB	Human	CCL 17			

Appendix III

FISH DIAGNOSTIC LABORATORIES

Alabama
Southern Cooperative Fish Disease Laboratory
Auburn University
Department of Fisheries and Allied Aquaculture
Auburn, AL 36830

(205) 826-4786

Alaska
Fish Pathology Section
Alaska Department of Fish and Game
333 Raspberry Road
Anchorage, AK 99502

(907) 344-0541

Arizona
Hatchery Biologist
U.S. Fish and Wildlife Service
P.O. Box 398
Whiteriver, AZ 85941

(602) 338-4765

Region 2 Fish Health Center
P.O. Box 39
Pinetop, AZ 85941

(602) 338-5119

Arkansas
Arkansas Game and Fish Commission
P.O. Box 178
Lonoke, AR 72086

(501) 676-7963

Fish Health Services
P.O. Box 674
Pocahontas, AR 72455

(501) 892-8357

Greers Ferry National Fish Hatchery
Rt. 3, Box 71
Heber Springs, AR 72160

(501) 362-6038

Lonoke Agricultural Center
Highway East
Lonoke, AR 72086

(501) 676-3124

U.S. Fish and Wildlife Service
Fish Farming Experimental Station
P.O. Box 860
Stuttgart, AR 72160

(501) 673-8761

California
Department of Medicine
School of Veterinary Medicine
University of California
Davis, CA 95616

(916) 752-3411

Fish Disease Laboratory
California Department of Fish and Game
407 West Line St.
Bishop, CA 93514

(714) 872-2791

Fish Disease Laboratory
California Department of Fish and Game
2111 Nimbus Rd.
Rancho Cordova, CA 95670

(916) 355-0809

Fish Disease Unit
California Department of Fish and Game
Mojave River Hatchery
Victorville, CA 92392

(714) 245-9981

Fish Health Center
Route 1, Box 2105
Anderson, CA 96007

(916) 365-4271

Colorado
Fish Disease Control Center
U.S. Fish and Wildlife Service
P.O. Box 917
Fort Morgan, CO 80701

(303) 867-9497

Florida
Central Florida Veterinary Laboratory
Rt. 2, Box 259
Archer, FL 32618

(904) 495-3105

Department of Fisheries and Aquaculture and
College of Veterinary Medicine
7922 NW 71 St.
Gainesville, FL 32606

(904) 392-9617

Table continued on following page

Florida *Continued*
Florida Department. of Agriculture and Consumer Service
Division of Animal Industry
Kissimmee Diagnostic Laboratory
P.O. Box 420460
Kissimmee, FL 34742-0460

(407) 847-3185

Florida Department of Agriculture and Consumer Service
Division of Animal Industry
Live Oak Diagnostic Laboratory
Drawer O
Live Oak, FL 32060

(904) 362-1218

Hillsborough County Extension Office
5339 St. Rt. 579
Seffner, FL 33584

(813) 621-5605

Northwest Florida Aquaculture
Demonstration Farm
P.O. Box 754, Rt. 1
Blountstown, FL 32434

(904) 674-3184

Georgia
Fish Health Center
Rt. 1, Box 105
Warm Springs, GA 31830

(404) 655-3620

North Georgia Diagnostic Assistance Laboratory
College of Veterinary Medicine
University of Georgia
Athens, GA 30602

(404) 542-5260

Hawaii
Hawaii Institute of Marine Biology
University of Hawaii at Monoa
P.O. Box 1246
Coconut Island, Kaneohe, HI 96744

Idaho
Department of Fish and Wildlife Resources
University of Idaho
Moscow, ID 83843

(208) 885-6336

Fish Health Center
P.O. Box 18
Ahsahka, ID 83520

(208) 476-4591

Idaho Department of Fish and Game
Fish Disease Laboratory
Hagerman State Hatchery
Hagerman, ID 83332

(208) 837-6672

Illinois
Fisheries Research Laboratory
Southern Illinois University
Carbondale, IL 62901

(618) 536-7761

Iowa
State Conservation Commission
Big Springs Hatchery
Elkader, IA 52043

(319) 245-2446

Louisiana
Aquatic Animal Diagnostic Laboratory
School of Veterinary Medicine
Louisiana State University
Baton Rouge, LA 70803

(504) 346-3312

Louisiana Wildlife and Fisheries Commission
P.O. Box 4004
District II
Monroe, LA 71203

(318) 343-4044

Maine
Department of Inland Fisheries and Wildlife
8 Federal St.
Augusta, ME 04330

(207) 289-2535

Fish Disease/Pathology Laboratory
Center for Environmental Sciences
Unity College
Unity, ME 04988

Maryland
Aquatic Toxicology and Pathology Facility
Department of Pathology, 711 MSTF
University of Maryland School of Medicine
10 S. Pine St.
Baltimore, MD 21201

(410) 328-7230
FAX (410) 328-8414

Fish Disease Laboratories
Cooperative Oxford Biological Laboratory
Oxford, MD 21654

(410) 226-5193

Fish Disease Laboratory
Microbiology Department
University of Maryland
College Park Campus
College Park, MD 20740

(410) 405-5465

Massachusetts
Laboratory for Marine Animal Health
Marine Biological Laboratories
Woods Hole, MA 02543

(617) 548-3705

Michigan
Michigan Department of Natural Resources
Wolf Lake State Fish Hatchery
Fish Pathology Lab, 34270 CR 652
Mattawan, MI 49071

(616) 668-2132

Minnesota
Fish and Wildlife Pathology
Department of Natural Resources
390 Centennial Office Building
St. Paul, MN 55155

(612) 296-3043

Mississippi
Extension Wildlife and Fisheries
Mississippi State University
P.O. Box 5405
Mississippi State, MS 39762

(601) 325-3174

Mississippi *Continued*
Fish Diagnostic Laboratory
College of Veterinary Medicine
Drawer V
Mississippi State, MS 39762

(601) 325-3432

Mississippi Cooperative Extension Service
Fish Disease Diagnostic Laboratory
Box 142
Stoneville, MS 38776

(601) 686-9311

Mississippi Cooperative Extension Service
Fish Disease Diagnostic Laboratory
Box 631
Belzoni, MS 39038

(601) 247-2917

Missouri
Missouri Department of Conservation
666 W. Primrose
Springfield, MO 65807

(417) 883-6677

Montana
U.S. Fish and Wildlife Service
Fish Cultural Development Center
Route 2, Box 333
Bozeman, MT 59715

(406) 586-5419

Nevada
University of Nevada—Reno
Max C. Fleischmann College of Agriculture
Division of Veterinary Medicine
5305 Mill Street
Reno, NV 89502

(702) 784-6135

New Hampshire
State of New Hampshire Fish and Game Department
34 Bridge Street
Concord, NH 03301

(603) 271-2503

New Jersey
Pequest State Fish Hatchery
Oxford, NJ 07863

New York
Department of Biological Sciences
State University of New York
College at Brockport
Brockport, NY 14420

(716) 395-2729

Fish Diagnostic Laboratory
Department of Avian and Aquatic Animal Medicine
College of Veterinary Medicine
Cornell University
Ithaca, NY 14853

(607) 253-3365

Fish Disease Control Unit
Rome Fish Hatchery
New York State Department of Environmental Conservation
8314 Fish Hatchery Road
Rome, NY 13440

(315) 337-0910

Pathology Laboratory
Osborn Laboratories of Marine Sciences
New York Aquarium, New York Zoological Society
Boardwalk & West 8th Street
Brooklyn, NY 11224

(718) 265-3417

North Carolina
Department of Companion Animal and Special Species Medicine
College of Veterinary Medicine
North Carolina State University
4700 Hillsborough St.
Raleigh, NC 27606

(919) 829-4200

Fish Hatchery Biologist
P.O. Box 158
Pisgah Forest, NC 28768

(704) 877-3122

Rollins Disease Diagnostic Laboratory
Blue Ridge Road
Raleigh, NC 27606

(919) 733-3986

Oklahoma
Warm Water Hatchery Biologist Center
National Fish Hatchery
Tishomingo, OK 73460

(405) 384-5463

Oregon
Department of Microbiology
Nash Hall, Oregon State University
Corvallis, OR 97331

(503) 754-4441

Oregon Department of Fish and Wildlife
17330 S.E. Evelyn St.
Clackamas, OR 97015

(503) 657-2014

Oregon State University
Marine Science Center
Newport, OR 97365

(503) 867-3011

Pennsylvania
Benner Springs Fishery Research Center
Pennsylvania Fish Commission
P.O. Box 200-C
Bellefonte, PA 16823

(814) 355-4837

Fish Health Unit
N.E. Fisheries Center
P.O. Box 155
Lamar, PA 16848

(717) 726-6611

Rhode Island
Marine Pathology Laboratory
University of Rhode Island
Kingston, RI 02881

(401) 792-2334

Table continued on following page

South Carolina
Cooperative Extension Service
Attn. Dr. T. E. Schwedler
Department of Aquaculture Fisheries and Wildlife
G08 Lehotsky Hall
Clemson University
Clemson, South Carolina 29634-0362

(803) 656-2810

South Dakota
Fisheries Management Specialist
3305 W. South Street
Rapid City, SD 57701

(605) 394-2391

Tennessee
Department of Biology
University of Tennessee
Martin, TN 38238

Texas
Aquatic Station
Southwestern Texas State University
San Marcos, TX 78666

(512) 245-2284

Department of Life Sciences
Sam Houston State University
Huntsville, TX 77341

(409) 295-6211, ext. 2495

Department of Veterinary Microbiology
College of Veterinary Medicine
Texas A & M University
College Station, TX 77843

(713) 845-5941

Extension Fish Disease Specialist
Department of Wildlife and Fisheries
Room 202, Nagle Hall
Texas A & M University
College Station, TX 77843

(409) 845-7471

Utah
Utah State Division of Wildlife Resources
Fisheries Experiment Station
Rt. 1, Box 254
Logan, UT 84321

(801) 752-1066

Zoology Department
153 WIDB
Brigham Young University
Provo, UT 84602

(801) 374-1211, ext. 2495

Vermont
White River National Fish Hatchery
Rt. 2, Box 107
Bethel, VT 05032

(802) 234-5241

Virginia
Department of Pathobiology
Virginia-Maryland Regional College of Veterinary Medicine
Virginia Polytechnic Institute and State University
Blacksburg, VA 24061

(704) 231-7666

Virginia Institute of Marine Sciences
P.O. Box 162
Gloucester Point, VA 23062

(804) 642-4083

Washington
Fish Health Center
MP61.75R
State Road 14
Underwood, WA 98651

(509) 493-3156

Fish Health Center
3704 Griffin Lane, S.E.
Suite 101
Olympia, WA 98501

(206) 753-9046

Lower Columbia Fish Health Center
U.S. Fish and Wildlife Service
Box 17
Cook, WA 98605

(509) 538-2232

Olympia National Fish Health Center
2625 Parkmont Lane, Bldg. A
Olympia, WA 98502

(206) 753-9460

School of Fisheries, WH-10
University of Washington
Seattle, WA 98195

(206) 543-4290

U.S. Fish and Wildlife Service
9317 Highway 99, Suite 1
Vancouver, WA 98665

(206) 696-7605

Western Fish Disease Laboratory
Building 204, Naval Support Activity
Seattle, WA 98115

(713) 845-5941

West Virginia
Eastern Fish Disease Laboratory
U.S. Fish and Wildlife Service
National Fish Health Research Laboratory
Box 700
Kearneysville, WV 25430

(304) 725-8461

Wisconsin
Fish Disease Control Center
U.S. Fish and Wildlife Service
P.O. Box 1595
LaCrosse, WI 54602-1595

(608) 783-6451

Wyoming
Wyoming Fish and Game Laboratory
University of Wyoming
P.O. Box 3312
Laramie, WY 82071

(307) 745-5865

Puerto Rico
Fish Parasitologist
Department of Marine Science
Mayaguez, Puerto Rico 00708

Australia
Fish Disease Specialist
Snobs Creek Freshwater Fisheries Research Station and Hatchery
Fisheries and Wildlife Division
Private Bag 20
Alexandria, Victoria
Australia 3714

Fish Parasitologist
Zoology Department
James Cook University
Townsville, Australia QLD 4811

Fisheries and Wildlife Department
605 Flinders Street Extension
Melbourne, Australia 3000

Austria
Institute de Ichthyopathology
Veterinary Medicine
Linke Bahngasse 11
A1030 Wien
Austria

Bangladesh
Director of Fisheries
Department of Fisheries
Dacca
Bangladesh

Zoology Department
University of Dacca
Dacca-2
Bangladesh

Brazil
Fish Parasitologist
UFRRJ KM 47 Antiga Rod
Rio-S Paulo 23.460
Seropedica
Rio de Janeiro
Brazil

Fish Parasitology
Instituto Oswaldo Cruz
Edo Guanavara
Rio de Janeiro
Brazil

Burma
FAO/TA Inland Fishery Biologist
c/o UNDP
P.O. Box 650
Rangoon
Burma

Canada
British Columbia
Aquatic Parasitology Identification Center
E.V.S. Consultants
Box 8
Marine Tech Center
9865 West Saanich Road
Sidney, British Columbia
V8L 3S1 Canada

(604) 656-0741

Fish Health Program
Pacific Biological Station
Department of Fisheries and Oceans
Nanaimo, British Columbia
V9R 5K6 Canada

(604) 756-7062

Ontario
Department of Biology and Pathology
McMaster University
Hamilton, Ontario
Canada

(416) 525-9140

Fish Pathology Laboratory
Department of Pathology
Ontario Veterinary College
University of Guelph
Guelph, Ontario
N1G 2W1 Canada

(519) 824-4120

Nova Scotia
Fish Health Unit Maritimes
Department of Fisheries and Oceans
Biological Sciences Branch
Benthic Fisheries and Aquaculture Section
P.O. Box 550
Halifax, Nova Scotia
B3J 2S7 Canada

(902) 426-8381

Quebec
Department of Pathology and Microbiology
Faculty of Veterinary Medicine
University of Montreal
P.O. Box 5000
St. Hyacinthe, PQ
J2S 7C6 Canada

(514) 773-8521

Denmark
Fish Pathology
Den Konglige Veterinær og Landbohøjskole
Ambulatorisk Klinisk
Bulowsvej 13
17K 1870 Copenhagen V
Denmark

Finland
Parasitological Institute
Abo Akademi
Porthansgatan 20500
Abo 50, Finland

France
Laboratoire d'Ichtyopathologie
Route de Thiverval
78 Thiverval-Griguan
France

Laboratoire de Parasitologie
Place E. Bataillon
F 34060 Montpellier
France

Germany
Arbeitsgruppe Biologie der Fische
Universitat Hohenheim
Stuttgart
Germany

Bayerische Lundesanstalt
fur Wasserforschung Versuchsanlage Wielenbach
8121 Wielenbach
Germany

Table continued on following page

Germany *Continued*
Fischkrankheiten und Fischhaltung
Tierartliche Hochschule Hannover
Bunteweg 17
Bischofsholer Damm 15
3000 Hannover 1
Germany

Forschungstelle fur Wirbeltierforschung
Tierpark Berlin
Am Tierpark 125
1136 Berlin
Germany

Institute fur Binnenfischerie
Muggelseedamm 310
1162 Berline-Friedrichshagen
Germany

Institute fur Pathologi
Friedrich-Schiller Universitat
Zugelmuhlenweg 1
Jena 69
Germany

Great Britain
Institute of Agriculture
University of Stirling
Stirling, Scotland FX9 4LA

National Fish Disease Laboratory
The Nothe
Weymouth, England

National Marine Laboratory
Box 101
Victoria Road
Aberdeen, Scotland AB9

India
Central Inland Fisheries Research Institute
1/644 Sidhnathghat
Buxar, India

Fish Pathology Unit
Central Indian Fisheries Research Sub Station
19 Cantoninent Roat
Cuttack, 1 Orissa
India

U.P. College of Veterinary Science and Animal Husbandry
Mathura, India

Japan
Department of Fisheries
Faculty of Agriculture
University of Tokyo
Yayoii 1-1-1
Bunkyo-ku
Tokyo 113
Japan

Laboratory of Fish Pathology
Hokkaido Fish Hatchery
Makanoshima
Toyohira-ku
Sapporo, Hokkaido
Japan

Korea
Laboratory of Fish Diseases
Pusan Fisheries College
Pusan 601-01
Korea

New Zealand
Fisheries Research
Box 19062
Ministry of Agriculture
Wellington, New Zealand

Norway
Zoologisk Laboratorium
Universitet Bergen
10A N-500 Bergen
Norway

Russia
Ichthyopathology
All Union Institute of Pond Fisheries
Dmitrowchi Raion
P/O Rybnoe
Moscow 141821
Russia

State Institute of Freshwater Fisheries
Smolonaja 2
St. Petersburg (Leningrad) C-124
Russia

Zoological Institute
Academy of Sciences
St. Petersburg (Leningrad) B-34
Russia

South Africa
Division of Inland Fisheries
Private Bag 5011
Stellenbosch
South Africa

Sudan
Fisheries and Hydrobiological Research Section
P.O. Box 1489
Khartoum
Sudan

Sweden
Zoologiska Institut
Box 6801
Radmansgaton 70A
Stockholm 113 86
Sweden

Appendix IV

SOURCES OF SUPPLIES

Supplier	Generic Agent	Trademark
Abbott Laboratories Veterinary Division P.O. Box 68 Abbott Park North Chicago, IL 60064	Erythromycin	Gallimycin
Aqua Health Ltd. 1755 Steeles Ave. West Willowdale, Ontario M2R 3T4 Canada (416) 667–2678	Bacterins	
Aquarium Systems 8141 Tyler Blvd. Mentor, OH 44060	Sea salts	Instant Ocean
Argent Chemical Labs 8702 152nd Ave. N.E. Redmond, WA 98052 (800) 426–6258	Tricaine methane sulfonate	Finquel
Beecham Laboratories 501 5th St. Bristol, TN 37620	Amoxicillin	Amoxi-drops Amoxi-tabs
BioMed 1720 130th Ave. NE Bellevue, WA 98005–2203 (206) 882–0448	Bacterins	
Boots Pharmaceutical 300 Tri-State International Center Suite 200 Lincolnshire, IL 60069–4415 (708) 405-7400	Sodium levothyroxine	Synthroid
Bristol Laboratories Veterinary Products Division P.O. Box 657 Syracuse, NY 13201	Ketamine HCl	Ketaset Ketaject
Dainippon Pharmaceutical Co. Ltd. Osaka, Japan	Nifurpirinol	Furanace
Fort Dodge Laboratories P.O. Box 518 Fort Dodge, IA 50501	Chlorhexidine	Nolvasan
Glaxo Laboratories Ltd. Glaxo Group Res. Ltd. Glaxochem, Ltd. 891–995 Greenford Rd. Greenford, Middlesex UB6 OHE, U.K.	Alphadolone/alphaxalone	Saffan
Hach Chemical Company P.O. Box 389 Loveland, CO 80539	Water-testing kits	
Haver-Lockhart Division of Bayvet Miles Laboratories Shawnee, KS 66201	Niclosamide Praziquantel Xylazine	Yomesan Droncit Rompun

Table continued on following page

Supplier	Generic Agent	Trademark
Hoechst-Roussel Pharmaceuticals, Inc. 202–206 North, Box 2500 Somerville, NJ 08876 (800) 451-4455	Fenbendazole	Panacur Susp. 10%
Janssen Pharmaceutica 40 Kingsbridge Rd. Piscataway, NJ 08854 (201) 524-9591	Fentanyl Ketoconazole Mebendazole Miconazole Itraconazole	Sublimaze Nizoral Telmin Monistat
Kirkegaard and Perry 2 Cessna Ct. Gaithersburg, MD 20879 (301) 948–7755 (800) 638–3167	Diagnostic antisera Goat anti-	
Lederle Laboratories American Cyanamid Pearl River, NY 10965	Chlortetracycline Nystatin	Aureomycin Nilstat
Eli Lilly and Co. P.O. Box 618 Indianapolis, IN 42606	Thiamine HCl	Betalin
Lynteq Inc. 598 S. Milledge Ave. Suite 8 Athens, GA 30605 (800) 233–9379	Red dietary pigments	Biored
MSD-AGVET Division of Merck and Co. Inc. Merck Chemical Division P.O. Box 2000 Rahway, NJ 07065	Amprolium Cambendazole Ivermectin Thiabendazole	Amprol Camvet Ivomec Omnizole
Marion Merrell Dow Pharmaceuticals, Inc. Subsidiary of Dow Chemical Co. 9300 Ward Pkwy. P.O. Box 8480 Kansas City, MO 64114–0480	Rifampin	Rifadin
Micrologix International 101–9865 West Saanich Rd. Sidney, British Columbia V8L 3Y3, Canada (604) 655–1455	Diagnostic antisera Rabbit anti- Mouse anti-	
Microtek Research and Development Ltd. P.O. Box 2460 100–9865 West Saanich Rd. Sidney, British Columbia V8L 3Y3 Canada (604) 655–1455	Diagnostic antisera Rabbit anti- Sheep anti-	
Norden Laboratories, Inc. P.O. Box 80809 Lincoln, NE 68521	Nitrofurazone	Furacin
Novalek, Inc. 2242 Davis Court Hayward, CA 94545	Water-testing kits	
Parke-Davis and Co. 201 Tabor Rd. Morris Plains, NJ 07950	Ketamine HCl Chloramphenicol Posterior pituitary injection	Ketalar Vetalar Chloromycetin Pituitrin
Pfizer, Inc. Agriculture Div. 235 E. 42nd St. New York, NY 10017	Neomycin sulfate Oxytetracycline	Neo-terramycin Soluble Powder Terramycin Soluble Powder
Pitman-Moore, Inc. P.O. Box 344 Washington Crossing, NJ 08560	Fentanyl citrate/droperidol Levamisole phosphate Mebendazole Rotenone	Innovar-Vet Levasole Telmin Canex

Supplier	Generic Agent	Trademark
A.H. Robins Co., Inc. 1407 Cummings Drive Richmond, VA 23220	Doxapram HCl	Dopram V
Roche Laboratories Hoffman-LaRoche, Inc. 340 Kingsland St. Nutley, NJ 07110	Diazepam 5-fluorocytosine Vitamins D_3 and A	Valium Ancoban Injecom
Salsbury Laboratories 2000 Rockford Rd. Charles City, IA 50616	Dimetridazole	Emtryl
Schering Corporation P.O. Box 529 Kenilworth, NJ 07033	Flunixin meglumine Gentamicin sulfate Melengestrol acetate Porcine follicle-stimulating hormone	Banamine Gentocin Ovaban Fsh-6
Searle Laboratories Div. of Searle Pharm. P.O. Box 5110 Chicago, IL 60680	Metronidazole	Flagyl
Shell Chemical Co. 235 Peachtree St. Atlanta, GA 30303	Dichlorvos	Atgard, Task
SmithKline & French Laboratories 1500 Spring Garden St. P.O. Box 7929 Philadelphia, PA 19101	Cimetidine	Tagamet
E.R. Squibb & Sons, Inc. Box 4000 Princeton, NJ 08540	Amphotericin B Nystatin, neomycin sulfate, thiostrepton, and triamcinolone acetonide	Fungizone Panalog
Upjohn Company 301 Henrietta St. Kalamazoo, MI 49001	Kaolin and pectin Methylprenisolone Neomycin sulfate	Kaopectate Depo-Medrol Biosol
West Chemical Products Inc. 42–16 West St. Long Island, NY 11101	Povidone-iodine	Prepodyne
Wildlife Laboratories Inc. 1322 Webster Ave. Ft. Collins, CO 80524 (800) 482–6267	Metomidate	Marinil
Winthrop Laboratories 90 Park Ave. New York, NY 10016	Benzalkonium chloride	Zephiran

Appendix V

CHEMOTHERAPEUTICS

This appendix is a compilation. Published information is included relatively uncritically. Unpublished personal communications have been solicited, but even so, numerous gaps remain. Most of the drugs in the tables are NOT approved by the U.S. Food and Drug Administration for use in food fish and represent extra label use.

The tabular format was selected for the convenience of clinicians needing information quickly to plan therapeutic regimens. There are advantages and limitations to this presentation. The primary advantage is easy accessibility. The primary weakness is the limited amount of information that can be presented with each entry. The tables cannot and are not intended to replace a strong background in clinical veterinary pharmacology.

Injectable Chemotherapeutics

Drug	Dose	Frequency	Route	Indication	Comment
Amikacin	5 mg/kg	BID	IM	Bacterial infections	No kinetics
Ampicillin	10 mg/kg	OID	IM	Bacterial infections	Sharks
Atropine	0.1 mg/kg	PRN	IM, IP, IV	Organophosphorus or chlorinated hydrocarbon toxicity	Sharks
BAL	4 mg/kg	QID, PRN	IM	Heavy metal toxicity	Until recovered
Calcium EDTA	25 mg/kg	QID	IP	Heavy metal toxicity	10 mg/ml in 5% dextrose
Chloramphenicol succinate	40 mg/kg	OID	IM	Bacterial infections	Sharks
Cloxacillin	10 mg/kg	BID	IM	Bacterial infections	
Dexamethasone	1–2 mg/kg	QID	IM, IP, IV	Shock, adrenal exhaustion	Sharks
Dextran	20 ml/kg	PRN	IV	Hypovolemia	To effect
Dextrose (5%)	20–30 ml/kg	PRN	IP, IV	Dehydration	Sharks
	40–50 ml/kg			Severe dehydration	Sharks
Diazepam	0.1–0.25 mg/kg	OID	IV	Appetite stimulant	Moray eels
Dihydrostreptomycin	10 mg/kg	OID	IM	Bacterial infections	Sharks
Dipyrone	25 mg/kg	OID	IM	Anti-inflammatory Analgesic	
Doxapram	5 mg/kg	PRN	IP, IV	Respiratory depression	Sharks
Epinephrine (1:1000)	0.2–0.5 ml		IP, IM, IV, IC	Cardiac arrest	
Flumequin	30 mg/kg	OID	IP	Furunculosis	
Flumethasone	0.2 mg	OID	IM	Immunosuppressant	
Flunixin meglumine	0.3 mg/kg	Once a week	IM	Adrenal exhaustion	Sharks
Furosemide	2–3 mg/kg	BID	IP, IM	Ascites, generalized edema	Sharks
Gentamicin	6 mg/kg	Every 6 days	IM	Gram-negative bacteria	Sharks, bioavailability in channel catfish is 60%
	1.6 mg/kg	Every 33 hours	IV		
	3 mg/kg	OID	IM		
Heparin	200 U/kg	Q4h, PRN	IV, IP	Disseminated intravascular coagulopathy	Sharks
Insulin	2 U/kg	Q2h	IV	Diabetes	To effect
Ivermectin	100 μg/kg	Once	IM	Nematode, cestode, crustacean parasitism	Toxicity can occur
Kanamycin	20 mg/kg	OID	IP	Bacterial infections	
Ketaconazole	5 mg/kg	OID	IM	Systemic fungal disease	Sharks
Lactated Ringer's	20–60 ml/kg/day	PRN	IV, IP	Dehydration	In divided doses
Lactolyl tetrapeptide	1 mg/kg	Once	IP	Immunostimulant	Rainbow trout, increased (FK 565) nonspecific phagocytosis
Levamisole	11 mg/kg	Twice, 1 week apart	IM	Nematode parasitism	
Lidocaine	1–2 mg/kg	PRN	IV	Cardiac arrhythmia	Bolus
Lincomycin	2.5 mg/kg	BID	IM	Bacterial infections	
Mannitol	1–2 g/kg	QID	IV	Diuresis	
Methicillin	10 mg/kg	QID	IM, IV	Gram-positive bacteria	
Miconazole	10 mg/kg	OID	IM	Systemic fungal disease	Sharks
	5 mg/kg		IP		
Minocycline	0.5 mg/kg	OID	IM	Bacterial infections— mycobacteria	
Nitrofurantoin	3 mg/kg	BID	IM	Bacterial infections	
Oxytetracycline	10 mg/kg	OID	IM	Bacterial infections	Sharks, goldfish peak 14 hr after IM injection, 80% bioavailable. Peak 10 hr after injection. Immunosuppressive at these doses
	10 mg/kg	OID	IM		
	40 mg/kg	OID	IP	Protozoan infections	

Injectable Chemotherapeutics *Continued*

	Dose	Frequency	Route	Indication	Comment
	40 mg/kg	PRN	IV, IP	Organophosphate or chlorinated hydrocarbon toxicity	Trout, half-life 80 hr
	0.15 mg/kg		IV	α-Adrenergic agonist vasoconstriction	African catfish, half-life 89 hr
	2 mg/kg	BID	IM	Bacterial infections	
Prednisolone	1 mg/kg	BID	IP, IV, IM	Shock	Sharks
Ringer's Solution	18 ml/kg	PRN	IV, IP	Dehydration	
Sulfadimethoxine	25 mg/kg	OID	IV, IM	Bacterial infections	
Sulfadimidine	75 mg/kg	Every 2 days	IP	Bacterial infections	Peak levels in 2 hr
Sulfamethazine	50 mg/kg	BID	IV	Bacterial infections	
Thiamine HCl	1 mg/kg	OID	IM	Vitamin B deficiency	Follow with oral
Thyroxine	20 μg/kg	OID	IM	Hypothyroidism	Sharks initial starting dose, titrate to serum levels
Tobramycin	6 μg/kg	Every 6 days	IM	Bacterial infections	Poorly absorbed from gut. Some resistant strains
Tylosin	5 mg/kg	BID	IM, IV	Bacterial infections	
Vitamin B$_{12}$	200 μg/day	OID	IM	Vitamin B deficiency	

Orally Administered Chemotherapeutics

Drug	Dose	Frequency	Indication	Comment
Acetylsalicylic acid	5 mg/kg	OID	Anti-inflammatory	Reduces leukotriene production
Acetarsone	1 g/kg food	OID for 3–4 days	*Eimeria* sp.	
Ampicillin	10 mg/kg	BID	Bacterial infections	Sharks
Amprolium	150 mg/kg	OID for 7–10 days	Protozoan infections— *Microsporidium* sp.	
	600 mg/kg	OID for 48 days		
Ascorbic Acid	700 mg/kg food	OID	Vitamin deficiency—Tang head erosions	
Aureomycin	10 mg/kg	OID	Bacterial infections	
Cambendazole	20 mg/kg	Q7D	Nematodes	Sharks, 3 doses
	10 mg/kg	Daily for 2 weeks		
Carbenicillin	200 mg/kg	OID	Bacterial infections	Sharks, poor acceptance, fouls the water
Cephalexin (Keflex)	40 mg/kg	BID	Bacterial infections	
Chloramphenicol palmitate	1 g/kg food	OID	Bacterial infections	Gray's syndrome in susceptible humans
	50–100 mg/kg fish			
Chlortetracycline	10–20 mg/kg	BID	Bacterial infections	
		OID		
Cimetidine	5–10 mg/kg	QID	Gastrointestinal distress	
Ciprofloxacin	5 mg/kg	OID	Bacterial infections	Quinalone
Clindamycin HCl	75 mg/kg	OID for 10 days	Bacterial infections	Prophylaxis *Renibacterium salmoninarum*
	150 mg/kg	OID for 14 days		Treatment Gram-positive bacteria
Dexamethasone	0.2–1.0 mg/kg	OID	Shock	
Diazepam	1–4 mg/kg	OID	Appetite stimulant	Large groupers
Dichlorvos	30 mg/kg	Once	Nematodes	
	20 mg/kg	Once		
Difloxacin	5 mg/kg	OID	Bacterial infections	Aryl-fluoroquinolone Low resistance potential
Dihydrostreptomycin	10 mg/kg	OID	Bacterial infections	
Dimetridazole	150 mg/100 g food	OID 5 days	*Hexamita* spp.	
Diphenhydramine	2–4 mg/kg	BID	Histamine antagonist	
Diphenylhydantoin	50–80 mg/kg	BID	Antiepileptic	
Doxycycline	2 mg/kg	OID	Streptococcosis	
Enrofloxacin	5 mg/kg	OID for 10 days	Bacterial septicemia	Quinalone
Erythromycin	20 mg/kg	Once	Prophylaxis against vertical transmission of *Renibacterium salmoninarum*	NOT EFFECTIVE Feed levels of 10 mg/g or higher are frequently rejected, palatability problems even at lower concentrations
	90–100 mg/kg	OID for 21 days		Australian recommendations for bacterial kidney disease in feed
Erythromycin thiocyanate	100 mg/kg	OID for 10 days	Prophylaxis *Renibacterium salmoninarum* treatment	In feed
	150 mg/kg	OID for 14 days		In feed
Erythromycin phosphate	100 mg/kg	OID for 10 days	Prophylaxis *Renibacterium salmoninarum* treatment	In feed
	150 mg/kg	OID for 14 days		In feed
Fenbendazole	11 mg/kg	OID twice	Nematodes	

Table continued on following page

Orally Administered Chemotherapeutics *Continued*

Drug	Dose	Frequency	Indication	Comment
Florfenicol	30 mg/kg	OID	Bacterial infections	Channel catfish, in feed
Fludrocortisone	0.5 mg	OID	Immunosuppressant	
Flumequine	0.5 g/kg	OID	Broad-spectrum antibacterial furunculosis, *Yersinia ruckeri*	Quinolone antibiotic ineffective against *Renibacterium salmoninarum* Residues out of flesh in 96 hr In feed
Flumethasone	0.2 mg	OID	Anti-inflammatory, long-acting	
Folic acid	5 mg/kg	OID	Vitamin deficiency	Sharks
Fumagillin	1 g/kg feed fed at 1% of body weight per day	OID for 5 weeks	Antimicrosporidial	Effective against *Sphaerospora* late stages only. Not effective against *Myxobolus cyprini* or *Thelohanellus nickolskii*. Arrests *Pleistophora* sp. development but does not effect cure. Also carcinogenic
	50 mg/kg	OID for 3 days	*Glugea* sp.	
	5 mg/kg	OID for 60 days	*Pleistophora* sp.	
	100 mg/kg food	OID for 14 days	*Sphaerospora* sp.	
Furazolidone	25 mg/kg	OID for 20 days	Antimicrosporidial	Inhibits spread and reduces severity of whirling disease but does not cure Mutagenic
Furosemide	2.5–5.0 mg/kg	BID	Edema, ascites	
Gentamicin	0.75 mg/kg		Bacterial infections	Poorly absorbed in gut
	2–3 mg/kg	OID		Some resistant strains
Glycerin	0.5 mg/kg	BID, TID	Constipation	
Griseofulvin	50 mg/kg	OID	Deep fungal infections	
Hetacillin	20 mg/kg	TID	Bacterial infections	
Hydrocortisone	4 mg/kg	BID	Anti-inflammatory	
Isoniazid	2 mg/kg	OID	Mycobacteriosis	
Isuprel (elixir)	0.4 mg/kg	BID, TID	Bradycardia, cardiac insufficiency	
Kanamycin	20 mg/kg	OID	Bacterial infections	Sharks
	10 mg/kg	QID		Poorly absorbed in gut Some resistant strains
Kaopectate	1 ml/kg	QID	Enteritis, gastritis	
Ketaconazole	5 mg/kg	OID	Systemic fungal disease	Sharks
Kitasamycin	125 mg/kg	OID for 10 days	Prophylaxis *Renibacterium salmoninarum*	In feed
	150 mg/kg	OID for 14 days	Treatment gram-positive bacteria	In feed
Levamisole	10 mg/kg	3 doses 7 days apart	Nematodes	Sharks
	400 mg in 100 g food	3 doses 7 days apart		
	5 g/L	3 doses 7 days apart		
	as soak for live food			
Levo-thyroxine	10 μg/kg	OID	Hypothyroidism	
Lincomycin	200 mg/kg food	OID for 14 days	Gram-positive bacteria	In feed
	2.5 mg/kg	BID	*Renibacterium salmoninarum*	Low cross-resistance
Mebendazole	20 mg/kg	Weekly for 3 treatments	Nematodes	
Methotrexate	0.05 mg/kg	OID	Immunosuppressant	
Metronidazol	50 mg/kg	OID for 5 days	Protozoan infection for flagellates, Hexamita	Sharks, angelfishes
	1 g/100 g food	OID for 5 days		
Miconazole	10 mg/kg	OID	Systemic fungal disease	Sharks
	5 mg/kg	OID		
Minocycline	0.5 mg/kg	OID	Bacterial infections, mycobacteriosis	
Nalidixic acid	20 mg/kg	OID	Bacterial infections	Quinolone
Neomycin	20 mg/kg	QID	Bacterial enteritis	Sharks, given once as a prophylaxis for transport bloat. Poorly absorbed from gut. Some resistant strains
Niclosamide	200 mg/kg	Twice 2 weeks apart	Cestodes	Repeat in 10 days
	5 g/kg diet		*Bothriocephalus* sp., *Khawia* sp.	
Nitrofurantoin	4 mg/kg	TID	Bacterial enteritis	
Nitrofurazone	50 mg/kg	OID	Bacterial enteritis	Sharks
	75–100 mg/kg	OID 5–15 days	Microsporidial infections	Controls but does not eliminate *Pleistophora* sp. in golden shiners. Stops fish reproduction
Nitrofurpuranol	2–4 mg/kg	OID	Bacterial infections	
Norfloxacin	8 mg/kg	OID	Bacterial infections	Quinolone
Nystatin	100,000 U	QID	Fungal infections	
Ofloxacin	10 mg/kg	OID	Bacterial infections	
Ormetoprim (see Sulfadimethoxine/Ormetoprim)				
Oxacillin	20 mg/kg	BID	Bacterial infections	

Orally Administered Chemotherapeutics *Continued*

Drug	Dose	Frequency	Indication	Comment
Oxolinic acid	8.5 mg/kg	OID for 7–10 days	Bacterial infections Furunculosis	Quinolone Resistant strains exist Residues 21 days in trout at 17°C
Oxytetracycline	60–75 mg/kg 20 mg/kg	OID TID	Bacterial infections *Aeromonas* sp., *Edwardsiella* sp., *Yersinia* sp.	Sharks Less than 1% bioavailable, generally more effective than chlortetracycline. Resistant strains common. Apparently not immunosuppressive at these doses
Penicillin G (Na)	125 mg/kg	OID for 21 days	Bacterial infections Bacterial kidney disease	
Penicillin (K)	40,000 U/kg	TID, QID	Bacterial infections	
Pepto-Bismol	2 ml/kg	QID	Gastritis, enteritis	
Piperazine	110 mg/kg	Once	Nematodes	
Praziquantel HCl	400 mg/100 g food 500 mg/kg	OID for 7 days Once	Trematodes *Diplostomum sanguinicola* Cestodes *Bothriocephalus* sp.	Sharks
Prednisolone	1 mg/kg 3 mg/kg	BID BID	Allergy therapy Immunosuppression for shock	
Pyridoxine	0.25 mg/kg	OID	Deficiency	
Quinacrine	75 mg	BID for 3 days	Protozoan infection	Repeat in 3 days
Riboflavin	10 mg/kg	OID	Deficiency	Sharks
Rifampicin	10 mg/kg 5 mg/kg 6 mg/100 g food	OID for 14 days OID OID	Gram-positive bacterial infections	In feed
Sarafoxacin	10–14 mg/kg	OID for 10 days	Bacterial infections	Aryl-fluoroquinolone Low resistance potential Channel catfish In feed
Spiramycin	200 mg/kg	OID for 14 days	Gram-positive bacterial infections	In feed
Streptomycin	25 mg/kg	OID	Broad-spectrum antibacterial	Poorly absorbed from gut Some resistant strains
Stanozolol	2–4 mg	BID	Appetite stimulant	
Styrid-caracide	0.1 ml/kg	OID	Filarial nematodes	
Sulfadiazine	220 mg/kg	Once, followed by 5 days at half of initial dose	Protozoan infections Bacterial infections	
Sulfadimethoxine/ ormetoprim	42/8 mg/kg	In feed	*Vibrio* spp., furunculosis, *Edwardsiella tarda*, *E. ictaluri* *Yersinia ruckeri*	Withdrawal 6 wk salmonids, 3 days catfish. Tissue tolerance 0.1 ppm. Resistant bacteria common. *Flexibacter* sp. often resistant. Peak levels at 20 hr. Bioavailability 38%
Sulfamerazine	42 mg/kg 220 mg/kg	OID OID, 14 days	Prophylaxis for bacterial kidney disease Furunculosis	In feed
Thyroxine	20 µg/kg	OID	Hypothyroidism	Sharks, initial starting dose titrate to serum levels
Thiabendazole	66 mg/kg	OID	Nematodes	Twice, 10 days apart
Thyroid (desiccated)	10 mg/kg	OID	Hypothyroidism	Possible renal toxicity in coho salmon
Tiamulin	5 mg/kg	OID for 14 days	*Yersinia ruckeri*. Gram-positive and some Gram-negative bacterial infections	15 times margin of safety in rainbow trout. Bacteriostatic. Not effective against *Pseudomonas* sp., *Proteus* sp., *Alcaligenes* sp.; is effective against spirochetes
Tribrissen	1 mg/kg	OID for 14 days	*Yersinia ruckeri*. Broad-spectrum antibacterial	(Trimethoprim-sulfadiazine) Effective against *Escherichia*, *Streptococcus*, *Proteus*, *Salmonella*, *Pasteurella*, *Shigella*, *Yersinia*
Trimethoprim- sulfadiazine (see Tribrissen)				
Tylosin	10 mg/kg	TID for 10 days	Bacterial infections	In feed
Vitamin A	500 U/kg	OID for 14 days	Vitamin A deficiency Wound healing	Sharks
Vitamin B$_{12}$	200 µg/day	Q3D	Deficiency Appetite stimulant	3 treatments
Vitamin D	30 U/kg	Q7D	Deficiency	3 treatments
Vitamin E	100 IU/kg	Q3D	Deficiency Oxidative stress	

Baths, Dips, and Water Treatments

Drug	Dose	Duration	Frequency	Indication	Comment
Acetic acid (glacial)	0.5 ml/L	30 sec	Every other day for 4 times	Protozoa, external Trematodes	
	2 ml/L	30 sec		Nematodes, crustaceans	
Acryflavin (neutral)	5–10 mg/L	Prolonged bath	Continuous	Protozoa	Kills plants
	500 mg/L	30 min	Daily	Bacteria	
Acyclovir (Acycloquanosine)	25 mg/L	30 min	Daily for 15 days	Antiviral	Effective against *Herpesvirus salmonis*. Not effective orally. Efficacy questionable
Amprolium	10 mg/L	Prolonged bath	Continuous 7–10 days	*Eimeria* sp.	
Antimycin A	20–200 μg/L	15 min	Once	Kill scaled fishes prior to stocking catfish in production ponds	TOXIC TO SCALED FISHES
	2–10 μg/L	Indefinite	Once	Pond treatment	
Atabrine	10 mg/L	48 hr	Once	Protozoa	Used in guppy, catfishes, trout
Aureomycin	13 mg/L	5 min	Once	*Oodinium* sp.	Question efficacy
Bacitracin	60–75 mg/L	Indefinite	Once	Bacteria	Not absorbed systemically
Basic bright green oxalate (Brilliant Green)	60 mg/L	45 sec	Once	Protozoa, fungi	
	1 mg/L	2.5 hr	Once	Protozoa, fungi	
Basic violet (Bayluscide)	0.1 mg/L	2 hr	Once	Protozoa	
Bayer 73	112–224 kg/ha	Indefinite	Once	Lampricide, molluscide	Non–food fish use only. Kills minnows, salmonids tilapia for up to 3 weeks after treatment
Baygon	1 mg/L	1 hr	Once	Crustaceans, leeches	Kills fish. Not effective against *Lernea* sp.
Benzalkonium chloride	1–2 mg/L	1 hr	Daily	Less effective in hard water	
Bithionol	20 mg/L	3 hr	Once	*Gyrodactylus* sp.	Trout
Calcium hypochlorite	200 mg/L	1 hr	Once	To sanitize and control algae and *Eimeria* sp.	Will kill fish at higher dose
	5–10 mg/L	12–24 hr	Once		
Chloramine-T	10 mg/L	1 hr	Once	Disinfectant treatment for *Pseudomonas* sp. Bacterial gill disease	Less toxic than other N-chloramines, registered under EPA 10575-1 as disinfectant but not for use with live fish. Currently under investigation, FDA INAD 4618
Chloramphenicol					Not effective as bath
Chloroquine	10 mg/L	Indefinite	Once	Protozoa	Used to control *Cryptocaryon irritans*
Closantel	0.125 mg/L	3 hr		*Gyrodactylus* sp.	Trout
Copper sulfate	0.0001 mg/L	Indefinite	Continuous	Protozoa	
	500 mg/L	1 min			
	2.3–4.0 mg/L	Indefinite		Algae control	
Dexamethasone	10 mg/L	1 hr			
Dichlobenil	7–17 kg/ha	Indefinite	Once	Herbicide	Not for use with food fish
Dichlone	55 μg/L	Continuous	Once	Algicide	Non–food fish only
Dichlorvos	0.2 mg/kg	Continuous	Weekly for 4 weeks	Monogenea, digenea Crustaceans	
Dimilin	0.01 mg/L	48 hr	3 treatments 6 days apart	Crustaceans	Chitin synthesis inhibitor. Kills nuplii, affects molt of adults. 76% of chemical persists at least 1 week in pond water
Diquat	5.4 mg/L	Prolonged bath	Once	Submerged weeds	
	3.4 kg/ha			Floating weeds	
Dylox (see Trichlorfon)					
Endothall	2.5–3.5 g/m³	Prolonged bath	Once	Herbicide	
Fenae	16.8–21.9 kg/ha			Herbicide	Non–food fish only
Flumequine	50 mg/L	1 hr	Once	Bacteria	Effective serum levels in brown trout and Atlantic salmon for 14 days at temperatures above 7°C. Absorption increased in lower pH. Calcium inhibits absorption
	50 mg/L	30 min		Furunculosis	
	100 mg/L	30 min			
Fluorescein sodium	0.1 mg/L			Check water flow	
Flumethasone	0.2 mg	OID	Once	Shock	

Baths, Dips, and Water Treatments *Continued*

Drug	Dose	Duration	Frequency	Indication	Comment
Formaldehyde (37%)	0.4 ml/L (softwater) 0.5 ml/L (hardwater) 2 ml/L (marine water)	Up to 1 hr	Every 3 days Up to 3 times if needed	Protozoa, monogenea, digenea, crustaceans	Effect on fish is highly species specific
Fresh water		5 min	Daily for 5 days	Protozoa, monogenea, digenea	For marine fishes
Furanace	0.05–0.1 mg/L 1 mg/L	Indefinite 5–10 min		Bacteria	Non–food fish only
Gentamicin					Not effective as bath
Gentian violet	0.3 mg/L	Indefinite	Continuous	Fungi, protozoa, *Cleidodiscus* sp.	Toxic to some fishes
Hyamine 3500	2 ppm	2 min	Once	Disinfectant treatment for bacterial gill disease, myxobacteria	FDA considers appropriate for routine disinfection of water, gear, tanks
Hydrocortisone	10 mg/L	10–30 min	As needed	Shock	
Hydrogen peroxide (3%)	17.5 ml/L	10 min	Once	Protozoa, monogenea	
Iodine	7% tincture			Paint on wound and rinse immediately	
Ipropran	3–4 mg/L	6–12 hr	Once	Hexamita	
Kanamycin	750 mg/L	2 hr	OID	Bacteria	Channel catfish
Lime (quick)	1165 kg/ha		Once	Pond sterilant	
Lime (slaked)	2002 kg/ha		Once		
Levamisol	2 mg/L	24 hr	Once	Nematodes Swimbladder worms	Most effective against larval nematodes, no
	50 mg/L	2 hr	Once	Trematodes	increase in effectiveness with higher dose. LD$_{50}$ for eels 250 mg/L. Single treatment kills about 50% of nematode load
Magnesium sulfate	70 g/L	5 min	Once	Cathartic	Freshwater only
Malachite green	0.1%	Paint on wound and rinse	Caution	Fungi	NOT approved by FDA, persistent tissue levels, mutagenic, teratogenic.
	67 mg/L	1 min			Toxic to tetras, gill
	0.2 mg/L	1 hr			damage, more toxic at
	0.1 mg/L	Indefinite			warm temperatures
	1.5 g/L	10 sec			Catfish
Mebendazole	1 mg/L	24 hr	Once	*Pseudodactylogyrus* sp.	
	100 mg/L	2 hr	Once		
6-Mercaptopurine	Not established			Antiviral	Prevents development of lymphocystis lesions, effective against IPN
Methylene blue	3 mg/L	Prolonged bath up to 5 days	Continuous	Cyanide toxicity	
	50 mg/L	10 sec		Fungi	
Metronidazole	50 mg/L	Up to 24 h	Repeat daily for 10 days	*Hexamita*	Change water with each treatment, poorly soluble
Neguvon (see Trichlorfon)					
Nitrofurpyrinol	2 mg/L	19 hr	Once	Antiprotozoan	Effective against *Chilodonella* but not *Ichthyophthirius*. Toxic to trout, not effective in salt water
	0.07 mg/L	Indefinite bath	Daily	*Aeromonas*, sp.	Cause skin and gill
	1 mg/L	1 hr		*Cytophaga*, sp. *Flexibacter*, sp. *Flavobacterium*, *Edwardsiella tarda*, sp.	lesions in catfish, mutagenic and carcinogenic. Use prohibited by FDA.
Nitroscanate	0.07 mg/L	3 hr	Once	*Gyrodactylus* sp. Trout	
Oxytetracycline	400 mg/L	1 hr	Daily for 7 days	Bacteria	Salt water
	100 mg/L	1 hr		Bacteria	Fresh water
Ozone	0.1 mg/L	60 sec	Daily for 7 days	Disinfectant	Effective against *Aeromonas salmonicida*,
	70 mg/L	10 min			*A. hydrophila, Yersinia ruckeri.* Destroys IHN
	90 mg/L	10 min			virus in hard water.
	90 mg/L	30 sec			Destroys IPN virus in hard water. May control myxosporidian infective stages. Destroys IPN virus in soft water. Controls *Saprolegnia* on eggs.

Table continued on following page

Baths, Dips, and Water Treatments *Continued*

Drug	Dose	Duration	Frequency	Indication	Comment
2-Phenoxytethanol	100 mg/L	1-hr bath	Once	Fungi	Can be toxic to goldfish.
Potassium permanganate	1 g/L	30–40 sec		Only in acid water	Food fish use
	20 mg/L	1 hr		Crustaceans, protozoa	
	2–5 mg/L	Indefinite			
Povidone-iodines	1:10 in water	Topical paint and rinse		Bacteria, fungi Disinfectant	Not effective controlling intraovum bacteria or as virucide
Praziquantel HCl	10 mg/L	3 hr		Trematodes Cestodes *Dactylogyrus* sp. *Diplozoon* sp. *Proteocephalus* sp.	Levels can cause toxicity in Corydoras catfishes. Repeat treatment at weekly intervals for 3 weeks for egg-laying monogenes
Quaternary ammonia	1 mg/L	10 min			
Quinine hydrochloride	30 mg/L	1 hr	Daily for 3 days continuous	Protozoa	Used to control *Cryptocaryon irritans*
	10 mg/L	3 days			
Quinine sulfate	30 mg/L	1 hr	Daily for 3 days	Protozoa	
Rhodamine B	20 μg/L			Check water flow	Food fish use
Ribavirin	20 mg/L		Prolonged bath continuous	Antiviral	Inhibits replication of IPN virus in vitro
Ribofuranosyl-6-mercaptopurine	Not established			Antiviral	Increased survival of steelhead infected with IHN virus
Ribofuranosyl-5-hydroxyuracil	Not established			Antiviral	Increased survival of steelhead infected with IHN virus
	2 mg/L	2 min	Daily for 3 days	Disinfectant treatment for bacterial gill disease, myxobacteria	FDA considers Roccal-D appropriate for routine disinfection of water, tools, and tanks. See Benzalkonium chloride
Ronidizole	500 mg/L	48 hr	Once	*Ichthyophthirius* sp.	
Rotenone	1–5 mg/L	Indefinite	Once	Fish toxicant	Non–food fish only
Sea salts	25 g/L	Up to 1 hr			
Silvex	2.2 g/m³	Indefinite	Once	Submerged weeds, emerged weeds	Not for food fish
	9 kg/ha				
Simazine	0.5–2.5 g/m³	Indefinite	Once	Herbicide, algacide	Food fish use. Will kill trees
Sodium chloride	22 g/L	30 min		Protozoa, fungi	Eliminates *Epistylis* sp.
	30 g/L	10 min		Osmoregulatory stress	
	1–3 g/L	Indefinite			Freshwater food fish use Time varies with fish species.
Sodium thiosulfate	100 mg/L	Indefinite	Once	Chlorine exposure	
Sulfamethazine	100 mg/L	1 hr	Daily for 7 days	Bacteria	
Toltrazuril	50 mg/ml	20 min	Once	*Trichodina*, sp. *Apiosoma*, sp.	May be effective for *Eimeria* sp. and *Haemogregarina* sp. at similar dose
	10 mg/L	2 hr initial	3 times 24-hr interval	*Ichthyophthirius* sp.	Follow with 2 daily baths 1 hr in 20 mg/L
	5–20 mg/L	4 hr initial	6 times 2-day intervals	*Glugea* sp.	1-hr baths after initial treatment
	10 mg/L	4 hr		*Myxobolus* sp. *Henneguya* sp. Monogenean flukes	
Tricaine methsulfonate	15–66 mg/L	6–48 hr		Sedation	21-day withdrawal for food fish
	50–330 mg/L	1–40 min		Anesthesia	
Trichlorfon	0.25 mg/L	1 hr	Every 5 days	Trematodes, crustaceans	Potentially carcinogenic but approved at low dose for food fish. Doses are in active ingredient. Measure in fume hood. Water to be discarded should be brought to pH 11
	0.5 mg/L	1 hr	Every 5 days		
	2.0 mg/L	1 hr	Once		
Trimethoprim sulfamethoxazole	28 mg/L	6–10 hr	Twice 24 hr apart	*Icthyobodo* sp. *Aeromonas salmonicida*	Bleeding heart tetras
Virazole (1-D-ribofluranosyl-1,2,4-triazole-3-carboxamide)	400 mg/L	Continuous	Change daily	Antiviral-IPN	Inhibits replication of IPN virus in vitro; some effect on mortality when given in vivo

Egg and Water Treatments

Drug	Dose	Frequency/Duration	Indication	Comment
Argentyne	100 mg/L	15 min	Antibacterial	Same egg mortality and deformities as povidone-iodine treatments
Erythromycin	50 mg/L	15 min	Antibacterial	NOT effective against *Renibacterium salmonarum*
Malachite green	5 mg/L	60 min	Antifungal	NOT approved by FDA; persistent tissue levels, mutagenic, teratogenic
Ozone	0.1 mg/L	60 sec	Antibacterial Antifungal	Effective against *Aeromonas salmonicida, A. hydrophila, Yersinia ruckeri*
	70 mg/L	10 min	Antiviral	Destroys IHN virus in hard water
	90 mg/L	10 min		Destroys IPN virus in hard water. May control myxosporidian infective stages
	90 mg/L	30 sec		Destroys IPN virus in soft water. Controls *Saprolegnia* on eggs
Povidone-iodine	100 mg/L	15 min	Antifungal Antibacterial	Some egg mortality and some fry deformities

Pharmacologic Abbreviations

BAL	British anti-lewisite
BID	Given twice daily
g	Gram
ha	Hectare
hr	Hour
IC	Intracardiac
ID	Intradermal
IM	Intramuscular
IP	Intraperitoneal
IT	Intratracheal
IU	International unit
IV	Intravenous
Kcal	Kilocalorie
kg	Kilogram (refers to body weight of the animal unless specified)
kunits	Thousand units
L	Liter
μg	Microgram
mEq	Milliequivalent
mg	Milligram
min	Minute
ml	Milliliter
OID	Given once daily
PO	Orally
Qnh	Given every n hours
QnD	Given every n days
SC	Subcutaneously
sec	Second
TID	Three times a day
U	Unit

Appendix VI

SCIENTIFIC NAMES AND THEIR COMMON EQUIVALENTS

Scientific Name	Common Name	Scientific Name	Common Name
Abramis brama	Bream	*Anguilla anguilla*	European eel
Abudefduf saxatilis	Sargent major	*Anguilla japonica*	Japanese eel
Acanthias vulgaris	Piked dogfish	*Anguilla rostrata*	American eel
Acanthogobius flavimanus	Yellowfin goby	*Anisotremus virginicus*	Porkfish
Acanthophthalmus kuhlii	Kuhlii loach	*Anoplopoma fimbria*	Sablefish, blackcod, coalfish
Acanthostracion quadricornis	Caribbean cowfish	Anoplopomatidae	Sablefishes
Acanthuridae	Tangs and surgeonfishes	*Anoptichthys jordani*	North American cavefish
Acanthurus achilles	Red-tailed surgeon, redspot tang	Anquillidae	Eels
Acanthurus bahianus	Ocean surgeon	Antennariidae	Anglerfishes and frogfishes
Acanthurus bleekeri	Striped surgeon	*Antennarius tridens*	Frogfish
Acanthurus chirurgus	Doctorfish	*Antimora rostrata*	Flatnose cod
Acanthurus coeruleus	Blue tang	*Apeltes quadracus*	Four-spine stickleback
Acanthurus glaucopareius	Gold-rimmed tang	*Aphredoderus sayanus*	Pirate perch
Acanthurus leucosternon	Powderblue surgeon	*Aphyosemion australe*	Lyretail panchax
Acanthurus lineatus	Clown tang	*Apistogramma ramirezi*	Ramirez' dwarf cichlid
Acanthurus triostegus	Convict tang, five-striped tang	*Aplodinotus grunniens*	Freshwater drum
Acipenser fulvescens	Lake sturgeon	Apogonidae	Cardinalfishes
Acipenser medirostris	Green sturgeon	*Amia calva*	Bowfin
Acipenser oxyrhynchus	Atlantic sturgeon	Apterontidae	Speckled knifefishes
Acipenser transmontanus	White sturgeon	*Archosargus probatocephalus*	Atlantic sheepshead, convictfish
Acipenseridae	Sturgeons	*Archosargus rhomboidalis*	Seabream
Aculeola nigra	Black shark	Argentinidae	Argentines
Aetobatus narinari	Spotted eagle ray	Ariidae	Sea catfishes and marine catfishes
Agonidae	Poachers	*Aristichthys nobilis*	Bighead
Agonus cataphractus	Hooknose	*Arius felis*	Hardhead sea catfish
Albula vulpes	Bonefish	*Arothron hispidus*	Balloonfish, rabbitfish
Alburnus alburnus	River bleak	*Artromotus ocellatus*	Oscar
Alopias superciliosis	Bigeye thresher shark	Aspredinidae	Banjo catfishes
Alopias vulpinus	Common thresher shark	Atherinidae	Silversides
Alosa aestivalis	Blueback herring	Aulostomidae	Trumpetfishes
Alosa mediocris	Hickory shad	Bagridae	Naked catfishes
Alosa pseudoharengus	Alewife	*Bairdiella chrysoura*	Silver perch
Alosa sapidissima	American shad, Atlantic shad	*Balistes bursa*	Whitelined triggerfish, humuhumu lei
Alphestes afer	Mutton hamlet		
Ambloplites rupestris	Rockbass, redeye	*Balistes capriscus*	Gray triggerfish
Amblycirrhitus pinos	Redspotted hawkfish	*Balistes vetula*	Queen triggerfish
Ammodytes americanus	American sand eel, glass eel	Balistidae	Filefishes and triggerfishes
Ammodytidae	Sand lances, glass eels	*Balistoides niger*	Clown triggerfish
Amphiprion akallopisos	Skunk-striped anemonefish	*Barbus barbus*	Barbel
Amphiprion bicinctus	Red sea anemonefish	*Barbus conchonius*	Rosy barb
Amphiprion clarkii	Yellow-tailed anemonefish	*Barbus tetrazona*	Tiger barb
Amphiprion chrysopterus	Orange-finned anemonefish	Bathylagidae	Deepsea smelts
Amphiprion frenatus	Black-backed anemonefish	*Bathylagus stilbius*	California smooth-tongued smelt
Amphiprion ocellaris	Clown anemonefish	Batrachoididae	Toadfishes
Amphiprioninae	Anemonefishes	*Bedotia geayi*	Madagascar rainbowfish
Anabantidae	Climbing perches	Belonidae	Needlefishes
Anabas testudineus	Climbing perch, climbing bass	Belontiidae	Bettas, paradisefishes, and gouramis
Anablepidae	Four-eyes		
Anableps anableps	Four-eyes	*Betta splendens*	Siamese fighting fish
Anarhichadidae	Wolffishes	Blenniidae	Combtooth blennies
Anarhichas latifrons	Broadheaded catfish	*Blennius pholis*	Blenny
Anchoa duodecim	New Jersey anchovy	*Blicca bjoerkna*	Silver bream, white bream
Ancylopsetta dilecta	Ocellated flounder	Bothidae	Lefteye flounders

Scientific Name	Common Name	Scientific Name	Common Name
Botia macracanthus	Clown loach	Chaenopsidae	Pike blennies
Brachaeluridae	Blind sharks	*Chaetodipterus faber*	Atlantic spadefish
Brachydanio rerio	Zebrafish, danio	*Chaetodon capistratus*	Four-eyed butterflyfish
Brama brama	Pomfret	*Chaetodon collare*	Collare butterflyfish
Bramidae	Pomfrets	*Chaetodon ocellatus*	Spotfin butterflyfish
Brevoortia patronus	Gulf menhaden	*Chaetodon striatus*	Banded butterflyfish
Brevoortia tyrannus	Atlantic menhaden, bughead, bunker, pogy	Chaetodontidae	Angelfishes and butterflyfishes
Bythitidae	Brotulas, viviparous	*Channa micropeltes*	Red snakehead
Calamus bajonado	Jolthead porgy	*Channa orientalis*	Brown snakehead
Calamus leucosteus	Whitebone porgy	*Channa punctatus*	Green snakehead
Calamus nodosus	Knobbed porgy	*Channa striata*	Striped snakehead
Callichthyidae	Armored catfishes. See also Loricariidae and *Coryodoras*.	Channidae	Snakeheads
Callionymidae	Dragonets	Characidae	Tetras and characins
Callorhynchus callorhynchus	Elephantfish	Cheilodactylidae	Morwongs
Callorhynchus capensis (old syn.)	Elephantfish	*Chiloscyllium griseum*	Gray bamboo shark, gray cat shark
Callorhynchus millii	Elephantfish	*Chiloscyllium indicum*	Slender bamboo shark
Cantherhines pullus	Tail-light filefish	*Chiloscyllium punctatum*	Brownbanded bamboo shark
Canthigaster jactator	White spotted pufferfish	*Chimaera monstrosa*	Ratfish
Canthigaster rostrata	Common sharpnose puffer	Chimaeridae	Chimeras
Canthigaster solandri	Red Sea sharpnose puffer	*Chlamydoselachus anguineus*	Frill shark
Canthigaster valentini	Indo-Pacific sharpnose puffer	*Chondrostoma nasus*	Nase
Canthigasteridae	Sharpnose puffers	*Chromis punctipinnis*	Blacksmith
Capoeta titteya	Cherry barb	*Chrysophrys major*	Red seabream
Carangidae	Jacks and pompano	*Cichlasoma cyanoguttatum*	Rio Grande perch
Caranx crysos	Bluerunner	*Cichlasoma nigrofasciatum*	Convict cichlid
Caranx latus	Horse-eye jack	Cichlidae	Cichlids
Caranx mate	Omaka	*Cirrhinus mrigala*	Indian carp
Carapidae	Pearlfishes	*Cirrhitichthys aprinus*	Spotted hawkfish
Carassius auratus	Goldfish	Cirrhitidae	Hawkfishes
Carassius auratus gibelio	Gibel	*Citharichthys spilopterus*	Bay whiff
Carassius carassius	Crucian carp	*Clarias batrachus*	Walking catfish, albino *Clarias* catfish
Carcharhinus brevipinna	Spinner shark	Clariidae	Labyrinth catfishes
Carcharhinus carcharias	White shark	*Clarias isheriensis*	Isher catfish
Carcharhinus falciforms	Silky shark	*Clarias mossambicus*	Mud barbel catfish
Carcharhinus galapagensis	Galapagos shark	Clinidae	Blennies
Carcharhinus hemiodon	Pondicherry shark	*Clupea harengus harengus*	Atlantic herring
Carcharhinus isodon	Finetooth shark	Clupeidae	Herrings
Carcharhinus leucas	Bull shark	Cobitidae	Loaches
Carcharhinus limbatus	Blacktip shark	*Conger oceanicus*	Conger eel
Carcharhinus longimanus	Ocean whitetip shark, whitetip shark	Congridae	Conger eels
Carcharhinus maculipinnis	Blacktip reef shark	*Corbicula* sp.	Asian clam
Carcharhinus melanopterus	Pacific blackfin reef shark, reef blacktip shark	*Coregonus artedii*	Cisco
Carcharhinus milberti	Sandbar shark	*Coregonus autumnalis*	Arctic cisco
Carcharhinus obscurus	Dusky shark	*Coregonus clupeaformis*	Lake whitefish
Carcharhinus plumbeus	Brown shark	*Coregonus lavaretus*	Pollan
Carcharias acutus	Lesser blue shark	*Coryodoras* (genus)	Armored catfishes. See also Callichthyidae and Loricariidae.
Carcharias gangeticus	Ganges shark	*Coryphaena hippurus*	Common dolphin, mahi-mahi
Carcharias walbeemi	Milk shark	*Coryphaenoides rupestris*	Rattail
Carcharhinidae	Requiem (family) sharks	Cottidae	Sculpins
Carcharhiniformes	Requiem (order) sharks	*Cottus cognatus*	Slimy sculpin
Carcinus maenas	Shore crab	*Cottus girardi*	Potomac sculpin
Catostomus ardens	Utah sucker	*Crassostrea gigas*	Pacific oyster
Catostomus commersoni	White sucker	*Crassostrea virginica*	American oyster
Catostomus discobolus	Chiselmouth sucker	*Crossocheilus siamensis*	Siamese algae eater
Catostomus platyrhynchus	Mountain sucker	Cryptacanthodidae	Wrymouths
Catyla catyla	Catyla carp	*Ctenacis fehlmanni*	Harlequin cat shark
Caulolatilus microps	Blueline tilefish	*Ctenopharyngodon idella*	Grass carp
Centrarchidae	Sunfishes	*Culaea inconstans*	Brook stickleback
Centrarchus macropterus	Flier	Cyclopteridae	Lumpfishes
Centrophorus granulosus	Granular dogfish	*Cyclopterus lumpus*	Lumpfish
Centropomus undecimalis	Snook	*Cyclopterus macalpini*	Arctic lumpsucker
Centropristis ocyurus	Bank sea bass, yellow sea bass	Cynoglossidae	Tonguefishes
Centropristis striata	Black sea bass	*Cynoglossus bengalensis*	Tongue sole
Centroscymnus coelolepis	Portuguese shark	*Cynoscion arenarius*	Sand sea trout
Cephalopholis miniatus	Miniatus grouper, red grouper	*Cynoscion nebulosus*	Spotted sea trout
Cephaloscyllium isabella	Carpet shark	*Cynoscion nothus*	Silver sea trout
Ceratias holboelli	Lanternfish	*Cynoscion regalis*	Weakfish
Cetorhinus maximus	Basking shark	*Cyphotilapia frontosa*	Frontosa cichlid
Chaenocephalus aceratus	Antarctic ice fish	*Cyprinodon macularius*	Desert pupfish
		Cyprinodon variegatus	Sheepshead minnow
		Cyprinodon sp.	Topminnows
		Cyprinodontidae	Killifishes

Table continued on following page

Scientific Name	Common Name	Scientific Name	Common Name
Cyprinus carpio	Koi, and common carp	Gadiformes	Brotulas and eelpouts, codfishes, grenadiers, and cusk-eels
Cyprinus carpio var. *specularis*	Mirror carp	*Gadus macrocephalus*	Pacific cod
Dactylopterus volitans	Flying gurnard	*Gadus morhua*	Atlantic cod
Dalatias licha	Black shark	*Galeocerdo cuvieri*	Tiger shark
Dasyatidae	Stingrays	*Galeorhinus australis*	School shark
Dasyatis akajei	Akaei stingray	*Galeorhinus zyopterus*	Soupfin shark
Dasyatis americana	Southern stingray	*Galeus canis*	Dogfish
Dasyatis brevis	Shorttail stingray	*Galeus inelastomus*	Blackmouth dogfish
Dasyatis centroura	Roughtail stingray	*Gambusia affinis*	Mosquitofish
Dasyatis imbricatus	Scaled stingray	Gasterosteidae	Sticklebacks
Dasyatis kuhluii	Bluespot stingray	*Gasterosteus aculeatus*	Three-spined stickleback
Dasyatis sabina	Atlantic stingray	*Gasterosteus wheatlandi*	Black-spotted stickleback
Dasyatis sayi	Bluntnose stingray	*Gila atraria*	Utah chub
Dasyatis sephan	Estuary stingray	*Ginglymostoma brevicaudatum*	Shorttailed nurse shark
Dasyatis uarnae	Coachwhip stingray	*Ginglymostoma cirratum*	Common nurse shark
Dasyatis violacea	Pelagic stingray	*Girella nigricans*	Opaleye
Dasyatis warnak	Warnak's stingray	*Glyphis gangeticus*	Ganges shark
Diodon holocanthus	Balloonfish	*Glyptocephalus cynoglossus*	Witch flounder
Diodon hystrix	Porcupinefish	*Gnathonemus petersii*	Peter's elephant-nose fish
Diodontidae	Porcupinefishes	Gobiesocidae	Clingfishes
Diplectrum formosum	Sand perch	Gobiidae	Gobies
Diplodus holbrooki	Spottail pinfish	*Gobiosoma evelynae*	Sharknose goby
Doradidae	Thorny catfishes	*Gobiosoma oceanops*	Neon goby (old syn.)
Dorosoma cepedianum	Gizzard shad	*Gomphosus varius*	Bird wrasse
Dorosoma petenense	Threadfin shad	*Gramma loreto*	Royal gramma and fairy basslet
Echinorhinus spinosus	Bramble shark	Grammidae	Basslets
Eigenmannia virescens	Green knifefish	Grammistidae	Soapfishes
Elacatinus oceanops	Neon goby	*Gymnothorax funebris*	Green moray eel
Electrophoridae	Electric eels	*Gymnothorax moringa*	Spotted moray eel
Electrophorus electricus	Electric eel	*Gymnothorax vicinus*	Purple mouth moray
Eleotridae	Sleeper gobies	Gymnotidae	Central and South American knifefishes
Elops saurus	Ladyfish		
Embiotocidae	Surfperches and seaperches	*Gymnotus carapo*	Banded knifefish
Engraulidae	Anchovies	*Gynmura bimaculata*	Two spotted skate
Engraulis eurystole	Silver anchovy	Gymnuridae	Butterfly rays
Engraulis mordax	Northern anchovy	Haemulidae	Grunts
Eopsetta jordani	Brill, petrale sole	*Haemulon album*	Margate
Epalzeorhynchus bicolor	Redtailed black shark	*Haemulon aurolineatum*	Tomtate
Ephippididae	Spadefishes	*Haemulon flavolineatum*	French grunt
Epinephelinae	Groupers	*Haemulon plumieri*	White grunt
Epinephelus drummondhayi	Speckled hind, calico grouper, strawberry grouper	*Haemulon sciurus*	Blue striped grunt
		Halichoeres maculipinna	Clown wrasse
Epinephelus flavolimbatus	Yellowedge grouper	*Haploblepharus edwardsii*	Skaamoong shark
Epinephelus guttatus	Red hind, strawberry grouper	*Haplochromis moffati*	Moffat's cichlid
Epinephelus itajara	Jewfish	*Haplochromis strigigena*	Egyptian cichlid
Epinephelus morio	Red grouper	*Helostoma temmincki*	Kissing gourami
Epinephelus nigritus	Warsaw grouper	Helostomatiidae	Kissing gouramis
Epinephelus niveatus	Snowy grouper, snowflake grouper	*Hemichromis bimaculatus*	Jewelfish
Eptatretus stouti	Pacific hagfish	Hemigaleidae	Snaggletoothed and weasel sharks
Equetus lanceolatus	Jackknifefish	*Hemipristis elongatus*	Snaggletoothed shark
Erilepis zonifer	Skilfish	*Hemipteronotus splendens*	Green razorfish
Erimyzon sucetta	Lake chubsucker	*Hemiramphus brasiliensis*	Ballyhoo
Erpetoichthys calabaricus	Snakefish	*Hemiscyllium ocellatum*	Epaulette shark
Esox americanus	Grass pickerel, banded pickerel, redfin pickerel	*Heptranchias cinereus*	Sevengill shark
		Heptranchias griseus	Sixgill shark
Esox lucius	Northern pike	*Heptranchias perlo*	Sharpnose sevengill shark
Esox masquinongy	Muskellunge	*Heterodontus francisci*	Horn shark
Esox niger	Chain pickerel	*Heterodontus mexicanus*	Mexican horn shark
Etmopterus lucifer	Blackbelly lantern shark	*Heterodontus philippi*	Bullhead shark
Etmopterus princeps	Rough sagre shark	*Heterodontus portjacksoni*	Port Jackson shark
Etmopterus spinax	Velvetbelly shark	*Heteropneustes fossilis*	Stinging catfish
Etroplus maculatus	Chromide cichlid	Hexagrammidae	Greenlings
Eupomacentrus leucostictus	Beau gregory	Hexanchiformes	Frill sharks and cow sharks
Euthynnus alletteratus	Spotted bonito, little tunny	*Hexanchus griseus*	Bluntnose sixgill shark, broadnose sixgill shark
Euthynnus solanderi	Wahoo		
Exocoetidae	Flyingfishes, halfbeaks	*Hexanchus vitulus*	Bigeye sixgill shark
Fistulariidae	Cornetfishes	*Hippocampus erectus*	Atlantic or northern sea horse
Fundulus diaphanus	Banded killifish	*Hippoglossoides elassodon*	Flathead sole
Fundulus grandis	Gulf killifish	*Hippoglossoides platessoides*	American plaice
Fundulus heteroclitus	Mummichog	*Hippoglossus hippoglossus*	Atlantic halibut
Fundulus kansae	Plains killifish	*Hippoglossus stenolepis*	Pacific halibut
Fundulus parvipinnis	California killifish	*Hirundichthys affinis*	Four wing flyingfish
Fundulus sp.	Topminnows	*Histiophryne bougainvilli*	Smooth anglerfish
Gadidae	Codfishes		

Scientific Name	Common Name	Scientific Name	Common Name
Holocanthus ciliaris	Queen angelfish	*Lophius piscatorius*	Anglerfish, goosefish
Holocanthus isabelita	Blue angelfish	*Lopholatilus chamaeleonticeps*	Rainbow tilefish
Holocanthus tricolor	Rock beauty	*Loricariidae*	Armored catfishes. See also
Holocentridae	Squirrelfishes and soldierfishes		Callichthyidas and *Coryodoras*.
Holocentrus ascensionis	Longjaw squirrelfish	*Lota lota*	Burbot
Holocentrus rufus	Common squirrelfish	*Lutjanidae*	Snappers
Hucho hucho	Huchen or Danube salmon	*Lutjanus apodus*	Schoolmaster
Hydrolagus affinis	Deep-water chimera	*Lutjanus campechanus*	Red snapper
Hydrolagus colliei	Spotted ratfish	*Lutjanus griseus*	Gray snapper, mangrove snapper
Hyphessobrycon erythrostigma	Bleeding-heart tetra	*Lutjanus jocu*	Dog snapper
Hyphessobrycon innesi	Neon tetra	*Lutjanus synagris*	Lane snapper
Hypophthalmichthys molitrix	Bighead carp	*Lutjanus vivanus*	Silk snapper
Hypophthalmichthys rabilis	Silver carp	*Luvaridae*	Louvars
Hypoprion signatus	Night shark	*Lythrypnus dalli*	Catalina goby
Ictaluridae	Bullhead catfishes	*Macropodus opercularis*	Paradisefish
Ictalurus catus	White catfish	*Macrouridae*	Grenadiers
Ictalurus furcatus	Blue catfish	*Macrozoarces americanus*	Ocean pout
Ictalurus melas	Black bullhead	*Makaira nigricans*	Blue marlin
Ictalurus natalis	Yellow bullhead	*Malacanthidae*	Tilefishes
Ictalurus nebulosus	Brown bullhead	*Malapteruridae*	Electric catfishes
Ictalurus punctatus	Channel catfish	*Malapterurus electricus*	African electric catfish, electric
Istiophorus platypterus	Sailfish		catfish
Isurus dekayi	Bonito shark	*Mallotus villosus*	Capelin
Isurus oxyrinchus	Shortfin mako shark	*Manta birostris*	Manta ray, giant devil ray
Isurus paucus	Longfin mako shark	*Mastacembelus armatus*	Spiny eel
Katsuwonus pelamis	Skipjack tuna	*Mastacembelus erythrotaenia*	Fire eel
Kryptopterus bicirrhis	Glass catfish	*Mastacemblidae*	Spiny eels
Labeo bicolor	Redtail shark	*Megachasma pelagios*	Megamouth shark
Labeo erythrurus	Rainbow shark	*Megalops atlanticus*	Tarpon
Labridae	Wrasses	*Melanogrammus aeglefinus*	Haddock
Lachnolaimus maximus	Hogfish	*Melanotaeniidae*	Rainbowfishes
Lactophrys quadricornis	Cowfish	*Menidia beryllina*	Inland silverside
Lactoria cornuata	Australian spotted trunkfish	*Menidia menidia*	Atlantic silverside
Lagocephalus lunau	Oopuhe puffer	*Menidia peninsulae*	Tidewater silverside
Lagodon rhomboides	Pinfish	*Menticirrhus americanus*	Southern kingfish
Lamna ditropis	Salmon shark	*Menticirrhus littoralis*	Gulf kingfish
Lamna nasus	Porbeagle	*Menticirrhus saxatilis*	Northern kingfish
Lamniformes	Mackerel sharks	*Menticirrhus sp.*	Whiting
Lampanyctus regalis	Pinpoint lampfish	*Mercenaria mercenaria*	Hard clam
Lampetra fluviatilis	River lamprey	*Metynnis argenteus*	Silver dollar
Lampridae	Opahs	*Microgadus proximus*	Pacific tomcod
Latimeria chalumnae	Coelacanth	*Microgadus tomcod*	Atlantic tomcod
Leionura atum	Australian barracouta	*Micropogonias undulatus*	Atlantic croaker
Leiostomus xanthurus	Spot	*Micropterus dolomieui*	Smallmouth bass
Lepidopsetta bilineata	Rock sole	*Micropterus punctulatus*	Spotted bass, Kentucky bass
Lepidorhombus whiffiagonis	Megrim	*Micropterus salmoides*	Largemouth bass, black bass
Lepidosiren paradoxa	South American lungfish	*Micropterus treculi*	Guadalupe bass
Lepisosteidae	Gars	*Microspathodon chrysurus*	Atlantic yellowtail damsel
Lepisosteus oculatus	Spotted gar	*Microstomus pacificus*	Dover sole
Lepisosteus osseus	Longnose gar	*Misgurnus fossilis*	Weather loach
Lepisosteus platostomus	Shortnose gar	*Mitsukurinidae*	Goblin sharks
Lepisosteus platyrhincus	Florida gar	*Mobula diabola*	Ox ray
Lepisosteus spatula	Alligator gar	*Mobula hypostoma*	Atlantic lesser devil ray, devil ray
Lepomis auritus	Redbreast sunfish	*Mobulidae*	Devil rays
Lepomis cyanellus	Green sunfish	*Mochocidae*	Upside-down catfishes and naked
Lepomis gibbosus	Pumpkinseed		catfishes
Lepomis gulosus	Warmouth	*Mola mola*	Ocean sunfish
Lepomis macrochirus	Bluegill	*Molidae*	Molas
Lepomis megalotis	Longear sunfish	*Monacanthidae*	Filefishes
Lepomis microlophus	Redear sunfish	*Moridae*	Moras
Lepomis punctatus	Spotted sunfish	*Morone americana*	White perch
Leptochariidae	Barbeled hound shark	*Morone chrysops*	White bass
Leuciscus (Squalius) cephalu	Chub	*Morone mississippiensis*	Yellow bass
Leuciscus idus	Golden ide	*Morone saxatilis*	Striped bass
Leuciscus rutilus	Roach	*Mugil capito*	Thinlip gray mullet, gray mullet
Limanda aspera	Yellowfin sole	*Mugil cephalus*	Striped mullet
Liminda ferruginea	Yellowtail flounder	*Mugil curema*	White mullet
Limanda limanda	Dab	*Mugilidae*	Mullets
Liopropoma rubre	Swissguard basslet	*Mullidae*	Goatfishes
Liopsetta putnami	Smooth flounder	*Mullus auratus*	Red goatfish
Liparididae	Snailfishes	*Mustelus antarcticus*	Gummy shark
Littorina littorea	Common periwinkle	*Mustelus californicus*	Gray smoothhound
Lobotes surinamensis	Tripletail	*Mustelus canis*	Smooth dogfish
Lophiidae	Goosefishes	*Mustelus henlei*	Brown smoothhound

Table continued on following page

Scientific Name	Common Name	Scientific Name	Common Name
Mustelus laevis	Smoothhound	Pantodontidae	Freshwater butterflyfishes
Mustelus lunulatus	Sicklefin smoothhound	*Paracanthurus hepatus*	Flag-tailed tang
Mustelus manazo	Hound	*Paracirrhites arcatus*	Arch-eyed hawkfish
Mustelus plebeius	Dogfish	*Paragaleus leucolomatus*	Whitetipped weasel shark
Mycteroperca microlepis	Gag grouper	*Paralabrax clathratus*	Bass, kelp
Mycteroperca phenax	Scamp	*Paralichthys albigutta*	Gulf flounder
Myctophidae	Lanternfishes	*Paralichthys dentatus*	Summer flounder
Myliobatidae	Eagle rays	*Paralichthys lethostigma*	Southern flounder
Myliobatis aquila	Whip ray	*Paralichthys olivaceus*	Japanese flounder, hirame
Myliobatis californica	Bat ray	*Parophrys vetulus*	English sole
Myliobatis freminvellei	Bullnose ray	*Patella vulgata*	European limpet
Myliobatis goodei	Bull ray	*Pelvicachromis pulcher*	Kribensis
Mylopharyngodon piceus	Black carp	*Pelvicachromis taeniatus*	Dwarf cichlid
Myripristis jacobus	Blackbar soldierfish	Pempheridae	Sweepers
Mystus gulio	Striped dwarf catfish	*Pempheris schomburgki*	Glassy sweeper
Mystus seenghala	Indian catfish	*Penaeus japonicus*	Kuruma shrimp
Mytilus edulis	Blue mussel	*Peprilus triacanthus*	Butterfish
Myxine glutinosa	Atlantic hagfish	*Perca flavescens*	Yellow perch, raccoon perch, redfin perch
Myxinidae	Hagfishes		
Narcine brasiliensis	Lesser electric ray	*Perca fluviatilis*	Redfish perch, Eurasian perch
Narke japonica	Electric ray	Percichthyidae	Temperate basses
Naso lituratus	Naso tang	Percidae	Perches
Nebrius ferrugineus	Tawny nurse shark	*Periophthalmus koelreuteri*	Mangrove mudskipper
Negaprion brevirostris	Lemon shark	*Petrometopon cruentatum*	Graysby
Neoceratodus forsteri	Australian lungfish	Pholidae	Gunnels
Notemigonus crysoleucas	Golden shiner	*Phoxinus phoxinus*	Minnow
Notobranchius rachovii	Fire killifish	*Phoxinus* spp.	Dace
Notopteridae	African knifefishes and featherbacks	*Pimephales promelas*	Fathead minnow
		Platacidae	Batfishes
Notopterus nigri	African knifefish	*Platax orbicularis*	Orbiculate batfish
Notopterus notopterus	Asian knifefish	*Platichthys stellatus*	Starry flounder
Notorynchus cepedianus	Broadsnouted sevengill shark	Pleuronectidae	Righteye flounders
Ocyurus chrysurus	Yellow snapper	*Platyrhina sinensis*	Chinese guitarfish
Odontaspis ferox	Smalltooth sand tiger shark	*Platyrhinoidis triseriata*	Thornback guitarfish
Odontaspis taurus	Sand tiger shark	*Plecoglossus altivelis*	Ayu
Ogcocephalus vespertilio	Longnosed batfish	*Plectorhynchus orientalis*	Oriental sweetlips
Oncorhynchus aguabonita	Golden trout	*Pleuronectes platessa*	Plaice
Oncorhynchus clarki	Cutthroat trout	*Pleuronectes quadrituberculatus*	Alaskan plaice
Oncorhynchus gorbuscha	Pink salmon, Pacific salmon	Pleuronectidae	Righteye flounders
Oncorhynchus keta	Chum salmon	Pleuronectiformes	Flatfishes
Oncorhynchus kisutch	Coho salmon	Plotosidae	Plotosid sea catfishes, eel tail catfishes
Oncorhynchus masou	Yamame salmon, Masou salmon		
Oncorhynchus mykiss	Rainbow trout	*Plotosus anguillaris*	Coral catfish
Oncorhynchus mykiss (marine)	Steelhead trout	*Poecilia formosa*	Amazon molly
Oncorhynchus mykiss kamloops	Kamloops trout	*Poecilia latipinna*	Sailfin molly
Oncorhynchus nerka	Sockeye salmon, kokanee salmon, Himemasu salmon	*Poecilia mexicana*	Shortfin molly
		Poecilia reticulata	Guppy
Oncorhynchus rhodurus	Amago trout, biwa salmon	*Poecilia sphenops*	Black molly, sphenops molly
Oncorhynchus tshawytscha	Chinook salmon	Poeciliidae	Mollies
Oophiocephalus striatus	Snakehead	*Pogonias cromis*	Black drum
Ophidiidae	Cusk-eels	*Pollachius virens*	Pollock
Ophidion beani	Longnosed cusk-eel	*Polyodon spathula*	Paddlefish
Ophiodon elongatus	Lingcod	*Polypterus dolloi*	Zaire polypterus
Ophidion holbrooki	Bank cusk-eel	*Polypterus ornatipinnis*	Spotted polypterus
Opistognathidae	Jawfishes	Pomacanthidae	Marine angelfishes
Opsanus tau	Oyster toadfish	*Pomacanthus arcuatus*	Gray angelfish
Orectolobus maculatus	Wobbegong	*Pomacanthus imperator*	Emperor angelfish
Orthopristis chrysoptera	Pigfish	*Pomacanthus paru*	French angelfish
Oryzias latipes	Medaka	Pomacentridae	Damselfishes and anemonefishes
Osmeridae	Smelts	*Pomacentrus partitus*	Bicolor damselfish
Osmerus eperlanus	European smelt	*Pomatomus saltatrix*	Bluefish, Boston bluefish
Osmerus mordax	Rainbow smelt	*Pomoxis annularis*	White crappie
Osphronemidae	Giant gouramis	*Pomoxis nigromaculatus*	Black crappie
Osphronemus gorami	Giant gourami, common gourami	Potamotrygonidae	River rays
Osteoglossidae	Boney-tongued fishes	*Potomotrygon laticeps*	Freshwater stingray
Osteoglossum bicirrhosum	Silver arowana	*Potomotrygon motoro*	Motoro ray
Osteoglossum ferreirai	Black arowana	Priacanthidae	Bigeyes
Ostraciidae	Trunkfishes	*Prionace glauca*	Blue shark
Ostracion meleagris	Spotted boxfish	*Prionotus carolinus*	Northern searobin
Ostrea edulis	Flat oyster	Pristidae	Sawfishes
Oxyeleotris marmoratus	Sand goby, marbled sleeper goby	Pristiophoriformes	Saw sharks
Oxynotus bruviensis	Prickly dogfish	*Pristiophorus cirratus*	Longnose saw shark
Pagrus pagrus	Red porgy	*Pristiophorus nudipinnis*	Shortnose saw shark
Pantodon buchholzi	Freshwater butterflyfish	*Pristis cusprodatus*	Thailand sawfish

Scientific Name	Common Name	Scientific Name	Common Name
Pristis microdon	Smalltooth sawfish	*Salmo trutta*	Brown trout
Pristis pectinata	Common sawfish	*Salvelinus alpinus*	Arctic char
Pristis perotteti	Largetooth sawfish	*Salvelinus fontinalis*	Brook trout
Pristis zijsron	Green sawfish	*Salvelinus malma*	Dolly Varden
Proscylliidae	Finback cat sharks	*Salvelinus namaycush*	Lake trout
Proscyllium habereri	Graceful cat shark	*Salvelinus pluvius*	Japanese char
Prosopium abyssicola	Bear Lake whitefish	*Sarda chiliensis*	Pacific bonito
Prosopium spilonotus	Bonneville whitefish	*Sarda sarda*	Atlantic bonito
Prosopium williamsoni	Mountain whitefish	*Sardina pilchardus*	Pilchard
Protopterus dolloi	African lungfish	*Sardinella aurita*	Spanish sardine
Pseudocarchariidae	Crocodile sharks	*Sardinops sagax*	Pacific sardine
Pseudochromuidae	Basslets	*Sarisoma aurofrenatum*	Redband parrotfish
Pseudopleuronectes americanus	Winter flounder	*Scaphirhynchus albus*	Pallid sturgeon
Pseudorasbora parva	Gudgeon	*Scaphirhynchus platorynchus*	Shovelnose sturgeon
Pseudotriakidae	False cat sharks	*Scardinius erythrophthalmus*	Rudd
Pseudotriakis microdon	False cat shark	Scaridae	Parrotfishes
Pterobobius elapoides	Serpentine goby	*Scarus chrysopterum*	Redtail parrotfish
Pteroidae	Lionfishes	*Scarus croicensis*	Striped parrotfish
Pterois antennata	Spotted lionfish	*Scarus guacamaia*	Rainbow parrotfish
Pterois lunulata	Lionfish	*Scarus taeniopterus*	Princess parrotfish
Pterois volitans	Turkeyfish	*Scatophagus argus*	Spotted scat
Pteromylaeus bovina	Tunisian butterfly ray	Sciaenidae	Drums, jacknife fishes, and croakers
Pterophyllum altum	Deep angelfish		
Pterophyllum scalare	Freshwater angelfish, scalare angelfish	*Sciaenops ocellatus*	Red drum
		Scoliodon laticaudus	Spadenose shark
Puntius conchonius	Rosy barb (old syn.)	*Scoliodon serrakowah*	Indian sharpnose shark
Pylodictis olivaris	Flathead catfish	*Scoliodon terraenovae*	Sharpnose shark
Rachycentron canadum	Cobia	*Scomber omorus maculatus*	Spanish mackerel
Raja batis	Gray skate, common skate	*Scomber scombrus*	Atlantic mackerel
Raja clavata	Thornback skate	Scomberesocidae	Sauries
Raja eglanteria	Clear-nosed skate	*Scomberomorus cavalla*	King mackerel
Raja ennacea	Little skate	Scombridae	Mackerels
Raja flavirostris	Yellownosed skate	*Scophthalmus aquosus*	Windowpane
Raja fullonica	Shagreen skate	*Scophthalmus maximus*	Turbot
Raja fyllae	Fylla's skate	*Scorpaena plumieri*	Spotted scorpionfish
Raja inornata	California skate	*Scorpaena porcus*	Scorpionfish
Raja kenojei	Kenoj's skate	Scorpaenidae	Lionfishes and scorpionfishes
Raja laevis	Barndoor skate	Scyliorhinidae	Cat sharks
Raja lebruni	Pale skate	*Scyliorhinus caniculus*	Mediterranean dogfish, lesser spotted dogfish
Raja maculata	Starry skate		
Raja miraletus	Miraletus skate	*Scyliorhinus torazame*	Sand shark
Raja naevus	Cuckoo skate	*Scyllium canicula*	European cat shark (nursehound)
Raja narce	Narce skate	*Scyllium stellare*	Stellar cat shark
Raja nasuta	Rough skate	*Scymnodon plunketi*	Plunket's shark
Raja ocellata	Winter skate	*Scymnorhinus licha*	European cat shark
Raja oxyrhynchus	Sharpnose skate	*Sebastes goodei*	Chilipepper
Raja porosa	Porosa skate	*Sebastes levis*	Cowcod
Raja radiata	Thorny skate	*Sebastes marinus*	Ocean perch or redfish
Raja rhina	Long-nosed skate	*Sebastes* spp.	Rockfish
Raja scabina	Scabina skate	*Selene peruviana*	Pacific moonfish
Raja senta	Smooth skate	*Selene setapinnis*	Atlantic moonfish
Rajidae	Skates	*Seriola dumerili*	Greater amberjack
Rajiformes	Batoids	*Seriola quinquerodiata*	Yellowtail
Rasbora daniconius	Common rasbora	*Seriola rivoliana*	Almaco jack
Reinhardtius hippoglossoides	Greenland halibut, Greenland turbot	Serranidae	Groupers and sea basses
		Serranus fasciatus	Orange-finned anemonefish, skunk-striped anemonefish
Rhamphichthyidae	American knifefishes		
Rhincodon typus	Whale shark	*Serranus subligarius*	Belted sandfish
Rhinesomus bicaudalis	Caribbean spotted trunkfish	*Serrasalmus calmoni*	Dusky piranha
Rhinobatidae	Guitarfishes, fiddler rays, banjo sharks	*Serrasalmus nattereri*	Red-bellied piranha
		Serrasalmus rhombeus	Spotted piranha
Rhinobatos djeddensis	White-spotted ray	Shilbeidae	Glass catfishes
Rhinobatos lentiginosus	Atlantic guitarfish	Siganidae	Rabbitfishes
Rhinobatos productus	Shovelnose guitarfish	Siluridae	True catfishes
Rhinochimaera atlantica	Knifenose chimera	*Siluris glanis*	Sheatfish
Rhinoptera bonasus	Atlantic cow-nosed ray	*Simochromis diagramma*	Diagramma
Rhinoptera javanica	Cownose ray	*Solea solea*	Sole
Rhinopteridae	Cow-nose rays	Soleidae	Soles
Rhizoprionodon terraenovae	Atlantic sharpnose shark	*Somniosus microcephalus*	Greenland shark
Rhomboplites aurorubens	Vermilion snapper	Sparidae	Porgies
Richardsonius balteatus	Redside shiner	*Sparisoma viride*	Stoplight parrotfish
Rivulus cylindraceus	Cuban killifish	*Sparus aurata*	Gilthead seabream
Rivulus marmoratus	Rivulus	*Sphoeroides maculatus*	Northern puffer
Salmo salar	Atlantic salmon	*Sphyraena barracuda*	Great barracuda

Table continued on following page

Scientific Name	Common Name	Scientific Name	Common Name
Sphyraenidae	Barracudas	*Tilapia aurea*	Blue tilapia
Sphyrna lewini	Scalloped hammerhead shark	*Tilapia mossambica*	Mozamabique tilapia
Sphyrna mokarran	Smalleye hammerhead shark	*Tilapia zilli*	Zilli cichlid
Sphyrna tiburo	Bonnethead shark	*Tinca tinca*	Tench
Sphyrna zygaena	Smooth hammerhead shark	Torpedinidae	Electric rays
Sphyrnidae	Hammerhead sharks	*Torpedo californica*	Pacific torpedo ray
Squaliformes	Dogfish sharks	*Torpedo fairchildi*	Fairchild's torpedo ray
Squalus acanthias	Spiny dogfish, spiked dogfish	*Torpedo marmorata*	Marbled torpedo ray
Squatina californica	Pacific angel shark	*Torpedo nobiliana*	Torpedo ray (old syn.)
Squatina nebulosa	Clouded angel shark	*Torpedo ocellata*	Ocellated torpedo ray
Squatina squatina	European angel shark	*Torpedo torpedo*	Torpedo ray
Squatiniformes	Angel sharks	*Toxotes jaculator*	Archerfish
Stegostoma fasciatum	Zebra shark	Trachinidae	Weevers
Stenotomus chrysops	Scup	*Trachinotus carolinus*	Florida pompano
Sternoptyx diaphana	Hatchetfish	*Triakis semifasciata*	Leopard shark
Stichaeidae	Pricklebacks	*Tribolomon hakonensis*	Japanese dace
Stizostedion lucioperca	Pike-perch	Trichiuridae	Cutlassfishes
Stizostedion vitreum vitreum	Walleye	*Trichogaster trichopterus*	Threespot gourami
Stromateidae	Butterfishes	Trichomycteridae	Parasitic catfishes
Strongylura marina	Atlantic needlefish	Triglidae	Searobins
Symphurus plagiusa	Blackcheek tonguefish	Trikidae	Hound sharks
Symphysodon discus	Discus	*Trinectes maculatus*	Hogchoker
Synaphobranchidae	Cutthroat eels	Tripterygiidae	Triplefin blennies
Synchiropus splendidus	Mandarinfish	*Trygon centroura*	Roughtail stingray
Syngnathidae	Sea horses and pipefishes	*Trygon walga*	Ceylonese stingray (old syn.)
Syngnathus schlegeli	Pipefish	*Trygonorrhina fasciata*	Fiddler ray
Synodontidae	Lizardfishes	Urolophidae	Round stingrays
Synodontis nigriventris	Upside-down catfish	*Urolophus jamaicensis*	Yellow stingray
Synodus foetens	Inshore lizardfish	*Urolophus testaceus*	Common stingray
Taeniura lymma	Queensland stingray	*Urophycis chuss*	Red hake
Tahifugu rubripes	Tiger puffer	*Urophycis regia*	Spotted hake
Tantogolabrus adspersus	Cunner	*Wallago attu*	Attu catfish
Tautoga onitis	Blackfish, tautog	*Xanthichthys ringens*	Sargassum triggerfish
Tellina tenuis	Tellina, tellin	*Xiphias gladius*	Broadbill swordfish
Tetraodontidae	Blowfishes and puffers	Xiphiidae	Swordfishes and platys
Tetrapturus albidus	White marlin	*Xiphophorus helleri* var. *ruber*	Red swordtail
Tetrapturus pflugeri	Hatchet marlin, longbill spearfish	*Xiphophorus helleri* var. *verdis*	Green swordtail
Thalassoma bifasciatum	Bluehead wrasse	*Xiphophorus maculatus*	Southern platyfish, platyfish
Thalassoma duperrey	Saddleback wrasse	*Xiphophorus variatus*	Variable platyfish
Thunnus alalunga	Albacore tuna	Zanclidae	Moorish idols
Thunnus albacares	Yellowfin tuna, yellowtail tuna	*Zanclus canescens*	Moorish idol
Thunnus atlanticus	Blackfin tuna	*Zapteryx exasperata*	Banded guitarfish
Thunnus obesus	Bigeye tuna	*Zebrasoma flavescens*	Yellow tang
Thunnus thynnus	Bluefin tuna	Zeidae	Dories
Thymallus arcticus	Arctic grayling	Zoarcidae	Eelpouts
Thymallus thymallus	Grayling		

Appendix VII

COMMON NAMES AND THEIR SCIENTIFIC EQUIVALENTS

Common Name	Scientific Name	Common Name	Scientific Name
Alewife	*Alosa pseudoharengus*	Bass, smallmouth	*Micropterus dolomieui*
Algae eater, Siamese	*Crossocheilus siamensis*	Bass, spotted	*Micropterus punctulatus*
Amberjack, greater	*Seriola dumerili*	Bass, striped	*Morone saxatilis*
Anchovies (family)	Engraulidae	Bass, white	*Morone chrysops*
Anchovy, New Jersey	*Anchoa duodecim*	Bass, yellow	*Morone mississippiensis*
Anchovy, northern	*Engraulis mordax*	Basses, temperate (family)	Percichthyidae
Anchovy, silver	*Engraulis eurystole*	Basslet, fairy	*Gramma loreto*
Anemonefish, black-backed	*Amphiprion frenatus*	Basslet, swissguard	*Liopropoma rubre*
Anemonefish, clown	*Amphiprion ocellaris*	Basslets (family)	Grammidae
Anemonefish, orange-finned	*Amphiprion chrysopterus*	Batfish, longnosed	*Ogcocephalus vespertilio*
Anemonefish, red sea	*Amphiprion bicinctus*	Batfish, orbiculate	*Platax orbicularis*
Anemonefish, skunk-striped	*Amphiprion akallopisos*	Batfishes (family)	Platacidae
Anemonefish, yellow-tailed	*Amphiprion clarkii*	Batoids (order)	Rajiformes
Anemonefishes (family)	Amphiprioninae	Bay whiff	*Citharichthys spilopterus*
Angelfish, blue	*Holocanthus isabelita*	Beau gregory	*Eupomacentrus leucostictus*
Angelfish, deep	*Pterophyllum altum*	Bettas (family)	Belontiidae
Angelfish, emperor	*Pomacanthus imperator*	Bigeyes (family)	Priacanthidae
Angelfish, French	*Pomacanthus paru*	Bighead	*Aristichthys nobilis*
Angelfish, freshwater	*Pterophyllum scalare*	Blackcod	*Anoplopoma fimbria*
Angelfish, gray	*Pomacanthus arcuatus*	Blackfish	*Tautoga onitis*
Angelfish, queen	*Holocanthus ciliaris*	Blacksmith	*Chromis punctipinnis*
Angelfish, scalare	*Pterophyllum scalare*	Bleak, river	*Alburnus alburnus*
Angelfishes, marine (family)	Pomacanthidae	Blennies (family)	Clinidae
Anglerfish, smooth	*Histiophryne bougainvilli*	Blennies, combtooth (family)	Blenniidae
Anglerfishes (family)	Antennariidae	Blennies, pike (family)	Chaenopsidae
Anglerfish	*Lophius piscatorius*	Blennies, triplefin (family)	Tripterygiidae
Antarctic ice fish	*Chaenocephalus aceratus*	Blenny	*Blennius pholis*
Archerfish	*Toxotes jaculator*	Blowfishes (family)	Tetraodontidae
Argentines (family)	Argentinidae	Bluefish	*Pomatomus saltatrix*
Arowana, black	*Osteoglossum ferreirai*	Bluefish, Boston	*Pomatomus saltatrix*
Arowana, silver	*Osteoglossum bicirrhosum*	Bluegill	*Lepomis macrochirus*
Ayu	*Plecoglossus altivelis*	Bluerunner	*Caranx crysos*
Balloonfish	*Diodon holocanthus*	Bonefish	*Albula vulpes*
Ballyhoo	*Hemiramphus brasiliensis*	Boney-tongued fishes (family)	Osteoglossidae
Barb, cherry	*Capoeta titteya*	Bonito, Atlantic	*Sarda sarda*
Barb, rosy	*Barbus conchonius* (*Puntius conchonius*, old syn.)	Bonito, Pacific	*Sarda chiliensis*
		Bonito, spotted	*Euthynnus alletteratus*
Barb, tiger	*Barbus tetrazona*	Bowfin	*Amia calva*
Barbel	*Barbus barbus*	Boxfish, spotted	*Ostracion meleagris*
Barracouta, Australian	*Leionura atum*	Bream	*Abramis brama*
Barracuda, great	*Sphyraena barracuda*	Bream, silver	*Blicca bjoerkna*
Barracudas (family)	Sphyraenidae	Bream, white	*Blicca bjoerkna*
Bass, black	*Micropterus salmoides*	Brill	*Eopsetta jordani*
Bass, climbing	*Anabas testudineus*	Brotulas and eelpouts (order)	Gadiformes
Bass, Guadalupe	*Micropterus treculi*	Brotulas, viviparous (family)	Bythitidae
Bass, kelp	*Paralabrax clathratus*	Bughead	*Brevoortia tyrannus*
Bass, Kentucky	*Micropterus punctulatus*	Bullhead, black	*Ictalurus melas*
Bass, largemouth	*Micropterus salmoides*	Bullhead, brown	*Ictalurus nebulosus*

Table continued on following page

Common Name	Scientific Name	Common Name	Scientific Name
Bullhead, yellow	*Ictalurus natalis*	Catsharks, finback	Proscylliidae
Bunker	*Brevoortia tyrannus*	Catsharks (family)	Scyliorhinidae
Burbot	*Lota lota*	Cavefish, North American	*Anoptichthys jordani*
Butterfish	*Peprilus triacanthus*	Char, arctic	*Salvelinus alpinus*
Butterfishes (family)	Stromateidae	Char, Japanese	*Salvelinus pluvius*
Butterfly fish, banded	*Chaetodon striatus*	Characins (family)	Characidae
Butterflyfish, Collare	*Chaetodon collare*	Chilipepper	*Sebastes goodei*
Butterflyfish, four-eyed	*Chaetodon capistratus*	Chimera, deep-water	*Hydrolagus affinis*
Butterflyfish, freshwater	*Pantodon buchholzi*	Chimera, knifenose	*Rhinochimaera atlantica*
Butterflyfish, spotfin	*Chaetodon ocellatus*	Chimeras (family)	Chimaeridae
Butterflyfishes (family)	Chaetodontidae	Chub	*Leuciscus (Squalius) cephalu*
Butterflyfishes, freshwater (family)	Pantodontidae	Chub, Utah	*Gila atraria*
Capelin	*Mallotus villosus*	Chubsucker, lake	*Erimyzon sucetta*
Cardinalfishes	Apogonidae	Cichlid, chromide	*Etroplus maculatus*
Caribbean cowfish	*Acanthostracion quadricornis*	Cichlid, convict	*Cichlasoma nigrofasciatum*
Carp, bighead	*Hypophthalmichthys molitrix*	Cichlid, dwarf	*Pelvicachromis taeniatus*
Carp, black	*Mylopharyngodon piceus*	Cichlid, Egyptian	*Haplochromis strigigena*
Carp, Catyla	*Catyla catyla*	Cichlid, Frontosa	*Cyphotilapia frontosa*
Carp, Chinese	See bighead carp, grass carp, and silver carp.	Cichlid, Moffat's	*Haplochromis moffati*
		Cichlid, Ramirez' dwarf	*Apistogramma ramirezi*
Carp, common	*Cyprinus carpio*	Cichlid, Zilli	*Tilapia zilli*
Carp, Crucian	*Carassius carassius*	Cichlids (family)	Cichlidae
Carp, grass	*Ctenopharyngodon idella*	Cisco, arctic	*Coregonus autumnalis*
Carp, Indian	*Cirrhinus mrigala*	Cisco	*Coregonus artedii*
Carp, mirror	*Cyprinus carpio* var. *specularis*	Clam, Asian	*Corbicula* sp.
Carp, silver	*Hypophthalmichthys rabilis*	Clam, hard	*Mercenaria mercenaria*
Catfish, African electric	*Malapterurus electricus*	Clingfishes (family)	Gobiesocidae
Catfish, albino Clarias	*Clarias batrachus*	Coalfish	*Anoplopoma fimbria*
Catfish, armored	*Coryodoras* sp. See also armored catfishes.	Cobia	*Rachycentron canadum*
		Cod, Atlantic	*Gadus morhua*
Catfish, Attu	*Wallago attu*	Cod, flatnose	*Antimora rostrata*
Catfish, blue	*Ictalurus furcatus*	Cod, Pacific	*Gadus macrocephalus*
Catfish, broadheaded	*Anarhichas latifrons*	Codfishes (family)	Gadidae
Catfish, bullhead	See bullhead.	Codfishes, cusk-eels, grenadiers (order)	Gadiformes
Catfish, channel	*Ictalurus punctatus*		
Catfish, coral	*Plotosus anguillaris*	Coelacanth	*Latimeria chalumnae*
Catfish, electric	*Malapterurus electricus*	Convictfish	*Archosargus probatocephalus*
Catfish, flathead	*Pylodictis olivaris*	Cornetfishes (family)	Fistulariidae
Catfish, glass	*Kryptopterus bicirrhis*	Cowcod	*Sebastes levis*
Catfish, hardhead sea	*Arius felis*	Cowfish	*Lactophrys quadricornis*
Catfish, Indian	*Mystus seenghala*	Crab, shore	*Carcinus maenas*
Catfish, Isher	*Clarias isheriensis*	Crappie, black	*Pomoxis nigromaculatus*
Catfish, mud barbel	*Clarias mossambicus*	Crappie, white	*Pomoxis annularis*
Catfish, stinging	*Heteropneustes fossilis*	Croaker, Atlantic	*Micropogonias undulatus*
Catfish, striped dwarf	*Mystus gulio*	Croakers (family)	Sciaenidae
Catfish, upside-down	*Synodontis nigriventris*	Cunner	*Tantogolabrus adspersus*
Catfish, walking	*Clarias batrachus*	Cusk-eel, bank	*Ophidion holbrooki*
Catfish, white	*Ictalurus catus*	Cusk-eel, longnosed	*Ophidion beani*
Catfishes, armored (families)	Callichthyidae and Loricariidae. See also armored catfish.	Cusk-eels (family)	Ophidiidae
		Cutlassfishes (family)	Trichiuridae
Catfishes, banjo (family)	Aspredinidae	Cutthroat eels (family)	Synaphobranchidae
Catfishes, bullhead (family)	Ictaluridae	Dab	*Limanda limanda*
Catfishes, electric (family)	Malapteruridae	Dace	*Phoxinus* spp.
Catfishes, glass (family)	Shilbeidae	Dace, Japanese	*Tribolomon hakonensis*
Catfishes, labyrinth (family)	Clariidae	Damsel, Atlantic yellowtail	*Microspathodon chrysurus*
Catfishes, marine (family)	Ariidae	Damselfish, bicolor	*Pomacentrus partitus*
Catfishes, naked (families)	Bagridae and Mochocidae	Damselfishes (family)	Pomacentridae
Catfishes, parasitic (family)	Trichomycteridae	Danio, zebra	*Brachydanio rerio*
Catfishes, plotosid sea (family)	Plotosidae	Danios	*Brachydanio* sp. and *Danio* sp.
Catfishes, sea (family)	Ariidae	Deepsea smelts (family)	Bathylagidae
Catfishes, thorny (family)	Doradidae	Devil rays (family)	Mobulidae
Catfishes, true (family)	Siluridae	Diagramma	*Simochromis diagramma*
Catfishes, upside-down (family)	Mochocidae	Discus	*Symphysodon discus*
		Doctorfish	*Acanthurus chirurgus*
Catshark, European (Nursehound)	*Scyllium canicula*	Dogfish	*Galeus canis*, *Mustelus plebeius*
		Dogfish, blackmouth	*Galeus inelastomus*
Catshark, European	*Scymnorhinus licha*	Dogfish, granular	*Centrophorus granulosus*
Catshark, false	*Pseudotriakis microdon*	Dogfish, lesser spotted	*Scyliorhinus caniculus*
Catshark, graceful	*Proscyllium habereri*	Dogfish, Mediterranean	*Scyliorhinus caniculus*
Catshark, gray	*Chiloscyllium griseum*	Dogfish, piked	*Acanthias vulgaris*
Catshark, harlequin	*Ctenacis fehlmanni*	Dogfish, prickly	*Oxynotus bruviensis*
Catshark, stellar	*Scyllium stellare*	Dogfish, smooth	*Mustelus canis*
Catsharks, false (family)	Pseudotriakidae	Dogfish, spiked	*Squalus acanthias*
		Dogfish, spiny	*Squalus acanthias*
		Dolly Varden	*Salvelinus malma*

Common Name	Scientific Name	Common Name	Scientific Name
Dolphin, common	*Coryphaena hippurus*	Goosefishes (family)	Lophiidae
Dories (family)	Zeidae	Gourami, common	*Osphronemus gorami*
Dragonets (family)	Callionymidae	Gourami, giant	*Osphronemus gorami*
Drum, freshwater	*Aplodinotus grunniens*	Gourami, kissing	*Helostoma temmincki*
Drum, red	*Sciaenops ocellatus*	Gourami, threespot	*Trichogaster trichopterus*
Drum, black	*Pogonias cromis*	Gouramis (family)	Belontiidae
Drums and jacknifefishes (family)	Sciaenidae	Gouramis, giant (family)	Osphronemidae
		Gouramis, kissing (family)	Helostomatiidae
Eel, American	*Anguilla rostrata*	Gramma, royal	*Gramma loreto*
Eel, American sand	*Ammodytes americanus*	Grayling	*Thymallus thymallus*
Eel, conger	*Conger oceanicus*	Grayling, arctic	*Thymallus arcticus*
Eel, electric	*Electrophorus electricus*	Graysby	*Petrometopon cruentatum*
Eel, European	*Anguilla anguilla*	Greenlings (family)	Hexagrammidae
Eel, fire	*Mastacembelus erythrotaenia*	Grenadiers (family)	Macrouridae
Eel, glass	*Ammodytes americanus*	Grouper, calico	*Epinephelus drummondhayi*
Eel, Japanese	*Anguilla japonica*	Grouper, gag	*Mycteroperca microlepis*
Eel, sand	*Ammodytes* spp.	Grouper, Miniatus	*Cephalopholis miniatus*
Eel, spiny	*Mastacembelus armatus*	Grouper, red	*Cephalopholis miniatus*
Eelpouts (family)	Zoarcidae	Grouper, red	*Epinephelus morio*
Eels (family)	Anquillidae	Grouper, snowflake	*Epinephelus niveatus*
Eels, conger (family)	Congridae	Grouper, snowy	*Epinephelus niveatus*
Eels, cutthroat (family)	Synaphobranchidae	Grouper, strawberry	*Epinephelus drummondhayi*
Eels, electric (family)	Electrophoridae	Grouper, strawberry	*Epinephelus guttatus*
Eels, spiny (family)	Mastacemblidae	Grouper, Warsaw	*Epinephelus nigritus*
Elephantfish	*Callorhynchus callorhynchus*	Grouper, yellowedge	*Epinephelus flavolimbatus*
Elephantfish	*Callorhynchus millii*	Groupers (family)	Serranidae
Elephant-nose fish, Peter's	*Gnathoneumus petersii*	Grunt, blue striped	*Haemulon sciurus*
Featherbacks	Notopteridae	Grunt, French	*Haemulon flavolineatum*
Fiddler rays (family)	Rhinobatidae	Grunt, white	*Haemulon plumieri*
Fighting fish, Siamese	*Betta splendens*	Grunts	Haemulidae
Filefish, tail-light	*Cantherhines pullus*	Gudgeon	*Pseudorasbora parva*
Filefishes (family)	Balistidae	Guitarfish, Atlantic	*Rhinobatos lentiginosus*
Flatfishes (order)	Pleuronectiformes	Guitarfish, banded	*Zapteryx exasperata*
Flier	*Centrarchus macropterus*	Guitarfish, Chinese	*Platyrhina sinensis*
Flounder, gulf	*Paralichthys albigutta*	Guitarfish, shovelnose	*Rhinobatos productus*
Flounder, Japanese	*Paralichthys olivaceus*	Guitarfish, thornback	*Platyrhinoidis triseriata*
Flounder, ocellated	*Ancylopsetta dilecta*	Guitarfishes (family)	Rhinobatidae
Flounder, smooth	*Liopsetta putnami*	Gunnels (family)	Pholidae
Flounder, southern	*Paralichthys lethostigma*	Guppy	*Poecilia reticulata*
Flounder, starry	*Platichthys stellatus*	Haddock	*Melanogrammus aeglefinus*
Flounder, summer	*Paralichthys dentatus*	Hagfish, Atlantic	*Myxine glutinosa*
Flounder, winter	*Pseudopleuronectes americanus*	Hagfish, Pacific	*Eptatretus stouti*
Flounder, witch	*Glyptocephalus cynoglossus*	Hagfishes (family)	Myxinidae
Flounder, yellowtail	*Limanda ferruginea*	Hake, red	*Urophycis chuss*
Flounders, lefteye (family)	Bothidae	Hake, spotted	*Urophycis regia*
Flounders, righteye (family)	Pleuronectidae	Halfbeaks (family)	Exocoetidae
Flying gurnard	*Dactylopterus volitans*	Halibut, Atlantic	*Hippoglossus hippoglossus*
Flyingfish, four wing	*Hirundichthys affinis*	Halibut, Greenland	*Reinhardtius hippoglossoides*
Flyingfishes (family)	Exocoetidae	Halibut, Pacific	*Hippoglossus stenolepis*
Four-eyes	*Anableps anableps*	Hamlet, mutton	*Alphestes afer*
Four-eyes (family)	Anablepidae	Hatchetfish	*Sternoptyx diaphana*
Frogfish	*Antennarius tridens*	Hawkfish, arch-eyed	*Paracirrhites arcatus*
Frogfishes (family)	Antennariidae	Hawkfish, redspotted	*Amblycirrhitus pinos*
Gar, alligator	*Lepisosteus spatula*	Hawkfish, spotted	*Cirrhitichthys aprinus*
Gar, Florida	*Lepisosteus platyrhincus*	Hawkfishes (family)	Cirrhitidae
Gar, longnose	*Lepisosteus osseus*	Herring, Atlantic	*Clupea harengus harengus*
Gar, shortnose	*Lepisosteus platostomus*	Herring, blueback	*Alosa aestivalis*
Gar, spotted	*Lepisosteus oculatus*	Herrings (family)	Clupeidae
Gars (family)	Lepisosteidae	Himemasu	*Oncorhynchus nerka*
Gibel	*Carassius auratus gibelio*	Hind, red	*Epinephelus guttatus*
Glassy sweeper	*Pempheris schomburgki*	Hind, speckled	*Epinephelus drummondhayi*
Goatfish, red	*Mullus auratus*	Hirame	*Paralichthys olivaceus*
Goatfishes (family)	Mullidae	Hogchoker	*Trinectes maculatus*
Gobies (family)	Gobiidae	Hogfish	*Lachnolaimus maximus*
Gobies, sleeper (family)	Eleotridae	Hooknose	*Agonus cataphractus*
Goby, Catalina	*Lythrypnus dalli*	Hornshark	*Heterodontus francisci*
Goby, marbled sleeper	*Oxyeleotris marmoratus*	Hornshark, Mexican	*Heterodontus mexicanus*
Goby, neon	*Elacatinus oceanops*	Hound	*Mustelus manazo*
Goby, sand	*Oxyeleotris marmoratus*	Houndshark, barbeled (family)	Leptochariidae
Goby, serpentine	*Pterobobius elapoides*	Houndsharks (family)	Trikidae
Goby, sharknose	*Gobiosoma evelynae*	Huchen	*Hucho hucho*
Goby, yellowfin	*Acanthogobius flavimanus*	Humuhumu lei	*Balistes bursa*
Goldfish	*Carassius auratus*	Ide, golden	*Leuciscus idus*
Goosefish	*Lophius piscatorius*	Jack, Almaco	*Seriola rivoliana*

Table continued on following page

Common Name	Scientific Name	Common Name	Scientific Name
Jack, horse-eye	*Caranx latus*	Molly, Amazon	*Poecilia formosa*
Jackknifefish	*Equetus lanceolatus*	Molly, black	*Poecilia sphenops*
Jacks and pompano (family)	Carangidae	Molly, sailfin	*Poecilia latipinna*
Jawfishes (family)	Opistognathidae	Molly, shortfin	*Poecilia mexicana*
Jewelfish	*Hemichromis bimaculatus*	Molly, Sphenops	*Poecilia sphenops*
Jewfish	*Epinephelus itajara*	Moonfish, Atlantic	*Selene setapinnis*
Killifish, banded	*Fundulus diaphanus*	Moonfish, Pacific	*Selene peruviana*
Killifish, California	*Fundulus parvipinnis*	Moorish idol	*Zanclus canescens*
Killifish, Cuban	*Rivulus cylindraceus*	Moorish idols (family)	Zanclidae
Killifish, fire	*Notobranchius rachovii*	Moras (family)	Moridae
Killifish, gulf	*Fundulus grandis*	Moray eel, green	*Gymnothorax funebris*
Killifish, plains	*Fundulus kansae*	Moray eel, purple mouth	*Gymnothorax vicinus*
Killifishes (family)	Cyprinodontidae	Moray eel, spotted	*Gymnothorax moringa*
Kingfish, gulf	*Menticirrhus littoralis*	Morwongs (family)	Cheilodactylidae
Kingfish, northern	*Menticirrhus saxatilis*	Mosquitofish	*Gambusia affinis*
Kingfish, southern	*Menticirrhus americanus*	Mudskipper, mangrove	*Periophthalmus koelreuteri*
Knifefish, African	*Notopterus nigri*	Mullet, gray	*Mugil capito*
Knifefish, Asian	*Notopterus notopterus*	Mullet, striped	*Mugil cephalus*
Knifefish, banded	*Gymnotus carapo*	Mullet, thinlip gray	*Mugil capito*
Knifefish, green	*Eigenmannia virescens*	Mullet, white	*Mugil curema*
Knifefishes, African (family)	Notopteridae	Mullets (family)	Mugilidae
Knifefishes, American (family)	Rhamphichthyidae	Mummichog	*Fundulus heteroclitus*
Knifefishes, Central and South American	Gymnotidae	Muskellunge	*Esox masquinongy*
		Muskellunge, tiger	Northern pike × muskellunge cross
Knifefishes, speckled (family)	Apterontidae		
Koi	*Cyprinus carpio*	Mussel, blue	*Mytilus edulis*
Kokanee	*Oncorhynchus nerka*	Nase	*Chondrostoma nasus*
Kribensis	*Pelvicachromis pulcher*	Needlefish, Atlantic	*Strongylura marina*
Labyrinthfishes (families)	Anabantidae, Belontiidae, Helostomatiidae, and Osphronemidae	Needlefishes (family)	Belonidae
		Nursehound	*Scyllium canicula*
		Ocean perch	*Sebastes marinus*
Ladyfish	*Elops saurus*	Ocean pout	*Macrozoarces americanus*
La morue	*Gadus* spp.	Omaka	*Caranx mate*
Lampfish, pinpoint	*Lampanyctus regalis*	Opaleye	*Girella nigricans*
Lamprey, river	*Lampetra fluviatilis*	Opahs (family)	Lampridae
Lanternfish	*Ceratias holboelli*	Orbiculate batfish	*Platax orbicularis*
Lanternfishes (family)	Myctophidae	Oscar	*Artromotus ocellatus*
Limpet	*Patella vulgata*	Oyster, American	*Crassostrea virginica*
Lingcod	*Ophiodon elongatus*	Oyster, flat	*Ostrea edulis*
Lionfish	*Pterois lunulata*	Oyster, Pacific	*Crassostrea gigas*
Lionfish, spotted	*Pterois antennata*	Paddlefish	*Polyodon spathula*
Lionfishes (family)	Scorpaenidae	Panchax, lyretail	*Aphyosemion australe*
Lizardfish, inshore	*Synodus foetens*	Paradisefishes (family)	Belontiidae
Lizardfishes (family)	Synodontidae	Paradisefish	*Macropodus opercularis*
Loach, clown	*Botia macracanthus*	Parrotfish, princess	*Scarus taeniopterus*
Loach, kuhlii	*Acanthophthalmus kuhlii*	Parrotfish, rainbow	*Scarus guacamaia*
Loach, weather	*Misgurnus fossilis*	Parrotfish, redband	*Sarisoma aurofrenatum*
Loaches (family)	Cobitidae	Parrotfish, redtail	*Scarus chrysopterum*
Louvars (family)	Luvaridae	Parrotfish, stoplight	*Sparisoma viride*
Lumpfish	*Cyclopterus lumpus*	Parrotfish, striped	*Scarus croicensis*
Lumpfishes (family)	Cyclopteridae	Parrotfishes (family)	Scaridae
Lumpsucker, arctic	*Cyclopterus macalpini*	Pearlfishes (family)	Carapidae
Lungfish, African	*Protopterus dolloi*	Perch, climbing	*Anabas testudineus*
Lungfish, Australian	*Neoceratodus forsteri*	Perch, Eurasian	*Perca fluviatilis*
Lungfish, South American	*Lepidosiren paradoxa*	Perch, ocean	*Sebastes marinus*
Mackerel, Atlantic	*Scomber scombrus*	Perch, pirate	*Aphredoderus sayanus*
Mackerel, king	*Scomberomorus cavalla*	Perch, raccoon	*Perca flavescens*
Mackerel, Spanish	*Scomber omorus maculatus*	Perch, redfin	*Perca flavescens*
Mackerels (family)	Scombridae	Perch, redfish	*Perca fluviatilis*
Mahi-mahi	*Coryphaena hippurus*	Perch, Rio Grande	*Cichlasoma cyanoguttatum*
Mandarinfish	*Synchiropus splendidus*	Perch, sand	*Diplectrum formosum*
Margate	*Haemulon album*	Perch, silver	*Bairdiella chrysoura*
Marlin, blue	*Makaira nigricans*	Perch, white	*Morone americana*
Marlin, hatchet	*Tetrapturus pfluegeri*	Perch, yellow	*Perca flavescens*
Marlin, white	*Tetrapturus albidus*	Perches (family)	Percidae
Medaka	*Oryzias latipes*	Perches, climbing (family)	Anabantidae
Megrim	*Lepidorhombus whiffiagonis*	Periwinkle, common	*Littorina littorea*
Menhaden, Atlantic	*Brevoortia tyrannus*	Pickerel, banded	*Esox americanus*
Menhaden, gulf	*Brevoortia patronus*	Pickerel, chain	*Esox niger*
Minnow, common	*Phoxinus phoxinus*	Pickerel, grass	*Esox americanus*
Minnow, fathead	*Pimephales promelas*	Pickerel, redfin	*Esox americanus*
Minnow, sheepshead	*Cyprinodon variegatus*	Pigfish	*Orthopristis chrysoptera*
Molas (family)	Molidae	Pike, blennies (family)	Chaenopsidae
Mollies	Poeciliidae	Pike, northern	*Esox lucius*

Common Name	Scientific Name	Common Name	Scientific Name
Pike-perch	*Stizostedion lucioperca*	Ray, torpedo	*Torpedo torpedo (Torpedo nobiliana* old syn.)
Pilchard	*Sardina pilchardus*	Ray, Tunisian butterfly	*Pteromylaeus bovina*
Pinfish	*Lagodon rhomboides*	Ray, whip	*Myliobatis aquila*
Pinfish, spottail	*Diplodus holbrooki*	Ray, white-spotted	*Rhinobatos djeddensis*
Pipefish	*Syngnathus schlegeli*	Rays, butterfly (family)	Gymnuridae
Pipefishes (family)	Syngnathidae	Rays, cow-nosed (family)	Rhinopteridae
Piranha, dusky	*Serrasalmus calmoni*	Rays, eagle (family)	Myliobatidae
Piranha, red-bellied	*Serrasalmus nattereri*	Rays, electric (family)	Torpedinidae
Piranha, spotted	*Serrasalmus rhombeus*	Rays, fiddler (family)	Rhinobatidae
Plaice	*Pleuronectes platessa*	Rays, river (family)	Potamotrygonidae
Plaice, Alaskan	*Pleuronectes quadrituberculatus*	Razorfish, green	*Hemipteronotus splendens*
Plaice, American	*Hippoglossoides platessoides*	Redeye	*Ambloplites rupestris*
Platyfish, variable	*Xiphophorus variatus*	Redfish	*Sebastes marinus*
Platyfish	*Xiphophorus maculatus*	Rivulus	*Rivulus marmoratus*
Platyfish, southern	*Xiphophorus maculatus*	Roach	*Leuciscus rutilus*
Platys	*Xiphophorus* sp.	Rock beauty	*Holocanthus tricolor*
Platys (family)	Xiphiidae	Rockbass	*Ambloplites rupestris*
Poachers (family)	Agonidae	Rockfish	*Sebastes* spp. or *Morone sexatilis*
Pogy	*Brevoortia tyrannus*	Rudd	*Scardinius erythrophthalmus*
Pollan	*Coregonus lavaretus*	Sablefish	*Anoplopoma fimbria*
Pollock	*Pollachius virens*	Sablefishes (family)	Anoplopomatidae
Polypterus, spotted	*Polypterus ornatipinnis*	Sailfish	*Istiophorus platypterus*
Polypterus, Zaire	*Polypterus dolloi*	Salmon, Atlantic	*Salmo salar*
Pomfret	*Brama brama*	Salmon, biwa	*Oncorhynchus rhodurus*
Pomfrets (family)	Bramidae	Salmon, Chinook	*Oncorhynchus tshawytscha*
Pompano, Florida	*Trachinotus carolinus*	Salmon, chum	*Oncorhynchus keta*
Porbeagle	*Lamna nasus*	Salmon, coho	*Oncorhynchus kisutch*
Porcupinefish	*Diodon hystrix*	Salmon, Danube	*Hucho hucho*
Porcupinefishes (family)	Diodontidae	Salmon, Himemasu	*Oncorhynchus nerka*
Porgies (family)	Sparidae	Salmon, Kokanee	*Oncorhynchus nerka*
Porgy, jolthead	*Calamus bajonado*	Salmon, Masou	*Oncorhynchus masou*
Porgy, knobbed	*Calamus nodosus*	Salmon, Pacific	*Oncorhynchus gorbuscha, O. keta, O. kisutch, O. nerka,* and *O. tshawytscha*
Porgy, red	*Pagrus pagrus*		
Porgy, whitebone	*Calamus leucosteus*		
Porkfish	*Anisotremus virginicus*	Salmon, pink	*Oncorhynchus gorbuscha*
Pricklebacks (family)	Stichaeidae	Salmon, sockeye	*Oncorhynchus nerka*
Puffer, Indo-Pacific sharpnose	*Canthigaster valentini*	Salmon, Yamame	*Oncorhynchus masou*
Puffer, northern	*Sphoeroides maculatus*	Sand lances (family)	Ammodytidae
Puffer, oopuhue	*Lagocephalus lunau*	Sandfish, belted	*Serranus subligarius*
Puffer, Red Sea sharpnose	*Canthigaster solandri*	Sardine, Pacific	*Sardinops sagax*
Puffer, tiger	*Tahifugu rubripes*	Sardine, Spanish	*Sardinella aurita*
Pufferfish, white spotted	*Canthigaster jactator*	Sargent major	*Abudefduf saxatilis*
Puffers (family)	Tetraodontidae	Sauries (family)	Scomberesocidae
Puffers, sharpnosed (family)	Canthigasteridae	Sawfish, common	*Pristis pectinata*
Pumpkinseed	*Lepomis gibbosus*	Sawfish, green	*Pristis zijsron*
Pupfish, desert	*Cyprinodon macularius*	Sawfish, largetooth	*Pristis perotteti*
Rabbitfish	*Arothron hispidus*	Sawfish, smalltooth	*Pristis microdon*
Rabbitfishes (family)	Siganidae	Sawfish, Thailand	*Pristis cusprodatus*
Rainbowfish, Madagascar	*Bedotia geayi*	Sawfishes (family)	Pristidae
Rainbowfishes (family)	Melanotaeniidae	Sawshark, longnose	*Pristiophorus cirratus*
Rasbora, common	*Rasbora daniconius*	Sawshark, shortnose	*Pristiophorus nudipinnis*
Ratfish	*Chimaera monstrosa*	Sawsharks (order)	Pristiophoriformes
Ratfish, spotted	*Hydrolagus colliei*	Scamp	*Mycteroperca phenax*
Rattail	*Coryphaenoides rupestris*	Scat, spotted	*Scatophagus argus*
Ray, Atlantic cownose	*Rhinoptera bonasus*	Schoolmaster	*Lutjanus apodus*
Ray, Atlantic lesser devil	*Mobula hypostoma*	Scorpionfish	*Scorpaena porcus*
Ray, bat	*Myliobatis californica*	Scorpionfish, spotted	*Scorpaena plumieri*
Ray, bull	*Myliobatis goodei*	Scorpionfishes (family)	Scorpaenidae
Ray, bullnose	*Myliobatis freminvellei*	Sculpin, Potomac	*Cottus girardi*
Ray, cow nose	*Rhinoptera javanica*	Sculpin, slimy	*Cottus cognatus*
Ray, devil	*Mobula hypostoma*	Sculpins (family)	Cottidae
Ray, electric	*Narke japonica*	Scup	*Stenotomus chrysops*
Ray, Fairchild's torpedo	*Torpedo fairchildi*	Sea bass, bank	*Centropristis ocyurus*
Ray, fiddler	*Trygonorrhina fasciata*	Sea bass, black	*Centropristis striata*
Ray, giant devil	*Manta birostris*	Sea bass, yellow	*Centropristis ocyurus*
Ray, lesser electric	*Narcine brasiliensis*	Sea basses (family)	Serranidae
Ray, manta	*Manta birostris*	Sea catfishes, plotosid (family)	Plotosidae
Ray, marbled torpedo	*Torpedo marmorata*	Sea perches	Embiotocidae
Ray, Motoro	*Potomotrygon motoro*	Sea horse, Atlantic	*Hippocampus erectus*
Ray, ocellated torpedo	*Torpedo ocellata*	Sea horse, lined	*Hippocampus* sp.
Ray, Ox	*Mobula diabola*	Sea horse, northern	*Hippocampus erectus*
Ray, Pacific torpedo	*Torpedo californica*	Sea horses (family)	Syngnathidae
Ray, spotted eagle	*Aetobatus narinari*		

Table continued on following page

Common Name	Scientific Name	Common Name	Scientific Name
Sea trout, sand	*Cynoscion arenarius*	Shark, redtailed black shark	*Epalzeorhynchus bicolor*
Sea trout, silver	*Cynoscion nothus*	Shark, reef blacktip	*Carcharhinus melanopterus*
Sea trout, spotted	*Cynoscion nebulosus*	Shark, rough sagre	*Etmopterus princeps*
Seabream	*Archosargus rhomboidalis*	Shark, salmon	*Lamna ditropis*
Seabream, gilthead	*Sparus aurata*	Shark, sand	*Scyliorhinus torazame*
Seabream, red	*Chrysophrys major*	Shark, sand tiger	*Odontaspis taurus*
Seaperches (family)	Embiotocidae	Shark, sandbar	*Carcharhinus milberti*
Searobin, northern	*Prionotus carolinus*	Shark, scalloped hammerhead	*Sphyrna lewini*
Searobins (family)	Triglidae	Shark, school	*Galeorhinus australis*
Shad, American	*Alosa sapidissima*	Shark, sevengill	*Heptranchias cinereus*
Shad, Atlantic	*Alosa sapidissima*	Shark, sharpnose	*Scoliodon terraenovae*
Shad, gizzard	*Dorosoma cepedianum*	Shark, sharpnose sevengill	*Heptranchias perlo*
Shad, hickory	*Alosa mediocris*	Shark, shortfin mako	*Isurus oxyrinchus*
Shad, threadfin	*Dorosoma petenense*	Shark, shortnose saw	*Pristiophorus nudipinnis*
Shark, Atlantic sharpnose	*Rhizoprionodon terraenovae*	Shark, shorttailed nurse	*Ginglymostoma brevicaudatum*
Shark, basking	*Cetorhinus maximus*	Shark, silky	*Carcharhinus falciformis*
Shark, bigeye sixgill	*Hexanchus vitulus*	Shark, sixgill	*Heptranchias griseus*
Shark, bigeye thresher	*Alopias superciliosis*	Shark, skaamoong	*Haploblepharus edwardsii*
Shark, black	*Dalatias licha*	Shark, slender bamboo	*Chiloscyllium indicum*
Shark, blackbelly lantern	*Etmopterus lucifer*	Shark, smalleye hammerhead	*Sphyrna mokarran*
Shark, blacktip	*Carcharhinus limbatus*	Shark, smalltooth sandtiger	*Odontaspis ferox*
Shark, blacktip reef	*Carcharhinus maculipinnis*	Shark, smooth hammerhead	*Sphyrna zygaena*
Shark, blue	*Prionace glauca*	Shark, snaggletoothed	*Hemipristis elongatus*
Shark, bluntnose sixgill	*Hexanchus griseus*	Shark, soupfin	*Galeorhinus zyopterus*
Shark, bonito	*Isurus dekayi*	Shark, spadenose	*Scoliodon laticaudus*
Shark, bonnethead	*Sphyrna tiburo*	Shark, spinner	*Carcharhinus brevipinna*
Shark, bramble	*Echinorhinus spinosus*	Shark, stellar cat	*Scyllium stellare*
Shark, broadnose sixgill	*Hexanchus griseus*	Shark, tawny nurse	*Nebrius ferrugineus*
Shark, broadsnouted sevengill	*Notorynchus cepedianus*	Shark, tiger	*Galeocerdo cuvieri*
Shark, brown	*Carcharhinus plumbeus*	Shark, velvetbelly	*Etmopterus spinax*
Shark, brownbanded bamboo	*Chiloscyllium punctatum*	Shark, whale	*Rhincodon typus*
Shark, bull	*Carcharhinus leucas*	Shark, white	*Caracharhinus carcharias*
Shark, bullhead	*Heterodontus philippi*	Shark, whitetip	*Carcharhinus longimanus*
Shark, carpet	*Cephaloscyllium isabella*	Shark, whitetipped weasel	*Paragaleus leucolomatus*
Shark, clouded angel	*Squatina nebulosa*	Shark, zebra	*Stegostoma fasciatum*
Shark, common nurse	*Ginglymostoma cirratum*	Sharks, angel (order)	Squatiniformes
Shark, common thresher	*Alopias vulpinus*	Sharks, banjo (family)	Rhinobatidae
Shark, dusky	*Carcharhinus obscurus*	Sharks, barbeled hound (family)	Leptochariidae
Shark, epaulette	*Hemiscyllium ocellatum*	Sharks, blind (family)	Brachaeluridae
Shark, European angel	*Squatina squatina*	Sharks, carpet (order)	Orectolobiformes
Shark, European cat	*Scymnorhinus licha*	Sharks, cat (family)	Scyliorhinidae
Shark, European cat (nursehound)	*Scyllium canicula*	Sharks, cow (order)	Hexanchiformes
Shark, false cat	*Pseudotriakis microdon*	Sharks, crocodile (family)	Pseudocarchariidae
Shark, finetooth	*Carcharhinus isodon*	Sharks, dogfish (order)	Squaliformes
Shark, frill	*Chlamydoselachus anguineus*	Sharks, false cat (family)	Pseudotriakidae
Shark, Galapagos	*Carcharhinus galapagensis*	Sharks, finback cat (family)	Proscylliidae
Shark, Ganges	*Carcharias gangeticus*	Sharks, frill (order)	Hexanchiformes
Shark, graceful cat	*Proscyllium habereri*	Sharks, goblin (family)	Mitsukurinidae
Shark, gray bamboo	*Chiloscyllium griseum*	Sharks, hammerhead (family)	Sphyrnidae
Shark, gray cat	*Chiloscyllium griseum*	Sharks, horn (order)	Heterodontiformes
Shark, Greenland	*Somniosus microcephalus*	Sharks, hound (family)	Trikidae
Shark, gummy	*Mustelus antarcticus*	Sharks, longtail carpet	*Chiloscyllium* spp.
Shark, harlequin cat	*Ctenacis fehlmanni*	Sharks, mackerel (order)	Lamniformes
Shark, horn	*Heterodontus francisci*	Sharks, requiem (family)	Carcharhinidae
Shark, Indian sharpnose	*Scoliodon serrakowah*	Sharks, requiem (order)	Carcharhiniformes
Shark, lemon	*Negaprion brevirostris*	Sharks, saw (order)	Pristiophoriformes
Shark, leopard	*Triakis semifasciata*	Sharks, snaggletoothed (family)	Hemigaleidae
Shark, lesser blue	*Carcharias acutus*	Sharks, weasel (family)	Hemigaleidae
Shark, longfin mako	*Isurus paucus*	Sharpnose puffer, common	*Canthigaster rostrata*
Shark, longnose saw	*Pristiophorus cirratus*	Sharpnose puffer, Indo-Pacific	*Canthigaster valentini*
Shark, Mexican horn	*Heterodontus mexicanus*	Sharpnose puffer, Red Sea	*Canthigaster solandri*
Shark, megamouth	*Megachasma pelagios*	Sharpnose puffers (family)	Canthigasteridae
Shark, milk	*Carcharias walbeemi*	Sheatfish	*Siluris glanis*
Shark, night	*Hypoprion signatus*	Sheepshead, Atlantic	*Archosargus probatocephalus*
Shark, ocean whitetip	*Carcharhinus longimanus*	Shiner, golden	*Notemigonus crysoleucas*
Shark, Pacific angel	*Squatina californica*	Shiner, redside	*Richardsonius balteatus*
Shark, Pacific blackfin reef	*Carcharhinus melanopterus*	Shiners	*Notropis* spp.
Shark, Plunket's	*Scymnodon plunketi*	Shrimp, kuruma	*Penaeus japonicus*
Shark, Pondicherry	*Carcharhinus hemiodon*	Siamese fighting fish	*Betta splendens*
Shark, Port Jackson	*Heterodontus port jacksoni*	Silver dollar	*Metynnis argenteus*
Shark, Portuguese	*Centroscymnus coelolepis*	Silverside, Atlantic	*Menidia menidia*
Shark, rainbow	*Labeo erythrurus*	Silverside, inland	*Menidia beryllina*
Shark, redtail	*Labeo bicolor*	Silverside, tidewater	*Menidia peninsulae*

Common Name	Scientific Name	Common Name	Scientific Name
Silversides (family)	Atherinidae	Squirrelfish, common	*Holocentrus rufus*
Skate, barndoor	*Raja laevis*	Squirrelfish, longjaw	*Holocentrus ascensionis*
Skate, big	*Raja binoculata*	Squirrelfishes (family)	Holocentridae
Skate, Burton	*Raja alba*	Stickleback, black spotted	*Gasterosteus wheatlandi*
Skate, California	*Raja inornata*	Stickleback, brook	*Culaea inconstans*
Skate, clear-nosed	*Raja eglanteria*	Stickleback, four-spined	*Apeltes quadracus*
Skate, common	*Raja batis*	Stickleback, three-spined	*Gasterosteus aculeatus*
Skate, cuckoo	*Raja naevus*	Sticklebacks (family)	Gasterosteidae
Skate, Fylla's	*Raja fyllae*	Stingray, Akaei	*Dasyatis akajei*
Skate, gray	*Raja batis*	Stingray, Atlantic	*Dasyatis sabina*
Skate, Kenoj's	*Raja kenojei*	Stingray, bluespot	*Dasyatis kuhluii*
Skate, little	*Raja ennacea*	Stingray, bluntnose	*Dasyatis sayi*
Skate, long-nosed	*Raja rhina*	Stingray, Ceylonese	*Trygon walga*
Skate, Miraletus	*Raja miraletus*	Stingray, coachwhip	*Dasyatis uarnae*
Skate, Narce	*Raja narce*	Stingray, common	*Urolophus testaceus*
Skate, pale	*Raja lebruni*	Stingray, estuary	*Dasyatis sephan*
Skate, Porosa	*Raja porosa*	Stingray, freshwater	*Potomotrygon laticeps*
Skate, rough	*Raja nasuta*	Stingray, pelagic	*Dasyatis violacea*
Skate, Scabina	*Raja scabina*	Stingray, Queensland	*Taeniura lymma*
Skate, shagreen	*Raja fullonica*	Stingray, roughtail	*Dasyatis centroura* (*Trygon centroura*, old syn.)
Skate, sharpnose	*Raja oxyrhynchus*		
Skate, smooth	*Raja senta*	Stingray, scaled	*Dasyatis imbricatus*
Skate, starry	*Raja maculata*	Stingray, shorttail	*Dasyatis brevis*
Skate, thornback	*Raja clavata*	Stingray, southern	*Dasyatis americana*
Skate, thorny	*Raja radiata*	Stingray, Warnak's	*Dasyatis warnak*
Skate, two spotted	*Gymnura bimaculata*	Stingray, yellow	*Urolophus jamaicensis*
Skate, winter	*Raja ocellata*	Stingrays (family)	Dasyatidae
Skate, yellownosed	*Raja flavirostris*	Stingrays, round (family)	Urolophidae
Skates (family)	Rajidae	Sturgeon, Atlantic	*Acipenser oxyrhynchus*
Skilfish	*Erilepis zonifer*	Sturgeon, green	*Acipenser medirostris*
Smelt, California smooth-tongued	*Bathylagus stilbius*	Sturgeon, lake	*Acipenser fulvescens*
		Sturgeon, pallid	*Scaphirhynchus albus*
Smelt, European	*Osmerus eperlanus*	Sturgeon, shovelnose	*Scaphirhynchus platorynchus*
Smelt, rainbow	*Osmerus mordax*	Sturgeon, white	*Acipenser transmontanus*
Smelts (family)	Osmeridae	Sturgeons (family)	Acipenseridae
Smoothhound	*Mustelus laevis*	Sucker, chiselmouth	*Catostomus discobolus*
Smoothhound, brown	*Mustelus henlei*	Sucker, mountain	*Catostomus platyrhynchus*
Smoothhound, gray	*Mustelus californicus*	Sucker, Utah	*Catostomus ardens*
Smoothhound, sicklefin	*Mustelus lunulatus*	Sucker, white	*Catostomus commersoni*
Snailfishes (family)	Liparididae	Sunfish, green	*Lepomis cyanellus*
Snakefish	*Erpetoichthys calabaricus*	Sunfish, longear	*Lepomis megalotis*
Snakehead	*Ophiocephalus striatus*	Sunfish, ocean	*Mola mola*
Snakehead, brown	*Channa orientalis*	Sunfish, redbreast	*Lepomis auritus*
Snakehead, green	*Channa punctatus*	Sunfish, redear	*Lepomis microlophus*
Snakehead, red	*Channa micropeltes*	Sunfish, spotted	*Lepomis punctatus*
Snakehead, striped	*Channa striata*	Sunfishes (family)	Centrarchidae
Snakeheads (family)	Channidae	Surfperches (family)	Embiotocidae
Snapper, dog	*Lutjanus jocu*	Surgeon, ocean	*Acanthurus bahianus*
Snapper, gray	*Lutjanus griseus*	Surgeon, powderblue	*Acanthurus leucosternon*
Snapper, lane	*Lutjanus synagris*	Surgeon, red-tailed	*Acanthurus achilles*
Snapper, mangrove	*Lutjanus griseus*	Surgeon, striped	*Acanthurus bleekeri*
Snapper, red	*Lutjanus campechanus*	Surgeonfishes (family)	Acanthuridae
Snapper, silk	*Lutjanus vivanus*	Sweepers (family)	Pempheridae
Snapper, vermilion	*Rhomboplites aurorubens*	Sweetlips, Oriental	*Plectorhynchus orientalis*
Snapper, yellow	*Ocyurus chrysurus*	Swordfish, broadbill	*Xiphias gladius*
Snappers (family)	Lutjanidae	Swordfishes	Xiphiidae
Snook	*Centropomus undecimalis*	Swordtail, green	*Xiphophorus helleri* var. *verdis*
Soapfishes (family)	Grammistidae	Swordtail, red	*Xiphophorus helleri* var. *ruber*
Soldierfish, blackbar	*Myripristis jacobus*	Swordtails (family)	Xiphiidae
Soldierfishes (family)	Holocentridae	Tang, blue	*Acanthurus coeruleus*
Sole	*Solea solea*	Tang, clown	*Acanthurus lineatus*
Sole, Dover	*Microstomus pacificus*	Tang, convict	*Acanthurus triostegus*
Sole, English	*Parophrys vetulus*	Tang, five-striped	*Acanthurus triostegus*
Sole, flathead	*Hippoglossoides elassodon*	Tang, flag-tailed	*Paracenthurus hepatus*
Sole, Petrale	*Eopsetta jordani*	Tang, goldrimmed	*Acanthurus glaucopareius*
Sole, rock	*Lepidopsetta bilineata*	Tang, Naso	*Naso lituratus*
Sole, tongue	*Cynoglossus bengalensis*	Tang, redspot	*Acanthurus achilles*
Sole, yellowfin	*Limanda aspera*	Tang, yellow	*Zebrasoma flavescens*
Soles (family)	Soleidae	Tangs (family)	Acanthuridae
Spadefish, Atlantic	*Chaetodipterus faber*	Tarpon	*Megalops atlanticus*
Spadefishes (family)	Ephippididae	Tautog	*Tautoga onitis*
Spearfish, longbill	*Tetrapturus pfluegeri*	Tellina	*Tellina tenuis*
Splake	*Hybrid brook trout × lake trout*	Tench	*Tinca tinca*
Spot	*Leiostomus xanthurus*	Tetra, bleeding-heart	*Hyphessobrycon erythrostigma*

Table continued on following page

Common Name	Scientific Name	Common Name	Scientific Name
Tetra, neon	*Hyphessobrycon innesi*	Tuna, albacore	*Thunnus alalunga*
Tetras (family)	Characidae	Tuna, bigeye	*Thunnus obesus*
Tilapia, blue	*Tilapia aurea*	Tuna, blackfin	*Thunnus atlanticus*
Tilapia, Mozambique	*Tilapia mossambica*	Tuna, bluefin	*Thunnus thynnus*
Tilefish, blueline	*Caulolatilus microps*	Tuna, skipjack	*Katsuwonus pelamis*
Tilefish, rainbow	*Lopholatilus chamaeleonticeps*	Tuna, yellowfin	*Thunnus albacares*
Tilefishes (family)	Malacanthidae	Tuna, yellowtail	*Thunnus albacares*
Toadfish, oyster	*Opsanus tau*	Tunny, little	*Euthynnus alletteratus*
Toadfishes (family)	Batrachoididae	Turbot	*Scophthalmus maximus*
Tomcod, Atlantic	*Microgadus tomcod*	Turbot, Greenland	*Reinhardtius hippoglossoides*
Tomcod, Pacific	*Microgadus proximus*	Turkeyfish	*Pterois volitans*
Tomtate	*Haemulon aurolineatum*	Wahoo	*Euthynnus solanderi*
Tonguefish, blackcheek	*Symphurus plagiusa*	Walleye	*Stizostedion vitreum vitreum*
Tonguefishes (family)	Cynoglossidae	Warmouth	*Lepomis gulosus*
Topminnows	*Fundulus* sp. and *Cyprinodon* sp.	Weakfish	*Cynoscion regalis*
Triggerfish, clown	*Balistoides niger*	Weevers (family)	Trachinidae
Triggerfish, gray	*Balistes capriscus*	White sucker	*Catostomus commersoni*
Triggerfish, queen	*Balistes vetula*	Whitefish, Bear Lake	*Prosopium abyssicola*
Triggerfish, sargassum	*Xanthichthys ringens*	Whitefish, Bonneville	*Prosopium spilonotus*
Triggerfish, whitelined	*Balistes bursa*	Whitefish, lake	*Coregonus clupeaformis*
Triggerfishes (family)	Balistidae	Whitefish, mountain	*Prosopium williamsoni*
Tripletail	*Lobotes surinamensis*	Whiting	*Menticirrhus* sp.
Trout, Amago	*Oncorhynchus rhodurus*	Windowpane	*Scophthalmus aquosus*
Trout, brook	*Salvelinus fontinalis*	Wobbegong	*Orectolobus maculatus*
Trout, brown	*Salmo trutta*	Wolffishes (family)	Anarhichadidae
Trout, cutthroat	*Oncorhynchus clarki*	Wrasse, bird	*Gomphosus varius*
Trout, golden	*Oncorhynchus aguabonita*	Wrasse, bluehead	*Thalassoma bifasciatum*
Trout, Kamloops	*Oncorhynchus mykiss kamloops*	Wrasse, clown	*Halichoeres maculipinna*
Trout, lake	*Salvelinus namaycush*	Wrasse, saddleback	*Thalassoma duperrey*
Trout, rainbow	*Oncorhynchus mykiss*	Wrasses (family)	Labridae
Trout, steelhead (Marine)	*Oncorhynchus mykiss*	Wrymouths (family)	Cryptacanthodidae
Trumpetfishes (family)	Aulostomidae	Yamame	*Oncorhynchus masou*
Trunkfish, Australian spotted	*Lactoria cornuata*	Yellowtail	*Seriola quinquerodiata*
Trunkfish, Caribbean spotted	*Rhinesomus bicaudalis*	Zebrafish	*Brachydanio rerio*
Trunkfishes (family)	Ostraciidae		

INDEX

Note: Page numbers in *italics* refer to illustrations;
page numbers followed by t refer to tables.

Quinaldine, 82t, *89*
 action of, 89
 chemical attributes of, 89
 dosage for, 82t, 89
 stability of, 89
Quinine, antiprotozoal action of, 838t
Quinolones, structure of, *435*
 treatment with, 435, 812t

Radiography, 68–69
 restraint chamber for, 68–69, *69*, *70*
 water blocking of, 69, *70*
 xerographic adaptation of, 71, *72*
Rainbow hemorrhagic disorder,
 erythrocyte virus in, 400
Rainbowfish, 538, *538*
Rancidity, 355, 695
Rapeseed meal, toxic ingredients in, 351
Rasboras, 534, *534*
 natural history of, 534
Rays, 738–816
 anatomy of, *28*, *29*, 744–748, *744–748*
 distribution of, 744–748, *744–748*
 electric, *744*, *745*
 electric receptors of, 46–47
 freshwater, 745
 fungal disease in, 776t, 777–779, *778*
 internal organs of, *10*, *28*, *29*
 natural history of, 744–748
 neoplasia in, 808
 parasitic disease in, 782–806, 783t–804t
 river, 745
 taxonomy of, 744–748
 types of, 744–748, *744–748*
 venom of, 745–748
Receptors, 53
 adrenergic, 680
 electric, 46–47, 56, 753, 762
 hearing and, 46
 lateral line, 46, 682
 smell and, 15, 47, 55
 taste and, 45, *45*
Rectal gland, electrolyte balance and, 50,
 50
 shark and, 26, 50, *50*
 skate and, 29
Red gland, swim bladder and, 37
Red pest disease, clinical signs in, 638
 culture in, 638
 marine tropical fish and, 638
 transmission of, 638
 treatment and control of, 638
 vibriosis causing, 638
Red tide, 195. See also *Phytoplankton*.
 human food poisoning and, 218
Red worms, freshwater temperate fish
 and, 302t
 freshwater tropical fish and, 586–587
Redmouth disease. See also *Hemorrhagic
 septicemia*.
 aeromoniasis and, 473t, 473–474
 enteric, 155–156, 365t, 366–367
 yersinial, 365t, 366–367
Redox potential, marine aquarium and,
 622, *622*
Red-sore disease. See *Heteropolarial
 infections*.
Reeling disease. See *Ichthyophoniasis*.
Refractometer, protein determination and,
 754
 specific gravity monitored with, *620*,
 620–621
Refrigeration, temperature control and,
 109–110, *110*

Rejection, allograft and, 152, *152*
Renibacterium, culture of, 369
 kidney disease due to, 365t, 368–370
 salmonid affected by, 365t, 368–370
Reovirus, bluegill and, 290–291
 catfish, 523
 grass carp, 482
 landlocked salmon, 389
 oyster and, 290
 salmonid hepatitis and, 389
Reproduction. See also *Broodfish*;
 Copulation; *Courtship*; *Spawning*.
 anatomy and, comparative, 3–29
 carp and, 470–472
 coral reef and, 628–633, *629*
 estuarine fish and, 241t, 251–266
 flatfish and, 671, 683
 freshwater bass and, 226
 freshwater temperate fish and, 241t,
 251–266
 freshwater tropical fish and, 554–558
 genetic factors and, 58–60
 goldfish and, 470–472
 inbreeding and, 60
 koi and, 470–472
 marine tropical fish and, 628–634, *629*,
 630t–632t
 ovoviviparous, 771t, 772–774
 parthenogenesis and, 60
 salmonid and, 358–363
 sexual differentiation and, 58–60
 shark and, 769–774, 771t
 skate and, 772, *772*
 temperature range and, 241t
 viviparous, 554–556, 771t, 772–774, *773*
Requiem sharks, 739–741, *740*
 attacks by, 739–741
 reproduction in, 771t
Reservoirs, aquarium and, *99*, 103, *104*
 brine, *104*
Respiration, 52, 679–680. See also *Gill
 system*.
 air breathing as, 537–538
 anesthesia and, 81–82
 comparative anatomy and, 8–29
 diphasic, 52
 fish out of water and, 64, 80–81
 gas exchange in, 52
 gill function and, 8–9, *9*, 323
 marine cold-water fish and, 679–680
 monophasic, 52
 patient examination and, 63
 ventilation and, 81–82, 679–680
Restraint, blinkering and, 79–80, *80*
 catfish and, 502
 chemical, 80–90
 life support chamber for, 73–74, *74*, 74t
 low temperature and, 79
 manual, 79, *79–80*
 MRI and, 73–74, *74*, 74t
 radiography chamber for, 68–69, *69*, *70*
 shark and, 809–810
Rete mirabile, eye and, 45
 swim bladder and, 11, 37
Retina, *14*
 detachment of, 77
 examination of, 77
 growth of, 55
 histology of, 45, *45*
 layers of, *45*
 ramp, 752
 riboflavin and, 347
 shark, 752
 tapetum of, 54–55, 347, 752
 vision and, 54

Retrovirus, freshwater temperate fish and,
 291–295
 Xiphophorus, 291–295
Rhabdovirus, angelfish encephalitis and,
 645
 carp affected by, 482–484
 codfish ulcus syndrome and, 700–701
 eel affected by, 704–705
 hepatitis and, 394
 pike head disease and, 284t, *296*, 296–
 297
 snakehead ulcerative disease and, 570–
 571
Rhodopsin, vision and, 54
Riboflavin, 346t, 347, 462t
 deficiency of, 356t
Right shift, differential cell count and, 118
Rock, 200
 acid, 200
 alkaline, 200
 carbonate, 174, 660–662
 copper therapy and, 660–662
 live, 623
 metals leaching from, 200
 pH and, 174
 soil properties and, 200
Rods, 45, *45*
 dark adaptation and, 54
 shark vision and, 752
Roe, lumpfish, 667
Rotenone, 838t
 structure of, *315*
 toxicity of, 315
Rotifers, 634
 fatty acids in, 690–691
 marine cold-water fish and, 690–691,
 693, 694
Round stingrays, *746*, 746–747
Round worms, freshwater tropical fish
 and, 586–587
 salmonid and, 424
Run-off, pollution and, 208, 312, 335
Rust disease. See also *Oodinium*.
 freshwater tropical fish and, 583, *583*

Sablefish, *667*
 age of, 667
 anatomy of, 673–674
 natural history of, 667
 reproduction in, 668, 682–683
 taxonomy of, 667
Saccule, ear and, 15, *16*
Sacculus vasculosus, *12*, 43
Saffan, *88*
 action of, 88–89
 chemical attributes of, 88
 dosage for, 89
Safranin, Gram stain and, 126t
Salinity, 242, 243t
 estuarine, 174
 estuarine fish and, 242, 243t
 freshwater temperate fish and, 242, 243t
 marine aquarium and, *620*, 620t, 620–
 621
 marine cold-water fish and, 680
 measurement of, 174
 monitoring of, *620*, 620t, 620–621
 MRI affected by, 74, 74t
 oxygen concentration and, 179t
 ranges of tolerance for, 174
 seawater, 174
 shark and, 762
 specific gravity conversion and, 620
 temperature and, 242, 243t